This book is dedicated to our families, friends and loved ones, who endured and assisted in the task of assembling this guide.

Contents

Section 1

Basic Info about PLAB and Current Training in UK

Section 2

Question Bank

Section 3
Explanatory Notes: Subject-wise

Section 4

Single Best Answers (Question Bank)

Section 5

Data Base of High Yield Study Material

Preface to the Third Edition

The current format of part one Professional and Linguistics Assessment Board (PLAB) Exam consists of 200 Extended Matching Questions (EMQ, 70%) and Single Best Answer (SBA, 30%) questions. Candidates are usually tested on a wide variety of skills, knowledge and professional attitudes in a systematic way. The scope of the test is usually limited to evaluate the clinical abilities relating to conditions commonly seen by Interns and fresh residents, the management of life-threatening situations and rarer, important, medical problems.

Since the last edition of this bestselling PLAB book, many subtle but important changes in exam format and skill assessment necessitated the introduction of a new edition. To make this well appreciated work even more useful, we have completely reworked the entire text while keeping the essence of the book intact. Main changes are:

1. Dr. Rashmi Yadav, PLAB Part 1 topper, June 2005, is now part of the *First Aid* Authors team. She has been especially instrumental in revalidating the text from the past editions and providing solutions to latest test papers.
2. To avoid unnecessary repetition of explanations and to make the book more useful at an early stage of your preparation, we have discarded the previously used paper based format in favour of a more practical and user friendly subject based format.
3. As there has been a gradual trend towards picture based questions and more questions pertaining to the knowledge of basic sciences, we have made a conscious effort throughout to include such information in our unparalleled explanations, which still remain as the USP of this book.
4. Addition of 431 explanatory answers to new EMQs and SBAs in recent examination papers.
5. Hundreds of minor changes have been incorporated based on your wonderful suggestions which we have been receiving via e-mails, letters and rxpg.com
6. Typographical errors have been given special attention.

Like the previous editions, this edition is also an end product of a continuous and painstaking process wherein we kept track of all the frequently tested facts, topic areas, questions and study strategies from a single computer database. The effort involved in maintaining and updating such a database has been overwhelming and time consuming, but to strive for perfection is never easy.

If you find this book useful, you might also benefit from peer discussions in PLAB forums at www.rxpg.com, which have been developed as an online support framework for all aspiring PLAB taking candidates. You can find study partners, read interviews of successful PLAB candidates (including the authors), get latest question papers and real time changes in the exam and errata of this book from RxPG website.

Good luck for your PLAB test.

Himanshu Tyagi
Ankush Vidyarthi
Rashmi Yadav

Preface to the Third Edition

The current format of part 1 of Professional and Linguistics Assessment Board (PLAB) Exam consists of 200 Extended Matching Questions (EMQs) and Single Best Answer (SBA) questions. Candidates are usually tested on a wide variety of skills, knowledge, and professional attitude, in a systematic way. The scope of the test is usually limited to evaluate the clinical abilities relating to conditions commonly seen by Interns and fresh residents, the management of life-threatening situations and rarer, important, medical problems.

Since the last edition of this best-selling PLAB book, many subtle but important changes in exam format and skill assessment necessitated the introduction of a new edition. To make this well appreciated work even more useful, we have completely reworked the entire text while keeping the essence of the book intact. Main changes are:

1. Dr. Rashmi Yadav, PLAB Part 1 topper June 2005, is now part of the First Aid Authors team, and has been especially instrumental in revalidating the text from the past editions and providing solutions to latest test papers.
2. To avoid unnecessary repetition of explanations and to make the book more useful at an early stage of your preparation, we have discarded the previously used paper based format in favour of a more practical and user friendly subject based format.
3. As there has been a gradual trend towards picture based questions and more questions pertaining to the knowledge of basic sciences, we have made a conscious effort throughout to include such information in our unparalleled explanations, which still remains the USP of this book.
4. Addition of 437 explanatory answers to new EMQs and SBAs in recent examination papers.
5. Hundreds of minor changes have been incorporated based on your wonderful suggestions which we have been receiving via e-mails, letters and expg.com.
6. Typographical errors have been given special attention.

Like the previous editions, this edition is also an end product of a continuous and painstaking process wherein we kept track of all the frequently tested facts, topic areas, questions and study strategies from a single computer database. The effort involved in maintaining and updating such a database has been overwhelming and time consuming, but to strive for perfection is never easy.

If you find this book useful, you might also benefit from peer discussions in PLAB forums at www.expg.com, which have been developed as an online support framework for all aspiring PLAB taking candidates. You can find study partners, read interviews of successful PLAB candidates (including the authors), get latest question papers and real time changes in the exam and errata of this book from ExPG website.

Good luck for your PLAB test.

Preface to the First Edition

The purpose of *First Aid for the PLAB Part I Exam* is to help medical students and international medical graduates review the clinical questions and prepare for the Professional and Linguistics Assessment Board Exam, Part I (PLAB Part I). Preparing for this examination can be a stressful, difficult and costly task. This book helps students make the most of their limited time, money and energy. As is often the case in medical college, we found that the best advice a student can receive is from other medical students. We also recognized that certain clinical topics and situations are 'popular' and appear frequently in examinations. With this in mind, *First Aid for the PLAB Part I Exam* was started in April, 2002.

As we studied for the PLAB Part I Exam, we examined and evaluated scores of books and thousands of sample EMQs. We kept track of useful study strategies, frequently tested facts, and helpful mnemonics through a simple computer database. This book is a culmination of that database.

The title reflects the potential value of this book as the "first" one to get before buying other, and the fact that PLAB Exams are stressful and unpleasant experiences that students may "aid" each other in overcoming. We feel that this study guide provides a unique and pragmatic approach to the PLAB PartI and that it contains useful text not found in current PLAB EMQ books.

Throughout the work a conscious motive has been kept by us not to provide solutions to the readers but to make him aware of the direction he or she may need to work into solve any question. Many controversial options or answers have been explicitly been told in the text and the readers are supposed to find or satisfy themselves about the correct answers on their own. We do not believe in spoon feeding as much as we do not believe in letting you wander aimlessly in the wild sea of these questions.

Entries in First Aid for the PLAB Part I Exam originated from hundreds of students who have appeared in previous PLAB Exams and reproduced those questions solely on the basis of their memory (Authors did not reproduce any questions themselves, they only solved the material available to them). Because of certain limitations of the method of reproducing question on the basis of memory, there can be wide variations from the actual questions or their options. So we along with the publishers are not claiming any responsibility for the accuracy or even existence of any question in this book in the exam quoted. Still this book is a necessecity as it teaches you to approach the frequently occurring PLAB EMQs in a clinical and systematic manner.

We and Jaypee Brothers Medical Publishers (P) Ltd intend to continue updating First Aid for the PLAB Part I Exam so that the book grows in quality and scope and continue to reflect the EMQs asked in the PLAB Part I Exam. If you have any study strategies, high yield facts with mnemonics, book reviews or previous questions of PLAB (should be strictly memory based), please use the forms inside to submit your contributions (See How to contribute, page *xvii*). Any one who submits material subsequently used in the next edition of First Aid for the PLAB Part I Exam receive personal acknowledgement in the next edition and a har.dsome cash reward per complete entry.

Good Luck for the PLAB

Dr. Himanshu Tyagi
Dr. Ankush Vidyarthi

Acknowledgements

Dr. Aditya Gupta
Maulana Azad Medical College
Helped us to compile question from the internet: RxPG thanks you for your contribution Adi.

Dr. Vikas Singhal
Maulana Azad Medical College
Helped us to sail past many a difficult questions. RxPG is highly obliged by your invaluable advises "Dosco"!

Dr. Sajat Agarwal
Maulana Azad Medical College
Helped us to develop a system of logical thinking and its practical application to the questions RxPG is grateful for your insights Sajat!

Dr. Mandeep Singh
Maulana Azad Medical College
Helped us to review the proofs of this book. RxPG salutes you for your enthusiasm Mandy!

Piku and Piggy
Our pets! RxPG is indebted to some of your excellent background works, dear!

Dr. M.C. Nath (H.O.D), Dr. Alok, Dr. Swagata and rest of the department, Blood bank
Lok Nayak Hospital
Helped us to complete this book by providing excellent working conditions, while we were busy with this book. RxPG would like to give its heart felt regards to them.

Mr. J.P.Vij, Chairman and Managing Director
Jaypee Brothers Medical Publishers (P) Ltd.
Helped us in this project with his underlying enthusiasm and support for us. RxPG will like to register its gratitude in highest terms for him. Without you this book would never have been possible, sir!

Ms Sunita
Jaypee Brothers Medical Publishers (P) Ltd.
Helped herself in understanding our illegible handwritings, while composing this book. RxPG is looking forward for tougher project with you. Sunita jee!

Acknowledgements

Dr Nitin Gupta
Maulana Azad Medical College
Helped us to compile questions from the internet. RxPG thanks you for your contribution [illegible]

Dr [illegible]
Maulana Azad Medical College
Helped us to sort out many a difficult questions. RxPG is highly obliged by your intuitiveness. [illegible]

Dr Sital Agarwal
Maulana Azad Medical College
Helped us to develop a system of medical thinking and its practical application to the questions. RxPG is grateful for your insightful support.

Dr [illegible]
Maulana Azad Medical College
Helped us to review the proofs of this book. RxPG salutes you for your enthusiasm. [illegible]

Our goal RxPG is indebted to some of your excellent background works done.

[illegible]
Lok Nayak Hospital
Helped us to complete this book by providing excellent working conditions, while we were busy with this book. RxPG would like to give its heartfelt regards to them.

Mr [illegible] Chairman and Managing Director
Jaypee Brothers Medical Publishers (P) Ltd.
Helped us in this project with his unflinching enthusiasm and support for us. RxPG will like to register its gratitude in highest terms for him. Without you this book would never have been possible.

[illegible]
Jaypee Brothers Medical Publishers (P) Ltd.
Helped us a lot in understanding our flexible handwritings while composing this book. RxPG is looking forward for another project with you. Sincere regards.

Why to Read this Book?

RxPG First Aid for the PLAB Part I Exam has been written keeping in mind the exact quantity and quality of knowledge required by any MBBS graduate to clear PLAB exam. This exam is conducted by General Medical Council (GMC) worldover. GMC has a questions bank of around 2000 questions out of which 200 questions are asked in any PLAB exam. The reason for GMC having such a small question bank is that they have a pains taking method to prepare new questions which are then tested and re-tested on SHOs and students to determine their level of difficulty. All this research consumes time and they are only able to increment their question bank by a few questions each year. Since around ten percent of the total question bank comes as a single question paper of PLAB exam, the frequency of repetition is one in ten, if you solve a single previous year question paper. That means out of 200 questions practised by you, around 20 questions stand a good chance of being repeated. Most of the students, who fail PLAB Part I, do so by a whisker and it is rare to fail by a margin of 20 marks. So practising even one previous question paper can change your fortune. This book contain seven previous PLAB papers, i.e. 1400 questions. This is about half of the GMC question bank. So if you practise these seven paper in advance you have a chance getting around 100 (20 × 5) repeat questions in your exam. That means you know about 50 percent of the paper in advance after doing this book. This would make not only passing but even scoring high in the PLAB Exam a cake walk. And believe us, when you will only apply for a job in UK. The score will certainly make a difference.

Features of This Book

Textbook type approach: Since passing the PLAB examination requires very specific knowledge about limited topics, we have deliberately kept the textbook type approach throughout to provide you a textbook that is specifically written for PLAB. This also eliminates the need to pains takingly filter bulky textbooks like Kumar and Clarke's for your preparation. Believe us, to pass the PLAB Exam even OHCM and OHCS are not required to be read completely. This exam has a very limited range of topics.

Intelligent format: The idea and the format of this book is based on our research conducting online at www.rxpg.com and offline at Maulana Azad Medical College. Several hundred previous students who have appeared for PLAB examination (including those who've failed it once), have contributed to our research and helped us evolve an intelligent and highly productive format. As per all the books of RxPG series, our format is a trademark for our success.

RxPG analysis: We have included a detailed analysis of every paper and every controversial point or question in this book. This will prove very helpful for those who want to maximize their efficiency and enhance their performance in this highly competitive exam.

Confusa: It is an integral part of almost all our explanatory answers. This helps you to understand the finer "traps" and "catches" in the question which are usually invisible to untrained minds and accounts for most of the wrong answers. By highlighting their points this book ensures that you won't commit simple mistakes in the actual exam.

Paper-wise approach: The biggest blunder that most of the students appearing for PLAB commit is that they study for it in a subject-wise fashions, i.e. the old Indian way to study for any exam. Studying for PLAB means studying all clinical subjects together and randomly. When you will go through the themes in these previous papers, you will realise that mostly these themes don't represent a subject but a clinical condition that overlaps through many subjects, e.g. in a single theme of acute abdomen, questions can be asked about ectopic pregnancy (Obstetrics), Renal colic (surgery, mesenteric ischaemia (medicine), vertebral column fracture (Orthopaedics) and laxatives (pharmacology). So one need to have an orientation of all the subjects for a single given prospective which is impossible if you study one subject at a time. To validate our hypothesis, we conducted a random case-control study amongst the students of Maulana Azad Medical College who appeared for PLAB April 2002 and July 2002 exams. It was found that students who did integrated study fared better by 5-15% marks than those who preferred the old subject-wise approach. Another significant observation

was that subject-based preparation gave the students a false feeling of over confidence which proved detrimental in their scores. So RxPG strictly advise you to follow an integrated paper based approach. Subject-wise approach is best left for examinations which are based upon reproducibility of facts and figures and PLAB is just not this kind of exam. (Note that even OHCM, in spite of being a book of medicine, has a big section on surgery. It is so because illness don't confine them according to subjects and the question setters of PLAB are more concerned about you having this understanding).

Perfect simulation: RxPG has tried its best to simulate the exact PLAB exam by giving all 200 questions separately and identical answersheets with them. This helps you to practise marking the answers with speed and precision. This is important because of two reasons. First is that scoring in PLAB exam also depends upon your speed (Three hours are not sufficient for 200 questions). Secondarily, probably you've never come across the whole breath of the paper (usually these are 12-16 option boxes per question). Adjusting to this unique answersheet takes time and practise, and examination hall is certainly not the first place to learn it. Practise marking with pencil on included answer-sheets and certainly you will be able to limit your "non-educational" mistakes in the actual paper.

Indexing: RxPG circulated a questionnaire, as a part of our offline and online research, among the students preparing PLAB. One of the question in it was "Mention the biggest short-coming of the EMQ books. They are referring to 74 percent of the students wrote "lack of index" or "lack of a table of contents where only the topics of theme are mentioned". RxPG has thus incorporated both these features in this book and certainly this makes RxPG PLAB-years the best buy you can get for PLAB.

Orientation: This book contains total 1000 questions, but the authors have managed to explain 4000. How is it possible? Actually there is a peculiar occurrence our research team has noted while it was going through the previous papers. That is whole themes are often repeated in PLAB exams with the same set of questions, but with a different header, i.e. "Diagnosis of a disease" can change to "Management of a disease". Since there are usually only four types of themes that are asked in PLAB exams (i.e. Diagnosis, Management, Investigation, Treatment), we have included all these four points in almost every explanation. So reading the explanation to one question makes you intelligent four times.

Most authentic questions: Though we are not claiming 100% authenticity, we have put in a lot of time in compiling these papers. Basically we scanned the internet, approached those who've already given the papers and launched a special drive to contribute previous PLAB questions on www.rxpg.com. Since all these three were independent sources with no overlapping between them, we made one complete independent set for each exam from all three sources. Thereafter our research team compared the three sets to reach the most authentic final set of questions. This process was long and tedious, but you will realise the high level of our accuracy in reproducibility, once you'll appear for the PLAB exam.

Online extension: To keep this book alive and interactive, we have an online section dedicated to this book, i.e.

http//www.rxpg.com/plab

Here you'll find any errata or additions to this book, a message board dedicated to PLAB part I and a serious plab e-group. Moreover any information about PLAB is available on www.rxpg.com.

Based exclusively on textbooks for PLAB exam: RxPG had contacted some PLAB coaching institutes about how to study, and all they said is "If you want to clear PLAB, throw all your books away and read only UK textbooks." You all should note that UK adopt quite a different approach about management and treatment of many diseases, so there is lot of unlearning that has to be done (as usually we read USA textbooks like Harrison's). It is true that by reading non-UK books you can indeed easily answer the themes based on "diagnosis", but of late the number of such themes in PLAB exam have consistently fallen and emphasis on "investigation" and "management" has increased. For example, most of us crammed throughout our college years that "amyl nitrite" is to be given in case of cyanide poisoning, in UK it is "Dicobalt edetate"- unheard of by most of us. So start un-learning today by following UK textbooks for even the most inconsequential fact. This book will simplify this process for you.

Send us a photocopy of your PLAB I result and get your name in the fourth edition of this book.

How to use this Book?

The Third Edition of First Aid for PLAB incorporates lots of changes, based on the requests and feedbacks of our previous users.

QUESTION BANK

The book starts with a Question Bank, which is composed of seven sets of Question Papers, simulated exactly to the original PLAB fashion, as format and difficulty levels. Each set of these papers contains 200 Questions, followed by a simulated answersheet and then the correct answers.

Each Question set starts with 'RxPG Analysis' which gives you an overview of the total number of themes asked in the paper, (new themes as well as repeated ones), the number of SBAs and also the Picture Slides. Note that, the pattern of the PLAB is gradually changing and the 1st appearance of Picture Slides in 13 July'05 exam was a surprise, with no previous warnings. The book gives you a good practice of the latest Picture Slides asked in the recent PLAB exams and to set your minds on what sort of questions can be asked 'picture-based'!

The SBAs, although not very new for PLAB, the proportion of SBAs is increasing with every passing exam. Hence, to give you thorough practice we have not only included the SBAs which have appeared as in the PLAB exams, but also included a separate SBAs Question Bank for your practice.

The basic format of questions appear under following subheadings:

THEME

Here is the theme of a set of EMQs. It could be a topic, subtopic or a condition. It tells you what the questions are about, in terms of both the clinical problem area, for example chronic joint pain and the skill required, for example diagnosis. Usually the themes are about only four skills, i.e. DIAGNOSIS, INVESTIGATION, MANAGEMENT, TREATMENT OR ANATOMY. It helps you to create a knowledge base on the basis of which you can attempt new questions on this very theme. This is important as themes are repeated more often than the exact questions in the PLAB I exam.

OPTIONS

Here is the list of options, usually of between 8 to twelve items, each of which is identified by a letter of the alphabet. You should look for the answer to any particular question under a theme in this list of options. If you cannot find the answer you have thought of, you should look for an option which, in your opinion is the best answer to the problem posed. Marks are not deducted for incorrect answers nor for failure to answer. The total score on the paper is the number of correct answers given. You should , therefore, attempt all items. Each option may be used once, more than once, or not at all. There may be two correct answers for a single question and marking anyone will fetch you the marks.

QUESTIONS

These are several numbered items concerning the theme, usually between three and six. These are the questions—the problems you have to solve. Read them carefully, consider each of the numbered item in the list of options and decide what you think the answer is.

ANSWERS

Here we provide the correct answers to each of the question. We have provided the list of answers after each set of paper.

EXPLANATORY NOTES: SUBJECT-WISE

After a high demand by the previous readers, we decided to undertake the tedious job of assorting all the explanatory notes in a subject-wise fashion. This gives you the flexibility to prepare your self subject-wise, especially when you are going through the OHCM/OHCS chapters, you can easily flip through the same topics in First Aid and not only assess your preparation level instantly, but also improve upon it. This section also gives a chance for last minute revision in a most concise and organized way. Here we provide you with text, tables, tips, mnemonics and other material helpful in creating an orientation and grasp of the theme itself. This provides you an advantage of learning a high yield topic in totalty instead of getting partial knowledge by solving the few questions only.

The section is subdivided subject-wise and each question is explained under following headings:

QUESTION
Here is the body of the actual question. There are usually three to six such questions under on theme. All this constitute one EMQ.

DIAGNOSIS: Here we provide you with the final diagnosis to the condition in the question.

CLINCHERS:
Here we provide the detailed explanations about the answer. We have divided the question stem into a number of parts [clinchers] for the purpose of better explanation and to simplify the process of reaching a final diagnosis. This is important as it will help you cultivate a logical approach to solve the questions.

CONFUSA: Here we will explain the most confusing aspects of the question that can be responsible for most errors in making the correct diagnosis.

INVESTIGATION OF CHOICE: Here we give the most important investigation required for the condition in question.

IMMEDIATE MANAGEMENT: Here we give the most important investigation required for the condition in question

TREATMENT OF CHOICE: Here we give the most important investigation required for the condition in question.

YOUR NOTES: This is your own personal space, to write down the most important points (I personally, used this space to write down the things which I thought, I am most likely to forget; and on the night just before the exam, all I needed was to go through these small notes, and I could revise the 'most forgotten' facts in a matter of minutes).

How to Start Preparing

Get Yourself Familiar with Medicine in UK

↓

Briefly go through the OHCM to get an air of UK medicine
(Do not spend more than 1 week on OHCM at this stage)

↓

Take each question paper one by one from the Question Bank

↓

Time and Score yourself
(Keep a record of this time and score)

↓

Go through the explanatory notes for the questions you went wrong

↓

Go through relevant pages in the OHCM/OHCS

↓

Discuss controversial questions in your study group and online at http://www.rxpg.com

↓

Go to the next question paper and repeat the above steps

↓

Solve the same question paper again and compare your score, time taken and mistakes

The above steps might look sort of time consuming, but we personally found it very useful in improving our scores. Don't get disheartened by the poor scores you achieve when you attempt the question papers for the first time. The first attempt is to make you aware of the fields you actually need to improve upon and also give you a real feel of what the exam is like. It is strongly recommended that you take each paper completely in one single sitting, with strict time limits, as one would take in a real exam *(see our next section on What is PLAB).*

How to Contribute?

This version of RxPG First Aid for the PLAB Part I exam incorporates hundreds of contributions suggested by faculty and student reviewers of Maulana Azad Medical College. We invite you to participate in this process to bring out a better book next time.

Please send us your suggestions for
- Study and test taking strategies for the PLAB exams (both parts).
- New facts, mnemonics, diagrams, and illustrations which help to simplify the process of learning and cramming for a medical student.
- High yield topics that may reappear in future in above mentioned exams.
- Extended match questions of recent exams.

For each entry incorporated into the next addition, you will receive a handsome cash reward per completed entry, as well as personal acknowledgement in the next edition. Diagrams, tables, partial entries, corrections, and study hints are also appreciated, and significant contributions will be compensated at the discretion of the authors.

The preferred way to submit entries, suggestions, or corrections is via e-mail. Please include name, address, school affiliation, phone number and e-mail address (if different from address of origin). If there are multiple entries, please consolidate into a single e-mail or file attachment. Please send submissions to

rxpgonline@gmail.com

Otherwise please send entries, neatly written or typed or on a disk (MS Word), to "RxPG series, **First Aid for the PLAB Part I Exam, Jaypee Brothers Medical Publishers (P) Ltd**, EMCA House, 23/23B Ansari Road, Daryaganj, New Delhi 110 002, India"

Note:

The reward will be given only to the first contributor, however, every contributor will get acknowledgement in this book.

Plate - 1

PREVIOUS YEAR PAPER: 1 (THEME 12)

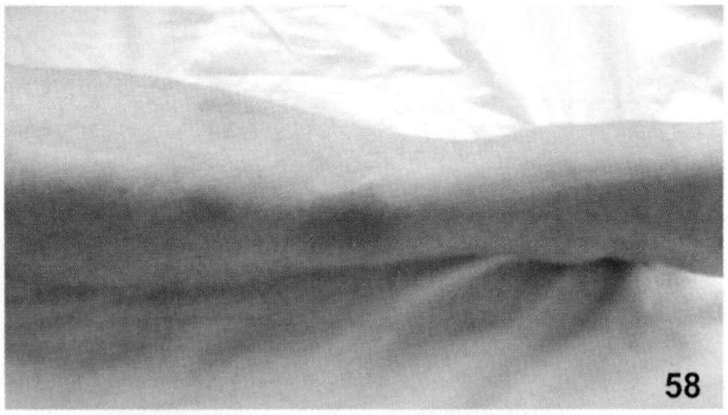

Figure 1

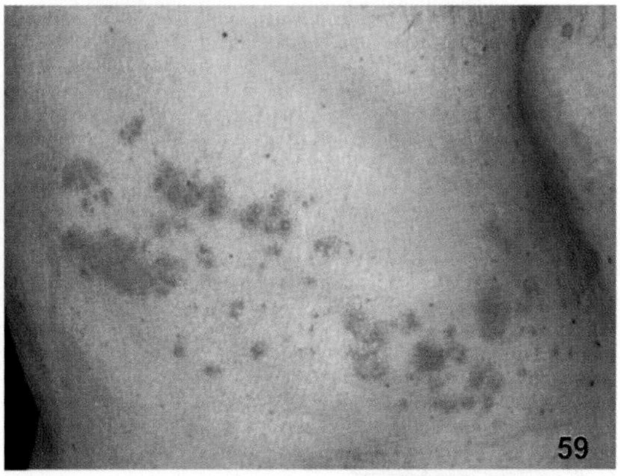

Figure 2

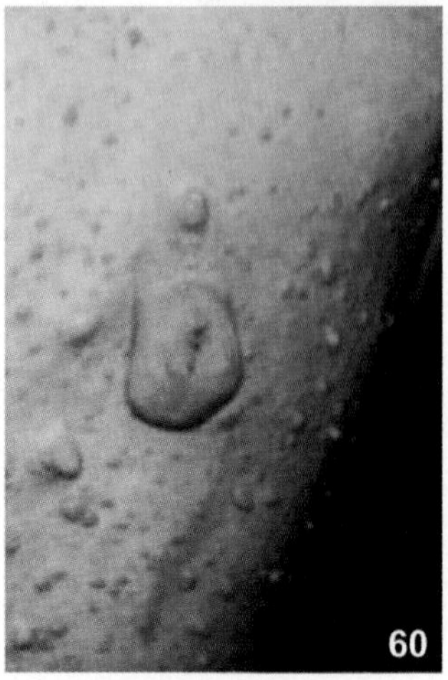

Figure 3

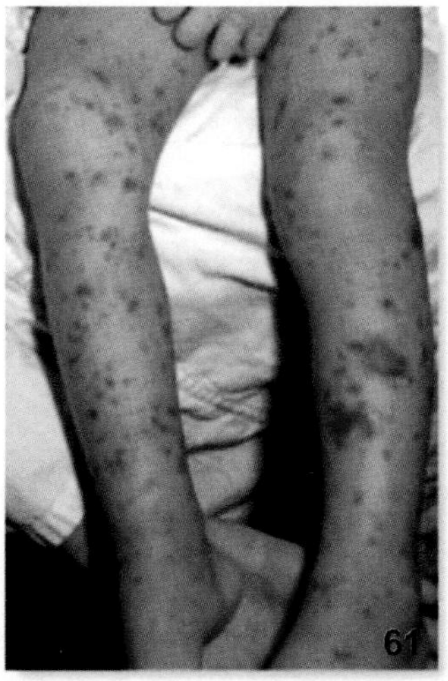

Figure 4

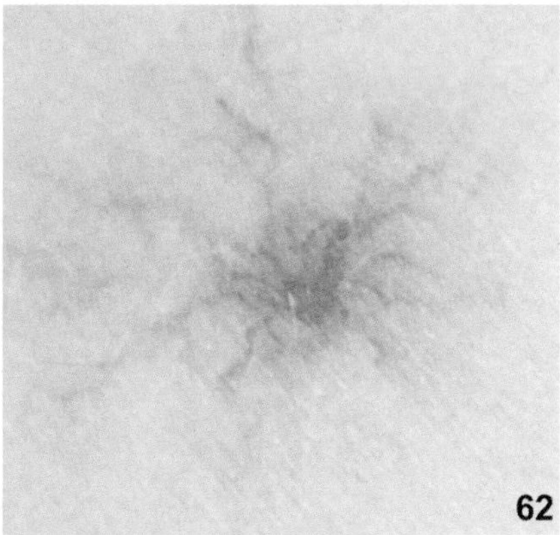

Figure 5

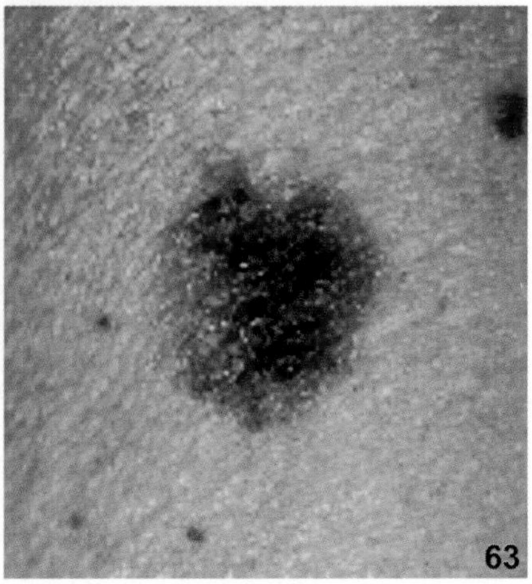

Figure 6

Plate - 2

PREVIOUS YEAR PAPER: 2 (THEME 33)

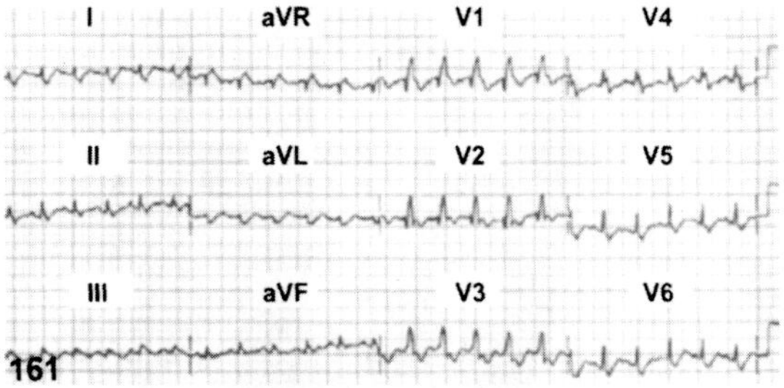

Figure 7

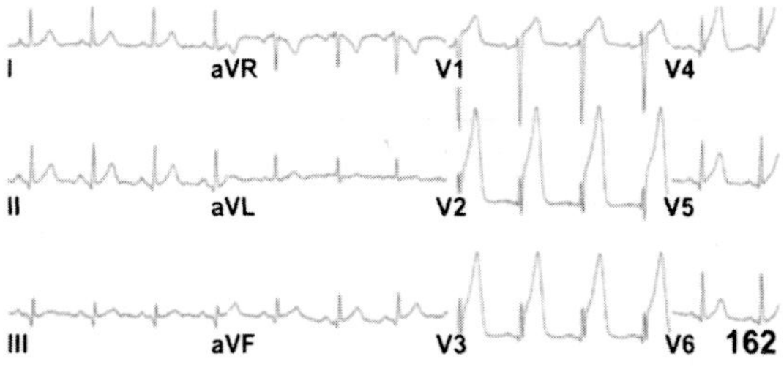

Figure 8

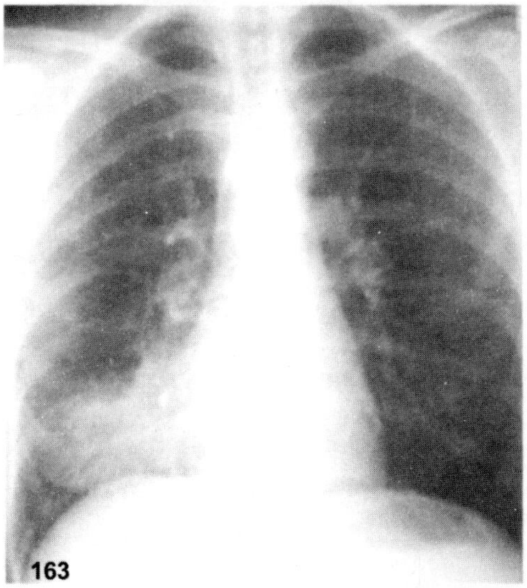

Figure 9

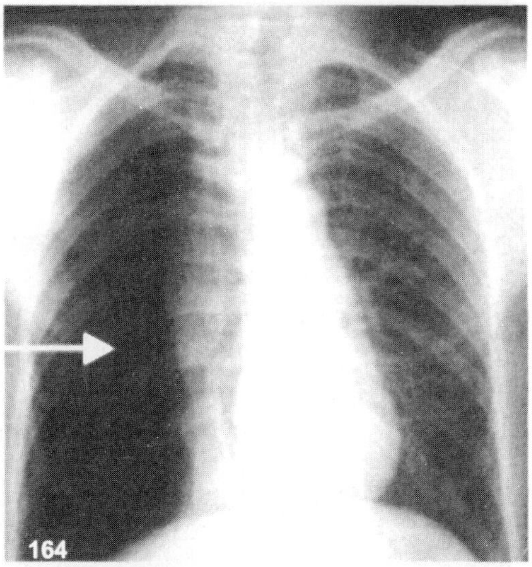

Figure 10

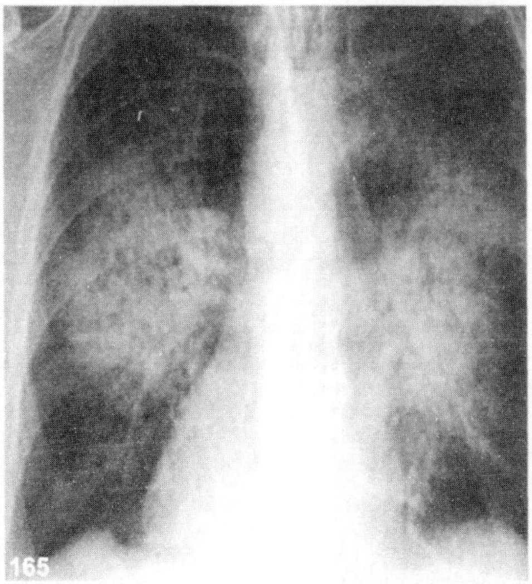

Figure 11

Section 1

Basic Info about PLAB and Current Training in UK

What is PLAB?

INTRODUCTION

For an overseas doctor in third world countries the UK degrees in medicine have always had a charm. Having MRCP (UK), MRCS (UK), MRCOG (UK), etc. have always been a ultimate desire for many a doctor. These degrees without any doubt enhance doctors credentials in laymans view compared to his colleagues. Also these degrees enhance one's ability to get better and best job internationally (particularly so in middle east). Having said all these everything boils down to being able to get these degrees. To get ultimately these degrees one has to work in UK (with exceptions in certain specialities). The UK government wants its people get medical services from a qualified doctors with professional knowledge and skill and knowledge of English. So there is the regulatory body for medical profession called general medical council (GMC) (similar to medical council of India). GMC is the body which allows the overseas doctor to practice in United Kingdom after limited registration. To get limited registration one has to pass PLAB test.

Purpose of the PLAB Test

Before granting limited registration to an overseas-qualified doctor, the GMC must be assured that the doctor has the knowledge of English and the professional knowledge and skill which are necessary for medical practice in the United Kingdom. One of the ways in which a doctor can satisfy the GMC that he or she has required abilities is by passing the test conducted by the professional and linguistic assessments board. This is known as the PLAB test. Having said this there are many different ways of obtaining limited registration which is discussed in a separate chapter.

Level of the PLAB Test

The standard required to pass the test is defined by the board in the following terms: "A candidate's command of the english language and professional knowledge and skill must be shown to be sufficient for him or her to undertake safely employment at first year senior house officer (SHO) level in a British hospital".

Qualification and Experience Needed

Admission to the PLAB test is open to doctors whose primary medical qualifications are accepted by the GMC for the purpose of limited registration. These include primary medical qualifications listed in the world directory of medical schools, which is published by the World Health Organization (WHO). In India it means MBBS degree of yours.

Evidence of Medical Qualification

A candidate will not be asked to provide proof of his/her qualification at the time of applying for admission to the PLAB test. However, before granting limited registration to doctors who have passed the test, the GMC will require the applicants to provide clear evidence that they hold an acceptable primary medical qualification.

The candidate should have a minimum of 12 months postgraduate clinical experience. This experience should be acquired in teaching hospitals or other hospitals which have been approved for internship training by the medical registration authorities concerned.

A doctor, who has not completed such experience, may be allowed by the GMC to enter the PLAB test. However, since the test is set at the level of senior house officer in the NHS, doctors without at least one year's experience of clinical practice are likely to be at a disadvantage. Doctors falling within this category who are able to pass the test will initially be granted limited registration only for employment at the grade of house officer (PRHO of UK), which is the NHS grade occupied by new medical graduates. After an appropriate period of satisfactory service as a house officer, the doctor would be able to apply for registration in respect of posts at a higher grade. The time spent as a House officer would be counted towards the total period of five years which the law permits for practice under limited registration and the number of PRHO is as much as the number of UK graduates, so overseas doctor will find it extremely difficult to obtain these posts. So it is advisable to complete internship and then write PLAB

test. The best will be for those who do not want to waste any time after internship can take this exam somewhere in between their internship program.

For applying for the PLAB test, one should have proved his linguistic capabilities with English as a language and for this one needs to take IELTS test. The minimum score for qualification in speaking: 7.0, listening: 6.0, academic reading: 6.0, academic writing: 6.0 and overall: 7.0. The IELTS is discussed in a separate chapter.

WHAT IT WILL COST

- The fee for taking part I (From 1st April 2001)
  145 pound sterlings
- The fee for taking part II (From 1st April 2001)
  430 pound sterlings
- The fee for checking your original documents when you apply for limited registration which is currently 100 pound sterlings
- The fee for limited registration(From January 2001)
  170 pound sterlings
- Air ticket (Return)
  500 pound sterlings
- Others
  300 pound sterlings

You have to consider the expenses involved in living in UK. Kindly multiply the total amout of money with the rupee value to get the exact amount of money involved in rupees in the process. (exchange rate as on 29th October, 2006 is 1 £ = 76.15 Rupees)

PLAB TEST PATTERN

This test refers to the whole **PLAB** test which is in **two** parts.

PART-I

An **extended matching questions (EMQ)** examination. The emphasis of this examination is on the clinical management and science as applied to clinical problems. It is confined to core knowledge, skills and attitudes relating to conditions commonly seen by SHO's, to the generic management of life-threatening situations and rarer, but important problems.

The examination paper will contain **200 questions** divided into a nubmer of themes. It will last **3 hours**. As per the GMC information the picture tests, clinical problem solving questions will no more be asked. These have not been asked in the the recent examinations, so student can be quite sure of these being not asked.

Syllabus (as outlined by the GMC in their information brochure).

Part I Assesses the ability to apply knowledge to the care of patients. The subject matter is defined in terms of the skill and of the content.

Skills

Four groups of skills will be tested in approximately equal proportions.

a. *Diagnosis* Given the important facts about a patient (such as age, sex, and nature of presenting symptoms, duration of symptoms) you are asked to select the most likely diagnosis from a range of possibilities.
b. *Investigations* This may refer to the selection or the interpretation of diagnostic tests. Given the important facts about a patient, you will be asked to select the investigation, which is most likely to provide the key to the diagnosis. Alternatively, you may be given the findings of investigations and asked to relate these to a patient's condition or to choose the most appropriate next course of action.
c. *Management* Given the important facts about a patient's condition, you will be asked to choose from a range of possibilities the most suitable course of treatment. In the case of medical treatments, you will be asked to choose the correct drug therapy and will be expected to know about side effects.
d. *Others:* These may include:
   i. Explanation of disease process: The natural history of disease will be tested with reference to basic physiology and pathology.
   ii. Legal/ethical: You are expected to know the major legal and ethical principles set out in the GMC publication- **Duties of a doctor.**
   iii. Practice of evidence based medicine: Questions on diagnosis, investigations and management may draw upon recent evidence published in peer-reviewed journals. In addition, there may be questions on the principles and practice of evidence-based medicine.
   iv. Understanding of epidemiology: You may be tested on the principles of epidemiology, and on the prevalence of important diseases in the UK.
   v. Health promotion: The prevention of disease through health promotion and knowledge of risk factors.
   vi. Awareness of multicultural society: You may be tested on your appreciation of the impact of the practice of medicine of the health beliefs and cultural values of the major cultural groups represented in the UK population.
   vii. Application of scientific understanding to medicine.

FREQUENTLY ASKED QUESTIONS

Below you will find the answers to a number of questions we are often asked.

Which qualifications are accepted? What if mine is not?
These include all the qualifications listed in the World Health Organisation's World Directory of Medical Schools (WHO WDMS). The General Medical Council holds copies and it is a widely available reference book. If your qualification is not in the WDMS, you will probably not be able to apply for registration after passing the PLAB test. The General Medical Council will not lobby the WHO on your behalf and you should contact your medical school or the WHO in Geneva.

What is the format of test?
Before entering Part I of the PLAB test, you must have obtained the required minimum scores in the IELTS test. The IELTS test report form is valid for up to two years from the date of the IELTS test to which it relates. The minimum IELTS scores are: Overall 7.0, Speaking 7.0, Listening 6.0, Academic Reading 6.0 and Academic Writing 6.0. PLAB Part I is in Extended Matching Question (EMQ) format. When you have passed PLAB Part 1, you must pass PLAB Part II—an Objective Structured Clinical Examination (OSCE) within two years.

Can I complete my internship in the UK? Do I need to pass the PLAB test for this?

Yes, you may undertake your internship in the UK, but you must pass the PLAB test first. Because the test is set at SHO level, it will be difficult to pass without any clinical experience.

How can I get a job when I have passed?

You should consult the British Medical Journal Classified Section (**www.bmj.com**) or get in touch with British Council National Advice Bureau (see Annex G for contact details). The General Medical Council is not linked to the Department of Health or the NHS and we have no information about job vacancies. Passing the PLAB test does not quarantee you a job.

Is Part 1 held overseas different from Part I in the UK?

No, they are identical papers, held as far as possible under identical conditions. All papers are marked at the same time in the UK.

How can I prepare for the PLAB test?

We have no recommended texts or specimen papers. There are details about the content and other helpful information for Part I in Annex A of this document. We are aware of the existence of preparatory courses, but we do not inspect them and can make no comment on them.

What sort of registration do I get when I pass PLAB and what sort of job can I do?

You may apply for limited registration, which enables you to apply for supervised, educationally approved posts in the NHS. It is granted for individual jobs up to a maximum total period of five years.

How do I get full (permanent) registration?

Full registration allows you to work in unsupervised posts outside the NHS and is not subject to a maximum period. You must have completed at least two years' limited registration before applying for full registration.

Can I have a reduction in the fee because of my special circumstances?

The PLAB test is self-financing and all candidates, except asylum seekers, must pay the full fee for each attempt.

Does a pass in Part 1 of the test entitle me to any sort of registration?

No. You must pass both parts of the test before applying for limited registration.

How long in my IELTS/Part I pass/Part II pass valid?

You must pass Part I within two years of the date of your IELTS report from and you must pass Part II within two years of passing Part I. You do not need a valid IELTS report to take Part II. At the moment, there is no limit on the time within which you must apply for registration after you have passed Part II.

What about exemption from the PLAB test?

You may be exempt from the PLAB test in certain circumstances. You should check this by contacting the General Medical Council's Registration Customer Services to ascertain your eligibility for registration.

If I cancel my test place, what happens?

If you want to cancel your place, please give the office which offered you the place as much notice as possible. You must return the letter offering you an Examination place. If you cancel early, we may be able to offer your place to another candidate waiting to take the Examination. You may not pass the letter offering you a place to anyone else.

If you cancel your place, you will be charged a fee. This will normally be deducted from the fee you paid to enter the Examination. The amount charged depends on the amount of notice you give.

Cancellation charges (2006 and 2007)

The current cancellation charges are as follows:

UK centres:

Period of notice	*Cancellation charge*
Four months or more	£ 87
Between 21 days and four months	£ 101
Less than 21 days	£ 145

If you do not want to re-book a place, we will refund the balance of your fee.

Overseas centres:

Period of notice	*Cancellation charge*
Before closing date	£ 20
After closing date	No refund

Can I take PLAB Part II outside the UK?

No. This is held only in the UK.

What is the pass rate?

There is no set pass rate.

What happens when I pass/fail Part 1/Part 2?

If you pass Part I, you will be sent an information pack and an application form for Part II. If you fail Part I, we will let you know in writing. We will not give results out

over the phone or by fax. We will send you further application papers for Part I if you took the test in the UK. If you took the test at an overseas centre, you should contact that centre for another application form (or another centre if you would like to take the Examination in a different place). If you fail Part II, the General Medical Council will send you a letter detailing your results and a further application form for Part II. If you pass Part II, you will be sent an application form and an information pack for limited registration.

What level is the PLAB test set at?

The PLAB test is set at the level of a SHO in a first appointment in a UK hospital. The emphasis of this Examination is on clinical management and science as applied to clinical problems. It is confined to core knowledge, skills and attitudes relating to conditions commonly seen by SHOs, the generic management of life-threatening situations and rarer, but important, problems.

How may times may I take Part I/Part II?

There is no limit to the number of times that you may take Part I, but you must have a valid IELTS report form dated not more than two years before each attempt. You may have four attempts at Part II, which must be within two years of your Part I pass. If you do not pass at your fourth attempt, you must re-take IELTS and Part I. There are no exceptions to this rule.

SYLLABUS FOR PLAB I

The PLAB test is designed to test the knowledge, skills and attitudes relating to conditions commonly seen by trainees entering the second year of the Foundation Programme (first year SHOs), the management of life-threatening situations and rarer, but important, medical problems. This means that UK-trained doctors and international medical graduates (IMGs) are expected to have the same level of knowledge and skills at this stage of their career.

You will not be expected to be familiar with NHS procedures or British culture other than in the way it might affect how you treat patients. You should be familiar with the GMC publication Good Medical Practice, and the other booklets in that series as you will be expected to answer questions in line with the advice they give. You should also make sure you are familiar with how people in the UK might behave: you should not make assumptions about a patient on the basis of gender or ethnic origin — for example, women may smoke and drink.

Skills

Four skill areas will be tested. Questions may draw upon recent evidence published in peer-reviewed journals. There may also be questions on the principles and practice of evidence-based medicine.

Diagnosis

Given the important facts about a patient (such as age, gender, nature of presenting symptoms and duration of symptoms) you will be asked to select the most likely diagnosis from a range of possibilities.

Investigations

This may refer to the selection or the interpretation of diagnostic tests. Given the important facts about a patient, you will be asked to select the investigation that is most likely to provide the key to the diagnosis. Or you may be given the findings of investigations and asked to relate these to a patient's condition, or to choose the most appropriate next course of action.

Management/Treatment

Given the important facts about a patient's condition, you will be asked to choose the most suitable treatment, including therapeutics, from a range of possibilities. In the case of medical treatments you will be asked to choose the correct drug therapy and will be expected to know about side effects. It also includes emergency and acute care, peri-operative care, pain relief, oncology, palliative care, terminal care and complementary therapy.

The context of clinical practice

This may include:

Explanation of the disease process: Disease factors and the natural history of the untreated disease.

Understanding of epidemiology: You may be tested on the principles of epidemiology, and on the prevalence of important diseases in the UK.

Health promotion: Promoting, monitoring and maintaining the health of individuals and groups.

Application of scientific understanding to medicine: You may be tested on the scientific disciplines that underpin medicine, such as anatomy, genetics and pathology.

Legal and ethical matters: You will be expected to know the major legal and ethical principles set out in good medical practice and supporting guidance.

Conditions

The content to be tested is, for the most part, defined by the symptoms with which the patient presents, and whether these symptoms are acute or chronic.

You will be expected to know about conditions that are common or important in the UK for all the areas outlined below. Examples of the conditions that may be asked about are given under each heading and may appear under more than one heading. Be aware that these examples are only for illustration. Other similar conditions might appear in the examination.

Blood and Lymphatic System

Examples: Abnormal blood film, bleeding/bruising/purpura, blood loss, enlarged lymph nodes, pallor.

Cardiovascular System

Examples: Chest pain (including acute myocardial infarction, acute coronary syndrome, coronary heart disease and angina), palpitations, peripheral arterial disease, peripheral oedema/breathlessness, peripheral venous problems.

Digestive System

Examples: Abdominal mass (generalised and localised), abdominal pain (acute and chronic), altered bowel habit

(including constipation), anorexia and weight loss, diarrhoea, dyspepsia, dysphagia, facial pain and swelling, gastrointestinal bleeding (lower and upper), jaundice, nausea and vomiting, nutrition, trauma.

ENT
Examples: Earache, hearing problems, hoarseness, nasal symptoms (including rhinorrhoea and epistaxis), speech disorder, vertigo.

Ophthalmology
Examples: Eye pain, orbital swelling, 'red eye', visual impairment.

Homeostasis
Examples: Abnormal blood sugar, acid-base imbalance, electrolyte abnormalities, shocked patient, thyroid abnormalities.

Infectious Diseases
Examples: Fever, serious infections (including meningitis, HIV, AIDS, Hepatitis B and TB), travel medicine and tropical infections (including malaria).

Mental Health
Examples: Alcohol and drug misuse and dependence, anxiety, confusion, poor concentration and memory loss (including dementia), deliberate selfharm, eating problems, learning and communication problems, mood (affective) problems (including depression, suicide risk), psychological problems, severe behavioural disturbance (including confusional states, psychoses and personality disorders).

Musculoskeletal System
Examples: Conditions relating to the back, neck, foot, ankle, hand, wrist, hip, knee, shoulder and upper limb, including fractures, dislocations, sprains, strains and rheumatological disease.

Neurological System
Examples: Coma, blackouts, cranial nerve problems, headache, faints and falls, movement disorders (including tremor and gait problems), peripheral nerve problems, seizures.

Renal System
Examples: Abnormalities of the urine, groin/scrotal pain and/or swelling, renal problems (including renal failure), urethral discharge (including STI), urinary symptoms, urinary tract obstruction (including prostate and calculus), fertility problems (male and female).

Respiratory System
Examples: Breathlessness (including pneumonia, bronchiolitis, COPD, asthma, sleep apnoea), chest pain, cough, haemoptysis (including pulmonary embolism), wheeze/stridor.

Seriously Ill Patient
Examples: Anaphylaxis, multiple trauma, septicaemia, serious infection.

Dermatology
Examples: Bites and stings, burns, infections, lumps, moles and pigmented lesions (including malignant melanoma), nail and/or hair problems, pruritis, rashes, ulcers.

Women's Health
Examples: Bleeding in pregnancy, breast lump and/or pain, contraception, irregular periods, normal pregnancy and care, pain and abnormal vaginal bleeding, pelvic mass, pelvic pain, problems in pregnancy (including ectopic, pre-eclampsia and eclampsia, hyperemesis), vaginal discharge.

Disorders Specific to Childhood
Examples: Congenital abnormalities, developmental delay and failure to thrive (including non-accidental injury and child sexual abuse).

HOW TO APPROACH THE EXTENDED MATCHING QUESTIONS EXAMINATION?

The examination paper will contain 200 questions in the extended matching format, divided into a number of themes.

Each theme has a heading which tells you what the questions are about, in terms both of the clinical problem area (e.g. chronic joint pain) and the skill required (e.g. diagnosis).

Within each theme there are several numbered items, usually between four and six. These are the questions- the problems you have to solve. These are examples below.

Begin by reading carefully the instruction which preceded the numbered items. The instruction is very similar throughout the paper and typically reads. 'For each scenario below, choose the **SINGLE** most discrimination investigation from the above list of options. Each option may be used once, more than once or not at all.'

Consider each of the numbered items and decide what you think the answer is. You should then look for that answer in the list of options (each of which is identified by a letter of the alphabet). If you cannot find the answer in the list you have thought of, you should look for the option which, in your opinion, is the best answer to the problem posed.

For each numbered item, you must choose ONE of the option. You may feel that there are several possible answers to an item, but you must choose the one most likely from the option list. **If you enter more than one answer on the answer sheet you will gain no mark** for the question even though you may have given the right answer along with one or more wrong ones.

In each theme there are more option than items, so not all the options will be used as answer. This is why the instruction says that some options may not be used at all.

A given option may provide the answer to more than one item. For example, there might be two items which contain descriptions of patients, and the most likely diagnosis could be the same in both instances. In these cases, the option would be used more than once.

You will be awarded one mark for each item answered correctly. Marks are **not** deducted for incorrect answers nor for failure to answer. The total score on the paper is the number of correct answers given. You should, therefore, attempt all items. Example of an EMQ:

THEME 1: DIAGNOSIS OF HEARING LOSS

OPTIONS

a. Acoustic neuroma
b. Blast injury
c. Petrous temporal bone fracture
d. Wax impaction
e. Acute otitis media
f. Ototoxicity
g. Fracture base of skull
h. CSOM
i. Glue ear
j. Herpes zoster
k. Foreign body

*For each presentation below, choose the **most likely dianosis** from the above list of options. Each option may be used once, more than once, or not at all.*

QUESTIONS

1. Man treated with gentamicin for peritonitis for 10 days presents with deafness.
2. Man with poor physical hygiene presents with pain and deafness after taking a shower.
3. Woman presents with deafness and corneal anaesthesia. On MRI, a widened internal auditory meatus is seen.
4. Male, 20 years, with history of head injury, bruising on the side of head complains of hearing loss.
5. A 54-year-old female develops mild fever, malaise and ear pain. 3 days later she developed multiple painful vesicles over her early canal and external meatus.

HOW TO STUDY FOR PLAB?

Note

All our conclusions given here are based on our research and feedback received in Maulana Azad Medical College and RxPG.com.

RxPG suggests you to opt for its unique strategy based on 5'P's. These are:

1. Plan
2. Pool
3. Prepare

4. Practise
5. Patience.

Now, these points in some detail are as follows.

Plan

A good plan is very important for your way to success. When you will start preparing for your PLAB exam, you will be more like an amateur in the world of PLAB professionals. By the time you will gain enough experience to play at a level field with them, time will deceive you. So here is where the advices of your seniors come in handy. Approach your seniors in the college, not only who came out with flying colours in the PLAB exam but also those who could not make it. Discuss in detail with the second or third attemptees. This is important as a successful student is usually not aware of the possible blunders anyone could make in their preparation. So do ask everybody about what not to do. Listen to everybody and make your own personalised plan. Do not follow anybody else plan blindly, however, successful it might have been for that person. This is because only you are the best judge of your shortcomings and plus points.

Pool

The next thing very important for your plan is to find a right kind of student or a pool of students as study partners. Remember if you study alone you are using only 10-20% of your brain faculties. But in a group study the process of gathering the information involves not only your eyes but ears, tongue and perhaps even hands sometimes! So you end up mobilising more of your brain in the same time span and this is very important as you have so little time on your hand. If you can't find a study partner (like if you stay at home in your hometown), then visit http://mediboard.meramamc.com. This page features message boards for PLAB exam from all websites.

Prepare

This needs a lot of consistency and regularity on your part. Believe us, it is not easy. So always have this thing playing in the back of your mind that you have to be regular. Study religiously every day for 5-8 hours. Set some punishments (like studying for more hours next day or mugging that impossible table from OHCM) for yourself if you cannot realise your targets. Set daily goals and allow a little flexibility in your goals and plan. Nothing can go strictly as per schedule, so even if you cannot make it for a few days, does not mean that you should drop the whole plan. Stick to it and see the result yourself. For PLAB, the optimum duration to revise whole syllabi once is 1 month.

Practice

Research showed that attempting mock tests is the best tool to practise for PLAB. Attempting mock tests fine tune your abilities to manage time, work out mistakes, minimising blunders, blunting the anxiety and stress and "gives you a feel" of the real exam. One cannot understand the difference until and unless one gives a mock test. Try these yourself online at

www.RxPG.com

The next most important thing is practise phase is to iron out your mistakes. Attempt tests, analyse your performances, spot the weaknesses, iron them out and then attempt more tests. Remember no one is perfect, but near perfection can be reached only by practise.

Note: You will need to revise selectively and not the whole course again. PLAB EMQs are from a very narrow pool of questions. So instead of wasting time on revising the whole syllabi, do PLAB questions in a retrograde way (like in this book).

Patience

This is the biggest virtue. Remember you will get everything only if you are through will all other 'Ps' and that need loads of patience. Don't be impatient to earn money (so do not do house jobs/residency because even if you get selected while doing them, you would have got a better seat had you opted for not doing it) or to start enjoying the role of a doctor. You are still a student and you are giving these exams as you want to remain as a student for next two/three years. Remember these lines by "Frost" to just keep yourself going:

"The woods are lovely, dark and deep,
But I have promise to keep
and miles to go, before I sleep."

WHAT SHOULD BE YOUR STRATEGY WHILE ATTEMPTING PLAB PART ONE EXAM?

Please read these instructions carefully and devise your own personalised strategy based on it. This strategy has been thoroughly researched and is found to be very effective.

Steps (after sitting on your seat in examination hall)

1. Read and listen to all instructions carefully.
2. Rapidly browse through the paper after opening the seal (when you are told to do so). Going through all the sheets in one minute helps you to:
   - Get a feel of the paper and therefore help you concentrate afterwards.

- Check out any missing pages and misprints in the paper.

3. Take a deep breath and concentrate
   - If you have any problem in concentration because of anxiety, close your eyes and count backwards from 100 to 1. This is a very effective method to get focussed in a very short time.

4. Start solving the paper. Take two rounds as follows:

FIRST ROUND: Answer all the questions as much as possible.

- Clearly mark the one you have left on question paper, (write all the probable options in front of them—this saves time and confusion in second round).
- Keep on tansferring the answers on the answer sheet at the same time. Never leave this for the end as this can be suicidal.
- Answering reflexly here is very important. One can develop these reflexes by practising on as many mock tests as one can. Online mock tests are available at www.rxpg.com.
- Don't do any hard thinking in this round. If you are forced to think long on any question then leave it for the next round. First round should be based on a quantitative approach as 3 hours is actually little time to solve 200 EMQs.
- Note the time taken to finish this round. Ideally you should be able to finish this round in first two hours.

Advantages: 120-130 questions in two-third of total time takes off the pressure, thereby you can:

- Relax and work efficiently to provide quality in the tougher questions left
- Not fall in danger of leaving the simple questions unattempted if time runs out.

SECOND ROUND: This round will decide your passing or failing the exam. So gather all your alertness and focus extra hard now. You should:

- Give maximum one minute to each question.
- If still there is confusion, mark the most probable answer according to you and move ahead. Don't get stuck any where.
- Do not leave any question unattempted as there is **No** negative marking.

After these if you still have time, tally your answers on the answer sheet with that of question paper randomly. This helps in exclusion of any inadvertent mistake by you while transferring the answers.

Ideal way to attempt a theme:

- Read the header and imbibe its relevance
- Go through all the options rapidly
- Read instructions before the questions especially what it is asking for, i.e. first investigation or most definitive investigation (both of these will result in different answers).
- Attempt questions one by one and simultaneously transfer your answers on answer sheet.
- Think on a SHO level only and never think like a theorist while solving EMQs.

Please note that this strategy is just like an ideal infrastructure on which your final strategy should be based. You should know or find what works best for you and thus fine tune this strategy to get your own customised version.

PLAB PART II (OSCE)

You may only enter part II of the test when you have passed part I. **You have to take part II within 2 years of passing part I.** This test is set at the following standard:

A candidate's command on English language and professional knowledge and skill must be shown to be sufficient for him or her to undertake safely, employment at first year Senior House officer level in a British hospital.

This test is a **14 station objective structured clinical examination (OSCE).**

The syllabus and format of this test as given in the GMC information brochure.

Aim

1. The aim of the OSCE is to test your clinical and communication skills. It is designed so that an examiner can observe you putting these skills into practice.

Overall Format

2. When you enter the examination, you find a series of 14 booths, known as 'station'. Each station requires you to undertake a particular task. Some tasks will involve talking to or examining patients, some will involve demonstrating a procedure on an anatomical model. Detail of the tasks are explained below under 'content'.
3. There will also be two rest stations in the circuit. At some tests one of these two station will contain instruction asking you to perform certain tasks as if you were at a real station. These are pilot stations and the results will not count towards your overall OSCE grades.
4. You will be required to perform all tasks. You will be told the number of the station at which you should begin when you enter the examination room. Each task will last five minutes.
5. Your instruction will be posted outside the station. You should read these instructions carefully to ensure that you follow them exactly. An example might be:
   'Mr McKenzie has been referred to you in a rheumatology clinic because he has joint pains. Please take a short history to establish supportive for a differential diagnosis.
6. A bell will ring. You may then enter the station. There will be an examiner in each station. However, unlike in the oral examination, you will not be required to have a conversation with the examiner; you should only direct your remarks to him or her if the instructions specifically ask you to do so. You should undertake the task as instructed. A bell will ring after four minutes 30 seconds to warn you that you are nearly out of time. Another bell will ring when the five minutes are up. At this point you must stop immediately and go and wait outside the next station. If you finish before the end, you must wait inside the station but you should not speak to the examiner or to the patient during this time.
7. You will wait outside the next station for minute. During this time you should read the instructions for the tasks in this station. After one minute, a bell will ring. You should then enter the station and undertake the task as instructed.
8. You should continue in this way until you have completed all 14 tasks. You will then have finished the OSCE.

Content of the Station

9. Each station consists of a scenario. An examiner will be present and will oserve you at work.
10. The scenario could be drawn from any medical speciality appropriate to a senior house officer (SHO).
11. Although the tasks you will be instructed to do will not necessarily be tested in the order given here. Under each skill area, you will find some examples. Please note that these are only examples; other topics will be tested.The main skills tested in OSCE examination are—**History taking, clinical examination skills, practical skills, communication and examination skills.**

A. History Taking

Your candidate instructions will set the scene. You will be asked to take a history from an actor pretending to be a patient (a stimulated patient). The actor will have been given all the necessary information to be able to answer your questions accurately. You should treat him or her as you would a real patient.

E.g: Diarrhoea, wheeze, vaginal bleeing, palpitations, abdominal pain, headache, anxiety.

B. Clinical Examination

You will be asked to examine a particular part of the body. You may have to examine a stimulated or real

patient or perform the examination on an anatomical model. Although you should talk to the patient as you would to a patient in real life. You should only take a history or give a diagnosis if the instructors require you to do so. You may be asked to explain your actions to the examiner as you go along.

Examples: Breast examination, cardiovascular examination, examination of abdomen, hip examination, knee examination, pervaginal examination, perrectal examination.

C. Practical Skills/Use of Equipment

This is to assess some of the practical skills an SHO needs. The stations concerned will normally involve anatomical models rather than patients.

Examples: IV cannulation, cervical smear, suturing, blood pressure.

D. Emergency Management

These stations will test whether you know what to do in an emergency situation. You may have to explain what you are doing to the patient or to the examiner. Your instructions will make this clear.

E. Communication Skills

There will be a communication skill element in most stations. However, in some stations this skill will be the principal skill tested. Areas tested may include interviewing (including appropriate questioning, active listening, explaining clearly, checking understanding) and building rapport (including showing empathy and respect, sensitivity to other's emotions and coping with strong emotions in others).

Examples: Instructions for discharge from hospital, explaining treatment, consent for autopsy, ectopic pregnancy explanation.

VENUES FOR EXAMINATIONS

You can take **part I** of the test in:
UK (Birmingham, Edinburgh, Glasgow, London).
Sydney, Australia
Bulgaria, Bulgaria
Cairo, Egypt
Calcutta, India
Chennai, India
Mumbai, India
NewDelhi, India
Bangalore, India
Iran, Iran
Lagos, Nigeria
Islamabad, Pakistan
Karachi, Pakistan
Johannesburg, SouthAfrica
Colombo, Sri Lanka
Dubai, United Arab Emirates
West Indies, West Indies

Part II of the test is available only in UK in London, Edinburgh, Leeds and Liverpool.

Details of dates are set out by the GMC at regular intervals the candidates are advised to get in contact with the office of the nearest British Council Divisions.

NOTIFICATION OF RESULTS

The part I paper is marked by computer. At the end of the part I test, you will be told the date on which your results will be available. Usually it takes about 4 weeks for the declaration of results.

For part II, you will be given grades for each station. However, the overall result of the examination is either pass or fail and this result is usually sent out 2 weeks after the date of the examination.

PLAB test dates and contacts

Part I and Part II

Note: Due to the high demand for places, you are strongly advised to allow at least four months from the time of submitting an application to getting a place. You may not hold a place in more than one examination.

Part I

Candidates for tests held outside the UK should apply to the local British Council office. Applications presented in person will not be given preference. For information about accommodation in the UK, visit the British Tourist Authority website. For the latest available dates refer to GMCs official website www.gmc-uk.org

The closing date for receipt of application forms tests overseas is six weeks before the test. If you wish to enquire about availability for test dates please fax +44 (0)20 7 915 3565 or telephone +44 (0)20 7915 3630. Applications presented in person will not be given preference.

Local British Council contacts

Country	City	Contact and email	Tel	Fax
Australia	Sydney (via Wellington, New Zealand office)	Richard Kyle	+64 (0) 4 924 2851	+64 (0) 4 473 6261
Bulgaria	Sofia	Nadya Ogorelkova	+359 2 9424200	+359 2 9424306
Egypt	Cairo	Hala Hamad	+20 2 3001666	+20 2 3443076
India	Kolkata	Suchitra Mukherjee	+91 33 282 9108/9144	+91 33 2282 4804
	Chennai	Nirupa Fernandez	+91 44 2852 5002 ext 304	+91 44 2852 3234
	Mumbai	Vivek Singh	+91 (0) 22 2282 3560/3530	+91 (0) 22 2285 2024 / 6619
	New Delhi	P V Chaary	+91 11 3710 111 / 555 ext 253 / 251	+91 11 331 8795
	Hyderabad	Nirupa Fernandez	+91 44 2852 5002 ext 304	+91 44 2852 3234
	Bangalore	Nirupa Fernandez	+91 44 2852 5002 ext 304	+91 44 2852 3234
Iran	Iran	Shiva Tohidi	+98 21 200 1222 Extension: 114	+98 21 200 7604
New Zealand	Wellington	Richard Kyle	+64 (0) 4 924 2851	+64 (0) 4 473 6261
Nigeria	Lagos	Bimbola Fashola	+234 1 2692188 / 2692189 / 2692190 / 2692191 / 2692192	+234 1 2692193 / 2690646
Pakistan	Islamabad	Shahnaz Farooq	+92 51 111 424 424	+92 51 111 425 425
	Karachi	Karima Kara	+92 21 111 424 424	+92 21 111 425 425
Russia	Moscow	Tanya Leonova	+007 095 782 0200	+007 095 782 0201
South Africa	Cape Town	Nazeema Saliemia	+27 21 460 6660	+27 21 460 6691
South Africa	Johannesburg	Shamima Jooma	+27 11 718 4300	+27 11 718 4401
Sri Lanka	Colombo	Panchalika Kulatunga	+94 4521 500	+94 1 587079
UAE	Dubai	Zara Khan	+971 4 3370109	+971 4 3370703
West Indies	Kingston, Jamaica	Nicola Johnson	+876 929 6915 / 7049	+876 960 3030

Part II

Tests with available places are listed below, although these may be filled before the closing date shown. From time to time Part II tests are added to or removed from the list of available dates. We may allocate you a place on any day within a block of consecutive tests at the same test centre.

Please note that if you have a confirmed booking on a test and wish to change to an earlier test which has been added to the list, you will still be charged a cancellation fee.

Due to the high demand for Part 2 places, you are strongly advised to allow at least four months from the time of submitting an application to getting a place. You should take this into account when applying for Part II, which you must pass within two years of passing Part I.

Maps of test locations appear below. For information about accommodation in the UK, visit the British Tourist Authority website.

Available PLAB II dates as on 29 October 2006

Date	Location	Availability	Closing Date
04 DEC 2006 (4 days)	London, United Kingdom	No Places Available	10 NOV 2006
08 JAN 2007 (4 days)	London, United Kingdom	Places Available	08 DEC 2006
12 FEB 2007 (4 days)	London, United Kingdom	Places Available	12 JAN 2007

RECOMMENDED BOOKS

MEDICINE
- OHCM, 5 edn—read it thoroughly with at least two revisions
- Kumar and Clark, 5 edn—Only for reference purposes.
- Lecture notes in emergency medicine—read selected topics from it like
  - Poisonings
  - Abdominal pain
  - Head injury

SURGERY
- OHCM, 5 edn—thorough reading
- Lecture notes, surgery—thorough reading with at least one revision
- Bailey and Love—Strictly for reference purposes

GYNAECOLOGY AND OBSTETRICS
- Lecture notes—thorough reading
- Ten teachers (Obs and Gynae) and Shaw's (Gyn)—Strictly for references

PSYCHIATRY
- Kumar and Clark, 5 edn + OHCS

ORTHOPEDICS
- OHCS, 5 edn

DERMATOLOGY
- Kumar and Clark, 5 edn + OHCS

OTHER
OHCS, 5 edn, Read thoroughly with at least one revision

EMQ
Nothing except fischtest and this book.

This is a review of books which we feel necessary for preparing for PLAB.

Medicine
1. "Oxford Handbook of Clinical Medicine" (OHCM) and 'Oxford Handbook of Clinical Specifications'(OHCS) published by the Oxford University Press are very important books for PLAB. They are like your bible (or Bhagvadgita!). Go through them at every single opportunity and learn them cover to cover. The years of experience of PLAB writing students is that this itself is enough to get you through the exam.
2. Davidson or Kumar and Clarke should form the basic textbook to prepare for medicine. There is no need to try and go through both of these books. A candidate should be thorough with either of the two books. It is better to go through the book one has read during his UG studies though some feel Kumar and Clarke is better option.
3. "Lecture Notes on Clinical Medicine". This book is optional. You may briefly go through this book. You do not have to read this book thoroughly if you have done the above reading for medicine.
4. Large textbooks of medicine and surgery like the Oxford Textbook of Medicine, Harrison's Principles of Internal Medicine and Sabiston's Textbook of Surgery are too large for study for this exam. However, these volumes are ideal for referring when one is solving EMQs.
5. "French Index of Differential Diagnosis" is a good reference book.

Paediatrics
6. Oxford handbooks cover this subject adequately, but "Essential Paediatrics" by David Hull published by Churchill Livingstone can be referred for important topics.

Dermatology
7. Go through OHCM and for very important topics please go through "Lecture Notes in Dermatology".

Surgery
8. Bailey and Love is very useful book containing all the information needed regarding for surgery
9. "Lecture Notes on General Surgery" is a good book for surgery reading.
10. Oxford handbooks contribute good supplementary reading, especially the "OHCM".
11. Orthopaedics is well covered in the "OHCM" but if time allows one should also read "Lecture Notes on Orthopedics" or Concise System of Orthopaedics and Fractures by Apley.

ENT and Ophthalmology
12. OHCS does contain ENT and Ophthalmology, ENT and Ophthalmology constitutes a very small portion of the PLAB test. The small coverage of this topic in this book is quite adequate to prepare for the PLAB test.

13. Lecture Notes in ENT and Ophthalmology can be referred to for some selected important topics.

Obstetrics and Gynaecology

13. Ten Teachers by is the one, which is commonly referred to by most of the students.
14. Lecture Notes on Obstetrics and Gynaecology can be another option but these subjects are also very well covered in the OHCS.

Psychiatry

15. The OHCM should suffice. For further reading one is advised to go through Davidson or Kumar and Clarke.

INTERNATIONAL ENGLISH LANGUAGE TESTING SYSTEM (IELTS)

Before attempting PLAB one has to prove his linguistic ability in English by getting adequate score in academic module of international English language testing system (IELTS). GMC has decided that adequate score in IELTS is a necessary prerequisite for attempting PLAB. IELTS is now an integral part of the PLAB and therefore no other English proficiency test is acceptable. PLAB and IELTS application forms should have identical details, especially the name and address as the two results will be joined together. So IELTS is the first hurdle one has to clear before attempting PLAB. The british council (which administers IELTS) requires ones identity. The only identify British council accepts valid PASSPORT or A NATIONAL IDENTITY CARD WITH A NUMBER. **Having a valid PASSPORT is the prerequisite for attempting IELTS so get a passport as the first step towards UK.**

INTRODUCTION

IELTS is a test of English language proficiency. It is a way of assessing the English of non-native speakers who want to study or train using English. The test is offered on demand and measures general language skills and also the skills needed for studying and training.

When can one take the Test?

Test centres have their own testing days in response to local demands. You have to apply 3-4 months in advance to be assured of a date of your choice.

What does the test consist of?

The candidates are tested in communication (written as well as oral) skills in the IELTS exam.

PLAB candidates shoud sit for the academic module. The test format is as follows:

I. *Listening*
4 sections, around 40 items
30 minutes

II. *Academic Reading*
3 sections, around 40 items
60 minutes

III. *Academic Writing*
2 tasks (150 to 250 words)
60 minutes

IV. *Speaking*
10-15 minutes

More details regarding each component of the exam is detailed in IELTS handbook which you will get when you apply for the test.

How long does it take to get the Result and What does it Mean?

- Your results are sent to you and can be sent direct to the GMC within two weeks of taking the test.
- Scores are recorded on a test report form.
- All scores are given on a scale ranging from 1 to 9; i.e. from non-user to expert user with fully operational command of the language.
- The GMC requirement is a minimum of Band 7.0 on the IELTS on a scale of 9 Bands.

Doctors taking PLAB need to get an overall IELTS score of at least 7 but must not score less than 6 in any section of the test. From June 2000 candidates must, in addition, score a minimum of 7 in the speaking section of the test.

Doctors with exemption from PLAB must not score less than 7 in any section of the test.

How can one Prepare for the Test?

An IELTS specimen material pack is available in British council and library. This includes a full practice test with a cassette and an answer key. One can gain experience in the format of the test and get an idea of ones competence. Another book called 'How to prepare for IELTS' is designed to help candidates prepare for the test. This book is available from the British council.

A study pack called 'Cambridge Practice Tests for IELTS T by Vanessa Jackman and Clare Mc-Dowell is available at the British library for reference.

Useful Tips

Instead of buying these expensive books, one may spend time at the British library reading the books for 3 to 5 days. One could also photocopy important sections from one's friend's copy. It is wise to go through these practice packs prior to taking the test (even if one thinks one is proficient with english language).

How do you Apply for IELTS?

One should write to the nearest test centre which is given below and ask them for an application form and IELTS Handbook. The names of test centres in UK, India, Pakistan, Bangladesh and Sri Lakna is given below:

Address

Bridgewater House
58 Whitworth Street
Manchester,
United Kingdom, M1 688
Tel: 44 1619577218
Fax: 441619577029
E-mail: ed@britcoun.org

India

In India there are 12 centres currently which offer IELTS. They are in Delhi, Mumbai, Kolkata, Chennai, Bangalore, Thiruvanthapuram, Hyderabad, Pune, Ahmedabad, Bhopal, Lucknow, Patna.

In North India
Examination Services Manager
New Delhi

Address
Name: Sanjay Patro
British High Commission
British Council Division
17 Kasturba Gandhi Marg
E-mail:sanjay.patro@in.britishcouncil.org. New Delhi 110 001
Tel: 91-3710111/37 10555
Fax: 91-3710717

The British Library
Mayfair Building,
Hazratganj
Lucknow 226 001
Telephone + 91 (0)522 22 2144
Fax + 91 (0)522 27 5426
E-mail bipin.kumar@in.britishcouncil.org.

The British Library
Guru Teg Bahadur Complex
Roshanpura Naka,
Bhopal 462 003
Telephone +91 (0)755 55 3767
Fax+91 (0)755 57 2797
E-mail girish.kunkur@in.britishcouncil.org.

In South India
Examination Services Manager
Chennai

Address
Name:Nirupa Fernandez
British Deputy High Commission
British Council Division
737 Anna Salai
E-mail:nirupa.fernandez@in.britishcouncil.org.
Chennai 600 002
Tel: 91-44-852-5002
Fax: 91-44-852-3234

The British Library
39, St. Mark's Road
Banglore 560 001
Telephone +91(0)80 2240763, 221 3485
Fax + 91(0) 80 224 0767
E-mail iqbal.jahagirdar@in.britishcouncil.org.

The British Library
Sarovar Centre, 5-9-22
Secretariat Road,
Hyderabad 500 063
Telephone+91(0)40 230774, 210267
Fax: +91(0)40 329 8273
E-mail sudhakar.goud@in.britishcouncil.org.

The British Library
YMCA Building,
Thiruvananthapuram 695 001
Telephone +91(0)471 330716
Fax +91(0)471 33 0717
E-mail tk.subramoni@in.britishcouncil.org.

Examination Services Manager
Kolkata

Address
Name: Suchitra Mukherjee
British Deputy Commission
British Council Division
5 Shakespeare Sarani
E-mail:suchitra.mukherjee@in.britishcouncil.org.
Kolkata 700071
Tel: 91-33-282-9108/9144
Fax: 91-33-282-4808

The British Library
BP Koirala Marg (Bank Rd.), Patna 800 001
Telephone +91(0)612 22 4198
Fax +91 (0)612 23 0798
E-mail dipak.goswami@in.britishcouncil.org.

Examinatination Services Manager
Mumbai

Address
Name: Kamal Taraparevala
British Deputy High Commission
British Council Division
Mittal Tower 'C' Wing
Nariman Point
Mumbai 400021
E-mail:kamal.taraporevala@in.britishcouncil.org.
Tel: 91-22-222-3560
Fax: 91-22-285-2024

The British Library
Bhaikaka Bhawan,
Law Garden Road,
Ahmedabad 380 006
Telephone +91(0)79 646 4693
Fax- +91 (0)79 646 9493
E-mail satish.deshpande@in.britishcouncil.org.

The British Library
917/1,
Fergusson College Road,
Pune 411 004
Telphone +91 (0)20 565 4352
Fax +91 (0)20 565 4351
E-mail.anil.bakshi@in.britishcouncil.org.

Pakistan
Examination Services Manager
Karachi

Address
Name: Irum Fawad
The British Council
20 Bleak House Road,
Near Cant's Station
E-mail:Irum.Fawad@bc-karachi.bcouncil.org.
(PO Box 10410), Karachi
Tel: 92215670391-7
Fax: 92215682694

Examination Services Manager
Islamabad

Address
Name: Shahnaz Farooq
The British Council
Block 14, Civic Centre — Tel: 9251111424424
G-6 — Fax: 9251276683
E-mail:shahnaz.farooq@bc.islamabad.bcouncil.org.
Islamabad

Bangladesh
Examination Services Manager
Dhaka

Address
Name: Saidur Rahman
The British Council — Tel: 8802868905-7
5 Fuller Road, — Fax: 8802863375
PO Box 161
E-mail:srhman@The British Council.net
Dhaka 1000

Sri Lanka
Examination Services Manager
Colombo

Address
Name: Ethel Nanayakkara — Tel:941581171
The British Council — Fax: 941587079
49 Alfred Gardens
E-mail:ethel.nanayakkara@britcoun.lk
(PO Box 753) Colombo 3
Sri Lanka

ROUTES OF EXEMPTION FROM THE PLAB TEST

INTRODUCTION

Doctors with a primary medical qualification accepted for limited registration must either have passed the PLAB test (a test of proficiency in the English language and knowledge of medicine), or be exempted from it before limited registration may be granted. Doctors may be granted exemption from the test if they qualify through one of the following routes. These doctors are not normally required to pass the test **unless they have previously failed it.** That means **once one attempts PLAB one cannot get limited registration through other routes.**

1. SPONSORSHIP ROUTE

This is for doctors who are sponsored for approved postgraduate training in the UK by one of the approved sponsoring bodies or the head of a university department.

To be eligible for restricted exemption a doctor must be sponsored for approved postgraduate training in the UK by one of the approved sponsoring bodies. The approved sponsoring bodies in the UK are the Medical Royal Colleges, the faculty of public health medicine, the British council, the commonwealth scholarship commission and the department of health (on behalf of the WHO).

Doctors who may be sponsored by the university head of department, are those who wish to undertake clinical duties in connection with or as a supplement to their academic training. In order to apply for such exemption the head of the university department should write to the GMC on behalf of the doctor setting out details of the post.

All doctors applying for exemption from the test by the sponsorship route must fulfil the following experience requirements. They must

- have completed overseas an acceptable internship of not less than twelve months, or other experience which the GMC regard as equivalent; and
- thereafter have completed not less than two years in medical practice overseas, of which not less than one year must have been spent in the specialty in which he or she wished to pursue further training in the UK; and
- the doctor must have been appointed, normally before arrival in the United Kingdom, either within the national health service to a supervised training post at the grade of senior house officer or higher or within a university, or comparable research body, to an appointment as lecturer or above, or to a clinical research position of equivalent status. In such cases there must be an honorary national health service contract and
- **he/she must have a minimum overall scale of 70 in IELTS academic modules with not less than 7.0 in each band.**

2. Higher Qualification Route

This is for doctors who, in addition to their primary overseas medical qualification, and 12 months internship also either hold or have passed all the examinations for a higher qualification granted by one of the medical royal colleges or faculties in the United Kingdom or the republic of Ireland (such as the MRCP (UK), FRCO path or FRCS Ireland) or have passed or been exempted from the primary examinations for the MRCPath or the FRCR. These doctors may be granted restricted exemption from the PLAB test in relation only to supervised appointments in the specialty or group of specialities covered by the higher qualification. A doctor applying for limited registration by this roue must first be offered a post for which limited registration may be granted, as explained above. They must meet the IELTS requirement described before.

3. Senior Doctor Route

The GMC will also accept an application from a doctor who has been qualified and has practised overseas for at least 10 years and reached consultant grade or equivalent. To be eligible a doctor should be intending to settle permanently in the UK and must have the support of UK consultant who can offer or arrange a post for which limited registration may be granted. The UK consultant must also be prepared to provide the necessary assurances as to the doctor's linguistic and professional ability as required by section 22 of the Medical Act 1983. For further information the consultant should write to the GMC enclosing the doctor's full curriculum vitae.

4. UK Qualification Route

Doctors who, in addition to their primary overseas medical qualification plus 12 months internship, also hold or have passed all the examinations for one of the following primary medical qualifications set by the united examining board:

- LRCS England, LRCP London
- LMSSA London

- LRCP Edinburgh, LRCS Edinburgh, LRCPS Glasgow are eligible for exemption from the PLAB test.

5. Irish Qualification Route

This is for doctors who are not EEA nationals and who qualified in the Republic of Ireland and have normally completed a one year internship.

Following a decision by overseas committee non-EEA nationals with Irish qualifications will, with effect from 1, January 2000, Cease to be except from the PLAB test solely by virtue of their primary qualifications. From this date, such doctors who wish to apply for limited registration will be required either to pass the PLAB test or to provide other objective evidence of their capability for medical practice in UK.

6. Temporary Full Registration: Visiting Overseas Doctors

Doctors who have a primary medical qualification and 12 months internship which is accepted for limited registration may under section 29 of the Medical Act 1983 apply for temporary full registration as a visiting overseas doctor. This type of registration is intended for doctors who are coming to the UK to demonstrate or provide specialist services in short-term appointments as visiting consultants or professors or at a similar academic level in a teaching hospital or medical school. Doctors wishing to apply should arrange for their prospective employer to write to the GMC for further details enclosing a full curriculum vitae and providing details of the post for which registration is required. All such initial applications are determined by a committee of the GMC.

7. Primary Medical Qualification Recognised for full/Provisional Registration

Doctors are exempt from the PLAB test because they qualified as follows:

a. in Australia, New Zealand, the West Indies; or
b. at the Universities of Cape Town, Natal or the Witwatersrand in South Africa; or
c. at certain universities in Hong Kong, or Singapore where the language of instruction is English; or
d. at the University of Malaya on or before 31 December 1987.

As from 1st January 1999, doctors who hold a qualification from the countries listed in sections (a) to (d) will be required to pass the IELTS test with a minimum overall score in 7.0 in the Academic module with not less than 7.0 in each band.

For further information and whether they qualify for these the candidates are advised to write to GMC directly.

OVERSEAS DOCTORS TRAINING SCHEME (ODTS)

What is the ODTS?

The overseas doctors training scheme (ODTS) is a formalised double sponsorship scheme initiated jointly by the department of health and the royal colleges and administered by the relevant royal college. The scheme grants acceptable candidates exemption from the professional and linguistic assessment board (PLAB) examination.

The scheme provides very able overseas-qualified doctors with postgraduate training posts to enable them to continue or complete their specialist training in the UK before returning home. It is not intended that overseas doctors remain in the UK on completion of their specialist training.

Why was the ODTS set up?

The Royal Colleges felt that a formalised scheme of this nature was needed to provide supervised specialist training of a consistently high standard for overseas-qualified doctors of quality who wished to complete their training in the UK. The aim of the scheme is to ensure that the training is of a high standard in order to prepare the overseas doctor for a specialist career in medicine in his/her own country.

Who is eligible?

The requirements are as follows

From January 1998, all overseas doctors must have passed the academic version of the IELTS test (international English language testing system) to be granted limited registration by the general medical council. Doctors with exemption from PLAB must score a minimum of 7 in each of the four bands of the test. This includes doctors from English speaking countries; USA, Australia New Zealand, Canada, South Africa, West Indies).

A primary medical qualification acceptable to the GMC for limited registration; plus one year's post-qualification experience (normally referred to as internship).

At least two years experience in the relevant speciality in which they wish to practice. An acceptable postgraduation qualification and/part-1of the relevant Royal College examination.

Canditates who do not meet the above requirements, would not be eligible for the ODTS scheme. Also excluded from applying would be the following:

- applicants who have previously failed the PLAB test.
- applicants who do not hold Part 1 of the relevant Royal College examination.
- applicants qualified in and/or nationals of an EEA country, or those with enforceable EC rights.
- applicants already working or who are resident in the UK, or another member state of the EU.

Which ODTS schemes exist?

Summary of recent information received from the Royal Colleges on the ODTS.

We have summarised below the current situation from information collected by the individual Royal Colleges. The situation is fluid and liable to change. **It is therefore important that you contact the relevant royal college for information and advice, before coming to the UK.**

The authors want the reader to write to respective Royal College to know the latest status.

Royal College of Anaesthetists

ODTS double-sponsorship scheme. The initial approach must be made by a senior medical practitioner from the UK. All appointments must be to substantive, approved training posts. Applications will also be considered from individual doctors whose medical background meets the criteria of the Royal College. They would be required to apply for advertised, approved training posts, in open competition.

Royal College of Obstetricians and Gynaecologists

The overseas doctors training scheme and double ended sponsorship scheme organised by the RCOG was abolished from February 2000. Requirements of a new unified scheme have been approved by the college council but the college is still waiting a final report from the department of health, reviewing of all the sponsorship schemes, before the RCOG will be in aposition to complement the new scheme. It is hoped that the new scheme will involve interviewing doctors overseas and numbers will be restricted to ensure that there is always a training programme available for every successful candidate (i.e. no waiting list). Until such time when the requirements for the new scheme are approved by department of health, the college will not be able to sponsor new doctors for exemption from the GMC's PLAB test. In the mean time the doctors who wish to apply for the new sponsorship scheme, should contact the college the details will be sent to them as soon as they become available.

E-mail:– cwood@rcog.org.uk

Royal College of Ophthalmologists

Dual sponsorship scheme is in operation. All posts must be approved for training by the college and postgraduate dean. Honorary SHO posts will be longer be accepted unless they have the approval of the postgraduate dean. For further information contact the Royal College. E-mail enquiries to **education@rcophth.btinternet.com.** Information can also be had from colleges website address.

Royal College of Paediatrics and Child Health

Double sponshorship scheme: Overseas sponsor and UK sponsor. The college will sponsor doctors for supernumerary posts that have been approved by the postgraduate dean and for approved substantive training posts. International Paediatric Training Scheme; information about the scheme is being updated, contact the Royal College for advice.

Royal College of Physicians of Edinburgh

The college has temporarily suspended the overseas doctors training double sponsorship scheme. Please contact the Royal College for updated information.

Royal College of Physicians and Surgeons of Glasgow

The college has advised that there are difficulties in placing people applying for the ODTS. Doctors applying must be funded/supported by their home country. Please contact the Royal College for updated information.

Royal College of Physicians of London

The Royal College of Physicians overseas doctors training scheme is closed. The college is awaiting the rsult of the current review of overseas doctors training being carried out by the department of health, before making a final decision on the development of any revised scheme. The college will consider applications for sponsorship for PLAB exemption from physicians who have been awarded an official scholarship or bursary for clinical training in the UK. Overseas training enquiries, telephone +44(0) 207935 1174;fax-+44(0)20 74864034 E-mail:international@rcplondon.ac.uk

Royal College of Psychiatrists

ODTS is closed indefinitely. Consultant assisted sponsorship scheme; Doctors applying for this scheme must have a UK sponsor who should be a consultant in the NHS and a member of the royal college of psychiatrists. Your UK sponsor must be able to offer you a training post within their own training scheme, which should be fully approved by the college. Your UK sponsor is also required to provide written confirmation that they know your overseas sponsor personally. For further information contact the Royal College of Psychiatrists.

Royal College of Radiologists

The initial application must be made by the UK Sponsor, not the trainee. An overseas sponsor is also required. The UK training post must be within a training scheme recognised by the Royal College of Radiologists, and a salaried, substantive NHS training post. For further information contact the Royal College of Radiologists.

Royal College of Edinburgh

The ODTS double sponsorship scheme is the only scheme operated at present. It is the responsibility of the overseas sponsor to set up a post for the application in the UK, in partnership with a UK consultant. The first contact with the Royal College must be made by the UK consultant who is offering the post.

Royal College and Surgeons of England

Applicants must be nominated by an approved sponsoring body in their home country. The Royal College of Surgeons of England will act as the UK sponsoring body. The college is not able to arrange training posts for sponsored doctors at present. Trainees must have an appointment arranged in the UK before applying to the college for double sponsorship. For further information, please contact the college.

Overview

- Applications direct from candidates will not be accepted by the Royal Colleges; only appropriate sponsors may apply on their behalf.
- Many more applications are received than there are training posts available.
- Detailed information on a particular overseas doctors training scheme is provided by the relevant college. If further information is required, please contact the college at the address given **in useful addresses chapter.** Applications from sponsors should be sent to the same address.

VISA MATTERS, TRAVEL AND STAY IN UK

Decide first whether you want to take part I in India or in UK, if you decide to take part I in India and after passing part I, after receiving hall ticket for part II, go to the British Embassy at Madras (Chennai) (for candidates from South India), Mumbai (for candidates from West Zone). Kolkata (East Zone), New Delhi for all others. There, one will be applying for a visa for a period of six months. One has to take these documents to be on the safe side.

1. PLAB hall ticket with passport.
2. Sponsor's letter from UK.
3. Bank statement showing finances of at least Rs. 2-2.5 lakhs.
4. A leave note from your present employer.

Visa Facts

1. Prior to October 2nd 2000, single entry VISA's were isued for 6 months, generally as a "tourist" or "for PLAB". Since then VISAs are being issued for upto 1 year or even 2 years, and are multiple-entry. This means that you can travel between India and UK as many times as you want, without having to get a new VISA.
2. The cost of the VISA is Rs.2300/- for a 6 month single entry but these are subject to change and should be found out from the British High Commission at the time of visa application.
3. On getting a job, you change your VISA to "permit free" VISA. Only then you can begin work in the hospital and be paid for it. The change of VISA happens within a day as soon as you produce the GMC registration and take it and your passport to the immigration office.
4. If you do not get a job in the first 6 months, your VISA has expired, you could extend it for another 6 months within the UK.

Experiences with Getting VISA from India

VISA is not a big problem, unlike the US VISA, only a few are refused VISA. The VISA form is available beforehand and you may fill it and take it with you. The officer mainly wants to confirm that you can fend for yourself in the months leading upto the examination and beyond before you get a job. They also would like to hear that you will return back to India when you are done with your training. You can show that you have reasons to return back (such a property in India, a promise of a job, etc.).

A PLAB admit card is almost a must. You do not need "no objection certificates" from anyone.

On some occasions the VISA officers have allegedly asked (unbecoming) questions, possibly due to a basic ignorance of the special VISA doctors have, to work in the UK. You should point out that doctors and dentists do not need a "work permit", they can work on a "Permit free training" type VISA. At heathrow, the VISA is but a formality, only those with forged documents are sent back.

The common mistakes doctors make:

1. Lying for anything to a VISA officer is a problem.
2. Do not produce any forged or wrong documents.
3. If they ask how long do you want to stay in UK, tell honestly that after the exam, I will be looking for a training post, and the earliest I return could be months or even a year odd.
4. No taking proper support letter from UK and PLAB entry letter is not helpful.
5. Refusal of VISA by the US on your passport is often counterproductive.

The cost of an air tickets to UK at present, is approximately Rs. 20000-30000 depending on the Air line (one-way). While travelling, take most of your clothing as buying these will entail extra expenses in England.

Pack lots of warm clothing, like thermal undergarments and sweaters. Take along packets of 'sambhar' powder and chilli powder to aid you in cooking.

Take a couple of blazers and ties along with formal showes. In hospitals in the UK, senior house officers wear formal outfits with a tie and the consultants wear suits. However, when you appear for PLAB part 2, you will have to wear a suit, preferably black. You will not need your white coats or your medical instruments when you appear for Part 2.

Before landing in England, have full knowledge of the place where you will be staying. It would be pertinent to note that paying guest accommodation in eastham is most suitable for Indian students. These houses are occupied by India families who will help in every way.

After landing in England and getting place of boarding, one would be benefitted immensely by joining the MMC flats (Madras Medical College, alumni flats). Here make a down payment of 100 pounds and use the material in the files for extensive revision. There is no need to pay for any subsequent attempts. The only disadvantage of this place is that one cannot xerox the files kept there.

REGISTRATION AND APPLYING FOR A JOB

The results of PLAB II (OSCE) examination will be declared within two to three weeks of the test. It will be either PASS or FAIL.

If one passes the OSCE one will be sent forms and details about applying for limited registration. Before you are granted limited registration your primary qualification must be checked. After passing the examination one will register with the general medical council after paying a registration fee. Then you should look for job opportunities in classified section of the BMJ and British Journal of Hospital Medicine.

The addresses and websites for looking for job is given in the end of the book.

Limited Registration

The information in this chapter will apply if one has taken and passed the PLAB test and hold a primary medical qualification accepted by the GMC for limited registration.

Applications, original documents and payments may be sent by post or submitted in person between 09:00 am and 16:30 pm Monday to Friday at the general medical council, reception, 5th floor, North entrance, 178 Great Portland street, London WlN 6 JE, please note that it is not possible for the reception staff to indicate whether or not registration will be granted.

The GMC authorities are not in position to answer questions relating to work permits or visas. One should direct such enquiries to the home office, immigration department, lunar house, wellesley road, Croydon Surrey.

Similarly, if one needs advice about postgraduate training, how to apply for jobs or clinical attachments one should contact the national advice centre for postgraduate medical education, central information service. The British council, Medlock Street, Manchester M15 4PR which is given separately.

BASIC REQUIREMENTS FOR LIMITED REGISTRATION

Qualifications

You must hold or have passed the final qualifying examinations for a primary medical qualifications accepted for limited registration. The GMC authorities normally accept primary medical qualifications awarded at universities listed in the world directory of medical schools published by the World Health Organisation as well as qualifications and universities which are not in the directory but which have, in the past, been accepted by the GMC. There are about 1400 universities awarding primary medical qualifications which are currently accepted.

Selection for Employment

By law, one must have been selected for employment before GMC can grant, one limited registration for the first time. Registration will normally be granted only for supervised employment in posts which afford education and training approved by a Royal College or faculty or joint higher committee or, in Scotland, by a regional postgraduate committee. The GMC authorities understand that normally only posts in the national health service training grades of senior house officer (SHO), specialist registrar (SpR) are educationally approved in this way, Positions such as a staff grade or consultant posts are not so approved.

Good Character

The medical act requires that the GMC is satisfied that an applicant for limited registration is of good character. One is asked to complete a declaration on the form and one should tell the GMC if one has any convictions or have had any restrictions placed on one's practice in another country.

Other types of employment one can hold under limited registration.

Honorary Posts

Limited registration may also be granted for an honorary, supernumerary or non-established hospital post which is not itself educationally approved but only if there is an equivalent established post in exactly the same grade and speciality which is educationally approved in the manner described above.

Clinical Assistant Posts

Limited registration may also be granted for a hospital post at clinical assistant grade. but only if the post is approved for training programmes under the auspices of a university faculty or university clinical department, and documentary evidence or this is provided by the head of the faculty or department concerned.

Posts at House Officer Level or in Family Planning Clinics

Please contact the board for individual advice if you wish to work in these posts.

Note-If one has taken the PLAB test without first completing a 12 month's internship or its equivalent one will have to complete the balance of experience in house officer posts, either in the UK or overseas. One can then apply to work at senior house officer level or higher.

Scope of Limited Registration

Once limited registration has been granted the board will send a certificate of limited registration which sets out the description of the employment which one may undertake. It you work in one post which are not covered by the description on one's certificate one may be practising illegally. It is one's responsibility to ensure that one holds registration which is appropriate to the employment in which one is engaged. Further advice on the scope of limited registration is given in the booklet 'limited registration' which will be sent with certificate of limited registration.

Guidance on the duties of a doctor will be sent with the first certificate issued. Additional specific guidance will be sent concerning the scope of limited registration.

Five Year Maximum Period

By law the maximum total period of limited registration which can be granted to a doctor is five years.

Limited registration will expire on the terminal date of registration shown on certificate of limited registration.

How to make an Application for Registration

Once one has passed the PLAB test a form LR/PLAB will be sent. One should complete part 1 oneself, and then ask an authorised officer of the autority or institution in which one is to be employed to complete part 2. This will normally be the medical, staffing officer, unit medical officer, personnel officer or cosultant in administrative charge.

If one is applying for a further period of limited registration one also needs to complete part 1, of form LR/PLAB. However, part 2 of the form need only be completed if one intends to renew or extend one's registration for employment as a house officer or clinical assistant.

Registration of Names

One will be registered in the names which appears on one's original diploma of qualification (or an English translation of it). Additional documentary evidence of your names may be required if:

a. One wishes to be registered in a name which is different from that which appears on one's diploma; or
b. One submits any other documents in support of one's application which refers by a name which does not appear on the original diploma.

One should bear in mind that, although initials can appear in doctor's entries in the limited register, all names must be shown in full in the 'main' register. If one was subsequently to apply for full registration at a later date, therefore, it may be necessary to provide further evidence of full names at that stage.

Where additional documentary evidence of a doctor's name is required the following is normally accepted provided that the document is original and gives in full both his name in which one wishes to be registered:

a. A further certificate from the university at which you obtained your primary medical qualification confirming the person who graduated and the person applying for registration are one and the same;
b. As evidence of a change of name on marriage, a marriage certificate.

One should give an address for entry in the register which is reliable and effective so that communications from the GMC can reach you without delay. Failure to maintain a reliable address may lead to delay in future grants of limited registration or to erasure from the register. Changes of address can be notified in writing (letter or fax) or by telephone.

Evidence of Qualifications

One will need to send original documentary evidence of one's primary medical qualification if not already produced. This evidence should comprise:

a. The original diploma issued by the university or other body which granted the medical qualification; or
b. An original certificate from that university or body stating the date on which the medical qualification was granted; or
c. An original certificate from that university or body stating that one passed the examinations and completed the curriculum necessary for obtaining the qualification and that one is eligible to receive the qualification.

Any certificate as described at a or b should bear the stamp or insign of the university or body by which it was first issued or give other acceptable evidence of authenticity. It should also be signed by a person whose name and official position at the university or body are clearly identified.

The GMC authorities accept only original documents: duplicate copies of university diplomas, including attested copies and photocopies are not accepted. If one cannot provide original documents, one should inform in writing of the circumstances why this is so. The

candidate will be advised on what other arrangement, if any, can be made.

Documents not in English must be accompanied by the original of a translation certified as correct by a government authority or an official translator.

Fees

The fees for an initial application for limited registration for up to 12 months and seven days is £ 300. In addition a scrutiny fee of £ 100 is also payable (making a total of £ 400) unless one has already paid this fee when applying to take the PLAB test. The fees for further grants of limited registration are as follows:

a. Renewal of limited registration for up to 12 months and seven days for the same description or range of employment as that or which limited registration was previously granted: £ 70.
b. Extension of limited registraion for up to 12 months and seven days for a different or additional description or range of employment from that for which limited registration was previously granted: £ 140.
c. Each additional year or part of a year, if more than 12 months and seven days registration is required at one time: £ 70 .

One can pay by cash, cheque, banker's draft or traveller's cheque provided that they are issued in sterling. Euro cheques up to a maximum value of £ 700 are also accepted.

How to Stop your Registration

Voluntary Erasure

The main advantage of voluntary erasure is to avoid using portions of the total period of five years, limited registration during periods when one does not need to be registered.

If one wishes to remove one's name from the register before the date on which one's limited registration expires one should complete the form on the back of all current certificates of limited registration.

If one proposes to apply for voluntary erasure while holding a contract of employment as a medical practitioner in the United Kingdom one is advised to discuss the matter with one's employing authority.

Voluntary erasure is not granted retrospectively. One should not assume that one's name has been removed from the register until one has received a letter confirming this.

No fee is charged for voluntary erasure but no refund is made for unused periods of limited registration, nor is credit given for registration.

When one wishes one's name to be returned to the register following voluntary erasure an application should be made on form LR/PLAB.

Notes on Moving from Limited to Full Registration

Please use of this chapter to help to make your application to move from limited to full registration.

Please note that this does not apply if one has requalified in the United Kingdom by obtaining one or more of the following qualifications:

1. LRCS England, LRCP London, LMSSA London; or
2. LRCP Edinburgh, LRCS Edinburgh, LRCPS Glasgow;

Please contact the GMC for the appropriate application form and guidance.

About this Guidelines

This guidelines is divided into the following sections:

A. What one should know about full registration.
B. Guidances used in deciding and application.
C. Other ways to move from limited to full registration.
D. What happens to an application.
E. How to make application.
F. Unsuccessful applications.

A. What one Should know about Full Registration

- The guidelines the board uses to decide whether one can move from limited to full registration are decribed in detail.
- The GMC authorities understand that the grant of full registration does not of itself have an effect an status under the immigration rules.
- If one's experience does not meet the guidelines please contact the authorities for advice before making an application.

B. Applications which do not Meet the Guidelines

1. Applications which do not meet the guidelines will be determined by the GMC's overseas committee.
2. However, it is open to apply if one has held limited registration with preserved rights that is, one's limited registration is not restricted to maximum of five years in aggregate and one has.

a. At least 10 years continuous service in the NHS in predominantly substantive or long-term (longer than six months) locum posts.
b. Recent clinical practice in the UK (at least two years practice during the previous three years) Plus.
c. Favourable reports from the UK consultants who have supervised one during the most recent two years practice.

The authorities will need to refer to the GMC's overseas committee applications from doctors with 'preserved rights' whose experience falls outside these guidelines.

One should inform if one has been offered a post as trainee in general practice and has obtained hospital experience accepted by the joint committee on postgraduate training for general practice as fulfilling the relevent requirements of the vocational training regulations. The Board will then tell what further documents one will need.

The overseas committee has indicated that, except in exceptional circumstances, it does not wish to consider applications where an applicant's experience falls substantially short of the guidelines. If one feels that one's circumstances are exceptional one must provide details of one's reasons for applying early.

E. How to make your Application

1. As the board has to gather a number of items to enable it to process one's application, one should make it well in advance of the date on which on would like full registration to begin.
2. Your application should consist of:
a. A completed application form to move from limited to full registration (Form LRFR);
b. A fee of £ 500 if one is making first application or £ 250 if one is re-applying;
c. The documents described in paragraphs D4 (if not already submitted) D6, and D10;
3. Please send application to the GMC. If one done not with to send original documents or payments through the post, one may bring them between 9.00 hours and 16.30 hours Monday to Friday to the GMC's reception on the fifth floor at 178 Great Portland street, London WIN6JE.

Documents Required

Primary Medical Qualifications

The GMC will normally have seen evidence of one's primary medical before one was the prefix 'p.e.' on one's certificate of limited registration this means that the GMC has received evidence only that one has passed the examinations for one's primary medical qualification. In this case, please submit additional evidence that the qualification was subsequently, conferred. The original diploma issued by the university or body stating the qualification and the date on which it was formally conferred. Such a certificate should bear the stamp of the university or body. It should also be signed by a person whose name and official position at the university body are clearly identified.

The board accepts only documents as evidence of one's primary qualification, not copies or photocopies. The evidence does not have diploma itself. It may be an original letter from the university or an original certificate. If one cannot provide original documents, please write and provide with details as to the reasons why. If the document is not in English, please provide an original translation certified as correct by a government authority or an official translator.

Evidence of Basic Specialist Training

If appropriate, please provide a document from the training body to confirm that one has completed basic specialist training. Photocopies and faxed copies are acceptable for this purpose.

Completing the Application Form

Applicant's name for entry in the register.

This will usually be the same as shown in the limited register (initials cannot be included in your register entry see d. below). If it is different you should send additional documentary evidence of the change. The following evidence is acceptable.

a. A further original certificate from the university at which you obtained your overseas primary medical qualification showing both the name in which you graduated and the name which you wish to be entered in the register of medical practitioners, with all names shown in full.
b. An original marriage certificate accompanied by a translation if necessary, provided that the certificate shows the name in which you have held limited registration and in full, the name which you are now using.
c. An affidavit or statutory declaration sworn before a notary public or oath commissioner.
d. Your passport as evidence of a name previously recorded by the GMC as an initial.

Address for Entry in the Register

It is important to choose for entry in the register of medical practitioners. It is reliable and effective. The board sends all communication to your registered address. If you do not respond to them, this may, in certain circumstances, lead to the erasure of your name from the register. You may wish to bear in mind that the whole of your register entry including your address is public information and, for this reason, you may prefer not to use your professional or private address for registration purposes.

While your application is being considered the board may wish to contact you by telephone. It would, therefore, be helpful if you could provide a daytime telephone and/or fax number. These will not form part of your register entry and will not be disclosed.

Consultant's Reports

You will need to provide in form LRFR the names and addresses of the consultants who have supervised you in every post at least for 3 months duration held in the UK during the last three years. Please forward to each of them a copy of the enclosed consultant report form (CRF) asking them to complete it and return it direct to the GMC. Further CRGs may be provided if required. Please do not ask your consultants to give their reports to you, the reports should be sent direct to the GMC.

Declaration

As an applicant for full registration you must satisfy the registrar of the GMC that you are of good character. You must declare on form LRER whether you have been convicted or found guilty by a court of law and whether you have been suspended or disqualified or prohibited from practicing medicine, or from being registered as a medical practitioner, in any country.

Information About Fees

The fee for an initial application is £ 500 pounds payable in advance. If the board does not approve your application, £ 250 pounds will be retained by the GMC to cover the cost of considering and determining your application; the remainder of the fee paid will be refunded to you. The fee for any subsequent application is £ 250 pounds.

Cheques or moneyorders for the appropriate fee should be made payable to the general medical council. Payments sent from overseas should be by bank draft or moneyorder payable in sterling in the United Kingdom or by a cheques on an account in the UK.

The board will send you a refund of any fees paid for whole years of unused limited registration which remain to you at the date on which full registration is granted.

Outcome of Your Application

If your application meets the guidelines, the board will send you a certificate of full registration and information booklet about full registration and a copy of the publication of duties of a doctor. When you are fully registered, your name will appear in the principal list of the register of medical practitioners. You will need to pay an annual fee of 80 £ on the anniversary of your date of full registration.

Not all applications received by the GMC meet the guidelines and you should not, therefore, work in any post for which full registration is required until the board have informed you that your application has been granted. If you currently hold limited registration for your present employment in the UK and are eligible to apply for it to be extended or renewed, you should do so if you need further registration while your application for full registration is being considered.

If your application is refused the board will notify you by letter as soon as the overseas committee has made its decision and the board will refund £ 250.

If you have held limited registration for a period of at least three years and six months at the time of the GMC's decision to refuse your application for full registration, you may apply to the review board for overseas qualified practitioners for a review of the decision. If you are eligible to apply to the board you will be given further information about this in the letter notifying you of the outcome of your application.

THE WORK PERMIT ISSUE

The Department of Health announced on 7 March 2006 that from 3 April 2006 International Medical Graduates (IMGs) - who are not UK or EEA nationals - wishing to work or train in the UK will need a work permit. To obtain a work permit an employer must show that a genuine vacancy exists, which cannot be filled by a doctor who is a UK or EEA national.

GMC mentions that the NHS will continue to need small numbers of specialist doctors, who can bring their skills and experience to the NHS. However, increasingly the NHS will be less reliant on international medical recruitment. This will obviously affect the number of posts available to IMGs.

According to the announcement, all doctors wishing to work in the UK from outside the European Union (EU) will be required to have a work permit from July 2006.

The move means that any NHS trust wishing to employ a doctor from outside the EU will have to prove that a 'home-grown' doctor cannot fill the vacant post, ending the current permit free training arrangement for international doctors.

Health Minister Lord Warner said:
"We now have more than 117,000 doctors working in the NHS, 27,400 more than in 1997 as well as record levels of doctors in training in UK medical schools.

"This investment and expansion, coupled with the reform of medical education, is leading to increased competition for medical posts as vacancy rates fall.

"Therefore, to ensure that we are only recruiting doctors to the UK where we have a genuine skills shortage NHS Trusts will be required to get a work permit for every doctor that they wish to employ from outside the EU.

"In future International Medical Graduates who wish to work or train in the NHS will need a work permit. To obtain a work permit an employer must show that a genuine vacancy exists, which cannot be filled with a resident worker."

"We recognise that international doctors have made a huge contribution to the NHS since it was founded in 1948 and there will still be opportunities for overseas staff to come to the UK. We will continue to need small numbers of specialist doctors, who can bring their skills and experience to the NHS. However, increasingly the NHS will be less reliant on international medical recruitment."

The only exception will be to allow two years of permit-free training for non-European Union nationals who have trained in a UK medical schools so that they can acquire full registration with the GMC.

Any doctor wishing to apply for postgraduate medical education training in the UK , whether at the Modernising Medical Careers Foundation Programme level or senior house officer stage, will be required to have a work permit.

Currently International Medical Graduates (IMGs) are able to undertake postgraduate medical education in the UK without needing a work permit.

Health Minister Lord Warner added:
"The Department of Health will continue to work with the General Medical Council to ensure that IMGs who are interested in working or training in the UK understand exactly what type of job and training opportunities exist. "

We anticipate International Medical Graduates' (IMGs) employment prospects will significantly worsen following the Department of Health announcement on 7 March 2006. This is in addition to the on-going difficulties IMGs have reported in seeking employment.

ABOLITION OF LIMITED REGISTRATION

The GMC plans to phase out limited registration.

The abolition of limited registration is a major step in achieving a single approach to the registration of all fully qualified doctors. It will mean that there will no longer be a separate probationary period for international medical graduates (IMGs).

IMGs who have completed an internship will in future be eligible to apply for full registration. They will no longer need to obtain an offer of employment in order to do so but they will need to satisfy a number of criteria before a grant of registration can be made.

All new full registrants - UK graduates as well as IMGs - will be restricted initially to working in practice settings recognised by the GMC as acceptable for a practitioner who is newly registered. There will be special arrangements for international medical graduates who have held limited registration and who have already undertaken an acceptable period of recent practice in the UK to allow them to reduce the amount of time that they must spend practising in an approved practice setting after first obtaining full registration. There will also be transitional arrangements which will allow doctors who hold limited registration at the time the changes come into effect to move to full registration, at no extra cost. These doctors will also have to work initially in approved practice settings. We envisage that approved practice settings will include organisations within and outside the NHS.

The Department of Health for England has already consulted on changes to the Medical Act which will, amongst other things, enable the abolition of limited registration, and Parliament and the Privy Council have now approved the necessary legislation. We will be discussing with the Department of Health the implementation time-table for its various provisions.

We will ensure that doctors, sponsors, employers and other interested stakeholders receive full information about the timing and implications of the abolition of limited registration as soon as we can.

More details at: http://www.gmc-uk.org/

FREQUENTLY ASKED QUESTIONS ABOUT CHANGES IN IMMIGRATION RULES

What are the new rules?

From 3rd April 2006, doctors and dentists in postgraduate training will be considered for immigration purposes to be in employment rather than in training. Permit-free training will no longer be available, and those who do not have right of residence in the UK or EEA will require a work permit to undertake employment.

The only exception is for those graduating from a UK medical school who will be allowed permit-free training in order to complete the 2-year Foundation Programme.

What will the changes mean for overseas students who have come to the UK to study medicine?

Overseas students will still be able to complete their undergraduate studies with a student visa. On graduation from a UK medical school they will be eligible to apply for leave to remain in the UK as a Postgraduate Doctor (permit-free training) to undertake a 2-year Foundation Programme and therefore to register with the General Medical Council.

They will compete on an equal footing with UK and EEA resident graduates in the allocation of posts. It is important that this provision remains so that they have a transferable professional registration on completion of their studies. Following completion of the Foundation Programme, if they want to remain in the UK then they will have to switch into another category of the Immigration Rules, such as the work permit system.

Does this stop doctors who have qualified overseas coming to train in the UK?

No. Overseas doctors will still be able to come and train in the UK. However, you will now be considered as being in employment for immigration purposes, and will therefore need to meet the requirements of an employment category of the Immigration Rules, such as the work permit system.

Work permits will only be issued where the post cannot be filled by someone with right of residence in the UK or Europe. The work permit is specific to the post and only for the duration of the post. Each new post will require a new work permit.

Will there still be opportunities for overseas doctors in the UK?

Competition for training posts is high, particularly in certain specialties and in certain parts of the country. Training posts in the popular specialties and in popular places are likely to be filled by UK or EEA resident doctors.

There will be some training posts available for overseas doctors because there is no suitable UK or EEA applicant. These posts will largely be in less popular specialties and/or in less popular parts of the country. There may also be opportunities in posts that are not approved training posts, designated service posts, which nonetheless may give useful experience and some training.

What will the process be?

Firstly, you should thoroughly research your employment prospects before you enter for the PLAB test. There is a significant cost associated with sitting PLAB, especially with coming to the UK to sit Part 2, and there is absolutely no guarantee of a job once you have passed.

Find out the likelihood of opportunities in the specialty you wish to pursue. Historical information is of somewhat limited value, because the situation will change significantly as a result of the changes to the immigration rules. Make sure that your information is right up to date.

Information on the number of applicants for each training post is becoming more readily available. Postgraduate Deaneries are beginning to publicise this information on their websites.

If posts have been popular in the past, you should assume that they will continue to be popular. In fact, employers will not consider applications from overseas doctors who do not already have the right to work in the UK unless they have insufficient applications from suitably qualified UK and EEA doctors.

Most training posts which begin in August 2006 have already been filled or will be filled very shortly. If you have not yet sat PLAB, you will not realistically be able to take up a training post until 2007.

We aim to recruit to most August 2007 training posts in England using a new electronic recruitment system. The recruitment will start towards the end of 2006 and further information will be available nearer the time at www.mmc.nhs.uk.

NHS Trusts are responsible for recruiting directly into their service posts. Again, electronic recruitment is being used more widely.

Electronic recruitment makes it easy for you to apply for posts from your home country. If you decide to take PLAB, you should seriously consider returning home after completion of Part 2 to apply for posts. Employers will be aware of where you are located and allow you sufficient time to travel to any interviews.

Will I be able to travel to the UK to look for jobs?
There are currently no provisions to enable overseas doctors to come to the UK solely to look for work. While sensible enquiry about posts is expected, this can be done at a distance, and there is no need to meet the consultants before applying.

You can come to the UK to take PLAB, and use any time remaining on your PLAB visa to seek a suitable training or service post (although you cannot take up such a post until you have switched to an appropriate category of leave to remain in the UK). However, the Immigration Rules are clear that you have to leave the UK if you do not find employment and switch into the appropriate immigration category by the time your leave to take the PLAB Test expires.

Can I cancel my PLAB Test?
PLAB candidates who have a place in either PLAB Part 1 or Part 2, but have not yet taken the exam, may cancel their place and receive a full refund of their fee provided the place was booked before the notice about these changes appeared on the GMC's website (17.00 on 17 March 2006).

Will doctors still be able to undertake clinical attachments?
Yes. Doctors can undertake short periods of clinical attachment in the UK. As these are unpaid and involve observation only and not treatment of patients, doctors will still be able to take these posts while they are in the UK to take PLAB.

There is also a specific category in the Immigration Rules for these posts. A restriction is being introduced on the amount of leave that can be granted specifically to undertake clinical attachments to 6 weeks at a time, or 6 months in total.

Why can SHO posts only be granted work permits until 10 August 2007?
Modernising Medical Careers is reforming the way doctors are trained in the UK. From August 2007, SHO posts will either be absorbed into the new run-through specialty training grade or will be converted to another kind of post. There will be no SHO posts as currently understood after August 2007, and so work permits for SHO posts will not be granted to extend beyond 10 August 2007.

Can I apply for Foundation Programmes?
To be eligible for the first year of Foundation Programmes, a doctor must hold provisional registration, or be eligible for limited registration but be required by the GMC to undertake a year in a properly supervised pre-registration post (F1 post).

This year there were sufficient applicants from the UK and Europe to fill the 2-year Foundation Programmes. This is likely to be the case in future years so, even if you are eligible, you are unlikely to be offered a post if you require a work permit to take it up.

A small number of Foundation posts may become available in the few weeks before 1st August because those appointed have failed to meet the entrance requirements, or have withdrawn. These posts will be advertised and it is unlikely that there will be sufficient UK and European applicants. For these posts, eligible candidates may also include those with full registration or limited registration with no restrictions.

In addition, there will be more posts in the second year of the Programmes than are needed by those completing the first year. To be eligible for these posts, you will have to hold full registration or be eligible for limited registration without the pre-registration restriction. These posts tend to be advertised in the Spring for an August start.

WHAT IS MMC?

Modernising Medical Careers (MMC) is a structured programme for reforming postgraduate medical training in UK. As it is a government led initiative, it has been the subject matter of intense debates, both inside and outside UK parliament. The scale and rate of introduction of the changes being introduced by MMC has cause anxiety both among the UK and overseas trainees.

Started as a phased pilot programme in 2005, it is due to fully replace the traditional grades of medical career before the level of Consultant from August 2007. The different stages of the programme will contribute towards a Certificate of Completion of Training (CCT) and will cut short the process of reaching a consultant grade by an average of two years.

MMC was proposed as an umbrella term for implementing many fundamental changes in British postgraduate medical training. The need for implementing these fundamental changes can be understood in terms of these two most common arguments in favour put forward by the decision makers.

1. The existing medical training system dates back to pre-information era and does not provide a scalable model of knowledge framework required to train tomorrow's doctors.
2. Some fundamental changes have been envisioned regarding the functioning of NHS which makes it absolutely necessary for doctors to possess a certain set of mobile and flexible skills.

A two-year foundation programme has now replaced the former one-year Pre-registration house officer term and the first year of the former senior house officer term. However, the title "Pre-registration house officer" is still used for doctors in the first year of the foundation programme, as they are still only provisionally registered with the General Medical Council during that year. Full registration takes place at the end of the first year of the foundation programme.

The foundation programme consists of two years training divided by rotations of 4 months in different groups. The two-year programme is marked by continuing assessments and intends to provide a more comprehensive exposure of different clinical/ academic fields in healthcare.

Graduates from the foundation programme are eligible to apply for either specialist or general practice CCT training. This will be divided into Basic Specialist Training programmes and Higher Specialist Training programmes. On completion of these, trainees will be awarded a CCT and will be entitled to enter the Specialist Register or the General Practitioner (GP) register as appropriate.

The programme is not fully supported by the medical profession. Grave concerns have been expressed by the British Medical Association, among others, that the reforms have not been fully thought through, and may worsen the training situation for many junior doctors.

Some problems facing the doctors due to MMC

1. It is uncertain what would happen to existing non-career grade doctors and how they would be integrated into the system.
2. Major concern exists that the doctors currently at SHO level may have difficulty entering the new MMC training programmes once the old style SpR training programmes are closed, and that they will therefore end up in the career (non-training) grade instead.
3. Some less desirable specialities may end up with recruitment difficulties as doctors may not have enough time to try the speciality out. Conversely, if the application system encourages people to put down these "shortage specialties" as a backup choice or fallback option, these specialties will end up being staffed by people for whom it is a frustration of their true ambition and a source of dissatisfaction.
4. Speciality changes will be difficult once someone has already started their specialty training, as the curricula for the different specialties lack overlap and shared competencies.
5. The application system (MTAS) will only run once a year, and therefore doctors will only have a single chance each year to apply for specialty training. If they are unsuccessful (and given the huge competition this year as the scramble to enter the training grade occurs) they must wait a whole year before they can try again. This contrasts with the current system where a failure to get into one region's specialty training programme does not stop the candidate from trying again in another region a few weeks later.

As you can see everyone must apply in open competition. This rules out any advantage for the doctors already in the system and makes future job scenario in UK a level playing field for a candidate who is in possession of the right kind of skills.

Applications will be made electronically and it seems as if you can apply for two eaneries and two specialties. There will be two recruitment rounds so, if you don't get an offer in round one, you can reapply in round two.

The latest provisional information about recruitment to the new specialty training programmes is as follows (all subject to confirmation of course so please just use this as a guide):

1-31 December 2006: information about programmes available on Deanery websites

22 January 2007: website open for electronic applications

2 February 2007: closing date

March 2007 onwards: 1st and 2nd round interviews taking place up

HOW TO APPLY FOR THE FOUNDATION PROGRAMME IN UK?

Applicants who have received their primary medical qualification from a medical school outside the UK must submit evidence of their eligibility before they can apply for the Foundation Programme.

First, visit the UK General Medical Council (GMC) website www.gmc-uk.org. Please review the flow chart about applying to join the register. Whether you are a graduate or a final year medical student, this will help guide you through what is required of doctors registering in the UK. Please contact the GMC if you have any questions on this chart and how it could apply to you.

If after looking at GMC registration, the eligibility criteria and person specification you wish us to consider your eligibility to apply, you will need to

1. Complete the Eligibility form for primary medical qualifications from an EEA or International Medical School. Click here for the form.

2. Provide hard copies * of
   - An original letter written in English and signed by the Dean (or Head) of your medical school, confirming their approval for you to make an application and confirming your academic rating (please click here for a copy of the template to be used)
   - A verifiable academic score. The academic score must be provided by your medical school by
     1. Compiling the overall academic performance for all final year students/graduates in your class for the entirety of the medical degree.
     2. Then dividing the class into four equal sized groups based on academic performance
     3. Assigning a score to you based on the academic group you are in. If you are in the top academic group you will receive a score of 45, the second group 40, the third group 35 and the fourth group 30.
   - A photocopy of your passport OR national identity card OR United Kingdom resident's permit OR a Home Office issued application registration card OR a birth certificate issued in the UK which specifies the names of the holder's parents OR certificate of Registration or Naturalisation as a British Citizen (if enclosing a copy of your passport please ensure the copy includes the pages upon which your name and photograph are shown. If you are providing one of the other documents, please attach a photo of yourself to the form).
   - Written evidence of English language proficiency (refer to eligibility criteria)
   - If you have, or are eligible for, provisional or limited restricted registration from the UK General Medical Council, you MUST provide a copy of the letter from the GMC confirming this. For more information visit www.gmc-uk.org.
   - A photocopy of your medical qualification, if you are a graduate
   - If you graduated more than two years ago, written evidence that you have maintained your clinical knowledge and skills since graduating

3. Mail the completed form and all documents to:
   MTAS Eligibility Office for Foundation Programme 2007
   Frenchay Hospital
   Frenchay Park Road
   Frenchay
   BRISTOL
   BS16 1LE
   United Kingdom
   Once we have received your form and relevant documents, we will endeavour to process them within ten (10) working days of receipt by the office. You will then be contacted via e-mail and informed of the outcome.

Your submission will not be processed if you do not complete and submit the form and provide all requested documents.

Please e-mail eligibility@mtas.org.uk if you have any questions relating to this process.

*electronic copies will not be accepted

USEFUL SITES

1. **www.RxPG.com** (contains more than 30,000 EMQs and more than 600 OSCE stations)
2. **www.RxPGnews.com** (keep yourself updated with latest research in medicine)
3. **www.mmc.nhs.uk** (latest news about changes in postgraduate training for doctors in UK)
4. **www.mtas.nhs.uk** (Medical Training and Application Service : The one point terminal for application for all the medical posts in UK)
5. **www.medicbyte.com** (free site offers paid online coaching and useful info)
6. **www.fischtest.co.uk** (free site and very useful information)
7. **www.plabpass.i-p.com** (free site with sample EMQ)
8. **www.plab.co.uk** (free site with information for part 1 coaching)
9. **www.pastest.co.uk** (pastest is known for its reputation)
10. **www.medical-library.org** (paid site £ 10 per year; very useful reading material given in form of themes and ideal preparatory material for PLAB 1 exam)
11. **www.bmj.com** (free site useful information on latest developments)
12. **www. overseasdoctors.com** (free with useful information but has to be updated)
13. **www.bnf.org** (must visit a week before PLAB exam to get aware about recent changes and developments)
14. **www.gmc-uk.org** (the GMC website).

Section 2

QUESTION BANK

Previous Year Paper 1

RxPG Analysis

Total Themes:	**36**
Total SBAs:	**31**
Picture Slides:	**6**
Repeat Themes:	**7**
Repeat Themes with a Different Header:	**11**

THEME 1: INVESTIGATIONS IN NONACCIDENTAL INJURY

OPTIONS
a. CT head
b. FBC and coagulation profile
c. Serial height and weight measurement
d. No investigations
e. MSU cytology and culture
f. Skeletal survey
g. Look for blue sclera
h. Nutritional survey
i. Toxicology screen
j. MRI
k. Barium enema

INSTRUCTIONS
*For each of the presentation given below choose the **single most likely investigation** from the above list of options. Each options may be used once, more than once or not at all.*

QUESTIONS
1. A child just started living with her foster mother was found have weight in the 3rd percentile. The child appears well and no abnormalities found.
2. A child with bleeding from mouth was found to have torn lingual frenulum.
3. An unconscious child is brought to accident and emergency with parents complaining that she suddenly stopped breathing. Ophthalmoscopy shows multiple retinal haemorrhages.
4. An 18-month baby brought to Accident and Emergency with bronchiolitis. He has 6 posterior rib healing fractures.
5. An 8-yr-old boy sustained a wrist fracture following a fall in rugby match. He has a history of 6 fractures in previous 3 years. Father is deaf.
6. A child attends A and E with multiple bruise on her body. Parents fail to explain the cause.

THEME 2: PATHOLOGY – CELLS OF ORIGIN

OPTIONS
a. Adipocyte
b. Ganglion cells
c. Plasma cells
d. Megakaryoblast
e. Skeletal muscle cell
f. Lymphocytes
g. Erythroblast
h. Monocytes
i. Schwann's cells
j. Neutrophil precursors
k. Astrocytes
l. Erythrocyte precursor
m. Lymphocyte precursor
n. Smooth muscle cell

INSTRUCTIONS
*For each of the presentation given below choose the **single most likely cells of origin** from the above list of options. Each options may be used once, more than once or not at all.*

QUESTIONS
7. An elderly with bone pain and visual loss. Pathologist gives a diagnosis of multiple myeloma after bone marrow biopsy.
8. A young male with recent onset seizures. Brain biopsy performed gives a diagnosis of glioblastoma multiforme.
9. A young female with lymph node enlargement and splenomegaly. Bone marrow examination confirms the diagnosis to be acute myeloid leukemia.
10. A paravaginal mass is noted in a baby. Biopsy of the mass was done to come to a diagnosis of rhabdomyosarcoma.

THEME 3: MECHANISM OF DISEASE

OPTIONS

a. Infection
b. Allergy
c. Genetic
d. Immune process
e. Chloride channel defect
f. Alpha-1 antitrypsin deficiency
g. Trinucleotide repeats
h. Ciliary Dyskinesia
i. Fibrosis
j. Hyperplasia
k. Surfactant deficiency

INSTRUCTIONS

*For each of the presentation given below choose the **single most likely mechanism of the disease** from the above list of options. Each options may be used once more than once, or not at all.*

QUESTIONS

11. Childhood asthma.
12. A child with malabsorption and bronchiectasis with progressive productive cough and green sputum.
13. Bronchiolitis.
14. A disease affecting premature babies due to inadvertent use of oxygen.
15. A boy with mental retardation and learning difficulites. Father and uncle had similar problems.
16. A young male with recurrent sinusitis and pneumonia, presents with infertility.
17. Respiratory distress. Syndrome of prematurity
18. An adult with childhood liver failure now comes with emphysema.

THEME 4: MANAGEMENT OF ACUTE EYE CONDITIONS –TOPICAL EYE DROPS

OPTIONS

a. Antibiotic
b. Mast cell stabilizer
c. Prednisolone
d. Mydriatic
e. Miotic
f. Prostaglandins
g. NSAIDs
h. Carbonic anhydrase inhibitor
i. Beta blockers
j. Pilocarpine

INSTRUCTIONS

*For each of the presentation given below choose the **single most appropriate eye drop** from the above list of options. Each options may be used once, more than once or not at all.*

QUESTIONS

19. Acute bacterial conjunctivitis.
20. Acute allergic conjunctivitis.
21. Acute angle closure glaucoma.
22. Keratitis (non-infective).
23. Corneal abrasion.
24. Uveitis.

THEME 5: OVERDOSAGES AND POISONING

OPTIONS

a. Paracetamol
b. Salicylate
c. Sodium hypochlorite (bleach)
d. Paraquat
e. Organophosphorus
f. Digoxin
g. Tricyclic antidepressant
h. Methanol
i. Ethanol

INSTRUCTIONS

For each of the presentation given below choose the ***single most likely cause of symptoms*** *from the above list of options. Each option may be used once, more than once or not at all.*

QUESTIONS

25. A child living with his grandmother presents with nausea, vomiting and features of heart block.
26. A farmer presents with excessive sweating, abdominal pain and has dilated pupils.
27. A man comes to accident and emergency with complains of sore mouth. He is also having pulmonary edema , raised creatinine and oliguria.
28. A 13-year-old girl with hyperventilation and acidosis.
29. A girl with right upper quadrant pain with raised liver enzymes.
30. A 25-year-old male presents with metabolic acidosis, dilated pupil, elevated serum amylase and hypoglycemia.

THEME 6: SIDE EFFECTS OF ANTIPSYCHOTICS

OPTIONS

a. Clozapine
b. Chlorpromazine
c. Amitryptiline
d. Fluoxetine
e. Lithium
f. Quetiapine
g. Sertinadole
h. Amisulpride
i. Haloperidol
j. Droperidol

INSTRUCTIONS

For each of the presentation given below choose the ***single most likely drug*** *from the above list of options. Each option may be used once, more than once, or not at all.*

QUESTIONS

31. A chronic schizophrenic on treatment develops sore throat and agranulocytosis.
32. A schizophrenic on treatment develops galactorrhoea and loss of libido.
33. A schizophrenic on treatment develops fever, stiffness of limbs and raised creatinine kinase.
34. A patient with long term treatment for bipolar disorder complains of lethargy, weight gain and hypothermia.
35. A 40-year-old lady on treatment for depression develops dry skin and mouth.

THEME 7: SIDE EFFECTS OF ANTI-EPILEPTICS

OPTIONS

a. Carbamazepine
b. Sodium valproate
c. Phenytoin
d. Ethosuximide
e. Vigabatrin
f. Tigabain
g. Vigabatrin
h. Phenobarbitone
i. Primidone
j. Clonazepam

INSTRUCTIONS

*For each of the presentation given below choose the **single most likely drug** from the above list of options. Each option may be used once, more than once or not at all.*

QUESTIONS

36. An epileptic patient on treatment develops nausea vomiting with oliguria and raised levels of urea, creatinine.
37. A boy on treatment for generalized tonic clonic epilepsy, develops features of hepatic failure in few weeks of starting treatment.
38. A lady on treatment for epilepsy develops ataxia and gum hypertrophy.

THEME 8: INVESTIGATION OF SEIZURES

OPTIONS

a. EEG
b. ECG
c. CT head
d. Serum calcium
e. Blood glucose
f. ESR
g. Serum potassium
h. Hematocrit
i. MRI
j. Angiography

INSTRUCTIONS

*For each of the presentation given below choose the **single most likely investigation** from the above list of options. Each option may be used once, more than once or not at all.*

QUESTIONS

39. An adult with recent onset seizure. Opthalomoscopy shows papilloedema.
40. A child with two episodes of jerking limb movements. Teacher says he does not concentrate in the class.
41. A 50-year-old lady with jerking of thumb followed by limb and then generalized convulsions.
42. A 65-year-old previously healthy man with sudden loss of consciousness followed by generalized tonic clonic convulsions. He appears flushed and pulse rate is 40 bpm.

THEME 9: DIAGNOSIS OF DEMENTIA

OPTIONS

a. Depression
b. Alzeihmer's disease
c. Frontal lobe dementia
d. Vascular dementia
e. Carbon monoxide poisoning
f. Huntington's disease
g. Pick's disease
h. Creutzfeldt Jacob syndrome
i. Delirium

INSTRUCTIONS

For each of the presentation given below choose the ***single most likely diagnosis*** *from the above list of options. Each option may be used once, more than once or not at all.*

QUESTIONS

43. A 55-year-old man with history of stroke and repeated falls, now confused and cannot remember things.

44. A 48-year-old man has normal memory on examination; wife complaints of him becoming aggressive lately and talking about their sexual life publicly.

45. A 65-year-old lady with no previous history of behaviour abnormality is found entering shop at odd hours of early morning.

46. A 68-year-old man refuses to talk. Says that there is no point talking to him as he is a complete failure and that his memory has given up.

47. A man admitted in hospital develops features of disorientation and visual hallucinations on third day of admission.

48. A man brought to OPD with features of disorientation and visual hallucinations. Wife says he was all right till few days before when he caught cold.

THEME 10: DIAGNOSIS OF INCONTINENCE

OPTIONS

a. Fistula
b. Pelvic floor weakness
c. Multiple sclerosis
d. UTI
e. Detrusor Instability
f. Spinal cord compression
g. Stroke
h. Cauda equina syndrome
i. Inter vertebral disc prolapse
j. Reflux
k. Diabetes mellitus

INSTRUCTIONS

For each of the presentation given below choose the ***single most likely diagnosis*** *from the above list of options. Each option may be used once, more than once or not at all.*

QUESTIONS

49. A 60-year-old lady complaints of continuous dribbling of urine. She underwent hysterectomy few months back.

50. A lady after child birth complains of passing urine on coughing and stressing

51. A young girl with history of visual loss and bilateral lower limb weakness, complains of not able to pass urine at all.

52. A 47-year-old lady with frequency and unavoidable desire to urinate at a few seconds notice but no dysuria.

THEME 11: DIAGNOSIS OF ENDOCRINE DISEASES

OPTIONS

a. Aldosterone
b. Cortisole
c. Erythropoetin
d. Parathormone
e. Prolactin
f. Thyroid stimulating hormone
g. T3, T4
h. FSH
i. LH
j. ACTH
k. Growth hormone
l. Blood glucose

INSTRUCTIONS

*For each of the presentation given below choose the **single most likely diagnosis** from the above list of options. Each option may be used once, more than once or not at all.*

QUESTIONS

53. A heavy smoker with raised hematocrit and hemoglobin.

54. A 30-year-old female presents with lethargy. Her BP is 160/100 with serum electrolytes Na^+ 149 mmol/L, K^+ 2.6 mmol/L and HCO_3^- 30mmol/L.

55. A 35-year-old female presents with hypotension and lethargy. She is noted to have hyperpigmentation of her oral mucosa.

56. A 40-year-old patient complaints of lethargy, bone pain, polyuria and polydyspia. His blood glucose level is 3.0mmol/L.

57. A 32-year-old female presents with galactorrhoea, amenorrhoea and infertility.

THEME 12: DERMATOLOGY COLORED SLIDES

OPTIONS

a. Herpes simplex
b. Herpes zoster
c. HIV
d. Varicella
e. Erythema multiforme
f. Erythema nodosum
g. Steven-Johnson's syndrome
h. Idiopathic thrombocytopenic purpura
i. Henoch-Schönlein Purpura
j. Malignant melanoma
k. Meningococcal septicemia
l. Neurofibromatosis
m. Lipoma
n. Fibroma
o. Spider nevi

INSTRUCTIONS

*For each of the presentation given below choose the **single most likely diagnosis** from the above list of options. Each option may be used once, more than once, or not at all.*

QUESTIONS

58. A 30-year-old lady presents with breathlessness and perihilar shadow. On examination she has red erythematous lesions on her shins (Fig. 1, Plate 1).

59. A 46-year-old man on steroids for his asthma comes with fever and chest pain. On examination he has a fine vesicular rash on his right thoracic dermatome (Fig. 2, Plate 1).

60. A 42-year-old male with multiple generalized soft hyperpigmented nodules associated with coffee colored patches throughout the body (Fig. 3, Plate 1).

61. A 4-year-old boy presents with fever, photophobia and neck stiffness. He has multiple petechial lesions scatterd throughout his body (Fig. 4, Plate 1).

62. A 48-year-old chronic alcoholic with history of hematemesis. Oesophgogastroscopy revealed esophageal varices (Fig. 5, Plate 1).

63. A 34-year-old woman had a pigmented lesion on her foot which has now rapidly increased in size and shows ulceration (Fig. 6, Plate 1).

THEME 13: TREATMENT OF PNEUMONIA

OPTIONS

a. Benzyl penicillin
b. Cotrimoxazole
c. Ciprofloxacin
d. Clarithromycin
e. Fluconazole
f. Griesofulvin
g. Salbutamol inhaler
h. Ipratropium inhaler
i. Flu vaccine
j. Antituberculous therapy

INSTRUCTIONS

*For each of the presentation given below choose the **single most appropriate treatment** from the above list of options. Each option may be used once, more than once, or not at all.*

QUESTIONS

64. Man with right lower lobe pneumonia, is allergic to pencillin.
65. A HIV positive drug abuser with shortness of breath and bilateral expanding shadows on CXR.
66. An alcoholic comes with hemoptysis and chronic cough; CXR shows right upper lobe consolidation.
67. A 53-year-old business executive develops acute onset breathlessness, myalgia and dry cough. Chest X-ray shows bibasal consolidation.
68. An elderly man with COPD having attacks of pnuemonia every winter for the past two years.He wants your advice for this winter.
69. An 18 year old girl comes with fever, myalgia and shortness of breath. Half of her hostel is similarly ill.

THEME 14: CHOICE OF ANAESTHESIA

OPTIONS

a. General Anaesthesia
b. Epidural anaesthesia
c. Ketamine
d. Intravenous anesthetics
e. Peribulbar infiltration with lignocaine
f. Lignocaine infiltration
g. Retrobulbar Bupivacaine infiltration
h. Topical Xylocaine

INSTRUCTIONS

*For each of the presentation given below choose the **single most appropriate type of anesthesia** from the above list of options. Each option may be used once, more than once or not at all.*

QUESTIONS

70. A patient with history of COPD, presently complaining of cough is posted for cataract extraction.
71. Removal of corneal foreign body.
72. A pregnant lady posted for elective caesarean section.
73. Anaesthesia required during excision of Meibomian cyst eye.

THEME 15: EPIDEMIOLOGY OF PSYCHIATRIC CONDITIONS

OPTIONS

a. Major depression
b. Acute psychosis
c. Bipolar affective disorder
d. Dysthymia
e. Cyclothymia
f. Recurrent brief depression
g. Seasonal affective disorder
h. Mixed anxiety and depression
i. Mania
j. Schizophrenia
k. Frontal lobe syndrome

INSTRUCTIONS

*For each of the presentation given below choose the **single most appropriate condition** from the above list of options. Each option may be used once, more than once, or not at all.*

QUESTIONS

74. More common in females; associated with low mood and recurring depression, which lasts for not more than two weeks.

75. More common in females; characterized by low mood, insomnia, palpitations and sweating.

76. More common in females: characterized by annual recurrence of depressive symptoms.

77. More common in females, characterized by profound depression that alternate with periods of excessively elevated and/or irritable mood.

78. More commonly seen in males; characterized by elevated mood inflated self-esteem, overspending grandiosity and increased libido.

THEME16: EPIDEMIOLOGY OF JOINT DISEASES

OPTIONS

a. Rheumatoid arthritis
b. Osteoarthritis
c. Osteoporosis
d. Osteomalacia
e. Ankylosing spondylitis
f. Benign backache
g. IVDP
h. Otseopetrosis
i. Gout
j. Pyrophosphate arthropathy
k. Still's disease

INSTRUCTIONS

*For each of the presentation given below choose the **single most appropriate condition** from the above list of options. Each option may be used once, more than once or not at all.*

QUESTIONS

79. More common in females; with incidence of 20% in elderly Caucasian females and associated with change in body shape.

80. More common in females; affecting 1% of population, associated with loss of activity within 10 years of onset of disease.

81. More common in males, associated with stiff back and joints and positive HLA B27.

82 Associated with heavy work; pulling and pushing and psychosocial factors.

83. Associated with incidence of more than 70% and more than 90% show complete recovery.

THEME 17: MANAGEMENT OF POST PARTUM HAEMORRHAGE

OPTIONS

a. IM synometrine
b. Prostaglandins
c. Synotocin drip
d. IV fluids
e. Blood transfusion
f. Laparotomy
g. Antibiotics
h. Fresh frozen plasma
i. Heparin
j. Vitamin K

INSTRUCTIONS

*For each of the presentation given below choose the **single best management** from the above list of options. Each option may be used once, more than once, or not at all.*

QUESTIONS

84. A primipara after instrumental delivery lost 800 ml blood. Uterus is well contracted.
85. A multipara with history of two previous PPH.
86. A lady on 10th day post LSCS, brought with bleeding per vaginum lasting for 24 hr. She has suprapubic tenderness.
87. A primipara after normal vaginal delivery bled 600 ml after removal of placenta.

THEME 18: DIAGNOSIS OF RENAL CONDITIONS

OPTIONS

a. Henoch-Sehönlein purpura
b. Hemolytic uremic syndrome
c. Chronic renal failure
d. Acute glomerulonephritis
e. Nephrotic syndrome
f. SLE
g. Haemolytic anaemia
h. Idiopathic thrombocytopenic purpura
i. Systemic sclerosis
j. CREST syndrome

INSTRUCTIONS

*For each of the lab values given below choose the **single best diagnosis** from the above list of options. Each option may be used once, more than once, or not at all.*

QUESTIONS

88. Normocytic normochromic anaemia (Hb- 8g/dl)
    Reticulocytosis
    Fragmented red cells
    Thrombocytopenia
    Urea 7.9 mmol/L; Creatinine 180 micromol/L
89. Normochromic Normocytic Anaemia
    Oliguria
    Hypertension
    Low erythropoetin
90. Urea 8.9 mmol/L; Creatinine 180 mmol/L
    positive ANA.
91. Proteinuria
    Hypercholesterolemia
    Generalised edema
92. Hematuria, proteinuria
    Raised urea and creatinine
    Hypertension

THEME 19: INVESTIGATIONS IN NEPHROLOGY

OPTIONS

a. Ultrasound abdomen
b. Catheterize
c. IVU
d. Cystoscopy
e. PSA
f. CT scan kidney
g. MRI
h. Diagnostic peritoneal lavage
i. Laparotomy
j. Suprapubic aspiration

INSTRUCTIONS

For each of the presentation given below choose the ***single best investigation*** *from the above list of options. Each option may be used once, more than once or not at all.*

QUESTIONS

93. A boy suffered a blow to his flank during a rugby match. He later complained of one episode of frank haematuria. He is normal otherwise.
94. A 67-year-old man with painless hematuria.
95. A 72-year-old man with poor stream, hesitancy and dribbling.
96. A man comes with acute retention of urine following blow to perineum. On examination, perineum is swollen and bruised.

THEME 20: DIAGNOSIS OF PELVIC INFLAMMATORY DISEASES

OPTIONS

a. Candidiasis
b. Gonorrhoea
c. Chlamydia
d. Herpes
e. Cervical ectropion
f. Trichomonas
g. Bacterial vaginosis
h. Actinobacter
i. *Myocobacterium tuberculosis*
j. Mycoplasma

INSTRUCTIONS

For each of the presentation given below choose the ***single best diagnosis*** *from the above list of options. Each option may be used once, more than once or not at all.*

QUESTIONS

97. A 26-year-old female with sore vagina and whitish discharge; smear shows mycelia.
98. A 27-year-old sexually active female on oral contraceptives for two years, complains of mucoid discharge per vaginum.
99. A 18-year-old girl with recently developed dysmenorrhoea and deep dyspareunia. Speculum examination reveals purulent discharge from cervical os. Tested negative for gonorrhoea.
100. A 37-year-old lady with multiple painful, vesicular lesions at the introitus with scanty offensive discharge.
101. A 34-year-old lady with discharge per vaginum. Wet mount shows clue cells.

THEME 21: BLOOD SUPPLY

OPTIONS

a. Cavernous sinus
b. Internal carotid artery
c. Superficial temporal artery
d. Middle meningeal artery
e. Central retinal artery
f. Facial artery
g. Middle cerebral artery
h. Vertebral artery
i. Central retinal vein
j. Ophthalmic artery
k. Ophthalmic vein
l. Mandibular artery
m. Lingual artery

INSTRUCTIONS

For each of the presentation given below choose the ***single most likely blood vessel affected*** *from the above list of options. Each option may be used once, more than once, or not at all.*

QUESTIONS

102. A young child with abscess near upper lip.

103. A diabetic and hypertensive with sudden painless loss of vision. On examination, fundus appears pale.

104. A laceration near the angle of mandible in front of masseter with profuse bleeding.

105. A 60-year-old man with transient loss of vision and dysphasia which improved completely without any residual neurological deficits.

106. A 42-year-old man with fracture petrous temporal bone and confusion.

THEME 22: NEXT STEP IN MANAGEMENT OF DYSPEPTIC SYMPTOMS

OPTIONS

a. Anti-helicobacter therapy
b. Esophagodudenoscopy
c. Measure serum gastrin
d. IV proton pump inhibitors
e. Oral proton pump inhibitors
f. Pancreatectomy
g. Antacids
h. H2 antagonists
i. Urea breath tests
j. Serology for helicobacter
k. Life style modification

INSTRUCTIONS

For each of the presentation given below choose the single best next step in management from the above list of options. Each option may be u sed once, more than once, or not at all.

QUESTIONS

107. A patient wid hematemesis following 40% burns. His vitals are stable;esophagoduodenoscopy shows multiple superficial ulcers in stomach.

108. A 47-year-old female comes with hematesis. Her vitals are now stable. She was on treatment for rheumatoid arthritis.

109. A 56-year-old male presents with dyspeptic symptoms. Cytological brushings from stomach postive for gram-negative spiral organisms.

110. A 34-year-old male with severe dyspepsia, not responding to usual anti-dyspeptic measures. Gastroduodenoscopy shows several ulcers in esophagus, stomach and small intestine.

THEME 23: INTERPRETATION OF CHEST FINDINGS

OPTIONS

a. Pulmonary embolism
b. Myocardial infarction
c. Simple pneumothorax
d. Tension pneumothorax
e. Pneumonia
f. Haemothorax
g. Pulmonary edema
h. Esophageal rupture

INSTRUCTIONS

*For each of the lab values given below choose the **single most likely diagnosis** from the above list of options. Each option may be used once, more than once or not at all.*

QUESTIONS

111. Temp 37°C
JVP raised
CXR normal
ECG–T inversion in L3
BP 100/60; PR 130 bpm

112. Temp 37°C
JVP normal
CXR normal
BP 120/80 PR 110 bpm
ECG–Q-waves in V1, 2, 3

113. Temp 39°C
JVP normal
CXR consolidation of right middle lobe
BP 120/90 PR 100 bpm/irregular.

114. Temp 37°C
JVP increased
CXR reduced markings on right side
BP 130/80 PR 90 bpm/regular.

115. Temp 37°C
JVP decreased
PR 120 bpm regular
BP 90/60
CXR shows left sided effusion
Surgical emphysema present on neck palpation.

116. Temp 37° C
JVP raised
PR 90 bpm /regular
BP 100/90
CXR bilateral shadows
Basal creptitions.

THEME 24: DIAGNOSIS OF NECK LUMPS

OPTIONS

a. Thyroid carcinoma
b. Goitre
c. Cystic hygroma
d. Branchial cyst
e. Tuberculous lymphadenitis
f. Lymphoma
g. Ca stomach
h. Ca lung
i. Mesothelioma

INSTRUCTIONS

*For each of the presentations given below choose the **single most likely diagnosis** from the above list of options. Each option may be used once, more than once or not at all.*

QUESTIONS

117. A 40-year-old lady from Asia with lumps in her neck, FNAC of which revealed center of casseous material surrounded by fibrosis.

118. A 60-year-old man with a lump in supra-clavicular region and decreased appetite. He has lost 5 kg weight recently.

119. A man comes with a lump in front of his neck which moves up on swallowing. Scan shows a mass replacing the left lobe of thyroid and spreading to sternomastoid and adjacent muscles.

120. An infant with brilliantly transilluminable swelling at the base of his neck.

121. A shipyard worker develops shortness of breath and a lump in his supraclavicular fossa.There is a small pleural effusion noted on the same side of the lump.

THEME 25: MANAGEMENT OF ELECTROLYTE IMBALANCES

OPTIONS

a. Insulin only
b. Insulin with normal saline
c. Normal saline with hydrocortisone
d. Oral potassium
e. IV potassium
f. Dialysis
g. Saline and potassium supplementation
h. Normal saline with potassium

INSTRUCTIONS

*For each of the presentations given below choose the **single most appropriate management** from the above list of options. Each option may be used once, more than once or not at all.*

QUESTIONS

122. A 20-yr-old girl with hypotension, hyperkalaemia and is mildly hyponatremic. She has recently lost weight and her skin appears hyperpigmented.
123. A young boy with polyuria, has very high blood glucose levels.
124. A patient has diarrhoea, appears to be dehydrated with low potassium levels.
125. A patient on vigorous diuretic therapy develops hypokalaemia.
126. A person develops anuria after severe crushing injuries. His blood urea level at 60 mmol/L and serum potassium 7.5 mmol/l.

THEME 26: MANAGMENT OF ARRYTHMIAS

OPTIONS

a. Adrenaline
b. Adenosine
c. Digoxin
d. Carbimazole plus beta-blockers
e. Implantable pace maker
f. External pacemaker
g. Atropine
h. Surgical resection

INSTRUCTIONS

*For each of the presentations given below choose the **single most appropriate management** from the above list of options. Each option may be used once, more than once or not at all.*

QUESTIONS

127. A man after falling unconscious on a number of occasions was found to have a heart rate of 40 bpm.
128. A 25-year-old female with sweaty palms, tremors and weight loss. Heart rate is 140 bpm/irregular.
129. A 32-year-old female complains of rapid palpitations and syncope. Her pulse rate is 160 bpm/regular.

THEME 27: INVESTIGATIONS OF PALPITATIONS

OPTIONS
a. ECG
b. ECHO
c. 24 hr Holter monitoring
d. Thyroid function tests
e. CXR
f. ESR
g. Serum potassium
h. Haematocrit
i. MRI
j. Angiography

INSTRUCTIONS
For each of the presentations given below choose the ***single most appropriate investigation*** *from the above list of options. Each option may be used once, more than once, or not at all.*

QUESTIONS
130. An 18-year-old girl, sweaty with tremors and weight loss, says that her heart races.

131. A woman experiences 'thumping' in her chest associated with breathlessness, while asleep. She sits up to get symptoms resolve in few minutes.

132. A woman with a family history of coronary artery disease. She has noticed palpitations especially during the night. She describes a sensation of her heartbeat momentarily stopping, and then racing.

133. A man complains of episodes of palpitations which last for few minutes and leave him dizzy. His pulse appears to be normal at the point of examination.

THEME 28: DIAGNOSIS OF PRENATAL CONDITIONS

OPTIONS
a. Fetal blood sampling
b. Chorionic villous sampling
c. Amniocentesis and karyotyping
d. USG
e. Check serum anti-D
f. Fetal ECHO
g. Fetal blood at birth
h. Triple test
i. Quadruple test
j. Fetal Doppler

INSTRUCTIONS
For each of the presentations given below choose the ***single most appropriate investigation*** *from the above list of options. Each option may be used once, more than once or not at all.*

QUESTIONS
134. A lady at 16 weeks gestation, scan shows nuchal folds and double bubble sign; the most reliable way to diagnose Down's syndrome.

135. Pregnant lady with previous baby affected with cystic fibrosis, wants to confirm if her present baby is alright.

136. Pregnant lady with previous baby with severe anaemia and jaundice.

137. A lady 24 weeks pregnant with a previous child dead from some congenital heart disease.

138. A pregnant lady wants to know if her baby will be suffering from hypothyroidism.

THEME 29: INVESTIGATIONS OF PELVIC INFLAMMATORY DISEASES

OPTIONS

a. Endocervical swab
b. High vaginal swab
c. Contact tracing
d. Laparoscopy
e. Pelvis ultrasound
f. Abdominal ultrasound
g. Pipelle sampling
h. Vaginal ultrasound
i. Urine microscopy
j. Cystoscopy
k. Colposcopy

INSTRUCTIONS

For each of the presentations given below choose the ***single most appropriate investigation*** *from the above list of options. Each option may be used once, more than once or not at all.*

QUESTIONS

139. A 24-year-old lady with pelvic pain and offensive vaginal discharge.

140. An asymptomatic 25-year-old lady says her husband had a purulent urethral discharge and does not wants to talk about it.

141. An elderly with bleeding per vaginum. USG shows thickened endometrium.

142. A 47-year-old female with bilateral pelvic masses and terminal haematuria.

THEME 30: DIAGNOSIS AND MANAGEMENT OF ABDOMINAL PAIN

OPTIONS

a. CXR
b. Abdominal X-ray
c. Barium enema
d. Laparotomy
e. USG
f. Laparoscopy
g. Colonoscopy
h. CT scan
i. Partial gastrectomy
j. Total gastrectomy

INSTRUCTIONS

For each of the presentations given below choose the ***single most appropriate diagnosis or management*** *from the above list of options. Each option may be used once, more than once, or not at all.*

QUESTIONS

143. A man underwent sigmoidoscopy after which he develops severe pain abdomen and guarding.

144. A man with features of peritonitis; erect CXR shows gas under diaphragm.

145. A child with abdominal pain and current jelly stools. A sausage shaped mass is palpable per abdomen.

146. A 55-year-old man with epigastric pain and haematemesis. Endoscopy confirms adenocarcinoma stomach.

THEME 31: INVESTIGATIONS IN OVARIAN CARCINOMA

OPTIONS

a. Pelvic USG
b. Pelvic CT
c. CA 125
d. CA 153
e. Laparotomy
f. Laparoscopy
g. Paracentesis
h. CA 199

INSTRUCTIONS

*For each of the presentations given below choose the **single most appropriate investigation** from the above list of options. Each option may be used once, more than once, or not at all.*

QUESTIONS

147. A lady with family history of ovarian carcinoma. Pelvic USG fails to reveal any abnormality.

148. A lady had undergone total abdominal hysterectomy with bilateral salpingo-oophorectomy and omentectomy for carcinoma ovary, now comes for follow up. Her CA 125 had come to normal levels after surgery.

149. A lady underwent debulking surgery for ovarian carcinoma now presents with signs of intestinal obstruction.

150. A lady with history of treated ovarain carcinoma, attends clinic to rule out recurrence.

THEME 32: DIAGNOSIS OF HEADACHE

OPTIONS

a. Petrous temporal fracture
b. Base of the skull fracture
c. Frontal bone fracture
d. Intracranial space occupying lesion
e. Migraine
f. Temporal arteritis
g. Takayasu's arteritis
h. Mandible fracture
i. Sub arachnoid hemorrhage
j. Temporal bone fracture

INSTRUCTIONS

*For each of the presentations given below choose the **single most likely diagnosis** from the above list of options. Each option may be used once, more than once, or not at all.*

QUESTIONS

151. A man involved in a road traffic accident comes with CSF rhinorrhoea.

152. A man after sustaining a fall comes with haemotympanum.

153. A patient presents with unilateral temporal headache.

THEME 33: DIAGNOSIS OF GASTROINTESTINAL DISEASES

OPTIONS

a. Irritable Bowel disease
b. Carcinoma caecum
c. Carcinoma rectum
d. Crohn's disease
e. Ulcerative colitis
f. Solitary rectal ulcer
g. Anorexia nervosa
h. Anal fissure
i. Anal fistula
j. Haemorrhoids

INSTRUCTIONS

*For each of the presentations given below choose the **single most likely diagnosis** from the above list of options. Each option may be used once, more than once or not at all.*

QUESTIONS

154. A 37-year-old lady with chronic history of constipation, diarrhoea and passing bloody stools. Barium enema shows rose thorn ulcers.

155. A 46-year-old man with recent change of bowel habits, weight loss and occult blood in stools positive.

156. An 18-year-old girl comes with complains of alternating diarrhoea and constipation. There is no weight loss.

157. A 42-year-old with recent change in bowel habits, tenesmus and bloody stools. Sigmoidoscopy shows ulcerative mass in rectum.

THEME 34: DIAGNOSIS OF COMA/UNCONSCIOUSNESS

OPTIONS

a. Extradural haemorrhage
b. Subdural haemorrhage
c. Heroine abuse
d. Plasma glucose levels
e. Vasovagal syncope
f. Stokes-adams attack
g. Pulmonary embolism
h. Shy dragger syndrome

INSTRUCTIONS

*For each of the presentations given below choose the **single most likely diagnosis** from the above list of options. Each option may be used once, more than once or not at all.*

QUESTIONS

158. Male with needle marks, is brought in coma state with pinpoint puplis.

159. A 70-year-old lady shopping in a supermarket fainted suddenly and sustained fracture neck of femur. Her daughter who was with her said she went pale before fainting.

160. An elderly traveling alone was brought to accident and emergency from the airport in unconscious state. There are needles and a syringe in his hand baggage.

161. A 52-year-old chronic alcoholic comes in a state of confusion. Wife gives history of repeated falls over last few months.

THEME 35: DIAGNOSIS OF ACCIDENTAL INJURIES

OPTIONS

a. Bronchial rupture
b. Aortic rupture
c. Cardiac tamponade
d. Pericarditis
e. Acute blood loss
f. Splenic rupture
g. Intracerebral bleed
h. Subdural haemorrhage
i. Exradural haemorrhage

INSTRUCTIONS

For each of the presentations given below choose the ***single most likely diagnosis*** *from the above list of options. Each option may be used once, more than once or not at all.*

QUESTIONS

162. A man comes to A and E after high speed automobile injury. CXR shows widened mediastinum.
163. A lady after road traffic accident comes with hypotension and rigid abdomen. She has broken left ribs 10-12.
164. A lady after road traffic accident presents with increased pulse decreased BP.
165. A man involved in an RTA, presents with headache and loss of consciousness after admission.

THEME 36: DIAGNOSIS OF CHEST PAIN

OPTIONS

a. Myocardial infarction
b. Cardiac tamponade
c. Pneumonia
d. SLE
e. Sarcoidosis
f. Gastro esophageal reflux disease
g. Aortic dissection
h. Pulmonary embolism
i. Bronchitis
j. Lung carcinoma
k. Reiter's syndrome
l. Sjögren's syndrome

INSTRUCTIONS

For each of the presentations given below choose the ***single most likely diagnosis*** *from the above list of options. Each option may be used once, more than once or not at all.*

QUESTIONS

166. A 27-year-old female with sharp chest pain which becomes worse on coughing or taking deep breaths. She has a red rash over her cheeks and nose.
167. A 45-year-old male presents with chest pain and joint pains. He also complains of dry gritty eyes.
168. A 39-year-old lady presents with dull ache in the chest and arthritis. Chest X-ray shows bilateral enlarged hilar lymph nodes.
169. A 40-year-old smoker presents with chest pain, haemoptysis and headache.

SBAs

170. A mentally retarded child puts a green pea in his ear while having his dinner. The carer confirms this. Otoscopy shows a green colored object in the ear canal.

Most appropriate single best approach to remove this:

a. By a magnet
b. Syringing
c. Under GA
d. By hook
e. By instilling olive oil

171. During laparoscopy the first trocar is inserted midway between umbilicus and anterior superior iliac spine.

The structures most likely to be pierced by the inserted trocar are:

a. Rectus abdominis muscle
b. Linea alba
c. External oblique aponerosis and internal oblique muscle
d. External oblique and internal oblique muscles
e. Conjoint tendon

172. A 47-year-old man comes with 2 episodes of grossly bloody stools. He is a chronic alcoholic taking 10 units of alcohol per day. On examination he has raised alkaline phosphtase and bilirubin.

Single most likely diagnosis could be:

a. Alcoholic hepatitis
b. Chronic hepatitis
c. Viral hepatitis
d. Primary sclerosing cholangitis
e. Autoimmune hepatitis

173. A boy is brought to A and E with complaints of barking cough associated with inspiratory and expiratory stridor; A diagnosis of laryngotrachebronchitis is reached.

What is the single most likely prognosis of the disease if left untreated ?

a. Bronchiectasis
b. Complete resolution
c. Lung abscess
d. Pneumonia
e. Bronchial asthma

174. A boy develops generalized edema with proteinuria +++1. He is started on steroids and improves.

What is the single best long-term prognosis of the disease?

a. Complete resolution
b. Recurrence with gradual resistant to steroids
c. Recurrence with full response to steroids
d. Chronic renal failure
e. Acute renal failure

175. A diabetic with blood pressure 140/90 and proteinuria 0.2 mg/day.

The single most likely agent to offer him benefit is:

a. ACE inhibitors
b. Angiotensin inhibitors
c. Beta-blockers
d. Fibrates
e. Statins

176. A 30-year-old lady was treated successfully for CIN 2 two years back. She was a heavy smoker and discontinued smoking few months back. She was on oral contraceptives all these years, but now her partner uses condoms. She is anxious as her aunt died of ovarian carcinoma at the age of 48.

The single most important factor which puts her at the risk of ovarian cancer is:

a. Age
b. Family history
c. CIN 2
d. Smoking
e. Oral contraceptives

177. A 59-year-old man underwent surgery for rectal carcinoma, has not yet opened his bowels. He complains of abdominal distension and NG tube is aspirating large amount of fluids.

Single most likely cause for his condition is:

a. Calcium 2.2 mmol/l
b. Potassium 2.4 mmol/litre
c. Sodium 128 mmol/litre
d. Chloride 94 mmol/litre
e. Bicarbonate 22.5 mmol/litre

178. A 62-year-old lady comes with unilateral weakness of arm and headache. On examination the affected arm has brisk reflexes and increased tone. Rest all examination appears normal.

The single best investigation required to be done here:

a. Skull X-ray
b. CT scan head
c. Lymphangiography
d. X-ray limb
e. Electromyography

179. A 47-year-old female with carcinoma breast complains of intense thirst, polyuria and confusion.

The single best way to manage:

a. Dexamethasone
b. Palmidronate
c. Fluid restriction
d. Insulin therapy
e. Calcium gluconate

180. A man fell from scaffold to injure his spine. Investigation revealed damage to S1.

Which single symptom will correspond to this level of injury:

a. Bladder dysfunction
b. Bowel dysfunction
c. Limb weakness
d. Numbness of sacral area
e. Loss of ankle jerk

181. A male complains of sudden onset dysphagia after eating bread which gets relieved by vomiting. He had 2 similiar episodes in last 3 years while having steaks. His BMI is 32.

The single most likely investigation which would lead to the diagnosis of his condition is:

a. Barium Swallow
b. Chest X-ray
c. Motility Studies
d. Esophgaoscopy
e. The 24-hour esophageal pH monitoring

182. A vagrant man, dishevelled, sweating and fizzy. He is brought to A and E with seizures, dilated pupil.

The most likely agent to cause these symptoms could be:

a. Alcohol
b. Heroine
c. Cocaine
d. Cannabis
e. Solvent abuse

183. A chronic alcoholic is brought to A/E in agitated state, picking at imaginary things. He is started on chlordiazepoxide.

The other single most important agent to be added to his treatment regimen should be:

a. Chlormethiazole
b. Thiamine
c. IV Glucose
d. Phenobarbitone
e. Phenothiazines

184. A female experienced intense headache, while painting her bathroom wall. She fainted and hit her head. She was brought to A and E, where she regained her consciousness and is well otherwise, except for a small laceration on her skull.

The single most important investigation to be done at this stage is:

a. CT scan
b. Skull X-ray
c. Doppler
d. EEG
e. ECG

185. A 27-year-old man is brought to A and E, with severe breathlessness following RTA. His breathlessness not relieved even after putting chest drain.

The single most likely cause could be:

a. Tension pneumothorax
b. Bronchial rupture
c. Aortic rupture
d. Simple pneumothorax
e. Haemothorax

186. A neonate is brought to A and E with temperature of 38.5°C. He is otherwise appearing normal.

The single best next step should be:

a. Reassurance
b. Discharge with broad spectrum antibiotics
c. Admit for full infection screen
d. Admit for full infection screen and start broad spectrum antibiotics
e. Admit and observe

187. A man with chronic atrial fibrillation develops features of pulmonary edema.

Single best next step would be:

a. DC cardioversion
b. Anticoagulation and digoxin
c. Digoxin
d. Frusemide
e. Dopamine

188. A patient with a long history of GORD, underwent esophago-duodenoscopy and a diagnosis of Barret's Esophagus was reached.

The single most appropriate term to define this condition would be:

a. Squamous Metaplasia
b. Columnar Metaplasia
c. Dysplasia
d. Neoplasia
e. Hyperplasia

189. A 30 year old heavy smoker with previous history of treatment for DVT and varicose veins develops swelling and ulcer just above her medial malleolus surrounded by lipodermarosclerosis and induration on her right foot . She is currently on OCPs.

The single most likely cause for her foot condition is:

a. Varicose veins
b. DVT
c. Peripehral vascular disease
d. OCPs
e. Smoking

190. A young girl complains of abdominal pain whenever in school. She is otherwise normal in public holidays and when her school is closed. Her epigastric pain is associated with nausea and no vomiting. She was also, needed to be sent home from school because of this abdominal pain on a number of occasions.

The single most likely diagnosis could be:

a. Abdominal Migraine
b. Coeliac disease
c. Appendicitis
d. Mesenteric adenitis.
e. Intusussception

191. A patient after a fall on his outstretched hands complains of pain in his wrist. X-ray of the wrist appears normal. No fracture is seen.

The single most appropriate next step should be:

a. Discharge with reassurance
b. Scaphoid cast for 6 weeks
c. Take X-ray at a later date
d. Plaster and review after 2 weeks
e. Open reduction

192. A 25-years-old man was recently admitted with severe depression complicated by psychosis now came in emergency because of worsening mental status and fever. He is unable to give history because he is profoundly confused and claimed to be on Mars. He was taking haloperidol and amitryptiline. On examination: temperature 105° C, muscle rigidity and dry skin. A cooling blanket is ordered.

Which single most important agent should be ordered at this time?

a. Bromocriptine
b. Atropine
c. Lavretrenol
d. Chlorpheniramine
e. Methyl-prednisolone

193. A man comes to OPD with earache. On examination his left tonsil is ulcerated with rolled out edges.

Single most likely diagnosis could be:

a. Tonsillar tumour
b. Quinsy
c. Lymphoma
d. Abscess
e. Follicular tonsilitis

194. A patient comes again and again to his general physician saying that he is suffering from AIDs. His all results for HIV are negative, checked thrice.

The single most likely condition which describes his symptoms best is:

a. OCD
b. Hypochondriasis
c. Munchhausen's syndrome
d. Body dysmorphic disorder
e. Briquet Syndrome

195. A 42-year-old man develops fever 48 hours after undergoing surgery. He has mild abdominal distension.

The single most likely cause for his fever could be:

a. Pleural effusion
b. UTI
c. Thrombophlebitis
d. Sepsis
e. DVT

196. A tall young guy is brought with acute onset scrotal pain associated with vomiting.

The single most likely diagnosis can be:

a. Testicular torsion
b. Torsion of appendicualr appendage
c. Epididymorchitis
d. UTI
e. Scrotal abscess

197. A women on postnatal period on being visited by midwife on the 4th day, is extremely worried about her kid. Her husband says she is showing mood changes and is extremely tearful sometimes.

The single most likely diagnosis is:

a. Postpartum psychosis
b. Postnatal blues
c. Postpartum depression
d. Mania
e. OCD

198. A 27-year-old female 7-10 days postpartum, is feeling depressed, worried and tearful. Recurring thoughts of harming baby disturbs her. She expresses her anxiety if she can take care of her baby properly.

The single most likely diagnosis is:

a. Postpartum psychosis
b. Postnatal blues
c. Postpartum depression
d. Mania
e. OCD

199. A 37-year-old lady experiences dizziness while looking back as she was reversing her car.

The single most likely cause for her presenting symptoms could be:

a. Vertebrobasilar insufficiency
b. Carotid artery insufficiency
c. Thoracic outlet syndrome
d. Migraine
e. Stroke

200. Child after taking his MMR vaccination 2 weeks back comes with fever, headache, photophobia and a rapidly spreading purpuric rash.

The single most likely diagnosis is:

a. Anaphylaxis
b. Meningococcemia
c. Vaccine side effect
d. Aseptic meningitis
e. Measles

General Medical Council PLAB Test Part 1

Full Name

Test Centre/Date

- Use pencil only • Make heavy marks that fill the lozenge completely
- Write your candidate number in the top row of the box to the right **AND** fill in the appropriate lozenge below each number
- Give **ONE** answer only for each question

0	0	0	0	0	0
1	1	1	1	1	1
2	2	2	2	2	2
3	3	3	3	3	3
4	4	4	4	4	4
5	5	5	5	5	5
6	6	6	6	6	6
7	7	7	7	7	7
8	8	8	8	8	8
9	9	9	9	9	9

1	A	B	C	D	E	F	G	H	I	J	K	L	M	N	O	P	Q	R	S	T	1
2	A	B	C	D	E	F	G	H	I	J	K	L	M	N	O	P	Q	R	S	T	2
3	A	B	C	D	E	F	G	H	I	J	K	L	M	N	O	P	Q	R	S	T	3
4	A	B	C	D	E	F	G	H	I	J	K	L	M	N	O	P	Q	R	S	T	4
5	A	B	C	D	E	F	G	H	I	J	K	L	M	N	O	P	Q	R	S	T	5
6	A	B	C	D	E	F	G	H	I	J	K	L	M	N	O	P	Q	R	S	T	6
7	A	B	C	D	E	F	G	H	I	J	K	L	M	N	O	P	Q	R	S	T	7
8	A	B	C	D	E	F	G	H	I	J	K	L	M	N	O	P	Q	R	S	T	8
9	A	B	C	D	E	F	G	H	I	J	K	L	M	N	O	P	Q	R	S	T	9
10	A	B	C	D	E	F	G	H	I	J	K	L	M	N	O	P	Q	R	S	T	10
11	A	B	C	D	E	F	G	H	I	J	K	L	M	N	O	P	Q	R	S	T	11
12	A	B	C	D	E	F	G	H	I	J	K	L	M	N	O	P	Q	R	S	T	12
13	A	B	C	D	E	F	G	H	I	J	K	L	M	N	O	P	Q	R	S	T	13
14	A	B	C	D	E	F	G	H	I	J	K	L	M	N	O	P	Q	R	S	T	14
15	A	B	C	D	E	F	G	H	I	J	K	L	M	N	O	P	Q	R	S	T	15
16	A	B	C	D	E	F	G	H	I	J	K	L	M	N	O	P	Q	R	S	T	16
17	A	B	C	D	E	F	G	H	I	J	K	L	M	N	O	P	Q	R	S	T	17
18	A	B	C	D	E	F	G	H	I	J	K	L	M	N	O	P	Q	R	S	T	18
19	A	B	C	D	E	F	G	H	I	J	K	L	M	N	O	P	Q	R	S	T	19
20	A	B	C	D	E	F	G	H	I	J	K	L	M	N	O	P	Q	R	S	T	20
21	A	B	C	D	E	F	G	H	I	J	K	L	M	N	O	P	Q	R	S	T	21
22	A	B	C	D	E	F	G	H	I	J	K	L	M	N	O	P	Q	R	S	T	22
23	A	B	C	D	E	F	G	H	I	J	K	L	M	N	O	P	Q	R	S	T	23
24	A	B	C	D	E	F	G	H	I	J	K	L	M	N	O	P	Q	R	S	T	24
25	A	B	C	D	E	F	G	H	I	J	K	L	M	N	O	P	Q	R	S	T	25
26	A	B	C	D	E	F	G	H	I	J	K	L	M	N	O	P	Q	R	S	T	26
27	A	B	C	D	E	F	G	H	I	J	K	L	M	N	O	P	Q	R	S	T	27
28	A	B	C	D	E	F	G	H	I	J	K	L	M	N	O	P	Q	R	S	T	28
29	A	B	C	D	E	F	G	H	I	J	K	L	M	N	O	P	Q	R	S	T	29
30	A	B	C	D	E	F	G	H	I	J	K	L	M	N	O	P	Q	R	S	T	30
31	A	B	C	D	E	F	G	H	I	J	K	L	M	N	O	P	Q	R	S	T	31
32	A	B	C	D	E	F	G	H	I	J	K	L	M	N	O	P	Q	R	S	T	32
33	A	B	C	D	E	F	G	H	I	J	K	L	M	N	O	P	Q	R	S	T	33
34	A	B	C	D	E	F	G	H	I	J	K	L	M	N	O	P	Q	R	S	T	34
35	A	B	C	D	E	F	G	H	I	J	K	L	M	N	O	P	Q	R	S	T	35
36	A	B	C	D	E	F	G	H	I	J	K	L	M	N	O	P	Q	R	S	T	36
37	A	B	C	D	E	F	G	H	I	J	K	L	M	N	O	P	Q	R	S	T	37
38	A	B	C	D	E	F	G	H	I	J	K	L	M	N	O	P	Q	R	S	T	38
39	A	B	C	D	E	F	G	H	I	J	K	L	M	N	O	P	Q	R	S	T	39
40	A	B	C	D	E	F	G	H	I	J	K	L	M	N	O	P	Q	R	S	T	40
41	A	B	C	D	E	F	G	H	I	J	K	L	M	N	O	P	Q	R	S	T	41
42	A	B	C	D	E	F	G	H	I	J	K	L	M	N	O	P	Q	R	S	T	42
43	A	B	C	D	E	F	G	H	I	J	K	L	M	N	O	P	Q	R	S	T	43
44	A	B	C	D	E	F	G	H	I	J	K	L	M	N	O	P	Q	R	S	T	44
45	A	B	C	D	E	F	G	H	I	J	K	L	M	N	O	P	Q	R	S	T	45
46	A	B	C	D	E	F	G	H	I	J	K	L	M	N	O	P	Q	R	S	T	46
47	A	B	C	D	E	F	G	H	I	J	K	L	M	N	O	P	Q	R	S	T	47
48	A	B	C	D	E	F	G	H	I	J	K	L	M	N	O	P	Q	R	S	T	48
49	A	B	C	D	E	F	G	H	I	J	K	L	M	N	O	P	Q	R	S	T	49
50	A	B	C	D	E	F	G	H	I	J	K	L	M	N	O	P	Q	R	S	T	50

DO NOT WRITE IN THIS SPACE

51	A	B	C	D	E	F	G	H	I	J	K	L	M	N	O	P	Q	R	S	T	51
52	A	B	C	D	E	F	G	H	I	J	K	L	M	N	O	P	Q	R	S	T	52
53	A	B	C	D	E	F	G	H	I	J	K	L	M	N	O	P	Q	R	S	T	53
54	A	B	C	D	E	F	G	H	I	J	K	L	M	N	O	P	Q	R	S	T	54
55	A	B	C	D	E	F	G	H	I	J	K	L	M	N	O	P	Q	R	S	T	55
56	A	B	C	D	E	F	G	H	I	J	K	L	M	N	O	P	Q	R	S	T	56
57	A	B	C	D	E	F	G	H	I	J	K	L	M	N	O	P	Q	R	S	T	57
58	A	B	C	D	E	F	G	H	I	J	K	L	M	N	O	P	Q	R	S	T	58
59	A	B	C	D	E	F	G	H	I	J	K	L	M	N	O	P	Q	R	S	T	59
60	A	B	C	D	E	F	G	H	I	J	K	L	M	N	O	P	Q	R	S	T	60
61	A	B	C	D	E	F	G	H	I	J	K	L	M	N	O	P	Q	R	S	T	61
62	A	B	C	D	E	F	G	H	I	J	K	L	M	N	O	P	Q	R	S	T	62
63	A	B	C	D	E	F	G	H	I	J	K	L	M	N	O	P	Q	R	S	T	63
64	A	B	C	D	E	F	G	H	I	J	K	L	M	N	O	P	Q	R	S	T	64
65	A	B	C	D	E	F	G	H	I	J	K	L	M	N	O	P	Q	R	S	T	65
66	A	B	C	D	E	F	G	H	I	J	K	L	M	N	O	P	Q	R	S	T	66
67	A	B	C	D	E	F	G	H	I	J	K	L	M	N	O	P	Q	R	S	T	67
68	A	B	C	D	E	F	G	H	I	J	K	L	M	N	O	P	Q	R	S	T	68
69	A	B	C	D	E	F	G	H	I	J	K	L	M	N	O	P	Q	R	S	T	69
70	A	B	C	D	E	F	G	H	I	J	K	L	M	N	O	P	Q	R	S	T	70
71	A	B	C	D	E	F	G	H	I	J	K	L	M	N	O	P	Q	R	S	T	71
72	A	B	C	D	E	F	G	H	I	J	K	L	M	N	O	P	Q	R	S	T	72
73	A	B	C	D	E	F	G	H	I	J	K	L	M	N	O	P	Q	R	S	T	73
74	A	B	C	D	E	F	G	H	I	J	K	L	M	N	O	P	Q	R	S	T	74
75	A	B	C	D	E	F	G	H	I	J	K	L	M	N	O	P	Q	R	S	T	75
76	A	B	C	D	E	F	G	H	I	J	K	L	M	N	O	P	Q	R	S	T	76
77	A	B	C	D	E	F	G	H	I	J	K	L	M	N	O	P	Q	R	S	T	77
78	A	B	C	D	E	F	G	H	I	J	K	L	M	N	O	P	Q	R	S	T	78
79	A	B	C	D	E	F	G	H	I	J	K	L	M	N	O	P	Q	R	S	T	79
80	A	B	C	D	E	F	G	H	I	J	K	L	M	N	O	P	Q	R	S	T	80
81	A	B	C	D	E	F	G	H	I	J	K	L	M	N	O	P	Q	R	S	T	81
82	A	B	C	D	E	F	G	H	I	J	K	L	M	N	O	P	Q	R	S	T	82
83	A	B	C	D	E	F	G	H	I	J	K	L	M	N	O	P	Q	R	S	T	83
84	A	B	C	D	E	F	G	H	I	J	K	L	M	N	O	P	Q	R	S	T	84
85	A	B	C	D	E	F	G	H	I	J	K	L	M	N	O	P	Q	R	S	T	85
86	A	B	C	D	E	F	G	H	I	J	K	L	M	N	O	P	Q	R	S	T	86
87	A	B	C	D	E	F	G	H	I	J	K	L	M	N	O	P	Q	R	S	T	87
88	A	B	C	D	E	F	G	H	I	J	K	L	M	N	O	P	Q	R	S	T	88
89	A	B	C	D	E	F	G	H	I	J	K	L	M	N	O	P	Q	R	S	T	89
90	A	B	C	D	E	F	G	H	I	J	K	L	M	N	O	P	Q	R	S	T	90
91	A	B	C	D	E	F	G	H	I	J	K	L	M	N	O	P	Q	R	S	T	91
92	A	B	C	D	E	F	G	H	I	J	K	L	M	N	O	P	Q	R	S	T	92
93	A	B	C	D	E	F	G	H	I	J	K	L	M	N	O	P	Q	R	S	T	93
94	A	B	C	D	E	F	G	H	I	J	K	L	M	N	O	P	Q	R	S	T	94
95	A	B	C	D	E	F	G	H	I	J	K	L	M	N	O	P	Q	R	S	T	95
96	A	B	C	D	E	F	G	H	I	J	K	L	M	N	O	P	Q	R	S	T	96
97	A	B	C	D	E	F	G	H	I	J	K	L	M	N	O	P	Q	R	S	T	97
98	A	B	C	D	E	F	G	H	I	J	K	L	M	N	O	P	Q	R	S	T	98
99	A	B	C	D	E	F	G	H	I	J	K	L	M	N	O	P	Q	R	S	T	99
100	A	B	C	D	E	F	G	H	I	J	K	L	M	N	O	P	Q	R	S	T	100

DO NOT WRITE IN THIS SPACE

101	A	B	C	D	E	F	G	H	I	J	K	L	M	N	O	P	Q	R	S	T	101
102	A	B	C	D	E	F	G	H	I	J	K	L	M	N	O	P	Q	R	S	T	102
103	A	B	C	D	E	F	G	H	I	J	K	L	M	N	O	P	Q	R	S	T	103
104	A	B	C	D	E	F	G	H	I	J	K	L	M	N	O	P	Q	R	S	T	104
105	A	B	C	D	E	F	G	H	I	J	K	L	M	N	O	P	Q	R	S	T	105
106	A	B	C	D	E	F	G	H	I	J	K	L	M	N	O	P	Q	R	S	T	106
107	A	B	C	D	E	F	G	H	I	J	K	L	M	N	O	P	Q	R	S	T	107
108	A	B	C	D	E	F	G	H	I	J	K	L	M	N	O	P	Q	R	S	T	108
109	A	B	C	D	E	F	G	H	I	J	K	L	M	N	O	P	Q	R	S	T	109
110	A	B	C	D	E	F	G	H	I	J	K	L	M	N	O	P	Q	R	S	T	110
111	A	B	C	D	E	F	G	H	I	J	K	L	M	N	O	P	Q	R	S	T	111
112	A	B	C	D	E	F	G	H	I	J	K	L	M	N	O	P	Q	R	S	T	112
113	A	B	C	D	E	F	G	H	I	J	K	L	M	N	O	P	Q	R	S	T	113
114	A	B	C	D	E	F	G	H	I	J	K	L	M	N	O	P	Q	R	S	T	114
115	A	B	C	D	E	F	G	H	I	J	K	L	M	N	O	P	Q	R	S	T	115
116	A	B	C	D	E	F	G	H	I	J	K	L	M	N	O	P	Q	R	S	T	116
117	A	B	C	D	E	F	G	H	I	J	K	L	M	N	O	P	Q	R	S	T	117
118	A	B	C	D	E	F	G	H	I	J	K	L	M	N	O	P	Q	R	S	T	118
119	A	B	C	D	E	F	G	H	I	J	K	L	M	N	O	P	Q	R	S	T	119
120	A	B	C	D	E	F	G	H	I	J	K	L	M	N	O	P	Q	R	S	T	120
121	A	B	C	D	E	F	G	H	I	J	K	L	M	N	O	P	Q	R	S	T	121
122	A	B	C	D	E	F	G	H	I	J	K	L	M	N	O	P	Q	R	S	T	122
123	A	B	C	D	E	F	G	H	I	J	K	L	M	N	O	P	Q	R	S	T	123
124	A	B	C	D	E	F	G	H	I	J	K	L	M	N	O	P	Q	R	S	T	124
125	A	B	C	D	E	F	G	H	I	J	K	L	M	N	O	P	Q	R	S	T	125
126	A	B	C	D	E	F	G	H	I	J	K	L	M	N	O	P	Q	R	S	T	126
127	A	B	C	D	E	F	G	H	I	J	K	L	M	N	O	P	Q	R	S	T	127
128	A	B	C	D	E	F	G	H	I	J	K	L	M	N	O	P	Q	R	S	T	128
129	A	B	C	D	E	F	G	H	I	J	K	L	M	N	O	P	Q	R	S	T	129
130	A	B	C	D	E	F	G	H	I	J	K	L	M	N	O	P	Q	R	S	T	130
131	A	B	C	D	E	F	G	H	I	J	K	L	M	N	O	P	Q	R	S	T	131
132	A	B	C	D	E	F	G	H	I	J	K	L	M	N	O	P	Q	R	S	T	132
133	A	B	C	D	E	F	G	H	I	J	K	L	M	N	O	P	Q	R	S	T	133
134	A	B	C	D	E	F	G	H	I	J	K	L	M	N	O	P	Q	R	S	T	134
135	A	B	C	D	E	F	G	H	I	J	K	L	M	N	O	P	Q	R	S	T	135
136	A	B	C	D	E	F	G	H	I	J	K	L	M	N	O	P	Q	R	S	T	136
137	A	B	C	D	E	F	G	H	I	J	K	L	M	N	O	P	Q	R	S	T	137
138	A	B	C	D	E	F	G	H	I	J	K	L	M	N	O	P	Q	R	S	T	138
139	A	B	C	D	E	F	G	H	I	J	K	L	M	N	O	P	Q	R	S	T	139
140	A	B	C	D	E	F	G	H	I	J	K	L	M	N	O	P	Q	R	S	T	140
141	A	B	C	D	E	F	G	H	I	J	K	L	M	N	O	P	Q	R	S	T	141
142	A	B	C	D	E	F	G	H	I	J	K	L	M	N	O	P	Q	R	S	T	142
143	A	B	C	D	E	F	G	H	I	J	K	L	M	N	O	P	Q	R	S	T	143
144	A	B	C	D	E	F	G	H	I	J	K	L	M	N	O	P	Q	R	S	T	144
145	A	B	C	D	E	F	G	H	I	J	K	L	M	N	O	P	Q	R	S	T	145
146	A	B	C	D	E	F	G	H	I	J	K	L	M	N	O	P	Q	R	S	T	146
147	A	B	C	D	E	F	G	H	I	J	K	L	M	N	O	P	Q	R	S	T	147
148	A	B	C	D	E	F	G	H	I	J	K	L	M	N	O	P	Q	R	S	T	148
149	A	B	C	D	E	F	G	H	I	J	K	L	M	N	O	P	Q	R	S	T	149
150	A	B	C	D	E	F	G	H	I	J	K	L	M	N	O	P	Q	R	S	T	150

DO NOT WRITE IN THIS SPACE

151	A	B	C	D	E	F	G	H	I	J	K	L	M	N	O	P	Q	R	S	T	151
152	A	B	C	D	E	F	G	H	I	J	K	L	M	N	O	P	Q	R	S	T	152
153	A	B	C	D	E	F	G	H	I	J	K	L	M	N	O	P	Q	R	S	T	153
154	A	B	C	D	E	F	G	H	I	J	K	L	M	N	O	P	Q	R	S	T	154
155	A	B	C	D	E	F	G	H	I	J	K	L	M	N	O	P	Q	R	S	T	155
156	A	B	C	D	E	F	G	H	I	J	K	L	M	N	O	P	Q	R	S	T	156
157	A	B	C	D	E	F	G	H	I	J	K	L	M	N	O	P	Q	R	S	T	157
158	A	B	C	D	E	F	G	H	I	J	K	L	M	N	O	P	Q	R	S	T	158
159	A	B	C	D	E	F	G	H	I	J	K	L	M	N	O	P	Q	R	S	T	159
160	A	B	C	D	E	F	G	H	I	J	K	L	M	N	O	P	Q	R	S	T	160
161	A	B	C	D	E	F	G	H	I	J	K	L	M	N	O	P	Q	R	S	T	161
162	A	B	C	D	E	F	G	H	I	J	K	L	M	N	O	P	Q	R	S	T	162
163	A	B	C	D	E	F	G	H	I	J	K	L	M	N	O	P	Q	R	S	T	163
164	A	B	C	D	E	F	G	H	I	J	K	L	M	N	O	P	Q	R	S	T	164
165	A	B	C	D	E	F	G	H	I	J	K	L	M	N	O	P	Q	R	S	T	165
166	A	B	C	D	E	F	G	H	I	J	K	L	M	N	O	P	Q	R	S	T	166
167	A	B	C	D	E	F	G	H	I	J	K	L	M	N	O	P	Q	R	S	T	167
168	A	B	C	D	E	F	G	H	I	J	K	L	M	N	O	P	Q	R	S	T	168
169	A	B	C	D	E	F	G	H	I	J	K	L	M	N	O	P	Q	R	S	T	169
170	A	B	C	D	E	F	G	H	I	J	K	L	M	N	O	P	Q	R	S	T	170
171	A	B	C	D	E	F	G	H	I	J	K	L	M	N	O	P	Q	R	S	T	171
172	A	B	C	D	E	F	G	H	I	J	K	L	M	N	O	P	Q	R	S	T	172
173	A	B	C	D	E	F	G	H	I	J	K	L	M	N	O	P	Q	R	S	T	173
174	A	B	C	D	E	F	G	H	I	J	K	L	M	N	O	P	Q	R	S	T	174
175	A	B	C	D	E	F	G	H	I	J	K	L	M	N	O	P	Q	R	S	T	175
176	A	B	C	D	E	F	G	H	I	J	K	L	M	N	O	P	Q	R	S	T	176
177	A	B	C	D	E	F	G	H	I	J	K	L	M	N	O	P	Q	R	S	T	177
178	A	B	C	D	E	F	G	H	I	J	K	L	M	N	O	P	Q	R	S	T	178
179	A	B	C	D	E	F	G	H	I	J	K	L	M	N	O	P	Q	R	S	T	179
180	A	B	C	D	E	F	G	H	I	J	K	L	M	N	O	P	Q	R	S	T	180
181	A	B	C	D	E	F	G	H	I	J	K	L	M	N	O	P	Q	R	S	T	181
182	A	B	C	D	E	F	G	H	I	J	K	L	M	N	O	P	Q	R	S	T	182
183	A	B	C	D	E	F	G	H	I	J	K	L	M	N	O	P	Q	R	S	T	183
184	A	B	C	D	E	F	G	H	I	J	K	L	M	N	O	P	Q	R	S	T	184
185	A	B	C	D	E	F	G	H	I	J	K	L	M	N	O	P	Q	R	S	T	185
186	A	B	C	D	E	F	G	H	I	J	K	L	M	N	O	P	Q	R	S	T	186
187	A	B	C	D	E	F	G	H	I	J	K	L	M	N	O	P	Q	R	S	T	187
188	A	B	C	D	E	F	G	H	I	J	K	L	M	N	O	P	Q	R	S	T	188
189	A	B	C	D	E	F	G	H	I	J	K	L	M	N	O	P	Q	R	S	T	189
190	A	B	C	D	E	F	G	H	I	J	K	L	M	N	O	P	Q	R	S	T	190
191	A	B	C	D	E	F	G	H	I	J	K	L	M	N	O	P	Q	R	S	T	191
192	A	B	C	D	E	F	G	H	I	J	K	L	M	N	O	P	Q	R	S	T	192
193	A	B	C	D	E	F	G	H	I	J	K	L	M	N	O	P	Q	R	S	T	193
194	A	B	C	D	E	F	G	H	I	J	K	L	M	N	O	P	Q	R	S	T	194
195	A	B	C	D	E	F	G	H	I	J	K	L	M	N	O	P	Q	R	S	T	195
196	A	B	C	D	E	F	G	H	I	J	K	L	M	N	O	P	Q	R	S	T	196
197	A	B	C	D	E	F	G	H	I	J	K	L	M	N	O	P	Q	R	S	T	197
198	A	B	C	D	E	F	G	H	I	J	K	L	M	N	O	P	Q	R	S	T	198
199	A	B	C	D	E	F	G	H	I	J	K	L	M	N	O	P	Q	R	S	T	199
200	A	B	C	D	E	F	G	H	I	J	K	L	M	N	O	P	Q	R	S	T	200

Answers

Serial No.	*Answer No.*	*Answer*
1.	c	Serial height and weight measurement
2.	a	CT head
3.	a	CT head
4.	f	Skeletal survey
5.	g	Look for Blue Sclera
6.	b	FBC and Coagulation profile
7.	c	Plasma cells
8.	k	Astrocytes
9.	j	Neutrophil precursors
10.	e	Skeletal muscle cells
11.	b	Allergy
12.	e	Chloride channel defect
13	a	Infection
14	i	Fibrosis
15	g	Trinucleotide repeats
16	h	Ciliary Dyskinesia
17	k	Surfactant deficiency
18	f	Alpha-1 antitrypsin deficiency
19	a	Antibiotic
20	b	Mast cell stabilizer
21	f	Carbonic anhydrase inhibitor
22	c	Prednisolone
23	d	Mydriatic
24	d	Mydraitic
25	f	Digoxin
26	e	Organophosphorus
27	d	Paraquat
28	b	Salicylate
29	a	Paracetamol
30	i	Ethanol
31	a	Clozapine
32	b	Chlorpromazine
33	b	Chlorpromazine
34	e	Lithium
35	c	Amitryptiline
36	a	Carbamazepine
37	b	Sodium valproate
38	c	Phenytoin
39	c	CT head
40	a	EEG
41	c	CT head
42	b	ECG
43	d	Vascular dementia
44	c	Frontal lobe dementia
45	b	Alzeihmer's disease
46	a	Depression
47	i	Delirium
48	i	Delirium
49	a	Fistula
50	b	Pelvic floor weakness
51	c	Multiple scleorsis
52	e	Detrusor instability
53	c	Erythropoetin
54	a	Aldosterone
55	j	ACTH
56	d	Parathormone
57	e	Prolactin

58	f	Erythema nodosum
59	b	Herpes zoster
60	L	Neurofibromatosis
61	k	Meningococcal septicemia
62	O	Spider nevi
63	j	Malignant melanoma
64	d	Clarithromycin
65	b	Cotrimoxazole
66	j	Anti-tuberculous therapy
67	d	Clarithromycin
68	i	Flu vaccine
69	a	Benzyl penicillin
70	d	Intravenous anaesthetics
71	f	Topical xylocaine
72	b	Epidural anaesthesia
73	f	Lignocaine infiltration
74	f	Recurrent brief depression
75	h	Mixed anxiety and depression
76	g	Seasonal affective disorder
77	c	Bipolar affective disorder
78	i	Mania
79	c	Osteoporosis
80	a	Rheumatoid arthritis
81	e	Ankylosing spondylitis
82	g	IVDP
83	f	Benign backache
84	d	IV fluids
85	c	Synotocin drip
86	g	Antibiotics
87	a	IM Synometrine
88	b	Haemolytic uremic syndrome
89	c	Chronic renal failure

90	f	SLE
91	e	Nephrotic syndrome
92	d	Acute glomerulonephritis
93	f	CT scan kidney
94	d	Cystoscopy
95	e	PSA
96	j	Suprapubic catheterization
97	a	Candidiasis
98	e	Cervical ectropion
99	c	Chlamydia
100	d	Herpes
101	g	Bacterial vaginosis
102	a	Cavernous sinus
103	e	Central retinal artery
104	f	Facial artery
105	b	Internal carotid artery
106	c	Superficial temporal artery
107	d	IV propton pump inhibitors
108	e	Oral proton pump inhibitors
109	a	Anti helicobacter therapy
110	c	Measure serum gastrin
111	a	Pulmonary embolism
112	b	Myocardial infarction
113	e	Pneumonia
114	c	Simple Pneumothorax
115	h	Esophageal rupture
116	g	Pulmonary edema
117	e	Tuberculous lymphadenitis
118	g	Ca Stomach
119	a	Thyroid carcinoma
120	c	Cystic hygroma
121	i	Mesothelioma

122	c	Normal saline with hydrocortisone
123	b	Insulin with normal saline
124	h	Normal saline with potassium
125	d	Oral potassium
126	f	Dialysis
127	e	Implantable pace maker
128	d	Carbimazole plus beta blockers
129	b	Adenosine
130	d	Thyroid Function tests
131	b	ECHO
132	a	ECG
133	c	The 24 hour Holter monitoring
134	c	Amniocentesis and karyotyping
135	b	Chorionic villous sampling
136	a	Fetal blood sampling
137	f	Fetal ECHO
138	g	Fetal blood at birth
139	a	Endocervical swab
140	c	Contact tracing
141	g	Pipelle sampling
142	f	Abdominal ultrasound
143	a	CXR
144	d	Laparotomy
145	c	Barium enema
146	h	CT Scan
147	c	CA 125
148	c	CA 125
149	e	Laparotomy
150	b	Pelvic CT
151	c	Frontal bone fracture
152	a	Petrous temporal fracture
153	f	Temporal arteritis

154	d	Crohn's disease
155	b	Carcinoma caecum
156	a	Irritable bowel disease
157	c	Carcinoma rectum
158	c	Heroine abuse
159	e	Vasovagal syncope
160	d	Plasma glucose levels
161	b	Subdural haemorrhage
162	b	Aortic rupture
163	f	Splenic rupture
164	e	Acute blood loss
165	i	Exradural haemorrhage
166	d	SLE
167	L	Sjögren's Syndrome
168	e	Sarcoidosis
169	j	Lung carcinoma
170	d	By hook
171	c	External oblique aponeurosis and internal oblique muscle
172	b	Chronic hepatitis
173	b	Complete resolution
174	c	Recurrence with full response to steroids
175	a	ACE inhibitors
176	b	Family history
177	b	Potassium 2.4 mmol/litre
178	b	CT scan head
179	b	Palmidronate
180	e	Loss of ankle jerk
181	a	Barium swallow
182	c	Cocaine
183	b	Thiamine
184	a	CT scan

185	b	Bronchial rupture
186	c	Admit for full infection screen
187	a	DC cardioversion
188	b	Columnar metaplasia
189	a	Varicose veins
190	a	Abdominal Migraine
191	d	Plaster and review after 2 weeks
192	a	Bromocriptine

193	a	Carcinoma Tonsil
194	b	Hypochondriasis
195	b	UTI
196	a	Testicular torsion
197	b	Postnatal blues
198	c	Postpartum depression
199	a	Vertebrobasilar insufficiency
200	b	Meningococcemia

Previous Year Paper 2

RxPG Analysis	
Total Themes:	34
Total SBAs:	30
Picture Slides:	5
Repeat Themes:	9
Repeat Themes with a Different Header:	13

THEME 1: COMPLICATIONS BREAST CANCER

OPTIONS
a. Pathological fracture
b. Cerebral metastases
c. Hypocalcaemia
d. Hypercalcaemia
e. Lymphoedema
f. Spinal cord compression
g. Pleural effusion
h. Liver metastasis
i. Peritoneal recurrence
j. Local recurrence
k. Diabetes mellitus
l. Lymphangitis carcinomatosis

INSTRUCTIONS
For each of the presentations given below choose the ***single most likely diagnosis*** *from the above list of options. Each option may be used once, more than once or not at all.*

QUESTIONS
1. Female with breast carcinoma 3 yr back, was treated with mastectomy and lymph node clearance on the left side. She now presents with a swollen left arm and decreased hand movements.

2. A 35-year-old female treated one year ago for breast carcinoma presents with 2-day history of confusion. She is drowsy and disoriented. Her husband reports that she had been complaining of severe thirst for past week.

3. A 45-year-old women treated 3-year ago for breast carcinoma presented with back pain and lack of sensation in legs. She says that even after evacuation she feels that her bladder is full. She has been constipated for last 24-hr.

4. A 43-year-old woman treated 2-years ago for grade 3 axillary node positive, breast carcinoma present with confusion, headache and vomiting.On examination she is drowsy but has no focal neurological sings. She has diplopia and O/E, papilloedema is present.

5. A 60-year-old woman is admitted to the accident and emergency department having fallen in the street. She is complaining of pain in the right hip and the right lower limb is lying in external rotation. She had breast conserving surgery, radiotherapy and chemotherapy eight years ago for breast cancer.

THEME 2: DIAGNOSIS OF HAEMATURIA

OPTIONS
a. Accelerated malignant hypertension
b. Chronic glomerulonephritis
c. Acute glomerulonephritis
d. Membranous nephropathy
c. Minimal change disease
e. Carcinoma bladder
f. Urinary calculus
g. Alport's syndrome
h. Polycystic kidney disease
i. Benign recurrent haematuria
j. Haemolytic uraemic syndrome
k. Renal cell carcinoma

INSTRUCTIONS
For each of the presentations given below choose the ***single most likely diagnosis*** *from the above list of options. Each option may be used once, more than once or not at all.*

QUESTIONS
6. A 40-year-old man was investigated with cystoscopy which was normal, for recurrent haematuria 15 years ago. He now presents with haematuria and his BP is found to be 180/110.

7. A 62-year-old man with recurrent painless haematuria and loss of weight.

8. A 4-year-old deaf child presents with recurrent haematuria.

9. A 42-year-old man presents with flank pain and gross haematuria. His left flank appears full.

10. A 6-year-old has a number of episodes of painless microscopic haematuria with no evidence of a UTI and a normal IVU.

THEME 3 : FEVER WITH RASH

OPTIONS

a. Infectious mononucleosis
b. Varicella
c. Measles
d. Kawasaki's disease
e. Staphylococcal scalded skin syndrome
f. Erythema infectiosum
g. Roseola infantum
h. Rubella
i. Lyme's disease
j. Drug reaction

INSTRUCTIONS

*For each of the presentations given below choose the **single most likely diagnosis** from the above list of options. Each option may be used once, more than once or not at all.*

QUESTIONS

11. A 7-year-old child with cervical lymphadenopathy, conjunctivitis and a rash on hand which started to peel after the fifth day.

12. A 12-year-old girl develops a fine macular rash after taking ampicillin prescribed to her for sore throat and fever. She has enlarged cervical lymph nodes.

13. A 7-month-old infant is brought with a rose-pink macular rash over the trunk. The baby was febrile before the onset of rash.

14. A 6-year-old child develops fever, arthralgias and a confluent rash on the face with a "slapped cheek" appearance.

15. A 4-year-old child presents with a generalised blanching and an erythematous rash. He also has fever, conjunctivitis, photophobia and coryza. Red lesions with white centers are present on the buccal mucosa.

THEME 4 : SCIENTIFIC BASIS OF DIABETES

OPTIONS

a. Absolute deficiency of insulin
b. Relative deficiency of insulin
c. Severe deficiency of insulin
d. Insulin excess
e. Insulin resistance
f. Endogenous insulin secretion
g. Exogenous insulin administration
h. Absolute deficiency of glucagon

INSTRUCTIONS

*For each of the presentations given below choose the **single most likely basis** of diabetic conditions from the above list of options. Each option may be used once, more than once or not at all.*

QUESTIONS

16. Diabetic ketoacidosis

17. Hyperosmolar nonketotic hyperglycaemia

18. Hypoglycaemia

19. Hyperglycaemia

20. Syndrome X

THEME 5: DIAGNOSIS OF ABDOMINAL INJURIES

OPTIONS

a. Aortic rupture
b. Bladder rupture
c. Bowel rupture
d. Cardiac tamponade
e. Diaphragmatic rupture
f. Liver rupture
g. Mesenteric vascular injury
h. Pancreatic contusion
i. Renal contusion
j. Renal pedicle avulsion
k. Splenic rupture
l. Urethral rupture

INSTRUCTIONS

*For each of the presentations given below choose the **single most likely diagnosis** from the above list of options. Each option may be used once, more than once or not at all.*

QUESTIONS

21. A boy was riding his bicycle when he was hit by a car. After examination in the A and E, he was found to have left upper quadrant tenderness.

22. A man fell off a ladder, has diffuse pain on right side of the trunk. IVU shows no excretion on right side.

23. A man was stabbed with a 10 cm knife in the left upper quadrant, stable for 20 minutes after which BP falls to 90/60 mmHg. On USG, no free fluid seen in abdomen.

24. A 25-year-old woman car driver is involved in a front impact accident. She develops central, epigastric and shoulder tip pain three hours later and is noted to have linear transverse bruising from the lap belt above the umbilicus.

25. A 32-year-old man has a kick in the loin region, developed haematuria.There is no blood seen at the uretheral meatus, no perineal injury seen.

THEME 6: DIAGNOSIS OF ANEMIA

OPTIONS

a. Hereditary spherocytosis
b. Haemolytic anaemia
c. Sickle cell anaemia
d. Beta thalassaemia
e. Chronic renal failure
f. Chronic liver failure
g. Pernicious anaemia
h. Megaloblastic anaemia
i. Sideroblastic anaemia
j. Fanconi's anaemia
k. Aplastic anaemia

INSTRUCTIONS

*For each of the presentation given below choose the **single most likely diagnosis** from the above list of options. Each option may be used once, more than once or not at all.*

QUESTIONS

26. A 5-year-old child from South Africa is brought to the accident and emergency department deeply jaundiced. He is found to have mildly swollen, tender feet and hands. His mucosae are pale.

27. A 7-year-old child had recurrent urinary tract infection in childhood. He looks pale with a yellowish complexion and his height is at present at the third centile.

28. A 28-year-old lady with history of intermittent jaundice, looks pale. Her spleen is palpable and USG abdomen shows gallstones.

29. A man is brought in with haematemesis and malena. He is anaemic, jaundiced, has spider naevi and gynaecomastia.

30. Following a mild viral illness, a 2-year-old child suddenly becomes severely pale. On examination there is no hepatosplenomegaly. Blood smear shows normocytic and normochromic RBCs and there are very few reticulocytes.

THEME 7: INVESTIGATION OF SIDE EFFECTS OF ANTI-EPILEPTICS

OPTIONS

a. Prothrombin time
b. Clotting time
c. FBC
d. Plasma drug level
e. White blood cell count
f. Renal function tests
g. Liver function tests
h. Visual acuity
i. Visual field mapping
j. Gum biopsy

INSTRUCTIONS

For each of the presentation given below choose the ***single most appropriate investigation*** *from the above list of options. Each option may be used once, more than once or not at all.*

QUESTIONS

31. An epileptic patient on treatment develops nausea vomiting with oliguria and raised levels of urea, creatinine.

32. A boy on treatment for generalized tonic clonic epilepsy, develops features of hepatic failure in few weeks of starting treatment.

33. A lady on treatment for epilepsy develops ataxia and gum hypertrophy.

34. A 12-year-old boy is started on anti-epileptic for his absence seizures. After few days he develops fever, sore throat and ataxia.

35. A known epileptic on treatment, is started on some antibiotic for upper respiratory tract infections. She is now extremely drowsy and develops a bout of seizure. Her plasma sodium level is found to be very low.

THEME 8: NATURAL HISTORY OF EPISTAXIS

OPTIONS

a. Anticoagulant overdosage
b. Coagulopathy
c. Hypertensive disease
d. Local infection
e. Maxillary antral carcinoma
f. Nasal polyposis
g. Nasopharyngeal angiofibroma
h. ORF
i. Sarcoidosis
j. Septal perforation
k. Trauma

INSTRUCTIONS

For each of the presentation given below choose the ***single best diagnosis*** *from the above list of options. Each option may be used once, more than once or not at all.*

QUESTIONS

36. A 50-year-old man presents with epistaxis. He has an artificial heart valve.

37. A 50-year-old furniture maker presents with anaesthesia of the left check and repeated left sided episodes of epistaxis.

38. An actor presents with repeated episodes of epistaxis as associated with whistling on breathing in through the nose.

39. A 45-year-old sheep farmer presents with unilateral epistaxis. Inspection reveals a bleeding polyp attached to the anterior nasal septum.

40. An 80-year-old man presents with epistaxis of two hours duration.

THEME 9: INVESTIGATIONS FOR ABDOMINAL CONDITIONS

OPTIONS

a. Plain X-ray abdomen
b. Chest X-ray
c. X-ray pelvis
d. Barium enema
e. Barium meal
f. Barium swallow
g. Upper GI endoscopy
h. Sigmoidoscopy
i. Colonoscopy
j. Proctoscopy
k. Mesenteric angiogram
l. Abdominal CT scan
m. Abdominal ultrasound

INSTRUCTIONS

For each of the presentation given below choose the ***single best investigation*** *from the above list of options. Each option may be used once, more than once or not at all.*

QUESTIONS

41. A patient presents with increasing constipation, and passing ribbon-like stools. He is well otherwise.

42. A 32-year-old female presents with acute onset constipation with abdominal pain and vomiting. She is noted to have a small swelling in her groin.

43. A 40-year-old patient comes with two year history of epigastric pain after food and tarry stools.

44. A 55-year-old woman presents with a six-month history of severe central abdominal pain, which comes on 30-minutes after meals. She has lost 10-kg in weight, and on examination of her abdomen there is a bruit in the epigastrium. She also suffers from intermittent claudication.

45. A 25-year-old teacher complains that she has had central abdominal discomfort of six-month duration, intermittent abdominal distension and alteration in bowel habit. On examination, there is a palpable swelling in the right iliac fossa. A barium enema carried out showed no abnormality.

THEME 10 : MANAGEMENT OF PSYCHOSIS

OPTIONS

a. TCA
b. Clozapine
c. Education
d. ECT
e. Family therapy
f. MAO inhibitor
g. Oral antipsychotics
h. Risk management strategy
i. Depot antipsychotics
j. Alternative housing
k. Detain under Mental Health Act
l. Rehabilitation ward
m. Hospital hostel
n. Voluntary inpatient admission

INSTRUCTIONS

For each of the presentation given below choose the ***single best treatment*** *option from the above list of options. Each option may be used once, more than once or not at all.*

QUESTIONS

46. A 26-year-old woman with established schizophrenia since age 15, lives with her very supportive parents, but has never fully recovered. She has been on a range of appropriate medication in adequate dosage since diagnosis.

47. A 28-year-old man has been detained in hospital and is being treated for paranoid schizophrenia with depot antipsychotic medication. He had stabbed his mother in the hand with a screwdriver. He is now symptom free and ready to be discharged home to live with his mother, who is worried.

48. A 64-year-old man with eight admissions to hospital in the last five years is again brought to hospital by his son. It is known that he always stops taking his antipsychotic tablets at home. His wife died 6 months ago and he has been depressed and threatening to kill himself and refused any treatment.

49. An 80-year-old man has a paranoid psychosis and mild cognitive decline. He is hard of hearing and says his neighbours are killing his chattels, but the authority has already announced that there is an outburst of some disease due to which cows are dying. He is continuously observing the neighbours by binoculars.

50. An 89-year -old woman presents with a three -week history of not eating and not sleeping. She is convinced that she is about to be investigated by the government for spying, which is not the case. She refuses to eat or drink and her physical state is deteriorating. She is agreeable to treatment.

THEME 11: DIAGNOSIS OF NEUROLOGICAL DISEASES

OPTIONS

a. Vertebrobasilar stroke
b. Carotid artery territory stroke
c. Motor neuron disease
d. Supranuclear palsy
e. Parietal lobe stroke
f. Temporal lobe stroke
g. Occipital lobe stroke
h. Multiple sclerosis
i. Alzheimer's disease
j. Korsakoff's psychosis

INSTRUCTIONS

*For each of the presentations given below choose the **single most appropriate diagnosis** from the above list of options. Each option may be used once, more than once or not at all.*

QUESTIONS

51. A 61-year-old man presents with sudden onset dysarthria, headache, vertigo and dysphagia. He gives history of myocardial infarction 8 months back.

52. A 20-year-old male with few days history of hoarseness and dysphagia, now develops paresis of both lower limbs.

53. A 32-year-old lady had been confined to the wheelchairs because of paraplegia for now almost 2 years. She now develops blurred vision leading to blindness.

54. A 72-year-old patient is now totally confined to the bed. He is getting increasingly forgetful within the last a few years.

55. A 65-year-old man had a transient loss of consciousness and weakness of left hand, from which he recovered completely. However, now he appears to always look towards right side while walking. His left eye vision is normal on testing.

THEME 12 : DIAGNOSIS OF DEMENTIA

OPTIONS

a. Alzheimer's dementia
b. Alcoholic dementia
c. Huntington's chorea
d. Crutzfeldt-Jakob's disease
e. Pick's disease
f. Lewy body dementia
g. Multi-infarct dementia
h. HIV
i. Frontotemporal dementia
j. Korsakoff's syndrome
k. Acute delirium

INSTRUCTIONS

*For each of the presentation given below choose the **single most likely diagnosis** from the above list of options. Each option may be used once, more than once, or not at all.*

QUESTIONS

56. A 40-year-old lady comes with gradual loss of memory. She has right handed involuntary writhing movement. Her father and uncle had similar problems.

57. A 55-year-old, otherwise healthy, man is brought to A and E by his wife who says that he has become progressively more forgetful. He also tends to lose his temper more often and is emotionally labile.

58. A 77-year-old man with weakness in his arm and leg, from which he recovered within few days. He now presents with short term memory loss. On examination he has extensor plantar response. He had similar episodes 2 years ago and became unable to identify objects and make proper judgements.

59. A 59-year-old man with early loss and speech and memory with visuospatial orientation preserved.

60. A 42-year-old man brought to OPD with features of disorientation and visual hallucinations. Wife says he was alright till few days before when he caught cold.

THEME 13: PRENATAL SCREENING

OPTIONS

a. Duchenne's muscular dystrophy
b. Spina bifida
c. Down's syndrome
d. Cystic fibrosis
e. Sickle cell anaemia
f. Beta thalassaemia
g. Congenital adrenal hyperplasia
h. Potter's syndrome
i. Trisomy 18
j. Congenital hypothyroidism

INSTRUCTIONS

*For each of the presentations given below choose the **single most appropriate diagnosis** from the above list of options. Each option may be used once, more than once or not at all.*

QUESTIONS

61. A pregnant lady with previous male child affected with this disorder want to know whether this child is also affected.

62. A pregnant lady with high alpha feto protein.

63. A pregnant lady with high HCG and low AFP.

64. A pregnant lady is advised to take folate prior to conception and during pregnancy to prevent this condition.

65. A pregnant lady with previous child affected with recurrent chest infections and diarrhoea wants to know whether this child is affected too.

THEME 14 : PRENATAL DIAGNOSIS

OPTIONS

a. Neural tube defects
b. Trisomy 18
c. Trisomy 21
d. Amniocentesis
e. Chorionic villous sampling
f. Foetal cordocentesis
g. Ultrasound
h. 17-hydroxyprogesterone
i. Serum estriol
j. Serum HCG
k. Fetal ECG
l. Fetal ECHO
m. Spina bifida

INSTRUCTIONS

*For each of the presentations given below choose the **single most appropriate investigation** from the above list of options. Each option may be used once more than once or not at all.*

QUESTIONS

66. A 30-year-old second gravida with previous child diagnosed with Duchenne's muscular dystrophy.

67. A 35-year-old pregnant at 16 weeks gestation was found to have a high hCG, low AFP and low oestriol.

68. A 27-year-old at 14 weeks gestation was found to have very high AFP.

69. A 32-year-old hypertensive with severe oilgohydramnios.

70. A 28-year-old pregnant lady with previous child diagnosed with congenital adrenal hyperplasia.

THEME 15: TREATMENT OF SEXUALLY TRANSMITTED DISEASES

OPTIONS

a. Erythromycin
b. Doxycycine
c. Metronidazole
d. Clotrimazole
e. Ciprofloxacin
f. Benzylpencillin
g. Cefixime
h. Ofloxacin
i. Ofloxacin + metronidazole
j. Fluconazole
k. Laparotomy
l. Wait and watch
m. Laparoscopy

INSTRUCTIONS

*For each of the presentation given below choose the **single best treatment** from the above list of options. Each option may be used once, more than once or not at all.*

QUESTIONS

71. A 25-year-old sexually active female comes with mucopurulent discharge per vaginum. She is febrile and noted to have a diffuse pustular erythematous rash.

72. A 32-year-old female complains of offensive white, fishy odor vaginal discharge. She has recently changed her partner.

73. A 23-year-old female comes with complains of dysuria. Bacterial culture of urine yields no growth. Cervical tenderness is elicited on per vaginum examination.

74. An 18-year-old girl on OCPs, with severe vaginal itching and cheese like discharge per vaginum.

75. A 27-year-old sexually active female on oral contraceptives for two years, with mucoid discharge per vaginum.

THEME 16: TREATMENT OF HEADACHE

OPTIONS

a. Antihypertensives
b. Burr holes
c. IV Mannitol
d. Low dose prednisolone
e. High dose prednisolone
f. Amitriptyline
g. Atenolol
h. Gabapentin
i. Lamotrigine
j. Sumatriptan
k. Ergotamine
l. Neurological opinion

INSTRUCTIONS

*For each of the presentations given below choose the **single most appropriate treatment** from the above list of options. Each option may be used once, more than once or not at all.*

QUESTIONS

76. A man involved in RTA, presents with headache and loss of consciousness after admission.

77. A 45-year-old man presents with unilateral temporal headache.

78. A 27-year-old female with recurrent unilateral headache and transient visual disturbances.

79. A 32-year-old man presents with bouts of intense headache everyday as soon as he wakes up. He is well otherwise.

80. A 22-year-old man complains of dull headache which is worst upon awakening. He also complains of defective vision left side and vomiting.

THEME 17: DIAGNOSIS OF INCONTINENCE

OPTIONS

a. Fistula
b. Stress incontinence
c. Multiple sclerosis
d. Urge incontinence
e. Detrusor instability
f. Spinal cord compression
g. Stroke
h. Cauda equina syndrome
i. Inter vertebral disc prolapse
j. Reflux
k. Diabetes Melitus
l. Autonomic bladder

INSTRUCTIONS

For each of the presentation given below choose the ***single most likely diagnosis*** *from the above list of options. Each option may be used once, more than once or not at all.*

QUESTIONS

81. A 47-year-old lady presents with urinary incontinence and recurrent urinary tract infections. She continues to soil her clothes with urine even after being catheterized.

82. A 28-year-old multipara complains of passing urine on coughing and stressing.

83. An 18-year-old girl comes with acute pain lower abdomen and difficulty in walking. She has not passed urine since 48 hr. She gives history of visual loss few years back, which has now resolved completely.

84. A 47-year-old lady with frequency and unavoidable desire to urinate at a few seconds' notice but no dysuria.

85. A 60-year-old lady complaints of continuous dribbling of urine. She underwent hysterectomy few months back.

THEME 18: TREATMENT OF CONJUNCTIVITIS

OPTIONS

a. Topical fusidic acid
b. Oral indomethacin
c. Oral tetracycline
d. Sodium chromoglycate
e. Oral acyclovir
f. Topical betamethasone
g. Topical atropine
h. Topical timolol
i. Topical acetazolamide
j. Oral acetazolamide
k. Oral chloramphenicol
l. Topical chloramphenicol

INSTRUCTIONS

For each of the presentation given below choose the ***single most appropriate treatment*** *from the above list of options. Each options may be used once more than once or not at all.*

QUESTIONS

86. Allergic conjunctivitis.

87. Ophthalmia neonatorum.

88. Trachoma.

89. Reiter's disease.

90. Bacterial conjunctivitis.

THEME 19: DIAGNOSIS OF INCONTINENCE

OPTIONS
a. Fistula
b. Pelvic floor weakness
c. Multiple sclerosis
d. UTI
e. Detrusor instability
f. Spinal cord compression
g. Stroke
h. Cauda equina syndrome
i. Intervertebral disc prolapse
j. Reflux
k. Diabetes melitus

INSTRUCTIONS
*For each of the presentation given below choose the **single most likely diagnosis** from the above list of options. Each option may be used once, more than once or not at all.*

QUESTIONS
91. A 60-year-old lady complains of continuous dribbling of urine. She underwent hysterectomy few months back.

92. A lady after child birth complains of passing urine on coughing and stressing.

93. A young girl with history of visual loss and bilateral lower limb weakness, complains of not able to pass urine at all.

94. A 47-year-old lady with frequency and unavoidable desire to urinate at a few seconds' notice but no dysuria.

95. A 47-year-old lady presents with urinary incontinence and recurrent urinary tract infections. She continues to soil her clothes with urine even after being catheterized.

THEME 20: DIFFERENTIAL DIAGNOSIS OF ACUTE URINARY RETENTION

OPTIONS
a. Ureteric colic
b. Carcinoma prostate
c. BPH
d. Urinary tract infection
e. Stricture
f. Periventricular region lesion
g. Brainstem lesion
h. Spinal cord lesion
i. Antidepressant
j. Urethral valves
k. Ruptured ureters

INSTRUCTIONS
*For each presentation below, choose the **single most likely diagnosis** from the above list of options. Each option may be used once, more than once or not at all.*

QUESTIONS
96. A patient of multiple sclerosis has had urinary catheterisation for 4 years with intermittent obstruction.

97. A 60-year-old with complaints of frequency and dysuria. PSA is 120 ng/ml. He also has back pain.

98. A 27-year-old female patient comes to A and E with complaints of severe flank pain. She is restless. The pain radiates to the groin.

99. A 65-year-old man presents with history of ferquency, urgency and decreased urinary flow.

100. A 39-year-old female presents with weakness of both legs, difficulty walking and urinary retention.

THEME 21: TREATMENT OF GYNAECOLOGICAL CONDITIONS

OPTIONS

a. Laparotomy
b. Laparoscopy
c. Endoscopy
d. Contact tracing
e. Oral ofloxacin
f. Oral erythromycin
g. Oral metronidazole
h. Blind therapy
i. Empirical therapy
j. Abdominal hysterectomy
k. Vaginal hysterectomy

INSTRUCTIONS

*For each of the presentations given below choose the **single most appropriate treatment** from the above list of options. Each option may be used once, more than once or not at all.*

QUESTIONS

101. A 24-year-old lady with pelvic pain and offensive vaginal discharge.

102. An asymptomatic 25-year-old lady says her husband had a purulent urethral discharge and does not wants to talk about it.

103. A 67-year-old lady with bleeding per vaginum. USG shows thickened endometrium.

104. A 47-year-old female with bilateral pelvic masses and terminal haematuria.

105. A 34-year-old lady comes with discharge per vaginum. Wet mount shows clue cells.

THEME 22: TREATMENT OF INFECTIONS

OPTIONS

a. None
b. Benzyl penicillin
c. Amoxycillin
d. Cefotaxime
e. Gentamicin
f. Metronidazole
g. Ciprofloxacin
h. Erythromycin
i. Trimethoprim
j. Doxycycline
k. Co-amoxiclav
l. Two or more antibiotics together

INSTRUCTIONS

*For each of the presentations given below choose the **single most likely antibiotic** from the above list of options. Each option may be used once, more than once, or not at all.*

QUESTIONS

106. A 30-year-old man complains of severe burning on passing urine like 'passing a broken glass.' He also has a penile discharge. Gram stain of the urethral swab is negative.

107. A 40-year-old man has cough, fever and mild dyspnoea. He has reduced air entry and is dull to percussion at the left lung base. He is neither systemically unwell nor hypoxic. He has a documented penicillin murmur.

108. A 40-year-woman presents with malaise and low-grade fever for 2 weeks. She recently had treatment for a dental abscess. On examination she has splinter haemorrhages and an early diastolic murmur.

109. A 2-year-old child presents with acute fever, drowsiness, stridor and drooling. He looks shocked and unwell.

110. A 60-year-old male smoker presents with severe dyspnoea, dry cough and fever. He is unwell, tachycardic and cyanosed.

THEME 23 : DIAGNOSIS OF INJURIES

OPTIONS

a. Liver
b. Pancreas
c. Spleen
d. Aorta
e. Kidney
f. Urethra
g. Uterus
h. Ureter
i. Diaphragm
j. Intestines

INSTRUCTIONS

*For each of the presentations given below choose the **single most likely diagnosis** from the above list of options. Each option may be used once, more than once or not at all.*

QUESTIONS

111. A 40-year-old man sitting in a passenger seat met an accident where the car is hit from the left side. He now complains of pain in the left side abdomen. There is also bruising of that side.

112. A patient involved in an RTA comes to A and E complaining of pain in upper abdomen and breathlessness. On X-ray the nasogastric tube is seen coiled up in the chest region.

113. A woman had met with an RTA in the car she was driving. She went and hit to the windscreen and now developed epigastric pain.

114. A man had met with an RTA and he developed shock and bruising of the flanks.

115. A man had fallen from scaffolding astride. He now complains of pain and swelling in the scrotum.

THEME 24: DIFFERENTIAL DIAGNOSIS OF ALTERED BOWEL HABIT

OPTIONS

a. Carcinoma rectum
b. Carcinoma caecum
c. IBS with diarrhoea
d. IBS with constipation
e. Faecal impaction
f. Diverticulosis
g. Ulcerative colitis
h. Crohn's disease
i. Fissure in ano
j. Paralytic ileus
k. Haemorrhoids
l. Acute haematoma around anal region

INSTRUCTIONS

*For each of the presentations given below choose the **single most likely diagnosis** from the above list of options. Each option may be used once, more than once or not at all.*

QUESTIONS

116. A 19-year-old female with complaint of a 1 year history of bloody diarrhoea and tenesmus. She has pale skin lesions. On examination, sigmoidoscopy shows inflammation and granulomata

117. A 65-year-old male with weight loss, right-sided pain and tenesmus. On examination, a granular mass is seen in the rectum.

118. An 18-year-old presents with frequent diarrhoea and gaseous distension of the abdomen which is relieved by defaecation. Sigmoidoscopy is normal.

119. An 80-year-old with complaint of diarrhoea and urinary retention.

120. After an abdominal operation, a patient presents with subfebrile state and abdominal distention. There is associated no abdominal tenderness and constipation is present. On auscultation no bowel sounds are heard.

THEME 25: MODES OF INHERITANCE

OPTIONS

a. X-linked recessive
b. Autosomal dominant
c. Autosomal co-dominance
d. Autosomal recessive
e. Polygenic
g. Single gene defect
h. X-linked dominant
i. Y-linked
j. Mismatch mutation

INSTRUCTIONS

For each of the presentations given below choose the ***single most likely mode of inheritance*** *from the above list of options. Each option may be used once, more than once or not at all.*

QUESTIONS

121. A 4-year-old boy gets haemarthrosis with trivial injury. He had similar episodes before maternal grand father and uncle had a similar problem.

122. A young girl with complaint of prolonged bleeding following dental extraction. Father had a work-up for anaemia and mother had multiple transfusions.

123. A 15-year-old girl with features of diabetes mellitus.

124. An 11-year-old boy presents with increasing difficulty walking, tremor and instability. Father died in his 40's with same disease.

125. An 18-year-old female underwent caries tooth extraction and developed profuse bleeding. On taking history she revealed menorrhagia. Her mother and her grand father had the same disease.

THEME 26: DIAGNOSIS OF ABDOMINAL CONDITIONS

OPTIONS

a. Strangulated hernia
b. Constipation–atonic
c. Intestinal obstruction
d. Paralytic ileus
e. Pyloric stenosis
f. Carcinoma rectum
g. Hirchsprung's disease
h. Constipation – spastic
i. Abdominal angina
j. Abdominal migraine
k. Mesenteric adenitis
l. Diverticulitis
m. Peptic ulcer

INSTRUCTIONS

For each of the presentation given below choose the ***single best diagnosis*** *from the above list of options. Each option may be used once, more than once or not at all.*

QUESTIONS

126. A patient presents with increasing constipation, and passing ribbon-like stools. He is well otherwise.

127. A 32-year-old female presents with acute onset constipation with abdominal pain and vomiting. She is noted to have a small swelling in her groin.

128. A 40-year-old patient comes with two year history of epigastric pain after food and tarry stools.

129. A 55-year-old woman presents with a six-month history of severe central abdominal pain, which comes on 30-minutes after meals. She has lost 10-kg in weight, and on examination of her abdomen there is a bruit in the epigastrium. She also suffers from intermittent claudication.

130. A 25-year-old teacher complains that she has had central abdominal discomfort of six-month duration, intermittent abdominal distension and alteration in bowel habit. On examination, there is a palpable swelling in the right iliac fossa. A barium enema carried out showed no abnormality.

THEME 27: DIAGNOSIS OF ENDOCRINE DISEASES

OPTIONS

a. Cushing's syndrome
b. Cushing's disease
c. Conn's syndrome
d. Addison's disease
e. Hyperparathyroidism
f. Polycythemia vera
g. Secondary polycythaemia
h. Hypothyroidism
i. Hyperthyroidism
j. Thyrotoxicosis
k. Microadenoma
l. Macroadenoma

INSTRUCTIONS

For each of the presentation given below choose the ***single most likely diagnosis*** *from the above list of options. Each option may be used once, more than once or not at all.*

QUESTIONS

131. A heavy smoker with raised haematocrit and haemoglobin.

132. A 30-year-old female presents with lethargy. Her BP is 160/100 with serum electrolytes Na^+ 149 mmol/L, K^+ 2.6 mmol/L and HCO^-_3 30 mmol/L.

133. A 35-year-old female presents with hypotension and lethargy. She is noted to have hyperpigmentation of her oral mucosa.

134. A 40-year-old patient complaints of lethargy, bone pain, polyuria and polydyspia. His blood glucose level is 3.0 mmol/L.

135. A 32-year-old female presents with galactorrhoea, amenorrhoea and infertility.

THEME 28: DIAGNOSIS OF PALPITATIONS

OPTIONS

a. Supraventricular tachycardia
b. Ventricular fibrillation
c. Atrial fibrillation
d. Ventricular asystole
e. Ventricular extrasystole
f. Cardiac arrest
g. Cardiac tumour
h. Ventricular tachycardia
i. Atrial flutter
j. Complete heart block

INSTRUCTIONS

For each of the presentations given below choose the ***single most appropriate diagnosis*** *from the above list of options. Each option may be used once, more than once or not at all.*

QUESTIONS

136. An 18-year-old girl, sweaty with tremors and weight loss, says that her heart races.

137. A woman experiences 'thumping' in her chest associated with breathlessness, while asleep. She sits up to get symptoms resolve in few minutes time.

138. A woman with a family history of coronary artery disease. She has noticed palpitations especially during the night. She describes a sensation of her heartbeat momentarily stopping, and then racing.

139. A man complains of episodes of palpitations which last for few minutes and leave him dizzy. His pulse appears to be normal at the point of examination.

140. A man after falling unconscious on a number of occasions was found to have a heart rate of 40 bpm.

THEME 29: DIFFERENTIAL DIAGNOSIS OF EPILEPSY

OPTIONS

a. Myoclonic epilepsy
b. Crutzfeldt-Jacobs Disease
c. Alcohol intoxication
d. ICSOL
e. Hyperglycaemia
f. Hypoglycaemia
g. Tuberculous meningitis
h. Pyogenic meningitis
i. Epilepsy
j. Subarachnoid haemorrhage
k. Subdural haematoma
l. Head injury

INTRUCTION

*For each of the presentations given below choose the **single most appropriate investigation** from the above list of options. Each option may be used once, more than once, or not at all.*

QUESTIONS

141. A 53-year-old non-alcoholic, obese man presents with sweating, tremor, drowsiness, fits and agitation.

142. A 12-year-old girl is brought to Accident and Emergency department by her parents complaining of a persistent rash, photophobia, and neck pain.

143. A 35-year-old mechanic has recurrent epileptiform attacks. He has no history of trauma.

144. An 18-year-old student is brought to the Accident and Emergency department by ambulance having been flung off his bicycle in a road traffic accident upon arrival, he is noted to have deterioration in consciousness.

145. A 32-year-old boxer presents with headache, drowsiness, seizures, and a rising blood pressure.

THEME 30: DIAGNOSIS OF NECK LUMPS

OPTIONS

a. Thyroid carcinoma
b. Goitre
c. Cystic hygroma
d. Branchial cyst
e. Tuberculous lymphadenitis
f. Lymphoma
g. Ca stomach
h. Ca lung
i. Mesothelioma

INSTRUCTIONS

*For each of the presentations given below choose the **single most likely diagnosis** from the above list of options. Each option may be used once, more than once or not at all.*

QUESTIONS

146. A 40-year-old lady from Asia with lumps in her neck, FNAC of which revealed center of casseous material surrounded by fibrosis.

147. A 60-year-old man with a lump in supra-clavicular region and decreased appetite. He has lost 5 kg weight recently.

148. A man comes with a lump in front of his neck which moves up on swallowing. Scan shows a mass replacing the left lobe of thyroid and spreading to sternomastoid and adjacent muscles.

149. An infant with brilliantly transilluminable swelling at the base of his neck.

150. A shipyard worker develops shortness of breath and a lump in his supraclavicular fossa.There is a small pleural effusion noted on the same side of the lump.

THEME 31: TREATMENT OF PELVIC INFLAMMATORY DISEASES

OPTIONS

a. Metronidazole 100 mg single dose
b. Metronidazole 400 mg 7 days
c. Vidarabine
d. Idoxuridine
e. Acyclovir
f. Single dose ofloxacin + metronidazole
g. Ofloxacin + metronodazole 14 days
h. Oral clotrimazole
i. Clotrimazole pessary
j. None

INSTRUCTIONS

For each of the presentation given below choose the ***single best diagnosis*** *from the above list of options. Each option may be used once, more than once or not at all.*

QUESTIONS

151. A 26-year-old female with sore vagina and whitish discharge; smear shows mycelia.

152. A 27-year-old sexually active female on oral contraceptives for two years, complains of mucoid discharge per vaginum.

153. A 18-year-old girl with recently developed dysmenorrhoea and deep dyspareunia. Speculum examination reveals purulent discharge from cervical os. Tested negative for gonorrhoea.

154. A 37-year-old lady with multiple painful, vesicular lesions at the introitus with scanty offensive discharge.

155. A 34-year-old lady with discharge per vaginum. Wet mount shows clue cells.

THEME 32 : DIAGNOSIS OF ELECTROLYTE IMBALANCES

OPTIONS

a. Hypokalaemia
b. Hyperkalaemia
c. Dehydration
d. Dehydration with hypokalaemia
e. Rhabdomyolysis
f. Diabetic ketoacidosis
g. Diuretic overuse
h. Type I diabetes mellitus
i. Type II diabetes mellitus
j. Diabetes insipidus
k. Addison's disease
l. Conn's syndrome

INSTRUCTIONS

For each of the presentations given below choose the ***single most appropriate diagnosis*** *from the above list of options. Each option may be used once, more than once or not at all.*

QUESTIONS

156. A 20-year-old girl with hypotension,hyperkalaemia and is mildly hyponatraemic. She has recently lost weight and her skin appears hyperpigmented.

157. A young boy with polyuria, has very high blood glucose levels.

158. A patient has diarrhoea, appears to be dehydrated with low potassium levels.

159. A patient on vigorous diuretic therapy develops hypokalaemia.

160. A person develops anuria after severe crushing injuries. His blood urea level at 60 mmol/L and serum potassium 7.5 mmol/L.

THEME 33: DIAGNOSIS OF CHEST CONDITIONS

OPTIONS

a. Pleural effusion
b. Lobar pneumonia
c. Bronchial pneumonia
d. Pulmonary embolism
e. Pneumothorax (Tension)
f. Pneumothorax (Simple)
g. Inferior wall myocardial infarction
h. Anterior wall myocardial infarction
i. Anteroseptal myocardial infarction
j. Pulmonary embolism
k. Pulmonary edema
l. Aortic dissection

INSTRUCTION

For each of the presentations given below choose the ***single most appropriate diagnosis*** *co-relating with the relevant slide, from the above list of options. Each option may be used once, more than once or not at all.*

QUESTIONS

161. A 47-year-old man was brought to the emergency room after having experienced chest discomfort and shortness of breath, followed by a syncopal episode. He was short of breath (breathing at 40 and requiring 100% oxygen to maintain an adequate saturation) and had a depressed level of consciousness. He was pale, diaphoretic, and in shock with a pulse of 120 bpm and a blood pressure of 70 mmHg systolic (Fig. 7, Plate 2).

162. A 56-year-old male presents with severe chest pain. His JVP is normal and no positive findings on the Chest X-ray. He is tachycardic with pule rate of 110 bpm and his BP is 120/80 PR 110 bpm. The ECG taken shows changes in V1, 2, 3 (Fig. 8, Plate 2).

163. A 40-year-old male presents with an irregular pulse rate (100 bpm). His BP is 120/90 mm Hg , JVP is not elevated and temperature is 39°C. The chest X-ray taken in the A and E shows positive findings (Fig. 9, Plate 2).

164. A 22-year-old tall male presents with acute onset breathlessness. His temperature is 37°C and his JVP appears to be normal. His BP is 130/80 PR 90 bpm/regular and the CXR taken shows reduced markings on right side (Fig. 10, Plate 2).

165. An 85-year-old female presents with brethlessness. On examination her temperature is 37°C and JVP is raised. Her PR is 90 bpm /regular and BP 100/90. CXR shows bilateral shadows. (Fig. 11, Plate 2)

THEME 34: DIAGNOSIS OF DEMENTIA

OPTIONS

a. Depression
b. Alzeihmer's disease
c. Frontal lobe dementia
d. Vascular dementia
e. Carbon monoxide poisoning
f. Huntington's disease
g. Pick's disease
h. Crutzfeldt-Jacob syndrome
i. Delirium

INSTRUCTIONS

For each of the presentation given below choose the ***single most likely diagnosis*** *from the above list of options. Each option may be used once, more than once or not at all.*

QUESTIONS

166. A 55-year-old man with history of stroke and repeated falls, now confused and cannot remember things.

167. A 48-year-old man has normal memory on examination; wife complaints of him becoming aggressive lately and talking about their sexual life publicly.

168. A 65-year-old lady with no previous history of behavior abnormality is found entering shop at odd hours of early morning.

169. A 68-year-old man refuses to talk. Says that there is no point talking to him, as he is a complete failure and that his memory has given up.

170. A man admitted in hospital develops features of disorientation and visual hallucinations on third day of admission.

SBAs

171. A 42-year-old male expatriate is admitted semi-conscious being feverish with sweats. He is noted to have a temperature of 39.0°C and some neck stiffness. Thick blood film is positive for falciparum malaria and he is started on medication.

The single most likely cause for his present condition is:

a. Septicaemia
b. Aspirin overdosage
c. Quinine therapy
d. Alcoholic binge
e. Postprandial hypoglycaemia

172. A 28-year-old lady in 20 weeks of gestation suffered a severe upper respiratory tract infection which she could manage to treat herself by taking high doses of azithromycin.

The single most likely theoretical risk to her baby could be:

a. VI nerve damage
b. VII nerve damage
c. VIII nerve damage
d. II nerve damage
e. I nerve damage

173. A 35-year-old man has an appendicectomy. Fourty eight hours late he becomes febrile, hypotensive and unwell. Hb 12.8 g/dl , WBC 19.4 x 109/L , platelets 48 x 109/L

Blood film shows a neutrophilia. The single most likely cause of the thrombocytopenia could be:

a. Immune thrombocytopaenia
b. Disseminated intravascular cougulation
c. Post-transfusion purpura
d. Heparin induce thrombocytopaenia
e. Aplastic anaemia

174. A 31-year-old woman complains of abdominal pain which seems to increase during her periods.Over the last year, she has noticed difficulty in breathing and chest pain associated with occasional haemoptysis, following her periods. She has been unable to conceive. On examination, she is found to have an enlarged and tender uterus. Her BMI is 20.

The single most likely diagnosis is:

a. Possible malignancy
b. Polycystic ovarian disease
c. Adenomyosis
d. Endometriosis
e. Pulmonary tuberculosis

175. A 45-year-old man complains of headaches, excessive thirst and frequent urination. On examination, he is noted to have bad acne, coarse skin and has a goitre. He has moved his wedding band to the 5th finger.

The single most likely diagnosis is:

a. Hypothyroidism
b. Cushing's syndrome
c. Hysterical neurosis
d. Autonomic side effects
e. Acromegaly

176. A 35-year-old lady delivered a baby at term. She had hepatitis B infection during pregnancy and is worried for the baby.

For the baby, it is required to give:

a. Hepatitis B immunoglobulin alone
b. Hepatitis B immunoglobulin and vaccine
c. Hepatitis B vaccine only
d. Interferon
e. None

177. A young thin man suddenly become breathless. On examination, air entry is reduced in left side and no movement in right side.Trachea is deviated to left.

The single most important initial management should be:

a. Chest drain to right lung
b. Chest drain to left lung
c. Wide bore needle to right pleural cavity
d. Wide bore needle to left pleural cavity
e. Take a chest X-ray immediately

178. An 18-year-old student has come back from Ghana. He was taking anti-malarials for 2 weeks after he returned home. He has a temp of 39.5 and is vomiting. He is now sensitive to light and has a stiff neck.

The single most useful investigation would be:

a. CT scan
b. MRI
c. Lumbar puncture
d. Thick and thin smear
e. Blood culture

179. A woman has had severe rheumatoid arthritis for 12 years. She has been on long term methotrexate and naproxen for years. Her blood investigations reveal Hb 9.8, MCV 72, reticulocytes 6%.
The most likely diagnosis is:
a. Macrocytic anaemia
b. Folic acid deficiency
c. Chronic gastro intestinal blood loss
d. Anaemia of chronic disease
e. Haemolytic Anaemia

180. A 4-week-old baby is noticed to have breast milk jaundice. Otherwise the baby is well and developing.
The single most appropriate mode of action would be to :
a. Continue breast milk
b. Increased fluid intake
c. Phototherapy
d. Exchange transfusion
e. Stop breast milk

181. A 24-years-old woman has had 24 hours of vomiting and diarrhoea 'which she thinks followed eating reheated take away food. There was fresh blood in the last three vomitus. Vital signs are stable.
The single most likely diagnosis is:
a. Gastric erosions
b. Acute gastroenteritis
c. Oesophageal varices
d. Mallory weiss tear
e. Bleeding diathesis

182. A female experienced sudden intense headache, while painting her bathroom wall. She fainted and hit her head. She was brought to A and E, where she regained her consciousness and is well otherwise, except for a small laceration on her skull.
The single most important investigation to be done at this stage is:
a. CT scan
b. Skull X-ray
c. Doppler
d. EEG
e. ECG

183. A 47-year-old female with carcinoma breast complains of intense thirst, polyuria and confusion.
The single best way to manage is by administrating:
a. Dexamethasone
b. Palmidronate
c. Fluid restriction
d. Insulin therapy
e. Calcium gluconate

184. A vagrant man, disheveled, sweating and fizzy. He is brought to A and E with seizures and dilated pupil.
Which is the single most likely substance he could be abusing:
a. Alcohol
b. Heroine
c. Cocaine
d. Cannabis
e. Solvent abuse

185. A man with chronic atrial fibrillation develops features of pulmonary edema.
Single best next step would be:
a. DC cardioversion
b. Anticoagulation and digoxin
c. Digoxin
d. Frusemide
e. Dopamine

186. A butcher cut himself in the groin area. He used a towel, which is full of blood. On examination, the BP was 80/60 and pulse rate 130.
The estimated amount of blood loss is:
a. 250 ml
b. 500 ml
c. 750 ml
d. 1000 ml
e. 1500 ml

187. A 45-year-old man has developed left ventricular failure 2 weeks after an attack of myocardial infarction, which was successfully controlled by diuretics. The ECHO shows poor left ventricular function.
The single most proven drug class beneficial for this patient would be:
a. Beta blockers
b. Calcium channel blockers
c. ACE inhibitors
d. Aspirin
e. Clopidogrel

188. A lady presents for follow up six months after cervical smear was done showing mild atypia (CIN II) on the previous smear. On examination, ulcerated cervix found.
The single most appropriate step at this stage would be to go for:
a. Another cervical smear
b. Colposcopy
c. Urgent colposcopy
d. Urgent biopsy
e. Urgent colposcopy and biopsy

189. A 60-year-old patient presents with fever and pain in the left iliac fossa. He appears flushed and takes care to remain still. On examination, there is a tender mass palpable in the left iliac fossa.

The single best procedure that would be of help to diagnose the condition would be:

a. Abdominal ultrasound
b. Sigmoidoscopy
c. Colonoscopy
d. CT scan abdomen and pelvis
e. Barium enema

190. Trimethoprim was advised for a child weighing 10 kg, in a dose 4 mg/kg twice daily. The available pharmacological preparation contains 50 mg/5 ml.

The single most appropriate prescription for the drug would be:

a. 0.4 ml twice daily
b. 4 ml twice daily
c. 0.8 ml twice daily
d. 1 ml twice daily
e. 2 ml twice daily

191. A 25-year-old farmer complains of redness and grittiness in his eyes. On examination, no foreign body is found.

The single most useful agent for him would be:

a. Local antibacterial
b. Local antihistaminic
c. Local antifungal
d. Local anaesthetic
e. Local antibiotic

192. A 38-year-old lady, mother of 4 children and now in 30th week of pregnancy, presents with blood tinged watery discharge from vagina 3 weeks duration. On examination, there appears a 'raw' ring around the Os.

The single most likely diagnosis is:

a. Cervical carcinoma
b. Genital herpes
c. Cervical ectropion
d. Vaginitis
e. Marginal sinus bleed

193. A 16-year-girl with multiple sexual partners presents with painless postcoital bleeding.

The single most important investigation required at this stage is:

a. Pap smear
b. Biopsy
c. Colposcopy and biopsy
d. Speculum examination
e. Gram staining

194. A lady over 40 years of age presents with repeated episodes of amaurosis fugax, with complete recovery after the attacks.

What is the single most appropriate investigation that would diagnose the condition:

a. CT scan
b. Carotid Doppler
c. Echocardiography
d. MRI
e. Transcranial Doppler

195. A 60-year-old man presents with progressive dyspnoea and massive left-sided pleural effusion.

The single best diagnostic procedure that would diagnose the condition is:

a. CXR
b. Pleural biopsy
c. Aspiration
d. Ultrasound
e. Bronchoscopy

196. A 20-year-old student after being transferred to a new school has insomnia and loses weight. He does not mix with people and does not attend programmes as he thinks there will be a lot of germs over there. He lags behind in school work as he does all his work very perfectly.

The single most likely diagnosis is:

a. Adjustment disorder
b. Obsessive compulsive disorder
c. Post-traumatic stress disorder
d. Depression
e. Autism

197. A 76-year-old known hypertensive comes to the casualty ward with a painful abdominal mass. On examination, he has a pulsatile abdominal mass and is having a BP of 70/40 and a pulse rate of 120 bpm.

The single most appropriate management option for this patient would be:

a. CT scan abdomen
b. Transfuse till systolic BP 90 mmHg
c. Transfuse till systolic BP 120 mmHg
d. Per abdomen examination
e. Diagnostic peritoneal lavage

198. A 14-year-old boy suddenly develops difficulty in breathing with red edematous lips after eating peanuts.

The single most likely diagnosis is:

a. Aspiration
b. Asthma
c. Meckel's syndrome
d. Anaphylaxis
e. Shock

199. A 25-year-old patient on lithium now comes to you with tremors of hand.

The single most helpful investigation would be:

a. Thyroid function test
b. Lithium levels
c. ECHO
d. Doppler
e. USG

200. A six months old child, can smile, but has head lag.

The single most likely diagnosis is:

a. Fragile x syndrome
b. Tay-Sachs disease
f. Ducchene's muscular atrophy
g. Fetus alcohol syndrome
e. Hypothyroidism

General Medical Council PLAB Test Part 1

Full Name

Test Centre/Date

- Use pencil only • Make heavy marks that fill the lozenge completely
- Write your candidate number in the top row of the box to the right **AND** fill in the appropriate lozenge below each number
- Give **ONE** answer only for each question

0	0	0	0	0	0
1	1	1	1	1	1
2	2	2	2	2	2
3	3	3	3	3	3
4	4	4	4	4	4
5	5	5	5	5	5
6	6	6	6	6	6
7	7	7	7	7	7
8	8	8	8	8	8
9	9	9	9	9	9

1	A	B	C	D	E	F	G	H	I	J	K	L	M	N	O	P	Q	R	S	T	1
2	A	B	C	D	E	F	G	H	I	J	K	L	M	N	O	P	Q	R	S	T	2
3	A	B	C	D	E	F	G	H	I	J	K	L	M	N	O	P	Q	R	S	T	3
4	A	B	C	D	E	F	G	H	I	J	K	L	M	N	O	P	Q	R	S	T	4
5	A	B	C	D	E	F	G	H	I	J	K	L	M	N	O	P	Q	R	S	T	5
6	A	B	C	D	E	F	G	H	I	J	K	L	M	N	O	P	Q	R	S	T	6
7	A	B	C	D	E	F	G	H	I	J	K	L	M	N	O	P	Q	R	S	T	7
8	A	B	C	D	E	F	G	H	I	J	K	L	M	N	O	P	Q	R	S	T	8
9	A	B	C	D	E	F	G	H	I	J	K	L	M	N	O	P	Q	R	S	T	9
10	A	B	C	D	E	F	G	H	I	J	K	L	M	N	O	P	Q	R	S	T	10
11	A	B	C	D	E	F	G	H	I	J	K	L	M	N	O	P	Q	R	S	T	11
12	A	B	C	D	E	F	G	H	I	J	K	L	M	N	O	P	Q	R	S	T	12
13	A	B	C	D	E	F	G	H	I	J	K	L	M	N	O	P	Q	R	S	T	13
14	A	B	C	D	E	F	G	H	I	J	K	L	M	N	O	P	Q	R	S	T	14
15	A	B	C	D	E	F	G	H	I	J	K	L	M	N	O	P	Q	R	S	T	15
16	A	B	C	D	E	F	G	H	I	J	K	L	M	N	O	P	Q	R	S	T	16
17	A	B	C	D	E	F	G	H	I	J	K	L	M	N	O	P	Q	R	S	T	17
18	A	B	C	D	E	F	G	H	I	J	K	L	M	N	O	P	Q	R	S	T	18
19	A	B	C	D	E	F	G	H	I	J	K	L	M	N	O	P	Q	R	S	T	19
20	A	B	C	D	E	F	G	H	I	J	K	L	M	N	O	P	Q	R	S	T	20
21	A	B	C	D	E	F	G	H	I	J	K	L	M	N	O	P	Q	R	S	T	21
22	A	B	C	D	E	F	G	H	I	J	K	L	M	N	O	P	Q	R	S	T	22
23	A	B	C	D	E	F	G	H	I	J	K	L	M	N	O	P	Q	R	S	T	23
24	A	B	C	D	E	F	G	H	I	J	K	L	M	N	O	P	Q	R	S	T	24
25	A	B	C	D	E	F	G	H	I	J	K	L	M	N	O	P	Q	R	S	T	25
26	A	B	C	D	E	F	G	H	I	J	K	L	M	N	O	P	Q	R	S	T	26
27	A	B	C	D	E	F	G	H	I	J	K	L	M	N	O	P	Q	R	S	T	27
28	A	B	C	D	E	F	G	H	I	J	K	L	M	N	O	P	Q	R	S	T	28
29	A	B	C	D	E	F	G	H	I	J	K	L	M	N	O	P	Q	R	S	T	29
30	A	B	C	D	E	F	G	H	I	J	K	L	M	N	O	P	Q	R	S	T	30
31	A	B	C	D	E	F	G	H	I	J	K	L	M	N	O	P	Q	R	S	T	31
32	A	B	C	D	E	F	G	H	I	J	K	L	M	N	O	P	Q	R	S	T	32
33	A	B	C	D	E	F	G	H	I	J	K	L	M	N	O	P	Q	R	S	T	33
34	A	B	C	D	E	F	G	H	I	J	K	L	M	N	O	P	Q	R	S	T	34
35	A	B	C	D	E	F	G	H	I	J	K	L	M	N	O	P	Q	R	S	T	35
36	A	B	C	D	E	F	G	H	I	J	K	L	M	N	O	P	Q	R	S	T	36
37	A	B	C	D	E	F	G	H	I	J	K	L	M	N	O	P	Q	R	S	T	37
38	A	B	C	D	E	F	G	H	I	J	K	L	M	N	O	P	Q	R	S	T	38
39	A	B	C	D	E	F	G	H	I	J	K	L	M	N	O	P	Q	R	S	T	39
40	A	B	C	D	E	F	G	H	I	J	K	L	M	N	O	P	Q	R	S	T	40
41	A	B	C	D	E	F	G	H	I	J	K	L	M	N	O	P	Q	R	S	T	41
42	A	B	C	D	E	F	G	H	I	J	K	L	M	N	O	P	Q	R	S	T	42
43	A	B	C	D	E	F	G	H	I	J	K	L	M	N	O	P	Q	R	S	T	43
44	A	B	C	D	E	F	G	H	I	J	K	L	M	N	O	P	Q	R	S	T	44
45	A	B	C	D	E	F	G	H	I	J	K	L	M	N	O	P	Q	R	S	T	45
46	A	B	C	D	E	F	G	H	I	J	K	L	M	N	O	P	Q	R	S	T	46
47	A	B	C	D	E	F	G	H	I	J	K	L	M	N	O	P	Q	R	S	T	47
48	A	B	C	D	E	F	G	H	I	J	K	L	M	N	O	P	Q	R	S	T	48
49	A	B	C	D	E	F	G	H	I	J	K	L	M	N	O	P	Q	R	S	T	49
50	A	B	C	D	E	F	G	H	I	J	K	L	M	N	O	P	Q	R	S	T	50

DO NOT WRITE IN THIS SPACE

101	A	B	C	D	E	F	G	H	I	J	K	L	M	N	O	P	Q	R	S	T	101
102	A	B	C	D	E	F	G	H	I	J	K	L	M	N	O	P	Q	R	S	T	102
103	A	B	C	D	E	F	G	H	I	J	K	L	M	N	O	P	Q	R	S	T	103
104	A	B	C	D	E	F	G	H	I	J	K	L	M	N	O	P	Q	R	S	T	104
105	A	B	C	D	E	F	G	H	I	J	K	L	M	N	O	P	Q	R	S	T	105
106	A	B	C	D	E	F	G	H	I	J	K	L	M	N	O	P	Q	R	S	T	106
107	A	B	C	D	E	F	G	H	I	J	K	L	M	N	O	P	Q	R	S	T	107
108	A	B	C	D	E	F	G	H	I	J	K	L	M	N	O	P	Q	R	S	T	108
109	A	B	C	D	E	F	G	H	I	J	K	L	M	N	O	P	Q	R	S	T	109
110	A	B	C	D	E	F	G	H	I	J	K	L	M	N	O	P	Q	R	S	T	110
111	A	B	C	D	E	F	G	H	I	J	K	L	M	N	O	P	Q	R	S	T	111
112	A	B	C	D	E	F	G	H	I	J	K	L	M	N	O	P	Q	R	S	T	112
113	A	B	C	D	E	F	G	H	I	J	K	L	M	N	O	P	Q	R	S	T	113
114	A	B	C	D	E	F	G	H	I	J	K	L	M	N	O	P	Q	R	S	T	114
115	A	B	C	D	E	F	G	H	I	J	K	L	M	N	O	P	Q	R	S	T	115
116	A	B	C	D	E	F	G	H	I	J	K	L	M	N	O	P	Q	R	S	T	116
117	A	B	C	D	E	F	G	H	I	J	K	L	M	N	O	P	Q	R	S	T	117
118	A	B	C	D	E	F	G	H	I	J	K	L	M	N	O	P	Q	R	S	T	118
119	A	B	C	D	E	F	G	H	I	J	K	L	M	N	O	P	Q	R	S	T	119
120	A	B	C	D	E	F	G	H	I	J	K	L	M	N	O	P	Q	R	S	T	120
121	A	B	C	D	E	F	G	H	I	J	K	L	M	N	O	P	Q	R	S	T	121
122	A	B	C	D	E	F	G	H	I	J	K	L	M	N	O	P	Q	R	S	T	122
123	A	B	C	D	E	F	G	H	I	J	K	L	M	N	O	P	Q	R	S	T	123
124	A	B	C	D	E	F	G	H	I	J	K	L	M	N	O	P	Q	R	S	T	124
125	A	B	C	D	E	F	G	H	I	J	K	L	M	N	O	P	Q	R	S	T	125
126	A	B	C	D	E	F	G	H	I	J	K	L	M	N	O	P	Q	R	S	T	126
127	A	B	C	D	E	F	G	H	I	J	K	L	M	N	O	P	Q	R	S	T	127
128	A	B	C	D	E	F	G	H	I	J	K	L	M	N	O	P	Q	R	S	T	128
129	A	B	C	D	E	F	G	H	I	J	K	L	M	N	O	P	Q	R	S	T	129
130	A	B	C	D	E	F	G	H	I	J	K	L	M	N	O	P	Q	R	S	T	130
131	A	B	C	D	E	F	G	H	I	J	K	L	M	N	O	P	Q	R	S	T	131
132	A	B	C	D	E	F	G	H	I	J	K	L	M	N	O	P	Q	R	S	T	132
133	A	B	C	D	E	F	G	H	I	J	K	L	M	N	O	P	Q	R	S	T	133
134	A	B	C	D	E	F	G	H	I	J	K	L	M	N	O	P	Q	R	S	T	134
135	A	B	C	D	E	F	G	H	I	J	K	L	M	N	O	P	Q	R	S	T	135
136	A	B	C	D	E	F	G	H	I	J	K	L	M	N	O	P	Q	R	S	T	136
137	A	B	C	D	E	F	G	H	I	J	K	L	M	N	O	P	Q	R	S	T	137
138	A	B	C	D	E	F	G	H	I	J	K	L	M	N	O	P	Q	R	S	T	138
139	A	B	C	D	E	F	G	H	I	J	K	L	M	N	O	P	Q	R	S	T	139
140	A	B	C	D	E	F	G	H	I	J	K	L	M	N	O	P	Q	R	S	T	140
141	A	B	C	D	E	F	G	H	I	J	K	L	M	N	O	P	Q	R	S	T	141
142	A	B	C	D	E	F	G	H	I	J	K	L	M	N	O	P	Q	R	S	T	142
143	A	B	C	D	E	F	G	H	I	J	K	L	M	N	O	P	Q	R	S	T	143
144	A	B	C	D	E	F	G	H	I	J	K	L	M	N	O	P	Q	R	S	T	144
145	A	B	C	D	E	F	G	H	I	J	K	L	M	N	O	P	Q	R	S	T	145
146	A	B	C	D	E	F	G	H	I	J	K	L	M	N	O	P	Q	R	S	T	146
147	A	B	C	D	E	F	G	H	I	J	K	L	M	N	O	P	Q	R	S	T	147
148	A	B	C	D	E	F	G	H	I	J	K	L	M	N	O	P	Q	R	S	T	148
149	A	B	C	D	E	F	G	H	I	J	K	L	M	N	O	P	Q	R	S	T	149
150	A	B	C	D	E	F	G	H	I	J	K	L	M	N	O	P	Q	R	S	T	150

DO NOT WRITE IN THIS SPACE

151	A	B	C	D	E	F	G	H	I	J	K	L	M	N	O	P	Q	R	S	T	151
152	A	B	C	D	E	F	G	H	I	J	K	L	M	N	O	P	Q	R	S	T	152
153	A	B	C	D	E	F	G	H	I	J	K	L	M	N	O	P	Q	R	S	T	153
154	A	B	C	D	E	F	G	H	I	J	K	L	M	N	O	P	Q	R	S	T	154
155	A	B	C	D	E	F	G	H	I	J	K	L	M	N	O	P	Q	R	S	T	155
156	A	B	C	D	E	F	G	H	I	J	K	L	M	N	O	P	Q	R	S	T	156
157	A	B	C	D	E	F	G	H	I	J	K	L	M	N	O	P	Q	R	S	T	157
158	A	B	C	D	E	F	G	H	I	J	K	L	M	N	O	P	Q	R	S	T	158
159	A	B	C	D	E	F	G	H	I	J	K	L	M	N	O	P	Q	R	S	T	159
160	A	B	C	D	E	F	G	H	I	J	K	L	M	N	O	P	Q	R	S	T	160
161	A	B	C	D	E	F	G	H	I	J	K	L	M	N	O	P	Q	R	S	T	161
162	A	B	C	D	E	F	G	H	I	J	K	L	M	N	O	P	Q	R	S	T	162
163	A	B	C	D	E	F	G	H	I	J	K	L	M	N	O	P	Q	R	S	T	163
164	A	B	C	D	E	F	G	H	I	J	K	L	M	N	O	P	Q	R	S	T	164
165	A	B	C	D	E	F	G	H	I	J	K	L	M	N	O	P	Q	R	S	T	165
166	A	B	C	D	E	F	G	H	I	J	K	L	M	N	O	P	Q	R	S	T	166
167	A	B	C	D	E	F	G	H	I	J	K	L	M	N	O	P	Q	R	S	T	167
168	A	B	C	D	E	F	G	H	I	J	K	L	M	N	O	P	Q	R	S	T	168
169	A	B	C	D	E	F	G	H	I	J	K	L	M	N	O	P	Q	R	S	T	169
170	A	B	C	D	E	F	G	H	I	J	K	L	M	N	O	P	Q	R	S	T	170
171	A	B	C	D	E	F	G	H	I	J	K	L	M	N	O	P	Q	R	S	T	171
172	A	B	C	D	E	F	G	H	I	J	K	L	M	N	O	P	Q	R	S	T	172
173	A	B	C	D	E	F	G	H	I	J	K	L	M	N	O	P	Q	R	S	T	173
174	A	B	C	D	E	F	G	H	I	J	K	L	M	N	O	P	Q	R	S	T	174
175	A	B	C	D	E	F	G	H	I	J	K	L	M	N	O	P	Q	R	S	T	175
176	A	B	C	D	E	F	G	H	I	J	K	L	M	N	O	P	Q	R	S	T	176
177	A	B	C	D	E	F	G	H	I	J	K	L	M	N	O	P	Q	R	S	T	177
178	A	B	C	D	E	F	G	H	I	J	K	L	M	N	O	P	Q	R	S	T	178
179	A	B	C	D	E	F	G	H	I	J	K	L	M	N	O	P	Q	R	S	T	179
180	A	B	C	D	E	F	G	H	I	J	K	L	M	N	O	P	Q	R	S	T	180
181	A	B	C	D	E	F	G	H	I	J	K	L	M	N	O	P	Q	R	S	T	181
182	A	B	C	D	E	F	G	H	I	J	K	L	M	N	O	P	Q	R	S	T	182
183	A	B	C	D	E	F	G	H	I	J	K	L	M	N	O	P	Q	R	S	T	183
184	A	B	C	D	E	F	G	H	I	J	K	L	M	N	O	P	Q	R	S	T	184
185	A	B	C	D	E	F	G	H	I	J	K	L	M	N	O	P	Q	R	S	T	185
186	A	B	C	D	E	F	G	H	I	J	K	L	M	N	O	P	Q	R	S	T	186
187	A	B	C	D	E	F	G	H	I	J	K	L	M	N	O	P	Q	R	S	T	187
188	A	B	C	D	E	F	G	H	I	J	K	L	M	N	O	P	Q	R	S	T	188
189	A	B	C	D	E	F	G	H	I	J	K	L	M	N	O	P	Q	R	S	T	189
190	A	B	C	D	E	F	G	H	I	J	K	L	M	N	O	P	Q	R	S	T	190
191	A	B	C	D	E	F	G	H	I	J	K	L	M	N	O	P	Q	R	S	T	191
192	A	B	C	D	E	F	G	H	I	J	K	L	M	N	O	P	Q	R	S	T	192
193	A	B	C	D	E	F	G	H	I	J	K	L	M	N	O	P	Q	R	S	T	193
194	A	B	C	D	E	F	G	H	I	J	K	L	M	N	O	P	Q	R	S	T	194
195	A	B	C	D	E	F	G	H	I	J	K	L	M	N	O	P	Q	R	S	T	195
196	A	B	C	D	E	F	G	H	I	J	K	L	M	N	O	P	Q	R	S	T	196
197	A	B	C	D	E	F	G	H	I	J	K	L	M	N	O	P	Q	R	S	T	197
198	A	B	C	D	E	F	G	H	I	J	K	L	M	N	O	P	Q	R	S	T	198
199	A	B	C	D	E	F	G	H	I	J	K	L	M	N	O	P	Q	R	S	T	199
200	A	B	C	D	E	F	G	H	I	J	K	L	M	N	O	P	Q	R	S	T	200

DO NOT WRITE IN THIS SPACE

101	A	B	C	D	E	F	G	H	I	J	K	L	M	N	O	P	Q	R	S	T	101
102	A	B	C	D	E	F	G	H	I	J	K	L	M	N	O	P	Q	R	S	T	102
103	A	B	C	D	E	F	G	H	I	J	K	L	M	N	O	P	Q	R	S	T	103
104	A	B	C	D	E	F	G	H	I	J	K	L	M	N	O	P	Q	R	S	T	104
105	A	B	C	D	E	F	G	H	I	J	K	L	M	N	O	P	Q	R	S	T	105
106	A	B	C	D	E	F	G	H	I	J	K	L	M	N	O	P	Q	R	S	T	106
107	A	B	C	D	E	F	G	H	I	J	K	L	M	N	O	P	Q	R	S	T	107
108	A	B	C	D	E	F	G	H	I	J	K	L	M	N	O	P	Q	R	S	T	108
109	A	B	C	D	E	F	G	H	I	J	K	L	M	N	O	P	Q	R	S	T	109
110	A	B	C	D	E	F	G	H	I	J	K	L	M	N	O	P	Q	R	S	T	110
111	A	B	C	D	E	F	G	H	I	J	K	L	M	N	O	P	Q	R	S	T	111
112	A	B	C	D	E	F	G	H	I	J	K	L	M	N	O	P	Q	R	S	T	112
113	A	B	C	D	E	F	G	H	I	J	K	L	M	N	O	P	Q	R	S	T	113
114	A	B	C	D	E	F	G	H	I	J	K	L	M	N	O	P	Q	R	S	T	114
115	A	B	C	D	E	F	G	H	I	J	K	L	M	N	O	P	Q	R	S	T	115
116	A	B	C	D	E	F	G	H	I	J	K	L	M	N	O	P	Q	R	S	T	116
117	A	B	C	D	E	F	G	H	I	J	K	L	M	N	O	P	Q	R	S	T	117
118	A	B	C	D	E	F	G	H	I	J	K	L	M	N	O	P	Q	R	S	T	118
119	A	B	C	D	E	F	G	H	I	J	K	L	M	N	O	P	Q	R	S	T	119
120	A	B	C	D	E	F	G	H	I	J	K	L	M	N	O	P	Q	R	S	T	120
121	A	B	C	D	E	F	G	H	I	J	K	L	M	N	O	P	Q	R	S	T	121
122	A	B	C	D	E	F	G	H	I	J	K	L	M	N	O	P	Q	R	S	T	122
123	A	B	C	D	E	F	G	H	I	J	K	L	M	N	O	P	Q	R	S	T	123
124	A	B	C	D	E	F	G	H	I	J	K	L	M	N	O	P	Q	R	S	T	124
125	A	B	C	D	E	F	G	H	I	J	K	L	M	N	O	P	Q	R	S	T	125
126	A	B	C	D	E	F	G	H	I	J	K	L	M	N	O	P	Q	R	S	T	126
127	A	B	C	D	E	F	G	H	I	J	K	L	M	N	O	P	Q	R	S	T	127
128	A	B	C	D	E	F	G	H	I	J	K	L	M	N	O	P	Q	R	S	T	128
129	A	B	C	D	E	F	G	H	I	J	K	L	M	N	O	P	Q	R	S	T	129
130	A	B	C	D	E	F	G	H	I	J	K	L	M	N	O	P	Q	R	S	T	130
131	A	B	C	D	E	F	G	H	I	J	K	L	M	N	O	P	Q	R	S	T	131
132	A	B	C	D	E	F	G	H	I	J	K	L	M	N	O	P	Q	R	S	T	132
133	A	B	C	D	E	F	G	H	I	J	K	L	M	N	O	P	Q	R	S	T	133
134	A	B	C	D	E	F	G	H	I	J	K	L	M	N	O	P	Q	R	S	T	134
135	A	B	C	D	E	F	G	H	I	J	K	L	M	N	O	P	Q	R	S	T	135
136	A	B	C	D	E	F	G	H	I	J	K	L	M	N	O	P	Q	R	S	T	136
137	A	B	C	D	E	F	G	H	I	J	K	L	M	N	O	P	Q	R	S	T	137
138	A	B	C	D	E	F	G	H	I	J	K	L	M	N	O	P	Q	R	S	T	138
139	A	B	C	D	E	F	G	H	I	J	K	L	M	N	O	P	Q	R	S	T	139
140	A	B	C	D	E	F	G	H	I	J	K	L	M	N	O	P	Q	R	S	T	140
141	A	B	C	D	E	F	G	H	I	J	K	L	M	N	O	P	Q	R	S	T	141
142	A	B	C	D	E	F	G	H	I	J	K	L	M	N	O	P	Q	R	S	T	142
143	A	B	C	D	E	F	G	H	I	J	K	L	M	N	O	P	Q	R	S	T	143
144	A	B	C	D	E	F	G	H	I	J	K	L	M	N	O	P	Q	R	S	T	144
145	A	B	C	D	E	F	G	H	I	J	K	L	M	N	O	P	Q	R	S	T	145
146	A	B	C	D	E	F	G	H	I	J	K	L	M	N	O	P	Q	R	S	T	146
147	A	B	C	D	E	F	G	H	I	J	K	L	M	N	O	P	Q	R	S	T	147
148	A	B	C	D	E	F	G	H	I	J	K	L	M	N	O	P	Q	R	S	T	148
149	A	B	C	D	E	F	G	H	I	J	K	L	M	N	O	P	Q	R	S	T	149
150	A	B	C	D	E	F	G	H	I	J	K	L	M	N	O	P	Q	R	S	T	150

Answers

Serial No.	*Answer No.*	*Answer*
1	e	Lymphedema
2	d	Hypercalcaemia
3	f	Spinal cord compresion
4	b	Cerebral metasatses
5	a	Pathological fracture
6	h	Polycystic kidney disease
7	e	Carcinoma bladder
8	g	Alport's syndrome
9	k	Renal cell carcinoma
10	i	Benign recurrent haematuria
11	d	Kawasaki's disease
12	a	Infectious mononucleosis
13	g	Roseola infantum
14	f	Erythema infectiosum
15	c	Measles
16	c	Severe deficiency of insulin
17	b	Relative deficiency of insulin
18	d	Insulin excess
19	b	Relative deficiency of insulin
20	e	Insulin resistance
21	k	Splenic rupture
22	j	Renal pedicle avulsion
23	k	Splenic rupture
24	g	Mesenteric vascular injury
25	i	Renal contusion
26	c	Sickle cell anaemia
27	e	Chronic renal failure
28	a	Hereditary spherocytosis
29	f	Chronic liver failure
30	k	Aplastic Anemia
31	d	Renal function Tests
32	a	Prothrombin Time
33	d	Plasma drug level
34	e	White blood cell count
35	d	Plasma drug level
36	a	Anticoagulant overdosage
37	e	Maxillary antral carcinoma
38	j	Septal perforation
39	h	ORF
40	c	Hypertensive disease
41	d	Barium enema
42	a	Plain X-ray abdomen
43	g	Upper GI endoscopy
44	k	Mesenteric angiogram
45	l	Abdominal CT scan
46	e	Family therapy
47	h	Risk management strategy
48	d	ECT
49	n	Voluntary inpatient admission
50	n	Voluntary inpatient admission
51	a	Vertebrobasilar stroke
52	c	Motor neuron disease
53	h	Multiple sclerosis
54	i	Alzheimer's disease
55	e	Parietal lobe stroke
56	c	Huntington's chorea
57	a	Alzheimer's dementia
58	g	Multi-infarct dementia
59	i	Frontotemporal dementia

60	k	Acute delirium	92	b	Pelvic floor weakness
61	a	Duchenne's muscular dystrophy	93	c	Multiple sclerosis
62	b	Spina bifida	94	e	Detrusor instability
63	c	Down's syndrome	95	a	Fistula
64	b	Spina bifida	96	e	Stricture
65	d	Cystic fibrosis	97	b	Carcinoma prostate
66	e	Chorionic villous sampling	98	a	Stricture
67	c	Trisomy 21	99	c	BPH
68	g	Ultrasound	100	h	Spinal cord lesion
69	g	Ultrasound	101	h	Blind therapy
70	h	17-hydroxyprogesterone	102	i	Empirical therapy
71	g	Cefixime	103	j	Abdominal hysterectomy
72	c	Metronidazole	104	c	Endoscopy
73	i	Ofloxacin + metronidazole	105	g	Oral metronidazole
74	d	Clotrimazole	106	g	Ciprofloxacin
75	l	Wait and watch	107	a	None
76	b	Burr holes	108	l	Two or more antibiotics together
77	e	High dose prednisolone	109	d	Cefotaxime
78	g	Atenolol	110	h	Erythromycin
79	j	Sumatriptan	111	c	Spleen
80	l	Neurological opinion	112	i	Diaphragm
81	a	Fistula	113	b	Pancreas
82	b	Stress incontinence	114	b	Pancreas
83	c	Multiple sclerosis	115	f	Urethra
84	e	Detrusor instability	116	g	Ulcerative colitis
85	a	Fistula	117	a	Carcinoma rectum
86	d	Sodium chromoglycate	118	c	IBS with diarrhoea
87	a	Topical fusidic acid	119	e	Faecal impaction
88	c	Oral tetracycline	120	j	Paralytic ileus
89	a	Topical fusidic acid	121	a	X-linked recessive
90	l	Topical chloramphenicol	122	b	Autosomal dominant
91	a	Fistula	123	e	Polygenic

124	b	Autosomal dominant	156	k	Addison's disease
125	b	Autosomal dominant	157	h	Type I diabetes mellitus
126	h	Constipation – spastic	158	d	Dehydration with hypokalaemia
127	c	Intestinal obstruction	159	g	Diuretic overuse
128	m	Peptic ulcer	160	e	Rhabdomyolysis
129	i	Abdominal angina	161	j	Pulmonary embolism
130	k	Mesenteric adenitis	162	i	Anteroseptal myocardial infarction
131	g	Secondary polycythaemia	163	b	Lobar pneumonia
132	c	Conn's syndrome	164	f	Pneumothorax (Simple)
133	d	Addison's disease	165	k	Pulmonary edema
134	e	Hyperparathyroidism	166	d	Vascular dementia
135	k	Microadenoma	167	c	Frontal lobe dementia
136	c	Atrial fibrillation	168	b	Alzeihmer's disease
137	g	Cardiac tumour	169	a	Depression
138	e	Ventricular extrasystole	170	i	Delirium
139	h	Ventricular tachycardia	171	c	Quinine therapy
140	j	Complete heart block	172	c	VIII Nerve damage
141	f	Hypoglycaemia	173	b	Disseminated intravascular cougulation
142	h	Pyogenic meningitis	174	d	Endometriosis
143	i	Epilepsy	175	e	Acromegaly
144	l	Head injury	176	b	Hepatitis B immunoglobulin and vaccine
145	j	Subdural haematoma	177	d	Wide bore needle to right pleural cavity
146	e	Tuberculous lymphadenitis	178	d	Thick and Thin smear
147	g	Ca stomach	179	c	Chronic gastrointestinal blood loss
148	a	Thyroid carcinoma	180	a	Continue breast milk
149	c	Cystic hygroma	181	d	Mallory weiss tear
150	i	Mesothelioma	182	a	CT scan
151	i	Clotrimazole pessary	183	b	Palmidronate
152	J	None	184	c	Cocaine
153	g	Ofloxacin + metronodazole 14 days	185	a	DC cardioversion
154	e	Acyclovir	186	e	1500 ml
155	b	Metronidazole 400 mg 7 days	187	c	ACE inhibitor

188	e	Urgent colposcopy and biopsy
189	d	CT scan abdomen and pelvis
190	b	4 ml twice daily
191	b	Local antihistaminic
192	a	Cervical ectropion
193	d	Speculum examination
194	b	Carotid Doppler

195	c	Aspiration
196	b	Obsessive compulsive disorder
197	b	Transfuse till systolic BP 90 mmHg
198	d	Anaphylaxis
199	b	Lithium levels
200	b	Tay-Sachs disease

Previous Year Paper 3

RxPG Analysis

Total Themes:	**40**
Repeat Themes:	**9**
Repeat Themes with a Different Header:	**7**

THEME 1: THE DIAGNOSIS OF NON-ACCIDENTAL INJURY

OPTIONS

a. Accidental injury
b. Emotional abuse
c. Physical abuse
d. Sexual abuse
e. Child neglect
f. Osteogenesis imperfecta
g. ITP
h. Normally present in a child.
i. Elderly abuse
j. Henoch-Schönlein purpura
k. Immune thrombocytopenia purpura

*For each presentation below, choose the **single most likely diagnosis** from the above list of options. Each option may be used once, more than once or not at all.*

QUESTIONS

1. A 16-year-old mother brings her baby for immunisation. The nurse notices the baby has multiple bruises along both arms and legs. The baby is crying excessively. The house officer notices multiple fractures and that the baby has blue sclerae.
2. A 70-year-old man is receiving treatment for Alzheimer's disease. He is looked after by a 23-year-old grand daughter. He has recently developed faecal incontinence. The SHO notices bruises on both wrists and back.
3. An anxious mother brings her 6-year-old daughter who is bleeding per vaginum. Six months prior to this presentation the girl had a confirmed streptococcal sore-throat infection. She is otherwise normal.
4. A 4-day-old girl is brought to casualty by the maternal grandparent who is worried about two dark bluish patches on the child's buttocks. Child's mother is white and the father is black.
5. An 8-year-old girl is noted to have fresh bloody staining of her pants. She also suffers from enuresis. She has recently started horse-riding lessons.

THEME 2: THE TREATMENT OF VISUAL IMPAIRMENT

OPTIONS

a. Intra-ocular steroids
b. Intravenous steroids
c. Oral steroids
d. Laser treatment
e. No treatment required
f. Tropicamide
g. Amethocaine
h. Timolol
i. Pilocarpine
j. Vitrectomy
k. Tetracycline ointment
l. ECCE with PCIOL

*For each presentation below, choose the **single most appropriate treatment** from the above list of options. Each option may be used once, more than once or not at all.*

QUESTIONS

6. A 73-year-old complains of a severe right-sided headache associated with an acute loss of right-sided vision. Urgent treatment is needed to prevent left sided vision loss.
7. A 75-year-old has difficulty watching television complaining of a peripheral constriction of vision. On examination, there is cupping of both optical discs.
8. A 50-year-old with a history of SLE complains of loss of vision. On examination, he is found to have multiple opacity in the lens of his eyes.
9. A diabetic on oral hypoglycaemics complains of sudden deterioration in vision of his right eye. On examination, he is found to have bilateral proliferative retinopathy with retinal haemorrhage on the right side.
10. An 80-year-old has markedly decreased visual acuity. On fundoscopy, she is found to have bilateral macular pigmentation.

THEME 3: THE TREATMENT OF SEPTICAEMIA

OPTIONS
a. Percutaneous drainage
b. Ventilatory support + IV fluids
c. Stent
d. Acyclovir
e. Open surgical debridement
f. Resection of superficial tissue with wide margin
g. Oral cefuroxamine
h. IV corticosteroids
i. Laparotomy
j. Intravenous catecholamines
k. Flucloxacillin

*For each presentation below, choose the **single most appropriate treatment** from the above list of options. Each option may be used once, more than once or not at all.*

QUESTIONS
11. A 28-year-old woman after cholecystectomy following a perforated gallbladder has a raised right diaphragm with a temperature of 38°C and a pulse of 120 beats per minute.
12. A febrile 39-year-old woman with hypertension, has a history of recurrent urinary tract infections. Abdominal ultrasound showed a dilated calyx.
13. A 32-year-old woman has chickenpox. She scratches herself excessively and develops a blue discolouration on the abdomen. She has a history of not passing urine in the last 24 hours. She continues to scratch herself and the discolouration increases in size.
14. A middle-aged man with acute pancreatitis develops hypotension. On CT, he is found to have peripancreatic fluid and a lack of enhancement of the pancreatic tail.
15. Following a perforated bowel, a middle-aged man develops severe shock and septicaemia as well as a central dark discolouration on his abdomen, which is growing larger.

THEME 4: INVESTIGATION OF NEUROLOGICAL COMPLAINTS

OPTIONS
a. Twenty-four hours holter monitor
b. EEG
c. Serum calcium
d. Random glucose
e. CT scan
f. MRI spine
g. Lateral cervical spine radiograph
h. Carotid doppler
i. ESR
j. MRI skull
k. None required

*For each presentation below, choose the **single most helpful investigation** from the above list of options. Each option may be used once, more than once or not at all.*

QUESTIONS
16. A 16-year-old girl suddenly collapses after standing for a while. Her limbs are flaccid and she is not incontinent. Following 30 seconds she recovers fully.
17. An 82-year-old has five episodes of loss of consciousness with no convulsions.
18. A 50-year-old male wakes up with a tingling and numbness in his right hand. This is accompanies by slurring of speech which recovers following about four hours complications and associations of blood dyscrasias.
19. A 34-year-old woman has 6 months history of on and off hemiparesis which resolves with no neurological deficits.
20. A 55-year-old woman treated for breast cancer with chemotherapy and radiotherapy presented with a history of confusion, tiredness, weakness and polyuria. On examination, no neurological deficits were found.

THEME 5: COMPLICATIONS OF BLOOD DYSCRASIAS

OPTIONS

a. Splenomegaly
b. Hepatomegaly
c. Generalised lymphadenopathy
d. Gingival hypertrophy
e. Macroglossia
f. Meningitis
g. Petechial rash
h. Subarachnoid haemorrhage
i. Intracerebral haemorrhage
j. Bone pain
k. Thrombophilia

For each presentation below, choose the ***single most common complication of given blood dyscrasias*** *from the above list of options. Each option may be used once, more than once or not at all.*

QUESTIONS

21. A 51-year-old is lethargic and found to be anaemic. his blood picture is found to have a granulocytic tendency with an increase in the platelet count.
22. A 5-year-old with generalised lymphadenopathy develops fever and neck stiffness and headache. He is found to have a lot of lymphoblasts in the blood picture.
23. 55-year-old man with history of hypertension untreated presents with hemiparesis.
24. A 72-year-old is having a routine examination. he is found to have a mild lymphocytosis and splenomegaly.
25. A 38-year-old woman presents with cervical lymphadenopahty. Mature lymphoblasts are seen on the blood film. Examination reveals a mild splenomegaly. She is on phenytoin for epilepsy.

THEME 6: DIFFERENTIAL DIAGNOSIS OF ECTOPIC PREGNANCY

OPTIONS

a. Appendicitis
b. Inevitable abortion
c. Missed abortion
d. Septic abortion
e. PID
f. Diverticular disease
g. Torsion of an ovarian mass
h. Irritable bowel syndrome (IBS)
i. Toxic shock syndrome
j. Inflammatory bowel disease
k. Incomplete abortion

For each presentation below, choose the ***single most likely diagnosis*** *from the above list of options. Each option may be used once, more than once or not at all.*

QUESTIONS

26. A pregnant woman with an LMP of 9 weeks and a positive home pregnancy test presents with an enlarged tender uterus and bright red bleeding per vagina. On examination, her cervical os is fully open.
27. A 16-year-old with right iliac fossa pain has a vaginal ulatrsound which demonstrates an echogenic cystic mass just superior ro the right fornix.
28. An 18-year-old girl is doing her exams and is very stressed. She has missed her last period. Her pregnacy test is negative. She complains of a three month hsitory of generalised abdominal pain and bloating.
29. A 22-year-old girl with a hitory of two terminations complains of right iliac fossa pain, a watery brownish vaginal discharge and fever. She is found to have an elevated white cell count. She uses tampons.
30. A 27-year-old girl reliably on oral contraceptives develops a high white cell count, fever and a malodourous vaginal discharge young woman with 9 weeks pregnancy presents with heavy bleeding and passage of clots. USG shows fetal heart activity. How to manage?

THEME 7: MANAGEMENT OF AN INJURED PATIENT

OPTIONS
a. Diagnostic needle thoracocentesis
b. CT scan
c. X-ray femur
d. Splinting of the femur
e. Auscultation
f. Chest X-ray
g. Fluid challenge
h. Blood transfusion
i. Suprapubic cystostomy
j. 500 ml IV mannitol
k. Walk around

For each presentation below, choose the ***single most likely diagnosis*** *from the above list of options. Each option may be used once, more than once or not at all.*

QUESTIONS
31. A young man involved in a motorcycle accident is stable in the casulaty department. His neck is cleared but when he sits up he develops sudden shortness of breath. His breath sounds are dimished on the right side.
32. A young man involved in a motorcycle accident has a secure airway and a normal Glasgow Coma Scale. He is noted to have a swollen right thigh.
33. A young man involved in a motorcycle accident has a secure airway, is ventilated, immobilised and anesthesized after admission with a Glasgow Coma Scale of 9. He is noted to have a swollen right thigh.
34. A man involved in a mining accident presents with oliguria and passing dark brown urine.
35. A 23-year-old man who sustained a pelvic fracture is unable to pass urine. On examination, he has abdominal tenderness and fullness and blood on the uretheral meatus.

THEME 8: DIFFERENTIAL DIAGNOSIS OF HYPERTENSION

OPTIONS
a. Conn's disease
b. Cushing's disease
c. Co-arctation of the aorta
d. Exerbation of chronic hypertension
e. Renal artery stenosis
f. Carcinoid syndrome
g. Essential hypertension
h. Phaeochromocytoma
i. Acromegaly
j. Addison's disease
k. Cushing's syndrome

For each presentation below, choose the ***single most likely diagnosis*** *from the above list of options. Each option may be used once, more than once or not at all.*

QUESTIONS
36. A 17-year-old girl with hypertension of 160/100 is found to have a femoral pulse delay.
37. A 40-year-old with a blood pressure of 180/115 is found to have a loud bruit in his right upper abdomen.
38. A 50-year-old male complains of flushing , tremor, palpitations. He is found to have a fluctuating blood pressure of 200/120.
39. A middle aged woman with a blood pressure of 160/110 is found to have abdominal striae and facial hirsutism.
40. A 42-year-old patient with prominent jaw and supraorbital ridges.

THEME 9: INVESTIGATION OF HOARSENESS

OPTIONS

a. Fibreoptic bronchoscopy
b. CT scan
c. Laparoscopic mediastinotomy
d. Surgical mediastinotomy
e. Laryngoscopy
f. No further investigation required
g. Chest X-ray
h. Throat swab
i. TSH
j. MRI
k. Sputum culture

For each presentation below, choose the ***single most appropriate investigation*** *from the above list of options. Each option may be used once, more than once or not at all.*

QUESTIONS

41. A patient is suspected of having bronchiectasis.
42. A patient with an area of consolidation and fever on his chest X-ray is treated with antibiotics. His fever resolves but four weeks later he still has a large area of consolidation.
43. A singer has a six-month history of hoarseness.
44. A 55-year-old smoker complains of shortness of breath and a cough. Laryngoscopy is normal.
45. A 30-year-old complains of hoarseness since he came back from a football match the day before.

THEME 10: DIFFERENTIAL DIAGNOSIS OF DEVELOPMENTAL DELAY

OPTIONS

a. Birth dysphyxia
b. Fragile X syndrome
c. Duchenne muscular dystrophy
d. Storage disorder
e. Hnter's disease
f. Hypothyroidism
g. Meningitis
h. Constitutional delay
i. Treatment of hyperthyroidism
j. Prematurity
k. Normal finding

For each presentation below, choose the ***single most likely diagnosis*** *from the above list of options. Each option may be used once, more than once or not at all.*

QUESTIONS

46. A four-year-old boy walks with a prominent lordosis. He has good speech, can build objects using blocks and has good social awareness.
47. A nine-month-old baby born at term has a weight in the 97th percentile. His development is delayed.
48. A nine-month-old baby born at term has a weight in the 3rd percentile. His development is delayed. His head and body size are both small.
49. A nine-year-old girl has difficulty with speech. She has recently been hospitalised for a medical reason. Her speech before hospitalisation was completely normal.
50. A four-year-old boy has delayed speech. Both his father and paternal uncle has the same problem.

THEME 11: MANAGEMENT OF COMA

OPTIONS

a. The 50% dextrose drip
b. The 5% dextrose drip
c. Naloxone
d. Direct intravenous insulin
e. Insulin through a drip
f. One litre of normal saline
g. Naltrexone
h. IV $CaCl_2$
i. IV bicarbonate
j. Calcium resonium
k. Dobutamine
l. CT scan

For each presentation below, choose the ***single most appropriate management*** *from the above list of options. Each option may be used once, more than once or not at all.*

QUESTIONS

51. A middle-aged woman remains unconcious 12 hours following a cholecystectomy. On examination, both pupils are seen to be pinpoint.
52. A young diabetic is admitted in a comatose state. His plasma glucose level is 2 mmols.
53. A young diabetic is admitted in a comatose state. his plasma glucose level is 17 mmol and he is dehydrated.
54. A 37-year-old alcoholic is found wandering in a park. His partner says he has had a number of falls recently and in the A and E the patient is confused. The blood sugar level is normal.
55. A 25-year-old found deeply unconscious is brought to the accident and emergency (A and E) department. He has an abrasion over his left temple and puncture marks on his left forearm.

THEME 12: MANAGEMENT OF DEPRESSION

OPTIONS

a. ECT
b. Amitryptyline
c. Tricyclics
d. Imipramine
e. Psychoanalysis
f. Marital counselling
g. Lithium
h. St. John's wart
i. MAO inhibitors
j. Fluoxetine
k. Lorazepam

For each presentation below, choose the ***single most likely diagnosis*** *from the above list of options. Each option may be used once, more than once or not at all.*

QUESTIONS

56. A middle-aged woman has had several admissions for severe depression. She now turns up with a very severe depression despite all treatment.
57. A woman has bouts of depression alternating with bouts of mania. She has had first line anti-depressants but they have not worked.
58. A young dentist, successful at work lacks confidence in himself. He finds that he is unable to socialise properly and has early morning waking. He is on no treatment.
59. A 44-year-old has repeated episodes of depressed mood in response to feeling rejected, and a craving for sweets and chocolate. These reactive mood changes are accompanied by lethargy and increased appetite, particularly with a preference for carbohydrates.
60. A 20-year-old previously healthy girl is waiting for her college exam result. The result is arriving that day by post and she is suffering from acute anxiety due to the importance of the results for her future career. Her mother consults their general practitioners.

THEME 13: INVESTIGATION OF HAEMOPTYSIS

OPTIONS

a. CT
b. MRI
c. Laryngoscopy
d. Sputum culture
e. Sputum cytology
f. Ventilation perfusion scan
g. Thoracoscopy
h. Pulmonary angiogram
i. Selective arteriogram
j. Mediastinoscopy
k. Fine needle aspiration
l. Fibreoptic bronchoscopy

*For each presentation below, choose the **single most definitive diagnosis investigation** from the above list of options. Each option may be used once more than once or not at all.*

QUESTIONS

61. Carcinoma of the right main bronchus.
62. Pulmonary embolism.
63. Bronchial carcinoid.
64. Bronchiectasis.
65. Tuberculosis.

THEME 14: THE DIAGNOSIS OF SHOCK

OPTIONS

a. Anaphylaxis
b. Septic shock
c. Cardiogenic shock
d. Hypovolaemic shock
e. Pulmonary embolism
f. Disseminated intravascular coagulation
g. Neurogenic shock
h. Spinal shock
i. Acute renal failure (ATN)
j. Third space sequesteration
k. CHF

*For each presentation below, choose the **single most likely diagnosis** from the above list of options. Each option may be used once, more than once or not at all.*

QUESTIONS

66. A middle-aged man has recently been operated after sustaining a perforated gallbladder. He becomes increasingly comatose and on examination is noted to have peripheral warming.
67. Following a motorcycle accident a young man has a pulse rate of 110 and a blood pressure that falls to 90/50. On examination of the CXR, he is noted to have fractures of the lower ribs on the left.
68. A 64-year-old patient on the surgical ward has been operated on for a hernia, he presents with warm extremities and a blood pressure of 90/60 mmHg.
69. A woman had a caesarean section done in the morning presented with a blood pressure of 80/65 mmHg and pulse rate of 120 beats/min.
70. A 23-year-old man is brought into the accident and emergency department from the local park, with a read swollen arm. He is found to have a blood pressure of 100/60 mmHg.

THEME 15: THE MANAGEMENT OF HEAD INJURY

OPTIONS

a. CT scan
b. Neck collar
c. MRI
d. Skull X-ray
e. Discharge home with head injury instructions
f. Admit overnight for observation
g. Suction of skull vault
h. Antibiotics
i. Intracranial pressure monitoring
j. Burr holes
k. IV mannitol

*For each presentation below, choose the **single most appropriate management** from the above list of options. Each option may be used once, more than once or not at all.*

QUESTIONS

71. Following an alcoholic binge a 36-year-old male falls and comes to casualty with a cut in his temporal region his Glasgow Coma Scale is normal and his neck is cleared by the orthopaedic SHO.
72. An 8-year-old boy falls off a swing at his school. He is brought to casualty by one of his teachers. He has a bruise over his right eye but the examination is otherwise normal. He is fully conscious with no history of blackouts since the accident. A skull X-ray is performed, which is normal.
73. A young woman is involved in an RTA and is brought in with a Glasgow Coma Scale of 6 . A CT scan shows evidence of diffuse cerebral oedema but no evidence of haemorrhage. She has bilateral papilloedema.
74. A young man is involved in a fight and suffers a blow to the back of the head. A skull X-ray reveals a depressed fracture of the occiput. His Glasgow Coma Scale on admission is 14 but falls rapidly within an hour.
75. A 24-year-old patient presents with RTA. The pupil on the left side is dilated and the patient is obtunded. CT scan of the head reveals a biconvex hyperdense lesion on the temporal region.

THEME 16: DIAGNOSIS OF STROKE / TIA

OPTIONS

a. Carotid artery stenosis
b. Cerebellar haemorrhage
c. Cerebral embolus
d. Cerebral haemorrhage
e. Cerebral vasculitis
f. Migraine
g. Subarachnoid haemorrhage
h. Subdural haematoma
i. Temporal arteritis
j. Vertebrobasilar TIA
k. Polymyalgia rheumatica (PMR)

*For each presentation below, choose the **single most likely diagnosis** from the above list of options. Each option may be used once, more than once or not at all.*

QUESTIONS

76. A 27-year-old woman has a long-standing history of headaches associated with nausea and vomiting. On this occasion she present with sudden loss of vision in the right half of the visual field. By the time you see her it has improved considerably.
77. An 82-year-old woman complains of increasing weakness and muscle pain to the point where she is finding it difficulty to brush her hair and get out of a chair. She now presents with sudden loss of vision in her left eye.
78. A woman previously in good health, presents with sudden onset of severe occipital headache and vomiting. Her only physical sign on examination is a stiff neck.
79. A 74-year-old woman had a fall two weeks ago. She is brought into the A and E department with slowly increasing drowsiness. On examination, you find mild hemiparesis and unequal pupils.
80. A 73-year-old man presents with hemianopia, hemi-sensory loss, hemiparesis and aphasia of 16 hour duration.

THEME 17: THE PREVENTION OF JAUNDICE/ HEPATITIS

OPTIONS:

a. Hepatitis A
b. Hepatitis B
c. Hepatitis C
d. Cirrhosis
e. Hepatocellular carcinoma
f. Sclerosing cholangitis
g. Infectious mononucleosis
h. Lyme disease
i. Leptrospirosis
j. Sclerosing cholangitis
k. Chronic active hepatitis

For each presentation below, choose the ***single most effective prevention*** *from the above list of options. Each option may be used once, more than once or not at all.*

QUESTIONS

81. Immunisation of health workers who are in contact with body fluid.
82. Mass immunisation of hepatitis B, besides preventing hepatitis B also prevents.
83. Avoidance of alcohol for six months after hepatitis A.
84. Counselling for intravenous (IV) drug users to use needle exchange facilities.
85. Immunisation of sewage workers.

THEME 18: THE MANAGEMENT OF EARACHE

OPTIONS

a. Removal of foreign body by suction under GA
b. Removal of foreign body using forceps under GA
c. Amoxycillin
d. Amoxicillin with clavulanic acid
e. Acyclovir
f. No specific treatment required
g. Paracetamol
h. Antibiotic against otitis externa
i. Metronidazole
j. Cefuroxime
k. Gentamycin
l. Myringotomy

For each presentation below, choose the ***single most appropriate management*** *from the above list of options. Each option may be used once, more than once or not at all.*

QUESTIONS

86. A 7-year-old has right sided earache and rhinorrhoea. On examination, his right sided tympanic membrane appears pink in colour.
87. A 4-year-old with right sided earache is examined using otoscopy. This reveals a red bulging tympanic membrane
88. An 8-year-old boy who has been playing outside now complains of right sided earache. On inspection a green bead is seen protruding into his ear canal. The walls of the canal are red.
89. A 9-year-old girl with a history of recurrent otitis media now complains of left sided earache. On examination the right sided tympanic membrane appears scarred. On examination of the left ear, pus is seen throughout the ear canal
90. A 54-year-old female develops mild fever, malaise and ear pain. 3 days later she developed multiple painful vesicles over her early canal and external meatus.

THEME 19: THE TYPES OF SKIN CANCER

OPTIONS
a. Kaposi's sarcoma
b. Lentigo maligna
c. Squamous cell carcinoma
d. Basal cell carcinoma
e. Melanoma
f. Keratosis
g. Acanthoma
h. Neurofibroma
i. Leukoplakia
j. Mycoses fungoides
k. Bowen's disease

*For each presentation below, choose the **single most likely diagnosis** from the above list of options. Each option may be used once, more than once or not at all.*

QUESTIONS

91. A fair 18-year-old girl has had dark black facial patches, one of which is now growing rapidly in size.
92. A 70-year-old bald gardener has had a brownish patch on his scalp which has been slowly growing for the last 30 years.
93. A young HIV positive man develops raised patches in his skin and in his mouth.
94. A builder has been exposed to sun for long periods of time devlops an ulcerated lesion on his face.
95. An 18-year-old girl with moles on her back of different colour and sizes.

THEME 20: MANAGEMENT OF DRUG DEPENDENCY

OPTIONS
a. Disulfiram
b. Methadone
c. Needle exchange programme
d. Intravenous vitamin B and thiamine
e. Gradual reducing course of diazepam
f. Outpatient referral to drug dependency team
g. Chlormethiazole
h. Chlordiazepoxide
i. Naloxone
j. Group psychotherapy
k. Hospital admission
l. Inform police

*For each presentation below, choose the **single most appropriate management** from the above list of options. Each option may be used once, more than once or not at all.*

QUESTIONS

96. A 70-year-old woman has taken 20 mg of temazepam at night for the last 30 years. She has begun to suffer with falls and has agreed that the temazepam might be contributing to the falls.
97. A 26-year-old heroin addict is worried because her partner has been diagnosed as having HIV infection. She is HIV negative. She does not feel able to stop using heroin currently.
98. A 40-year-old man has become increasingly dependent on alcohol since his wife died last year. He admits that he has a problem and wishes to stop drinking. He does not with to take antidepressants.
99. A 63-year-old retired surgeon is admitted with a short history of bizarre behaviour. He claims that GMC are investigating him for murder and have hired a private detective to follow him. He has evidence of a coarse tremor, horizontal nystagmus and an ataxic gait. His wife says that the story about GMC is untrue but is worried about the amount of gin that her husband has drunk since retirement.
100. A 37-year-old retired professional footballer admits of using cocaine and heroin for the last three years. He has recently signed a contract to present a sports show on television and wishes to 'clean his life up' first. His wife and family are very supportive of this.

THEME 21: CAUSES OF PNEUMONIA

OPTIONS

a. Bronchiectasis
b. *Haemophilus influenzae*
c. *Mycoplasma pneumoniae*
d. *Staphyloccus aureus*
e. *Streptococcus pneumoniae*
f. *Pneumocystis carinii*
g. Acid fast bacillus
h. Candidiasis
i. *Legionella pneumophila*
j. *Chlamydia psittaci*
k. *Chlamydia trachomatis*

For each presentation below, choose the ***single most likely diagnosis*** *from the above list of options. Each option may be used once, more than once, or not at all.*

QUESTIONS

101. A middle-aged woman develops a purulent cough with some hemoptysis. A chest X-ray reveals right upper lobe consolidation.
102. A young woman with no relevant medical history develops a severe purulent cough. A chest X-ray reveals multiple cavitating bilateral lung lesions.
103. A young male prostitute develops a dry cough. A chest X-ray reveals bilateral interstitial infiltrates.
104. A young man has recently suffers from a bout of influenza. He now develops a purulent cough.
105. Man comes back from a holiday in Malaysia and he develops malaise, fever and dry cough.

THEME 22: DIFFERENTIAL DIAGNOSIS OF RECTAL LESIONS

OPTIONS

a. Amoebic dysentery
b. Pseudomembranous colitis
c. Crohn's involvement of the colon
d. Ulcerative proctitis
e. Ulcerative pancolitis
f. Diverticular disease
g. Caecal carcinoma
h. Sigmoid carcinoma
i. Condyloma accuminatum
j. Anal fissure
k. Sigmoid volvulus

For each presentation below, choose the ***single most likely diagnosis*** *from the above list of options. Each option may be used once, more than once or not at all.*

QUESTIONS

106. A businessperson has just returned from a business trip to Asia. He now develops copious watery and bloody diarrhoea.
107. A middle-aged man develops constipation with overflow diarrhoea and bright red bleeding per rectum. A barium enema reveals an ulcerated stricture in the sigmoid colon.
108. A young man develops bloody diarrhoea. A rigid sigmoidoscopy examination revealed granular ulceration in the sigmoid colon with proximal sparing.
109. A middle-aged woman has been on several antibiotic treatments recently because of a persistent pneumonia. She now develops a severe watery diarrhoea. Colonoscopy reveals whitish plaques scattered throughout the colon.
110. An elderly woman is found anaemic. As part of her examination, she has a barium enema, which reveals a mass lesion in the ascending colon.

THEME 23: INVESTIGATION OF JOINT PAIN

OPTIONS

a. Serum uric acid
b. Joint fluid uric acid crystals
c. Plain radiograph of the knee
d. Plasma rheumatoid factor
e. Joint fluid rheumatoid factor
f. ESR
g. Antinuclear DNA antibody
h. Joint fluid culture
i. Joint fluid crystal examination
j. Plain radiograph of hip
k. Blood culture
l. X-ray femur

For each presentation below, choose the ***single most likely investigation*** *from the above list of options. Each option may be used once, more than once or not at all.*

QUESTIONS

111. A middle-aged woman with a history of rheumatoid arthritis develops sudden swelling in one of her knees. This knee is swollen and hot to touch.
112. An elderly man with recently diagnosed heart failure has been treated with diuretics. He now develops severe joint pain in his left ankle with swelling and redness.
113. A 78-year-old woman complains of a stiff left hip joint after walking some distance. This is most evident when she attempts to abduct the hip joint with limited abduction.
114. A 34-year-old woman complains of bilateral stiff and painful joints in her hands and feet.
115. A 67-year-old woman complains of right hip pain. On examination the right hip is adducted, externally rotated and flexed.

THEME 24: DIAGNOSIS OF CENTRAL CHEST PAIN

OPTIONS

a. Dissecting aortic aneurysm
b. Myocardial infarction
c. Osteochondritis
d. Achalasia
e. Pericarditis
f. Pulmonary embolism
g. Reflux oesophagitis
h. Lung fibrosis
i. Spontaneous pneumothorax
j. Pleural effusion
k. Tension pneumothorax
l. Oesophageal candidiasis

For each presentation below, choose the ***single most likely diagnosis*** *from the above list of options. Each option may be used once, more than once or not at all.*

QUESTIONS

116. A tall 34-year-old man develops severe central chest pain radiating to his back. He soon develops a dense haemiplegia.
117. An elderly gentleman suffers a sudden severe crushing central chest pain radiating to his neck
118. A middle-aged man has severe chest pain. Repeated St elevation patterns are seen and a Pericardial rub is heard.
119. A woman 10 days following hysterectomy complaints of severe left sided chest pain and breathlessness. Chest X-ray and ECG failed to relieve any abnormality.
120. A young homosexual man complains of central chest pain. On examination of his mouth, he has white granular lesions on the buccal mucal which is red.

THEME 25: INVESTIGATION OF MISCARRIAGE

OPTIONS

a. Serum HCG levels
b. Lupus plasma marker
c. Hysteroscopy
d. Colposcopy
e. Ultrasound examination
f. MRI
g. Hysterosalpingogram
h. Abdominal X-ray
i. Cardiotocogram
j. Serum AFP levels
k. Kliehauer's test

For each presentation below, choose the ***single most likely investigation*** *from the above list of options. Each option may be used once, more than once or not at all.*

QUESTIONS

121. A woman in the eight-week of her pregnancy develops bright red bleeding of four hours duration. On examination, her cervical os is completely closed.

122. A woman in the twelfth week of her pregnancy develops bright red bleeding of four hours duration with large clots. On examination the cervical os is wide open.

123. A woman in the tenth week of her pregnancy develops bright red bleeding of one day duration. Her Gp organises an ultrasound examination which reveals heart contractions.

124. A 23-year-old woman has a history of a termination of pregancy at 12 weeks. She subsequently suffers a spontaneous misacarriage after 22 weeks of pregnancy. She has a history of DVT.

125. A young lady had a miscarriage in her second trimester following which she bleed profusely, needing 6 units of blood and had to be taken for surgical evacuation of her uterus. She needed medical treatment as she had milk secretion for a few days, but since she has had no periods.

THEME 26: THE DISEASE PROCESS IN ASTHMA

OPTIONS

a. IgA
b. IgM
c. IgE
d. IgG
e. T cells
f. Histamine
g. Improvement of FEV of 5% after treatment
h. Improvement of FEV of 15% after treatment
i. Vital capacity
j. Antigen provocation test
k. Raised eosinophil count
l. Beta-2 receptors

For each presentation below, choose the ***single most likely cause*** *from the above list of options. Each option may be used once, more than once or not at all.*

QUESTIONS

126. This test of lung function is characteristically not involved in asthmatic patients.

127. This substance is released by mast cells and causes flushing.

128. This substance is characteristically found in the saliva of most asthma patients IgE.

129. This test is done as a diagnostic test for asthma.

130. Blocking of these can cause worsening of asthma.

THEME 27: MANAGEMENT OF MENINGITIS

OPTIONS
a. Lumbar puncture
b. CT skull
c. X-ray
d. Immunisation
e. Immediated hydration
f. Rifampicin prophylaxis
g. Immediate hydration
h. Contact tracing
i. Isoniazid prophylaxis
j. Transfer to ITU
k. Reassure
l. Serum urate

For each presentation below, choose the ***single most appropriate management*** *from the above list of options. Each option may be used once, more than once or not at all.*

QUESTIONS
131. An HIV patient develops a severe headache and confusion. She is discovered to have bilateral papilloedema.
132. An 8-year-old boy with acute leukaemia is admitted in a comatose state. He is found to have lymphoblast depletion prevention.
133. A 14-year-old boy presents with drowsiness and generalised headache. He is recovering from a bilateral parotitis. His CT scan is normal.
134. An intravenous drug abuser presents with suspected meningitis. The organism is confirmed in the CSF by India ink preparation.
135. An anxious mother called you to say that her son's best friend in school has caught meningitis.

THEME 28: IMPORTANT SIDE EFFECTS OF COMMON DRUGS

OPTIONS
a. Impotence
b. Wasting
c. Deep vein thrombosis
d. Bronchospasm
e. Pseudomembranous colitis
f. Haemorrhagic cystitis
g. Constipation
h. Retrobulbar neuritis
i. Endometrial carcinoma
j. Stevens-Johnson syndrome
k. Retroperitoneal fibrosis

For each presentation below, choose the ***single most important side effects*** *from the above list of options. Each option may be used once, more than once or not at all.*

QUESTIONS
136. Cimetidine.
137. Cyclophosphamide.
138. Diamorphine.
139. Amoxicillin.
140. Oral contraceptive pill.

THEME 29: INVESTIGATION OF ACUTE ABDOMEN

OPTIONS

a. Serum amylase levels
b. CT scan
c. Ultrasound
d. Erect chest X-ray
e. Plain film of the kidneys, ureter and bladder
f. Stent
g. Barium enema
h. Sigmoidoscopy
i. Diagnostic laparoscopy
j. Arterial blood gases
k. Urgent operation

*For each presentation below, choose the **single most appropriate investigation** from the above list of options. Each option may be used once, more than once or not at all.*

QUESTIONS

141. Middle-aged man with haematuria and colicky left loin pain.

142. An elderly gentleman with left iliac fossa pain and tenderness and rectal bleeding.

143. A middle-aged woman with recurrent right upper abdominal pain radiating to the right shoulder. She is tender in this region.

144. Middle-aged chronic alcoholic presents with severe pain in upper abdomen, radiating to the back.

145. A fit 17-year-old man present with a 12-hour history of central abdominal pain localising to his right iliac fossa. He is pyrexical with tenderness, guarding and rebound tenderness in the right iliac fossa.

THEME 30: TESTS IN DIABETES

OPTIONS

a. Glucose tolerance test
b. Random glucose level
c. Fasting glucose level
d. Determination of diurnal steroid level pattern
e. Serum insulin levels
f. Haemoglobin A/C
g. Dietary adjustment
h. Twice daily long/short mixed insulin injections
i. Subcutaneous insulin sliding scale
j. Insulin tolerance test

*For each presentation below, choose the **single most likely diagnosis** from the above list of options. Each option may be used once, more than once or not at all.*

QUESTIONS

146. A 35-year-old female with a high blood glucose level is noted to be obese and has abdominal striae.

147. An elderly gentleman with frequency is found to have a raised random blood glucose level.

148. An elderly gentleman with polyuria is found to have a raised fasting blood glucose level.

149. A known diabetic on treatment has several episodes of hypoglycaemia.

150. A 27-year-old woman was found to have glycosuria at a routine antenatal clinic visit. A glucose tolerance test confirmed the diagnosis of gestational diabetes. What will be your like of action.

THEME 31: TREATMENT OF ANXIETY DISORDERS

OPTIONS
a. Fluoxetine
b. Amitryptaline
c. Tricyclics
d. Behaviour therapy
e. Marriage counselling
f. Psychoanalysis
g. ECT (electro convulsive therapy)
h. Desensitisation
i. Counselling
j. Systemic relaxation
k. No treatment required
l. MAO inhibitors

*For each presentation below, choose the **single most appropriate treatment** from the above list of options. Each option may be used once, more than once or not at all.*

QUESTIONS
151. A female lawyer is becoming increasing anxious when she has to speak in front of people. This is affecting her work as she needs to speak out in court.

152. A student approaching her secondary level exams is becoming increasingly anxious a few days ahead of her exam.

153. A 20-year-old woman attends A and E complaining of sudden breathlessness and anxiety. She describes palpitations and paraesthesiae of her hands, feet and lips. ECG shows sinus tachycardia and O_2 saturation is normal.

154. This treatment is very effective in endogenous anxiety and phobias.

155. A 25-year-old woman finds it difficult to leave her house. She becomes very agitated in supermarkes and describes palpitations and difficult breathing when in crowds.

THEME 32: DIAGNOSIS OF VAGINAL DISCHARGE

OPTIONS
a. Cervical epithelial conversion (cervical erosion)
b. Candidiasis
c. Herpes simplex
d. Gonorrhoea
e. Syphilis
f. *Chlamydia*
g. Endometriosis
h. Endometritis
i. *Gardnerella vaginalis*
j. Bacterial vaginosis
k. Pelvic inflammatory disease

*For each presentation below, choose the **single most likely diagnosis** from the above list of options. Each option may be used once, more than once or not at all.*

QUESTIONS
156. A pregnant woman has a vaginal discharge. The pH is 2 and mycelia are seen.

157. A woman has a vaginal discharge. The pH is 8 and clue cells are seen.

158. A woman has severe right sided abdominal pain and fever. She has a foul smelling vaginal discharge. She has a palpable right sided firmness.

159. A woman on the contraceptive pill for several years has a slight whitish vaginal discharge. On inspection she is found to have a pinkish colouration of the outer cervix.

160. A middle-aged woman with a vaginal disharge is found to have several ulcers at the vaginal introitus.

THEME 33: MANAGEMENT/INVESTIGATION OF LIMB ISCHAEMIA

OPTIONS

a. Amputation
b. Arteriography
c. Bypass graft
d. Intra-arterial vasodilator
e. Femoral embolectomy
f. Advise stop smoking and exercise
g. Fasciotomy
h. Venography
i. Compartmental manometry
j. Ankle-branchial index measurement (ABPI)
k. None of the above

*For each presentation below, choose the **single most appropriate answer** from the above list of options. Each option may be used once, more than once or not at all.*

QUESTIONS

161. Man involved in road traffic accident is found to have comminuted fractures of the tibia and fibula. He develops rapid swelling of the lower limb below the knee. Arterial pulses are absent below the knee.

162. An elderly male develops pain in his thigh and leg when walking for approximately 20 metres. This pain resolves with rest. He is a long-time smoker. In examination his dorsalis pedis pulse on the affected side is absent.

163. A 70-year-old with known atrial fibrillation on treatment dvelops a sudden cold leg. Pulses are absent in the level at and below the knee.

164. A 67-year-old male with a history of peripheral vascular disease develops sever ulceration and cellulitis in his left foot and extending up his left leg above the left ankle. The popliteal pulse is absent on that side. He has a history of ulceration on the contralateral side which resolved following a bypass graft operation on that side.

165. A 55-year-old man complains of intermittent pain in his toe on walking. He says that in addition it looks 'white.'

THEME 34: INVESTIGATION OF TRAUMA

OPTIONS

a. Chest X-ray
b. CT head scan
c. Lateral cervical spine X-ray
d. Lumbar spine X-ray
e. MRI thoracolumbar spine
f. Shoulder X-ray
g. Skull X-ray
h. USG abdomen
i. MRI skull
j. Peritoneal lavage
k. Nerve conduction studies

*For each presentation below, choose the **single most helpful investigation** from the above list of options. Each option may be used once, more than once or not at all.*

QUESTIONS

166. A 33-year-old boxer who complains of left sided weakness 24 hours after a boxing match.

167. An 18-year-old man who has sustained stab wounds to his abdomen and trunk. His respiratory rate is 23 breaths/min, his breath sounds appear normal but his pulse is 142/min and his BP is only 80/40 mmHg.

168. A 48-year-old woman complains of left shoulder and neck pain after having fallen off her bicycle. She has a graze on her forehead and also complains of tingling in her left ring and little fingers [digits IV and V].

169. A 28-year-old motorcyclist has been involved in an accident and complains of loss of sensation below the umbilicus and paralysis of both legs. His BP is 80/50 mmHg with a pulse rate of 72/min.

170. A 55-year-old roofer complains of lower back pain radiating into the right leg having fallen from a scaffold. He has no loss of power or sensation when examined.

THEME 35: MANAGEMENT OF INFERTILITY

OPTIONS

a. Bacteriological examination of urine
b. Day 21 progesterone
c. Semen analysis
d. Tubal patency test
e. Wait and see
f. Karyotyping
g. TSH
h. USG abdomen
i. Serum prolactin
j. Urinary B-HCG
k. Urinary FSH/LH

*For each presentation below, choose the **single most appropriate management** from the above list of options. Each option may be used once, more than once or not at all.*

QUESTIONS

171. A couple aged 25 years have been trying for a baby for six months.
172. Useful in determining ovulation.
173. An essential investigation for all heterosexual infertile couples.
174. This investigation is of little value in infertility.
175. It is an essential investigation of the female partner.

THEME 36: DIAGNOSIS OF ACUTE CHEST PAIN

OPTIONS

a. Acute pancreatitis
b. Angina pectoris
c. Aortic dissection
d. Trigeminal neuralgia
e. Herpes zoster
f. Lobar pneumonia
g. Ruptured oesophagus
h. Herpes simplex
i. Acute myocardial infarction
j. Spontaneous pneumothorax
k. Acute cholecystitis
l. Bornholm disease
m. Tietze's syndrome
n. Oesophageal spasm
o. Fracture rib

*For each presentation below, choose the **single most likely diagnosis** from the above list of options. Each option may be used once, more than once or not at all.*

QUESTIONS

176. A 23-year-old woman develops an acute pain in her right chest radiating to her right shoulder associated with a fever. She is vomiting and has mild yellowing of her skin.
177. A tall young man developed sharp chest pain on his right, following a road traffic accident. On palpation, this area is tender. A chest X-ray shows his lungs are not injured.
178. A 23-year-old male prostitute develops severe chest pain. This area of chest pain corresponds to an area with an erythematous rash.
179. A 69-year-old man develops crushing chest pain associated with nausea and profuse sweating radiating to the neck. By the time he gets to the hospital [quarter of an hour later] the pain is gone.
180. Minutes after upper GI endoscopy a 57-year-old man develops chest pain. When you examine him, he has a crackling feeling under the skin around his upper chest and neck.

THEME 37: DIFFERENTIAL DIAGNOSIS OF ABDOMINAL PAIN IN A WOMAN

OPTIONS

a. Uterine rupture
b. Ulcerative colitis
c. Twisted ovarian mass
d. Threatened miscarriage
e. Irritable bowel syndrome
f. Pelvic inflammatory disease
g. Renal colic
h. Endometriosis
i. Appendicitis
j. Acute pancreatitis
k. Ectopic pregnancy
l. Septic abortion
m. Break through bleeding
n. Inevitable miscarriage
o. Missed abortion
p. Bowel carcinoma

*For each presentation below, choose the **single most likely diagnosis** from the above list of options. Each option may be used once, more than once or not at all.*

QUESTIONS

181. A 35-year-old woman complains of abdominal discomfort relieved by passing flatus or defecation. Over the last 6 months she has had episodes of diarrhoea and constipation, but denied she had lost weight.

182. A 37-year-old woman presents with a sudden onset of severe left iliac fossa pain. On vaginal USG, 2 cm echogenic masses are seen in the broad ligament. She says this pain seems to come on every month.

183. A 23-year-old woman just had an intrauterine device fitted. She complains of a watery brown vaginal discharge and abdominal pain.

184. An 18 weeks pregnant female presents with lower abdominal pain and tenderness, with offensive vaginal discharge. She has high grade fever since last two days.

185. A 32-year-old woman who conscientiously uses the oral contraceptive pill, has experienced monthly vaginal bleeding. On abdominal examination, she is uncomfortable. Her temperature is 37°C. She is otherwise healthy.

THEME 38: THE MANAGEMENT OF HYPERTENSION IN PREGNANCY

OPTIONS

a. Low dose aspirin
b. A period of observation for blood pressure
c. Twenty-four hours urinary protein
d. Foetal ultrasound
e. Retinoscopy
f. Induction of labour
g. Renal function tests
h. Intravenous antihypertensive
i. Intravenous benzodiazepine
j. Magnesium hydroxide
k. Oral antihypertensive
l. Oral diuretic
m. Recheck blood pressure in seven days
n. Complete neurological exam
o. Immediate caesarian section

*For each presentation below, choose the **single most appropriate action** from the above list of options. Each option may be used once, more than once or not at all.*

QUESTIONS

186. A patient in her third pregnancy presents to her GP at 12 weeks gestation. She was mildly hypertensive in both of her previous pregnancies. Her BP is 150/100 mmHg. Two weeks later at the hospital antenatal clinic her BP is 150/95 mmHg.

187. A 22-year-old Nigerian woman has an uneventful first pregnancy to 30 weeks. She is then admitted as an emergency with epigastric pain. During the first two hours her BP rises from 150/105 to 170/120 mmHg. On dipstick she is found to have 3+ proteinuria. The fetal cardiotocogram (CTG) is normal.

188. At an antenatal clinic visit at 38 weeks gestation, a 36-year-old multiparous woman has a BP of 140/90 mmHg. She has no proteinuria and is otherwise well.

189. At 32 weeks, a 22-year-old primigravida is found to have a BP of 145/100 mmHg. She has no proteinuria but is found to have oedema of her knees.

190. At 34 weeks, a 86 kg woman complains of persistent headaches and 'flashing lights.' There is no hyper-reflexia and her BP is 150/100 mmHg. Urinalysis is negative but she has finger oedema.

THEME 39: DIAGNOSIS OF VISUAL LOSS

OPTIONS

a. Acute glaucoma
b. Central retinal vein occlusion
c. Central retinal artery occlusion
d. Cranial arteritis
e. Uveitis
f. Occipital lobe infarct
g. Direct trauma
h. Retrobulbar neuritis
i. Retinal detachment

For each presentation below, choose the ***single most likely cause of visual loss*** *from the above list of options. Each option may be used once, more than once or not at all.*

QUESTIONS

191. A 35-year-old man presents with pain in the right eye, vomiting and loss of vision.
192. A 55-year-old known diabetic and hypertensive wakes up in the morning with diminished vision.
193. A 25-year-old man presents to the accident and emergency department with pain in the right eye associated with backache.
194. An elderly woman presents with a history of visual loss and scalp soreness.
195. An elderly man who is an inpatient (for hypertension) wakes in the morning note that he cannot see his breakfast. He has no other complaints. He has a carotid bruit.

THEME 40: THE PAINFUL HIP IN CHILDREN

OPTIONS

a. Developmental dysplasia of the hip (CDH)
b. Irritable hip syndrome
c. Osteomyelitis
d. Perthes' disease
e. Septic arthritis
f. Slipped upper femoral epiphysis (SUFE)
g. Osteogenesis imperfecta
h. Fracture femur
i. Osteogenic sarcoma
j. Ewing's sarcoma
k. Juvenile rheumatoid arthritis

For each presentation below, choose the ***single most likely condition*** *from the above list of options. Each option may be used once, more than once or not at all.*

QUESTIONS

196. A six-year-old boy complains of intermittent hip pain for several months. Haematological investigations are normal. X-rays show flattening of the femoral head.
197. A two-year-old girl with one day history of increasing hip pain has become unable to weight bear. Her WCC is 21/fl, with an ESR of 89 mm/hr and a CRP of 300 mg/L. A radiograph of the hip shows a widened jaoint space.
198. A 12-year-old boy with left groin pain for 6 weeks is noticed to stand with the left leg externally rotated. Examination reveals negligible internal rotation of the hip.
199. A four-year-old boy complains of right hip pain a few days following an upper respiratory tract infection. Blood tests are as follows: WCC 12/fl, ESR 10 mm/hr and CRP 2 mg/L
200. A five-year-old girl complains of progressively increasing severe pain in her left hip and upper leg for 6 days. She is able to walk but limps visibly. Blood tests are as follows: WCC 19/fl, ESR 72 mm/hr and CRP 94 mg/L. X-rays and ultrasound scans of the hip are normal.

General Medical Council PLAB Test Part 1

0	0	0	0	0	0
1	1	1	1	1	1
2	2	2	2	2	2
3	3	3	3	3	3
4	4	4	4	4	4
5	5	5	5	5	5
6	6	6	6	6	6
7	7	7	7	7	7
8	8	8	8	8	8
9	9	9	9	9	9

Full Name

Test Centre/Date

- Use pencil only • Make heavy marks that fill the lozenge completely
- Write your candidate number in the top row of the box to the right **AND** fill in the appropriate lozenge below each number
- Give **ONE** answer only for each question

1	A	B	C	D	E	F	G	H	I	J	K	L	M	N	O	P	Q	R	S	T	1
2	A	B	C	D	E	F	G	H	I	J	K	L	M	N	O	P	Q	R	S	T	2
3	A	B	C	D	E	F	G	H	I	J	K	L	M	N	O	P	Q	R	S	T	3
4	A	B	C	D	E	F	G	H	I	J	K	L	M	N	O	P	Q	R	S	T	4
5	A	B	C	D	E	F	G	H	I	J	K	L	M	N	O	P	Q	R	S	T	5
6	A	B	C	D	E	F	G	H	I	J	K	L	M	N	O	P	Q	R	S	T	6
7	A	B	C	D	E	F	G	H	I	J	K	L	M	N	O	P	Q	R	S	T	7
8	A	B	C	D	E	F	G	H	I	J	K	L	M	N	O	P	Q	R	S	T	8
9	A	B	C	D	E	F	G	H	I	J	K	L	M	N	O	P	Q	R	S	T	9
10	A	B	C	D	E	F	G	H	I	J	K	L	M	N	O	P	Q	R	S	T	10
11	A	B	C	D	E	F	G	H	I	J	K	L	M	N	O	P	Q	R	S	T	11
12	A	B	C	D	E	F	G	H	I	J	K	L	M	N	O	P	Q	R	S	T	12
13	A	B	C	D	E	F	G	H	I	J	K	L	M	N	O	P	Q	R	S	T	13
14	A	B	C	D	E	F	G	H	I	J	K	L	M	N	O	P	Q	R	S	T	14
15	A	B	C	D	E	F	G	H	I	J	K	L	M	N	O	P	Q	R	S	T	15
16	A	B	C	D	E	F	G	H	I	J	K	L	M	N	O	P	Q	R	S	T	16
17	A	B	C	D	E	F	G	H	I	J	K	L	M	N	O	P	Q	R	S	T	17
18	A	B	C	D	E	F	G	H	I	J	K	L	M	N	O	P	Q	R	S	T	18
19	A	B	C	D	E	F	G	H	I	J	K	L	M	N	O	P	Q	R	S	T	19
20	A	B	C	D	E	F	G	H	I	J	K	L	M	N	O	P	Q	R	S	T	20
21	A	B	C	D	E	F	G	H	I	J	K	L	M	N	O	P	Q	R	S	T	21
22	A	B	C	D	E	F	G	H	I	J	K	L	M	N	O	P	Q	R	S	T	22
23	A	B	C	D	E	F	G	H	I	J	K	L	M	N	O	P	Q	R	S	T	23
24	A	B	C	D	E	F	G	H	I	J	K	L	M	N	O	P	Q	R	S	T	24
25	A	B	C	D	E	F	G	H	I	J	K	L	M	N	O	P	Q	R	S	T	25
26	A	B	C	D	E	F	G	H	I	J	K	L	M	N	O	P	Q	R	S	T	26
27	A	B	C	D	E	F	G	H	I	J	K	L	M	N	O	P	Q	R	S	T	27
28	A	B	C	D	E	F	G	H	I	J	K	L	M	N	O	P	Q	R	S	T	28
29	A	B	C	D	E	F	G	H	I	J	K	L	M	N	O	P	Q	R	S	T	29
30	A	B	C	D	E	F	G	H	I	J	K	L	M	N	O	P	Q	R	S	T	30
31	A	B	C	D	E	F	G	H	I	J	K	L	M	N	O	P	Q	R	S	T	31
32	A	B	C	D	E	F	G	H	I	J	K	L	M	N	O	P	Q	R	S	T	32
33	A	B	C	D	E	F	G	H	I	J	K	L	M	N	O	P	Q	R	S	T	33
34	A	B	C	D	E	F	G	H	I	J	K	L	M	N	O	P	Q	R	S	T	34
35	A	B	C	D	E	F	G	H	I	J	K	L	M	N	O	P	Q	R	S	T	35
36	A	B	C	D	E	F	G	H	I	J	K	L	M	N	O	P	Q	R	S	T	36
37	A	B	C	D	E	F	G	H	I	J	K	L	M	N	O	P	Q	R	S	T	37
38	A	B	C	D	E	F	G	H	I	J	K	L	M	N	O	P	Q	R	S	T	38
39	A	B	C	D	E	F	G	H	I	J	K	L	M	N	O	P	Q	R	S	T	39
40	A	B	C	D	E	F	G	H	I	J	K	L	M	N	O	P	Q	R	S	T	40
41	A	B	C	D	E	F	G	H	I	J	K	L	M	N	O	P	Q	R	S	T	41
42	A	B	C	D	E	F	G	H	I	J	K	L	M	N	O	P	Q	R	S	T	42
43	A	B	C	D	E	F	G	H	I	J	K	L	M	N	O	P	Q	R	S	T	43
44	A	B	C	D	E	F	G	H	I	J	K	L	M	N	O	P	Q	R	S	T	44
45	A	B	C	D	E	F	G	H	I	J	K	L	M	N	O	P	Q	R	S	T	45
46	A	B	C	D	E	F	G	H	I	J	K	L	M	N	O	P	Q	R	S	T	46
47	A	B	C	D	E	F	G	H	I	J	K	L	M	N	O	P	Q	R	S	T	47
48	A	B	C	D	E	F	G	H	I	J	K	L	M	N	O	P	Q	R	S	T	48
49	A	B	C	D	E	F	G	H	I	J	K	L	M	N	O	P	Q	R	S	T	49
50	A	B	C	D	E	F	G	H	I	J	K	L	M	N	O	P	Q	R	S	T	50

DO NOT WRITE IN THIS SPACE

51	A	B	C	D	E	F	G	H	I	J	K	L	M	N	O	P	Q	R	S	T	51
52	A	B	C	D	E	F	G	H	I	J	K	L	M	N	O	P	Q	R	S	T	52
53	A	B	C	D	E	F	G	H	I	J	K	L	M	N	O	P	Q	R	S	T	53
54	A	B	C	D	E	F	G	H	I	J	K	L	M	N	O	P	Q	R	S	T	54
55	A	B	C	D	E	F	G	H	I	J	K	L	M	N	O	P	Q	R	S	T	55
56	A	B	C	D	E	F	G	H	I	J	K	L	M	N	O	P	Q	R	S	T	56
57	A	B	C	D	E	F	G	H	I	J	K	L	M	N	O	P	Q	R	S	T	57
58	A	B	C	D	E	F	G	H	I	J	K	L	M	N	O	P	Q	R	S	T	58
59	A	B	C	D	E	F	G	H	I	J	K	L	M	N	O	P	Q	R	S	T	59
60	A	B	C	D	E	F	G	H	I	J	K	L	M	N	O	P	Q	R	S	T	60
61	A	B	C	D	E	F	G	H	I	J	K	L	M	N	O	P	Q	R	S	T	61
62	A	B	C	D	E	F	G	H	I	J	K	L	M	N	O	P	Q	R	S	T	62
63	A	B	C	D	E	F	G	H	I	J	K	L	M	N	O	P	Q	R	S	T	63
64	A	B	C	D	E	F	G	H	I	J	K	L	M	N	O	P	Q	R	S	T	64
65	A	B	C	D	E	F	G	H	I	J	K	L	M	N	O	P	Q	R	S	T	65
66	A	B	C	D	E	F	G	H	I	J	K	L	M	N	O	P	Q	R	S	T	66
67	A	B	C	D	E	F	G	H	I	J	K	L	M	N	O	P	Q	R	S	T	67
68	A	B	C	D	E	F	G	H	I	J	K	L	M	N	O	P	Q	R	S	T	68
69	A	B	C	D	E	F	G	H	I	J	K	L	M	N	O	P	Q	R	S	T	69
70	A	B	C	D	E	F	G	H	I	J	K	L	M	N	O	P	Q	R	S	T	70
71	A	B	C	D	E	F	G	H	I	J	K	L	M	N	O	P	Q	R	S	T	71
72	A	B	C	D	E	F	G	H	I	J	K	L	M	N	O	P	Q	R	S	T	72
73	A	B	C	D	E	F	G	H	I	J	K	L	M	N	O	P	Q	R	S	T	73
74	A	B	C	D	E	F	G	H	I	J	K	L	M	N	O	P	Q	R	S	T	74
75	A	B	C	D	E	F	G	H	I	J	K	L	M	N	O	P	Q	R	S	T	75
76	A	B	C	D	E	F	G	H	I	J	K	L	M	N	O	P	Q	R	S	T	76
77	A	B	C	D	E	F	G	H	I	J	K	L	M	N	O	P	Q	R	S	T	77
78	A	B	C	D	E	F	G	H	I	J	K	L	M	N	O	P	Q	R	S	T	78
79	A	B	C	D	E	F	G	H	I	J	K	L	M	N	O	P	Q	R	S	T	79
80	A	B	C	D	E	F	G	H	I	J	K	L	M	N	O	P	Q	R	S	T	80
81	A	B	C	D	E	F	G	H	I	J	K	L	M	N	O	P	Q	R	S	T	81
82	A	B	C	D	E	F	G	H	I	J	K	L	M	N	O	P	Q	R	S	T	82
83	A	B	C	D	E	F	G	H	I	J	K	L	M	N	O	P	Q	R	S	T	83
84	A	B	C	D	E	F	G	H	I	J	K	L	M	N	O	P	Q	R	S	T	84
85	A	B	C	D	E	F	G	H	I	J	K	L	M	N	O	P	Q	R	S	T	85
86	A	B	C	D	E	F	G	H	I	J	K	L	M	N	O	P	Q	R	S	T	86
87	A	B	C	D	E	F	G	H	I	J	K	L	M	N	O	P	Q	R	S	T	87
88	A	B	C	D	E	F	G	H	I	J	K	L	M	N	O	P	Q	R	S	T	88
89	A	B	C	D	E	F	G	H	I	J	K	L	M	N	O	P	Q	R	S	T	89
90	A	B	C	D	E	F	G	H	I	J	K	L	M	N	O	P	Q	R	S	T	90
91	A	B	C	D	E	F	G	H	I	J	K	L	M	N	O	P	Q	R	S	T	91
92	A	B	C	D	E	F	G	H	I	J	K	L	M	N	O	P	Q	R	S	T	92
93	A	B	C	D	E	F	G	H	I	J	K	L	M	N	O	P	Q	R	S	T	93
94	A	B	C	D	E	F	G	H	I	J	K	L	M	N	O	P	Q	R	S	T	94
95	A	B	C	D	E	F	G	H	I	J	K	L	M	N	O	P	Q	R	S	T	95
96	A	B	C	D	E	F	G	H	I	J	K	L	M	N	O	P	Q	R	S	T	96
97	A	B	C	D	E	F	G	H	I	J	K	L	M	N	O	P	Q	R	S	T	97
98	A	B	C	D	E	F	G	H	I	J	K	L	M	N	O	P	Q	R	S	T	98
99	A	B	C	D	E	F	G	H	I	J	K	L	M	N	O	P	Q	R	S	T	99
100	A	B	C	D	E	F	G	H	I	J	K	L	M	N	O	P	Q	R	S	T	100

DO NOT WRITE IN THIS SPACE

101	A	B	C	D	E	F	G	H	I	J	K	L	M	N	O	P	Q	R	S	T	101
102	A	B	C	D	E	F	G	H	I	J	K	L	M	N	O	P	Q	R	S	T	102
103	A	B	C	D	E	F	G	H	I	J	K	L	M	N	O	P	Q	R	S	T	103
104	A	B	C	D	E	F	G	H	I	J	K	L	M	N	O	P	Q	R	S	T	104
105	A	B	C	D	E	F	G	H	I	J	K	L	M	N	O	P	Q	R	S	T	105
106	A	B	C	D	E	F	G	H	I	J	K	L	M	N	O	P	Q	R	S	T	106
107	A	B	C	D	E	F	G	H	I	J	K	L	M	N	O	P	Q	R	S	T	107
108	A	B	C	D	E	F	G	H	I	J	K	L	M	N	O	P	Q	R	S	T	108
109	A	B	C	D	E	F	G	H	I	J	K	L	M	N	O	P	Q	R	S	T	109
110	A	B	C	D	E	F	G	H	I	J	K	L	M	N	O	P	Q	R	S	T	110
111	A	B	C	D	E	F	G	H	I	J	K	L	M	N	O	P	Q	R	S	T	111
112	A	B	C	D	E	F	G	H	I	J	K	L	M	N	O	P	Q	R	S	T	112
113	A	B	C	D	E	F	G	H	I	J	K	L	M	N	O	P	Q	R	S	T	113
114	A	B	C	D	E	F	G	H	I	J	K	L	M	N	O	P	Q	R	S	T	114
115	A	B	C	D	E	F	G	H	I	J	K	L	M	N	O	P	Q	R	S	T	115
116	A	B	C	D	E	F	G	H	I	J	K	L	M	N	O	P	Q	R	S	T	116
117	A	B	C	D	E	F	G	H	I	J	K	L	M	N	O	P	Q	R	S	T	117
118	A	B	C	D	E	F	G	H	I	J	K	L	M	N	O	P	Q	R	S	T	118
119	A	B	C	D	E	F	G	H	I	J	K	L	M	N	O	P	Q	R	S	T	119
120	A	B	C	D	E	F	G	H	I	J	K	L	M	N	O	P	Q	R	S	T	120
121	A	B	C	D	E	F	G	H	I	J	K	L	M	N	O	P	Q	R	S	T	121
122	A	B	C	D	E	F	G	H	I	J	K	L	M	N	O	P	Q	R	S	T	122
123	A	B	C	D	E	F	G	H	I	J	K	L	M	N	O	P	Q	R	S	T	123
124	A	B	C	D	E	F	G	H	I	J	K	L	M	N	O	P	Q	R	S	T	124
125	A	B	C	D	E	F	G	H	I	J	K	L	M	N	O	P	Q	R	S	T	125
126	A	B	C	D	E	F	G	H	I	J	K	L	M	N	O	P	Q	R	S	T	126
127	A	B	C	D	E	F	G	H	I	J	K	L	M	N	O	P	Q	R	S	T	127
128	A	B	C	D	E	F	G	H	I	J	K	L	M	N	O	P	Q	R	S	T	128
129	A	B	C	D	E	F	G	H	I	J	K	L	M	N	O	P	Q	R	S	T	129
130	A	B	C	D	E	F	G	H	I	J	K	L	M	N	O	P	Q	R	S	T	130
131	A	B	C	D	E	F	G	H	I	J	K	L	M	N	O	P	Q	R	S	T	131
132	A	B	C	D	E	F	G	H	I	J	K	L	M	N	O	P	Q	R	S	T	132
133	A	B	C	D	E	F	G	H	I	J	K	L	M	N	O	P	Q	R	S	T	133
134	A	B	C	D	E	F	G	H	I	J	K	L	M	N	O	P	Q	R	S	T	134
135	A	B	C	D	E	F	G	H	I	J	K	L	M	N	O	P	Q	R	S	T	135
136	A	B	C	D	E	F	G	H	I	J	K	L	M	N	O	P	Q	R	S	T	136
137	A	B	C	D	E	F	G	H	I	J	K	L	M	N	O	P	Q	R	S	T	137
138	A	B	C	D	E	F	G	H	I	J	K	L	M	N	O	P	Q	R	S	T	138
139	A	B	C	D	E	F	G	H	I	J	K	L	M	N	O	P	Q	R	S	T	139
140	A	B	C	D	E	F	G	H	I	J	K	L	M	N	O	P	Q	R	S	T	140
141	A	B	C	D	E	F	G	H	I	J	K	L	M	N	O	P	Q	R	S	T	141
142	A	B	C	D	E	F	G	H	I	J	K	L	M	N	O	P	Q	R	S	T	142
143	A	B	C	D	E	F	G	H	I	J	K	L	M	N	O	P	Q	R	S	T	143
144	A	B	C	D	E	F	G	H	I	J	K	L	M	N	O	P	Q	R	S	T	144
145	A	B	C	D	E	F	G	H	I	J	K	L	M	N	O	P	Q	R	S	T	145
146	A	B	C	D	E	F	G	H	I	J	K	L	M	N	O	P	Q	R	S	T	146
147	A	B	C	D	E	F	G	H	I	J	K	L	M	N	O	P	Q	R	S	T	147
148	A	B	C	D	E	F	G	H	I	J	K	L	M	N	O	P	Q	R	S	T	148
149	A	B	C	D	E	F	G	H	I	J	K	L	M	N	O	P	Q	R	S	T	149
150	A	B	C	D	E	F	G	H	I	J	K	L	M	N	O	P	Q	R	S	T	150

DO NOT WRITE IN THIS SPACE

151	A	B	C	D	E	F	G	H	I	J	K	L	M	N	O	P	Q	R	S	T	151
152	A	B	C	D	E	F	G	H	I	J	K	L	M	N	O	P	Q	R	S	T	152
153	A	B	C	D	E	F	G	H	I	J	K	L	M	N	O	P	Q	R	S	T	153
154	A	B	C	D	E	F	G	H	I	J	K	L	M	N	O	P	Q	R	S	T	154
155	A	B	C	D	E	F	G	H	I	J	K	L	M	N	O	P	Q	R	S	T	155
156	A	B	C	D	E	F	G	H	I	J	K	L	M	N	O	P	Q	R	S	T	156
157	A	B	C	D	E	F	G	H	I	J	K	L	M	N	O	P	Q	R	S	T	157
158	A	B	C	D	E	F	G	H	I	J	K	L	M	N	O	P	Q	R	S	T	158
159	A	B	C	D	E	F	G	H	I	J	K	L	M	N	O	P	Q	R	S	T	159
160	A	B	C	D	E	F	G	H	I	J	K	L	M	N	O	P	Q	R	S	T	160
161	A	B	C	D	E	F	G	H	I	J	K	L	M	N	O	P	Q	R	S	T	161
162	A	B	C	D	E	F	G	H	I	J	K	L	M	N	O	P	Q	R	S	T	162
163	A	B	C	D	E	F	G	H	I	J	K	L	M	N	O	P	Q	R	S	T	163
164	A	B	C	D	E	F	G	H	I	J	K	L	M	N	O	P	Q	R	S	T	164
165	A	B	C	D	E	F	G	H	I	J	K	L	M	N	O	P	Q	R	S	T	165
166	A	B	C	D	E	F	G	H	I	J	K	L	M	N	O	P	Q	R	S	T	166
167	A	B	C	D	E	F	G	H	I	J	K	L	M	N	O	P	Q	R	S	T	167
168	A	B	C	D	E	F	G	H	I	J	K	L	M	N	O	P	Q	R	S	T	168
169	A	B	C	D	E	F	G	H	I	J	K	L	M	N	O	P	Q	R	S	T	169
170	A	B	C	D	E	F	G	H	I	J	K	L	M	N	O	P	Q	R	S	T	170
171	A	B	C	D	E	F	G	H	I	J	K	L	M	N	O	P	Q	R	S	T	171
172	A	B	C	D	E	F	G	H	I	J	K	L	M	N	O	P	Q	R	S	T	172
173	A	B	C	D	E	F	G	H	I	J	K	L	M	N	O	P	Q	R	S	T	173
174	A	B	C	D	E	F	G	H	I	J	K	L	M	N	O	P	Q	R	S	T	174
175	A	B	C	D	E	F	G	H	I	J	K	L	M	N	O	P	Q	R	S	T	175
176	A	B	C	D	E	F	G	H	I	J	K	L	M	N	O	P	Q	R	S	T	176
177	A	B	C	D	E	F	G	H	I	J	K	L	M	N	O	P	Q	R	S	T	177
178	A	B	C	D	E	F	G	H	I	J	K	L	M	N	O	P	Q	R	S	T	178
179	A	B	C	D	E	F	G	H	I	J	K	L	M	N	O	P	Q	R	S	T	179
180	A	B	C	D	E	F	G	H	I	J	K	L	M	N	O	P	Q	R	S	T	180
181	A	B	C	D	E	F	G	H	I	J	K	L	M	N	O	P	Q	R	S	T	181
182	A	B	C	D	E	F	G	H	I	J	K	L	M	N	O	P	Q	R	S	T	182
183	A	B	C	D	E	F	G	H	I	J	K	L	M	N	O	P	Q	R	S	T	183
184	A	B	C	D	E	F	G	H	I	J	K	L	M	N	O	P	Q	R	S	T	184
185	A	B	C	D	E	F	G	H	I	J	K	L	M	N	O	P	Q	R	S	T	185
186	A	B	C	D	E	F	G	H	I	J	K	L	M	N	O	P	Q	R	S	T	186
187	A	B	C	D	E	F	G	H	I	J	K	L	M	N	O	P	Q	R	S	T	187
188	A	B	C	D	E	F	G	H	I	J	K	L	M	N	O	P	Q	R	S	T	188
189	A	B	C	D	E	F	G	H	I	J	K	L	M	N	O	P	Q	R	S	T	189
190	A	B	C	D	E	F	G	H	I	J	K	L	M	N	O	P	Q	R	S	T	190
191	A	B	C	D	E	F	G	H	I	J	K	L	M	N	O	P	Q	R	S	T	191
192	A	B	C	D	E	F	G	H	I	J	K	L	M	N	O	P	Q	R	S	T	192
193	A	B	C	D	E	F	G	H	I	J	K	L	M	N	O	P	Q	R	S	T	193
194	A	B	C	D	E	F	G	H	I	J	K	L	M	N	O	P	Q	R	S	T	194
195	A	B	C	D	E	F	G	H	I	J	K	L	M	N	O	P	Q	R	S	T	195
196	A	B	C	D	E	F	G	H	I	J	K	L	M	N	O	P	Q	R	S	T	196
197	A	B	C	D	E	F	G	H	I	J	K	L	M	N	O	P	Q	R	S	T	197
198	A	B	C	D	E	F	G	H	I	J	K	L	M	N	O	P	Q	R	S	T	198
199	A	B	C	D	E	F	G	H	I	J	K	L	M	N	O	P	Q	R	S	T	199
200	A	B	C	D	E	F	G	H	I	J	K	L	M	N	O	P	Q	R	S	T	200

Answers

Serial No.	Answer No.	Answer
1	f	Osteogenesis imperfecta
2	g	Elderly abuse
3	d	Sexual abuse
4	c	Physical abuse
5	a	Accidental injury
6	b	IV steroids
7	h	Timolol
8	l	ECCE with PCIOL
9	J	Vitrectomy
10	d	Laser treatment
11	a	Percutaneous drainage
12	a	Percutaneous drainage
13	k	Flucloxacillin
14	b	Ventilatory support + IV fluids
15	i	Laparotomy
16	k	None required
17	a	The 24 hours holter monitor
18	h	Carotid doppler
19	j	MRI skull
20	c	Serum calcium
21	k	Thrombophilia
22	f	Meningitis
23	i	Intracerebral haemorrhage
24	a	Splenomegaly
25	d	Gingival hypertrophy
26	b	Inevitable abortion
27	g	Torsion
28	h	IBS
29	e	PID
30	i	Toxic shock syndrome
31	a	Diagnostic needle thoracocentesis
32	d	Splinting
33	d	Splinting
34	g	IV mannitol
35	i	Suprapubic systostomy
36	c	Coarctation of aorta
37	e	Renal artery stenosis
38	h	Phacochromocytoma
39	k	Cushing's syndrome
40	i	Acromegaly
41	b	CT scan
42	a	Fibreoptic bronchoscopy
43	e	Laryngoscopy
44	g	Chest X-ray
45	e	Laryngoscopy
46	c	Duchenne muscular dystrophy
47	f	Hypothyroidism
48	h	Constitutional delay
49	g	Meningitis
50	k	Normal finding
51	c	Naloxone
52	a	The 50% dextrose drip
53	e	Insulin through a drip
54	l	CT scan
55	c	Naloxone
56	a	ECT
57	g	Lithium

58	c	Tricyclics
59	j	Fluoxetine
60	k	Lorazepam
61	l	Fibreoptic bronchoscopy
62	h	Pulmonary angiogram
63	a	CT
64	a	CT
65	d	Sputum culture
66	b	Septic shock
67	d	Hypovolaemic shock
68	b	Septic shock
69	d	Hypovolaemic shock
70	a	Anaphylaxis
71	d	Skull X-ray
72	f	Admit overnight for observation
73	k	IV mannitol
74	a	CT scan
75	j	Burr holes
76	f	Migraine
77	k	PMR
78	g	Subarachnoid haemorrhage
79	h	Subdural haematoma
80	a	Carotid artery stenosis
81	b	Hepatitis B
82	e	Hepatocellular carcinoma
83	d	Cirrhosis
84	b	Hepatitis B
85	a	Hepatitis A
86	g	Paracetamol
87	l	Myringotomy
88	a	Removal of foreign body by suction under GA
89	d	Amoxicillin with clavulinic acid

90	e	Acyclovir
91	b	Lentigo maligna
92	f	Keratosis
93	a	Kaposi's sarcoma
94	c	Squamous cell carcinoma
95	e	Melanoma
96	e	Gradual reducing course of dizepam
97	c	Needle exchange programme
98	j	Group psychotherapy
99	d	IV vitamin B and thiamine
100	f	Outpatient referral to dry depending team
101	e	*Streptococcus*
102	d	*Staphylococcus*
103	f	*Pneumocystis carinii*
104	d	*Staphylococcus*
105	i	*Legionella*
106	a	Amoebic dysentery
107	h	Sigmoid carcinoma
108	c	Crohn's involvement of colon
109	b	Pseudomembranous colitis
110	g	Caecal carcinoma
111	i	Joint fluid crystal examination
112	b	Joint fluid uric acid crystals
113	j	Plain radiograph of hip
114	d	Plasma rheumatoid factor
115	j	Plain radiograph of hip
116	a	Dissecting aortic aneurysm
117	b	Myocardial infaction
118	e	Pericarditis
119	f	Pulmonary embolism
120	g	Reflux oesophagitis
121	e	USG

122	e	USG
123	d	Colposcopy
124	b	Lupus plasma marker
125	f	MRI
126	i	Vital capacity
127	f	Histamine
128	k	Raised eosinophil count
129	h	Improvement of FEV, of 15% after treatment
130	l	Beta-2-receptors
131	b	CT skull
132	l	Serum urate
133	a	Lumbar puncture
134	a	Lumbar puncture
135	k	Reassure
136	a	Impotence
137	f	Haemorrhagic cystitis
138	g	Constipation
139	j	Stevens-Johnson syndrome
140	c	Deep vein thrombosis
141	e	Plain film of kidneys, ureter and bladder
142	h	Sigmoidscopy
143	c	USG
144	a	Serum amylase levels
145	i	Diagnostic laparoscopy
146	d	Determination of diurnal steroid level pattern
147	c	Fasting glucose
148	a	GT T
149	f	Haemoglobin A/C
150	a	GT T
151	h	Desensitisation

152	j	Systemic relaxation
153	k	No treatment required
154	l	MAO inhibitors
155	d	Behaviour therapy
156	b	Candidiasis
157	j	Bacterial vaginosis
158	k	PID
159	a	Cervical erosion
160	c	Herpes simplex
161	i	Compartmental manometry
162	b	Arteriography
163	e	Femoral embolectomy
164	a	Amputation
165	j	ABPI
166	b	CT head scan
167	h	USG abdomen
168	c	Lateral cervical spine X-ray
169	e	MRI thoracolumbar spine
170	d	Lumbar spine X-ray
171	e	Wait and see
172	b	Day 21 progesterone
173	c	Seman analysis
174	a	Bacteriological examination of urine
175	d	Tubal patency test
176	k	Acute cholecytitis
177	o	Fracture rib
178	e	Herpes zoster
179	b	Angina pectoris
180	g	Ruptured oesophagus
181	e	IBS

182	h	Endometriosis
183	f	PID
184	l	Septic abortion
185	m	Break through bleeding
186	k	Oral antihypertensive
187	h	IV antihypertensive
188	b	A period of observation for BP
189	d	Foetal USG
190	c	The 24 hours urinary protein
191	a	Acute glaucoma

192	i	Retinal detachment
193	e	Uveitis
194	d	Cranial arteritis
195	f	Occipital lobe infarcts
196	d	Perthes' disease
197	e	Septic arthritis
198	f	SUFE
199	b	Irritable hip syndrome
200	c	Osteomyelitis

Previous Year Paper 4

RxPG Analysis

Total Themes:	**40**
Repeat Themes:	**4**
Repeat Themes with a Different Header:	**9**

THEME 1: DIAGNOSIS OF HEARING LOSS

OPTIONS

a. Acoustic neuroma
b. Blast injury
c. Petrous temporal bone fracture
d. Wax impaction
e. Acute otitis media
f. Ototoxicity
g. Fracture base of skull
h. CSOM
i. Glue ear
j. Herpes zoster
k. Foreign body

*For each presentation below, choose the **most likely diagnosis** from the above list of options. Each option may be used once, more than once or not at all.*

QUESTIONS

1. Man treated with gentamicin for peritonitis for 10 days presents with deafness.
2. Man with poor physical hygiene presents with pain and deafness after taking a shower.
3. Woman presents with deafness and corneal anaesthesia. On MRI, a widened internal auditory meatus is seen.
4. Male, 20 years, with history of head injury, bruising on the side of head complains of hearing loss.
5. A 54-year-old female develops mild fever, malaise and ear pain. Three days later she developed multiple painful vesicles over her ear canal and external auditory meatus.

THEME 2: DIAGNOSIS OF EPISTAXIS

OPTIONS

a. Nasopharyngeal angiofibroma
b. Carcinoma maxillary antrum
c. Nasal polyposis
d. ORF (Cutaneous pustules-sheep)
e. Septal perforation
f. Coagulopathy
g. Anticoagulant overdose
h. Sarcoidosis
i. Trauma
j. HTN

*For each presentation below, choose the **single most likely diagnosis** from the above list of options. Each option may be used once, more than once or not at all.*

QUESTIONS

6. A sheep farmer with a bleeding polyp on anterior part of nasal septum.
7. Man working in a chrome factory presents with whistling sound on talking
8. Man with prosthetic heart valve presents with epistaxis.
9. Man who is involved in furniture making presents with recurrent epistaxis and anaesthesia of right cheek.
10. An 80-year-old man with history of epistaxis since 2 hours.

THEME 3: MECHANISM OF ACTION OF DRUGS

OPTIONS

a. Ipratropium
b. Amoxycillin
c. Salbutamol
d. Doxapram
e. Theophylline
f. Trimethoprim

*For each presentation below, choose the **correct answer** from the above list of options. Each option may be used once, more than once or not at all.*

QUESTIONS

11. β_2 agonist
12. Antimuscarinic
13. Interferes with cell wall synthesis
14. Increases the activity of respiratory muscles
15. Urinary antiseptic

THEME 4: DRUGS USED IN MANAGEMENT OF ASTHMA

OPTIONS

a. Nebulised β_2-agonist
b. Inhaled short-acting β_2
c. Inhaled long-acting β_2
d. Oral short-acting β_2
e. Oral long-acting β_2
f. Leukotriene antagonist
g. Na cromoglycate
h. Oral theophylline
i. Paracetamol
j. β-blocker
k. Carcinoma channel antagonists

*For each presentation below, choose the **correct answer** from the above list of options. Each option may be used once, more than once or not at all.*

QUESTIONS

16. First line drug used in treating mild asthma.
17. Not given in a chronic asthmatic after a myocardial infarction.
18. Used to control acute severe asthma in a 15-year old with severe breathlessness in A and E.
19. Used to control intermittent night wheeze in a person using inhaled high dose steroids presently.
20. A nine-year-old boy has a mild cough and wheeze after playing football in the cold weather.

THEME 5: DIAGNOSIS OF ELECTROLYTE DISTURBANCES

OPTIONS

a. Metabolic acidosis
b. Metabolic alkalosis
c. Renal failure
d. Fluid overload
e. Hypokalaemia
f. Respiratory acidosis
g. Hyperkalaemia

*For each presentation below, choose the **most likely diagnosis** from the above list of options. Each option may be used once, more than once, or not at all.*

QUESTIONS

21. Man with pyloric stenosis, profuse vomiting, hypokalaemia and increased bicarbonate.
22. Man who is not able to pass urine, tired, complains of hiccups.
23. Man with villous adenoma, profuse diarrhoea.
24. Female, 24 hours after hysterectomy complains of breathlessness, increased JVP.
25. A patient in severe renal failure has potassium level of 2. 5 mmol/L.

THEME 6: DIAGNOSIS OF UNCONSCIOUS PATIENTS

OPTIONS

a. Subdural haematoma
b. Extradural haematoma
c. Mild injury
d. Moderate injury
e. Fracture base of skull
f. Fracture cervical spine
g. Meningitis

*For each presentation below, choose the **most likely diagnosis** from the above list of options. Each option may be used once, more than once, or not at all.*

QUESTIONS

26. A chronic alcoholic with history of recurrent falls comes to A and E with complaint of ataxia. Blood glucose is 7.
27. A 17-year-old rugby player becomes unconscious after a fall. After sometime, he recovers, gives his name and address to the people in the ambulance. Later condition deteriorates.
28. A child becomes unconscious after falling off his bicycle, later he is better and active. Only complaint is headache.
29. Man with head trauma—GCS found to be 12.
30. Man with GCS=5, hemotympanum.

THEME 7: INVESTIGATION OF UNCONSCIOUS PATIENTS

OPTIONS

a. CT skull
b. Blood glucose
c. Lumbar puncture
d. Full blood count
e. Serum urea electrolytes
f. MRI scan
g. Toxicology screen
h. X-ray skull
i. Blood alcohol
j. Plasma osmolarity
k. Arterial blood gases

*For each presentation below, choose the **most appropriate answer** from the above list of options. Each option may be used once, more than once, or not at all.*

QUESTIONS

31. A 10-year-old girl, unconscious, brought to A and E. She is found to be dehydrated on examination and respiratory rate is 40/min.
32. A young boy is brought to A and E by his grandparents. He is unconscious with a bruise on the temporal area.
33. A 10-year-old boy is drowsy, febrile with a rash.
34. A old lady fell and broke her hand one week back. After that slowly increasing confusion. Today her relatives could not wake her up from sleep.
35. A 21-year-old female found unconscious next to her 22-year-old husband, who was found dead. Her ECG shows evidence of acute MI.

THEME 8: MANAGEMENT OF BURNS

OPTIONS

a. Referral to burns unit
b. IV opioid
c. Dressing
d. Escharotomy + referral to burns unit
e. Anaesthesia and intubation
f. IV fluids in A and E before discharge
g. Reassure
h. Deroof blisters
i. Aspirate blisters
j. Antibiotics
k. Fasciotomy
l. IV fluids + referral for admission to burns unit

*For each presentation below, choose the **most appropriate management** from the above list of options. Each option may be used once, more than once, or not at all.*

QUESTIONS

36. Man rescued from burning building. Burns on face and anterior chest, soot in pharynx and singed nasal hair, asking about his family members.
37. Baby with less than 3% burns on chest and shoulders [scald due to tea falling on him] is irritable, crying, not allowing examination.
38. Man was electrocuted. Full thickness burn on fingers complaining of pain.
39. Man with 40% burns over trunk an limbs.
40. Man, slept while sunbathing comes with redness, pain all over his body, otherwise well.

THEME 9: VACCINES

OPTIONS

a. Delay by 2 weeks
b. Omit pertussis and meningitis
c. Give vaccine in hospital
d. Continue as per schedule
e. Give inactivated vaccines
f. Omit pertussis, Hib, measles
g. Do not give any vaccines
h. Omit pertussis only
i. Omit meningitis only
j. Omit measles only
k. Delay by 2 months

*For each presentation below, choose the **correct answer** from the above list of options. Each option may be used once, more than once, or not at all.*

QUESTIONS

41. Child who is HIV positive is due for MMR.
42. Child due for Hib, DPT, etc. suffering from acute febrile illness.
43. Child cried for 2 hours after Hib, DPT, etc.
44. Family history of egg allergy. Child due for MMR.
45. History of convulsions. Child due for Hib, DPT, etc.

THEME 10: INVESTIGATIONS IN POSTOPERATIVE PATIENTS

OPTIONS

a. Pulse oximetry
b. Wound swab
c. V/Q scan
d. ECG
e. Ultrasound abdomen + pelvis
f. Coronary angiogram
g. Serum urea, electrolytes
h. Blood culture
i. MSU
j. Chest X-ray

*For each presentation below, choose the **correct answer** from the above list of options. Each option may be used once, more than once, or not at all.*

QUESTIONS

46. Woman after open cholecystectomy presents with fever, redness, tenderness of wound.
47. Chronic smoker 1 day after splenectomy presents with chest pain and dyspnoea.
48. Female after anterior resection of rectum complains of anterior chest pain radiating to her left arm.
49. Man with COPD presents with central cyanosis.
50. Man after appendicectomy presents with spiking fever with rigors, tenesmus, diarrhoea.

THEME 11: CONTRACEPTION

OPTIONS
a. Condoms
b. COCP
c. POPs
d. OCPs + condom
e. Depovera
f. Mirena coil
g. Diaphragm
h. IUCD
i. Abstinence

*For each presentation below, choose the **best answer** from the above list of options. Each option may be used once, more than once, or not at all.*

QUESTIONS

51. A 14-year-old girl has just started having sexual relationship with her boyfriend of 2 months.
52. A 35-year-old female after her third child wants reliable contraception. She is a smoker and does not want to gain weight.
53. An 18-year-old girl has been on OCPs since 2 years, has to have rifampicin prophylaxis since her roommate has meningitis.
54. Girl with learning disorder begins to find males attractive. Her parents and teachers are worried.
55. Female after her first child wants reliable contraception but wants no chemicals in her body, complains of heavy periods and dysmenorrhoea, husband does not want to use condoms.

THEME 12: DEMENTIA DIAGNOSIS

OPTIONS
a. Alzheimer's
b. Multi infarct
c. Lewy body
d. Pseudodementia
e. Frontal dementia
f. CJD
g. Alcoholic dementia

*For each presentation below, choose the **single most likely diagnosis** from the above list of options. Each option may be used once, more than once, or not at all.*

QUESTIONS

56. Most common form of dementia in the UK.
57. Characterised by neurofibrillary tangles and senile plaques.
58. May respond to antidepressants.
59. Increased disinhibition, preservation of intellect
60. An elderly hypertensive with recurrent faints presents with deteriorating mental functions.

THEME 13: SIDE EFFECTS OF ANTIPSYCHOTIC DRUGS

OPTIONS
a. Chlorpromazine
b. Phenelezine
c. Lithium
d. Fluoxetine
e. Haloperidol
f. Amitryptyline
g. Clozapine

For each presentation below, choose the ***correct answer*** *from the above list of options. Each option may be used once, more than once, or not at all.*

QUESTIONS

61. A schizophrenic on long-term treatment complains of impotence, has high prolactin levels, extrapyramidal side effects.
62. Drug with anticholinergic side effects, dry mouth, blurred vision, tremor.
63. Patient on treatment for bipolar disorder, hypothyroidism features.
64. Schizophrenic patient under treatment presents with sore throat, decreased WBC, agranulocytosis.
65. Schizophrenic patient under treatment presents with fever, increased WBC, increased muscle creatinine kinase levels.

THEME 14: DEMENTIA DIAGNOSIS

OPTIONS
a. Alzheimer's
b. Delirium
c. Depression
d. Late onset schizophrenia
e. Frontal dementia
f. Chronic anxiety state
g. Vascular dementia

For each presentation below, choose the ***most likely diagnosis*** *from the above list of options. Each option may be used once, more than once, or not at all.*

QUESTIONS

66. Man living in a hostel, brought to hospital after he collapsed. On the 3rd day, he points out things other people cannot see, disorientation in time and place.
67. An 80-year-old female is on no medication. Cause of concern is that she was trying to get into a shop at 6:00 AM. Neighbours say she is ok except her memory is not as good as it used to be since 2 years. She is otherwise well.
68. Female brings her husband to A and E, says he talks about their sex life in public. There is loss of inhibition, (intellect normal) in him.
69. Man has cough and fever since 2 days. Wife notices he has disorientation in time and place, decreased concentration and confused. He was ok mentally 1 day before.
70. A 70-year-old man says his life is not worth living, his existence is a waste, he performs all his work very slowly, he has lost weight.

THEME 15: DIAGNOSIS IN TRAUMA PATIENTS

OPTIONS

a. Aortic rupture
b. Splenic rupture
c. Diaphragmatic rupture
d. Cardiac tamponade
e. Renal contusion
f. Renal pedicle avulsion
g. Bladder rupture
h. Pancreatic rupture
i. Tension pneumothorax

For each presentation below, choose the ***most likely diagnosis*** *from the above list of options. Each option may be used once, more than once, or not at all.*

QUESTIONS

71. Boy was riding his bicycle when he was hit by a car. After examination in A and E, he was found to have left upper quadrant tenderness. He is pale.
72. Man fell off a ladder, has diffuse pain on right side of the trunk. IVU shows no excretion on right side.
73. Man was stabbed with a 10 cm knife in the left upper quadrant, stable for 20 min after which BP falls to 90/60 mmHg. On ultrasound, no free fluid seen in abdomen.
74. Known asthmatic patient involved in road traffic accident (RTA). Has a right-sided chest pain. On auscultation right side is hyper-resonant. Trachea is deviated to the left.
75. A 19-year-old girl has fallen off her horse. Neck is immobilised + 100% oxygen. Has left upper abdominal pain, is pale and tachycardiac.

THEME 16: CRANIAL NERVE PALSIES

OPTIONS

a. I cranial nerve
b. II cranial nerve
c. III cranial nerve
d. IV cranial nerve
e. V cranial nerve
f. VI cranial nerve
g. VII cranial nerve
h. VIII cranial nerve
i. IX cranial nerve
j. X cranial nerve
k. XI cranial nerve
l. XII cranial nerve

For each presentation below, choose the ***correct answer*** *from the above list of options. Each option may be used once, more than once, or not at all.*

QUESTIONS

76. Fracture of anterior cranial fossa, rhinorrhoea, anosmia.
77. Cavernous sinus affected, pupil not responding to light and accommodation, ptosis present.
78. After head trauma, patient cannot shrug his shoulder.
79. Forehead sparing, lower face no voluntary movements. Involuntary movements possible.
80. Fracture of base of skull, loss of taste in anterior two-thirds of tongue, deviation of angle of mouth.

THEME 17: MANAGEMENT OF FRACTURES

OPTIONS

a. Strapping and discharge
b. Strapping and review in hospital
c. Urgent orthopaedic referral
d. X-ray wrist including oblique scaphoid view
e. Isotope scan of the wrist

For each presentation below, choose the ***most appropriate step in management*** *from the above list of options. Each option may be used once, more than once, or not at all.*

QUESTIONS

81. A 16-year-old boy falls from a tree. Complains of pain in left anatomical fossa. X-rays are normal.
82. Man falls on hand. X-ray shows perilunate dislocation.
83. A 43-year-old man after a fall, pain in anatomical snuff box and X-ray shows impacted distal radius fracture.
84. Man falls on hand, pain in anatomical fossa.
85. Young girl tripped while holding mother's hand. Now cannot use arm at all.

THEME 18: CHILD CARE

OPTIONS

a. Child protection conference
b. Nutritional assessment
c. CT skull
d. Skeletal survey
e. Coagulation profile
f. Continue regular health care
g. Examine under anaesthesia
h. High vaginal swab
i. Gluten free diet

For each presentation below, choose the ***correct answer*** *from the above list of options. Each option may be used once, more than once, or not at all.*

QUESTIONS

86. A 12-month-old child of unemployed parents, did not gain weight from 6 months.
87. Child brought to A and E, age 6 months, swollen thigh, X-ray shows transverse fracture of shaft of femur.
88. A nine-year-old female child with itching, sore vagina, perineum is red and excoriated.
89. An 18-year-old female brings her baby unconscious to A and E, cyanosed, dilated fixed left pupil.
90. Child with forearm bruise, brought by teacher, Mom says she held her to prevent her from running across the road.

THEME 19: DIAGNOSIS OF CONFUSION

OPTIONS

a. Schizophrenia
b. Substance abuse
c. Opiate abuse
d. Opiate withdrawal
e. Generalised tonic clonic seizure
f. Panic attack

*For each presentation below, choose the **single most likely diagnosis** from the above list of options. Each option may be used once, more than once, or not at all.*

QUESTIONS

91. A 40-year-old lady stops talking suddenly, says someone took away her thoughts.
92. A 17-year-old girl comes anxious and tearful to A and E. She is unkept and dishevelled, says she lost her medication, says she aches all over and demand immediate pain relief.
93. Unconscious boy with pinpoint pupils, respiratory rate 4/min.
94. Boy brought by his friend to the A and E. History of suddenly falling to the ground, jerky movements, urine incontinence. He is confused now but neurological examination is normal.
95. A 20-year-old woman attends A and E complaining of sudden breathlessness and anxiety. She describes palpitations and paraesthesiae of her hands, feet and lips. ECG shows sinus tachycardia and O_2 saturation is normal.

THEME 20: MANAGEMENT OF ECZEMA

OPTIONS

a. Emollient with 1% hydrocortisone
b. Emollient with 3% beclomethasone
c. Admit in hospital
d. Oral antihistamine
e. Desensitisation
f. Oral prednisolone
g. Steroids and flucloxacillin
h. Breastfeeding
i. Emollient with 2.5% hydrocortisone
j. Psychiatric referral
k. None required

*For each presentation below, choose the **most appropriate management** from the above list of options. Each option may be used once, more than once, or not at all.*

QUESTIONS

96. A bottle-fed baby has developed flexural eczema. His brother has the same history. Family history of asthma. Mom is presently avoiding using soap.
97. Young girl with eczema, treated with emollient and topical hydrocortisone, did not get better.
98. Young girl with severe eczema, weeping vesicles, skin swab was taken, topical steroids did not work.
99. A 49-year-old woman complains of itchy blisters, which are occurring in groups on her knees and elbows. The itch is becoming unbearable and she is contemplating suicide. She responds to 180 mg of dapsone within 48 hours of treatment.
100. An 18-month-old baby, red swollen lips after eating egg. Presently under treatment with emollients and topical hydrocortisone three times a day.

THEME 21: INVESTIGATIONS OF INECTIOUS DISEASES

OPTIONS

a. Lyme disease serology
b. Leptospirosis serology
c. Viral serology
d. Wound swab
e. Lumbar puncture
f. MSU
g. LFTs [liver function tests]
h. Serum urea and electrolytes
i. Well-Felix test
j. Ultrasound abdomen
k. Blood culture

*For each presentation below, choose the **most appropriate investigation** from the above list of options. Each option may be used once, more than once, or not at all.*

QUESTIONS

101. Girl goes into a forest, remembers getting bitten by a tick, redness near the bite is slowly increasing in size.
102. A policeman bit on his hand by a heroin addict while arresting him. He comes to the A and E, on examination, a deep wound seen on his hand.
103. An 18-month-old baby, drowsy, febrile, headache, CT normal.
104. A chronic alcoholic presents with flapping tremors and confusion.
105. A 70-year-old woman, confusion, constipation, frequency of urine.

THEME 22: MECHANISMS OF HYPERTENSION

OPTIONS

a. Renal artery stenosis
b. Conn's syndrome
c. Cushing's syndrome
d. Chronic pyelonephritis
e. Phaeochromocytoma
f. Glomerulonephritis
g. Polycystic kidney disease
h. Acromegaly
i. Coarctation of aorta
j. Systemic sclerosis
k. Diabetic neuropathy

*For each presentation below, choose the **most likely cause of hypertension** from the above list of options. Each option may be used once, more than once, or not at all.*

QUESTIONS

106. Due to increased catecholamines.
107. Autosomal dominant.
108. Increased production of aldosterone.
109. Deposition of immune complexes on basement membrane.
110. A 17-year-old girl with hypertension of 160/100 is found to have a femoral pulse delay.

THEME 23: DIFFERENTIAL DIAGNOSIS OF HAEMOPTYSIS

OPTIONS

a. Bronchiectasis
b. TB (tuberculosis)
c. Inhaled foreign body
d. Pneumonia
e. Pulmonary embolism
f. Pulmonary oedema
g. Goodpasture's syndrome
h. Wegener's granulomatosis
i. Mitral stenosis
j. Hereditary haemorrhagic telaengiectasia
k. Coagulation disorders
l. Carcinoma of lung

*For each presentation below, choose the **most likely cause of haemoptysis** from the above list of options. Each option may be used once, more than once, or not at all.*

QUESTIONS

111. A 40-year-old man underwent removal of tooth under anaesthesia, presents after one month with coughing up of blood.
112. Female with cough, copious blood tinged sputum for more than a month. She is from south-east Asia.
113. Female presents with acute pleuritic chest pain, haemoptysis after undergoing hysterectomy.
114. A middle-aged woman develops a purulent cough with some haemoptysis. A chest X-ray reveals right upper lobe shadows.
115. A patient with an area of consolidation and fever on his chest X-ray is treated with antibiotics. His fever resolves but four weeks later he still has a large area of consolidation.

THEME 24: COMPLICATIONS OF MYOCARDIAL INFARCTION

OPTIONS

a. Papillary muscle rupture
b. Acute pericarditis
c. PE
d. Acute atrial fibrillation
e. Ventricular fibrillation
f. Congestive cardiac failure
g. Complete heart block
h. Ventricular free wall rupture
i. Ventricular aneurysm
j. Cardiac tamponade
k. Dressler's syndrome

*For each presentation below, choose the **most likely complication** from the above list of options. Each option may be used once, more than once, or not at all.*

QUESTIONS

116. Patient, 12 hours after MI presents with recurrent chest pain, breathlessness, heart rate—40/min.
117. Patient with pulmonary oedema features presents with irregular pulse, heart rate—140/bpm.
118. A woman 10 days following hysterectomy complains of severe left sided chest pain and breathlessness. Chest X-ray and ECG failed to relieve any abnormality.
119. Ten days after MI, female presents with chest pain on inspiration, persistently elevated ST segment on ECG.
120. Patient after MI found to have a harsh pansystolic murmur at the apex.

THEME 25: INVESTIGATIONS OF NEUROLOGICAL COMPLAINTS

OPTIONS

a. Carotid Doppler
b. MRI temporal lobe
c. MRI occipital lobe
d. CT scan
e. ESR
f. Echocardiography
g. MRI pituitary fossa
h. Skull X-ray
i. MRI cervical spine
j. MRI lumbar spine
k. Tensilon test

*For each presentation below, choose the **most appropriate investigation** from the above list of options. Each option may be used once, more than once, or not at all.*

QUESTIONS

121. Man with recurrent amaurosis fugax of right eye.
122. An elderly female with scalp tenderness on both sides of the head, complains of headache, sudden loss of vision in one eye.
123. A 40-year-old female comes with complaints of headache, bitemporal hemianopia, increase in shoe size.
124. Patient with attacks of numbness in left hand and right sided headache.
125. Patient gets diplopia when he works very hard.

THEME 26: INVESTIGATION OF COMPLICATIONS OF PROSTATIC CARCINOMA

OPTIONS

a. PSA
b. Serum acid phosphatase
c. Serum alkaline phosphatase
d. Transrectal ultrasound
e. Abdominal ultrasound
f. Serum calcium
g. Gallium scan
h. Technitium scan
i. Thallium scan
j. Transrectal biopsy
k. HLA status
l. Urodynamic studies

*For each presentation below, choose the **most appropriate investigation** from the above list of options. Each option may be used once, more than once, or not at all.*

QUESTIONS

126. An 80-year-old with prostatic carcinoma comes with 4 month history of low backache.
127. Patient with prostatic cancer has been treated, now complains of confusion, thirst, bodyaches, constipation.
128. Man on GnRHs for prostate cancer comes after 2 months for a follow-up.
129. Man with prostate carcinoma which has extended outside the capsule presenting with features of renal failure.
130. A man having adenocarcinoma prostate which has already spread to pelvic side walls has to be given chemotherapy.

THEME 27: DIAGNOSIS OF ALTERED BOWEL HABIT

OPTIONS

a. Irritable bowel syndrome
b. Inflammatory bowel disease
c. Acute gastroenteritis
d. Faecal impaction
e. Carcinoma colon
f. Diverticular disease
g. Diverticulitis

For each presentation below, choose the ***most likely diagnosis*** *from the above list of options. Each option may be used once, more than once, or not at all.*

QUESTIONS

131. An elderly female has history of uncontrollable loose stools many times a day. On examination, packed solid faeces in rectum.

132. A 30-year-old female has history of alternating constipation and diarrhoea for 7 months. She told that she is passing hard pellet like stools.

133. Female, 22-year-old, with bleeding and mucus per rectum, fever, loss of weight, has never been abroad.

134. An 80-year-old woman, fever 39 degrees centigrade, acute generalised abdominal pain, diarrhoea and vomiting, slightly dehydrated.

135. A 55-year-old man, history of altered bowel habit from 2 months, anaemia, loss of weight.

THEME 28: MANAGEMENT OF EPILEPSY

OPTIONS

a. EEG
b. CT skull
c. Add 2nd drug
d. Check drug levels
e. IV lorazepam
f. Give rectal diazepam to parents and teach them how to use it
g. Evaluate dose of drug

For each presentation below, choose the ***most appropriate management*** *from the above list of options. Each option may be used once, more than once, or not at all.*

QUESTIONS

136. A 4-year-old boy has fever since 2 days, presents with convulsions since 5 min, still convulsing in the ambulance, IV line has been established.

137. A 2-year-old boy with past and family history of febrile convulsions. He is ok now.

138. Young girl on Na valproate, parents come with complaints of increased seizure frequency and frequent absences from school. On examination, she is mildly obese.

139. A 12-year-old girl, one episode of grand mal seizure of 3 min duration in her sleep.

140. A 14-year-old girl has had been academically brilliant, lately has had difficult with her schoolwork. She has been caught day dreaming in class on a number of occasions.

THEME 29: DIAGNOSIS OF GYNAECOLOGICAL CONDITIONS

OPTIONS

a. Endometrial carcinoma
b. Cervical ectropion
c. Polycystic ovarian disease
d. Cervical carcinoma
e. Pregnancy
f. Hypothalamus related disorder
g. Trauma

For each presentation below, choose the ***most likely diagnosis*** *from the above list of options. Each option may be used once, more than once, or not at all.*

QUESTIONS

141. A 55-year-old lady with history of intermittent postmenopausal bleeding. Vaginal and speculum examinations are normal.

142. Young girl has put on weight, hirsutism, oligomenorrhoea

143. Female on OCPs complains of postcoital bleeding.

144. An 18-year-old university student with history of 3 months of amenorrhoea and starvation.

145. A woman on the contraceptive pill for several years has a slight whitish vaginal discharge. On inspection she is found to have a pinkish colouration of the outer cervix.

THEME 30: FEEDING

OPTIONS

a. PEG feeding (gastrostomy)
b. Nasogastric tube feeding
c. Parenteral feeding
d. Gluten free diet
e. Low protein diet
f. Low calorie diet
g. Lactose free diet

For each presentation below, choose the ***most appropriate feeding modality*** *from the above list of options. Each option may be used once, more than once, or not at all.*

QUESTIONS

146. Patient with long-standing Parkinson's disease with intractable dysphagia.

147. Patient after a stroke, 5 days later, fluids still being aspirated from stomach.

148. Man after large bowel resection and ileostomy is septicaemic.

149. Man with jaundice and ascites suddenly deteriorates.

150. Girl with diarrhoea and jejunal villous atrophy.

THEME 31: PAIN RELIEF

OPTIONS

a. NSAIDs
b. Methotrexate
c. Home exercises
d. Local steroid injection
e. Splinting
f. IV biphosphonates
g. Oral steroids
h. Physiotherapy
i. Exercise training

*For each presentation below, choose the **most appropriate way of pain relief** from the above list of options. Each option may be used once, more than once, or not at all.*

QUESTIONS

151. An elderly busy man with indigestion, acute pain lateral side of hip.

152. Patient with symmetrical polyarthritis, pain does not decrease with simple analgesia.

153. Patient with hot swollen MT joint, pain does not decrease with paracetamol.

154. Pregnant woman with numbness, tingling on lateral side of hand.

155. A 35-year-old woman treated one year ago for a breast cancer with 12/20 nodes positive, presents with a two days history of increasing confusion, She is drowsy and disoriented. Her husband reports that she has been complaining of severe thirst for the past week.

THEME 32: PALLIATIVE CARE

OPTIONS

a. Cyclizine
b. Haloperidal
c. Hyoscine
d. Oral dexamethasone
e. Oral beclamethasone
f. Per rectal predisolone
g. Metronidazole gel
h. Long-term catheterisation
i. Intermittent self-catheterisation

*For each presentation below, choose the **most appropriate palliative method** from the above list of options. Each option may be used once, more than once, or not at all.*

QUESTIONS

156. Patient with intractable hiccups.

157. Patient cannot cough up bronchial secretions. Noise is distressing to attendants.

158. Patient after radiotherapy for bowel adenocarcinoma comes with bright red rectal bleeding.

159. Patient with superior vena cava obstruction after radiotherapy.

160. Female with fungating breast carcinoma with a bad odour.

THEME 33: ANAEMIA INVESTIGATIONS

OPTIONS

a. Blood film for parasites
b. Serum B_{12}
c. Schilling test
d. Bone marrow biopsy
e. Serum/gel electrophoresis
f. Mesenteric angiogram

*For each presentation below, choose the **most appropriate investigation** from the above list of options. Each option may be used once, more than once, or not at all.*

QUESTIONS

161. A middle-aged man with hepatosplenomegaly, fatigue, immature cells seen in blood film.
162. Man returns from Ghana presents with fever with rigors.
163. A 60-year-old man presents with fatigue and backache with localised tenderness. He also has decreased visual acuity.
164. Old lady with Hb is 3g/dl, MCV is 120 fl, family history presents with fatigue, lethargy.
165. An elderly female with past history of rectal bleeding, normal on endoscopy and enema studies done previously presents with profuse fresh rectal bleeding.

THEME 34: MANAGEMENT OF GYNAECOLOGY CONDITIONS

OPTIONS

a. Vaginal estrogens
b. Infection control
c. Prophylactic antibiotic treatment
d. Ring pessary
e. High fibre diet
f. Surgery

*For each presentation below, choose the **most appropriate step in management** from the above list of options. Each option may be used once, more than once, or not at all.*

QUESTIONS

166. 85-year-old with 14 children, severe heart failure, complains of dysuria, feeling of pressure in lower abdomen.
167. Female with well-controlled diabetes mellitus type 2 with recurrent UTI.
168. A young female with long-standing irregular bowel habit and persistent UTI.
169. An 80-year-old sexually active woman with dyspareunia and recurrent dysuria.
170. A middle-aged woman with a vaginal discharge is found to have several ulcers at the vaginal introitus.

THEME 35: MANAGEMENT OF VARICOSE VEINS

OPTIONS

a. Injection sclerotherapy
b. Graded compression stockings
c. Operation for varicose veins
d. Reduce weight
e. Prophylactic anticoagulation

For each presentation below, choose the most appropriate management from the above list of options. Each option may be used once, more than once, or not at all.

QUESTIONS

171. Female with bilateral varicose veins, lipodermatosclerosis. She is using compression stockings. Despite that increase in itching and eczema. BMI is 27.

172. A 75-year-old, underwent 2 operations for varicose veins, presents with painful legs, has history of heart failure. On examination bilateral gross varicose veins, lipodermatosclerosis, no ulcers.

173. Female with BMI 33, comes with complaints of varicose veins and eczema.

174. Man with varicose veins has to fly for 20 hours . His father has a history of pulmonary embolism after flying.

175. A patient presents with a shallow ulcer, with no inrolled edges, situated over the medical malleolus. It has been reducing in size with compression bandaging. There is some evidence of lipodermatosclerosis and varicose veins in the distribution of the greater saphenous veins.

THEME 36: INVESTIGATIONS IN JAUNDICE

OPTIONS

a. Liver biopsy
b. Liver ultrasound
c. Oral cholecystography
d. Viral serology
e. ERCP
f. Percutaneous transhepatic cholangiography
g. Serum AMAs

For each presentation below, choose the ***most appropriate investigation*** *from the above list of options. Each option may be used once, more than once, or not at all.*

QUESTIONS

176. Man returned from trip to Asia, complains of anorexia, malaise, dark urine, pale stools.

177. An 80-year-old man has never been out of UK, one month history of epigastric pain, dark urine, pale stools, jaundice.

178. Female with fever, rigors, right upper quadrant pain, jaundice, ultrasound is normal.

179. Female, 50-year-old, 5 years history of mild pruritus. History of pale stools, dark urine, jaundice.

180. Man with history of haemochromatosis and alcohol addiction presents with jaundice, ascites, variceal bleed. USG is unequivocal, high ferritin level.

THEME 37: INVESTIGATION OF SCROTAL PAIN

OPTIONS

a. MSU
b. Urethral swab
c. Urgent surgical exploration
d. IVU
e. Ultrasound
f. Syphilis serology
g. Three glass test
h. CT scan
i. Laparoscopy
j. Testicular biopsy
k. None required

*For each presentation below, choose the **most appropriate investigation** from the above list of options. Each option may be used once, more than once, or not at all.*

QUESTIONS

181. Man after trip to Asia presents with red, swollen scrotum.
182. Man with painful red scrotum and vomiting.
183. Man with painless testicular swelling since 2 months.
184. Man with a swelling of scrotum since 3 years.
185. Man with no history of unsafe sex presents with dysuria and urinary frequency.

THEME 38: DIAGNOSIS OF ABDOMINAL CONDITIONS

OPTIONS

a. Acute pancreatitis
b. Chronic pancreatitis
c. *H. pylori* infection
d. Pernicious anaemia
e. Barrett's oesophagus
f. Prostatic carcinoma
g. Acute cholecystitis
h. Hepatitis
i. Chronic cholecystitis
j. Duodenal ulcer
k. Aplastic anaemia

*For each presentation below, choose the **most likely diagnosis** from the above list of options. Each option may be used once, more than once, or not at all.*

QUESTIONS

186. Condition that can cause necrosis, formation of fluid-filled spaces that can get infected.
187. Condition associated with gastroesophageal reflux, epithelial metaplasia, increased risk of carcinoma.
188. Condition associated with epigastric pain radiating to the back, pale loose stools, associated with alcohol consumption.
189. Condition associated with persistent inflammation, can cause lymphoma.
190. Condition associated with megaloblastic anaemia, increased risk of carcinoma.

THEME 39: DIFFERENTIAL DIAGNOSIS OF THYROID DISORDERS

OPTIONS

a. Anaplastic carcinoma
b. Follicular carcinoma
c. Papillary carcinoma
d. Hashimoto's thyroiditis
e. Thyrotoxic goitre
f. Autoimmune hypothyroidism
g. Drug-induced thyrotoxicosis
h. Graves' disease
i. Riedel's thyroiditis
j. de Quervain thyroiditis
k. Small bowel lymphoma

*For each presentation below, choose the **most likely diagnosis** from the above list of options. Each option may be used once, more than once, or not at all.*

QUESTIONS

191. Female, 41-year-old, presents with hard, irregular fixed swelling, stridor, dysphagia since 3 months.

192. Old lady with smooth neck swelling, bradycardia, spare coarse hair, macrocytic anaemia.

193. Female on treatment for supraventricular tachycardia complains of seeing dots and glare on driving at night, exophthalmos, no goitre.

194. Female, swelling in the neck, tremor irritability, diarrhoea, bruit.

195. A 35-year-old woman who was diagnosed as having coeliac disease at the age of 12 years has had good control of her abdominal symptoms for a number of years. She presents with a recent history of weight loss, tiredness, diarrhoea and abdominal pain.

THEME 40: COMPLICATIONS OF BREAST CARCINOMA

OPTIONS

a. Pathological fracture
b. Cerebral metastases
c. Hypocalcaemia
d. Lymphoedema
e. Spinal cord compression
f. Hypercalcaemia
g. Hyperparathyroidism

*For each presentation below, choose the **most common complication** from the above list of options. Each option may be used once, more than once, or not at all.*

QUESTIONS

196. Female with breast carcinoma 3 years back, was treated with mastectomy and lymph node clearance on the left side, presents with a swollen limb and decreased hand movements.

197. Presents with thirst, confusion, constipation.

198. Presents with weakness of both legs, difficulty walking, urine retention.

199. Presents with headache, confusion. On examination, papilloedema present.

200. Presents with features of fracture femur.

General Medical Council PLAB Test Part 1

Full Name

Test Centre/Date

- Use pencil only
- Make heavy marks that fill the lozenge completely
- Write your candidate number in the top row of the box to the right **AND** fill in the appropriate lozenge below each number
- Give **ONE** answer only for each question

0	0	0	0	0	0
1	1	1	1	1	1
2	2	2	2	2	2
3	3	3	3	3	3
4	4	4	4	4	4
5	5	5	5	5	5
6	6	6	6	6	6
7	7	7	7	7	7
8	8	8	8	8	8
9	9	9	9	9	9

1	A	B	C	D	E	F	G	H	I	J	K	L	M	N	O	P	Q	R	S	T	1
2	A	B	C	D	E	F	G	H	I	J	K	L	M	N	O	P	Q	R	S	T	2
3	A	B	C	D	E	F	G	H	I	J	K	L	M	N	O	P	Q	R	S	T	3
4	A	B	C	D	E	F	G	H	I	J	K	L	M	N	O	P	Q	R	S	T	4
5	A	B	C	D	E	F	G	H	I	J	K	L	M	N	O	P	Q	R	S	T	5
6	A	B	C	D	E	F	G	H	I	J	K	L	M	N	O	P	Q	R	S	T	6
7	A	B	C	D	E	F	G	H	I	J	K	L	M	N	O	P	Q	R	S	T	7
8	A	B	C	D	E	F	G	H	I	J	K	L	M	N	O	P	Q	R	S	T	8
9	A	B	C	D	E	F	G	H	I	J	K	L	M	N	O	P	Q	R	S	T	9
10	A	B	C	D	E	F	G	H	I	J	K	L	M	N	O	P	Q	R	S	T	10
11	A	B	C	D	E	F	G	H	I	J	K	L	M	N	O	P	Q	R	S	T	11
12	A	B	C	D	E	F	G	H	I	J	K	L	M	N	O	P	Q	R	S	T	12
13	A	B	C	D	E	F	G	H	I	J	K	L	M	N	O	P	Q	R	S	T	13
14	A	B	C	D	E	F	G	H	I	J	K	L	M	N	O	P	Q	R	S	T	14
15	A	B	C	D	E	F	G	H	I	J	K	L	M	N	O	P	Q	R	S	T	15
16	A	B	C	D	E	F	G	H	I	J	K	L	M	N	O	P	Q	R	S	T	16
17	A	B	C	D	E	F	G	H	I	J	K	L	M	N	O	P	Q	R	S	T	17
18	A	B	C	D	E	F	G	H	I	J	K	L	M	N	O	P	Q	R	S	T	18
19	A	B	C	D	E	F	G	H	I	J	K	L	M	N	O	P	Q	R	S	T	19
20	A	B	C	D	E	F	G	H	I	J	K	L	M	N	O	P	Q	R	S	T	20
21	A	B	C	D	E	F	G	H	I	J	K	L	M	N	O	P	Q	R	S	T	21
22	A	B	C	D	E	F	G	H	I	J	K	L	M	N	O	P	Q	R	S	T	22
23	A	B	C	D	E	F	G	H	I	J	K	L	M	N	O	P	Q	R	S	T	23
24	A	B	C	D	E	F	G	H	I	J	K	L	M	N	O	P	Q	R	S	T	24
25	A	B	C	D	E	F	G	H	I	J	K	L	M	N	O	P	Q	R	S	T	25
26	A	B	C	D	E	F	G	H	I	J	K	L	M	N	O	P	Q	R	S	T	26
27	A	B	C	D	E	F	G	H	I	J	K	L	M	N	O	P	Q	R	S	T	27
28	A	B	C	D	E	F	G	H	I	J	K	L	M	N	O	P	Q	R	S	T	28
29	A	B	C	D	E	F	G	H	I	J	K	L	M	N	O	P	Q	R	S	T	29
30	A	B	C	D	E	F	G	H	I	J	K	L	M	N	O	P	Q	R	S	T	30
31	A	B	C	D	E	F	G	H	I	J	K	L	M	N	O	P	Q	R	S	T	31
32	A	B	C	D	E	F	G	H	I	J	K	L	M	N	O	P	Q	R	S	T	32
33	A	B	C	D	E	F	G	H	I	J	K	L	M	N	O	P	Q	R	S	T	33
34	A	B	C	D	E	F	G	H	I	J	K	L	M	N	O	P	Q	R	S	T	34
35	A	B	C	D	E	F	G	H	I	J	K	L	M	N	O	P	Q	R	S	T	35
36	A	B	C	D	E	F	G	H	I	J	K	L	M	N	O	P	Q	R	S	T	36
37	A	B	C	D	E	F	G	H	I	J	K	L	M	N	O	P	Q	R	S	T	37
38	A	B	C	D	E	F	G	H	I	J	K	L	M	N	O	P	Q	R	S	T	38
39	A	B	C	D	E	F	G	H	I	J	K	L	M	N	O	P	Q	R	S	T	39
40	A	B	C	D	E	F	G	H	I	J	K	L	M	N	O	P	Q	R	S	T	40
41	A	B	C	D	E	F	G	H	I	J	K	L	M	N	O	P	Q	R	S	T	41
42	A	B	C	D	E	F	G	H	I	J	K	L	M	N	O	P	Q	R	S	T	42
43	A	B	C	D	E	F	G	H	I	J	K	L	M	N	O	P	Q	R	S	T	43
44	A	B	C	D	E	F	G	H	I	J	K	L	M	N	O	P	Q	R	S	T	44
45	A	B	C	D	E	F	G	H	I	J	K	L	M	N	O	P	Q	R	S	T	45
46	A	B	C	D	E	F	G	H	I	J	K	L	M	N	O	P	Q	R	S	T	46
47	A	B	C	D	E	F	G	H	I	J	K	L	M	N	O	P	Q	R	S	T	47
48	A	B	C	D	E	F	G	H	I	J	K	L	M	N	O	P	Q	R	S	T	48
49	A	B	C	D	E	F	G	H	I	J	K	L	M	N	O	P	Q	R	S	T	49
50	A	B	C	D	E	F	G	H	I	J	K	L	M	N	O	P	Q	R	S	T	50

DO NOT WRITE IN THIS SPACE

51	A	B	C	D	E	F	G	H	I	J	K	L	M	N	O	P	Q	R	S	T	51
52	A	B	C	D	E	F	G	H	I	J	K	L	M	N	O	P	Q	R	S	T	52
53	A	B	C	D	E	F	G	H	I	J	K	L	M	N	O	P	Q	R	S	T	53
54	A	B	C	D	E	F	G	H	I	J	K	L	M	N	O	P	Q	R	S	T	54
55	A	B	C	D	E	F	G	H	I	J	K	L	M	N	O	P	Q	R	S	T	55
56	A	B	C	D	E	F	G	H	I	J	K	L	M	N	O	P	Q	R	S	T	56
57	A	B	C	D	E	F	G	H	I	J	K	L	M	N	O	P	Q	R	S	T	57
58	A	B	C	D	E	F	G	H	I	J	K	L	M	N	O	P	Q	R	S	T	58
59	A	B	C	D	E	F	G	H	I	J	K	L	M	N	O	P	Q	R	S	T	59
60	A	B	C	D	E	F	G	H	I	J	K	L	M	N	O	P	Q	R	S	T	60
61	A	B	C	D	E	F	G	H	I	J	K	L	M	N	O	P	Q	R	S	T	61
62	A	B	C	D	E	F	G	H	I	J	K	L	M	N	O	P	Q	R	S	T	62
63	A	B	C	D	E	F	G	H	I	J	K	L	M	N	O	P	Q	R	S	T	63
64	A	B	C	D	E	F	G	H	I	J	K	L	M	N	O	P	Q	R	S	T	64
65	A	B	C	D	E	F	G	H	I	J	K	L	M	N	O	P	Q	R	S	T	65
66	A	B	C	D	E	F	G	H	I	J	K	L	M	N	O	P	Q	R	S	T	66
67	A	B	C	D	E	F	G	H	I	J	K	L	M	N	O	P	Q	R	S	T	67
68	A	B	C	D	E	F	G	H	I	J	K	L	M	N	O	P	Q	R	S	T	68
69	A	B	C	D	E	F	G	H	I	J	K	L	M	N	O	P	Q	R	S	T	69
70	A	B	C	D	E	F	G	H	I	J	K	L	M	N	O	P	Q	R	S	T	70
71	A	B	C	D	E	F	G	H	I	J	K	L	M	N	O	P	Q	R	S	T	71
72	A	B	C	D	E	F	G	H	I	J	K	L	M	N	O	P	Q	R	S	T	72
73	A	B	C	D	E	F	G	H	I	J	K	L	M	N	O	P	Q	R	S	T	73
74	A	B	C	D	E	F	G	H	I	J	K	L	M	N	O	P	Q	R	S	T	74
75	A	B	C	D	E	F	G	H	I	J	K	L	M	N	O	P	Q	R	S	T	75
76	A	B	C	D	E	F	G	H	I	J	K	L	M	N	O	P	Q	R	S	T	76
77	A	B	C	D	E	F	G	H	I	J	K	L	M	N	O	P	Q	R	S	T	77
78	A	B	C	D	E	F	G	H	I	J	K	L	M	N	O	P	Q	R	S	T	78
79	A	B	C	D	E	F	G	H	I	J	K	L	M	N	O	P	Q	R	S	T	79
80	A	B	C	D	E	F	G	H	I	J	K	L	M	N	O	P	Q	R	S	T	80
81	A	B	C	D	E	F	G	H	I	J	K	L	M	N	O	P	Q	R	S	T	81
82	A	B	C	D	E	F	G	H	I	J	K	L	M	N	O	P	Q	R	S	T	82
83	A	B	C	D	E	F	G	H	I	J	K	L	M	N	O	P	Q	R	S	T	83
84	A	B	C	D	E	F	G	H	I	J	K	L	M	N	O	P	Q	R	S	T	84
85	A	B	C	D	E	F	G	H	I	J	K	L	M	N	O	P	Q	R	S	T	85
86	A	B	C	D	E	F	G	H	I	J	K	L	M	N	O	P	Q	R	S	T	86
87	A	B	C	D	E	F	G	H	I	J	K	L	M	N	O	P	Q	R	S	T	87
88	A	B	C	D	E	F	G	H	I	J	K	L	M	N	O	P	Q	R	S	T	88
89	A	B	C	D	E	F	G	H	I	J	K	L	M	N	O	P	Q	R	S	T	89
90	A	B	C	D	E	F	G	H	I	J	K	L	M	N	O	P	Q	R	S	T	90
91	A	B	C	D	E	F	G	H	I	J	K	L	M	N	O	P	Q	R	S	T	91
92	A	B	C	D	E	F	G	H	I	J	K	L	M	N	O	P	Q	R	S	T	92
93	A	B	C	D	E	F	G	H	I	J	K	L	M	N	O	P	Q	R	S	T	93
94	A	B	C	D	E	F	G	H	I	J	K	L	M	N	O	P	Q	R	S	T	94
95	A	B	C	D	E	F	G	H	I	J	K	L	M	N	O	P	Q	R	S	T	95
96	A	B	C	D	E	F	G	H	I	J	K	L	M	N	O	P	Q	R	S	T	96
97	A	B	C	D	E	F	G	H	I	J	K	L	M	N	O	P	Q	R	S	T	97
98	A	B	C	D	E	F	G	H	I	J	K	L	M	N	O	P	Q	R	S	T	98
99	A	B	C	D	E	F	G	H	I	J	K	L	M	N	O	P	Q	R	S	T	99
100	A	B	C	D	E	F	G	H	I	J	K	L	M	N	O	P	Q	R	S	T	100

DO NOT WRITE IN THIS SPACE

101	A	B	C	D	E	F	G	H	I	J	K	L	M	N	O	P	Q	R	S	T	101
102	A	B	C	D	E	F	G	H	I	J	K	L	M	N	O	P	Q	R	S	T	102
103	A	B	C	D	E	F	G	H	I	J	K	L	M	N	O	P	Q	R	S	T	103
104	A	B	C	D	E	F	G	H	I	J	K	L	M	N	O	P	Q	R	S	T	104
105	A	B	C	D	E	F	G	H	I	J	K	L	M	N	O	P	Q	R	S	T	105
106	A	B	C	D	E	F	G	H	I	J	K	L	M	N	O	P	Q	R	S	T	106
107	A	B	C	D	E	F	G	H	I	J	K	L	M	N	O	P	Q	R	S	T	107
108	A	B	C	D	E	F	G	H	I	J	K	L	M	N	O	P	Q	R	S	T	108
109	A	B	C	D	E	F	G	H	I	J	K	L	M	N	O	P	Q	R	S	T	109
110	A	B	C	D	E	F	G	H	I	J	K	L	M	N	O	P	Q	R	S	T	110
111	A	B	C	D	E	F	G	H	I	J	K	L	M	N	O	P	Q	R	S	T	111
112	A	B	C	D	E	F	G	H	I	J	K	L	M	N	O	P	Q	R	S	T	112
113	A	B	C	D	E	F	G	H	I	J	K	L	M	N	O	P	Q	R	S	T	113
114	A	B	C	D	E	F	G	H	I	J	K	L	M	N	O	P	Q	R	S	T	114
115	A	B	C	D	E	F	G	H	I	J	K	L	M	N	O	P	Q	R	S	T	115
116	A	B	C	D	E	F	G	H	I	J	K	L	M	N	O	P	Q	R	S	T	116
117	A	B	C	D	E	F	G	H	I	J	K	L	M	N	O	P	Q	R	S	T	117
118	A	B	C	D	E	F	G	H	I	J	K	L	M	N	O	P	Q	R	S	T	118
119	A	B	C	D	E	F	G	H	I	J	K	L	M	N	O	P	Q	R	S	T	119
120	A	B	C	D	E	F	G	H	I	J	K	L	M	N	O	P	Q	R	S	T	120
121	A	B	C	D	E	F	G	H	I	J	K	L	M	N	O	P	Q	R	S	T	121
122	A	B	C	D	E	F	G	H	I	J	K	L	M	N	O	P	Q	R	S	T	122
123	A	B	C	D	E	F	G	H	I	J	K	L	M	N	O	P	Q	R	S	T	123
124	A	B	C	D	E	F	G	H	I	J	K	L	M	N	O	P	Q	R	S	T	124
125	A	B	C	D	E	F	G	H	I	J	K	L	M	N	O	P	Q	R	S	T	125
126	A	B	C	D	E	F	G	H	I	J	K	L	M	N	O	P	Q	R	S	T	126
127	A	B	C	D	E	F	G	H	I	J	K	L	M	N	O	P	Q	R	S	T	127
128	A	B	C	D	E	F	G	H	I	J	K	L	M	N	O	P	Q	R	S	T	128
129	A	B	C	D	E	F	G	H	I	J	K	L	M	N	O	P	Q	R	S	T	129
130	A	B	C	D	E	F	G	H	I	J	K	L	M	N	O	P	Q	R	S	T	130
131	A	B	C	D	E	F	G	H	I	J	K	L	M	N	O	P	Q	R	S	T	131
132	A	B	C	D	E	F	G	H	I	J	K	L	M	N	O	P	Q	R	S	T	132
133	A	B	C	D	E	F	G	H	I	J	K	L	M	N	O	P	Q	R	S	T	133
134	A	B	C	D	E	F	G	H	I	J	K	L	M	N	O	P	Q	R	S	T	134
135	A	B	C	D	E	F	G	H	I	J	K	L	M	N	O	P	Q	R	S	T	135
136	A	B	C	D	E	F	G	H	I	J	K	L	M	N	O	P	Q	R	S	T	136
137	A	B	C	D	E	F	G	H	I	J	K	L	M	N	O	P	Q	R	S	T	137
138	A	B	C	D	E	F	G	H	I	J	K	L	M	N	O	P	Q	R	S	T	138
139	A	B	C	D	E	F	G	H	I	J	K	L	M	N	O	P	Q	R	S	T	139
140	A	B	C	D	E	F	G	H	I	J	K	L	M	N	O	P	Q	R	S	T	140
141	A	B	C	D	E	F	G	H	I	J	K	L	M	N	O	P	Q	R	S	T	141
142	A	B	C	D	E	F	G	H	I	J	K	L	M	N	O	P	Q	R	S	T	142
143	A	B	C	D	E	F	G	H	I	J	K	L	M	N	O	P	Q	R	S	T	143
144	A	B	C	D	E	F	G	H	I	J	K	L	M	N	O	P	Q	R	S	T	144
145	A	B	C	D	E	F	G	H	I	J	K	L	M	N	O	P	Q	R	S	T	145
146	A	B	C	D	E	F	G	H	I	J	K	L	M	N	O	P	Q	R	S	T	146
147	A	B	C	D	E	F	G	H	I	J	K	L	M	N	O	P	Q	R	S	T	147
148	A	B	C	D	E	F	G	H	I	J	K	L	M	N	O	P	Q	R	S	T	148
149	A	B	C	D	E	F	G	H	I	J	K	L	M	N	O	P	Q	R	S	T	149
150	A	B	C	D	E	F	G	H	I	J	K	L	M	N	O	P	Q	R	S	T	150

DO NOT WRITE IN THIS SPACE

151	A	B	C	D	E	F	G	H	I	J	K	L	M	N	O	P	Q	R	S	T	151
152	A	B	C	D	E	F	G	H	I	J	K	L	M	N	O	P	Q	R	S	T	152
153	A	B	C	D	E	F	G	H	I	J	K	L	M	N	O	P	Q	R	S	T	153
154	A	B	C	D	E	F	G	H	I	J	K	L	M	N	O	P	Q	R	S	T	154
155	A	B	C	D	E	F	G	H	I	J	K	L	M	N	O	P	Q	R	S	T	155
156	A	B	C	D	E	F	G	H	I	J	K	L	M	N	O	P	Q	R	S	T	156
157	A	B	C	D	E	F	G	H	I	J	K	L	M	N	O	P	Q	R	S	T	157
158	A	B	C	D	E	F	G	H	I	J	K	L	M	N	O	P	Q	R	S	T	158
159	A	B	C	D	E	F	G	H	I	J	K	L	M	N	O	P	Q	R	S	T	159
160	A	B	C	D	E	F	G	H	I	J	K	L	M	N	O	P	Q	R	S	T	160
161	A	B	C	D	E	F	G	H	I	J	K	L	M	N	O	P	Q	R	S	T	161
162	A	B	C	D	E	F	G	H	I	J	K	L	M	N	O	P	Q	R	S	T	162
163	A	B	C	D	E	F	G	H	I	J	K	L	M	N	O	P	Q	R	S	T	163
164	A	B	C	D	E	F	G	H	I	J	K	L	M	N	O	P	Q	R	S	T	164
165	A	B	C	D	E	F	G	H	I	J	K	L	M	N	O	P	Q	R	S	T	165
166	A	B	C	D	E	F	G	H	I	J	K	L	M	N	O	P	Q	R	S	T	166
167	A	B	C	D	E	F	G	H	I	J	K	L	M	N	O	P	Q	R	S	T	167
168	A	B	C	D	E	F	G	H	I	J	K	L	M	N	O	P	Q	R	S	T	168
169	A	B	C	D	E	F	G	H	I	J	K	L	M	N	O	P	Q	R	S	T	169
170	A	B	C	D	E	F	G	H	I	J	K	L	M	N	O	P	Q	R	S	T	170
171	A	B	C	D	E	F	G	H	I	J	K	L	M	N	O	P	Q	R	S	T	171
172	A	B	C	D	E	F	G	H	I	J	K	L	M	N	O	P	Q	R	S	T	172
173	A	B	C	D	E	F	G	H	I	J	K	L	M	N	O	P	Q	R	S	T	173
174	A	B	C	D	E	F	G	H	I	J	K	L	M	N	O	P	Q	R	S	T	174
175	A	B	C	D	E	F	G	H	I	J	K	L	M	N	O	P	Q	R	S	T	175
176	A	B	C	D	E	F	G	H	I	J	K	L	M	N	O	P	Q	R	S	T	176
177	A	B	C	D	E	F	G	H	I	J	K	L	M	N	O	P	Q	R	S	T	177
178	A	B	C	D	E	F	G	H	I	J	K	L	M	N	O	P	Q	R	S	T	178
179	A	B	C	D	E	F	G	H	I	J	K	L	M	N	O	P	Q	R	S	T	179
180	A	B	C	D	E	F	G	H	I	J	K	L	M	N	O	P	Q	R	S	T	180
181	A	B	C	D	E	F	G	H	I	J	K	L	M	N	O	P	Q	R	S	T	181
182	A	B	C	D	E	F	G	H	I	J	K	L	M	N	O	P	Q	R	S	T	182
183	A	B	C	D	E	F	G	H	I	J	K	L	M	N	O	P	Q	R	S	T	183
184	A	B	C	D	E	F	G	H	I	J	K	L	M	N	O	P	Q	R	S	T	184
185	A	B	C	D	E	F	G	H	I	J	K	L	M	N	O	P	Q	R	S	T	185
186	A	B	C	D	E	F	G	H	I	J	K	L	M	N	O	P	Q	R	S	T	186
187	A	B	C	D	E	F	G	H	I	J	K	L	M	N	O	P	Q	R	S	T	187
188	A	B	C	D	E	F	G	H	I	J	K	L	M	N	O	P	Q	R	S	T	188
189	A	B	C	D	E	F	G	H	I	J	K	L	M	N	O	P	Q	R	S	T	189
190	A	B	C	D	E	F	G	H	I	J	K	L	M	N	O	P	Q	R	S	T	190
191	A	B	C	D	E	F	G	H	I	J	K	L	M	N	O	P	Q	R	S	T	191
192	A	B	C	D	E	F	G	H	I	J	K	L	M	N	O	P	Q	R	S	T	192
193	A	B	C	D	E	F	G	H	I	J	K	L	M	N	O	P	Q	R	S	T	193
194	A	B	C	D	E	F	G	H	I	J	K	L	M	N	O	P	Q	R	S	T	194
195	A	B	C	D	E	F	G	H	I	J	K	L	M	N	O	P	Q	R	S	T	195
196	A	B	C	D	E	F	G	H	I	J	K	L	M	N	O	P	Q	R	S	T	196
197	A	B	C	D	E	F	G	H	I	J	K	L	M	N	O	P	Q	R	S	T	197
198	A	B	C	D	E	F	G	H	I	J	K	L	M	N	O	P	Q	R	S	T	198
199	A	B	C	D	E	F	G	H	I	J	K	L	M	N	O	P	Q	R	S	T	199
200	A	B	C	D	E	F	G	H	I	J	K	L	M	N	O	P	Q	R	S	T	200

Answers

Serial No.	Answer No.	Answer
1	f	Ototoxicity
2	d	Wax impaction
3	a	Acoustic neuroma
4	c	Petrous temporal bone fracture
5	j	Herpes zoster
6	d	ORF
7	e	Nasal perforation
8	g	Anticoagulant overdose
9	b	Carcinoma of maxillary antrum
10	j	Hypertension
11	c	Salbutamol
12	a	Impratropium bromide
13	b	Amoxycillin
14	d	Doxapram
15	f	Trimethoprim
16	b	Inhaled short-acting β_2-agonist
17	j	Beta-blockers
18	a	Nabulised β_2-agonist
19	c	Inhaled long-acting β_2-agonist
20	g	Na cromoglycate
21	b	Metabolic alkalosis
22	c	Renal failure
23	e	Hypokalaemia
24	d	Fluid overload
25	e	Hypokalaemia
26	a	Subdural haematoma
27	b	Extradural haematoma
28	c	Mild injury
29	d	Moderate injury
30	e	Fracture base of skull
31	b	Blood glucose
32	a	CT skull
33	c	Lumbar puncture
34	a	CT skull
35	g	Toxicology screen
36	e	Anaesthesia and intubation
37	b	IV opioid
38	d	Escharotomy
39	l	IV fluids + referral for admission to burns unit
40	g	Reassure
41	d	Continue as her schedule
42	a	Delay by 2 weeks
43	d	Continue as per schedule
44	d	Continue as per schedule
45	d	Continue as per schedule
46	b	Wound swab
47	a/j	Chest X-ray/pulse oximetry
48	d	ECG
49	a	Pulse oximetry
50	e	USG abdomen + pelvis
51	d	OCP + Condom
52	h	IUCD
53	d	OCP+Condom
54	e	Depovera
55	f	Mirena coil
56	a	Alzheimer's
57	a	Alzheimer's
58	d	Pseudodementia
59	e	Frontal dementia

60	b	Multi infarct
61	a	Chlorpromazine
62	f	Amitryptyline
63	c	Lithium
64	g	Clozapine
65	e	Haloperidol
66	b	Delirium
67	a	Alzheimer's
68	e	Frontal dementia
69	b	Delirium
70	c	Depression
71	b	Splenic rupture
72	f	Renal pedicle avulsion
73	d	Cardiac tamponade
74	i	Tension pneumothorax
75	b	Splenic rupture
76	a	I cranial nerve
77	c	III cranial nerve
78	k	XI cranial nerve
79	g	VII cranial nerve
80	g	VII cranial nerve
81	e	Isotope scan
82	c	Urgent orthopaedic referral
83	c	Urgent orthopaedic referral
84	d	X-ray wrist including oblique view of scaphoid
85	c	Urgent orthopaedic referral
86	b	Nutritional assessment
87	d	Skeletal surgery
88	g	Examine under anaesthesia
89	c	CT skull
90	e	Coagulation profile
91	a	Schizophrenia
92	d	Opiate withdrawl
93	c	Opiate abuse
94	e	GTCS
95	f	Panic attack
96	a	Emollient with 1% hydrocortisone
97	i	Emollient with 25% hydrocortisone
98	g	Steroids and flucloxacillin
99	j	Psychiatric referral
100	c	Admit in hospital
101	a	Lyme disease serology
102	d	Wound swab
103	e	Lumbar puncture
104	g	LFT
105	f	MSU
106	e	Phaeochromocytoma
107	g	Polycystic kidney disease
108	b	Conn's syndrome
109	f	Glomerulonephritis
110	i	Coarctation of aorta
111	c	Inhaled foreign body
112	b	TB
113	e	Pulmonary embolism
114	b	TB
115	l	Carcinoma
116	g	Complete heart block
117	d	Acute AF
118	c	PE
119	b	Acute pericarditis
120	a	Papillary muscle rupture
121	a	Carotid Doppler

122	e	ESR
123	g	MRI pituitary fossa
124	d	CT scan
125	k	Tensilon test
126	h	Technitium scan
127	f	Serum calcium
128	a	PSA
129	l	Urodynamic studies
130	d	Transrectal USG
131	d	Faecal impaction
132	a	IBS
133	b	IBD
134	c	Acute gastroenteritis
135	e	Carcinoma colon
136	e	IV lorazepam
137	f	Give rectal
138	d	Check dry levels
139	a	EEG
140	a	EEG
141	a	Endemetrial carcinoma
142	c	Polycystic ovarian disease
143	b	Cervical ectropion
144	f	Hypothalamus related disorders
145	b	Cervical ectropion
146	a	PEG feeding
147	c	Parenteral feeding
148	c	Parenteral feeding
149	e	Low protein diet
150	d	Gluten free diet
151	d	Local steroid
152	a	NSAID
153	a	NSAID

154	e	Splinting
155	f	IV bisphosphonates
156	b	Haloperidol
157	c	Hyoscine
158	f	Per rectal diazepam
159	d	Oral dexamethasone
160	g	Metronidazole gel
161	d	Bone marrow biopsy
162	a	Blood film for parasites
163	e	Serum/gel electrophoresis
164	c	Schilling test
165	f	Mesenteric angiogram
166	d	Ring pessary
167	b	Infection control
168	f	Surgery
169	a	Vaginal estrogens
170	b	Infection control
171	d	Reduce weight
172	b	Graded compression stockings
173	d	Reduce weight
174	b	Graded compression stockings
175	a	Injection sclerotherapy
176	d	Viral serology
177	e	ERCP
178	c	Oral cholecystography
179	a	Liver biopsy
180	a	Liver biopsy
181	b	Uretheral swab
182	c	Urgent surgical exploration
183	e	USG
184	k	None required
185	a	MSU

186	a	Acute pancreatitis
187	e	Bargets's oesophagus
188	b	Chronic pancreatitis
189	c	*H. pylori* infection
190	d	Pernicious anaemia
191	a	Anaplastic carcinoma
192	d	Hashimoto's thyroiditis
193	g	Drug induced thyrotoxiosis
194	h	Graves' disease
195	k	Small bowel lymphoma
196	d	Lymphoedema
197	f	Hypercalcaemia
198	e	Spinal cord compression
199	b	Cerebral metastases
200	a	Pathological fracture

Previous Year Paper 5

RxPG Analysis

Total Themes:	**40**
Repeat Themes:	**4**
Repeat Themes with a Different Header:	**7**

THEME 1: DIAGNOSIS OF PERSONALITY DISORDERS

OPTIONS

a. Histrionic personality disorder
b. Borderline personality disorder
c. Schizotypal personality disorder
d. Schizoid personality disorder
e. Panic attack disorder
f. Paranoid personality disorder
g. Obsessive-compulsive personality disorder
h. Avoidant personality disorder
i. Antisocial personality disorder
j. Dependent personality disorder
k. Manic-depressive illness

INSTRUCTIONS

For each patient described below choose the ***single most likely diagnosis*** *from the list of options above. Each option may be used once, more than once or not at all.*

QUESTIONS

1. A 20-year-old man keeps cleaning his hands every time he shakes his partners hands. He was a high achiever in high school.
2. A 56-year-old farmer believes his 34-year-old neighbour is killing his farm animals despite the local veterinary's advice that the death is due to an outbreak of anthrax. He spends hours watching his neighbour through pair of binocular lens, hoping to catch in the act.
3. A 16-year-old girl is described as 'queer' by her mates. She is unfriendly and has no close friends despite numerous attempts by boys in her college. She lacks empathy and is largely introspective.
4. A 16-year-old girl in high school always comes late to class wearing strong perfume in a vain attempt to attract attention. She laughs loudly at jokes, many of her mates do not find particularly hilarious.
5. A 32-year-old man always gives in to his wife over any decision even when he knows this is not right. He insists on having his wife prepare his every meal, wash him and put him to sleep. He cries whenever his wife is away.

THEME 2: DIAGNOSIS OF DIABETIC COMPLICATIONS

OPTIONS

a. Hyperglycaemia
b. Hypoglycaemia
c. Urinary tract infection
d. Somatic neuropathy
e. Autonomic neuropathy
f. Intermittent claudication
g. Atherosclerosis
h. Possible infection
i. Lactic acidosis
j. Ketoacidosis
k. Amyotrophy

INSTRUCTIONS

For each of the patients listed below, choose the **most likely complication** *from the list of options above. Each option may be used once, more than once, or not at all.*

QUESTIONS

6. A 48-year-old female, insulin dependent diabetic, who has been on treatment for 20-year presents with a history of three episodes of severe hypoglycaemia. She has not changed her insulin requirement, diet or exercise pattern.
7. A 48-year-old female, insulin dependent diabetic, who has been on treatment for 20 years, presents with urinary frequency but no dysuria or urgency. Her blood glucose is 17.5 mmol/L.
8. A 30-year-old female, insulin dependent diabetic, presents with failure to pass urine.
9. A 68-year-old diabetic on treatment for the last 5-year presents with calf pain exacerbated by movement.
10. A 70-year-old diabetic on treatment with metformin presents with severe epigastric pain, drowsiness and confusion.

THEME 3: DIAGNOSIS OF PNEUMONIA ORGANISMS

OPTIONS
a. Aspiration
b. Bronchiectasis
c. Fungal
d. *Haemophilus influenzae*
e. *Klebsiella*
f. Lung cancer
g. *Mycoplasma pneumoniae*
h. *Pneumocystitis carinii*
i. *Staphylococcus aureus*
j. *Streptococcus pneumoniae*
k. Tuberculosis

INSTRUCTIONS
For each patient described below, choose the **single most likely** *underlying cause from the above list of options. Each option may be used once, more than once, or not at all.*

QUESTIONS
11. A 35-year-old woman presents with a four-month history of cough, productive of sputum, and recent haemoptysis. She has lost 5 kg in weight. The chest X-ray shows right upper lobe consolidation.
12. A previously well 18-year-old girl has had influenzae for the last two weeks. She is deteriorating and has a swinging fever. She is coughing up copious purulent sputum. Chest X-ray shows cavitating lesions.
13. A 65-year-old man, currently undergoing chemotherapy for chronic leukaemia, has felt unwell with fever and an unproductive cough for two weeks despite treatment with broad spectrum intravenous antibiotics. The chest X-ray shows an enlarging right sided, mid-zone consolidation.
14. A 27-year-old male prostitute has felt generally unwell for two months with some weight loss. Over the last three weeks he has noticed a dry cough with increasing breathlessness. Two courses of antibiotics from his GP has produced no improvement. The chest X-ray shows bilateral interstitial infiltrates.
15. On return to university, a 20-year-old student presented with the onset of fever, malaise and a dry cough. The student health service gave him amoxycillin. After a week he felt no better and his chest X-ray showed patchy bilateral consolidation.

THEME 4: DIAGNOSIS OF SUDDEN VISUAL LOSS

OPTIONS
a. Acute glaucoma
b. Cataract
c. Central retinal artery occlusion
d. Cerebral embolism
e. Cerebral haemorrhage
f. Chronic (simple) glaucoma
g. Hypertensive encephalopathy
h. Polymyalgia rheumatica
i. Retinal detachment
j. Temporal arteritis
k. Uveitis

INSTRUCTIONS
For each patient described below, choose the **single most likely diagnosis** *from the above list of options. Each option may be used once, more than once, or not at all.*

QUESTIONS
16. A 78-year-old man has had a painful scalp and headache for three weeks, and is generally unwell, complains of acute onset of blindness in his right eye.
17. A 50-year-old woman complains of sudden loss of vision in one eye. She describes the incident, like a curtain coming down.
18. An 84-year-old woman notices sudden increased visual impairment. She is found to have homonymous hemianopia.
19. A 68-year-old smoker suddenly notices markedly reduced vision in one eye. He cannot read any letter on visual acuity chart but can count fingers. The fundus is pale.
20. A 30-year-old man has recurrent episodes of an acutely painful red eye with reduced vision.

THEME 5: DIFFERENTIAL DIAGNOSIS OF DEMENTIA

OPTIONS

a. Alcoholic dementia
b. Alzheimer's dementia
c. Creutzfeldt-Jakob's disease
d. Head trauma
e. Human immunodeficiency virus (HIV)
f. Huntington's chorea
g. Parkinsonism
h. Pick's disease
i. Repeated trauma
j. Vascular dementia
k. Substance induced dementia

INSTRUCTIONS

For each patient described below, choose the ***single most likely diagnosis*** *from the above lists of options. Each option may be used once, more than once or not at all.*

QUESTIONS

21. A 56-year-old man with no previous history is brought to the accident and emergency department by his wife who says that he has become progressively more forgetful, tends to lose his temper and is emotionally labile. There is no history of infectious diseases or trauma.
22. A 74-year-old man presents with weakness in his arm and leg (from which he recovered within a few days) and short-term memory loss. He has an extensor plantar response. He had a similar episode two years ago and became unable to identify objects and to make proper judgements.
23. A 38-year-old haemophiliac who received several blood transfusions a few years ago presents with irritability and increasing memory deficit. He is unable to speak properly. He is on antitubercular treatment.
24. A 34-year-old woman presents with memory loss, poor concentration and inability to recognise household objects. On examination she has a right handed involuntary writhing movement. There is a strong family history of similar complaints.
25. A 62-year-old patient with chronic schizophrenia presents with mask-like face and involuntary pill rolling movement in both hands. He complains of chronic cough and forgetfulness.

THEME 6: PRESCRIBING AND RENAL FAILURE

OPTIONS

a. Cyclosporine
b. Bendrofluazide
c. Spirinolactone
d. Cyclophosphamide
e. Captopril
f. Gentamicin
g. Calcium
h. Magnesium
i. Metoprolol
j. Furosemide
k. Paracetamol

INSTRUCTIONS

For each patient described below, choose the single most **appropriate drug** *to prescribe from the above list of options. Each option may be used once, more than once, or not at all.*

QUESTIONS

26. A 60-year-old woman hypertensive was started on antihypertensive 2 weeks ago. Now has a creatinine level of 500 micromol/L
27. A child with recurrent nephrotic syndrome is brought for treatment. Three weeks after start of treatment, he now has massive haematuria.
28. A patient in severe renal failure has potassium level of 2. 5 mmol/L.
29. Patient with complaint of ataxia and tinnitus and mild hearing loss. He has moderate renal failure.
30. A fit 50-year-old man is prescribed oral acetazolamide by an ophthalmologist for suspected glaucoma. He presents with lethargy and shortness of breath on exertion. Sodium 140 mmol/L, potassium 3.2 mmol/L, bicarbonate 18 mmol/L, chloride 115 mmol/L, urea 6.7 mmol/L, creatinine 114 μmol/L.

THEME 7: IMMEDIATE MANAGEMENT IN TRAUMA

OPTIONS

a. Plain abdominal X-ray
b. Assess airway and stabilise spine
c. CT scan of abdomen
d. Transfer to operating theatre
e. Burr hole(s) should be drilled
f. Chest drain after needle thoracocentesis
g. Normal saline infusion
h. Immediate blood transfusion
i. Splint limb
j. Bolus of 50% dextrose followed by a saline infusion
k. Computed tomography (CT) brain scan

INSTRUCTIONS

For each patient described below choose the **single most likely immediate action** *from the above options. Each option may be used once, more than once, or not at all.*

QUESTIONS

31. A 43-year-old man is brought to the accident and emergency department delirious, following and injury at a rugby match. His Glasgow Coma Scale (GCS) at the scene of injury is 13. On examination, his right pupil is fixed and dilated and GCS is now 7. Initial resuscitation has been done. The neurosurgeon is 30 minutes away.
32. A 22-year-old motorist arrives in the accident and emergency department after an accident. His airway is patent. He is noted to have a splinted right leg.
33. A 30-year-old man is involved in a fight. He has a bruise on the cheek. He complains of an acute abdominal pain and is vomiting. He had a herniorraphy two weeks ago. He is conscious and fundoscopy has not been done.
34. A 29-year-old motorist, in the accident and emergency department resuscitation room, appears to be stable after an accident. While standing up, he becomes progressively dyspnoeic. There is reduced air entry on the left side of his chest.
35. An 18-year-old girl is being resuscitated after an accident. Her airway is secure. She complains of neck pain. Her pulse rate is 100 beats/min and blood pressure is 110/70 mmHg. Glasgow Coma Scale is 13. She has a deformed left thigh.

THEME 8 : TREATMENT OF ASTHMA IN CHILDHOOD

OPTIONS

a. As required oral bronchodilator
b. Adrenaline
c. Desensitisation
d. Inhaled long-acting bronchodilator
e. Inhaled sodium cromoglycate
f. Inhaled steroid
g. Intermittent inhaled bronchodilation
h. Intravenous (IV) aminophylline
i. Milk-free diet
j. Oral steroids
k. Nebulised bronchodilators

INSTRUCTIONS

For each condition described below, choose the **single most appropriate treatment** *from the above list of options. Each option may be used once, more than once, or not at all.*

QUESTIONS

36. A nine-year-old boy has a mild cough and wheeze after playing football in the cold weather.
37. A six-year-old girl with asthma uses her bronchodilator twice a day to relieve her mild wheeze. Her parents refuse to give her any treatment containing corticosteroids.
38. A nine-year-old girl with chronic asthma presents to the A and E department with rapidly worsening wheeze not relieved with inhaled bronchodilators.
39. A four-year-old boy with eczema and recurrent wheeze whenever he gets a viral infection has now developed night cough, there has been no improvement in spite of using inhaled bronchodilator twice each night.
40. A 14-year-old boy, with well-controlled asthma, using inhaled steroids and a bronchodilator comes to the A and E department with breathlessness and swollen lips after eating a peanut, butter-sandwich.

THEME 9: DIAGNOSIS OF COMPLICATIONS OF CHOLECYSTECTOMY

OPTIONS

a. Acute pancreatitis
b. Acute renal failure
c. Biliary peritonitis
d. Inferior vena cava thrombosis
e. Myocardial infarction
f. Pulmonary embolism
g. Small bowel obstruction
h. Stone in common bile duct
i. Subphrenic abscess

INSTRUCTIONS

For each test result below, choose the single most likely complication of cholecystectomy from the above list of options. Each option may be used once, more than once or not at all.

QUESTIONS

41. Chest X-ray shows raised right diaphragm with small pleural effusion above.
42. Ultrasound scan shows intra-abdominal free fluid with paralytic ileus.
43. Liver function tests show raised alkaline phosphates, raised bilirubin, normal albumin and normal hepatocellular enzymes.
44. Ultrasound scan shows dilated common bile duct with no free intra-abdominal fluid or bowel distension.
45. Chest X-ray shows signs of left ventricular dilatation and an electrocardiograph (ECG) shows Q waves with ST elevation.

THEME 10: POSTOPERATIVE COMPLICATIONS

OPTIONS

a. DVT
b. Septicaemia
c. Impending wound dehiscence
d. Wound infection
e. Urinary tract infection
f. Myocardial infarction
g. Acute tubular necrosis
h. Transfusion reaction
i. Cardiac failure
j. Pelvic abscess
k. Pulmonary collapse

INSTRUCTIONS

For each patient described below, choose the single most likely postoperative complication from the above list of options. Each option may be used once, more than once, or not at all.

QUESTIONS

46. A 50-year-old woman underwent an anterior resection for carcinoma of the rectum one week ago. Has low grade fever and with complaint of pain in the calf + tenderness in the calf.
47. A young woman underwent emergency appendicectomy days ago for perforated appendix. She appeared to be making a good recovery but has developed intermittent pyerexia (up to 39 deg. C). On examination—no obvious cause found, but he is tender anteriorly on rectal examination.
48. An elderly man underwent an emergency repair of an abdominal aortic aneurysm. Had been severely hypotensive before and during surgery. After surgery, his blood pressure was satisfactory, but urine output only 5 ml/hr in the first 2 hours.
49. An elderly woman underwent emergency laparotomy for peritonitis. Fourth postoperative day she is noted to have sero-sanuinous discharge from the wound, but there is no erythema or tenderness around the wound.
50. A 60-year-old with features of septicaemia (warm peripheries, low BP, etc.)

THEME 11 : THE DIAGNOSIS OF ABDOMINAL PAIN

OPTIONS

a. Familial polyposis
b. Food poisoning
c. Anorexia-bulaemia
d. Irritable bowel syndrome
e. Crohn's disease
f. Ulcerative colitis
g. Diverticular disease
h. Gallstone ileus
i. Rectal carcinoma
j. Colonic cancer
k. Pelvic abscess

INSTRUCTIONS

From the list of options given above choose the **diagnosis that fully and accurately** *reflects the details of the presentations given below. You may use each option once, more than once, or not at all.*

QUESTIONS

51. For the past two weeks a middle-aged railway engineer has complained of acute constipation. His stools are dark, but not apparently blood stained. Abdominal palpation detects a mass with moderate tenderness.
52. A 43-year-old man says he cannot finish his stool and that what he does pass is streaked with blood. He says he has always been regular. He wants to know if a laxative will help.
53. A 49-year-old lawyer complains of blood and diarrhoea. She is also suffering from abdominal pain, fever, and general ill-health. On palpation you find tenderness in the lower abdomen.
54. A young woman presents with recurrent abdominal pain, episodic diarrhoea, malaise, and fever. Over the past few years she has felt her health to be declining. At presentation she complains of severe abdominal pain and constipation.
55. A young woman complains of cramp like abdominal pain, and difficulties with bowel movements. Acute abdominal pain is frequently relieved by embarrassing flatulence. Barium studies and sigmoidoscopy have proved inconclusive.

THEME 12: DIAGNOSIS OF HIP PAIN

OPTIONS

a. Fracture neck of femur
b. Perthes disease
c. Slipped femoral epiphysis
d. Osteoarthritis
e. Septic arthritis
f. Congenital dislocation of the hip
g. Transient synovitis
h. Osteogenesis imperfecta
i. Osteomyelitis

INSTRUCTIONS

For each of the patients described below, choose the **single most likely diagnosis** *from the list of options above. Each option may be used once, more than once or not at all.*

QUESTIONS

56. A 7-year-old boy presents with a history of acute onset of pain in the knee. On examination, the left lower limb is flexed, abducted, internally rotated.
57. A 67-year-old woman complains of right hip pain. On examination the right hip is adducted, externally rotated and flexed.
58. A 10-year-old girl is febrile. On examination it is difficult to abduct the thighs.
59. A child presents with right hip pain. On examination the hip is flexed, abducted and externally rotated.
60. A five-year-old girl complains of progressively increasing severe pain in her left hip and upper leg for 6 days. She is able to walk but limps visibly. Blood tests are as follows: WCC 19/fl, ESR 72 mm/hr and CRP 94 mg/L. X rays and ultrasound scans of the hip are normal.

THEME 13: THE MANAGEMENT OF RED EYE

OPTIONS

a. No treatment
b. Check blood pressure and do coagulation studies
c. Immediate antibiotic therapy
d. Enucleation
e. 0.5% prednisolone drops 4 hourly
f. 0.5% prednisolone drops 2 hourly and cyclopentolate drops
g. 3% pilocarpine drops and acetazolamide
h. 500 mg acetazolamide
i. Acyclovir drops
j. Total iridectomy 15% flourescein drops

INSTRUCTIONS

For each patient described below, choose the single **most appropriate mode of management** *from the above list of options. Each option may be used once more than once or not at all.*

QUESTIONS

61. A 69-year-old patient presented to his GP with sudden onset of redness in the right eye. There was no pain and vision was unaffected.
62. A 60-year-old patient complains of severe pain in his left eye with severe deterioration of vision. He had noticed haloes around street lights at night for a few days before the onset of the pain.
63. A mother brings her 2-year-old child with a squint. On examination a leucokoric right pupil is seen with an absent red reflex.
64. A 12-year-old Libyan boy gave a two weeks history of discomfort, redness and mucopurulent discharge affecting both eyes. His two siblings have a similar problem.
65. A 23-year-old man has a history of recurrent attacks of blurring of vision associated with redness, pain and photophobia. Both eyes have been affected in the past. His brother is currently being investigated for bowel disease and a severe backache.

THEME 14: THE DIAGNOSIS OF WEAKNESS AND ILL HEALTH

OPTIONS

a. Teratoma
b. Seminoma
c. Chronic infection
d. Multiple myeloma
e. Burkitt's lymphoma
f. Non-Hodgkin's lymphoma
g. Hodgkin's disease
h. Thrombocytopenia
i. Chronic myeloid leukaemia
j. Waldenstrom's macroglobinaemia
k. Acute lymphoblastic leukaemia

INSTRUCTIONS

From the list of options given above choose the **diagnosis that most fully and accurately** *corresponds to the clinical details of the individual presentations given below. You may use each option once, more than once, or not at all.*

QUESTIONS

66. A child is brought to you with weakness, malaise, and bone pain. On physical examination you find painfully enlarged lymph nodes and hard and enlarged testicles. He has a history of sore throats and chest infections.
67. A 51-year-old lecturer presents with lethargy, abdominal pain, fever, and weight loss. On physical examination you find a large spleen. A blood examination shows normocytic normochromic anaemia with a very high white cell count.
68. An elderly man presents with backache, pallor, and shortness of breath. He has suddenly had some difficulties with his vision. Blood examination demonstrates a high ESR, and normochromic normocytic anaemia. There is rouleux formation.
69. A young woman complains of weakness, fatigue, and anorexia. Her cervical lymph nodes are enlarged, painless, and rubbery. Her skin itches and she sometimes has night sweats. On physical examination you find her spleen and liver to be enlarged.
70. A 44-year-old man presents with ill-health. He complains of wasting, fever and sweats. He does not have a skin rash, but he does have skin nodules. On physical examination you find disparate groups of lymph nodes to be enlarged.

THEME 15: PHARMACOLOGY AND TOXICOLOGY

OPTIONS
a. Tricyclic antidepressants
b. Opiate
c. Naloxone
d. Warfarin
e. Specific antidote
f. Heparin
g. Cyanide
h. Ethanol
i. Vitamin A
j. Paracetamol
k. 100% O_2

INSTRUCTIONS
Choose the most appropriate answer. You may use each option once, more than once, or not at all.

QUESTIONS
71. A homeless patient presents to A and E with drowsiness. On examination, abrasions and puncture marks were found on his arm. He has pin point pupil. What would you give?
72. This drug competes with vitamin K.
73. A man was found in his car with a hose directed from the exhaust. What would you give?
74. A patient who has overdosed on an unknown medication presents with palpitations. What is the most likely cause?
75. This interferes with metabolism at the mitochondrial level.

THEME 16: DIAGNOSIS OF MALABSORPTION AND DIARRHOEA IN CHILDREN

OPTIONS
a. Lactose intolerance
b. Chronic disease
c. Acrodermatitis enteropathica
d. Chronic nonspecific diarrhoea
e. Coeliac disease
f. Ulcerative colitis
g. *Giardia lamblia* infection
h. *Enterobius vermicularis* infection
i. *Ascaris lumbricoides*
j. Hirschsprungs's disease
k. Irritable bowel syndrome

INSTRUCTIONS
For each patient described below, choose the **single most likely diagnosis** *from the options listed above. Each option may be used once, more than once, or not at all.*

QUESTIONS
76. A 4-year-old Irish girl looks wasted and appears short for her age. The mother reports the daughter has been vomiting on several occasions in the past, with associated diarrhoea. The SHO thinks he has an enteropathy and on serology IgA gliadin and Endomysial antibodies are found.
77. A mother brings her 5-year-old son who has been passing bloody stool associated with severe abdominal pain. On examination he is found to have mildly swollen tender wrists and red nodular tender lesions were found on his forearms.
78. An 8-year-old girl has got repeated episodes of diarrhoea. On each occasion the stool contains segments of undigested vegetables. The paediatrician recommends restricting fluids to meal times. The girl's condition improves and she is thriving.
79. A mother and her daughter have just returned from a tropical holiday and is concerned that her daughter has an STD, since she complains of constant perianal and vulval irritation. There is no associated vaginal discharge. She has worms coming out of her bottom at night.
80. A 15-year-old girl complains of episodic diarrhoea which typically starts in the morning with a constant urge to go to the toilet on waking, and after breakfast. She says there is associated abdominal pain in the right iliac fossa relieved by defaecation or flatus. She has had the symptoms for 3 months.

THEME 17 : MANAGEMENT OF PAIN IN LABOUR

OPTIONS

a. Spinal anaesthesia
b. Epidural anaesthesia
c. Pudendal nerve block
d. General anaesthesia
e. Pethidine injection
f. Nitrous oxide
g. Local anaesthesia
h. Naloxane
i. Transcutaneous electrical nerve stimulation (TNES)
j. Aspirin
k. Omeprazole

INSTRUCTIONS

For each of the patients described below, **choose the most appropriate option,** *from the list of options above. Each option may be used once, more than once or not at all.*

QUESTIONS

81. A 20-year-old primigravida at 40 weeks, is 6 cm dilated and she requests pain relief. She dislikes injections.
82. A 39-year gravida 3 para 2 + 0, presents at 39 weeks. Her cervix is 8 cm dilated but she complains of severe pain. Her baby is in occipito-posterior position.
83. A 28-year-old woman wants to be able to move around during labour, pain free.
84. A gravida 4 para 2 + 1, has been in labour for 4 hours. She is 3 cm dilated and has already received 2 injections of pethidine. She stills complains of pain.
85. A 31-year-old woman has a retained placenta, following a spontaneous vaginal delivery.

THEME 18: THE DIAGNOSIS OF FACIAL PAIN

OPTIONS

a. Migraine
b. Abscess
c. Coryza
d. Serous otitis media
e. Glaucoma
f. Iritis
g. Trigeminal neuralgia
h. Sinusitis
i. Systemic lupus erythematosus
j. Temporal arteritis
k. Herpes zoster
l. Cluster headache

INSTRUCTIONS

Examine the following five cases of facial pain and decide which of the above mentioned diagnoses is most likely given the somewhat limited information you have before you. You may use each diagnosis once, more than once, or not at all.

QUESTIONS

86. A 53-year-old nurse complains of facial pain. A week earlier she had a red rash and blisters around her right eye. This area of her face has now become acutely painful.
87. A 31-year-old man complains of facial pain between the eyes and on one side of the face. His nose and the affected eye are congested. He says the pain is severe.
88. A 20-year-old man says his face hurts, especially around the eyes and cheeks. When he bends forwards it worsens and makes him cry.
89. A 57-year-old teacher says she has facial pain, especially in the temples at night. On the right side of her face it throbs. For the past three weeks she has felt unwell and had to miss classes. Also, combing her hair has become painful.
90. A 43-year-old mechanic complains of left sided facial pain. The pain is stabbing and runs up and down his face, especially at meal times. He has been to the dentist, but the dentist has found his teeth to be in good order.

THEME 19: THE DIAGNOSIS OF DIFFICULTIES WITH MICTURITION

OPTIONS

a. Pregnancy
b. Infection
c. Gylcosuria
d. Congenital abnormalities
e. Bladder tumour
f. Childbirth
g. Urethral syndrome
h. Urge incontinence
i. Stress incontinence
j. True incontinence
k. Vesicovaginal fistula

INSTRUCTIONS

For each of the patient cases given below choose an **appropriate and accurate diagnosis** *from the list of options given above. You may use each options once, more than once, or not at all.*

QUESTIONS

91. An overweight woman complains of having to go to the toilet more than usual. She says she does drink a lot of tea but that she is always thirsty and tired. She needs the energy.
92. A young mother with chronic bronchitis says that every time she coughs, she pees, and she would like you to do something about it. She is on a course of antibiotics at the moment.
93. A middle-aged woman complains of having to urinate frequently. She says that unless she rushes to the toilet she wets herself and she finds wetting herself most embarrassing.
94. A 36-year-old sales executive says she wets herself without warning all the time. Before the birth of her third child she had no complaints but now she says she has no control whatsoever.
95. A 27-year-old travel guide wants something done about the pain she feels on micturition, especially when it is cold. Repeated urine cultures have all been negative. Sometimes, she says, going to the toilet is very painful for her.

THEME 20: INVESTIGATION OF BREAST DISEASE

OPTIONS

a. Open biopsy
b. Fine-needle aspiration cytology
c. Ultrasound
d. Reassurance
e. Mammography
f. Wide excision
g. Computed tomography (CT)
h. Magnetic resonance imaging (MRI)
i. Lymphangiography

INSTRUCTIONS

For each of the patients described below, **choose the single most useful option** *from the list above. Each option may be used once, more than once, or not at all.*

QUESTIONS

96. A 35-year-old woman comes to the clinic for screening of her breasts.
97. A 45-year-old woman presents with a mass in the right upper quadrant of her right breast. A round smooth mass is found in the axilla.
98. A 36-year-old woman comes with a hard mass in her breast. The skin is tethered. Ultrasound and mammography were inconclusive. The patient wants to be satisfied that this is not malignant.
99. A 36-year-old woman presents with itching of her left nipple. On examination, no ulceration is seen, but a scaly lesion around the nipple is observed.
100. A 23-year-old woman says she feels lumps in her breasts during the time of her periods. She also feels anxious and irritable.

THEME 21: THE MANAGEMENT OF PATIENTS IN A COMA

OPTIONS

a. Alcohol level
b. Angiography
c. Arterial blood gases
d. Blood cultures
e. Blood sugar
f. Computed tomography (CT)
g. Naloxone
h. Paracetamol screen
i. Plasma osmolality
j. Toxicology
k. Urea and electrolytes

INSTRUCTIONS

For each patient described below, **choose the single most appropriate intervention** *from the options above. Each option may be used once, more than once, or not at all.*

QUESTIONS

101. A 25-year-old found deeply unconscious is brought to the accident and emergency department. He has an abrasion over his left temple and puncture marks on his left forearm.

102. A 37-year-old alcoholic is found wandering in a park. His partner says he has had a number of falls recently and in the accident and emergency the patient is confused. The blood sugar level is normal.

103. A young diabetic is admitted in a comatose state, his plasma glucose level is 17 mmol and he is dehydrated.

104. A middle-aged woman remains unconscious 12 hours following a cholecystectomy. On examination both pupils are seen to be pinpoint.

105. A young diabetic is admitted in a comatose state. His plasma glucose level is 2 mmol.

THEME 22: TRANSMISSION OF DISEASE

OPTIONS

a. Brucellosis
b. *Staphylococcus aureus*
c. *Escherichia coli*
d. *Klebsiella pneumoniae*
e. Hepatitis C
f. *Pseudomonas aeruginosa*
g. *Neisseria meningitidis*
h. Typhoid
i. Scabies
j. Hepatitis A
k. Tuberculosis

INSTRUCTIONS

For each of the conditions below, **choose the most likely answer** *from the list of options above. Each option may be used once, more than once or not at all.*

QUESTIONS

106. A 45-year-old sheep farmer complains of headache, anorexia, muscle and joint pain. He has as 'undulating' fever.

107. It is a skin to skin contact disease.

108. A 32-year-old woman presents with dysuria, swinging fever and loin pain.

109. It spreads by faecal-oral route.

110. A 67-year-old man has lost 10 kg in weight, over the last 6 months. ln addition he has a 5 months history of a productive cough.

THEME 23: ECG INTERPRETATION

OPTIONS

a. Hypothermia
b. Pyrexia
c. Right atrial hypertrophy
d. Left atrial hypertrophy
e. Right ventricular hypertrophy
f. Left ventricular hypertrophy
g. Conduction defect
h. Myocardial infarction
i. Ischaemic heart disease
j. Pulmonary hypertension
k. Myocarditis

INSTRUCTIONS

Choose an option from the above list of diagnoses that most fully and accurately corresponds to the ECG changes described below. You may use each option once, more than once, or not at all.

QUESTIONS

111. A teenage boy with dyspnoea and chest pain is brought into accident and emergency. He has a history of rheumatic fever. An ECG demonstrates left atrial hypertrophy and left ventricular hypertrophy. It also demonstrates Q waves and raised ST segment.
112. An elderly woman is found unconscious at home. An ECG demonstrates sinus bradycardia. J waves, ST depression, and flattened T waves.
113. A patient's ECG shows a biphasic P wave.
114. A patient's ECG shows T wave inversion and ST depression.
115. A 25-year-old woman complains of tiredness and malaise. Her T waves are widespread and deep.

THEME 24: DIZZINESS, FITS AND CONFUSION

OPTIONS

a. Nephrotic syndrome
b. Tuberculosis
c. Intestinal hurry
d. Recurrence of carcinoma
e. Glucose-6-phosphatase deficiency
F Pernicious anaemia
g. Nephroblastoma
h. Wilms' tumour
i. Secondaries
j. Benign postural hypotension
k. Alkalosis

INSTRUCTIONS

Choose an option from the list of diagnoses given above that accurately and fully captures the details of the presentations given below. You may use each option once, more than once, or not at all.

QUESTIONS

116. A 45-year-old man is diagnosed as having a kidney condition and treated. He soon develops postural hypotension with ankle oedema. His serum sodium is high, his potassuim normal, his urea normal, and he has heavy proteinuria.
117. A 20-year-old teacher is restless and confused. She is pale and sweaty and tachyapnoeic. Her arterial oxygen is high and her carbon dioxide is low.
118. A baby has a number of fits, each occurring in the morning on four consecutive days. On physical examination you find the liver to be enlarged. His fasting blood sugar is low and his uric acid is high.
119. A 30-year-old salesman complains of night sweats and dizziness. His ESR is high and his blood sugar is low. He has a normocytic anaemia and sterile pyuria.
120. A 50-year-old man is brought in by his wife who says he is always fatting. He has a fresh abdominal scar. His haemoglobin is low. His mean corpuscular volume is low. His mean corpuscular haemoglobin concentration is low, and his glucose tolerance test shows lag storage.

THEME 25: NON-ACCIDENTAL INJURY

OPTIONS

a. Elderly abuse
b. Child physical abuse
c. Child sexual abuse
d. Emotional abuse
e. Henoch-Schonlein purpura
f. Immune thrombocytopenic purpura
g. Child neglect
h. Coeliac disease
i. Osteogenesis imperfecta
j. Osteoporosis
k. Sickle cell anaemia
l. Accidental injury

INSTRUCTIONS

For each patient described below, choose the **single most likely diagnosis** *from the above list of options. Each option may be used once, more than once, or not at all.*

QUESTIONS

121. A mother 16 years, brings her baby for immunisation. The nurse notices the baby has multiple bruises along both arms and legs and is crying excessively. The house officer notices multiple fractures and that the baby has blue sclerae.

122. A 70-year-old man is receiving treatment for Alzheimer's disease. A 23-year-old granddaughter looks him after. He has recently developed faecal incontinence. The SHO notices bruises on both wrists and back.

123. An anxious mother brings her 6-year-old daughter who is bleeding per vaginum. Six months prior to this presentation the girl had a confirmed streptococcal sore-throat infection. She is otherwise normal.

124. A 4-day-old girl is brought to casualty by the maternal grandparent who is worried about two dark bluish patches on the child's buttocks. Child's mother is white and the father is black.

125. An 8-year-old girl is noted to have fresh bloody staining of her pants. She also suffers from enuresis. She has recently started horse-riding lessons.

THEME 26: DIFFERENTIAL DIAGNOSIS OF ANGINA

OPTIONS

a. Unstable angina
b. Stable angina
c. Syndrome X
d. Myocardial infarction
e. Pericarditis
f. Peptic ulcer disease
g. Arrhythmia
h. Spontaneous pneumothorax
i. Acute cholecystitis
j. Chronic pancreatitis
k. Tuberculosis

INSTRUCTIONS

For each of the patients below, choose the **single most appropriate diagnosis** *from the list of options above. Each option may be used once, more than once or not at all.*

QUESTIONS

126. An obese 34-year-old man complains of epigastric pain, which seems to exacerbated by eating his favourite meal, fish and chips. He gets temporary relief when hungry.

127. An obese 45-year-old man complains of recurring chest pain which radiates to his neck lasting 20 minutes. It coincides with his weekly executive board meetings.

128. An obese 29-year-old woman complains of with a cough of two weeks complains of right upper quadrant pain. She is mildly febrile. There was no abdominal tenderness on examination.

129. Condition associated with epigastric pain radiating to the back, pale loose stools, associated with alcohol consumption.

130. Female with fever, rigors, right upper quadrant pain, jaundice, ultrasound is normal.

THEME 27: THE IMMEDIATE MANAGEMENT OF MENINGITIS

OPTIONS

a. Lumbar puncture
b. CT skull
c. X-ray
d. Immunisation
e. Immediated hydration
f. Rifampicin prophylaxis
g. MRI spine
h. Contact tracing
i. Isoniazid prophylaxis
j. Transfer to ITU
k. Reassure
l. Serum urate

INSTRUCTIONS

For each patient described below, **choose the single most urgent first step** *from the above list of options. Each option may be used once, more than once or not at all.*

QUESTIONS

131. An HIV patient develops a severe headache and confusion. She is discovered to have bilateral papilloedema.

132. An 8-year-old boy with acute leukaemia is admitted in a comatose state. He is found to have lymphoblast depletion prevention.

133. A 14-year-old boy presents with drowsiness and generalised headache. He is recovering from a bilateral parotitis. His CT scan is normal.

134. An intravenous drug abuser presents with suspected meningitis. The organism is confirmed in the CSF by India ink preparation.

135. An anxious mother called you to say that her son's best friend in school has caught meningitis.

THEME 28: PRESCRIPTION AND DISEASE

OPTIONS

a. Vancomycin
b. Benzyl penicillin
c. Erythromycin
d. Actinomycin
e. Metronidazole
f. Amoxycillin
g. Glyceryl trinitrate (GTN)
h. Co-trimoxazole
i. Zidovudine (AZT)
j. Ondansetron
k. Trimethoprim

INSTRUCTIONS

For each of the disease conditions mentioned below, **choose the drug of choice** *from the above list of possible options. Each option may be used once, more than once or not at all.*

QUESTIONS

136. Uncomplicated urinary tract infection (UTI).

137. Pseudomembranous colitis (Patient allergic to vancomycin).

138. Sinusitis in patient allergic to penicillin.

139. Acute otitis media.

140. Acute streptococcal sore throat (patient allergic to penicillin).

THEME 29: CLINICAL MANAGEMENT OF HYPERTENSION IN PREGNANCY

OPTIONS

a. Low dose aspirin
b. A period of observation for blood pressure
c. 24 hour urinary protein
d. Foetal ultrasound
e. Retinoscopy
f. Induction of labour
g. Renal function tests
h. Intravenous antihypertensive
i. Recheck blood pressure in seven days
J. Immediate caesarean section
k. Oral antihypertensive

INSTRUCTIONS

For each patient described below, **choose the single most appropriate action** *from the above list of options. Each option may be used once, more than once or not at all.*

QUESTIONS

141. A patient in her third pregnancy presents to her GP at 12-weeks gestation. She was mildly hypertensive in both of her previous pregnancies. Her BP is 150/100 mmHg. Two weeks later at the hospital antenatal clinic her BP is 150/95 mmHg.

142. A 22-year-old Nigerian woman has an uneventful first pregnancy to 30 weeks. She is then admitted as an emergency with epigastric pain. During the first 2 hours her BP rises from 150/105 to 170/120 mmHg. On dipstick she is found to have 3+ proteinuria. The foetal cardiotocogram (CTG) is normal.

143. At an antenatal clinic visit at 38-weeks gestation, a 36-year-old multiparous woman has a BP of 140/90 mmHg. She has no proteinuria, and is otherwise well.

144. At 32 weeks, a 22-year-old primigravida is found to have a BP of 145/100 mmHg. She has no proteinuria, but she is found to have oedema to her knees.

145. At 34 weeks, a 86 kg woman complains of persistent headaches and 'flashing lights'. There is no hyperreflexia and her BP is 150/100 mmHg. Urinalysis is negative but she has finger oedema.

THEME 30: DIAGNOSIS OF CONSTIPATION

OPTIONS

a. Carcinoma of the colon
b. Parkinsonism
c. Anorexia nervosa
d. Myxoedema
e. Bulimia
f. Diverticulosis
g. Chronic pseudo-obstruction
h. Systemic sclerosis
i. Hypercalcaemia
j. Diabetic neuropathy
k. Irritable bowel syndrome

INSTRUCTIONS

For each patient described below, choose the **single most likely diagnosis** *from the above list of option. Each option may be used once, more than once, or not at all.*

QUESTIONS

146. A 42-year-old woman complains of excessive thirst, polyuria, polydipsia and constipation. She admits to losing weight. Her fasting blood glucose is 5.4 mmol/L.

147. A 23-year-old man being treated for myeloma is brought to the A and E department, confused. This followed a hour history of severe abdominal pain, vomiting. Prior to this, the patient had complained of polyuria, polydipsia and constipation.

148. A 16-year-old frail girl complains of constipation. Her body mass index (BMI) is found to be 17. She is extremely afraid of eating and admits to sticking a finger down her throat to induce vomiting after meals. She is unusually sensitive to cold.

149. A 60-year-old man with a history of weight loss, presents with bleeding per rectum. He also reports a history of diarrhoea which seems to alternate with constipation. His haemoglobin is 10 g/dl.

150. A 65-year-old woman presents with constipation, and reports difficulty in starting or stopping to walk. She has dysarthria and dribbling.

THEME 31: HUMAN IMMUNODEFICIENCY VIRUS

OPTIONS

a. Prophylactic AZT
b. Needle exchange
c. Refer to social worker
d. Refer to your consultant
e. Methadone
f. Counselling
g. Condoms
h. Combination therapy
i. Pentamidine
j. Pyridoxine and sulphadiazine
k. Cotrimoxazole

INSTRUCTIONS

For each of the patients described **choose the single most appropriate intervention** *from the list of options above. Each option may be used once, more than once or not at all.*

QUESTIONS

151. A 23-year-old woman has been using heroin (IV) for 4 years. She is not willing to stop using the heroin.
152. A third-year medical student was drawing blood from a known HIV positive patient gets a needle stick injury.
153. A healthy 20-year-old pregnant woman whose partner is a haemophiliac.
154. A 28-year-old haemophiliac with a history of 20 previous blood transfusions presents with a dry cough and fever. His chest X-ray shows widespread mottling.
155. A 20-year-old sexually active woman who is going to Thailand for a holiday.

THEME 32: DIAGNOSIS OF RENAL DISEASE

OPTIONS

a. Acute hypothyroidism
b. Type IV renal tubular acidosis
c. Acute adrenal insufficiency
d. Central nervous lesion with panhypopituitarism
e. Cytomegalovirus disease
f. Type I renal tubular acidosis
g. Syndrome of inappropriate ADH secretion (SIADH) with nephrotic syndrome
h. None of the answers
i. Membranous nephropathy
j. Type II Renal tubular acidosis

INSTRUCTIONS

For each patient described low, **choose the single most appropriate diagnosis** *from the above list of options. Each option may be used once, more than once or not used at all.*

QUESTIONS

156. A 30-year-old man with AIDS presented in shock. Serum biochemistry reveals: Potassium 6.7 mmol/L, bicarbonate 20 mmol/L, chloride 84 mmol/L, creatinine 160 μmol/L.
157. A 41-year-old Londoner developed a temperature of 41°C, 5 weeks after cadaveric renal transplantation. WBC is 2.1 × 1,000,000,000/L, Hb is 8.8 g/dl, creatinine 177 μmol/L. Aspartate aminotransferase (AST) 82 U/L. Alanine aminotransferase (ALT) 132 U/L.
158. A 36-year-old woman with leukaemia has been treated with Amphotericin B for a fungal pneumonia. She presents with muscle weakness. Sodium 137 mmol/L, potassium 2.7 mmol/L , bicarbonate 19 mmol/L, chloride 110 mmol/L, creatinine 84 μmol/L, urine pH 6.8 mmol/L.
159. An 83-year-old woman with small cell lung cancer presents with ankle oedema and is found to have 8 g/day, urine proteinuria. He is started on frusemide. Ten days later his blood pressure is 115/75 mmHg lying and 85/65 mmHg standing. Serum biochemistry was; sodium 121 mmol/L, bicarbonate 24 mmol/L, potassium 3.6 mmol/L, creatinine 113 μmol/L, chloride 95 mmol/L, urea 11.5 mmol/L, glucose 5.7 mmol/L , albumin 27g, osmolality 263 mOs m/L, urine osmolality 417 mOs m/L.
160. A fit 50-year-old man is prescribed oral acetazolamide by an ophthalmologist for suspected glaucoma. He presents with lethargy and shortness of breath on exertion. Sodium 140 mmol/L, potassium 3.2 mmol/L, bicarbonate 18 mmol/L, chloride 115 mmol/L, urea 6.7 mmol/L, creatinine 114 μmol/L.

THEME 33: RISK FACTORS FOR DEEP VEIN THROMBOSIS (DVT)

OPTIONS

a. Dehydration
b. Hormone replacement therapy (HRT)
c. Immobility
d. Inherited clotting abnormality
e. Malignancy
f. Multiple myeloma
g. Polycythaemia rubra vera
h. Pregnancy
i. Varicose veins

INSTRUCTIONS

For each patient described below who presents with a DVT, choose the **single most likely underlying risk factors** *from the above lists of options. Each option may be used once, more than once or not at all.*

QUESTIONS

161. A 60-year-old man presents with malaise and back pain which has been present for three months. He is found to have significant proteinuria.

162. A 30-year-old woman presents with a three month history of amenorrhoea.

163. A 60-year-old man with a plethoric appearance presents with pleuritic chest pain. He has palpable splenomegaly.

164. A 70-year-old man presents with back pain and jaundice.

165. A 25-year-old woman with a family history of deep vein thrombosis was prescribed a combined oral contraceptive pill six months ago and has not missed any tablets.

THEME 34: DIAGNOSIS OF A RASH

OPTIONS

a. Pulmonary tuberculosis
b. Sarcoidosis
c. Reiter's syndrome
d. Urticaria
e. Lyme disease
f. Dystonia myotonica
g. Herpes simplex
h. Behcet's syndrome
i. Myasthenia
j. Dermatomyositis
k. Smallpox

INSTRUCTIONS

For each of the patients with a rash described below, choose the **single most likely diagnosis** *from the above list of options.*

QUESTIONS

166. A 29-year-old man with known arthritis presented with a painful red eye and a brownish rash on his feet. He has recently been treated for dysentery.

167. A 30-year-old woman presented to the family GP complaining of difficulty in lifting her arms up. She also reported having difficulty getting up and down stairs. A scaly, erythematous rash was noticed on the dorsum of the hand, and knuckles. She had earlier complained dysphagia.

168. A mother brought her 10-year-old son to the GP, with a history of joint pains and recurrent oral ulcers. On examination the boy had hypopyon and mild conjunctivitis.

169. A 40-year-old sheep farmer from Kent presented to her GP complaining of muscle and joint pain with an associated chronic headache, which has been present for 3 weeks. On examination, she had an erythematous annular rash with a central clear area, on her abdomen.

170. A 30-year-old woman presented with tender, red nodules on both lower limbs and forearms. She had painful joints and was febrile. She had a month history of a productive cough and investigations revealed raised, angiotensin converting enzyme levels.

THEME 35: ASSOCIATION OF SKIN LESIONS AND SPECIFIC DISEASE

OPTIONS

a. Hyperthyroidism
b. Diabetes mellitus
c. Liver disease
d. Coeliac disease
e. Hypogonadism
f. *Borrelia burgdorferi* infection
g. Carcinoma of tail of pancreas
h. Measles
i. Deep vein thrombosis
j. Psoriasis
k. Leptospirosis

INSTRUCTIONS

For each of the patients described below, choose the **most likely association** *from the options given above. Each option may be used once, more than once, or not at all.*

QUESTIONS

171. A fit 55-year-old gentleman, complains of recurrent episodes of 'seeing visible veins on his body', which are tender. He has started to lose weight and attributes this to his diarrhoea. The consultant dermatologist thinks he has thrombophlebitis migrans.

172. A 49-year-old woman complains of itchy blisters, which are occurring in groups on her knees and elbows. The itch is becoming unbearable and she is contemplating suicide. She responds to 180 mg of dapsone within 48 hours of treatment.

173. A Welsh farmer with malaise and arthralgia is increasingly anxious about a skin lesion which started as a papule (Diameter approx 1 mm) which has progressed to a red ring (Diameter approx 50 mm) with central fading.

174. A 42-year-old woman who reports a loss in weight, presents with a shiny erythematous lesion on her skin. Its centre appears yellowish and edges are beginning to ulcerate with undermining. (Fasting blood glucose is 5.3 mmol/L).

175. A 32-year-old woman complains of palpitations and is found to have red oedematous swellings above both lateral malleoli, which she says are beginning to affect her feet. She is found to have digital clubbing and periorbital puffiness.

THEME 36: NATURAL HISTORY CERVICAL CANCER

OPTIONS

a. 3-6 months
b. 12 months
c. 24-36 months
d. 3-10 years
e. 20 years
f. 30 years
g. 45 years
h. 50 years
i. 55 years
j. 65 years
K. 80 years

INSTRUCTIONS

For each scenario below, choose the **single most likely time or time interval** *from the above list of options. Each option may be used once, more than once, or not at all.*

QUESTIONS

176. The time span over which a percentage of women with cervical intraepithelial neoplasia (CIN) untreated will develop cancer.

177. The age at which the peak incidence of cervical carcinoma occurs.

178. The interval for cervical smears to be taken in a woman treated one year previously for cervical intraepithelial neoplasia.

179. The age at which screening stops for women with a normal smear history.

180. The timescale within which the 50% of patients with recurrent disease will present, following treatment for stage 1B cervical cancer.

THEME 37: DIAGNOSIS OF COMMON GENETICAL DISORDERS

OPTIONS

a. Klinefelter's syndrome
b. Patau syndrome
c. Down's syndrome
d. Turner's syndrome
e. Cri-du-chat syndrome
f. Fragile X-syndrome
g. Sickle cell disease
h. Sickle cell trait
i. Beta thalassaemia
j. Williams syndrome
k. Prader-Willi syndrome
l. DiGeorge syndrome
m. Acute myeloid leukaemia
n. Edward's syndrome

INSTRUCTIONS

For each patient described below choose the **single most appropriate diagnosis** *from the list of options above. Each option may be used once, more than once, or not at all.*

QUESTIONS

181. A 15-year-old boy has very poor grades at school despite being very attentive and hard working. His mother reckons its because he is teased at school because his breasts look like a girl's. On further examination he is found to have small firm testes. He is mildly asthmatic.

182. A 5-year-old South African boy is brought to the accident and emergency department deeply jaundiced. He is found to have mildly swollen, tender feet and hands. His mucosae are pale.

183. A 6-year-old Asian boy gets regular blood transfusion for his haematological abnormality. His mucosae are pale and skull is grossly bossed. Haematological investigations were done and showed; MCHC 25g/dl, Hb 8g/dl , MCV 74fl.

184. A 10-year-old boy is brought to the accident and emergency department with a swollen right arm. His temperature is 38.5ºC and is unable to move his arm due to severe pain. Blood culture confirms *Salmonella typhi* osteomyelitis. This is his second presentation this month and earlier presented with an acute onset hepatosplenomegaly associated with severe pallour. The SHO does a Sodium metabisulphite test on the patient's blood which turns out to be positive.

185. A 39-year-old male is getting progessively forgetful and is later found to have Alzheimer's disease. He has small ears and an IQ score of 67.

THEME 38: MANAGEMENT OF ACUTE CHEST PAIN

OPTIONS

a. Glyceryl trinitrate (0.5 mg) sublingually
b. IV 50 ml of 50% dextrose
c. High flow O_2 and ramipril 2.5 mg/12 hr PO
d. High flow O_2, 10 mg IV morphine + anticoagulation
e. Cross-match blood and inform surgeons
f. Insert a 16 G cannula in second intercostal space
g. IV heparin 5000-10,000 iu over 5 min
h. Underwater seal drainage
i. 10 mg IV diamorphine
j. Nifedine
k, Ramipril

INSTRUCTIONS

For each patient described below, choose the **single most appropriate immediate measure** *to take from the above list of options. Each option may be used once, more than once or not at all.*

QUESTIONS

186. A tall young man developed sharp pain on one side of his chest two days ago. Since then he has been short of breath on exertion.

187. After a heavy bout of drinking a 56-year-old man vomits several times and develops chest pain. When you examine him, he has a crackling feeling under the skin around his neck.

188. A 23-year-old woman on the oral contraceptive pill suddenly gets tightness in her chest and becomes very breathless.

189. A 30-year-old man with Marfan's syndrome has sudden central chest pain going through to the back.

190. A 57-year-old man develops crushing pain in the chest associated with nausea and profuse sweating. The pain is still present when he arrives in hospital an hour later.

THEME 39: INVESTIGATIONS OF PATIENT WITH HAEMOPTYSIS

OPTIONS

a. Computed tomography
b. Fibreoptic bronchoscopy
c. Fine-needle aspiration
d. Mediastinoscopy
e. Mediastinotomy
f. Magnetic resonance imaging (MRI)
g. Pulmonary angiogram
h. Selective arteriogram
i. Sputum culture
j. Sputum cytology
k. Ventilation perfusion scan

INSTRUCTIONS

For each suspected diagnosis below, choose the **single most definitive investigation** *from the above list of options. Each option may be used once, more than once, or not at all.*

QUESTIONS

191. Tuberculosis.
192. Carcinoma of the right main bronchus.
193. Pulmonary embolism
194. Bronchiectasis.
195. Bronchial carcinoid.

THEME 40: ANTIBIOTIC PROPHYLAXIS OF SURGICAL PATIENTS

OPTIONS

a. Angiography
b. Bronchoscopy
c. Colle's fracture
d. Dental treatment of a cardiac patient
e. Dislocated shoulder
f. Emergency appendicectomy
g. Heart valve replacement
h. Sigmoid colectomy
i. Splenectomy
j. Thyroidectomy

INSTRUCTIONS

For each prophylactic regimen given below, choose the **single most likely indication** *from the above list of options. Each option may be used once, more than once or not at all.*

QUESTIONS

196. 3 gm sachet of amoxicillin one hour before the procedure.
197. Three days of intravenous broad spectrum antibiotics beginning with induction of anaesthesia.
198. Clear fluids by mouth and two sachets of sodium picosulphate on the day before the operation plus broad spectrum intravenous antibiotics at induction.
199. Long-term oral penicillin and immunisation against pneumococcal infection.
200. One dose of metronidazole at induction of anaesthesia.

General Medical Council PLAB Test Part 1

Full Name

Test Centre/Date

- Use pencil only • Make heavy marks that fill the lozenge completely
- Write your candidate number in the top row of the box to the right **AND** fill in the appropriate lozenge below each number
- Give **ONE** answer only for each question

0	0	0	0	0	0
1	1	1	1	1	1
2	2	2	2	2	2
3	3	3	3	3	3
4	4	4	4	4	4
5	5	5	5	5	5
6	6	6	6	6	6
7	7	7	7	7	7
8	8	8	8	8	8
9	9	9	9	9	9

1	A	B	C	D	E	F	G	H	I	J	K	L	M	N	O	P	Q	R	S	T	1
2	A	B	C	D	E	F	G	H	I	J	K	L	M	N	O	P	Q	R	S	T	2
3	A	B	C	D	E	F	G	H	I	J	K	L	M	N	O	P	Q	R	S	T	3
4	A	B	C	D	E	F	G	H	I	J	K	L	M	N	O	P	Q	R	S	T	4
5	A	B	C	D	E	F	G	H	I	J	K	L	M	N	O	P	Q	R	S	T	5
6	A	B	C	D	E	F	G	H	I	J	K	L	M	N	O	P	Q	R	S	T	6
7	A	B	C	D	E	F	G	H	I	J	K	L	M	N	O	P	Q	R	S	T	7
8	A	B	C	D	E	F	G	H	I	J	K	L	M	N	O	P	Q	R	S	T	8
9	A	B	C	D	E	F	G	H	I	J	K	L	M	N	O	P	Q	R	S	T	9
10	A	B	C	D	E	F	G	H	I	J	K	L	M	N	O	P	Q	R	S	T	10
11	A	B	C	D	E	F	G	H	I	J	K	L	M	N	O	P	Q	R	S	T	11
12	A	B	C	D	E	F	G	H	I	J	K	L	M	N	O	P	Q	R	S	T	12
13	A	B	C	D	E	F	G	H	I	J	K	L	M	N	O	P	Q	R	S	T	13
14	A	B	C	D	E	F	G	H	I	J	K	L	M	N	O	P	Q	R	S	T	14
15	A	B	C	D	E	F	G	H	I	J	K	L	M	N	O	P	Q	R	S	T	15
16	A	B	C	D	E	F	G	H	I	J	K	L	M	N	O	P	Q	R	S	T	16
17	A	B	C	D	E	F	G	H	I	J	K	L	M	N	O	P	Q	R	S	T	17
18	A	B	C	D	E	F	G	H	I	J	K	L	M	N	O	P	Q	R	S	T	18
19	A	B	C	D	E	F	G	H	I	J	K	L	M	N	O	P	Q	R	S	T	19
20	A	B	C	D	E	F	G	H	I	J	K	L	M	N	O	P	Q	R	S	T	20
21	A	B	C	D	E	F	G	H	I	J	K	L	M	N	O	P	Q	R	S	T	21
22	A	B	C	D	E	F	G	H	I	J	K	L	M	N	O	P	Q	R	S	T	22
23	A	B	C	D	E	F	G	H	I	J	K	L	M	N	O	P	Q	R	S	T	23
24	A	B	C	D	E	F	G	H	I	J	K	L	M	N	O	P	Q	R	S	T	24
25	A	B	C	D	E	F	G	H	I	J	K	L	M	N	O	P	Q	R	S	T	25
26	A	B	C	D	E	F	G	H	I	J	K	L	M	N	O	P	Q	R	S	T	26
27	A	B	C	D	E	F	G	H	I	J	K	L	M	N	O	P	Q	R	S	T	27
28	A	B	C	D	E	F	G	H	I	J	K	L	M	N	O	P	Q	R	S	T	28
29	A	B	C	D	E	F	G	H	I	J	K	L	M	N	O	P	Q	R	S	T	29
30	A	B	C	D	E	F	G	H	I	J	K	L	M	N	O	P	Q	R	S	T	30
31	A	B	C	D	E	F	G	H	I	J	K	L	M	N	O	P	Q	R	S	T	31
32	A	B	C	D	E	F	G	H	I	J	K	L	M	N	O	P	Q	R	S	T	32
33	A	B	C	D	E	F	G	H	I	J	K	L	M	N	O	P	Q	R	S	T	33
34	A	B	C	D	E	F	G	H	I	J	K	L	M	N	O	P	Q	R	S	T	34
35	A	B	C	D	E	F	G	H	I	J	K	L	M	N	O	P	Q	R	S	T	35
36	A	B	C	D	E	F	G	H	I	J	K	L	M	N	O	P	Q	R	S	T	36
37	A	B	C	D	E	F	G	H	I	J	K	L	M	N	O	P	Q	R	S	T	37
38	A	B	C	D	E	F	G	H	I	J	K	L	M	N	O	P	Q	R	S	T	38
39	A	B	C	D	E	F	G	H	I	J	K	L	M	N	O	P	Q	R	S	T	39
40	A	B	C	D	E	F	G	H	I	J	K	L	M	N	O	P	Q	R	S	T	40
41	A	B	C	D	E	F	G	H	I	J	K	L	M	N	O	P	Q	R	S	T	41
42	A	B	C	D	E	F	G	H	I	J	K	L	M	N	O	P	Q	R	S	T	42
43	A	B	C	D	E	F	G	H	I	J	K	L	M	N	O	P	Q	R	S	T	43
44	A	B	C	D	E	F	G	H	I	J	K	L	M	N	O	P	Q	R	S	T	44
45	A	B	C	D	E	F	G	H	I	J	K	L	M	N	O	P	Q	R	S	T	45
46	A	B	C	D	E	F	G	H	I	J	K	L	M	N	O	P	Q	R	S	T	46
47	A	B	C	D	E	F	G	H	I	J	K	L	M	N	O	P	Q	R	S	T	47
48	A	B	C	D	E	F	G	H	I	J	K	L	M	N	O	P	Q	R	S	T	48
49	A	B	C	D	E	F	G	H	I	J	K	L	M	N	O	P	Q	R	S	T	49
50	A	B	C	D	E	F	G	H	I	J	K	L	M	N	O	P	Q	R	S	T	50

DO NOT WRITE IN THIS SPACE

51	A	B	C	D	E	F	G	H	I	J	K	L	M	N	O	P	Q	R	S	T	51
52	A	B	C	D	E	F	G	H	I	J	K	L	M	N	O	P	Q	R	S	T	52
53	A	B	C	D	E	F	G	H	I	J	K	L	M	N	O	P	Q	R	S	T	53
54	A	B	C	D	E	F	G	H	I	J	K	L	M	N	O	P	Q	R	S	T	54
55	A	B	C	D	E	F	G	H	I	J	K	L	M	N	O	P	Q	R	S	T	55
56	A	B	C	D	E	F	G	H	I	J	K	L	M	N	O	P	Q	R	S	T	56
57	A	B	C	D	E	F	G	H	I	J	K	L	M	N	O	P	Q	R	S	T	57
58	A	B	C	D	E	F	G	H	I	J	K	L	M	N	O	P	Q	R	S	T	58
59	A	B	C	D	E	F	G	H	I	J	K	L	M	N	O	P	Q	R	S	T	59
60	A	B	C	D	E	F	G	H	I	J	K	L	M	N	O	P	Q	R	S	T	60
61	A	B	C	D	E	F	G	H	I	J	K	L	M	N	O	P	Q	R	S	T	61
62	A	B	C	D	E	F	G	H	I	J	K	L	M	N	O	P	Q	R	S	T	62
63	A	B	C	D	E	F	G	H	I	J	K	L	M	N	O	P	Q	R	S	T	63
64	A	B	C	D	E	F	G	H	I	J	K	L	M	N	O	P	Q	R	S	T	64
65	A	B	C	D	E	F	G	H	I	J	K	L	M	N	O	P	Q	R	S	T	65
66	A	B	C	D	E	F	G	H	I	J	K	L	M	N	O	P	Q	R	S	T	66
67	A	B	C	D	E	F	G	H	I	J	K	L	M	N	O	P	Q	R	S	T	67
68	A	B	C	D	E	F	G	H	I	J	K	L	M	N	O	P	Q	R	S	T	68
69	A	B	C	D	E	F	G	H	I	J	K	L	M	N	O	P	Q	R	S	T	69
70	A	B	C	D	E	F	G	H	I	J	K	L	M	N	O	P	Q	R	S	T	70
71	A	B	C	D	E	F	G	H	I	J	K	L	M	N	O	P	Q	R	S	T	71
72	A	B	C	D	E	F	G	H	I	J	K	L	M	N	O	P	Q	R	S	T	72
73	A	B	C	D	E	F	G	H	I	J	K	L	M	N	O	P	Q	R	S	T	73
74	A	B	C	D	E	F	G	H	I	J	K	L	M	N	O	P	Q	R	S	T	74
75	A	B	C	D	E	F	G	H	I	J	K	L	M	N	O	P	Q	R	S	T	75
76	A	B	C	D	E	F	G	H	I	J	K	L	M	N	O	P	Q	R	S	T	76
77	A	B	C	D	E	F	G	H	I	J	K	L	M	N	O	P	Q	R	S	T	77
78	A	B	C	D	E	F	G	H	I	J	K	L	M	N	O	P	Q	R	S	T	78
79	A	B	C	D	E	F	G	H	I	J	K	L	M	N	O	P	Q	R	S	T	79
80	A	B	C	D	E	F	G	H	I	J	K	L	M	N	O	P	Q	R	S	T	80
81	A	B	C	D	E	F	G	H	I	J	K	L	M	N	O	P	Q	R	S	T	81
82	A	B	C	D	E	F	G	H	I	J	K	L	M	N	O	P	Q	R	S	T	82
83	A	B	C	D	E	F	G	H	I	J	K	L	M	N	O	P	Q	R	S	T	83
84	A	B	C	D	E	F	G	H	I	J	K	L	M	N	O	P	Q	R	S	T	84
85	A	B	C	D	E	F	G	H	I	J	K	L	M	N	O	P	Q	R	S	T	85
86	A	B	C	D	E	F	G	H	I	J	K	L	M	N	O	P	Q	R	S	T	86
87	A	B	C	D	E	F	G	H	I	J	K	L	M	N	O	P	Q	R	S	T	87
88	A	B	C	D	E	F	G	H	I	J	K	L	M	N	O	P	Q	R	S	T	88
89	A	B	C	D	E	F	G	H	I	J	K	L	M	N	O	P	Q	R	S	T	89
90	A	B	C	D	E	F	G	H	I	J	K	L	M	N	O	P	Q	R	S	T	90
91	A	B	C	D	E	F	G	H	I	J	K	L	M	N	O	P	Q	R	S	T	91
92	A	B	C	D	E	F	G	H	I	J	K	L	M	N	O	P	Q	R	S	T	92
93	A	B	C	D	E	F	G	H	I	J	K	L	M	N	O	P	Q	R	S	T	93
94	A	B	C	D	E	F	G	H	I	J	K	L	M	N	O	P	Q	R	S	T	94
95	A	B	C	D	E	F	G	H	I	J	K	L	M	N	O	P	Q	R	S	T	95
96	A	B	C	D	E	F	G	H	I	J	K	L	M	N	O	P	Q	R	S	T	96
97	A	B	C	D	E	F	G	H	I	J	K	L	M	N	O	P	Q	R	S	T	97
98	A	B	C	D	E	F	G	H	I	J	K	L	M	N	O	P	Q	R	S	T	98
99	A	B	C	D	E	F	G	H	I	J	K	L	M	N	O	P	Q	R	S	T	99
100	A	B	C	D	E	F	G	H	I	J	K	L	M	N	O	P	Q	R	S	T	100

DO NOT WRITE IN THIS SPACE

101	A	B	C	D	E	F	G	H	I	J	K	L	M	N	O	P	Q	R	S	T	101
102	A	B	C	D	E	F	G	H	I	J	K	L	M	N	O	P	Q	R	S	T	102
103	A	B	C	D	E	F	G	H	I	J	K	L	M	N	O	P	Q	R	S	T	103
104	A	B	C	D	E	F	G	H	I	J	K	L	M	N	O	P	Q	R	S	T	104
105	A	B	C	D	E	F	G	H	I	J	K	L	M	N	O	P	Q	R	S	T	105
106	A	B	C	D	E	F	G	H	I	J	K	L	M	N	O	P	Q	R	S	T	106
107	A	B	C	D	E	F	G	H	I	J	K	L	M	N	O	P	Q	R	S	T	107
108	A	B	C	D	E	F	G	H	I	J	K	L	M	N	O	P	Q	R	S	T	108
109	A	B	C	D	E	F	G	H	I	J	K	L	M	N	O	P	Q	R	S	T	109
110	A	B	C	D	E	F	G	H	I	J	K	L	M	N	O	P	Q	R	S	T	110
111	A	B	C	D	E	F	G	H	I	J	K	L	M	N	O	P	Q	R	S	T	111
112	A	B	C	D	E	F	G	H	I	J	K	L	M	N	O	P	Q	R	S	T	112
113	A	B	C	D	E	F	G	H	I	J	K	L	M	N	O	P	Q	R	S	T	113
114	A	B	C	D	E	F	G	H	I	J	K	L	M	N	O	P	Q	R	S	T	114
115	A	B	C	D	E	F	G	H	I	J	K	L	M	N	O	P	Q	R	S	T	115
116	A	B	C	D	E	F	G	H	I	J	K	L	M	N	O	P	Q	R	S	T	116
117	A	B	C	D	E	F	G	H	I	J	K	L	M	N	O	P	Q	R	S	T	117
118	A	B	C	D	E	F	G	H	I	J	K	L	M	N	O	P	Q	R	S	T	118
119	A	B	C	D	E	F	G	H	I	J	K	L	M	N	O	P	Q	R	S	T	119
120	A	B	C	D	E	F	G	H	I	J	K	L	M	N	O	P	Q	R	S	T	120
121	A	B	C	D	E	F	G	H	I	J	K	L	M	N	O	P	Q	R	S	T	121
122	A	B	C	D	E	F	G	H	I	J	K	L	M	N	O	P	Q	R	S	T	122
123	A	B	C	D	E	F	G	H	I	J	K	L	M	N	O	P	Q	R	S	T	123
124	A	B	C	D	E	F	G	H	I	J	K	L	M	N	O	P	Q	R	S	T	124
125	A	B	C	D	E	F	G	H	I	J	K	L	M	N	O	P	Q	R	S	T	125
126	A	B	C	D	E	F	G	H	I	J	K	L	M	N	O	P	Q	R	S	T	126
127	A	B	C	D	E	F	G	H	I	J	K	L	M	N	O	P	Q	R	S	T	127
128	A	B	C	D	E	F	G	H	I	J	K	L	M	N	O	P	Q	R	S	T	128
129	A	B	C	D	E	F	G	H	I	J	K	L	M	N	O	P	Q	R	S	T	129
130	A	B	C	D	E	F	G	H	I	J	K	L	M	N	O	P	Q	R	S	T	130
131	A	B	C	D	E	F	G	H	I	J	K	L	M	N	O	P	Q	R	S	T	131
132	A	B	C	D	E	F	G	H	I	J	K	L	M	N	O	P	Q	R	S	T	132
133	A	B	C	D	E	F	G	H	I	J	K	L	M	N	O	P	Q	R	S	T	133
134	A	B	C	D	E	F	G	H	I	J	K	L	M	N	O	P	Q	R	S	T	134
135	A	B	C	D	E	F	G	H	I	J	K	L	M	N	O	P	Q	R	S	T	135
136	A	B	C	D	E	F	G	H	I	J	K	L	M	N	O	P	Q	R	S	T	136
137	A	B	C	D	E	F	G	H	I	J	K	L	M	N	O	P	Q	R	S	T	137
138	A	B	C	D	E	F	G	H	I	J	K	L	M	N	O	P	Q	R	S	T	138
139	A	B	C	D	E	F	G	H	I	J	K	L	M	N	O	P	Q	R	S	T	139
140	A	B	C	D	E	F	G	H	I	J	K	L	M	N	O	P	Q	R	S	T	140
141	A	B	C	D	E	F	G	H	I	J	K	L	M	N	O	P	Q	R	S	T	141
142	A	B	C	D	E	F	G	H	I	J	K	L	M	N	O	P	Q	R	S	T	142
143	A	B	C	D	E	F	G	H	I	J	K	L	M	N	O	P	Q	R	S	T	143
144	A	B	C	D	E	F	G	H	I	J	K	L	M	N	O	P	Q	R	S	T	144
145	A	B	C	D	E	F	G	H	I	J	K	L	M	N	O	P	Q	R	S	T	145
146	A	B	C	D	E	F	G	H	I	J	K	L	M	N	O	P	Q	R	S	T	146
147	A	B	C	D	E	F	G	H	I	J	K	L	M	N	O	P	Q	R	S	T	147
148	A	B	C	D	E	F	G	H	I	J	K	L	M	N	O	P	Q	R	S	T	148
149	A	B	C	D	E	F	G	H	I	J	K	L	M	N	O	P	Q	R	S	T	149
150	A	B	C	D	E	F	G	H	I	J	K	L	M	N	O	P	Q	R	S	T	150

DO NOT WRITE IN THIS SPACE

151	A	B	C	D	E	F	G	H	I	J	K	L	M	N	O	P	Q	R	S	T	151
152	A	B	C	D	E	F	G	H	I	J	K	L	M	N	O	P	Q	R	S	T	152
153	A	B	C	D	E	F	G	H	I	J	K	L	M	N	O	P	Q	R	S	T	153
154	A	B	C	D	E	F	G	H	I	J	K	L	M	N	O	P	Q	R	S	T	154
155	A	B	C	D	E	F	G	H	I	J	K	L	M	N	O	P	Q	R	S	T	155
156	A	B	C	D	E	F	G	H	I	J	K	L	M	N	O	P	Q	R	S	T	156
157	A	B	C	D	E	F	G	H	I	J	K	L	M	N	O	P	Q	R	S	T	157
158	A	B	C	D	E	F	G	H	I	J	K	L	M	N	O	P	Q	R	S	T	158
159	A	B	C	D	E	F	G	H	I	J	K	L	M	N	O	P	Q	R	S	T	159
160	A	B	C	D	E	F	G	H	I	J	K	L	M	N	O	P	Q	R	S	T	160
161	A	B	C	D	E	F	G	H	I	J	K	L	M	N	O	P	Q	R	S	T	161
162	A	B	C	D	E	F	G	H	I	J	K	L	M	N	O	P	Q	R	S	T	162
163	A	B	C	D	E	F	G	H	I	J	K	L	M	N	O	P	Q	R	S	T	163
164	A	B	C	D	E	F	G	H	I	J	K	L	M	N	O	P	Q	R	S	T	164
165	A	B	C	D	E	F	G	H	I	J	K	L	M	N	O	P	Q	R	S	T	165
166	A	B	C	D	E	F	G	H	I	J	K	L	M	N	O	P	Q	R	S	T	166
167	A	B	C	D	E	F	G	H	I	J	K	L	M	N	O	P	Q	R	S	T	167
168	A	B	C	D	E	F	G	H	I	J	K	L	M	N	O	P	Q	R	S	T	168
169	A	B	C	D	E	F	G	H	I	J	K	L	M	N	O	P	Q	R	S	T	169
170	A	B	C	D	E	F	G	H	I	J	K	L	M	N	O	P	Q	R	S	T	170
171	A	B	C	D	E	F	G	H	I	J	K	L	M	N	O	P	Q	R	S	T	171
172	A	B	C	D	E	F	G	H	I	J	K	L	M	N	O	P	Q	R	S	T	172
173	A	B	C	D	E	F	G	H	I	J	K	L	M	N	O	P	Q	R	S	T	173
174	A	B	C	D	E	F	G	H	I	J	K	L	M	N	O	P	Q	R	S	T	174
175	A	B	C	D	E	F	G	H	I	J	K	L	M	N	O	P	Q	R	S	T	175
176	A	B	C	D	E	F	G	H	I	J	K	L	M	N	O	P	Q	R	S	T	176
177	A	B	C	D	E	F	G	H	I	J	K	L	M	N	O	P	Q	R	S	T	177
178	A	B	C	D	E	F	G	H	I	J	K	L	M	N	O	P	Q	R	S	T	178
179	A	B	C	D	E	F	G	H	I	J	K	L	M	N	O	P	Q	R	S	T	179
180	A	B	C	D	E	F	G	H	I	J	K	L	M	N	O	P	Q	R	S	T	180
181	A	B	C	D	E	F	G	H	I	J	K	L	M	N	O	P	Q	R	S	T	181
182	A	B	C	D	E	F	G	H	I	J	K	L	M	N	O	P	Q	R	S	T	182
183	A	B	C	D	E	F	G	H	I	J	K	L	M	N	O	P	Q	R	S	T	183
184	A	B	C	D	E	F	G	H	I	J	K	L	M	N	O	P	Q	R	S	T	184
185	A	B	C	D	E	F	G	H	I	J	K	L	M	N	O	P	Q	R	S	T	185
186	A	B	C	D	E	F	G	H	I	J	K	L	M	N	O	P	Q	R	S	T	186
187	A	B	C	D	E	F	G	H	I	J	K	L	M	N	O	P	Q	R	S	T	187
188	A	B	C	D	E	F	G	H	I	J	K	L	M	N	O	P	Q	R	S	T	188
189	A	B	C	D	E	F	G	H	I	J	K	L	M	N	O	P	Q	R	S	T	189
190	A	B	C	D	E	F	G	H	I	J	K	L	M	N	O	P	Q	R	S	T	190
191	A	B	C	D	E	F	G	H	I	J	K	L	M	N	O	P	Q	R	S	T	191
192	A	B	C	D	E	F	G	H	I	J	K	L	M	N	O	P	Q	R	S	T	192
193	A	B	C	D	E	F	G	H	I	J	K	L	M	N	O	P	Q	R	S	T	193
194	A	B	C	D	E	F	G	H	I	J	K	L	M	N	O	P	Q	R	S	T	194
195	A	B	C	D	E	F	G	H	I	J	K	L	M	N	O	P	Q	R	S	T	195
196	A	B	C	D	E	F	G	H	I	J	K	L	M	N	O	P	Q	R	S	T	196
197	A	B	C	D	E	F	G	H	I	J	K	L	M	N	O	P	Q	R	S	T	197
198	A	B	C	D	E	F	G	H	I	J	K	L	M	N	O	P	Q	R	S	T	198
199	A	B	C	D	E	F	G	H	I	J	K	L	M	N	O	P	Q	R	S	T	199
200	A	B	C	D	E	F	G	H	I	J	K	L	M	N	O	P	Q	R	S	T	200

Answers

Serial No.	Answer No.	Answer
1	g	Obsessive-compulsive personality disorders
2	f	Paranoid personality disorders
3	d	Schizoid personality disorder
4	a	Histrionic personality disorder
5	j	Dependent personality disorder
6	h	Possible infection
7	a	Hyperglycaemia
8	e	Autonomic neuropathy
9	f	Intermittent claudication
10	i	Lactic acidosis
11	k	Tuberculosis
12	i	*Staphylococcus aureus*
13	c	Fungal pneumonia
14	h	*Pneumocystitis carinii* pneumonia
15	g	*Mycoplasma pneumoniae*
16	j	Temporal arteritis
17	i	Retinal detachment
18	e	Cerebral haemorrhage
19	c	Central retinal artery occulsion
20	k	Uveitis
21	b	Alzheimer's dementia
22	j	Vascular dementia
23	e	HIV
24	f	Huntington's chorea
25	g	Parkinsonim (drug induced)
26	e	Captopril
27	d	Cyclophosphamide
28	j	Frusemide
29	f	Gentamicin
30	i	Acetazolamide
31	e	Burr hole(s) should be drilled
32	g	Normal saline infusion
33	d	Transfer to operating theatre
34	f	Chest drain after needle thoracocentesis
35	i	Splint limb
36	g	Intermittent inhaled bronchodilation
37	e	Inhaled sodium chromoglycate
38	k	Nebulised Bronchodilator
39	e	Inhaled sodium chromoglycate
40	b	Adrenaline
41	i	Subphrenic abscess
42	c	Biliary peritonitis
43	h	Stone in common bile duct
44	h	Stone in common bile duct
45	e	Myocardial infarction
46	a	DVT
47	j	Pelvic abscess
48	g	Acute tubular necrosis
49	c	Impending wound dehiscence
50	b	Septicaemia
51	j	Colonic cancer (left side)
52	i	Rectal carcinoma
53	f	Severe ulcerative colitis
54	e	Crohn's disease
55	d	Irritable bowel syndrome (IBS)
56	b	Perthes disease
57	a	Fracture neck of femur
58	e	Septic arthritis

59	c	Slipped femoral epiphyses
60	i	Osteomyelitis
61	a	No treatment
62	g	3% pilocarpine and acetazolamide
63	d	Enucleation
64	c	Immediate antibiotic therapy
65	f	05% prednisolone drops 2 hourly and cyclopentolate drops
66	k	Acute lymphoblastic leukaemia
67	i	Chronic myeloid leukaemia
68	d	Multiple myeloma
69	g	Hodgkin's disease
70	f	Non-Hodgkin's lymphoma
71	c	Naloxone
72	d	Warfarin
73	k	100% O_2
74	a	Tricyclic antidepressants
75	g	Cyanide
76	e	Coeliac disease
77	f	Ulcerative colitis
78	d	Chronic non-specific diarrhoea
79	h	Entrobius vermicularis
80	k	IBS
81	f	Nitrous oxide
82	b	Epidural anaesthesia
83	c	Pudendal nerve block
84	b	Epidural anaesthesia
85	d	General anaesthesia
86	k	Herpes zoster
87	l	Cluster headache
88	h	Sinusitis
89	j	Temporal arteritis

90	g	Trigeminal neualgia
91	c	Glycosuria
92	i	Stress incontinence
93	h	Urge incontinence
94	j	True incontinence
95	g	Urethral syndrome
96	e	Mammography
97	b	Fine-needle aspiration cytology
98	b	Fine-needle aspiration cytology
99	e	Mammogram
100	d	Reassurance
101	g	Naloxone
102	f	CT scan
103	i	Plasma osmolality
104	g	Nalaxone
105	k	Urea and electrolytes
106	a	Brucellosis
107	i	Scabies
108	c	*Escherichia coli*
109	j	Hepatitis A
110	k	Tuberculosis
111	h	Myocardial infarction
112	a	Hypothermia
113	d	LAH
114	i	IHD
115	k	Myocarditis
116	a	Nephrotic syndrome
117	k	Alkalosis
118	e	G6PD deficiency
119	b	Tuberculosis
120	c	Intestinal hurry
121	i	Osteogenesis imperfecta
122	a	Elderly abuse
123	c	Child sexual abuse
124	b	Child physical abuse

125	l	Accidental injury
126	f	Peptic ulcer disease
127	b	Stable angina
128	k	Tuberculosis
129	j	Chronic pancreatitis
130	i	Acute cholecystitis
131	b	CT skull
132	g	Immediate hydration
133	a	Lumbar puncture
134	j	Transfer to ITU
135	k	Reassure
136	k	Trimethoprim
137	e	Metronidazole
138	c	Erythromycin
139	f	Amoxycillin
140	c	Erythromycin
141	k	Oral hypotensive drugs
142	h	IV antihypertensive
143	b	A period of observation of BP
144	i	Recheck blood pressure in seven days
145	c	24 hours urinary protein
146	i	Hypercalcaemia
147	i	Hypercalcaemia
148	c	Anorexia nervosa
149	a	Carcinoma colon
150	b	Parkinsonism
151	b	Needle exchange
152	h	Combination therapy
153	f	Counselling
154	k	Cotrimoxazole
155	g	Condoms
156	c	Acute adrenal insufficiency

157	e	CMV disease
158	f	Type I RTA
159	h	None of the answers
160	j	Type II RTA
161	f	Multiple myeloma
162	h	Pregnancy
163	g	Polycythemic rubra vera
164	e	Malignancy
165	d	Inherited clotting abnormality
166	c	Reiter's syndrome
167	j	Dermatomyositis
168	h	Behcet's syndrome
169	e	Lyme's disease
170	b	Sarcoidosis
171	g	Carcinoma of tail of pancreas
172	d	Coeliac disease
173	f	*Borrelia burghdorferi*
174	b	Diabetes mellitus
175	a	Hyperthyroidism
176	d	3-10 years
177	f	30 years
178	b	12 months
179	j	65 years
180	b	12 months
181	a	Klinefelters's syndrome
182	g	Sickle cell disease
183	i	Beta thalassaemia
184	g	Sickle cell disease
185	c	Down's syndrome
186	h	Underwater seal drainage
187	e	Cross match blood and inform surgeons

188	c	High flow O_2 + 10 mg IV morphine + anticoagulation
189	e	Cross-match blood and inform surgeons
190	c	High flow O_2 + 10 mg IV morphine + anticoagulation
191	i	Sputum culture
192	b	Fibreoptic bronchoscopy
193	g	Pulmonary angiogram

194	a	CT
195	a	CT
196	d	Dental treatment of a cardiac patient
197	g	Heart value replacement
198	h	Sigmoid colectomy
199	i	Splenectomy
200	f	Emergency appendicectomy

Previous Year Paper 6

RxPG Analysis

Total Themes:	**40**
Repeat Themes:	**7**
Repeat Themes with a Different Header:	**16**

THEME 1: INVESTIGATION OF RED EYE

OPTIONS

a. Eye washing
b. Intraocular pressure
c. Flourescein stain
d. Eye secretion swap culture
e. Acrocyst drainage
f. X-ray of orbit
g. Conjunctival cytology
h. MRI
i. Gonioscopy
j. CT
k. None required

For each presentation below, choose the ***most appropriate investigation*** *from the above list of OPTIONS. Each option may be used once, more than once, or not at all.*

QUESTIONS

1. A 69-year-old patient presented to his GP with sudden onset of redness in the right eye. There was no pain and vision was unaffected.
2. A patient presents with metal pieces to his eyes.
3. A mother brings her 2-year-old child with a squint. On examination a leucokoric right pupil is seen with an absent red reflex.
4. A 12-year-old Libyan boy gave a two weeks history of discomfort, redness and mucopurulent discharge affecting both eyes. His two siblings have a similar problem.
5. A 23-year-old man has a history of recurrent attacks of blurring of vision associated with redness, pain and photophobia. Both eyes have been affected in the past. His brother is currently being investigated for bowel disease and a severe backache.

THEME 2: MANAGEMENT OF SUDDEN VISUAL LOSS

OPTIONS

a. Do nothing
b. Steroids
c. Laser photocoagulation
d. Pilocarpine
e. Lens transplantation
f. Eye surgery
g. Admit for specialist neurosurgical evaluation
h. IV mannitol
i. 1% atropine sulphate ointment
j. LASIK
k. Cataract surgery

For each presentation below, choose the ***most appropriate management*** *from the above list of OPTIONS. Each option may be used once, more than once, or not at all.*

QUESTIONS

6. A 78-year-old man has had a painful scalp and headache for three weeks, and is generally unwell, complains of acute onset of blindness in his right eye.
7. A 50-year-old woman complains of sudden loss of vision in one eye. She describes the incident, like a curtain coming down.
8. An 84-year-old woman notices sudden increased visual impairment. She is found to have homonymous hemianopia.
9. A 68-year-old smoker suddenly notices markedly reduced vision in one eye. He cannot read any letter on visual acuity chart but can count fingers. The fundus is pale.
10. A 30-year-old man has recurrent episodes of an acutely painful red eye with reduced vision.

THEME 3: DIAGNOSIS OF HEAD INJURY

OPTIONS

a. Diffuse brain damage
b. Cerebral haematoma
c. Extradural haematoma
d. Subdural haematoma
e. Temporal linear fracture
f. Subarachnoid haematoma
g. Epilepsy
h. Depression
i. Superficial head injury
j. Insignificant head injury
k. Vasogenic cerebral oedema

For each presentation below, choose the ***single most likely diagnosis*** *from the above list of OPTIONS. Each option may be used once, more than once, or not at all.*

QUESTIONS

11. Following an alcoholic binge a 36-year-old male falls and comes to casualty with a cut in his temporal region his Glasgow Coma Scale is normal and his neck is cleared by the orthopaedic SHO.
12. An 8-year-old boy falls off a swing at his school. He is brought to casualty by one of his teachers. He has a bruise over his right eye but the examination is otherwise normal. He is fully conscious with no history of blackouts since the accident. A skull X-ray is performed, which is normal.
13. A young woman is involved in an RTA and is brought in with a Glasgow Coma Scale of 6 . A CT scan shows evidence of diffuse cerebral oedema but no evidence of haemorrhage. She has bilateral papilledema.
14. A young man is involved in a fight and suffers a blow to the back of the head. A skull X-ray reveals a depressed fracture of the occiput. His Glasgow Coma Scale on admission is 14 but falls rapidly within an hour.
15. A 24-year-old patient presents with RTA. The pupil on the left side is dilated and the patient is obtunded. CT scan of the head reveals a biconvex hyperdense lesion on the temporal region.

THEME 4: POISONING MANAGEMENT

OPTIONS

a. Carbon monooxide
b. Warfarin
c. Heparin
d. Ethyl alcohol
e. Quinine
f. Paracetamol
g. Carbamazepine
h. Tricyclic antidepressants
i. Cyanide
j. Aspirin
k. Ecstacy

For each presentation below, choose the ***single most likely diagnosis management*** *from the above list of OPTIONS. Each option may be used once, more than once, or not at all.*

QUESTIONS

16. Condition in which patient was found with nasal involvement and nasal hairs sighing. He presents with myalgia, malaise and headache.
17. Condition in which vitamin K is given to improve patient.
18. A 7-year-old boy accidentally swallowed some unknown white tablets and now complaining of right hypochondrial pain after 12 hours.
19. The side effect is urinary retention, heart block and ringing of ear.
20. A patient who has overdosed on an unknown medication presents with palpitations. What is the most likely cause?

THEME 5: DRUGS

OPTIONS

a. Opioid overdose
b. Opioid withdrawal
c. Tricyclic intoxication
d. Carbamazepine
e. Lithium
f. Haloperidol
g. Clozapine
h. Naloxone
i. Natrexone
j. Paracetamol
k. Aspirin

For each presentation below, choose the ***single most likely cause*** *from the above list of OPTIONS. Each option may be used once, more than once, or not at all.*

QUESTIONS

21. Schizophrenic patient under treatment presents with fever, increased WBC, increased muscle creatinine kinase levels.
22. A homeless patient presents to A and E with drowsiness. On examination, abrasions and puncture marks were found on his arm. He has pinpoint pupil. What would you give?
23. Schizophrenic patient under treatment presents with sorethroat, decreased WBC, agranulocytosis.
24. Patient on treatment for bipolar disorder, hypothyroidism features.
25. A patient who has overdosed on an unknown medication presents with palpitations. What is the most likely cause?

THEME 6: INVESTIGATION IN GASTROINTESTINAL DISEASE

OPTIONS

a. Chest X-ray
b. Abdominal USG
c. Amylase level
d. Brain CT
e. Barium enema
f. Laparotomy
g. Stool culture
h. Blood culture
i. Bulk laxatives
j. Stimulant laxatives
k. Colonoscopy
l. Sigmoidoscopy

For each presentation below, choose the ***most appropriate investigation*** *from the above list of OPTIONS. Each option may be used once, more than once, or not at all.*

QUESTIONS

26. For the past two weeks a middle-aged railway engineer has complained of acute constipation. His stools are dark, but not apparently blood stained. Abdominal palpation detects a mass with moderate tenderness.
27. A 43-year-old man says he cannot finish his stool and that what he does pass is streaked with blood. He says he has always been regular. He wants to know if a laxative will help.
28. A 49-year-old lawyer complains of blood and diarrhoea. She is also suffering from abdominal pain, fever, and general ill-health. On palpation you find tenderness in the lower abdomen.
29. A young woman presents with recurrent abdominal pain, episodic diarrhoea, malaise, and fever. Over the past few years she has felt her health to be declining. At presentation she complains of severe abdominal pain and constipation.
30. A young woman complains of cramp like abdominal pain, and difficulties with bowel movements. Acute abdominal pain is frequently relieved by embarrassing flatulence. Barium studies and sigmoidoscopy have proved inconclusive.

THEME 7: DIFFERENTIAL DIAGNOSIS OF DYSPHAGIA

OPTIONS

a. Candidiasis
b. Ebstein-Barr
c. Diffuse oesophageal spasm
d. Achalasia
e. Oesophageal carcinoma
f. Pharyngeal pouch
g. Barret's oesophagus
h. Carcinoma stomach
i. Gastrectomy
j. Sialadenitis
k. Schatzki's rings

For each presentation below, choose the ***most likely diagnosis*** *from the above list of OPTIONS. Each option may be used once, more than once, or not at all.*

QUESTIONS

31. A known HIV (+) patient presents with pain in swallowing and some lesion in the mouth. The underlying tissue is red when the lesion is taken off.
32. A patient comes with dysphagia for solids for 5 years and now presents with regurgitation when he eats, it relieves a few hours after meal.
33. A 65-year-old male presents with weight loss, difficulty in swallowing solid. Dysphagia is getting worse.
34. A patient presents with intermittent dysphagia for both solids and liquids and chest pain. No weight loss.
35. A patient with difficulty in swallowing, filling defect. He has a long standing history of Barret's oesophagus.

THEME 8: DIAGNOSIS OF HEPATOBILIARY DISEASE

OPTIONS

a. Chronic pancreatitis
b. Acute pancreatitis
c. Duodenal ulcer
d. Gastric ulcer
e. Gallstones
f. Hepatitis B
g. CBD obstruction
h. Hereditary haemochromatosis (HHC)
i. Acute cholecystitis
j. Primary biliary cirrhosis (PBC)
k. Hepatoma

For each presentation below, choose the ***single most likely diagnosis*** *from the above list of OPTIONS. Each option may be used once, more than once, or not at all.*

QUESTIONS

36. Man returned from trip to Asia, complains of anorexia, malaise, dark urine, pale stools.
37. An 80-year-old man has never been out of UK, one month history of epigastric pain, dark urine, pale stools, jaundice.
38. Female with fever, rigors, right upper quadrant pain, jaundice, ultrasound is normal.
39. Female, 50-year-old, 5 years history of mild pruritus. History of pale stools, dark urine, jaundice.
40. Man with history of haemochromatosis and alcohol addiction presents with jaundice, ascites, variceal bleed. USG is unequivocal, high ferritin level.

THEME 9: DIAGNOSIS OF SCROTAL PAIN

OPTIONS

a. Acute epidydimo-orchitis
b. Chronic epididimo-orchitis
c. Hydrocoele
d. Varicocoele
e. Teratoma
f. Seminoma
g. Testicular torsion
h. Lymphoma
i. UTI
j. Sebaceous cyst
k. Seminoma or teratoma

*For each presentation below, choose the **single most likely diagnosis** from the above list of OPTIONS. Each option may be used once, more than once, or not at all.*

QUESTIONS

41. Man after trip to Asia presents with red, swollen scrotum.
42. Man with painful red scrotum and vomiting.
43. Man with painless testicular swelling since 2 months.
44. Man with a swelling of scrotum since 3 years.
45. Man with no history of unsafe sex presents with dysuria and urinary frequency.

THEME 10: MANAGEMENT OF DIABETIC COMPLICATIONS

OPTIONS

a. Hyperglycaemia
b. Hypoglycaemia
c. Urinary tract infection
d. Somatic neuropathy
e. Autonomic neuropathy
f. Intermittent claudication
g. Atherosclerosis
h. Possible infection
i. Lactic acidosis
j. Ketoacidosis
k. Amyotrophy

INSTRUCTIONS

For each of the patients listed below, choose the **most likely complication** *from the list of options above. Each option may be used once, more than once, or not at all.*

QUESTIONS

46. A 48-year-old female, insulin dependent diabetic, who has been on treatment for 20-year presents with a history of three episodes of severe hypoglycaemia. She has not changed her insulin requirement, diet or exercise pattern.
47. A 48-year-old female, insulin dependent diabetic, who has been on treatment for 20 years, presents with urinary frequency but no dysuria or urgency. Her blood glucose is 17.5 mmol/L.
48. A 30-year-old female, insulin dependent diabetic, presents with failure to pass urine.
49. A 68-year-old diabetic on treatment for the last 5-year presents with calf pain exacerbated by movement.
50. A 70-year-old diabetic on treatment with metformin presents with severe epigastric pain, drowsiness and confusion.

THEME 11: INVESTIGATION OF THYROID DISORDERS

OPTIONS
a. Serum TSH levels
b. Serum T_4 levels
c. Skull X-ray
d. Serum T_3 levels
e. Contrast radiographs
f. FNAC
g. USG
h. MRI
i. Biopsy
j. Thyroglobulin autoantibodies
k. TSH receptor autoantibodies

*For each presentation below, choose the **most appropriate investigation** from the above list of OPTIONS. Each option may be used once, more than once, or not at all.*

QUESTIONS
51. Female, 41-year-old, presents with hard, irregular fixed swelling, stridor, dysphagia since 3 months.
52. Old lady with smooth neck swelling, bradycardia, spare coarse hair, macrocytic anaemia.
53. Female on treatment for supraventricular tachycardia complains of seeing dots and glare on driving at night, exophthalmos, no goitre.
54. Female, swelling in the neck, tremor irritability, diarrhoea, bruit.
55. A 35-year-old woman who was diagnosed as having coelic disease at the age of 12 years has had good control of her abdominal symptoms for a number of years. She presents with a recent history of weight loss, tiredness, diarrhoea and abdominal pain.

THEME 12: INVESTIGATION OF ABDOMINAL PAIN IN A WOMAN

OPTIONS
a. Transvaginal USG
b. Cervical os examination
c. Laparotomy
d. Colposcopic examination
e. Abdominal USG + high vaginal swab
f. Lupus factor
g. Fibroid study
h. Flexible sigmoidoscopy
i. Laparoscopy
j. None required
k. Endocervical swab

*For each presentation below, choose the **single most appropriate investigation** from the above list of OPTIONS. Each option may be used once, more than once, or not at all.*

QUESTIONS
56. A 35-year-old woman complains of abdominal discomfort relieved by passing flatus or- defaecation. Over the last 6 months she has had episodes of diarrhoea and constipation, but denied she had lost weight.
57. A 37-year-old woman presents with a sudden onset of severe left iliac fossa pain. On vaginal USG, 2 cm echogenic masses are seen in the broad ligament. She says this pain seems to come on every month.
58. A 23-year-old woman just had an intrauterine device fitted. She complains of a watery brown vaginal discharge and abdominal pain.
59. An 18 weeks pregnant female presents with lower abdominal pain and tenderness, with offensive vaginal discharge. She has high grade fever since last two days.
60. A 32-year-old woman who consciously uses the oral contraceptive pill, has experienced monthly vaginal bleeding. On abdominal examination she is uncomfortable. Her temperature is 37°C. She is otherwise healthy.

THEME 13: MANAGEMENT OF RENAL DISEASE

OPTIONS

a. IV hydrocortisone
b. Oral prednisolone
c. Indinavir
d. Frusemide
e. Sodium bicarbonate
f. Fluid restriction
g. Potassium supplements
h. Acetazolamide
i. Amphotericin
j. Ganciclovir IV
k. Shohl's solution

For each presentation below, choose the ***most appropriate management*** *from the above list of OPTIONS. Each option may be used once, more than once, or not at all.*

QUESTIONS

61. A 30-year-old man with AIDS presented in shock. Serum biochemistry reveals: Potassium 6.7 mmol/L, bicarbonate 20 mmol/L, chloride 84 mmol/L, creatinine 160 μmol/L.
62. A 41-year-old Londoner developed a temperature of 41°C, 5 weeks after cadaveric renal transplantation. WBC is 2.1 × 1,000,000,000/L, Hb is 8.8 g/dl, creatinine 177 μmol/L. Aspartate aminotransferase (AST) 82 U/L. Alanine aminotransferase (ALT) 132 U/L.
63. A 36-year-old woman with leukaemia has been treated with Amphotericin B for a fungal pneumonia. She presents with muscle weakness. Sodium 137 mmol/L, potassium 2.7 mmol/L , bicarbonate 19 mmol/L, chloride 110 mmol/L, creatinine 84 μmol/L, urine pH 6.8 mmol/L.
64. An 83-year-old woman with small cell lung cancer presents with ankle oedema and is found to have 8 g/day, urine proteinuria. He is started on frusemide. Ten days later his blood pressure is 115/75 mmHg lying and 85/65 mmHg standing. Serum biochemistry was; sodium 121 mmol/L, bicarbonate 24 mmol/L, potassium 3.6 mmol/L, creatinine 113 μmol/L, chloride 95 mmol/L, urea 11.5 mmol/L, glucose 5.7 mmol/L , albumin 27g, osmolality 263 mOs m/L, urine osmolality 417 mOs m/L.
65. A fit 50-year-old man is prescribed oral acetazolamide by an ophthalmologist for suspected glaucoma. He presents with lethargy and shortness of breath on exertion. Sodium 140 mmol/L, potassium 3.2 mmol/L, bicarbonate 18 mmol/L, chloride 115 mmol/L, urea 6.7 mmol/L, creatinine 114 μmol/L

THEME 14: IMMEDIATE MANAGEMENT OF ELECTROLYTE DISTURBANCES

OPTIONS

a. ACE inhibitors
b. Decrease insulin dose
c. Increase insulin dose
d. Thiazides
e. Beta-blockers
f. Frusemide
g. Potassium supplements
h. $NaHCO_3$
i. $NaCl + K^+$ supplements
j. 5% dextrose solution
k. Calcium resonium

For each presentation below, choose the ***most important step in immediate management*** *from the above list of OPTIONS. Each option may be used once, more than once, or not at all.*

QUESTIONS

66. Man with pyloric stenosis, profuse vomiting, hypokalaemia and increased bicarbonate.
67. Man who is not able to pass urine, tired, complains of hiccups.
68. Man with villous adenoma, profuse diarrhoea.
69. Female, 24 hours after hysterectomy complains of breathlessness, increased JVP.
70. A patient in severe renal failure has potassium level of 2. 5 mmol/L.

THEME 15: INVESTIGATION OF PULMONARY DISEASES

OPTIONS
a. Pleural biopsy
b. V/Q scan
c. Chest X-ray
d. Echocardiography
e. Mediastinoscopy
f. Bronchoscopy
g. Sputum culture and microscopy
h. ECG
i. Brochial lavage
j. Pulmonary function tests
k. Exercise ECG

*For each presentation below, choose the **most descriptive investigations** from the above list of OPTIONS. Each option may be used once, more than once, or not at all.*

QUESTIONS
71. A man who has been worked as boiler worker for 20 years presents with dyspnoea and pleurisy.
72. Female with cough, copious blood tinged sputum for more than a month. She is from south-east Asia.
73. A middle-aged woman develops a purulent cough with some haemoptysis. A chest X-ray reveals right upper lobe shadows.
74. Female presents with acute pleuritic chest pain, haemoptysis after undergoing hysterectomy.
75. A patient with an area of consolidation and fever on his chest X-ray is treated with antibiotics. His fever resolves but four weeks later he still has a large area of consolidation.

THEME 16: DIAGNOSIS OF PULMONARY DISEASES

OPTIONS
a. Sarcoidosis
b. COPD
c. Allergic rhinitis
d. Anxiety
e. Pulmonary oedema
f. Mitral stenosis
g. Pulmonary embolism
h. Pneumothorax-spontaneous
i. Pneumothorax-tension
j. Aspiration pneumonitis
k. Asthma

*For each presentation below, choose the **single most likely diagnosis** from the above list of OPTIONS. Each option may be used once, more than once, or not at all.*

QUESTIONS
76. Patient with acute shortness of breath, wheeze. chest X-ray—normal, low oxygen, low $PaCO_2$. PEFR-120 ml/minute.
77. Bilateral hilar opacities, ACE is high.
78. A 20-year-old woman attends A and E complaining of sudden breathlessness and anxiety. She describes palpitations and paraesthesiae of her hands, feet and lips. ECG shows sinus tachycardia and O_2 saturation is normal.
79. An alcoholic admitted semi-comatose. ABG shows low oxygen saturation.
80. Patient with recent MI, develops acute breathlessness with haemoptysis. CXR shows dilated pulmonary artery and wedge-shaped area of infarction. Decreased PaO_2 and $PaCO_2$.

THEME 17: MANAGEMENT OF ACUTE CHEST PAIN

OPTIONS
a. Glyceryl trinitrate (0.5 mg) sublingually
b. IV 50 ml of 50% dextrose
c. High flow O_2 and ramipril 2.5 mg/12 hr PO
d. High flow O_2, 10 mg IV morphine + anticoagulation
e. Crossmatch blood and inform surgeons
f. Insert a 16 G cannula in second intercostal space
g. IV heparin 5000-10,000 iu over 5 min
h. Underwater seal drainage
i. 10 mg IV diamorphine
j. Nifedine
k. Ramipril

*For each presentation below, choose the **best management** from the above list of OPTIONS. Each option may be used once, more than once, or not at all.*

QUESTIONS

81. A tall young man developed sharp pain on one side of his chest two days ago. Since then he has been short of breath on exertion.
82. After a heavy bout of drinking a 56-year-old man vomits several times and develops chest pain. When you examine him, he has a crackling feeling under the skin around his neck.
83. A 23-year-old woman on the oral contraceptive pill suddenly gets tightness in her chest and becomes very breathless.
84. A 30-year-old man with Marfan's syndrome has sudden central chest pain going through to the back.
85. A 57-year-old man develops crushing pain in the chest associated with nausea and profuse sweating. The pain is still present when he arrives in hospital an hour later.

THEME 18: COMPLICATIONS OF BREAST CARCINOMA

OPTIONS
a. Pathological fracture
b. Cerebral metastases
c. Hypocalcaemia
d. Lymphoedema
e. Spinal cord compression
f. Hypercalcaemia
g. Hyperparathyroidism

*For each presentation below, choose the **most common complication** from the above list of options. Each option may be used once, more than once, or not at all.*

QUESTIONS

86. Female with breast carcinoma 3 years back, was treated with mastectomy and lymph node clearance on the left side, presents with a swollen limb and decreased hand movements.
87. Presents with thirst, confusion, constipation.
88. Presents with weakness of both legs, difficulty walking, urine retention.
89. Presents with headache, confusion. On examination, papilloedema present.
90. Presents with features of fracture femur.

THEME 19: THE DIAGNOSIS OF NON-ACCIDENTAL INJURY

OPTIONS

a. Accidental injury
b. Emotional abuse
c. Physical abuse
d. Sexual abuse
e. Child neglect
f. Osteogenesis imperfecta
g. ITP
h. Normally present in a child
i. Elderly abuse
j. Henoch-Schönlein purpura
k. Immune thrombocytopenia purpura

*For each presentation below, choose the **single most likely diagnosis** from the above list of options. Each option may be used once, more than once, or not at all.*

QUESTIONS

91. A 16-year-old mother brings her baby for immunisation. The nurse notices the baby has multiple bruises along both arms and legs. The baby is crying excessively. The house officer notices multiple fractures and that the baby has blue sclerae.

92. A 70-year-old man is receiving treatment for Alzheimer's disease. He is looked after by a 23-year-old granddaughter. He has recently developed faecal incontinence. The SHO notices bruises on both wrists and back.

93. An anxious mother brings her 6-year-old daughter who is bleeding per vaginum. Six months prior to this presentation the girl had a confirmed streptococcal sore-throat infection. She is otherwise normal.

94. A 4-day-old girl is brought to casualty by the maternal grandparent who is worried about two dark bluish patches on the child's buttocks. Child's mother is white and the father is black.

95. An 8-year-old girl is noted to have fresh bloody staining of her pants. She also suffers from enuresis. She has recently started horse-riding lessons.

THEME 20: INVESTIGATION OF NECK LUMPS

OPTIONS

a. USG
b. Technetium scan
c. Aspiration and microscopy
d. CT scan
e. MRI scan
f. Chest X-ray
g. Digital substraction angiography
h. FNAC
i. Transillumination test
j. Biopsy

*For each presentation below, choose the **single most appropriate investgation** from the above list of OPTIONS. Each option may be used once, more than once, or not at all.*

QUESTIONS

96. Patient with a pulsatile hard mass fixed under the upper one-third of the sternomastoid muscle.

97. A 40-year-old male has a lump in the supero-posterior area of the anterior triangle.

98. A 16-year-old female has a midline lump in the neck which moves on protrusion of the tongue and is below the hyoid bone.

99. A 19-year-old male has a cystic mass under the anterior border of sternomastoid at the junction of upper one-third and middle one-third of the muscle. Aspiration revealed fluid containing cholesterol crystals.

100. An infant present with a transilluminant swelling in the lower third of neck.

THEME 21: IMMEDIATE MANAGEMENT OF BURNS

OPTIONS

a. IV fluids
b. Escharotomy
c. Admit to hospital
d. Carboxyhaemoglobin level
e. IV blood transfusion
f. Deroof blister
g. Aspirate blister
h. Blood transfusion
i. Skin grafting
j. Antibiotics
k. Fasciotomy
l. Reassure

For each presentation below, choose the ***most appropriate immediate management*** *from the above list of OPTIONS. Each option may be used once, more than once, or not at all.*

QUESTIONS

101. Patient after escaping from fire in a building has singed nostrils.

102. Patient has a large tense blister.

103. An adult patient has partial thickness burns on the anterior chest and upper thighs.

104. An adult patient has full thickness circumferential burns from the elbow to the fingers, covering them completely.

105. Man, slept while sunbathing comes with redness, pain all over his body. otherwise well.

THEME 22: DEVELOPMENTAL MILESTONES

OPTIONS

a. One week
b. 2 weeks
c. 6 weeks
d. 2 months
e. 6 months
f. 9 months
g. 1 year
h. 2 years
i. 3 years
j. 4 years
k. 4½ years

For each presentation below, choose the ***most appropriate answer*** *from the above list of OPTIONS. Each option may be used once, more than once, or not at all.*

QUESTIONS

106. Copies circle, can say 4 words,

107. Smiles responsively, head lags

108. Can walk 4 steps upstairs

109. Holds head up at 45° when prone, vocalise

110. Pincer grip; can say "Mummy" ± "Daddy"

THEME 23: ANATOMICAL LOCALISATION OF MULTIPLE SCLEROSIS

OPTIONS
a. Cerebrum
b. Optic disc
c. Optic nerve
d. Optic radiation
e. Cerebral cortex
f. Brainstem and its cerebellar connections
g. Cervical spinal cord
h. Thoracic spinal cord
i. Facial nerve
j. Trigeminal nerve
k. Fascial nucleus

*For each presentation below, choose the **best answer** from the above list of OPTIONS. Each option may be used once, more than once, or not at all.*

QUESTIONS

111. Known patient of multiple sclerosis now with complaint of urinary incontinence, weakness in all 4 limbs and difficulty walking.

122. Patient has nystagmus, diplopia, and positive past-pointing.

113. Patient has repeated attacks of multiple sclerosis, and now has pale temporal disc.

114. Patient with complaint of blurring of vision, papilloedema, pain in eye.

115. A known patient of multiple sclerosis with unilateral facial paralysis with no loss of taste.

THEME 24: ROLE OF IMMUNISATION AND PREVENTION IN LIVER DISEASES

OPTIONS
a. Hepatitis A immunisation
b. Hepatitis B immunoglobulin
c. Hepatitis B vaccine
d. Leptospirosis
e. Hepatitis A infection
f. Hepatocellular carcinoma
g. Schistosomiasis
h. Lyme disease
i. Cirrhosis
j. Haemangioma
k. Chronic active hepatitis

*For each presentation below, choose the **single most appropriate** from the above list of OPTIONS. Each option may be used once, more than once, or not at all.*

QUESTIONS

116. Not eating sea shell products prevents.

117. Immunisation of sewage workers.

118. Not swimming in foreign lakes prevents.

119. Immunisation of health workers who are in contact with body fluid.

120. Mass immunisation of hepatitis B, besides preventing hepatitis B also prevents.

THEME 25: DIAGNOSIS OF HEARING LOSS

OPTIONS

a. Acoustic neuroma
b. Blast injury
c. Petrous temporal bone fracture
d. Wax impaction
e. Acute otitis media
f. Ototoxicity
g. Fracture base of skull
h. CSOM
i. Glue ear
j. Herpes zoster
k. Foreign body

*For each presentation below, choose the **most likely diagnosis** from the above list of OPTIONS. Each option may be used once, more than once, or not at all.*

QUESTIONS

121. Man treated with gentamicin for peritonitis for 10 days presents with deafness.
122. A patient with poor hygenic condition presents with hearing loss after taking a shower.
123. Woman presents with deafness and corneal anaesthesia. On MRI, a widened internal auditory meatus is seen.
124. Male, 20 years, with history of head injury, bruising on the side of head complains of hearing loss.
125. A 54-year-old female develops mild fever, malaise and ear pain. Three days later she developed multiple painful vesicles over her early canal and external meatus.

THEME 26: INVESTIGATION OF PAINFUL JOINTS IN CHILDREN

OPTIONS

a. Serology for autoantibodies
b. Diagnostic aspiration for WBC demonstration
c. MRI
d. Diagnostic aspiration for culture
e. CT scan
f. Diagnostic aspiration for RBC
g. Serum urate
h. X-ray knee joint
i. Therapeutic aspiration of joint
j. AP X-ray—hip joint
k. Lateral X-ray—hip joint

*For each presentation below, choose the **single most appropriate** from the above list of OPTIONS. Each option may be used once, more than once, or not at all.*

QUESTIONS

126. A six-year-old boy complains of intermittent hip pain for several months. Haematological investigations are normal. X-rays show flattening of the femoral head.
127. A two-year-old girl with one day history of increasing hip pain has become unable to weight bear. Her WCC is 21/fl, with an ESR of 89 mm/hr and a CRP of 300 mg/L. A radiograph of the hip shows a widened joint space.
128. A 12-year-old boy with left groin pain for 6 weeks is noticed to stand with the left leg externally rotated. Examination reveals negligible internal rotation of the hip.
129. A four-year-old boy complains of right hip pain a few days following an upper respiratory tract infection. Blood tests are as follows: WCC 12/fl, ESR 10 mm/hr and CRP 2 mg/L.
130. A five-year-old girl complains of progressively increasing severe pain in her left hip and upper leg for 6 days. She is able to walk but limps visibly. Blood tests are as follows: WCC 19/fl, ESR 72 mm/hr and CRP 94 mg/L. X-rays and ultrasound scans of the hip are normal.

THEME 27: AETIOLOGY OF ANAEMIA

OPTIONS
a. Chronic blood loss
b. Rheumatoid arthritis
c. Pernicious anaemia
d. Haemolysis
e. Beta-thalassaemia
f. Alcoholism
g. Sickle cell anaemia
h. B_{12} deficiency
i. Scurvy
j. Nutritional deficit
k. Malabsorption

For each presentation below, choose the ***single most likely cause of the given profile*** *from the above list of OPTIONS. Each option may be used once, more than once, or not at all.*

QUESTIONS
131. Patient with atrophic gastritis has megaloblastic anaemia.
132. Patient who is a strict vegetarian has an MCV of 110.
133. Patient has both iron and folate deficiency radiology and sigmoidoscopy—normal, has pale stools which is difficult to flush away.
134. Elderly patient with complaint of anaemia and has bleeding gum.
135. Elderly patient in residential home stay with complaint of tiredness.

THEME 28: MANAGEMENT OF EPISTAXIS

OPTIONS
a. Anterior pack
b. Posterior pack
c. Anterior pack and posterior pack
d. Electrocautery
e. Surgery
f. Review anticoagulation
g. Antihypertensives
h. Embolisation of feeding vessel
i. Cocaine spray
j. Ice pack
k. Cryotherapy

For each presentation below, choose the ***most appropriate step in management*** *from the above list of OPTIONS. Each option may be used once, more than once, or not at all.*

QUESTIONS
136. There is just blood clotting in the nostrils bleeding has stopped.
137. A patient with nose bleeding, on exam vascular damage is found, there is still some leakage.
138. Man with prosthetic heart valve presents with epistaxis.
139. Man who is involved in furniture making presents with recurrent epistaxis and anaesthesia of right cheek.
140. An 80-year-old man with history of epistaxis since 2 hours.

THEME 29: IMMEDIATE MANAGEMENT OF COMMON HAEMATOLOGICAL COMPLICATIONS

OPTIONS
a. Central venous line
b. Intraosseous fluid injection
c. Fresh frozen plasma
d. Blood transfusion
e. Blood and platelet transfusion
f. Chemotherapy
g. CT scan skull
h. Hydroxyurea
i. Systemic steroids
j. Anticoagulation
k. Allogenic transplantation

For each presentation below, choose the ***most appropriate first step*** *from the above list of OPTIONS. Each option may be used once, more than once, or not at all.*

QUESTIONS
141. A 51-year-old is lethargic and found to be anemic. his blood picture is found to have a granulocytic tendency with an increase in the platelet count.

142. A 5-year-old with generalised lymphadenopathy develops fever and neck stiffness and headache. he is found to have a lot of lymphoblasts in the blood picture.

143. 55-year-old man with history of hypertension untreated presents with hemiparesis.

144. A 72-year-old is having a routine examination. He is found to have a mild lymphocytosis and splenomegaly.

145. A 38-year-old woman presents with cervical lymphadenopathy. Mature lymphoblasts are seen on the blood film. Examination reveals a mild splenomegaly. She is on phenytoin for epilepsy.

THEME 30: FIRST INVESTIGATION OF POSSIBLE THROMBOEMBOLIC DISEASE

OPTIONS
a. Muscle biopsy
b. Carotid Doppler
c. Retinoscopy
d. MRI
e. ESR
f. Lumbar puncture
g. Peripheral smear
h. CT scan
i. INR
j. Carotid angiography
k. Routine screen

For each presentation below, choose the ***most appropriate first investigation*** *from the above list of OPTIONS. Each option may be used once, more than once, or not at all.*

QUESTIONS
146. A 27-year-old woman has a long-standing history of headaches associated with nausea and vomiting. On this occasion she presents with sudden loss of vision in the right half of the visual field. By the time you see her it has improved considerably.

147. An 82-year-old woman complains of increasing weakness and muscle pain to the point where she is finding it difficulty to brush her hair and get out of a chair. She now presents with sudden loss of vision in her left eye.

148. A woman previously in good health, presents with sudden onset of severe occipital headache and vomiting. Her only physical sign on examination is a stiff neck.

149. A 74-year-old woman had a fall two weeks ago. She is brought into the A and E department with slowly increasing drowsiness. On examination you find mild hemiparesis and unequal pupils.

150. A 73-year-old man presents with hemianopia, hemi-sensory loss, hemiparesis and aphasia of 16 hour duration.

THEME 31: INVESTIGATION OF COMPLICATIONS OF PROSTATIC CARCINOMA

OPTIONS

a. PSA
b. Serum acid phosphatase
c. Serum alkaline phosphatase
d. Transrectal ultrasound
e. Abdominal ultrasound
f. Serum calcium
g. Gallium scan
h. Technitium scan
i. Thallium scan
j. Transrectal biopsy
k. HLA status
l. Urodynamic studies

For each presentation below, choose the ***most appropriate investigation*** *from the above list of OPTIONS. Each option may be used once, more than once, or not at all.*

QUESTIONS

151. 80-year-old with prostatic carcinoma comes with 4 month history of low backache.

152. Patient with prostatic cancer has been treated, now complains of confusion, thirst, bodyaches, constipation.

153. Man on GnRHs for prostate cancer comes after 2 months for a follow-up.

154. Man with prostate carcinoma which has extended outside the capsule presenting with features of renal failure.

155. A man having adenocarcinoma prostate which has already spread to pelvic side walls has to be given chemotherapy.

THEME 32: ANALGESIA

OPTIONS

a. IV opiate
b. Subcutaneous opiate infusion
c. Acupuncture
d. Carbamazepine
e. Hypnotherapy
f. NSAIDs IM
g. Oral NSAIDs
h. Oral opiates
i. Proton pump inhibitors
j. SSRI, e.g. fluoxetine

For each presentation below, choose the ***single most appropriate method of pain relief*** *from the above list of OPTIONS. Each option may be used once, more than once, or not at all.*

QUESTIONS

156. A 65-year-old man presents with severe, retrosternal chest pain and sweating. An ECG shows an acute anterolateral myocardial infarction.

157. A 70-year-old man inoperable gastric cancer causing obstruction, and multiple liver metastases, is taking a large dose of oral analgesia. Despite this, his pain is currently unrelieved.

158. A 25-year-old woman has just been diagnosed a having rheumatoid arthritis and her rheumatologists has begun giving her gold injections. She continues to complain of joint pain and stiffnesss, particularly for the first two hours of each day.

159. A 50-year-old obese man with a known hiatus hernia, presents with recurrent, severe, burning retrosternal chest pain associated with acid regurgitation and increased oral flatulence.

160. A 67-year-old woman reports severe paroxysms of knife-like or electric shock-like pain, lasting seconds in the lower part of the right side of her face.

THEME 33: DIAGNOSIS OF GYNAECOLOGICAL CONDITIONS

OPTIONS
a. Crohn's disease
b. Ulcerative colitis
c. *Chlamydia*
d. *E. coli*
e. Genital prolapse
f. Procidentia
g. Herpes labialis
h. Chancre
i. Atrophic vaginitis
j. Chancroid
k. Cervicitis

For each presentation below, choose the ***best diagnosis*** *from the above list of OPTIONS. Each option may be used once, more than once, or not at all.*

QUESTIONS
161. An 85-year-old with 14 children, severe heart failure, complains of dysuria, feeling of pressure in lower abdomen.

162. Female with well-controlled diabetes mellitus type 2 with recurrent UTI.

163. A young female with long-standing irregular bowel habit and persistent UTI.

164. An 80-year-old sexually active woman with dyspareunia and recurrent dysuria.

165. A middle-aged woman with a vaginal discharge is found to have several ulcers at the vaginal introitus.

THEME 34: VAGINAL BLEEDING—MEDICAL TREATMENT

OPTIONS
a. Medroxyprogesterone (depot form)
b. Combined oral contraceptive pill
c. Danazol
d. GNRH
e. Antifibrinolytics
f. Prostaglandin synthetase antagonist
g. Optional hormone replacement therapy
h. Minipill
i. Total hysterectomy ± Radiotherapy
j. Uterine curettage
k. None required

For each presentation below, choose the ***most appropriate treatment modality*** *from the above list of OPTIONS. Each option may be used once, more than once, or not at all.*

QUESTIONS
166. A 20-year-old woman who has been on oral contraceptive develops bright red postcoital bleeding (PCB).

167. A 55-year-old female develops a single episode of PMB. She stopped menstruation 7 years ago. Ultrasound shows endometrial thickness.

168. A 49-year-old woman with complaint of hot flushes, vaginal dryness and her menstruation become irregular 5 months ago.

169. A 14-year-old woman with painless vaginal bleeding.

170. A woman with painful vaginal bleeding with brown clots. She feels embarrassed going to parties and wants a solution to her problem. Normal remedies over the counter did not help her.

THEME 35: DIAGNOSIS OF VISUAL IMPAIRMENT

OPTIONS
a. Conjunctivitis
b. Blepharitis
c. Dacryocystitis
d. Giant cell arteritis
e. Chronic simple glaucoma
f. Closed angle glaucoma
g. Vitreous haemorrhage
h. Cataract
i. Retinal detachment
j. Cerebral haemorrhage
k. Senile macular degeneration

For each presentation below, choose the ***single most likely diagnosis*** *from the above list of OPTIONS. Each option may be used once, more than once, or not at all.*

QUESTIONS

171. A 73-year-old complains of a severe right-sided headache associated with an acute loss of right-sided vision. Urgent treatment is needed to prevent left sided vision loss.

172. A 75-year-old has difficulty watching television complaining of a peripheral constriction of vision. On examination, there is cupping of both optical discs.

173. A 50-year-old with a history of SLE complains of loss of vision. On examination, he is found to have multiple opacity in the lens of his eyes.

174. A diabetic on oral hypoglycaemics complains of sudden deterioration in vision of his right eye. On examination, he is found to have bilateral proliferative retinopathy with retinal haemorrhage on the right side.

175. An 80-year-old has markedly decreased visual acuity. On fundoscopy, she is found to have bilateral macular pigmentation.

THEME 36: RHEUMATOLOGY—DIAGNOSIS

OPTIONS
a. Perthes disease
b. Slipped femoral epiphysis
c. Septic arthritis
d. Osteomyeltis
e. Pelvic fracture
f. Pseudogout
g. Osteoarthritis
h. Fracture femur—intertrochanteric
i. Fracture neck of femur
j. Rheumatoid arthritis
k. Gout

For each presentation below, choose the ***single most likely diagnosis*** *from the above list of OPTIONS. Each option may be used once, more than once, or not at all.*

QUESTIONS

176. A middle-aged woman with a history of rheumatoid arthritis develops sudden swelling in one of her knees. This knee is swollen and hot to touch.

177. An elderly man with recently diagnosed heart failure has been treated with diuretics. He now develops severe joint pain in his left ankle with swelling and redness.

178. A 78-year-old woman complains of a stiff left hip joint after walking some distance. This is most evident when she attempts to abduct the hip joint with limited abduction.

179. A 34-year-old woman complains of bilateral stiff and painful joints in her hands and feet.

180. A 67-year-old woman complains of right hip pain. On examination the right hip is adducted, externally rotated and flexed.

THEME 37: FIRST STEP IN MANAGEMENT OF MI COMPLICATIONS

OPTIONS

a. Tissue plasminogen activation
b. Heparin
c. Heparin and DC cardioversion
d. Streptokinase
e. Warfarin
f. IV atropine
g. IV digoxin
h. Intra-aortic balloon counter pulsation
i. IV fluids
j. Surgery
k. NSAIDs

For each presentation below, choose the ***most appropriate first step in management*** *from the above list of OPTIONS. Each option may be used once, more than once, or not at all.*

QUESTIONS

181. Patient, 12 hours after MI presents with recurrent chest pain, breathlessness, heart rate—40/min.
182. Patient with pulmonary oedema features presents with irregular pulse, heart rate—140/bpm.
183. A woman 10 days following hysterectomy complaints of severe left sided chest pain and breathlessness. Chest X-ray and ECG failed to relieve any abnormality.
184. Ten days after MI, female presents with chest pain on inspiration, persistently elevated ST segment on ECG.
185. Patient after MI found to have a harsh pansystolic murmur at the apex.

THEME 38: FLUID RESUSCITATION IN CHILDREN

OPTIONS

a. Do not do anything
b. IV saline 0.9%
c. IV saline 9%
d. IV Dextrose 5%
e. Water to sip
f. ORS 90 Na mEq/L
g. ORS 150 mEq of Na
h. Haemaccel
i. Ringer lactate
j. Intraosseous infusion
k. Oral opiates

For each presentation below, choose the ***most appropriate resuscitation modality*** *from the above list of OPTIONS. Each option may be used once, more than once, or not at all.*

QUESTIONS

186. A 24-month-old child, brought with a history of having been accidentally locked up in a car for about 3 hours. On examination in the A and E child is crying but his vitals are stable. What is the next step.
187. Female child from Ghana, brought to the A and E with a history of nausea and vomiting. On investigations Ketone 1+, Na 148 mEq, Glucose 18 mmol/L.
188. Mother comes to the A and E with her child of 3 years, history of D and V. On examination the child appears mildly dehydrated.
189. Boy has been brought to the A and E following a traffic accident. He has suffered from moderate blood loss. What is the most optimum method of fluid resuscitation.
190. A 2-year-old child with history of diarrhoea for 18 hours present and A to E. He is drowsy with cold extremities.

THEME 39: ANTIBIOTIC PROPHYLAXIS FOR SURGICAL PATIENTS

OPTIONS

a. Angiography
b. Bronchoscopy
c. Colles' fracture
d. Dental treatment of a cardiac patient
e. Dislocated shoulder
f. Emergency appendicectomy
g. Heart valve replacement
h. Sigmoid colectomy
i. Splenectomy
j. Thyroidectomy

INSTRUCTIONS

*For each prophylactic regimen given below, **choose the single most likely indication** from the above list of options. Each option may be used once, more than once or not at all.*

QUESTIONS

191. Three gm sachet of amoxicillin one hour before the procedure.

192. Three days of intravenous broad spectrum antibiotics beginning with induction of anaesthesia.

193. Clear fluids by mouth and two sachets of sodium picosulphate on the day before the operation plus broad spectrum intravenous antibiotics at induction.

194. Long-term oral penicillin and immunisation against pneumococcal infection.

195. One dose of metronidazole at induction of anaesthesia.

THEME 40: IMMUNISATION IN CHILDREN

OPTIONS

a. Delay by 2 weeks
b. Omit pertussis and meningitis
c. Give vaccine in hospital
d. Continue as per schedule
e. Give inactivated vaccines
f. Omit pertussis, Hib, measles
g. Don't give any vaccines
h. Omit pertussis only
i. Omit meningitis only
j. Omit measles only
k. Delay by 2 months

*For each presentation below, choose the **correct answer** from the above list of options. Each option may be used once, more than once, or not at all.*

QUESTIONS

196. Child who is HIV+ is due for MMR.

197. Child due for Hib, DPT, etc. suffering from acute febrile illness.

198. Child cried for 2 hours after Hib, DPT, etc.

199. Family history of egg allergy. Child due for MMR.

200. History of convulsions. Child due for HiB, DPT, etc.

General Medical Council PLAB Test Part 1

Full Name

Test Centre/Date

- Use pencil only • Make heavy marks that fill the lozenge completely
- Write your candidate number in the top row of the box to the right **AND** fill in the appropriate lozenge below each number
- Give **ONE** answer only for each question

0	0	0	0	0	0
1	1	1	1	1	1
2	2	2	2	2	2
3	3	3	3	3	3
4	4	4	4	4	4
5	5	5	5	5	5
6	6	6	6	6	6
7	7	7	7	7	7
8	8	8	8	8	8
9	9	9	9	9	9

1	A	B	C	D	E	F	G	H	I	J	K	L	M	N	O	P	Q	R	S	T	1
2	A	B	C	D	E	F	G	H	I	J	K	L	M	N	O	P	Q	R	S	T	2
3	A	B	C	D	E	F	G	H	I	J	K	L	M	N	O	P	Q	R	S	T	3
4	A	B	C	D	E	F	G	H	I	J	K	L	M	N	O	P	Q	R	S	T	4
5	A	B	C	D	E	F	G	H	I	J	K	L	M	N	O	P	Q	R	S	T	5
6	A	B	C	D	E	F	G	H	I	J	K	L	M	N	O	P	Q	R	S	T	6
7	A	B	C	D	E	F	G	H	I	J	K	L	M	N	O	P	Q	R	S	T	7
8	A	B	C	D	E	F	G	H	I	J	K	L	M	N	O	P	Q	R	S	T	8
9	A	B	C	D	E	F	G	H	I	J	K	L	M	N	O	P	Q	R	S	T	9
10	A	B	C	D	E	F	G	H	I	J	K	L	M	N	O	P	Q	R	S	T	10
11	A	B	C	D	E	F	G	H	I	J	K	L	M	N	O	P	Q	R	S	T	11
12	A	B	C	D	E	F	G	H	I	J	K	L	M	N	O	P	Q	R	S	T	12
13	A	B	C	D	E	F	G	H	I	J	K	L	M	N	O	P	Q	R	S	T	13
14	A	B	C	D	E	F	G	H	I	J	K	L	M	N	O	P	Q	R	S	T	14
15	A	B	C	D	E	F	G	H	I	J	K	L	M	N	O	P	Q	R	S	T	15
16	A	B	C	D	E	F	G	H	I	J	K	L	M	N	O	P	Q	R	S	T	16
17	A	B	C	D	E	F	G	H	I	J	K	L	M	N	O	P	Q	R	S	T	17
18	A	B	C	D	E	F	G	H	I	J	K	L	M	N	O	P	Q	R	S	T	18
19	A	B	C	D	E	F	G	H	I	J	K	L	M	N	O	P	Q	R	S	T	19
20	A	B	C	D	E	F	G	H	I	J	K	L	M	N	O	P	Q	R	S	T	20
21	A	B	C	D	E	F	G	H	I	J	K	L	M	N	O	P	Q	R	S	T	21
22	A	B	C	D	E	F	G	H	I	J	K	L	M	N	O	P	Q	R	S	T	22
23	A	B	C	D	E	F	G	H	I	J	K	L	M	N	O	P	Q	R	S	T	23
24	A	B	C	D	E	F	G	H	I	J	K	L	M	N	O	P	Q	R	S	T	24
25	A	B	C	D	E	F	G	H	I	J	K	L	M	N	O	P	Q	R	S	T	25
26	A	B	C	D	E	F	G	H	I	J	K	L	M	N	O	P	Q	R	S	T	26
27	A	B	C	D	E	F	G	H	I	J	K	L	M	N	O	P	Q	R	S	T	27
28	A	B	C	D	E	F	G	H	I	J	K	L	M	N	O	P	Q	R	S	T	28
29	A	B	C	D	E	F	G	H	I	J	K	L	M	N	O	P	Q	R	S	T	29
30	A	B	C	D	E	F	G	H	I	J	K	L	M	N	O	P	Q	R	S	T	30
31	A	B	C	D	E	F	G	H	I	J	K	L	M	N	O	P	Q	R	S	T	31
32	A	B	C	D	E	F	G	H	I	J	K	L	M	N	O	P	Q	R	S	T	32
33	A	B	C	D	E	F	G	H	I	J	K	L	M	N	O	P	Q	R	S	T	33
34	A	B	C	D	E	F	G	H	I	J	K	L	M	N	O	P	Q	R	S	T	34
35	A	B	C	D	E	F	G	H	I	J	K	L	M	N	O	P	Q	R	S	T	35
36	A	B	C	D	E	F	G	H	I	J	K	L	M	N	O	P	Q	R	S	T	36
37	A	B	C	D	E	F	G	H	I	J	K	L	M	N	O	P	Q	R	S	T	37
38	A	B	C	D	E	F	G	H	I	J	K	L	M	N	O	P	Q	R	S	T	38
39	A	B	C	D	E	F	G	H	I	J	K	L	M	N	O	P	Q	R	S	T	39
40	A	B	C	D	E	F	G	H	I	J	K	L	M	N	O	P	Q	R	S	T	40
41	A	B	C	D	E	F	G	H	I	J	K	L	M	N	O	P	Q	R	S	T	41
42	A	B	C	D	E	F	G	H	I	J	K	L	M	N	O	P	Q	R	S	T	42
43	A	B	C	D	E	F	G	H	I	J	K	L	M	N	O	P	Q	R	S	T	43
44	A	B	C	D	E	F	G	H	I	J	K	L	M	N	O	P	Q	R	S	T	44
45	A	B	C	D	E	F	G	H	I	J	K	L	M	N	O	P	Q	R	S	T	45
46	A	B	C	D	E	F	G	H	I	J	K	L	M	N	O	P	Q	R	S	T	46
47	A	B	C	D	E	F	G	H	I	J	K	L	M	N	O	P	Q	R	S	T	47
48	A	B	C	D	E	F	G	H	I	J	K	L	M	N	O	P	Q	R	S	T	48
49	A	B	C	D	E	F	G	H	I	J	K	L	M	N	O	P	Q	R	S	T	49
50	A	B	C	D	E	F	G	H	I	J	K	L	M	N	O	P	Q	R	S	T	50

DO NOT WRITE IN THIS SPACE

51	A	B	C	D	E	F	G	H	I	J	K	L	M	N	O	P	Q	R	S	T	51
52	A	B	C	D	E	F	G	H	I	J	K	L	M	N	O	P	Q	R	S	T	52
53	A	B	C	D	E	F	G	H	I	J	K	L	M	N	O	P	Q	R	S	T	53
54	A	B	C	D	E	F	G	H	I	J	K	L	M	N	O	P	Q	R	S	T	54
55	A	B	C	D	E	F	G	H	I	J	K	L	M	N	O	P	Q	R	S	T	55
56	A	B	C	D	E	F	G	H	I	J	K	L	M	N	O	P	Q	R	S	T	56
57	A	B	C	D	E	F	G	H	I	J	K	L	M	N	O	P	Q	R	S	T	57
58	A	B	C	D	E	F	G	H	I	J	K	L	M	N	O	P	Q	R	S	T	58
59	A	B	C	D	E	F	G	H	I	J	K	L	M	N	O	P	Q	R	S	T	59
60	A	B	C	D	E	F	G	H	I	J	K	L	M	N	O	P	Q	R	S	T	60
61	A	B	C	D	E	F	G	H	I	J	K	L	M	N	O	P	Q	R	S	T	61
62	A	B	C	D	E	F	G	H	I	J	K	L	M	N	O	P	Q	R	S	T	62
63	A	B	C	D	E	F	G	H	I	J	K	L	M	N	O	P	Q	R	S	T	63
64	A	B	C	D	E	F	G	H	I	J	K	L	M	N	O	P	Q	R	S	T	64
65	A	B	C	D	E	F	G	H	I	J	K	L	M	N	O	P	Q	R	S	T	65
66	A	B	C	D	E	F	G	H	I	J	K	L	M	N	O	P	Q	R	S	T	66
67	A	B	C	D	E	F	G	H	I	J	K	L	M	N	O	P	Q	R	S	T	67
68	A	B	C	D	E	F	G	H	I	J	K	L	M	N	O	P	Q	R	S	T	68
69	A	B	C	D	E	F	G	H	I	J	K	L	M	N	O	P	Q	R	S	T	69
70	A	B	C	D	E	F	G	H	I	J	K	L	M	N	O	P	Q	R	S	T	70
71	A	B	C	D	E	F	G	H	I	J	K	L	M	N	O	P	Q	R	S	T	71
72	A	B	C	D	E	F	G	H	I	J	K	L	M	N	O	P	Q	R	S	T	72
73	A	B	C	D	E	F	G	H	I	J	K	L	M	N	O	P	Q	R	S	T	73
74	A	B	C	D	E	F	G	H	I	J	K	L	M	N	O	P	Q	R	S	T	74
75	A	B	C	D	E	F	G	H	I	J	K	L	M	N	O	P	Q	R	S	T	75
76	A	B	C	D	E	F	G	H	I	J	K	L	M	N	O	P	Q	R	S	T	76
77	A	B	C	D	E	F	G	H	I	J	K	L	M	N	O	P	Q	R	S	T	77
78	A	B	C	D	E	F	G	H	I	J	K	L	M	N	O	P	Q	R	S	T	78
79	A	B	C	D	E	F	G	H	I	J	K	L	M	N	O	P	Q	R	S	T	79
80	A	B	C	D	E	F	G	H	I	J	K	L	M	N	O	P	Q	R	S	T	80
81	A	B	C	D	E	F	G	H	I	J	K	L	M	N	O	P	Q	R	S	T	81
82	A	B	C	D	E	F	G	H	I	J	K	L	M	N	O	P	Q	R	S	T	82
83	A	B	C	D	E	F	G	H	I	J	K	L	M	N	O	P	Q	R	S	T	83
84	A	B	C	D	E	F	G	H	I	J	K	L	M	N	O	P	Q	R	S	T	84
85	A	B	C	D	E	F	G	H	I	J	K	L	M	N	O	P	Q	R	S	T	85
86	A	B	C	D	E	F	G	H	I	J	K	L	M	N	O	P	Q	R	S	T	86
87	A	B	C	D	E	F	G	H	I	J	K	L	M	N	O	P	Q	R	S	T	87
88	A	B	C	D	E	F	G	H	I	J	K	L	M	N	O	P	Q	R	S	T	88
89	A	B	C	D	E	F	G	H	I	J	K	L	M	N	O	P	Q	R	S	T	89
90	A	B	C	D	E	F	G	H	I	J	K	L	M	N	O	P	Q	R	S	T	90
91	A	B	C	D	E	F	G	H	I	J	K	L	M	N	O	P	Q	R	S	T	91
92	A	B	C	D	E	F	G	H	I	J	K	L	M	N	O	P	Q	R	S	T	92
93	A	B	C	D	E	F	G	H	I	J	K	L	M	N	O	P	Q	R	S	T	93
94	A	B	C	D	E	F	G	H	I	J	K	L	M	N	O	P	Q	R	S	T	94
95	A	B	C	D	E	F	G	H	I	J	K	L	M	N	O	P	Q	R	S	T	95
96	A	B	C	D	E	F	G	H	I	J	K	L	M	N	O	P	Q	R	S	T	96
97	A	B	C	D	E	F	G	H	I	J	K	L	M	N	O	P	Q	R	S	T	97
98	A	B	C	D	E	F	G	H	I	J	K	L	M	N	O	P	Q	R	S	T	98
99	A	B	C	D	E	F	G	H	I	J	K	L	M	N	O	P	Q	R	S	T	99
100	A	B	C	D	E	F	G	H	I	J	K	L	M	N	O	P	Q	R	S	T	100

DO NOT WRITE IN THIS SPACE

101	A	B	C	D	E	F	G	H	I	J	K	L	M	N	O	P	Q	R	S	T	101
102	A	B	C	D	E	F	G	H	I	J	K	L	M	N	O	P	Q	R	S	T	102
103	A	B	C	D	E	F	G	H	I	J	K	L	M	N	O	P	Q	R	S	T	103
104	A	B	C	D	E	F	G	H	I	J	K	L	M	N	O	P	Q	R	S	T	104
105	A	B	C	D	E	F	G	H	I	J	K	L	M	N	O	P	Q	R	S	T	105
106	A	B	C	D	E	F	G	H	I	J	K	L	M	N	O	P	Q	R	S	T	106
107	A	B	C	D	E	F	G	H	I	J	K	L	M	N	O	P	Q	R	S	T	107
108	A	B	C	D	E	F	G	H	I	J	K	L	M	N	O	P	Q	R	S	T	108
109	A	B	C	D	E	F	G	H	I	J	K	L	M	N	O	P	Q	R	S	T	109
110	A	B	C	D	E	F	G	H	I	J	K	L	M	N	O	P	Q	R	S	T	110
111	A	B	C	D	E	F	G	H	I	J	K	L	M	N	O	P	Q	R	S	T	111
112	A	B	C	D	E	F	G	H	I	J	K	L	M	N	O	P	Q	R	S	T	112
113	A	B	C	D	E	F	G	H	I	J	K	L	M	N	O	P	Q	R	S	T	113
114	A	B	C	D	E	F	G	H	I	J	K	L	M	N	O	P	Q	R	S	T	114
115	A	B	C	D	E	F	G	H	I	J	K	L	M	N	O	P	Q	R	S	T	115
116	A	B	C	D	E	F	G	H	I	J	K	L	M	N	O	P	Q	R	S	T	116
117	A	B	C	D	E	F	G	H	I	J	K	L	M	N	O	P	Q	R	S	T	117
118	A	B	C	D	E	F	G	H	I	J	K	L	M	N	O	P	Q	R	S	T	118
119	A	B	C	D	E	F	G	H	I	J	K	L	M	N	O	P	Q	R	S	T	119
120	A	B	C	D	E	F	G	H	I	J	K	L	M	N	O	P	Q	R	S	T	120
121	A	B	C	D	E	F	G	H	I	J	K	L	M	N	O	P	Q	R	S	T	121
122	A	B	C	D	E	F	G	H	I	J	K	L	M	N	O	P	Q	R	S	T	122
123	A	B	C	D	E	F	G	H	I	J	K	L	M	N	O	P	Q	R	S	T	123
124	A	B	C	D	E	F	G	H	I	J	K	L	M	N	O	P	Q	R	S	T	124
125	A	B	C	D	E	F	G	H	I	J	K	L	M	N	O	P	Q	R	S	T	125
126	A	B	C	D	E	F	G	H	I	J	K	L	M	N	O	P	Q	R	S	T	126
127	A	B	C	D	E	F	G	H	I	J	K	L	M	N	O	P	Q	R	S	T	127
128	A	B	C	D	E	F	G	H	I	J	K	L	M	N	O	P	Q	R	S	T	128
129	A	B	C	D	E	F	G	H	I	J	K	L	M	N	O	P	Q	R	S	T	129
130	A	B	C	D	E	F	G	H	I	J	K	L	M	N	O	P	Q	R	S	T	130
131	A	B	C	D	E	F	G	H	I	J	K	L	M	N	O	P	Q	R	S	T	131
132	A	B	C	D	E	F	G	H	I	J	K	L	M	N	O	P	Q	R	S	T	132
133	A	B	C	D	E	F	G	H	I	J	K	L	M	N	O	P	Q	R	S	T	133
134	A	B	C	D	E	F	G	H	I	J	K	L	M	N	O	P	Q	R	S	T	134
135	A	B	C	D	E	F	G	H	I	J	K	L	M	N	O	P	Q	R	S	T	135
136	A	B	C	D	E	F	G	H	I	J	K	L	M	N	O	P	Q	R	S	T	136
137	A	B	C	D	E	F	G	H	I	J	K	L	M	N	O	P	Q	R	S	T	137
138	A	B	C	D	E	F	G	H	I	J	K	L	M	N	O	P	Q	R	S	T	138
139	A	B	C	D	E	F	G	H	I	J	K	L	M	N	O	P	Q	R	S	T	139
140	A	B	C	D	E	F	G	H	I	J	K	L	M	N	O	P	Q	R	S	T	140
141	A	B	C	D	E	F	G	H	I	J	K	L	M	N	O	P	Q	R	S	T	141
142	A	B	C	D	E	F	G	H	I	J	K	L	M	N	O	P	Q	R	S	T	142
143	A	B	C	D	E	F	G	H	I	J	K	L	M	N	O	P	Q	R	S	T	143
144	A	B	C	D	E	F	G	H	I	J	K	L	M	N	O	P	Q	R	S	T	144
145	A	B	C	D	E	F	G	H	I	J	K	L	M	N	O	P	Q	R	S	T	145
146	A	B	C	D	E	F	G	H	I	J	K	L	M	N	O	P	Q	R	S	T	146
147	A	B	C	D	E	F	G	H	I	J	K	L	M	N	O	P	Q	R	S	T	147
148	A	B	C	D	E	F	G	H	I	J	K	L	M	N	O	P	Q	R	S	T	148
149	A	B	C	D	E	F	G	H	I	J	K	L	M	N	O	P	Q	R	S	T	149
150	A	B	C	D	E	F	G	H	I	J	K	L	M	N	O	P	Q	R	S	T	150

DO NOT WRITE IN THIS SPACE

151	A	B	C	D	E	F	G	H	I	J	K	L	M	N	O	P	Q	R	S	T	151
152	A	B	C	D	E	F	G	H	I	J	K	L	M	N	O	P	Q	R	S	T	152
153	A	B	C	D	E	F	G	H	I	J	K	L	M	N	O	P	Q	R	S	T	153
154	A	B	C	D	E	F	G	H	I	J	K	L	M	N	O	P	Q	R	S	T	154
155	A	B	C	D	E	F	G	H	I	J	K	L	M	N	O	P	Q	R	S	T	155
156	A	B	C	D	E	F	G	H	I	J	K	L	M	N	O	P	Q	R	S	T	156
157	A	B	C	D	E	F	G	H	I	J	K	L	M	N	O	P	Q	R	S	T	157
158	A	B	C	D	E	F	G	H	I	J	K	L	M	N	O	P	Q	R	S	T	158
159	A	B	C	D	E	F	G	H	I	J	K	L	M	N	O	P	Q	R	S	T	159
160	A	B	C	D	E	F	G	H	I	J	K	L	M	N	O	P	Q	R	S	T	160
161	A	B	C	D	E	F	G	H	I	J	K	L	M	N	O	P	Q	R	S	T	161
162	A	B	C	D	E	F	G	H	I	J	K	L	M	N	O	P	Q	R	S	T	162
163	A	B	C	D	E	F	G	H	I	J	K	L	M	N	O	P	Q	R	S	T	163
164	A	B	C	D	E	F	G	H	I	J	K	L	M	N	O	P	Q	R	S	T	164
165	A	B	C	D	E	F	G	H	I	J	K	L	M	N	O	P	Q	R	S	T	165
166	A	B	C	D	E	F	G	H	I	J	K	L	M	N	O	P	Q	R	S	T	166
167	A	B	C	D	E	F	G	H	I	J	K	L	M	N	O	P	Q	R	S	T	167
168	A	B	C	D	E	F	G	H	I	J	K	L	M	N	O	P	Q	R	S	T	168
169	A	B	C	D	E	F	G	H	I	J	K	L	M	N	O	P	Q	R	S	T	169
170	A	B	C	D	E	F	G	H	I	J	K	L	M	N	O	P	Q	R	S	T	170
171	A	B	C	D	E	F	G	H	I	J	K	L	M	N	O	P	Q	R	S	T	171
172	A	B	C	D	E	F	G	H	I	J	K	L	M	N	O	P	Q	R	S	T	172
173	A	B	C	D	E	F	G	H	I	J	K	L	M	N	O	P	Q	R	S	T	173
174	A	B	C	D	E	F	G	H	I	J	K	L	M	N	O	P	Q	R	S	T	174
175	A	B	C	D	E	F	G	H	I	J	K	L	M	N	O	P	Q	R	S	T	175
176	A	B	C	D	E	F	G	H	I	J	K	L	M	N	O	P	Q	R	S	T	176
177	A	B	C	D	E	F	G	H	I	J	K	L	M	N	O	P	Q	R	S	T	177
178	A	B	C	D	E	F	G	H	I	J	K	L	M	N	O	P	Q	R	S	T	178
179	A	B	C	D	E	F	G	H	I	J	K	L	M	N	O	P	Q	R	S	T	179
180	A	B	C	D	E	F	G	H	I	J	K	L	M	N	O	P	Q	R	S	T	180
181	A	B	C	D	E	F	G	H	I	J	K	L	M	N	O	P	Q	R	S	T	181
182	A	B	C	D	E	F	G	H	I	J	K	L	M	N	O	P	Q	R	S	T	182
183	A	B	C	D	E	F	G	H	I	J	K	L	M	N	O	P	Q	R	S	T	183
184	A	B	C	D	E	F	G	H	I	J	K	L	M	N	O	P	Q	R	S	T	184
185	A	B	C	D	E	F	G	H	I	J	K	L	M	N	O	P	Q	R	S	T	185
186	A	B	C	D	E	F	G	H	I	J	K	L	M	N	O	P	Q	R	S	T	186
187	A	B	C	D	E	F	G	H	I	J	K	L	M	N	O	P	Q	R	S	T	187
188	A	B	C	D	E	F	G	H	I	J	K	L	M	N	O	P	Q	R	S	T	188
189	A	B	C	D	E	F	G	H	I	J	K	L	M	N	O	P	Q	R	S	T	189
190	A	B	C	D	E	F	G	H	I	J	K	L	M	N	O	P	Q	R	S	T	190
191	A	B	C	D	E	F	G	H	I	J	K	L	M	N	O	P	Q	R	S	T	191
192	A	B	C	D	E	F	G	H	I	J	K	L	M	N	O	P	Q	R	S	T	192
193	A	B	C	D	E	F	G	H	I	J	K	L	M	N	O	P	Q	R	S	T	193
194	A	B	C	D	E	F	G	H	I	J	K	L	M	N	O	P	Q	R	S	T	194
195	A	B	C	D	E	F	G	H	I	J	K	L	M	N	O	P	Q	R	S	T	195
196	A	B	C	D	E	F	G	H	I	J	K	L	M	N	O	P	Q	R	S	T	196
197	A	B	C	D	E	F	G	H	I	J	K	L	M	N	O	P	Q	R	S	T	197
198	A	B	C	D	E	F	G	H	I	J	K	L	M	N	O	P	Q	R	S	T	198
199	A	B	C	D	E	F	G	H	I	J	K	L	M	N	O	P	Q	R	S	T	199
200	A	B	C	D	E	F	G	H	I	J	K	L	M	N	O	P	Q	R	S	T	200

Answers

Serial No.	Answer No.	Answer
1	k	None required
2	f	X-ray orbit
3	f	X-ray orbit
4	g	Conjunctival cytology
5	h	MRI
6	b	Steroids
7	c	Laser photocoagulation
8	g	Admit for..........
9	h	IV mannitol
10	i	Atropine sulphate
11	i	Superficial head injury
12	j	Insignificant head injury
13	k	Vasogenic cerebral oedema
14	d	Subdural haematoma
15	c	Extradural haematoma
16	a	Carbon monoxide
17	b	Warfarim
18	f	Paracetamol
19	e	Quinine
20	h	Tricyclic antidepressants
21	f	Haloperidol
22	a	Opioid overdose
23	g	Clozapine
24	e	Lithium
25	c	Tricyclic intoxication
26	k	Colonoscopy
27	l	Sigmoidoscopy
28	e	Barium enema
29	e	Barium enema
30	g	Stool culture
31	a	Candidiasis
32	d	Achalasia
33	e	Oesophageal carcinoma
34	c	Diffuse oesophageal spasm
35	e	Oesophageal carcinoma
36	f	Hepatitis B
37	g	CBD obstruction
38	i	Acute cholecystitis
39	j	PBC
40	h	HHC
41	a	Acute epididimo-orchitis
42	g	Testicular torsion
43	k	Seminoma or teratoma
44	j	Sebaceous cyst
45	i	UTI
46	h	Possible infection
47	a	Hyperglycaemia
48	e	Autonomic neuropathy
49	f	Intermittent claudication
50	i	Lactic acidosis
51	i	Biopsy
52	j	Thyroglobulin autoantibodies
53	g	Dry induced thyrotoxiosis
54	k	TSH receptor autoantibodies
55	e	Contrast radiographs
56	h	Flexible sigmoidoscopy
57	i	Laparoscopy
58	k	Endocervical swab
59	e	Abdominal USG + High vaginal swab

60	j	None required
61	a	IV hydrocortisone
62	j	Ganciclovir IV
63	k	Shohl's solution
64	f	Fluid restriction
65	e	Sodium bicarbonate
66	i	NaCl+K^+ supplements
67	h	$NaHCO_3$
68	g	Potassium supplements
69	f	Frusemide
70	g	Potassium supplements
71	a	Pleural biopsy
72	c	Chest X-ray
73	g	Sputum culture and microscopy
74	b	V/Q scan
75	f	Bronchoscopy
76	k	Asthma
77	a	Sarcoidosis
78	d	Anxiety
79	j	Aspiration pneumonitis
80	g	Pulmonary embolism
81	h	Underwater seal drainage
82	e	Cross-match blood and inform surgeons
83	d	High flow O_2 + 10 mg IV morphine + anticoagulation
84	e	Cross-match blood and inform surgeons
85	d	High flow O_2 + 10 mg IV morphine + anticoagulation
86	d	Lymphoedema
87	f	Hypercalcaemia
88	e	Spinal cord compression
89	b	Cerebral metastases
90	a	Pathological fracture

91	f	Osteogenesis imperfecta
92	i	Elderly abuse
93	d	Sexual abuse
94	c	Physical abuse
95	a	Accidental injury
96	g	Digital substraction angiography
97	j	Biopsy
98	a	USG
99	c	Aspiration and microscopy
100	i	Transillumination test
101	d	Carboxyhaemoglobin level
102	g	Aspirate blister
103	a	IV fluids
104	b	Escharotomy
105	l	Discharge after dressing
106	i	3 years
107	c	6 weeks
108	h	2 years
109	d	2 months
110	g	1 year
111	g	Cervical spinal cord
112	f	Brainstem and its cerebellar connections
113	c	Optic nerve
114	c	Optic nerve
115	i	Facial nerve
116	e	Hepatitis A infection
117	a	Hepatitis A immunisation
118	g	Schistosomiasis
119	c	Hepatitis B vaccine
120	f	Hepatocellular carcinoma
121	f	Ototoxicity
122	d	Wax impaction

123	a	Acoustic neuroma
124	c	Petrous temporal bone fracture
125	j	Herpes zoster
126	k	Lateral X-ray-hip joint
127	d	Diagnostic aspiration for culture
128	k	Lateral X-ray-hip joint
129	b	Diagnostic aspiration for WBC demonstration
130	c	MRI
131	c	Pernicious anaemia
132	h	B_{12} deficiency
133	k	Malabsorption
134	i	Scurvy
135	j	Nutritional deficit
136	a	Anterior pack
137	d	Electrocautery
138	f	Review anticoagulation
139	h	Embolisation
140	g	Antihypertensives
141	d	Blood transfusion
142	e	Blood and platelet transfusion
143	g	CT scan skull
144	h	Hydroxyurea
145	i	Systemic steroids
146	b	Carotid Doppler
147	e	ESR
148	h	CT scan
149	h	CT scan
150	j	Carotid angiography
151	h	Technitium scan
152	f	Serum calcium
153	a	PSA

154	l	Urodynamic studies
155	d	Transrectal USG
156	a	IV opiate
157	b	SC opiate infusion
158	g	Oral NSAIDs
159	i	Proton pump inhibitors
160	d	Carbamazepine
161	e	Genital prolapse
162	c	*Chlamydia*
163	a	Crohn's disease
164	i	Atrophic vaginitis
165	g	Herpes labialis
166	k	None required
167	i	Total hysterectomy ± radiotherapy
168	g	Optional hormone replacement therapy
169	k	None required
170	i	Total hysterectomy ± radiotherapy
171	d	Giant cell arteritis
172	e	Chronic simple glaucoma
173	h	Cataract
174	g	Vitreous haemorrhage
175	k	Senile macular degeneration
176	f	Pseudogout
177	k	Gout
178	g	Osteoarthritis
179	j	Rheumatoid arthritis
180	i	Fracture neck femur
181	f	IV atropine
182	g	IV digoxin
183	b	Heparin
184	k	NSAIDs
185	h	Aortic balloon counter pulsation
186	e	Water to sip

187	b	IV saline 0.9%
188	f	ORS 90 Na MEq/L
189	h	Haemaccel
190	i	Ringer lactate
191	d	Dental treatment of a cardiac patient
192	g	Heart valve replacement
193	h	Sigmoid colectomy

194	I	Splenectomy
195	f	Emergency appendicectomy
196	d	Continue as per schedule
197	a	Delay by 2 weeks
198	d	Continue as per schedule
199	d	Continue as per schedule
200	d	Continue as per schedule

Previous Year Paper 7

RxPG Analysis

Total Themes:	**40**
Repeat Themes:	**5**
Repeat Themes with a Different Header:	**11**

THEME 1: PRESCRIPTION AND RENAL FAILURE

OPTIONS

a. Cyclosporine
b. Bendrofluazide
c. Spirinolactone
d. Cyclophosphamide
e. Captopril
f. Gentamicin
g. Calcium
h. Magnesium
i. Acetazolamide
j. Furosemide
k. Paracetamol

For each presentation below, choose the ***most appropriate drug producing the given condition*** *from the above list of OPTIONS. Each option may be used once, more than once, or not at all.*

QUESTIONS

1. A 60-year-old woman hypertensive was started on antihypertensive 2 weeks ago. Now has a creatinine level of 500 micromol/L.
2. A child with recurrent nephrotic syndrome is brought for treatment. Three weeks after start of treatment, he now has massive haematuria.
3. A patient in severe renal failure has potassium level of 2. 5 mmol/L.
4. Patient with complaint of ataxia and tinnitus and mild hearing loss. He has moderate renal failure.
5. A fit 50-year-old man is prescribed oral Acetazolamide by an ophthalmologist for suspected glaucoma. He presents with lethargy and shortness of breath on exertion. Sodium 140 mmol/L, potassium 3.2 mmol/L, bicarbonate 18 mmol/L, chloride 115 mmol/L, Urea 6.7 mmol/L, creatinine 114 μmol/L.

THEME 2: INVESTIGATION/ MANAGEMENT OF CYSTITIS

OPTIONS

a. IVU
b. Cystoscopy
c. Ultrasound kidney and bladder
d. MSU after 3 weeks
e. MSU monthly for 6 months
f. MSU culture
g. ^{99}Technetium renography
h. Urine culture and sensitivity
i. Catheter culture
j. Suprapubic aspiration
k. Urethral culture

For each presentation below, choose the ***most appropriate investigation*** *from the above list of OPTIONS. Each option may be used once, more than once, or not at all.*

QUESTIONS

6. A 3-year-old boy has a first confirmed urinary tract infection. Abdominal ultrasound is normal.
7. A female presents with frequent dysuria. This is the third episode. At this time *E. coli* confirmed.
8. A 70-year-old with prostatic symptoms. Urine culture is negative.
9. A 25-year-old male has a first confirmed urinary tract infection. IVU is normal.
10. A one and half year old girl, was brought with complaint of dysuria. Culture of urine reveals mixed bacteria.

THEME 3: DIFFERENTIAL DIAGNOSIS OF VOMITING IN CHILDREN

OPTIONS

a. Gastro-oesophageal reflux (physiological)
b. Gastroenteritis
c. Pyloric stenosis
d. Intussusception
e. Urinary tract infection
f. Diabetes mellitus
g. Gatro-oesophageal reflux (pathological) (UTI)
h. Meconium ileus
i. Necrotising enterocolitis
j. Poisoning
k. Septicaemia

For each presentation below, choose the ***single most likely diagnosis*** *from the above list of OPTIONS. Each option may be used once, more than once, or not at all.*

QUESTIONS

11. A 3-week-old child presents with projectile vomiting, appearing hungry after each emesis. On examination dehydration is present and there is a mass in abdomen.
12. A 1-year-old child presents with vomiting, crying and lifting her legs. Nappy is stained red. On examination sausage-shaped mass is palpated per abdominally.
13. A 3-month-old child is brought with recurrent vomiting, but is otherwise thriving well and healthy. The symptom seems to subside when the child is strapped in baby's seat.
14. A 6-year-old girl presents with fever, frequency, dysuria and abdominal pain.
15. Child with vomiting and diarrhoea. Brother had a similar problem 2 weeks ago.

THEME 4: DIFFERENTIAL DIAGNOSIS OF ACUTE DYSPNOEA (DATA INTERPRETATION- CO_2, OXYGEN, CHEST X-RAY, ECG)

OPTIONS

a. Panic attacks
b. Asthma
c. Pulmonary embolism
d. Cor pulmonale
e. Aspiration pneumonia
f. Alcohol withdrawal
g. Hypoglycaemia
h. Depression
i. Pulmonary oedema
j. Pneumothorax
k. Mitral stenosis

For each presentation below, choose the ***most likely diagnosis*** *from the above list of OPTIONS. Each option may be used once, more than once, or not at all.*

QUESTIONS

16. Patient had bilateral fluffy opacities and increased interstitial markings. Had low oxygen, normal CO_2.
17. Patient with acute shortness of breath, wheeze. chest X-ray—normal, low oxygen, low $PaCO_2$. PEFR-120 ml/minute.
18. A 20-year-old woman attends A and E complaining of sudden breathlessness and anxiety. She describes palpitations and paresthesiae of her hands, feet and lips. ECG shows sinus tachycardia and O_2 saturation is normal.
19. An alcoholic admitted semi-comatose. ABG shows low oxygen saturation.
20. Patient with recent MI, develops acute breathlessness with hemoptysis. CXR shows dilated pulmonary artery and wedge-shaped area of infarction. Decreased PaO_2 and $PaCO_2$.

THEME 5: MANAGEMENT OF MULTIPLE TRAUMA

OPTIONS
a. Gain IV access + normal saline/Haemaccel
b. Gain IV access + blood transfusion
c. Apply external pressure
d. Needle thoracostomy
e. Chest drain
f. Maintain open airway
g. Intubation and ventilation
h. Splint fracture
i. Urgent blood transfusion
j. Chest strapping
k. Analgesics

For each presentation below, choose the ***next most appropriate action*** *from the above list of OPTIONS. Each option may be used once, more than once, or not at all.*

QUESTIONS
21. Patient involved in road traffic accident (RTA), neck immobilised. Has massive head and facial injuries, together with noisy breathing despite administration of 100% oxygen.
22. Girl in road traffic accident (RTA). Neck is immobilised and line established. Has deformed, swollen thigh, pale.
23. Known asthmatic patient involved in road traffic accident (RTA). Has a right-sided chest pain. On auscultation right side is hyper-resonant. Trachea is deviated to the left.
24. A 19-year-old girl has fallen off her horse. Neck is immobilised + 100% oxygen. Has left upper abdominal pain, is pale and tachycardiac.
25. A 15-year-old girl has cut her wrist and bled profusely. She is pale, tachycardiac and does not want to live.

THEME 6: DIFFERENTIAL DIAGNOSIS OF ALTERED BOWEL HABIT

OPTIONS
a. Carcinoma rectum
b. Carcinoma caecum
c. IBS with diarrhoea
d. IBS with constipation
e. Faecal impaction
f. Diverticulosis
g. Ulcerative colitis
h. Crohn's disease
i. Fissure *in ano*
j. Paralytic ileus
k. Haemorrhoids
l. Acute haematoma around anal region

For each presentation below, choose the ***single most likely diagnosis*** *from the above list of OPTIONS. Each option may be used once, more than once, or not at all.*

QUESTIONS
26. A 19-year-old female with complaint of a 1 year history of bloody diarrhoea and tenesmus. Has pale skin lesions. On examination-sigmoidoscopy shows inflammation and granulomata.
27. A 65-year-old male with weight loss, right-sided pain, tenesmus. On examination-mass in the rectum
28. An 18-year-old presents with frequent diarrhoea for about 3/52, relieved by defaecation. Sigmoidoscopy is normal.
29. An 80-year-old with complaint of diarrhoea and urinary retention
30. After an abdominal operation, a patient presents with subfebrile state and abdominal distension. There is associated abdominal tenderness, constipation. On auscultation no bowel sounds are heard.

THEME 7: DIFFERENTIAL DIAGNOSIS OF ACUTE URINARY RETENTION

OPTIONS

a. Ureteric colic
b. Carcinoma prostate
c. BPH
d. Urinary tract infection
e. Stricture
f. Periventricular region lesion
g. Brainstem lesion
h. Spinal cord lesion
i. Antidepressant
j. Urethral valves
k. Ruptured ureters

*For each presentation below, choose the **single most likely diagnosis** from the above list of OPTIONS. Each option may be used once, more than once, or not at all.*

QUESTIONS

31. A patient of multiple sclerosis has had urinary catheterisation for 4 years with intermittent obstruction
32. A 60-year-old with complaint of frequency, dysuria. PSA is 120 ng/ml, also has back pain
33. Female patient with complaint of severe flank pain, is restless and the pain radiates to the groin.
34. A 65-year-old man presents with history of ferquency, urgency and decreased urinary flow.
35. A 39-year-old female presents with weakness of both legs, difficulty walking and urinary retention.

THEME 8 INVESTIGATION/MANAGEMENT OF MENINGITIS

OPTIONS

a. ZN staining
b. Serum urate
c. CT skull
d. Parenteral penicillin
e. IV acyclovir
f. Rifampicin
g. IV mannitol
h. Lumbar puncture
i. Blood culture
j. IV fluids
k. Hib vaccine

*For each presentation below, choose the **next most appropriate action** from the above list of OPTIONS. Each option may be used once, more than once, or not at all.*

QUESTIONS

36. A young boy back from holiday in North Africa presents with night fever, weight loss. Began on antibiotics with minimal improvement. CSF shows:protein-960 mg/dl, glucose-2 mmol/L, cells-lymphocytes.
37. An 8-year-old boy with acute leukaemia is admitted in a comatose state. He is found to have lymphoblast depletion prevention.
38. A 14-year-old boy presents with drowsiness and generalised headache. He is recovering from a bilateral parotitis. His CT scan is normal.
39. An intravenous drug abuser presents with suspected meningitis. The organism is confirmed in the CSF by India ink preparation.
40. An anxious mother called you to say that her son's best friend in school has caught meningitis.

THEME 9: DIFFERENTIAL DIAGNOSIS OF SHOCK

OPTIONS

a. Anaphylaxis
b. Tension pneumothorax
c. Aortic aneurysm
d. Ruptured ectopic pregnancy
e. Salpingitis
f. Acute pancreatitis
g. Adrenal insufficiency
h. Simple pneumothorax
i. Surgical emphysema
j. Haemoperitoneum
k. Haemothorax

*For each presentation below, choose the **most likely diagnosis** from the above list of OPTIONS. Each option may be used once, more than once, or not at all.*

QUESTIONS

41. Patient stabbed in right chest. ultrasound showed no free fluid per abdominally, patient is breathless, pale.
42. woman history of 8/52 amenorrhoea presents with abdominal pain rigidity and is pale.
43. Patient with history of suggestive of atherosclerosis, now presenting with shock.
44. Patient admitted with suspected tetanus and is given tetanus immunoglobulin and an antibiotic to which he is not allergic. Ten minutes later the patient is breathless with tachycardia
45. A known asthmatic on treatment with inhaled Beta-2-agonist and steroid. Now presents with hypotension.

THEME 10: INVESTIGATION OF AORTIC ANEURYSM

OPTIONS

a. Abdominal ultrasound
b. Spiral CT
c. IVU
d. Coronary angiography
e. Echocardiography
f. Plain abdomen X-ray
g. Chest X-ray
h. MRI
i. Only ECG
j. DTPA scan
k. High resolution CT

*For each presentation below, choose the **most appropriate investigation** from the above list of OPTIONS. Each option may be used once, more than once, or not at all.*

QUESTIONS

46. A 60-year-old attends A and E and it is thought he may have aortic aneurysm.
47. A tall 34-year-old man develops severe central chest pain radiating to his back. He soon develops a dense hemiplegia.
48. A patient is to have a repair of his aortic aneurysm but also has severe myocardial ischaemia.
49. Patient with aortic aneurysm has unstable angina.
50. Elderly patient suspected of having aortic dissection with complaint of abdominal pain yesterday, but is now haemodynamically stable.

THEME 11: INVESTIGATION/DIFFERENTIAL DIAGNOSIS OF ABDOMINAL PAIN

OPTIONS
a. Mesenteric angiogram
b. Perforated peptic ulcer
c. Nonulcer dyspepsia
d. Retrocaecal appendicitis
e. Ureteric colic
f. Carcinoma of stomach
g. Oesophagitis
h. Hepatitis
i. Acute pancreatitis
j. Acute cholecystitis
k. Myocardial infarction

*For each presentation below, choose the **single most likely diagnosis or investigation** from the above list of OPTIONS. Each option may be used once, more than once, or not at all.*

QUESTIONS

51. A patient presents with intermittent abdominal pain for about 30 minutes after meals. Also has history of abdominal pain radiating to the back. On examination-abdominal bruit. Also has intermittent claudication.

52. Patient on antacids for extensive epigastric pain presents with acute abdominal pain, rigidity and is pale.

53. Female patient with 24 hour history of severe abdominal pain and vomiting. She is restless and afebrile. She has a history of chronic alcoholism.

54. Patient with presenting complaint of severe flank pain. He is now restless. He says that the pain is radiating to the groin he is passing reddish urine.

55. A 50-year-old chronic alcoholic presents with a sudden onset diffuse abdominal pain. It is radiating to the back. He has generalised abdominal tenderness with vomiting and rigidity.

THEME 12: DIFFERENTIAL DIAGNOSIS OF FRACTURES IN CHILDREN

OPTIONS
a. Green stick fracture
b. Fracture shaft radius
c. Fracture ulna
d. Fracture shaft of femur
e. Pulled elbow
f. Fracture supracondylar
g. Slipped upper femoral epiphysis
h. Fracture neck of femur
i. Fracture scaphoid
j. Colles' fracture
k. Gallezzi fracture.

*For each presentation below, choose the **single most likely** diagnosis from the above list of OPTIONS. Each option may be used once, more than once, or not at all.*

QUESTIONS

56. A 7-day-old baby cries whenever lifted. Labour was difficult.

57. Young girl tripped while holding mother's hand. Now cannot use arm at all.

58. Young boy fell off horse onto his hand. Now with complaint of mild tenderness over the clavicle but able to use forearm.

59. Young child fell on outstretched hand and now has absent radial pulse.

60. A 12-year-old boy with left groin pain for 6 weeks is noticed to stand with the left leg externally rotated. Examination reveals negligible internal rotation of the hip.

THEME 13: MULTIPLE SCLEROSIS—ANATOMICAL SITES INVOLVED

OPTIONS
a. Cerebrum
b. Optic disc
c. Optic nerve
d. Optic radiation
e. Cerebral cortex
f. Brainstem and its cerebellar connections
g. Cervical spinal cord
h. Thoracic spinal cord
i. Facial nerve
j. Trigeminal nerve
k. Fascial nucleus

For each presentation below, choose the ***most likely anatomical site involved*** *from the above list of OPTIONS. Each option may be used once, more than once, or not at all.*

QUESTIONS

61. Known patient of multiple sclerosis now with complaint of urinary incontinence, weakness in all 4 limbs and difficulty walking.
62. Patient has nystagmus, diplopia, and positive past-pointing.
63. Patient has repeated attacks of multiple sclerosis, and now has pale temporal disc.
64. Patient with complaint of blurring of vision, papilledema, pain in eye.
65. A known patient of multiple sclerosis with unilateral facial paralysis with no loss of taste.

THEME 14: DIFFERENTIAL DIAGNOSIS OF CHRONIC NEUROLOGICAL DISEASES

OPTIONS
a. Alzheimer's
b. Multiple sclerosis
c. Myasthaenia gravis
d. Space occupying lesion
e. Acromegaly
f. Polymyositis
g. Dermatomyositis
h. Polymyalgia rheumatica
i. Parkinsonism
j. Dermatomyositis
k. Fibromyosis

For each presentation below, choose the ***single most likely diagnosis*** *from the above list of OPTIONS. Each option may be used once, more than once, or not at all.*

QUESTIONS

66. Patient gets diplopia when he works very hard.
67. Patient with attacks of numbness in left hand and right sided headache.
68. This disease is characterised by neurofibrillary tangels and sinel plaques.
69. A 40-year-old female comes with complaints of headache, bitemporal hemianopia, increase in shoe size.
70. A middle-aged woman presents with recurrent nausea, weight loss and fever. She has pain, stiffness and weakness in her hips and shoulders. She does not have a rash, but the skin around the neck and shoulders appears thickened.

THEME 15: IMMEDIATE MANAGEMENT OF BURNS

OPTIONS
a. IV fluids
b. Escharotomy
c. Admit to hospital
d. Carboxyhaemoglobin level
e. IV blood transfusion
f. Deroof blister
g. Aspirate blister
h. Blood transfusion
i. Skin grafting
j. Antibiotics
k. Fasciotomy
l. Reassure

*For each presentation below, choose the **most appropriate management** from the above list of OPTIONS. Each option may be used once, more than once, or not at all.*

QUESTIONS
71. Patient after escaping from fire in a building has singed nostrils.
72. Patient has a large tense blister.
73. An adult patient has partial thickness burns on the anterior chest and upper thighs.
74. An adult patient has full thickness circumferential burns from the elbow to the fingers, covering them completely.
75. Man, slept while sunbathing comes with redness, pain all over his body. Otherwise well.

THEME 16: DIFFERENTIAL DIAGNOSIS OF HEARING TESTS

OPTIONS
a. Bilateral sensory neural deafness
b. Bilateral conductive deafness
c. Bilateral total deafness
d. Unilateral sensory neural deafness
e. Unilateral conductive deafness
f. Threshold shift
g. High compliance on tympanogram
h. Absent recruitment
i. Mixed deafness
j. 50% SISI score
k. Cortical pathology

*For each presentation below, choose the **single most likely diagnosis** from the above list of OPTIONS. Each option may be used once, more than once, or not at all.*

QUESTIONS
76. Otosclerosis.
77. Presbycusis.
78. Otitis media with effusion.
79. Acoustic neuroma.
80. Noise-induced hearing loss (NIHL).

THEME 17: BIOSTATISTICS

OPTIONS

a. Specificity
b. Sensitivity
c. Mode
d. Mean
e. Median
f. Chi-square
g. Standard deviation
h. Cohort studies
i. Case control studies
j. Range
k. Random deviation

For each presentation below, choose the ***single most appropriate answer*** *from the above list of OPTIONS. Each option may be used once, more than once, or not at all.*

QUESTIONS

81. The ability of a test to detect people who do have the disease.
82. Measure of dispersion.
83. Relative risk can be obtained from these studies.
84. The best indicator of central value when one or more of the lowest or the highest observations are wide apart or not so evenly distributed.
85. The most frequently occurring observation in a series.

THEME 18: EPIDEMIOLOGY IN CARDIAC CONDITIONS

OPTIONS

a. IHD
b. Atrial fibrillation
c. Warfarin
d. Angina
e. Congenital aortic stenosis
f. Aortic regurgitation
g. Pericarditis
h. Hypertension
i. Rheumatic fever
j. HOCM
k. Aortic stenosis

For each presentation below, choose the ***correct answer*** *from the above list of OPTIONS. Each option may be used once, more than once, or not at all.*

QUESTIONS

86. The single largest cause of death in adults in the UK.
87. Warfarin decreases the incidence of stroke by about 30%.
88. Interferes with the function of vitamin K.
89. Probably most important public health problem in developed countries. Its ratio of frequency in women verses men increases from 0.6 to 0.7 at age 30 to 1.1 to 1.2 at age 65.
90. Its incidence in industrialized countries of the world has declined markedly. Peak age-related incidence is between 5 and 15 years.

THEME 19: MANAGEMENT OF MYOCARDIAL INFARCTION

OPTIONS

a. Diuretic
b. Thrombolysis
c. Beta-blockers
d. Nitrates
e. Oxygen
f. Cardiac pacing
g. High flow oxygen and morphine
h. Heparin
i. Digoxin
j. Adrenalin IM
k. Warfarin

*For each presentation below, choose the **most appropriate management** from the above list of OPTIONS. Each option may be used once, more than once, or not at all.*

QUESTIONS

91. A patient who developed myocardial infarction one month ago is now breathless and has basal crackles.
92. Patient presents with one and a half hours of epigastric pain radiating to his arm. ECG shows acute inferior myocardial infarction. Oxygen + analgesia have already been given.
93. Patient recovering from myocardial infarction has a heart rate of 36/minute.
94. A 57-year-old man develops crushing pain in the chest associated with nausea and profuse sweating. The pain is still present when he arrives in hospital an hour later.
95. Not given in a chronic asthmatic after a myocardial infarction.

THEME 20: CAUSATION OF DISEASES

OPTIONS

a. Skin-to-skin
b. Close community contact
c. Animal to human
d. Tinea
e. Female mite
f. Immunodeficiency
g. Blood
h. Mosquito bite
i. Deer tick
j. Allergens
k. Rat-flea

*For each presentation below, choose the **most likely route of transmission** from the above list of OPTIONS. Each option may be used once, more than once, or not at all.*

QUESTIONS

96. Scabies.
97. Candidial nappy rash.
98. Impetigo.
99. Toxoplasmosis.
100. A first year university student develops headache, fever, photophobia, in the 1st week of term.

THEME 21: MANAGEMENT AND INVESTIGATIONS OF SPEECH DISORDERS

OPTIONS

a. Hearing test
b. Speech therapy
c. Reassure
d. Refer to ENT
e. Milestone assessment
f. Carotid Doppler
g. EEG
h. USG
i. CT
j. Polysomnography
k. Adenoidectomy

*For each presentation below, choose the **most appropriate step in management** from the above list of OPTIONS. Each option may be used once, more than once, or not at all.*

QUESTIONS

101. Male patient has nasal speech, snores at night. Day time he is sleepy.
102. A 2-year-old been developing well, but now has decreased hearing. Motor function is normal.
103. An 18-month-old patient can still says a few words, ...mother is worried.
104. A 50-year-old male wakes up with a tingling and numbness in his right hand. This is accompanied by slurring of speech which recovers following about four hours.
105. A 3-year-old with a persistent and rough voice.

THEME 22: TRANSMISSION OF DISEASES

OPTIONS

a. Mite
b. Faecal-oral
c. Blood-borne
d. Tick-borne
e. Louse-borne
f. Air-borne
g. Fomites
h. Sexual transmission
i. Animal to man
j. Dog bite
k. Spores

*For each presentation below, choose the **most likely route of transmission** from the above list of OPTIONS. Each option may be used once, more than once, or not at all.*

QUESTIONS

106. Warts.
107. Typhoid fever.
108. Hepatitis C.
109. HIV.
110. Lyme disease.

THEME 23: MANAGEMENT OF ACUTE PSYCHOSES

OPTIONS
a. Hospital hostel
b. Family therapy
c. Supportive
d. Education
e. Rehabilitation
f. Cognitive therapy
g. Oral antipsychotic
h. Risk management strategy
i. Detention under mental health act
j. Electroconvulsive treatment (ECT)
k. Psychiatric general wards
l. Sedation

*For each presentation below, choose the **most appropriate step in management** from the above list of OPTIONS. Each option may be used once, more than once, or not at all.*

QUESTIONS

111. A schizophrenic who stabbed his mother's hand with a screw driver was recently admitted and treated with depot injection antipsychotic. He is now symptom-free and ready for discharge.

112. Patient (schizophrenia) has had about 8 admissions in the last 5 years. He is uncompliant with drugs.

113. Young patient now 25 years was diagnosed with schizophrenia. At 15, but despite different medications has not recovered fully. The family is very supportive.

114. Patient 35-year-old is admitted depressed and has not been eating /drinking for many days. Has lost weight.

115. A 40-year-old patient with features of paranoid schizophrenia.

THEME 24: MANAGEMENT OF ANXIETY

OPTIONS
a. Cognitive and behavioural therapy (CBT)
b. Psychoanalysis
c. Desensitisation
d. Supportive therapy
e. Interpersonal therapy
f. Relation therapy
g. Electroconvulsive therapy
h. Alprazolam
i. Amitryptyline
j. MAO inhibitors
k. Lorazepam

*For each presentation below, choose the **most definitive management** from the above list of OPTIONS. Each option may be used once, more than once, or not at all.*

QUESTIONS

116. Arachnophobia

117. Post-traumatic stress disorder (PTSD)

118. Bereavement

119. A female lawyer is becoming increasing anxious when she has to speak in front of people. This is affecting her work as she needs to speak out in court.

120. This treatment is very effective in endogenous anxiety and phobias.

THEME 25: BASICS OF POISONING

OPTIONS

a. CO
b. TCA
c. Paracetamol
d. Digoxin
e. Aspirin
f. Organophosphate
g. Paraquat
h. Ectasy
i. Cyanide
j. Botulinum toxin
k. β-blockers

For each presentation below, choose the ***single most likely cause*** *from the above list of OPTIONS. Each option may be used once, more than once, or not at all.*

QUESTIONS

121. Interferes with glutathione (reversible by methionine and acetylcysteine).
122. Interferes with haemoglobin.
123. Anticholinergic effects arrhythmias.
124. Patient on treatment for atrial fibrillation, now has palpitations.
125. This interferes with metabolism at the mitochondrial level.

THEME 26: INVESTIGATION OF ANAEMIA

OPTIONS

a. Dietary history
b. B_{12} levels
c. Folate
d. FBC
e. Schilling's test
f. Barium meal
g. Barium enema
h. LFT
i. Isotope scan of liver
j. Alcohol history
k. Vitamin C levels

For each presentation below, choose the ***most appropriate initial investigation*** *from the above list of OPTIONS. Each option may be used once, more than once, or not at all.*

QUESTIONS

126. Patient with atrophic gastritis has megaloblastic anaemia.
127. Patient who is a strict vegetarian has an MCV of 110.
128. Patient has both Iron and Folate deficiency radiology and sigmoidoscopy—normal, has pale stools which is difficult to flush away.
129. Elderly patient with complaint of anaemia and has bleeding gum.
130. Elderly patient in residential home stay with complaint of tiredness.

THEME 27: MANAGEMENT OF ASTHMA

OPTIONS

a. Inhaled long-acting β_2 agonists
b. Inhaled short-acting β_2 agonists
c. Nebulised β_2 agonists
d. Oral theophylline
e. Oral steroid
f. IV hydrocortisone
g. IV aminophylline
h. Inhaled steroid
i. Inhaled cromolyn
j. Reduce steroid dose
k. Aspiration

*For each presentation below, choose the **most appropriate management** from the above list of OPTIONS. Each option may be used once, more than once, or not at all.*

QUESTIONS

131. A 25-year-old patient now has to use inhaled β_2 2-3 times a day.

132. A 35-year-old uses β_2 agonist + lowdose steroid but symptoms still uncontrolled.

133. A 37-year-old female presents with breathlessness, high RR.

134. A patient who was on 1000 microgram of beclomethasone has now developed oral thrush.

135. An asthmatic patient presents to A and E department with sudden onset dyspnoea. On examination there is reduce expansion, and diminished breath sounds on one side of chest. Trachea is deviated towards otherside.

THEME 28: INITIAL MANAGEMENT/INVESTIGATION IN EYE CONDITIONS

OPTIONS

a. ESR
b. CT
c. Intraocular pressure
d. Artificial tears
e. Visual acuity assessment
f. Visual field mapping
g. Pilocarpine
h. Blood sugar
i. Conjunctival cytology
j. Lumbar puncture
k. X-ray orbit

*For each presentation below, choose the **most appropriate answer** from the above list of OPTIONS. Each option may be used once, more than once, or not at all.*

QUESTIONS

136. A 70-year-old with complaint of malaise, weight-loss, anorexia. Then develops sudden left-sided visual loss.

137. A 60-year-old develops tunnel vision, there is enlargement of the optic cup.

138. A 50-year-old woman with history of symmetrical joint pains complains of eye symptoms and Schirmer's test is positive.

139. Woman, 30-year-old with complaint of blurred vision. CT is normal but she has bilateral papilloedema.

140. A woman who is a Visual Display Operator develops headache when she works several hours.

THEME 29: MANAGEMENT/INVESTIGATION OF HEAD INJURY

OPTIONS
a. Admit to hospital
b. Discharge
c. Discharge with advice after normal skull X-ray
d. CT
e. IV mannitol
f. IV dexamethasone
g. Burr hole
h. MRI
i. Refer to social services
j. Skull X-ray
k. Dipstick glucose test

*For each presentation below, choose the **most appropriate next step in management** from the above list of OPTIONS. Each option may be used once, more than once, or not at all.*

QUESTIONS
141. A 2-year-old boy ran and hit his forehead on the door. No history of loss of consciousness, and since then is playing well. No neurological signs.

142. An 8-year-old boy falls off a swing at his school. He is brought to casualty by one of his teachers. He has a bruise over his right eye but the examination is otherwise normal. He is fully conscious with no history of blackouts since the accident. A skull X-ray is performed, which is normal.

143. A 19-year-old involved in an road traffic accident (RTA). He is talking, responding and smells of alcohol.

144. A 74-year-old woman had a fall two weeks ago. She is brought into the A and E department with slowly increasing drowsiness. On examination you find mild hemiparesis and unequal pupils.

145. A 24-year-old patient presents with RTA. The pupil on the left side is dilated and the patient is obtunded. CT scan of the head reveals a biconvex hyperdense lesion on the temporal region.

THEME 30: DIFFERENTIAL DIAGNOSIS OF JOINT DISEASE

OPTIONS
a. Gout
b. Pseudogout
c. Osteoarthritis (OA)
d. Rheumatoid arthritis
e. Enteropathic arthritis
f. Septic arthritis
g. SUFE
h. Reiter's disease
i. Perthes' disease
j. Congenital dysplasia of hip
k. SLE

*For each presentation below, choose the **single most likely diagnosis** from the above list of OPTIONS. Each option may be used once, more than once, or not at all.*

QUESTIONS
146. A 40-year-old hypertensive male with complaint of left knee pain. Also history of similar attacks. Joint aspirate is cloudy.

147. A patient's ECG shows T wave inversion and ST depression.

148. Three days of intravenous broad spectrum antibiotics beginning with induction of anaesthesia.

149. A middle-aged woman with a history of rheumatoid arthritis develops sudden swelling in one of her knees. This knee is swollen and hot to touch.

150. A 78-year-old woman complains of a stiff left hip joint after walking some distance. This is most evident when she attempts to abduct the hip joint with limited abduction.

THEME 31: CAUSES OF CONFUSION IN THE ELDERLY

OPTIONS
a. Subdural haematoma
b. Infection toxicity
c. Hyperthyroidism
d. Hypothyroidism
e. Acute pancreatitis
f. Hypoglycaemia
g. Korsakoff's psychosis
h. Wernikes-Korsakoff's syndrome (WKS)
i. Wernike's encephalopathy
j. Acute psychiatric disturbance
k. Hypopituitarism

For each presentation below, choose the ***single most likely diagnosis*** *from the above list of OPTIONS. Each option may be used once, more than once, or not at all.*

QUESTIONS

151. A chronic alcoholic presents with increasing confusion and confabulation.
152. A patient presents with weight gain, hypothermia and confusion.
153. Elderly patient with complaint of fever and increasing confusion.
154. A 57-year-old male comes to the A and E with his daughter, in a confused state. The daughter said that her father was started on some medication by his GP.
155. An elderly man found wandering aimlessely, brought to the A and E by neighbours, who inform that his GP had called on him yesterday.

THEME 32: INVESTIGATION OF VAGINAL BLEEDING

OPTIONS
a. Endometrial sampling
b. Urinary FSH
c. Serum LH
d. Vaginal ultrasound
e. Pregnancy test
f. Colposcopy
g. Per speculum examination
h. Laparoscopy
i. None required
j. Oestrogen levels
k. Blood culture

For each presentation below, choose the ***most appropriate investigation*** *from the above list of OPTIONS. Each option may be used once, more than once, or not at all.*

QUESTIONS

156. Female on OCPs complains of postcoital bleeding.
157. A 55-year-old female develops a single episode of PMB. She stopped menstruation 7 years ago. ultrasound shows endometrial thickness.
158. A 49-year-old woman with complaint of hot flushes, vaginal dryness and her menstruation become irregular 5 months ago.
159. A 14-year-old woman with painless vaginal bleeding.
160. A 55-year-old lady with history of intermittent postmenopausal bleeding. Vaginal and speculum examinations are normal.

THEME 33: INVESTIGATION OF THYROID DISEASE

OPTIONS

a. FNAC
b. Ultrasound thyroid
c. Thyroid scan
d. Serum TSH
e. Serum T_3 and T_4
f. Radioactive iodine uptake
g. USG
h. Chest X-ray
i. Isthmusectomy
j. Free T_3 and T_4
k. TSH and T_4

For each presentation below, choose the ***most appropriate next investigation*** *from the above list of OPTIONS. Each option may be used once, more than once, or not at all.*

QUESTIONS

161. A 39-year-old woman on thyroxine replacement comes for first check-up.
162. A 40-year-old woman, euthyroid (TSH normal) complains of palpitations, weight loss and diarrhoea.
163. A 13-year-old woman, euthyroid has a soft diffuse swelling that moves with swallowing.
164. An elderly woman presents with a hard fixed lump ultrasound shows no cystic spaces.
165. An elderly man presents with hoarse voice. On examination he has dilated chest vessels and engorged neck veins.

THEME 34: DIAGNOSIS OF LUMPS OF THE HEAD AND NECK

OPTIONS

a. Cystic hygroma
b. Carotid body tumour
c. Brachial cyst
d. Lymph node
e. Carotid artery aneurysm
f. Cx rib
g. Subclavian aneurysm
h. Branchial fistula
i. Thyroglossal cyst
j. Thyroglossal fistula
k. Parotid tumour

For each presentation below, choose the ***most appropriate investigation*** *from the above list of OPTIONS. Each option may be used once, more than once, or not at all.*

QUESTIONS

166. Patient with a pulsatile hard mass fixed under the upper one-third of the sternomastoid muscle.
167. A 40-year-old male has a lump in the supero-posterior area of the anterior triangle.
168. A 16-year-old female has a midline lump in the neck which moves on protrusion of the tongue and is below the hyoind bone.
169. A 19-year-old male has a cystic mass under the anterior border of sternomastoid at the junction of upper one-third and middle one-third of the muscle. Aspiration revealed fluid containing cholesterol crystals.
170. An infant present with a transilluminant swelling in the lower third of neck.

THEME 35: POSTOPERATIVE COMPLICATIONS

OPTIONS

a. DVT
b. Septicaemia
c. Impending wound dehiscence
d. Wound infection
e. Urinary tract infection
f. Myocardial infarction
g. Acute tubular necrosis
h. Transfusion reaction
i. Cardiac failure
j. Pelvic abscess
k. Pulmonary collapse

*For each presentation below, choose the **single most likely diagnosis** from the above list of OPTIONS. Each option may be used once, more than once, or not at all.*

QUESTIONS

171. A 50-year-old woman underwent an anterior resection for carcinoma of the rectum one week ago. Has low grade fever and with complaint of pain in the calf + tenderness in the calf.

172. A young woman underwent emergency appendicectomy 6 days ago for perforated appendix. She appeared to be making a good recovery but has developed intermittent pyrexia (up to 39 deg. C). On examination—no obvious cause found, but he is tender anteriorly on rectal examination

173. An elderly man underwent an emergency repair of an abdominal aortic aneurysm. Had been severely hypotensive before and during surgery. After surgery, his blood pressure was satisfactory, but urine output only 5 ml/hr in the first 2 hours.

174. An elderly woman underwent emergency laparotomy for peritonitis. Fourth postoperative day she is noted to have sero-sanuinous discharge from the wound, but there is no erythema or tenderness around the wound.

175. A 60-year-old with features of septicaemia (warm peripheries, low BP, etc.).

THEME 36: MODE OF INHERITANCE

OPTIONS

a. X-linked recessive
b. Autosomal dominant
c. Autosomal co-dominance
d. Autosomal recessive
e. Polygenic
f. Single gene defect
g. X-linked dominant
h. Y-linked
i. Mismatch mutation

*For each presentation below, choose the **most appropriate answer** from the above list of OPTIONS. Each option may be used once, more than once, or not at all.*

QUESTIONS

176. A 4-year-old boy gets haemarthrosis with trivial injury. He had similar episodes before maternal grandfather and uncle had a similar problem.

177. A young girl with complaint of prolonged bleeding following dental extraction. Father had a work-up for anaemia and mother had multiple transfusion.

178. A 15-year-old girl with features of diabetes mellitus.

179. An 11-year-old boy presents with increasing difficulty walking, tremor and instability. Father died in his 40's with same disease.

180. An 18-year-old female underwent caries tooth extraction and developed profuse bleeding. On taking history she revealed menorrhagia. Her mother and her grandfather had the same disease.

THEME 37: PROGRESSION OF CARCINOMA BREAST

OPTIONS

a. Asthma
b. Axillary recurrence
c. Bone marrow infiltration
d. Bony metastasis
e. Cerebral metastasis
f. Hypercalcaemia
g. Left ventricular failure
h. Liver metastasis
i. Local recurrence
j. Spinal cord compression
k. Pleural effusion

For each presentation below, choose the ***single most like diagnosis*** *from the above list of OPTIONS. Each option may be used once, more than once, or not at all.*

QUESTIONS

181. A 56-year-old woman who underwent mastectomy for a breast tumour four years ago, now complains of increasing breathlessness. On examination of her respiratory system, she is noted to have decreased movement of the left hemithorax which is dull to percussion and has absent breath sounds.

182. A 60-year-old woman is admitted to the accident and emergency department having fallen in the street. She is complaining of pain in the right hip and the right lower limb is lying in external rotation. She had breast conserving surgery, radiotherapy and chemotherapy eight years also for breast cancer.

183. A 43-year-old woman treated two years ago for a grade 3 axillary node positive breast cancer presents with increasing confusion, headache and vomiting. On examination, she is drowsy but has no focal neurological signs. She does have blurring of the optic disc margins.

184. A 35-year-old woman treated one year ago for a breast cancer with 12/20 nodes positive, presents with a two days history of increasing confusion, She is drowsy and disoriented. Her husband reports that she has been complaining of severe thirst for the past week.

185. A 45-year-old woman treated three years ago for breast cancer is unable to walk. She complains of increasing weakness in her leg for the last seven days. She has been constipated and unable to pass urine for the last 24 hours.

THEME 38: PRESCRIBING FOR PAIN RELIEF

OPTIONS

a. IV opiate
b. Subcutaneous opiate infusion
c. Acupuncture
d. Carbamazepine
e. Hypnotherapy
f. NSAIDs IM
g. Oral NSAIDs
h. Oral opiates
i. Proton pump inhibitors
j. SSRI, e.g. fluoxetine

For each presentation below, choose the ***single most appropriate method of pain relief*** *from the above list of OPTIONS. Each option may be used once, more than once, or not at all.*

QUESTIONS

186. A 65-year-old man presents with severe, retrosternal chest pain and sweating. An ECG shows an acute anterolateral myocardial infarction.

187. A 70-year-old man inoperable gastric cancer causing obstruction, and multiple liver metastases, is taking a large dose of oral analgesia. Despite this, his pain is currently unrelieved.

188. A 25-year-old woman has just been diagnosed a having rheumatoid arthritis and her rheumatologists has begun giving her gold injections. She continues to complain of joint pain and stiffnesss, particularly for the first two hours of each day.

189. A 50-year-old obese man with a known hiatus hernia, presents with recurrent, severe, burning retrosternal chest pain associated with acid regurgitation and increased oral flatulence.

190. A 67-year-old woman reports severe paroxysms of knife-like or electric shock-like pain, lasting seconds in the lower part of the right side of her face.

THEME 39: DIFFERENTIAL DIAGNOSIS OF ACUTE ABDOMINAL PAIN IN A YOUNG WOMAN

OPTIONS

a. Acute gastroenteritis
b. Acute pancreatitis
c. Appendicitis
d. Biliary colic
e. Cholecystitis
f. Ectopic pregnancy
g. Mesenteric thrombosis
h. Perforated peptic ulcer
i. Renal colic
j. Salpingitis
k. Strangulated hernia

For each presentation below, choose the ***single most likely diagnosis*** *from the above list of OPTIONS. Each option may be used once, more than once, or not at all.*

QUESTIONS

191. A 20-year-old married woman presents in the accident and emergency department with the onset of acute lower abdominal pain. Her past menstrual period was six weeks previously. She has pain radiating to the left shoulder.

192. A 15-year-old girl presents with a 24 hours history of central abdominal pain, followed by the right iliac fossa pain, worse on coughing. She has fever and rebound in the right iliac fossa.

193. A 30-year-old woman has severe colic and upper abdominal pain radiating to her right scapula and is vomiting.

194. A 12-year-old girl has central abdominal pain and is vomiting. On examination, her abdomen is found to be distended with no rebound and a tender lump in the right groin.

195. A 31-year-old woman has severe colic and upper abdominal pain. She is febrile and vomiting. Haematological investigations show a moderate leukocytosis.

THEME 40: ETHICAL PRACTICE OF MEDICINE IN UK

OPTIONS

a. Report him to trust managers.
b. Do not do anything, since the actions of your consultant do not seem to be affecting the progress of patient's condition.
c. Call police and inform them at once.
d. Give her the pills after explaining risks to her and disregard her mother completely.
e. Carry out the termination even without the parent's knowledge.
f. Carry out operation to save at least one baby.
g. Repect parents decision and let nature take its course, even if this means certain death for both babies.
h. Carry out the sterilisation.
i. Tell her you cannot give her the pills without mother's consent.
j. Give her pills and phone the mother and tell her about the pills.
k. Tell the parents and only carry out termination, with their consent.
l. Get partners written and informed consent before carrying out sterilisation.
m. Inform Health Minister, as situation is complicated
n. Seek a judicial review

For each presentation below, choose the ***correct answer*** *from the above list of OPTIONS. Each option may be used once, more than once, or not at all.*

QUESTIONS

196. You are the SHO on the psychiatry ward. Your consultant is having a sexual relationship with a widow. She has been treated for depression. The lady is getting better and is awaiting discharge.

197. A 34-year-old woman wants to have a sterilisation. Her last born child has cerebral palsy and her partner strongly objects to the procedure. They are married.

198. A mother has siamese twins. One of the twins has no heart and liver and depends on the other for survival, and as such without an operation to save the one with major organs they will both perish. Since having the operation means certain death of one of the babies, the parents who are staunch christians oppose the operation. What should be done?

199. A 12-year-old girl wants oral contraceptive pills. She does not want her parents to know about this.

200. A 9-year-old girl wants to have a termination of pregnancy. She is 14 weeks pregnant. The procedure to terminate is not without complications. She does not want her mother informed about the termination.

General Medical Council PLAB Test Part 1

Full Name

Test Centre/Date

- Use pencil only • Make heavy marks that fill the lozenge completely
- Write your candidate number in the top row of the box to the right **AND** fill in the appropriate lozenge below each number
- Give **ONE** answer only for each question

0	0	0	0	0	0
1	1	1	1	1	1
2	2	2	2	2	2
3	3	3	3	3	3
4	4	4	4	4	4
5	5	5	5	5	5
6	6	6	6	6	6
7	7	7	7	7	7
8	8	8	8	8	8
9	9	9	9	9	9

1	A	B	C	D	E	F	G	H	I	J	K	L	M	N	O	P	Q	R	S	T	1
2	A	B	C	D	E	F	G	H	I	J	K	L	M	N	O	P	Q	R	S	T	2
3	A	B	C	D	E	F	G	H	I	J	K	L	M	N	O	P	Q	R	S	T	3
4	A	B	C	D	E	F	G	H	I	J	K	L	M	N	O	P	Q	R	S	T	4
5	A	B	C	D	E	F	G	H	I	J	K	L	M	N	O	P	Q	R	S	T	5
6	A	B	C	D	E	F	G	H	I	J	K	L	M	N	O	P	Q	R	S	T	6
7	A	B	C	D	E	F	G	H	I	J	K	L	M	N	O	P	Q	R	S	T	7
8	A	B	C	D	E	F	G	H	I	J	K	L	M	N	O	P	Q	R	S	T	8
9	A	B	C	D	E	F	G	H	I	J	K	L	M	N	O	P	Q	R	S	T	9
10	A	B	C	D	E	F	G	H	I	J	K	L	M	N	O	P	Q	R	S	T	10
11	A	B	C	D	E	F	G	H	I	J	K	L	M	N	O	P	Q	R	S	T	11
12	A	B	C	D	E	F	G	H	I	J	K	L	M	N	O	P	Q	R	S	T	12
13	A	B	C	D	E	F	G	H	I	J	K	L	M	N	O	P	Q	R	S	T	13
14	A	B	C	D	E	F	G	H	I	J	K	L	M	N	O	P	Q	R	S	T	14
15	A	B	C	D	E	F	G	H	I	J	K	L	M	N	O	P	Q	R	S	T	15
16	A	B	C	D	E	F	G	H	I	J	K	L	M	N	O	P	Q	R	S	T	16
17	A	B	C	D	E	F	G	H	I	J	K	L	M	N	O	P	Q	R	S	T	17
18	A	B	C	D	E	F	G	H	I	J	K	L	M	N	O	P	Q	R	S	T	18
19	A	B	C	D	E	F	G	H	I	J	K	L	M	N	O	P	Q	R	S	T	19
20	A	B	C	D	E	F	G	H	I	J	K	L	M	N	O	P	Q	R	S	T	20
21	A	B	C	D	E	F	G	H	I	J	K	L	M	N	O	P	Q	R	S	T	21
22	A	B	C	D	E	F	G	H	I	J	K	L	M	N	O	P	Q	R	S	T	22
23	A	B	C	D	E	F	G	H	I	J	K	L	M	N	O	P	Q	R	S	T	23
24	A	B	C	D	E	F	G	H	I	J	K	L	M	N	O	P	Q	R	S	T	24
25	A	B	C	D	E	F	G	H	I	J	K	L	M	N	O	P	Q	R	S	T	25
26	A	B	C	D	E	F	G	H	I	J	K	L	M	N	O	P	Q	R	S	T	26
27	A	B	C	D	E	F	G	H	I	J	K	L	M	N	O	P	Q	R	S	T	27
28	A	B	C	D	E	F	G	H	I	J	K	L	M	N	O	P	Q	R	S	T	28
29	A	B	C	D	E	F	G	H	I	J	K	L	M	N	O	P	Q	R	S	T	29
30	A	B	C	D	E	F	G	H	I	J	K	L	M	N	O	P	Q	R	S	T	30
31	A	B	C	D	E	F	G	H	I	J	K	L	M	N	O	P	Q	R	S	T	31
32	A	B	C	D	E	F	G	H	I	J	K	L	M	N	O	P	Q	R	S	T	32
33	A	B	C	D	E	F	G	H	I	J	K	L	M	N	O	P	Q	R	S	T	33
34	A	B	C	D	E	F	G	H	I	J	K	L	M	N	O	P	Q	R	S	T	34
35	A	B	C	D	E	F	G	H	I	J	K	L	M	N	O	P	Q	R	S	T	35
36	A	B	C	D	E	F	G	H	I	J	K	L	M	N	O	P	Q	R	S	T	36
37	A	B	C	D	E	F	G	H	I	J	K	L	M	N	O	P	Q	R	S	T	37
38	A	B	C	D	E	F	G	H	I	J	K	L	M	N	O	P	Q	R	S	T	38
39	A	B	C	D	E	F	G	H	I	J	K	L	M	N	O	P	Q	R	S	T	39
40	A	B	C	D	E	F	G	H	I	J	K	L	M	N	O	P	Q	R	S	T	40
41	A	B	C	D	E	F	G	H	I	J	K	L	M	N	O	P	Q	R	S	T	41
42	A	B	C	D	E	F	G	H	I	J	K	L	M	N	O	P	Q	R	S	T	42
43	A	B	C	D	E	F	G	H	I	J	K	L	M	N	O	P	Q	R	S	T	43
44	A	B	C	D	E	F	G	H	I	J	K	L	M	N	O	P	Q	R	S	T	44
45	A	B	C	D	E	F	G	H	I	J	K	L	M	N	O	P	Q	R	S	T	45
46	A	B	C	D	E	F	G	H	I	J	K	L	M	N	O	P	Q	R	S	T	46
47	A	B	C	D	E	F	G	H	I	J	K	L	M	N	O	P	Q	R	S	T	47
48	A	B	C	D	E	F	G	H	I	J	K	L	M	N	O	P	Q	R	S	T	48
49	A	B	C	D	E	F	G	H	I	J	K	L	M	N	O	P	Q	R	S	T	49
50	A	B	C	D	E	F	G	H	I	J	K	L	M	N	O	P	Q	R	S	T	50

DO NOT WRITE IN THIS SPACE

51	A	B	C	D	E	F	G	H	I	J	K	L	M	N	O	P	Q	R	S	T	51
52	A	B	C	D	E	F	G	H	I	J	K	L	M	N	O	P	Q	R	S	T	52
53	A	B	C	D	E	F	G	H	I	J	K	L	M	N	O	P	Q	R	S	T	53
54	A	B	C	D	E	F	G	H	I	J	K	L	M	N	O	P	Q	R	S	T	54
55	A	B	C	D	E	F	G	H	I	J	K	L	M	N	O	P	Q	R	S	T	55
56	A	B	C	D	E	F	G	H	I	J	K	L	M	N	O	P	Q	R	S	T	56
57	A	B	C	D	E	F	G	H	I	J	K	L	M	N	O	P	Q	R	S	T	57
58	A	B	C	D	E	F	G	H	I	J	K	L	M	N	O	P	Q	R	S	T	58
59	A	B	C	D	E	F	G	H	I	J	K	L	M	N	O	P	Q	R	S	T	59
60	A	B	C	D	E	F	G	H	I	J	K	L	M	N	O	P	Q	R	S	T	60
61	A	B	C	D	E	F	G	H	I	J	K	L	M	N	O	P	Q	R	S	T	61
62	A	B	C	D	E	F	G	H	I	J	K	L	M	N	O	P	Q	R	S	T	62
63	A	B	C	D	E	F	G	H	I	J	K	L	M	N	O	P	Q	R	S	T	63
64	A	B	C	D	E	F	G	H	I	J	K	L	M	N	O	P	Q	R	S	T	64
65	A	B	C	D	E	F	G	H	I	J	K	L	M	N	O	P	Q	R	S	T	65
66	A	B	C	D	E	F	G	H	I	J	K	L	M	N	O	P	Q	R	S	T	66
67	A	B	C	D	E	F	G	H	I	J	K	L	M	N	O	P	Q	R	S	T	67
68	A	B	C	D	E	F	G	H	I	J	K	L	M	N	O	P	Q	R	S	T	68
69	A	B	C	D	E	F	G	H	I	J	K	L	M	N	O	P	Q	R	S	T	69
70	A	B	C	D	E	F	G	H	I	J	K	L	M	N	O	P	Q	R	S	T	70
71	A	B	C	D	E	F	G	H	I	J	K	L	M	N	O	P	Q	R	S	T	71
72	A	B	C	D	E	F	G	H	I	J	K	L	M	N	O	P	Q	R	S	T	72
73	A	B	C	D	E	F	G	H	I	J	K	L	M	N	O	P	Q	R	S	T	73
74	A	B	C	D	E	F	G	H	I	J	K	L	M	N	O	P	Q	R	S	T	74
75	A	B	C	D	E	F	G	H	I	J	K	L	M	N	O	P	Q	R	S	T	75
76	A	B	C	D	E	F	G	H	I	J	K	L	M	N	O	P	Q	R	S	T	76
77	A	B	C	D	E	F	G	H	I	J	K	L	M	N	O	P	Q	R	S	T	77
78	A	B	C	D	E	F	G	H	I	J	K	L	M	N	O	P	Q	R	S	T	78
79	A	B	C	D	E	F	G	H	I	J	K	L	M	N	O	P	Q	R	S	T	79
80	A	B	C	D	E	F	G	H	I	J	K	L	M	N	O	P	Q	R	S	T	80
81	A	B	C	D	E	F	G	H	I	J	K	L	M	N	O	P	Q	R	S	T	81
82	A	B	C	D	E	F	G	H	I	J	K	L	M	N	O	P	Q	R	S	T	82
83	A	B	C	D	E	F	G	H	I	J	K	L	M	N	O	P	Q	R	S	T	83
84	A	B	C	D	E	F	G	H	I	J	K	L	M	N	O	P	Q	R	S	T	84
85	A	B	C	D	E	F	G	H	I	J	K	L	M	N	O	P	Q	R	S	T	85
86	A	B	C	D	E	F	G	H	I	J	K	L	M	N	O	P	Q	R	S	T	86
87	A	B	C	D	E	F	G	H	I	J	K	L	M	N	O	P	Q	R	S	T	87
88	A	B	C	D	E	F	G	H	I	J	K	L	M	N	O	P	Q	R	S	T	88
89	A	B	C	D	E	F	G	H	I	J	K	L	M	N	O	P	Q	R	S	T	89
90	A	B	C	D	E	F	G	H	I	J	K	L	M	N	O	P	Q	R	S	T	90
91	A	B	C	D	E	F	G	H	I	J	K	L	M	N	O	P	Q	R	S	T	91
92	A	B	C	D	E	F	G	H	I	J	K	L	M	N	O	P	Q	R	S	T	92
93	A	B	C	D	E	F	G	H	I	J	K	L	M	N	O	P	Q	R	S	T	93
94	A	B	C	D	E	F	G	H	I	J	K	L	M	N	O	P	Q	R	S	T	94
95	A	B	C	D	E	F	G	H	I	J	K	L	M	N	O	P	Q	R	S	T	95
96	A	B	C	D	E	F	G	H	I	J	K	L	M	N	O	P	Q	R	S	T	96
97	A	B	C	D	E	F	G	H	I	J	K	L	M	N	O	P	Q	R	S	T	97
98	A	B	C	D	E	F	G	H	I	J	K	L	M	N	O	P	Q	R	S	T	98
99	A	B	C	D	E	F	G	H	I	J	K	L	M	N	O	P	Q	R	S	T	99
100	A	B	C	D	E	F	G	H	I	J	K	L	M	N	O	P	Q	R	S	T	100

DO NOT WRITE IN THIS SPACE

101	A	B	C	D	E	F	G	H	I	J	K	L	M	N	O	P	Q	R	S	T	101
102	A	B	C	D	E	F	G	H	I	J	K	L	M	N	O	P	Q	R	S	T	102
103	A	B	C	D	E	F	G	H	I	J	K	L	M	N	O	P	Q	R	S	T	103
104	A	B	C	D	E	F	G	H	I	J	K	L	M	N	O	P	Q	R	S	T	104
105	A	B	C	D	E	F	G	H	I	J	K	L	M	N	O	P	Q	R	S	T	105
106	A	B	C	D	E	F	G	H	I	J	K	L	M	N	O	P	Q	R	S	T	106
107	A	B	C	D	E	F	G	H	I	J	K	L	M	N	O	P	Q	R	S	T	107
108	A	B	C	D	E	F	G	H	I	J	K	L	M	N	O	P	Q	R	S	T	108
109	A	B	C	D	E	F	G	H	I	J	K	L	M	N	O	P	Q	R	S	T	109
110	A	B	C	D	E	F	G	H	I	J	K	L	M	N	O	P	Q	R	S	T	110
111	A	B	C	D	E	F	G	H	I	J	K	L	M	N	O	P	Q	R	S	T	111
112	A	B	C	D	E	F	G	H	I	J	K	L	M	N	O	P	Q	R	S	T	112
113	A	B	C	D	E	F	G	H	I	J	K	L	M	N	O	P	Q	R	S	T	113
114	A	B	C	D	E	F	G	H	I	J	K	L	M	N	O	P	Q	R	S	T	114
115	A	B	C	D	E	F	G	H	I	J	K	L	M	N	O	P	Q	R	S	T	115
116	A	B	C	D	E	F	G	H	I	J	K	L	M	N	O	P	Q	R	S	T	116
117	A	B	C	D	E	F	G	H	I	J	K	L	M	N	O	P	Q	R	S	T	117
118	A	B	C	D	E	F	G	H	I	J	K	L	M	N	O	P	Q	R	S	T	118
119	A	B	C	D	E	F	G	H	I	J	K	L	M	N	O	P	Q	R	S	T	119
120	A	B	C	D	E	F	G	H	I	J	K	L	M	N	O	P	Q	R	S	T	120
121	A	B	C	D	E	F	G	H	I	J	K	L	M	N	O	P	Q	R	S	T	121
122	A	B	C	D	E	F	G	H	I	J	K	L	M	N	O	P	Q	R	S	T	122
123	A	B	C	D	E	F	G	H	I	J	K	L	M	N	O	P	Q	R	S	T	123
124	A	B	C	D	E	F	G	H	I	J	K	L	M	N	O	P	Q	R	S	T	124
125	A	B	C	D	E	F	G	H	I	J	K	L	M	N	O	P	Q	R	S	T	125
126	A	B	C	D	E	F	G	H	I	J	K	L	M	N	O	P	Q	R	S	T	126
127	A	B	C	D	E	F	G	H	I	J	K	L	M	N	O	P	Q	R	S	T	127
128	A	B	C	D	E	F	G	H	I	J	K	L	M	N	O	P	Q	R	S	T	128
129	A	B	C	D	E	F	G	H	I	J	K	L	M	N	O	P	Q	R	S	T	129
130	A	B	C	D	E	F	G	H	I	J	K	L	M	N	O	P	Q	R	S	T	130
131	A	B	C	D	E	F	G	H	I	J	K	L	M	N	O	P	Q	R	S	T	131
132	A	B	C	D	E	F	G	H	I	J	K	L	M	N	O	P	Q	R	S	T	132
133	A	B	C	D	E	F	G	H	I	J	K	L	M	N	O	P	Q	R	S	T	133
134	A	B	C	D	E	F	G	H	I	J	K	L	M	N	O	P	Q	R	S	T	134
135	A	B	C	D	E	F	G	H	I	J	K	L	M	N	O	P	Q	R	S	T	135
136	A	B	C	D	E	F	G	H	I	J	K	L	M	N	O	P	Q	R	S	T	136
137	A	B	C	D	E	F	G	H	I	J	K	L	M	N	O	P	Q	R	S	T	137
138	A	B	C	D	E	F	G	H	I	J	K	L	M	N	O	P	Q	R	S	T	138
139	A	B	C	D	E	F	G	H	I	J	K	L	M	N	O	P	Q	R	S	T	139
140	A	B	C	D	E	F	G	H	I	J	K	L	M	N	O	P	Q	R	S	T	140
141	A	B	C	D	E	F	G	H	I	J	K	L	M	N	O	P	Q	R	S	T	141
142	A	B	C	D	E	F	G	H	I	J	K	L	M	N	O	P	Q	R	S	T	142
143	A	B	C	D	E	F	G	H	I	J	K	L	M	N	O	P	Q	R	S	T	143
144	A	B	C	D	E	F	G	H	I	J	K	L	M	N	O	P	Q	R	S	T	144
145	A	B	C	D	E	F	G	H	I	J	K	L	M	N	O	P	Q	R	S	T	145
146	A	B	C	D	E	F	G	H	I	J	K	L	M	N	O	P	Q	R	S	T	146
147	A	B	C	D	E	F	G	H	I	J	K	L	M	N	O	P	Q	R	S	T	147
148	A	B	C	D	E	F	G	H	I	J	K	L	M	N	O	P	Q	R	S	T	148
149	A	B	C	D	E	F	G	H	I	J	K	L	M	N	O	P	Q	R	S	T	149
150	A	B	C	D	E	F	G	H	I	J	K	L	M	N	O	P	Q	R	S	T	150

DO NOT WRITE IN THIS SPACE

151	A	B	C	D	E	F	G	H	I	J	K	L	M	N	O	P	Q	R	S	T	151
152	A	B	C	D	E	F	G	H	I	J	K	L	M	N	O	P	Q	R	S	T	152
153	A	B	C	D	E	F	G	H	I	J	K	L	M	N	O	P	Q	R	S	T	153
154	A	B	C	D	E	F	G	H	I	J	K	L	M	N	O	P	Q	R	S	T	154
155	A	B	C	D	E	F	G	H	I	J	K	L	M	N	O	P	Q	R	S	T	155
156	A	B	C	D	E	F	G	H	I	J	K	L	M	N	O	P	Q	R	S	T	156
157	A	B	C	D	E	F	G	H	I	J	K	L	M	N	O	P	Q	R	S	T	157
158	A	B	C	D	E	F	G	H	I	J	K	L	M	N	O	P	Q	R	S	T	158
159	A	B	C	D	E	F	G	H	I	J	K	L	M	N	O	P	Q	R	S	T	159
160	A	B	C	D	E	F	G	H	I	J	K	L	M	N	O	P	Q	R	S	T	160
161	A	B	C	D	E	F	G	H	I	J	K	L	M	N	O	P	Q	R	S	T	161
162	A	B	C	D	E	F	G	H	I	J	K	L	M	N	O	P	Q	R	S	T	162
163	A	B	C	D	E	F	G	H	I	J	K	L	M	N	O	P	Q	R	S	T	163
164	A	B	C	D	E	F	G	H	I	J	K	L	M	N	O	P	Q	R	S	T	164
165	A	B	C	D	E	F	G	H	I	J	K	L	M	N	O	P	Q	R	S	T	165
166	A	B	C	D	E	F	G	H	I	J	K	L	M	N	O	P	Q	R	S	T	166
167	A	B	C	D	E	F	G	H	I	J	K	L	M	N	O	P	Q	R	S	T	167
168	A	B	C	D	E	F	G	H	I	J	K	L	M	N	O	P	Q	R	S	T	168
169	A	B	C	D	E	F	G	H	I	J	K	L	M	N	O	P	Q	R	S	T	169
170	A	B	C	D	E	F	G	H	I	J	K	L	M	N	O	P	Q	R	S	T	170
171	A	B	C	D	E	F	G	H	I	J	K	L	M	N	O	P	Q	R	S	T	171
172	A	B	C	D	E	F	G	H	I	J	K	L	M	N	O	P	Q	R	S	T	172
173	A	B	C	D	E	F	G	H	I	J	K	L	M	N	O	P	Q	R	S	T	173
174	A	B	C	D	E	F	G	H	I	J	K	L	M	N	O	P	Q	R	S	T	174
175	A	B	C	D	E	F	G	H	I	J	K	L	M	N	O	P	Q	R	S	T	175
176	A	B	C	D	E	F	G	H	I	J	K	L	M	N	O	P	Q	R	S	T	176
177	A	B	C	D	E	F	G	H	I	J	K	L	M	N	O	P	Q	R	S	T	177
178	A	B	C	D	E	F	G	H	I	J	K	L	M	N	O	P	Q	R	S	T	178
179	A	B	C	D	E	F	G	H	I	J	K	L	M	N	O	P	Q	R	S	T	179
180	A	B	C	D	E	F	G	H	I	J	K	L	M	N	O	P	Q	R	S	T	180
181	A	B	C	D	E	F	G	H	I	J	K	L	M	N	O	P	Q	R	S	T	181
182	A	B	C	D	E	F	G	H	I	J	K	L	M	N	O	P	Q	R	S	T	182
183	A	B	C	D	E	F	G	H	I	J	K	L	M	N	O	P	Q	R	S	T	183
184	A	B	C	D	E	F	G	H	I	J	K	L	M	N	O	P	Q	R	S	T	184
185	A	B	C	D	E	F	G	H	I	J	K	L	M	N	O	P	Q	R	S	T	185
186	A	B	C	D	E	F	G	H	I	J	K	L	M	N	O	P	Q	R	S	T	186
187	A	B	C	D	E	F	G	H	I	J	K	L	M	N	O	P	Q	R	S	T	187
188	A	B	C	D	E	F	G	H	I	J	K	L	M	N	O	P	Q	R	S	T	188
189	A	B	C	D	E	F	G	H	I	J	K	L	M	N	O	P	Q	R	S	T	189
190	A	B	C	D	E	F	G	H	I	J	K	L	M	N	O	P	Q	R	S	T	190
191	A	B	C	D	E	F	G	H	I	J	K	L	M	N	O	P	Q	R	S	T	191
192	A	B	C	D	E	F	G	H	I	J	K	L	M	N	O	P	Q	R	S	T	192
193	A	B	C	D	E	F	G	H	I	J	K	L	M	N	O	P	Q	R	S	T	193
194	A	B	C	D	E	F	G	H	I	J	K	L	M	N	O	P	Q	R	S	T	194
195	A	B	C	D	E	F	G	H	I	J	K	L	M	N	O	P	Q	R	S	T	195
196	A	B	C	D	E	F	G	H	I	J	K	L	M	N	O	P	Q	R	S	T	196
197	A	B	C	D	E	F	G	H	I	J	K	L	M	N	O	P	Q	R	S	T	197
198	A	B	C	D	E	F	G	H	I	J	K	L	M	N	O	P	Q	R	S	T	198
199	A	B	C	D	E	F	G	H	I	J	K	L	M	N	O	P	Q	R	S	T	199
200	A	B	C	D	E	F	G	H	I	J	K	L	M	N	O	P	Q	R	S	T	200

Answers

Serial No.	Answer No.	Answer
1	e	Captopril
2	d	Cyclophosphamide
3	j	Frusemide
4	f	Genatamicin
5	i	Acetazolamide
6	d	MSU after 3 weeks
7	a	IVU
8	c	USG kidney and bladder
9	d	MSU after 3 weeks
10	f	MSU culture
11	c	Pyloric stenosis
12	d	Intussusception
13	a	GER (physiological)
14	e	UIL
15	b	Gastroenteritis
16	i	Pulmonary edema
17	b	Asthma
18	a	Panic attacks
19	e	Aspiration pneumonia
20	c	Pulmonary embolism
21	g	Intubation and ventilation
22	i	Urgent blood transfusion
23	d	Needle thoracostomy
24	a	Gain IV access + normal saline/Haemaccel
25	c	Apply external pressure
26	g	Ulcerative colitis
27	a	Carcinoma rectum
28	c	IBS with diarrhoea
29	e	Faecal impaction
30	j	Paralytic ileus
31	h	Multiple sclerosis with spinal cord lesion
32	b	Carcinoma prostate
33	a	Ureteric colic
34	c	BPH
35	h	Spinal cord lesion
36	a	ZN staining
37	b	Serum urate
38	h	Lumbar puncture
39	h	Lumbar puncture
40	f	Rifampicin
41	k	Haemothorax
42	d	Ruptured ectopic pregnancy
43	c	Aortic aneurysm
44	a	Anaphylaxis
45	b	Tension pneumothorax
46	a	Abdominal USG
47	h	MRI
48	d	Coronary angiography
49	d	Coronary angiography
50	e	Echocardiography
51	a	Mesenteric angiogram
52	b	Perforated peptic ulcer
53	i	Acute pancreatitis
54	e	Ureteric colic
55	i	Acute pancreatitis
56	d	Fracture shaft of femur
57	e	Pulled elbow

58	a	Green stick fracture
59	f	Supracondylar fracture
60	g	Slipped upper femoral epiphysis
61	g	Cervical spinal cord
62	f	Brainstem and its cerebellar connections
63	c	Optic nerve
64	c	Optic nerve
65	i	Facial nerve
66	c	Myasthaenia gravis
67	d	Space occupying lesion
68	a	Alzheimer's disease
69	e	Acromegaly
70	f	Polymyositis
71	d	Carboxyhaemoglobin level
72	g	Aspirate blister
73	c	Admit to hospital
74	b	Escharotomy
75	l	Reassure
76	b	Bilateral conductive deafness
77	a	Bilateral sensory neural deafness
78	e	Unilateral conductive deafness
79	d	Unilateral sensory neural deafness
80	f	Threshold shift
81	b	Sensitiving
82	g	Standard derivation
83	h	Cohort studies
84	e	Median
85	c	Mode
86	a	IHD
87	b	Atrial fibrillation
88	c	Warfarin

89	h	Hypertension
90	i	Rheumatic fever
91	a	Diuretic
92	b	Thrombolysis
93	f	Cardiac pacing
94	g	High flow O_2 and morphine
95	c	β-blockers
96	e	Female mite
97	f	Immunodeficiency
98	b	Close community contact
99	c	Animal to human
100	b	Close community contact
101	j	Polysomnography
102	d	Refer to ENT
103	c	Reassure
104	f	Carotid Doppler
105	d	Refer to ENT
106	h	Sexual transmission
107	b	Faeco-oral
108	c	Blood borne
109	h/c	Sexual transmission or blood borne
110	d	Tick borne
111	b	family therapy
112	f	Cognitive therapy
113	d	Education
114	j	ECT
115	l	Sedation
116	a/j	CBT/MAO inhibitors
117	a	CBT
118	d	Supportive therapy
119	c	Densensitisation
120	j	MAO inhibitors

121	c	Paracetamol
122	a	CO
123	b	TCA
124	d	Digoxin
125	i	Cyanide
126	e	Schilling's test
127	b	B_{12} levels
128	j	Alcohol history
129	k	Vitamin C levels
130	a	Dietary history
131	h	Inhaled steroid
132	a	Inhaled long-acting B_2 agonist
133	c	Nebulised B_2-agonist
134	j	Reduce steroids
135	k	Aspiration
136	a	ESR
137	f	Visual field mapping
138	d	Artificial tears
139	j	Lumbar puncture
140	e	Visual acuity assessment
141	b	Discharge
142	j	Skull X-ray
143	a	Admit to hospital
144	d	CT
145	g	Burr hole
146	a	Gout
147	d	Rheumatoid arthritis
148	f	Septic arthritis
149	b	Pseudogout
150	c	Osteoarthritis
151	h	WKS
152	d	Hypothyroidism

153	b	Infection toxicity
154	f	Hypoglycaemia
155	j	Acute psychiatric disturbance
156	g	Per speculum examination
157	a	Endometrial sampling
158	b	Urinary FSH
159	i	None required
160	a	Endometrial sampling
161	d	Serum TSH
162	e	Serum T_3 and T_4
163	k	TSH and T_4
164	i	Isthmusectomy
165	h	Chest X-ray
166	b	Carotid body tumour
167	k	Parotid tumour
168	i	Thyroglossal cyst
169	c	Brachial cyst
170	a	Cystic hygroma
171	a	DVT
172	j	Pelvic abscess
173	g	Acute tubular necrosis
174	c	Impending wound dehiscence
175	b	Septicaemia
176	a	X-linked recessive
177	b	Autosomal dominant
178	e	Polygenic
179	b	Autosomal dominant
180	d	Autosomal recessive
181	k	Pleural effusion
182	d	Bony metastases
183	e	Cerebral metastases
184	f	Hypercalcaemia

185	j	Spinal cord compression
186	a	IV opiate
187	b	Subcutaneous opiate infusion
188	g	Oral NSAID
189	i	Proton pump inhibitors
190	d	Carbamazepine
191	f	Ectopic pregnancy
192	c	Appendicitis

193	d	Biliary colic
194	k	Strangulated hernia
195	e	Cholecystitis
196	a	Report him to trust managers
197	n	Seek a judicial review
198	n	Seek a judicial review
199	d	Give her the pills after...
200	e	Carry out...

Section 3

EXPLANATORY NOTES (SUBJECT-WISE)

1 Acid Base Balance

PAPER 1

Serial No.124

Subject: Medicine

Topic: Electrolyte Imbalance

Question: A patient has diarrhoea, appears to be dehydrated with low serum potassium levels.

Diagnosis: Dehydration with hypokalaemia

Clinchers

- *Has diarrhoea:* Passage of more than 300 g of stool per day or a change in frequency of defaecation or loosening of the consistency is defined as diarrhoea.
- *Dehydrated:*Gastrointestinal secretions are a heavy reservoir of fluid and rich in electrolytes. Loss of this in the form of diarrhoea or vomiting lead to rapid loss of third space fluid causing dehydration and severe electrolyte imbalance.
- *With low serum potassium levels:* Most cases of hypokalaemia are the result of either diuretic consumption or loss of GI fluids either through persistent vomiting, chronic diarrhoea or laxative abuse. In diarrhoea, loss of bicarbonate may cause metabolic acidosis which causes a shift of potassium into the cells so that serum concentration may not reflect total potassium levels.

CONFUSA

Fluids of Choice:

- Fluid of choice in hypovolaemic shock: normal saline, ringer lactate.
- Fluid of choice in shock due to blood loss: whole blood transfusion.
- Fluid of choice in a dehydrated individual: 5% glucose.
- Fluid of choice in a patient with dehydration due to hypertrophic pyloric stenosis/repeated vomiting/ diarrhoea: normal saline/with or without supplemental potassium depending on the patient requirement.
- Fluid of choice in hypoglycaemia: 10-25% glucose.

Investigation of Choice

- Urea and electrolytes, blood glucose
- Extensive investigations to look into the cause for diarrhoea if persists more than 14 days.
  (Most diarrhoea are self-limiting and caused by viruses)

Immediate Management

- Maintain proper hydration and electrolyte balance.
- ORS is most appropriate, providing with all the major electrolytes in right proportion.
- If IV fluids needed, normal saline with/without potassium supplementation may be considered.

Treatment of Choice

According to the cause identified.

Your notes:

Serial No. 125

Subject: Medicine

Topic: Electrolyte Imbalance

Question: A patient on vigorous diuretic therapy develops hypokalaemia.

Diagnosis: Diuretic induced hypokalaemia

Clinchers

- *On vigorous diuretic therapy:* Most cases of hypokalaemia are iatrogenic, diuretics being the most common group of drugs involved.
- *Develops hypokalaemia:* Aggressive use of diuretics especially, the thiazide or loop diuretics, is associated with hypokalaemia. It is not seen with potassium sparing diuretics. Hypokalaemia is defined as serum concentration of potassium <3.5 mmol/L.
  - Mild hypokalaemia - K^+ 3.0-3.5 mmol/L
  - Severe hypokalaemia < 3.0 mmol/L
  - Very severe hypokalaemia < 2.5 mmol/L

CONFUSA

- Suspect hypokalaemia from the patient's clinical context, e.g. diuretics, copious vomiting, prolonged diarrhoea.
- Patients usually conceal their abuse of diuretics or laxatives and self-induced vomiting (Bulimia and Anorexia Nervosa).
- Potassium levels of less than 2.5 mmol/L require urgent treatment. In patients on diuretics, aim to maintain the potassium above 3.5 mmol/L.

Investigation of Choice

Check the plasma levels of potassium

Rule out the cause of low potassium by clinical history, do a possible diuretic screen.

Immediate Management

- If levels more than 2.5 mmol/L - Give oral potassium
- If less than 2.5 mmol/L then cautiously administer potassium IV.
- Note that potassium should not be administered at more than 20 mmol/h, and not more than 40 mmol/L. Potassium should not be given if the patient is oliguric.
- Treatment of hypokalaemic periodic paralysis is with carbonic anhydrase inhibitor and potassium supplements.

Treatment of Choice

- Treat the cause.
- Replace thiazide/loop diuretics with with potassium-sparing one, e.g. sprionolactone, amiloride trimterene.

Note: Combination diuretics and potassium contain insufficient potassium to prevent significant hypokalaemia and there exists no rational indication for prescibing such drugs.

Your notes:

PAPER 2

Serial No. 2

Questions: A 35-year-old woman treated one year ago for a breast cancer with 12/20 nodes positive, presents with a two day history of increasing confusion. She is drowsy and disoriented. Her husband reports that she has been complaining of severe thirst for the past week.

Diagnosis: Hypercalcaemia.

Clinchers

- *35-year-old woman treated one year ago for a breast cancer with 12/20 nodes positive:* This status suggest a high risk of recurrence as nodal status is the best indicator of metastatic disease.
- *Two day history of increasing confusion ...... severe thirst:* Signs and symptoms of hypercalcaemia of malignancy are:
  - Lethargy
  - Anorexia
  - Nausea
  - Polydipsia
  - Polyuria
  - Constipation
  - Dehydration
  - Confusion
  - Weakness.

CONFUSA

The signs and symptoms of hypercalcaemia of malignancy are most obvious with serum calcium > 3 mmol/L. Diuretics should always be avoided in it. It is caused by:

- Lytic bone metastases
- Production of osteoclast activating factor by tumour
- PTH like hormones by tumour.

Investigation of Choice

Serum calcium.

Immediate Management

Bisphosphonate IV (if resistant: calcitonin).

Treatment of Choice

Control of underlying malignancy.

Your notes:

Serial No.158

Subject: Medicine

Topic: Electrolyte Imbalance

Question: A patient has diarrhoea, appears to be dehydrated with low serum potassium levels.

Diagnosis: Dehydration with hypokalaemia

Clinchers

- *Has diarrhaea:* Passage of more than 300 g of stool per day or a change in frequency of defaecation or loosening of the consistency is defined as diarrhaea.
- *Dehydrated:* Gastrointestinal secretions are a heavy reservoir of fluid and rich in electrolytes. Loss of this in the form of diarrhoea or vomiting lead to rapid loss of third space fluid causing dehydration and severe electrolyte imbalance.
- *With low serum potassium levels:* Most cases of hypokalaemia are the result of either diuretic consumption or loss of GI fluids either through persistent vomiting, chronic diarrhoea or laxative abuse. In diarrhoea, loss of bicarbonate may cause metabolic acidosis which causes a shift of potassium into the cells so that serum concentration may not reflect total potassium levels.

CONFUSA

Fluids of Choice:

- Fluid of choice in hypovolaemic shock: normal saline, Ringer lactate.
- Fluid of choice in shock due to blood loss: whole blood transfusion.
- Fluid of choice in a dehydrated individual: 5% glucose.
- Fluid of choice in a patient with dehydration due to hypertrophic pyloric stenosis/repeated vomiting/ diarrhoea: normal saline/with or without supplemental potassium depending on the patient requirement.
- Fluid of choice in hypoglycaemia: 10-25% glucose.

Investigation of Choice

Urea and electrolytes, blood glucose

Extensive investigations to look into the cause for diarrhoea if persists more than 14 days.

(Most diarrhoea are self-limiting and caused by viruses)

Immediate Management

Maintain proper hydration and electrolyte balance.

ORS is most appropriate, providing with all the major

electrolytes in right proportion.

If IV fluids needed, normal saline with/without potassium supplementation may be considered.

Treatment of Choice

According to the cause identified.

Your notes:

Serial No. 159

Subject: Medicine

Topic: Electrolyte Imbalance

Question: A patient on vigorous diuretic therapy develops hypokalaemia.

Diagnosis: Diuretic induced hypokalaemia

Clinchers

- *On vigorous diuretic therapy:* Most cases of hypokalaemia are iatrogenic, diuretics being the most common group of drugs involved.
- *Develops hypokalaemia:* Aggressive use of diuretics especially, the thiazide or loop diuretics, is associated with hypokalaemia. It is not seen with potassium sparing diuretics. Hypokalaemia is defined as serum concentration of potassium <3.5 mmol/L.
  - Mild hypokalaemia - K^+ 3.0-3.5 mmol/L
  - Severe hypokalemia <3.0 mmol/L
  - Very severe hypokalaemia <2.5 mmol/L

CONFUSA

- Suspect hypokalaemia from the patient's clinical context, e.g. diuretics, copious vomiting, prolonged diarrhoea.
- Patients usually conceal their abuse of diuretics or laxatives and self-induced vomiting (Bulimia and Anorexia Nervosa).
- Potassium levels of less than 2.5 mmol/L require urgent treatment. In patients on diuretics, aim to maintain the potassium above 3.5 mmol/L.

Investigation of Choice

- Check the plasma levels of potassium
- Rule out the cause of low potassium by clinical history, do a possible diuretic screen.

Immediate Management

- If levels more than 2.5 mmol/L - Give oral potassium
- If less than 2.5 mmol/L then cautiously administer potassium IV.
- Note that potassium should not be administered at more than 20 mmol/h, and not more than 40 mmol/L. Potassium should not be given if the patient is oliguric.
- Treatment of hypokalaemic periodic paralysis is with carbonic anhydrase inhibitor and potassium supplements.

Treatment of Choice

- Treat the cause.
- Replace thiazide/loop diuretics with potassium-sparing one, e.g. sprionolactone, amiloride triamterene.

Note: Combination diuretics and potassium contain insufficient potassium to prevent significant hypokalaemia and there exists no rational indication for prescribing such drugs.

Your notes:

Serial No. 160

Subject: Surgery

Topic: Crush Injuries

Question: A person develops anuria and pulmonary oedema after severe crushing injuries. His blood urea level at 60 mmol/L and serum potassium 7.5 mmol/L.

Diagnosis: Rhabdomyolysis (Crush syndrome or Bywater's syndrome)

Clinchers

- *Severe crushing injuries:*Rhabdomyolysis is breakdown of muscle fibres and leakage of toxic contents from injured myocytes into the systemic circulation. It most commonly follows severe crush injuries, but may also be an important side effect of statins. It may also occur in infants with inherited enzyme deficiencies of carbohydrate or lipid metabolism.
- *Develops anuria:* Liberated myocyte contents are severely toxic (especially cytochrome c) which kidney tubules or cause renal artery spasm, precipitating acute renal failure.
- *Blood urea level at 60 mmol/L:* such severely raised urea signify severe renal injury demanding emergency treatment.
- *Serum potassium 7.5 mmol/L:* This level of hyperkalaemia is a medical emergency capable of producing life threatening arrhythmias. It occurs due to relase of intracellular potassium into the systemic circulation.

CONFUSA

- In case of proceeding for amputation of the involved limb in the crush injury, remember that any amputation must be carried out above the site of compression and before the crushing force is removed.
- In case, the compression force has already be removed then the limb must be cooled and the patient first treated for renal failure and shock.
- A limb which has had a tourniquet on for more than 6 hours also needs to be amputated.

Investigation of Choice

Serum creatinine kinase is the most useful investigation.
Monitor serum potassium levels closely.
Blood urea and electrolytes to monitor renal functions.

Immediate Management

Immediate renal dialysis

Indications for haemodialysis:

- Hyperkalaemia >7.0 mmol/L
- Severe acid-base disturbances
- Refractory pulmonary oedema
- Progressive renal failure

Get Venous Access

Start saline infusion of 1000-1500 ml/h.

When a urine flow has been established, a forced mannitol-alkaline diuresis up to 8 L/day should be maintained (urine pH greater than 6.5).

Once the patient reaches hospital, 5% dextrose should be alternated with normal saline to reduce the potential sodium load.

Treatment of Choice

Fasciotomy in case of compartment syndrome. It may be necessary to amputate the crushed limbs.

Your notes:

PAPER 3

20. A 55-year-old woman treated for breast cancer with chemotherapy and radiotherapy presented with a history of confusion, tiredness, weakness and polyuria. On examination no neurological deficits were found.

Diagnosis: Hypercalcaemia.

Clinchers

- *55-year-old woman:* The age is conducive with the incidence of breast malignancies.
- *Chemotherapy and radiotherapy treatment:* It means that the tumour is inoperable with metastatic spread out palliative treatment is being given. Breast cancer commonly metastasise to bone (lytic metastases), brain and liver.
- *Confusion, tiredness, weakness and polyuria:* These are a characteristic group of symptoms in hypercalcaemia. Other features can be anorexia, polydipsia, nausea, constipation, dehydration, etc. These signs and symptoms are most obvious with serum calcium more than 3 mmol/L.

CONFUSA

A brain metastases might also produce similar symptoms and signs. But since on examination no neurological deficits are found, it can be safely excluded.

Investigation of Choice

Serum calcium.

Immediate Management

Rehydrate with 3-4 litres of 0.9% saline IV over 24 hours.

Treatment of Choice

- Bisphosphonate IV (60 mg IV pamidronate)
- Best treatment is control of underlying malignancy
- In resistant hypercalcaemia consider calcitonin.

Hypercalcaemia causes dehydration by creating a secondary type of nephrogenic diabetes insipidus.

PAPER 4

21. Man with pyloric stenosis, profuse vomiting, hypokalaemia and increased bicarbonate.

Diagnosis: Metabolic alkalosis.

Clinchers

- *Pyloric stenosis:* Presents with vomiting of large amounts of food some hours after meal. Metabolic alkalosis develops as a result of net gain of (HCO_3^-) or loss of nonvotile acid (usually HCl by vomiting) from extracellular flush.
- *Profuse vomiting:* Which is a sign of pyloric stenosis will lead to loss of acid (HCl). Vomiting/pyloric stenosis is an important cause of hypokalaemia.

The combination of hypokalaemia and alkalosis in a normotensive, nonedematous patient can be due to Bartter's syndrome, magnesium deficiency, vomiting, evogenosis alkali or diuretic ingestion.

Gastrointestinal loss of H^+ results in retention of HCO_3^-. Increased H^+ loss through gastric secretions can be caused by vomiting, gastric aspiration, or gastric fistula. This loss of fluid and NaCl in vomitus, results in contraction of extracellular fluid volume (ECFV) and increased in secretion of renin and aldosterone. Volume contraction causes a reduction in GFR and an enhanced capacity of the renal tubule to reabsorb HCO_3^-. Thus during active vomiting, there is continued addition of HCO_3^- to plasma in exchange for Cl^-.

CONFUSA

Presence of hypertension and hypokalaemia in an alkalotic patient suggests either mineralocorticoid excess or a hypertensive patient receiving diuretics.

Investigation of Choice

ABG and serum electrolytes (already done in the patient).

Immediate Management

Correct contracted extracellular fluid volume (ECFV) with NaCl, along with K^+ supplements.

Your notes:

23. Man with villous adenoma, profuse diarrhoea.

Diagnosis: Hypokalaemia.

Clinchers

Diarrhoea may be associated with villous adenoma (usually with large tumours, more than 3-4 cm in diameter). Here hypokalaemia due to potassium loss is common.

Acute diarrhoea is generally infectious. Chronic diarrhoea can be inflammatory, osmotic (malabsorption) or secretory due to intestinal dysmotility.

In cases of villous adenoma, diarrhoea is secretory in nature, caused by abnormal fluid and electrolyte transport not necessarily related to ingestion of food.

Vomiting, diarrhoea, villous adenoma rectum, pyloric stenosis, diuretics, Cushing's syndrome, alkalosis, all are important causes of hypokalaemia. Normal potassium levels in serum: 3.5-5 mmol/L.

CONFUSA

Metabolic alkalosis has been described in cases of villous adenoma, but this is most likely the result of potassium depletion.

Investigation of Choice

Serum electrolytes.

Immediate Management

In mild cases (>2.5 mmol/L, no symptoms) give oral K^+ supplement. If no thiazide diuretic, hypokalaemia > 3.0 mmol/L rarely needs treating. In severe cases (< 2.5 mmol/L, dangerous symptoms) give IV potassium cautiously, not more that 20 mmol/h, and not more concentrated than 40 mmol/L. Do not give K^+ if oliguric.

Your notes:

24. Female, 24 hours after hysterectomy complains of breathlessness, increased JVP.

Diagnosis: Fluid overload.

Clinchers

- *24 hours after hysterectomy:* Intravenous fluid and blood components that may have been transfused to this female in this whole process of hysterectomy, may have lead to these signs of fluid overload (breathlessness and increased JVP).

  Blood components are excellent volume expanders and transfusion may quickly lead to volume overload.
- *Breathlessness and increased JVP:* JVP is best indicator of estimating the central venous pressure (CVP), which is no doubt raised in fluid overload. Fluid overload will lead to elevated pulmonary capillary pressure, which may be due to left ventricular dysfunction. This elevation of hydrostatic pressure in the pulmonary vascular bed leads to dyspnoea by multiple mechanisms like pulmonary oedema.

Investigation of Choice

Central line to measure CVP.

Immediate Management

Treatment is aimed by reducing extracellular fluid volume by lowering total body Na^+ stores by following mechanisms:

- Reducing dietary intake of Na^+
- Increasing its urinary excretion with the aid of diuretics.

Treatment of Choice

Monitoring the rate and volume of transfusion, along with the use of a diuretic, can minimise this problem of fluid overload.

Your notes:

25. A patient in severe renal failure has potassium level of 2.5 mmol/L.

Diagnosis: Hypokalaemia (Answer: frusemide)

Clinchers

- *Severe renal failure:* May be due to glomerulonephritis, pyelonephritis, interstitial nephritis, DM, hypertension, cystic diseases, etc. In CRF there is usually, irreversible and long-standing loss of renal function. In CRF treatment is aimed at treating reversible causes (relieve obstruction, stop nephrotoxic drugs, treat hypercalcaemia). High does of loop diuretics (furosemide) are used to treat edema.
- *Potassium level of 2.5:* Normal range of potassium is 3.5-5 mmol/L. Hypokalaemia is the most significant problem with high ceiling diuretics (frusemide) and thiazides. Usual manifestations of hypokalaemia are weakness, fatigue, muscle cramps and cardiac arrhythmias.

CONFUSA

Hypokalaemia is less common with standard doses of high ceiling diuretics (frusemide), than with thiazides, possibly because of shorter duration of action of the former which permits intermittent operation of compensatory reflection mechanism.

Investigation of Choice

- Blood: FBC, ESR, U and E, Creatinine, S calcium
- Urine: Microscopy, creatinine clearance
- Renal ultrasound.

Immediate Management

Change furosemid with potassium sparing diuretics.

Treatment of Choice

For hypokalaemia: Attempt to maintain serum K^+ at or above 3.5 mEq/L, by:

- High dietary K^+ intake
- Supplements of KCl (24-72 mEq/day) or
- Concurrent use of K^+ sparing diuretics

Your notes:

127. Patient with prostatic cancer has been treated, now complains of confusion, thirst, body aches, constipation.

Diagnosis: Hypercalcaemia

Clinchers

- *Prostate carcinoma:* It produces osteoblastic metastases to the bone.
- *Has been treated:* The patient might have been operated upon to remove the local disease. The metastases to bone would either have been missed then or have now presented as a recurrence.
- *Confusion, thirst, body aches, constipation:* These all are symptoms of hypercalcaemia. Other symptoms and signs can be:
  - Lethargy
  - Anorexia
  - Nausea
  - Polydipsia
  - Polyuria
  - Dehydration
  - Weakness.

CONFUSA

Hypercalcaemia is produced by following cancers:
- Myeloma (40% cases of hypercalcaemia in malignancy)
- Breast
- Prostate
- Bronchus
- Kidney
- Thyroid

Investigation of Choice

Serum calcium.

Immediate Management

Rehydrate (3-4 litres of 0.9% saline IV over 24 hours)

Treatment of Choice

Bisphosphonate IV
- Best treatment is control of underlying malignancy
- Resistant hypercalcaemia—calcitonin

Your notes:

147. Patient after a stroke, 5 days later, fluids still being aspirated from stomach.

Diagnosis: Paralytic ileus.

Clinchers

- *Fluid still being aspirated from stomach:* This mean that there is no functioning bowel obstruction due to reduced bowel motility. It can be differentiated clinically from mechanical obstruction as there is no pain and bowel sounds are absent (hyperdynamic bowel sounds in mechanical obstruction). This adynamic bowel leads to no drainage of secretions of stomach and hence fluid can be aspirated from stomach. This sign along with no passage of any flatus are the clinical hallmarks of paralytic ileus. Postsurgical paralytic ileus can improve in 24-48 hours but in post-stroke patients (as is this case) it can extend for longer periods.

CONFUSA

The main confusion is among choosing between enteral and parenteral feedings. The criteria is quite clear cut, i.e. for enteral feeding to be successful, a dynamic and functioning GIT is required. That means if there is a paralytic ileus or bowel obstruction, parenteral feeding is the only choice.

Investigation of Choice

Serum electrolytes (to rule out hyperkalaemia, which also causes paralytic ileus)

Immediate Management

NG aspiration of stomach contents.

Treatment of Choice

Correction of electrolyte balance IV

+

Parenteral feeding.

Your notes:

155. A 35-year-old woman treated one year ago for a breast cancer with 12/20 nodes positive, presents with a two day history of increasing confusion. She is drowsy and disoriented. Her husband reports that she has been complaining of severe thirst for the past week.

Diagnosis: Hypercalcaemia.

Clinchers

➢ *35-year-old woman treated one year ago for a breast cancer with 12/20 nodes positive:* This status suggest a high risk of recurrence as nodal status is the best indicator of metastatic disease.

➢ *Two day history of increasing confusion ...... severe thirst:* Signs and symptoms of hypercalcaemia of malignancy are:

- Lethargy
- Anorexia
- Nausea
- Polydipsia
- Polyuria
- Constipation
- Dehydration
- Confusion
- Weakness.

CONFUSA

The signs and symptoms of hypercalcaemia of malignancy are most obvious with serum calcium > 3 mmol/L. Diuretics should always be avoided in it. It is caused by:

- Lytic bone metastases
- Production of osteoclast activating factor by tumuor
- PTH like hormones by tumour.

Investigation of Choice

Serum calcium.

Immediate Management

Bisphosphonate IV (if resistant: calcitonin).

Treatment of Choice

Control of underlying malignancy.

Your notes:

156. Patient with intractable hiccups.

Diagnosis: Intractable hiccups.

Clinchers

➢ *Intractable hiccups:* Hiccups are due to involuntary diaphragmatic contraction with closure of the glottis and are extremely common. Occasionally, patients present with persistent hiccups. This can be result of:

- Diaphragmatic irritation (e.g. subphrenic abscess)
- Metabolic cause (e.g. uraemia)

In palliative care hiccups are seen more commonly after chemotherapy as a side effects (mechanism metabolic).

CONFUSA

Hiccups are also a feature of vertebrobasilar circulation emboli. But it will be accompanied by more prominent focal defects. For it remember that vomiting, hiccup and excessive yawning indicate a lower brainstem lesion in a stuporose patient.

Investigation of Choice

Serum electrolytes, urea and uric acid.

Immediate Management

Adequate hydration if chemotherapy is the cause.

Treatment of Choice

- Chlorpromazine 50 mg TDS
  +
  Diazepam 5 mg TDS
- Haloperidol if it due to metabolic causes (as in this case).

Your notes:

PAPER 5

28. A patient in severe renal failure has potassium level of 2.5 mmol/L.

Diagnosis: Hypokalemia (Answer: Frusemide)

Clinchers

- *Severe renal failure:* May be due to glomerulonephritis, pyelonephritis, interstitial nephritis, DM, hypertension, cystic diseases, etc. In CRF there is usually, irreversible and long-standing loss of renal function. In CRF treatment is aimed at treating reversible causes (relieve obstruction, stop nephrotoxic drugs, treat hypercalcaemia). High does of loop diuretics (frusemide) are used to treat edema.
- *Potassium level of 2.5:* Normal range of potassium is 3.5-5 mmol/L. Hypokalaemia is the most significant problem with high ceiling diuretics (frusemide) and thiazides. Usual manifestations of hypokalaemia are weakness, fatigue, muscle cramps and cardiac arrhythmias.

CONFUSA

Hypokalaemia is less common with standard doses of high ceiling diuretics (frusemide), than with thiazides, possibly because of shorter duration of action of the former which permits intermittent operation of compensatory reflection mechanism.

Investigation of choice

- Blood: FBC, ESR, U and E, Creatinine, Serum calcium
- Urine: Microscopy, creatinine clearance
- Renal ultrasound

Immediate management

Change frusemide with potassium sparing Diuretics

Treatment of choice

For hypokalaemia: Attempt to maintain serum K^+ at or above 3.5 mEq/L, by:

- High dietary K^+ intake
- Supplements of KCl (24-72 mEq/day) or
- Concurrent use of K^+ sparing diuretics

Your notes:

30. A fit 50-year-old man is prescribed oral Acetazolamide by an Ophthalmologist for suspected glaucoma. He presents with lethargy and shortness of breath on exertion. Sodium 140 mmol/L, Potassium 3.2 mmol/L, Bicarbonate 18 mmol/L, Chloride 115 mmol/L, Urea 6.7 mmol/L, Creatinine 114 mmol/L.

Diagnosis: Type II renal tubular acidosis (Proximal RTA)

Clinchers

- *Fit 50-year-old man:* Excludes any pre-existing pathology to be the cause of this condition.
- *Oral acetazolamide:* Acetazolamide causes increased renal bicarbonate losses. Hence it is the most probable cause in this case.
- *Lethargy and shortness of breath on exertion:* These are due to hypokalaemia and acidosis respectively.
- *Sodium 140 mmol/L:* Normal.
- *Potassium 3.5 mmol/L:* Low, as hypokalaemia is a feature.
- *Bicarbonate 18 mmol/L:* Low as acetazolamide - renal losses.
- *Urea 6.7 mmol/L:* Normal, but still on higher side (range 2.5-6.7 mmol/L).
- *Creatinine 114 mmol/L:* Normal.

CONFUSA

Renal tubular acidosis generally may be secondary to immunological drug-induced or structural damage to the tubular cells, an inherited abnormality, or an isolated (primary) abnormality. As with most disorders which are not well understood, the nomenclature is confusing.

Investigation of Choice

Urinary pH and serum electrolytes

Immediate Management

Discontinue acetazolamide if still taking

Treatment of Choice

Sodium bicarbonate (massive doses may be required to overcome the renal 'leak').

Your notes:

117. A 20-year-old teacher is restless and confused. She is pale and sweaty and tachypnoeic. Her arterial oxygen is high and her carbon dioxide is low.

Diagnosis: Alkalosis (Hyperventilation)

Clinchers

- *20-year-old teacher:* Hyperventilation syndrome due to panic attacks is very common in young females.
- *Pale:* Due to sympathetic activation that decreases blood flow to skin and peripheries.
- *Confused:* The alkalaemia associated with hypocapnia due to hyperventilation may produce neurologic symptoms (however in panic attacks usually the consciousness is preserved).
- *Tachypnoeic:* This confirms hyperventilation to be the cause of her symptoms.
- *Arterial oxygen is high and CO_2 low:* Due to hyperventilation itself.

CONFUSA

Alveolar hyperventilation decreases $PaCO_2$ and increases the $HCO_3^-/PaCO_2$ ratio, thus increasing pH. Nonbicarbonate cellular buffers respond by consuming HCO_3^-. Hypocapnia develops when a sufficiently strong ventilatory stimulus causes CO_2 output in the lungs to exceed its metabolic production by tissues. Plasma pH and (HCO_3^-) appear to vary proportionately with $PaCO_2$ over a range from 15 to 40 mmHg. Alkalosis thus produces also causes hypocalcaemia.

Investigation of Choice

ABG

Immediate Management

Reassurance + rebreathing from paper bag

Treatment of Choice

Correct alkalosis (+ hypocalcaemia if present).

Your notes:

146. A 42-year-old woman complains of excessive thirst, polyuria, polydipsia and constipation. She admits to losing weight. Her fasting blood glucose is 5.4 mmol/L.

Diagnosis: Hypercalcaemia

Clinchers

- *Excessive thirst, polyuria, polydipsia and constipation:* All these along with abdominal pain, vomiting, depressions, anorexia, weight loss, tiredness, weakness, BP -, confusion, pyrexia, renal stones, corneal calcification and cardiac arrest are the symptoms of hypercalcaemia.
- *Admits to losing weight:* Already disccused above, weight loss is also seen in hypercalcaemia.
- *Fasting glucose of 5.4 mmol/L:* This is normal. Normal range of fasting glucose ranges between 3.5 and 5.5 mmol/L. Fasting glucose of $\geq$ 7 mmol/L, is diagnostic of diabetes mellitus. A glucose of 6-7 mmol/L implies impaired fasting glucose.

CONFUSA

Since fasting blood glucose level of this patient is 5.4 mmol/L, (i.e. well within normal limits) these signs and symptoms should not be confused with diabetes mellitus.

Investigation of Choice

- Blood tests: U and E, Mg^{2+}, Ca^{2+}, PO_4^{3-}
- ECG: Q-T interval

Immediate Management

Monitor U and E

Aim to Reduce Serum Calcium as Follows:

- Rehydrate with 0.9% salive (IVI) as needed
- Correct hypokalaemia/hypomagnesaemia, as this will reduce symptoms and renal Ca^{2+} loss.

Treatment of Choice

Once rehydrated

- Give diuretics (Frusemide) avoid thiazide
- Bisphosphate: acts over 2-3 day. Maximum effect is at 1 week. It lowers serum Ca^{2+}.

Your notes:

147. A 23-year-old man being treated for myeloma is brought to the A and E Department, confused. This followed an hour history of severe abdominal pain, vomiting. Prior to this, the patient had complained of polyuria, polydipsia and constipation.

Diagnosis: Hypercalcaemia

Clinchers

- *Being treated for myeloma:* Most common cause of hypercalcaemia is malignancy (myeloma, bone metastases, PTH - P-) and 1° hyperparathyroidism.
- *Brought to A and E department, confused:* Confusion, pyreixa, depression are the important presenting symptoms of hypercalcaemia.
- *History of severe abdominal pain, vomiting:* These along with constipation, polyuria, polydipsia, weight loss, are important signs and symptoms of hypercalcaemia.

CONFUSA

Malignancy and 1° hyperparathyroidism are the most common cause of hypercalcaemia. Always rule out DM.

Investigation of Choice

- Serum calcium (normal — 2.12-2.65 mmol/L)
- Blood sugar
- ECG.

Immediate Management

- Monitor U and E
- Aim to reduce serum (Ca^{2+} as follow
  - Rehydrate with 0.9% saline (IVI) as needed
  - Correct hypokalaemia/hypomagnesaemia as this will reduce symptoms and serum Ca^{2+} loss.

Treatment of Choice

Once rehydrated:

- Give diuretics (frusemide) avoid thiazides
- Bisphonoate: acts over 2-3 days. Maximum effect is at 1 week. It lowers serum Ca^{2+}.

Your notes:

158. A 36-year-old woman with leukaemia has been treated with amphotericin B for a fungal pneumonia. She presents with muscle weakness. Sodium 137 mmol/L, potassium 2.7 mmol/L , bicarbonate 19 mmol/L, Chloride 110 mmol/L , creatinine 84 mmol/L, urine pH 6.8 mmol/L

Diagnosis: Type I renal tubular acidosis (Distal RTA).

Clinchers

- *36-year-old woman with leukaemia:* Adult onset leukaemia usually affect patients in 30's and 40's. Distal RTA may occur in association with a systemic illness such as Sjögren's syndrome, multiple myeloma or rarely leukaemias.
- *Treated with amphotericin B for a fungal pneumonia:* Amphotericin B poisoning can cause distal RTA due to an ability to maintain a pH gradient across the collecting duct.
- *Muscle weakness:* It is due to hypokalaemia
- *Sodium 137 mmol/L:* Normal
- *Potassium 2-7 mmol/L:* Low, and is characteristic
- *HCO_3^- 19 mmol/L:* Low as alkali is lost from kidneys.
- *Chloride 110 mmol/L:* high, RTA is hyperchloraemic acidosis.
- *Creatinine 84 mmol/L:* Normal
- *Urine pH 6.8 mmol/L:* Inappropriately high. Such patients are unable to acidify urine below pH = 5.5.

CONFUSA

These abnormalities suggest that one or both of the active proton pumps present in the collecting duct (the H^+-ATPase or the H^+, K^+-ATPase is defective. In addition, excretory rates of NH_4^+ are uniformly low when the degree of systemic acidosis is taken into account, indicating that the kidney is responsible for the metabolic acidosis. Ammonium excretion is low because of failure to trap NH_4^+ in the medullary collecting duct, as a result of higher than normal tubular fluid pH in this segment and the urine pH is high because of impaired H^+ secretion

Investigation of Choice

Urinary pH + serum electrolytes.

Immediate Management

Discontinue amphotericin is still taking.

Treatment of Choice

Oral alkali (Shohl's solution).

Note: Potassium supplements are not required in distal RTA as correction of acidosis resolves hypokalaemia.

160. A fit 50-year-old man is prescribed oral acetazolamide by an ophthalmologist for suspected glaucoma. He presents with lethargy and shortness of breath on exertion. Sodium 140 mmol/L, potassium 3.2 mmol/L, bicarbonate 18 mmol/L, chloride 115 mmol/L, urea 6.7 mmol/L, creatinine 114 mmol/L.

Diagnosis: Type II renal tubular acidosis (Proximal RTA).

Clinchers

- *Fit 50-year-old man:* Excludes any pre-existing pathology to be the cause of this condition.
- *Oral acetazolamide:* Acetazolamide causes increased renal bicarbonate losses. Hence it is the most probable cause in this case.
- *Lethargy and shortness of breath on exertion:* These are due to hypokalaemia and acidosis respectively.
- *Sodium 140 mmol/L:* Normal.
- *Potassium 3.5 mmol/L:* Low, as hypokalaemia is a feature.
- *Bicarbonate 18 mmol/L:* Low as acetazolamide - renal losses.
- *Urea 6.7 mmol/L:* Normal, but still on higher side (range 2.5-6.7 mmol/L).
- *Creatinine 114 mmol/L:* Normal.

CONFUSA

Renal tubular acidosis generally may be secondary to immunological drug-induced or structural damage to the tubular cells, an inherited abnormality, or an isolated (primary) abnormality. As with most disorders which are not well-understood, the nomenclature is confusing.

Investigation of Choice

Urinary pH and serum electrolytes.

Immediate Management

Discontinue acetazolamide if still taking.

Treatment of Choice

Sodium bicarbonate (massive doses may be required to overcome the renal 'leak').

Your notes:

PAPER 6

63. A 36-year-old woman with leukaemia has been treated with amphotericin B for a fungal pneumonia. She presents with muscle weakness. Sodium 137 mmol/L, potassium 2.7 mmol/L , bicarbonate 19 mmol/L, Chloride 110 mmol/L , creatinine 84 mmol/L, urine pH 6.8 mmol/L.

Diagnosis: Type I renal tubular acidosis (Distal RTA).

Clinchers

- *36-year-old woman with leukaemia:* Adult onset leukaemia usually affect patients in 30's and 40's. Distal RTA may occur in association with a systemic illness such as Sjögren's syndrome, multiple myeloma or rarely leukemias.
- *Treated with amphotericin B for a fungal pneumonia:* Amphotericin B poisoning can cause distal RTA due to an ability to maintain a pH gradient across the collecting duct.
- *Muscle weakness:* It is due to hypokalemia
- *Sodium 137 mmol/L:* Normal
- *Potassium 2-7 mmol/L:* Low, and is characteristic
- *HCO_3^- 19 mmol/L:* Low as alkali is lost from kidneys.
- *Chloride 110 mmol/L:* high, RTA is hyperchloremic acidosis.
- *Creatinine 84 mmol/L:* Normal
- *Urine pH 6.8 mmol/L:* Inappropriately high. Such patients are unable to acidify urine below pH = 5.5.

CONFUSA

These abnormalities suggest that one or both of the active proton pumps present in the collecting duct (the H^+-ATPase or the H^+, K^+-ATPase is defective. In addition, excretory rates of NH_4^+ are uniformly low when the degree of systemic acidosis is taken into account, indicating that the kidney is responsible for the metabolic acidosis. Ammonium excretion is low because of failure to trap NH_4^+ in the medullary collecting duct, as a result of higher than normal tubular fluid pH in this segment and the urine pH is high because of impaired H^+ secretion

Investigation of Choice

Urinary pH + serum electrolytes.

Immediate Management

Discontinue amphotericin is still taking.

Treatment of Choice

Oral alkali (Shohl's solution).

Note: Potassium supplements are not required in distal RTA as correction of acidosis resolves hypokalaemia.

64. An 83-year-old man with small cell lung cancer presents with ankle oedema and is found to have 8 g/ day, urine proteinuria. He is started on frusemide. 10 days later his blood pressure is 115/75 mmHg lying and 85/65 mmHg standing. Serum biochemistry was; Sodium 121 mmol/L, bicarbonate 24 mmol/L, potassium 3.6 mmol/L, Creatinine 113 mmol/L, chloride 95 mmol/L, Urea 11.5 mmol/L, Glucose 5.7 mmol/L, albumin 27g, osmolality 263 mOs m/L, urine osmolality 417 mOsm/L.

Diagnosis: Dilutional hyponatraemia with nephrotic syndrome.

Clinchers

- *83-year-old woman:* Incidence of most of the malignancies increases with increasing age.
- *Small cell lung cancer:* SIADH is mostly associated with four malignancies, i.e.
  - Small cell lung carcinoma
  - Pancreas
  - Prostate
  - Lymphoma
- *Ankle oedema + 8 g/day urine proteinuria:* Daily urinary protein excretion is < 150 mg in normal persons. This massive proteinuria along with ankle oedema is characteristic of nephrotic syndrome.
- *Frusemide:* Excess diuretics administration can produce a dilutional hyponatraemia with electrolyte profile similar to SIADH.
- *10 days later:* Dilutional hyponatraemia develops after repeated administration of the offending diuretic over days.
- *Sodium 121 mmol/L:* Low, as it is dilutional hyponatraemia.
- *BP 115/75 mmHg lying and 85/65 mmHg standing:* Orthostatic hypotension is present in nephrotic syndrome usually.
- *Bicarbonate 24 mmol/L:* Normal.
- *Potassium 3.6 mmol/L:* Normal.
- *Creatinine 113 µmol/L:* Normal.
- *Chloride 95 mmol/L:* Normal.
- *Urea 11.5 mmol/L:* Increased owing to nephrotic syndrome.
- *Glucose 5.7 mmol/L:* Normal.
- *Albumin 27 g:* Low, owing to nephrotic syndrome.
- *Serum osmolality 263 mOsm/L:* Low (normal 278-305) but do not quality for SIADH which is < 260 Osmol/ L. It is low because of dilutional hyponatraemia.
- *Urine osmolality 417 mOsm/L:* It suggest concentrated urine but not > 500 mOsm/L to suggest SIADH.

CONFUSA

SIADH is an important, but overdiagnosed, caused of hyponatraemia. The diagnosis of SIADH requires, the absence of hypovolaemia oedema, or diuretics. SIADH must always be distinguished from dilutional hyponatraemia.

Investigation of Choice

Serum electrolytes.

Immediate Management

Stop diuretics or reset their dose.

Treatment of Choice

Treat the cause + fluid restriction.

Your notes:

65. A fit 50-year-old man is prescribed oral acetazolamide by an ophthalmologist for suspected glaucoma. He presents with lethargy and shortness of breath on exertion. Sodium 140 mmol/L, potassium 3.2 mmol/L, bicarbonate 18 mmol/L, chloride 115 mmol/L, urea 6.7 mmol/L, creatinine 114 mmol/L.

Diagnosis: Type II renal tubular acidosis (Proximal RTA).

Clinchers

- *Fit 50-year-old man:* Excludes any pre-existing pathology to be the cause of this condition.
- *Oral acetazolamide:* Acetazolamide causes increased renal bicarbonate losses. Hence it is the most probable cause in this case.
- *Lethargy and shortness of breath on exertion:* These are due to hypokalaemia and acidosis respectively.
- *Sodium 140 mmol/L:* Normal.
- *Potassium 3.5 mmol/L:* Low, as hypokalaemia is a feature.
- *Bicarbonate 18 mmol/L:* Low as acetazolamide - renal losses.
- *Urea 6.7 mmol/L:* Normal, but still on higher side (range 2.5-6.7 mmol/L).
- *Creatinine 114 mmol/L:* Normal.

CONFUSA

Renal tubular acidosis generally may be secondary to immunological drug-induced or structural damage to the tubular cells, an inherited abnormality, or an isolated (primary) abnormality. As with most disorders which are not well-understood, the nomenclature is confusing.

Investigation of Choice

Urinary pH and serum electrolytes.

Immediate Management

Discontinue acetazolamide if still taking.

Treatment of Choice

Sodium bicarbonate (massive doses may be required to overcome the renal 'leak').

Your notes:

66. Man with pyloric stenosis,profuse vomiting, hypokalaemia and increased bicarbonate.

Diagnosis: Metabolic alkalosis.

Clinchers

- *Pyloric stenosis:* Presents with vomiting of large amounts of food some hours after meal. Metabolic alkalosis develops as a result of net gain of (HCO_3^-) or loss of nonvotile acid (usually HCl by vomiting) from extracellular flush.
- *Profuse vomiting:* Which is a sign of pyloric stenosis will lead to loss of acid (HCl). Vomiting/pyloric stenosis is an important cause of hypokalaemia..

The combination of hypokalaemia and alkalosis in a normotensive, nonedematous patient can be due to Bartter's syndrome, magnesium deficiency, vomiting, evogenosis alkali or diuretic ingestion.

Gastrointestinal loss of H^+ results in retention of HCO_3^-. Increased H^+ loss through gastric secretions can be caused by vomiting, gastric aspiration, or gastric fistula. This loss of fluid and NaCl in vomitus, results in contraction of extracellular fluid volume (ECFV) and increased in secretion of renin and aldosterone. Volume contraction causes a reduction in GFR and an enhanced capacity of the renal tubule to reabsorb HCO_3^-. Thus during active vomiting, there is continued addition of HCO_3^- to plasma in exchange for Cl^-.

CONFUSA

Presence of hypertension and hypokalaemia in an alkalotic patient suggests either mineralocorticoid excess or a hypertensive patient receiving diuretics.

Investigation of Choice

ABG and serum electrolytes (already done in the patient).

Immediate Management

Correct contracted extracellular fluid volume (ECFV) with NaCl, along with K^+ supplements.

Your notes:

68. Man with villous adenoma, profuse diarrhoea.

Diagnosis: Hypokalaemia.

Clinchers

Diarrhoea may be associated with villous adenoma (usually with large tumours, more than 3-4 cm in diameter). Here hypokalaemia due to potassium loss is common.

Acute diarrhoea is generally infectious. Chronic diarrhoea can be inflammatory, osmotic (malabsorption) or secretory due to intestinal dysmotility.

In cases of villous adenoma, diarrhoea is secretory in nature, caused by abnormal fluid and electrolyte transport not necessarily related to ingestion of food.

Vomiting, diarrhoea, villous adenoma rectum, pyloric stenosis, diuretics, Cushing's syndrome, alkalosis, all are important causes of hypokalaemia. Normal potassium levels in serum: 3.5-5 mmol/L.

CONFUSA

Metabolic alkalosis has been described in cases of villous adenoma, but this is most likely the result of potassium depletion.

Investigation of Choice

Serum electrolytes.

Immediate Management

In mild cases (>2.5 mmol/L, no symptoms) give oral K^+ supplement. If no thiazide diuretic, hypokalaemia > 3.0 mmol/L rarely needs treating. In severe cases (< 2.5 mmol/L, dangerous symptoms) give IV potassium cautiously, not more that 20 mmol/h, and not more concentrated than 40 mmol/L. Do not give K^+ if oliguric.

Your notes:

69. Female, 24 hours after hysterectomy complains of breathlessness, increased JVP.

Diagnosis: Fluid overload.

Clinchers

- *24 hours after hysterectomy:* Intravenous fluid and blood components that may have been transfused to this female in this whole process of hysterectomy, may have lead to these signs of fluid overload (breathlessness and increased JVP).

  Blood components are excellent volume expanders and transfusion may quickly lead to volume overload.
- *Breathlessness and increased JVP:* JVP is best indicator of estimating the central venous pressure (CVP), which is no doubt raised in fluid overload. Fluid overload will lead to elevated pulmonary capillary pressure, which may be due to left ventricular dysfunction. This elevation of hydrostatic pressure in the pulmonary vascular bed leads to dyspnoea by multiple mechanisms like pulmonary oedema.

Investigation of Choice

Central line to measure CVP.

Immediate Management

Treatment is aimed by reducing extracellular fluid volume by lowering total body Na^+ stores by following mechanisms:

- Reducing dietary intake of Na^+
- Increasing its urinary excretion with the aid of diuretics

Treatment of Choice

Monitoring the rate and volume of transfusion, along with the use of a diuretic, can minimise this problem of fluid overload.

Your notes:

70. A patient in severe renal failure has potassium level of 2.5 mmol/L.

Diagnosis: Hypokalaemia (Answer: frusemide)

Clinchers

- *Severe renal failure:* May be due to glomerulonephritis, pyelonephritis, interstitial nephritis, DM, hypertension, cystic diseases, etc. In CRF there is usually, irreversible and long-standing loss of renal function. In CRF treatment is aimed at treating reversible causes (relieve obstruction, stop nephrotoxic drugs, treat hypercalcaemia). High does of loop diuretics (furosemide) are used to treat oedema.
- *Potassium level of 2.5:* Normal range of potassium is 3.5-5 mmol/L. Hypokalaemia is the most significant problem with high ceiling diuretics (frusemide) and thiazides. Usual manifestations of hypokalaemia are weakness, fatigue, muscle cramps and cardiac arrhythmias.

CONFUSA

Hypokalaemia is less common with standard doses of high ceiling diuretics (frusemide), than with thiazides, possibly because of shorter duration of action of the former which permits intermittent operation of compensatory reflection mechanism.

Investigation of Choice

- Blood: FBC, ESR, U and E, creatinine, S calcium
- Urine: Microscopy, creatinine clearance
- Renal ultrasound.

Immediate Management

Change furosemid with potassium sparing Diuretics

Treatment of Choice

For hypokalaemia: Attempt to maintain serum K^+ at or above 3.5 mEq/L, by:

- High dietary K^+ intake
- Supplements of KCl (24-72 mEq/day) or
- Concurrent use of K^+ sparing diuretics

Your notes:

189. Boy has been brought to the A and E following a traffic accident. He has suffered from moderate blood loss. What is the most optimum method of fluid resuscitation.

Diagnosis: Moderate blood loss

Clinchers

- *Boy*: Blood loss in children do not alter the vitals until and unless it is severe.
- *Moderate blood loss*: Even if the vitals are looking stable, the blood loss should be replaced immediately. However tachycardia is a common finding in such cases.

CONFUSA

The assessment of hypovolaemia in the trauma patient is notoriously difficult for the following reasons:

- The interaction of autonomic reflexes, head injury, pain, drugs and blood loss is complex and still not fully elucidated.
- Rapid blood loss may produce a reflex bradycardia.
- Haematocrit is an unreliable index of shock; a nearly normal value does not rule out significant blood loss.

So all abnormalities of colour, pulse, BP and consciousness should be regarded with suspicion in such cases.

Investigation of Choice

Urine output

Immediate Management

Control external blood loss

Treatment of Choice

Commence rapid fluid replacement with a bolus of 20 ml/kg. After reassessment of the patient this can be repeated. In small children, if venous access is not achieved within a few minutes, the intra-osseous route is most suitable (femoral venous access is an alternative). Cross-matched blood (whether by urgent or full cross match) is seldom available within 1 hour (even in UK) and is therefore not normally appropriate for unstable hypovolaemic patients (So use plasma expanders like Haemaccel).

Your notes:

190. A 2-year-old child with history of diarrhoea for 18 hours present to A and E. He is drowsy with cold extremities.

Diagnosis: Severe dehydration

Clinchers

- *2-year-old child:* Dehydration in a child is a potentially fatal condition and is a medical emergency.
- *Diarrhoea:* It is the main cause of dehydration in children. It can be due to infections or nutritional causes. Rotavirus is the most common infection causing diarrhoea in children.
- *For 18 hours:* It indicates a prolonged diarrhoea and hence is producing the serious state of dehydration, the child is currently in.
- *Drowsy with cold extremities:* A severely dehydrated patient appears drowsy, is apathetic and becomes moribund. As he goes into peripheral circulatory failure, extremities appear cold, though the body may be warm.

CONFUSA

If a child develops severe dehydration, it is prudent to start and IV drip of Ringer's lactate solution, given at a rate of 30 ml/kg of body weight in the first hour. The rate of drip is slowed to 20 ml/kg per hour in the next 2 hours. If the child does not pass urine within three hours of starting IV infusion, acute renal failure must be suspected.

Investigation of Choice
Urinary output

Immediate Management
Refer to ICU under paediatric supervision

Treatment of Choice
Ringer lactate infusion

Your notes:

2 Anaesthesia

PAPER 1

Serial No. 70

Subject: Anaesthesia

Topic: Eye surgery

Question: A patient with history of COPD, presently complaining of cough is posted for intracapsular cataract extraction (ICCE) and intraocular lens (IOL) implantation.

Diagnosis: ICCE with IOL implantation

Clinchers

- *History of COPD:* The main problems with COPD and general anaesthesia, are airflow obstruction (usually irreversible), mucus hypersecretion and repeated infections. The ASA grade correlates with the risk of postoperative pulmonary problems. Hence, regional anaesthesia is the usual preferred technique employed in COPD patients, wherever possible.
- *Complaining of cough:* This indicates infection, he should be treated before undergoing elective surgery as there is an increased risk of postoperative pulmonary complications.This puts him at the risk of vitreous leak during surgery, if performed under local infiltration, due to his cough which can cause sudden drastic rise in intraocular pressure.
- *Posted for ICCE and IOL implantation:* General anaesthesia would have been ideal but for his respiratory problems, we need to opt for something else which does not interfere with his respiratory functions and decreases intraocular pressure as well. Ketamine could have been a good choice considering its bronchidilatory effect, but disadvantage being the raised intraocular tension which is undesirable here. Hence, the most suitable option for this patient would be IV inducing agents which can cause supression of his cough reflexes, doesn't hamper his COPD status and help get a lowered intraocular pressure, as well.

CONFUSA

- Local anaesthesia is always the preferred technique for ophthalmic surgery. However, general anaesthesia may be indicated in certain cases of un cooperative patients, allergy to local anaesthetics or a case like above.
- Total intravenous anaesthesia (TIVA) fulfils many of the requirements for the ideal anaesthetic technique for ophthalmic surgery. Blood pressure, heart rate and intraocular pressure are lowered. It is rapidly titratable and recovery is fast. Postoperative nausea is reduced and TIVA works well in renal and hepatic disease. Remifentanil infusion allows nitrous oxide to be avoided and top up doses of muscle relaxants to be minimised during drug ventilation.

Investigation of Choice

Pre-op investigations.
Pulmonary function tests.

Immediate Management

Start antibiotics to treat his respiratory tract infections

Treatment of Choice

ICCE with IOL under TIVA is the procedure of choice.

Your notes:

Serial No.71

Subject: Opthalmology

Topic: Cornea

Question: Removal of corneal foreign body.

Diagnosis: Corneal foreign body (FB)

Clinchers

- *Removal of corneal foreign body:* The eye is instilled with a drop of local anaesthetic and the foreign body removed.
  - Various methods have been employed to remove a foreign body, e.g. using a triangle of clean card, or a moistened cotton bud.
  - If these methods do not work then a needle tip (or a special rotary drill) can be used; however great care must be taken when using these as the eye can easily be damaged.
  - A painful eye with vertically linear corneal abrasions may indicate a subtarsal foreign body. The upper eye should be everted and the body removed. Antibiotic ointment is instilled but a pad is unnecessary.

CONFUSA

- After trauma, especially with a foreign body, the eye should be evaluated for a ruptured globe and an intraocular foreign body.
- When a corneal foreign body encroaches on the visual axis, tell the patient about potential loss of visual acuity due to unavoidable scarring. This should be documented for medico-legal purposes.

Investigation of Choice

- Most superficial foreign bodies require no special investigations.
- If a penetrating foreign body is suspected it may be apparent on X-ray but that depends upon its composition. CT is sometimes used but avoid MRI, if there is any chance that the body may be metallic. Ultrasound can be used.
- Evert the upper eyelid and look for subtarsal foreign body.

Immediate Management

Remove the foreign body carefully.

Intraocular foreign bodies must be removed in the operating theatre using a microscope. These injuries are often vision threatening and should be treated quickly.

Treatment of Choice

Antibiotic ointment, e.g. chloramphenicol, and a cyclopegic drop e.g. cyclopentolate are applied after removing foreign body. The eye is covered with a pad until the epithelium has healed.

Your notes:

Serial No. 72

Subject: Obstetrics

Topic: Anaesthesia

Question: A pregnant lady posted for elective caesarean section.

Diagnosis: Elective caesarean section

Clinchers

- *Posted for elective caesarian section:* Regional anaesthesia is the preferred technique for caesarean section in a healthy parturient. General anaethesia is associated with high mortality because of high risk of aspiration, difficult intubation in pregnant ladies, increased incidence of postpartal haemorrhage. Regional anaesthesia also has the advantage of allowing the mother to participate actively in the procedure.
- Indications for general anaesthesia:
  1. Contraindications to regional anaesthesia including massive haemorrhage and haemodynamic instability.
  2. Significant coagulopathy and recent intake of low molecular weight heparin.
  3. Severe foetal "distress" in the absence of a pre-existing epidural or spinal catheter.
  4. Failure of regional technique intraoperatively.
  5. Cardiac diseases that would not tolerate acute sympathectomy.
  6. Patient refusal.

CONFUSA

- Single-shot spinal (SSS), combined spinal-epidural (CSE), and epidural may be used as regional anaesthesia.
- SSS is simple and quick to perform.
- CSE is associated with the lowest rate of conversion to general anaesthesia and greater haemodynamic stability than SSS.
- Epidural anaesthesia has the highest failure rate, but if an epidural has been placed for labour, it is always better to use this rather than resorting to intrathecal anaesthesia.

Investigation of Choice

Rule out contraindications for regional anaesthesia, viz major coagulopathy, spinal deformities and the like. Montior foetal well being

Immediate Management: None

Treatment of Choice

Combined spinal-epidural is the procedure of choice.

Serial No. 73

Subject: Ophthalmology

Topic: Anaesthesia

Question: Anaesthesia required during excision of meibomian cyst eye.

Diagnosis: Meibomian cyst (also known as chalazion/ tarsal cyst)

Clinchers

- *Meibomian cyst:* This is a retention cyst of the Meibomian gland. It may become infected or may develop into a sterile chronic granuloma in which case it is called a meibomian cyst or chalazion.
- It usually presents as a firm, painless lump in the lid which gradually enlarges. Initially, it may resemble a stye but lacks acute inflammatory signs.
- The majority point towards the conjunctival surface which may be slightly reddened or elevated. Occasionally, it may result in astigmatism due to direct pressure on the eyeball.

CONFUSA

- Internal stye is an acute inflammation of the meibomian glands; the infection is in the tarsal plate and the skin is not primarily involved. Usually, it is due to *Staphylococcus aureus*.
- While the internal stye is painful, meibomian cyst or chalazion presents as a painless lump.
- External stye is essentially a staphylococcal infection of a lash follicle possibly involving the glands of Zeis' or the glands of Moll. It corresponds to a boil of the skin elsewhere. Initially, the whole of the lid may be affected; soon, the swelling becomes localised, and a yellow, pus filled lesion may be seen near the lid margin associated with an eyelid.

Investigation of Choice

None; its usually easily recognised as a buish swelling on the undersurface of the lid.

Immediate Management

Hot compresses help to ease irritation.

An antibiotic ointment may be needed if it becomes infected.

Treatment of Choice

Treated by surgical incision under local anaesthesia into the tarsal gland followed by curettage of the glandular material and glandular epithelium.

3 Cardiovascular Medicine

PAPER 1

Serial No. 42

Subject: Medicine

Topic: Cardiovascular medicine

Question: A 65-year-old previously healthy man with sudden loss of consciousness followed by generalised tonic clonic convulsions. He appears flushed and pulse rate is 40 bpm.

Diagnosis: Stokes Adams attack

Clinchers

- *65-year-old:* The incidence of AV block increases with age. The incidence of third-degree AV block is highest in people older than 70 years.
- *Previously healthy:* This rules out possibility of any seizure disorder in the patient.
- *Sudden loss of consciousness:* The attack usually presents with sudden loss of consciousness without any apparent warning except for palpitations with slow or absent pulse. Patient may appear pale just before the attack.
- *Followed by generalised tonic clonic convulsions:* Cerebral anoxia caused due to sudden cardiac arrest can cause muscle twitching which can even progress to generalised convulsions.
- *Appears flushed:* On recovery the patient becomes flushed; this is due to well-oxygenated blood which has been in the pulmonary capillaries during the period of circulatory arrest being flung into systemic capillaries which are widely dilated as a result of the accumulation of vasodilator metabolites.
- *Pulse rate 40 bpm:* The bradycardia confirms that original pathology behind all the symptoms above was cardiac in origin.

CONFUSA

- Sudden loss of consciousness in an elderly can also be due to vasovagal syncope or orthostatic hypotension. However, in both these cases posture is an important factor.
- While Stokes Adams attack can occur in any posture (even during sleep), vasovagal or orthostatic hypotension usually follow sudden standing or prolonged standing. Also,it may be reproduced by a prolonged head-up tilt test.

Investigation of Choice

Routine ECG recording and cardiac monitoring with careful evaluation of the relationship between P waves and QRS complexes are the standard tests leading to proper diagnosis of AV blocks.

Immediate Management

IV Atropine; External pacemaker

Treatment of Choice

Permanent pacemaker

Your notes:

Serial No. 112

Subject: Medicine

Topic: Cardiology

Question:
Temp 37°C
JVP normal
CXR normal
BP 120/80 PR 110 bpm
ECG Q waves in V1, 2, 3

Diagnosis: Myocardial infarction (Anteroseptal)

Clinchers

- *Temp 37°C:* Normal temperature rules out infectious aetiologies. Low grade fever may be present in the cases of MI due to release of cytokines in the circulation.
- *JVP normal:* JVP is usually normal in isolated cases of myocardial infarction, however, its usually raised in cases of posterior wall infarction which is usually associated with right ventricular infarction and dysfunction.
- *CXR normal:* Chest X ray is usually normal in early cases of infarction, however, it is usually taken to assess the patient's heart size and the presence or absence of decompensated CHF with or without pulmonary oedema. A CXR may also assist in ruling out concomitant disease, such as pneumonia or aortic dissection.
- *BP 120/80 PR 110 bpm:* The tachycardia is usually due to agitation caused by intense chest pain. Both hypertension and hypotension can be present in MI depending on the extent of infarct and presence of cardiac failure.
- *ECG Q waves in V1, 2, 3:* Definitive diagnosis of myocardial infarction requires the presence of Q waves in the ECG. It takes hours to weeks to develop. Pathological Q waves are defined as duration beyond 40 msec or >¼ of R-wave amplitude. Over the next few hours after infarction, the ST segments return to normal and shortly after, the T waves become inverted but Q waves remain. If occlusion of the coronary artery is incomplete infarction can occur without Q waves.

CONFUSA

- The ECG changes of myocardial infarction vary according to the site of the infarction and whether it is partial or full thickness.
- Changes in Leads I and aVR signify anterior wall involvement.
- Typical changes in leads II, III, and aVF suggest inferior wall infarction.
- The V leads will show if it is anterior-septal with early V leads(V1,2,3) affected or anterior-lateral with late V(V4,5,6) leads involved.
- If there is ST depression in V1 and 2 but no other signs always check changes in V7,8,9 to rule out a posterior infarct.

Investigation of Choice

Diagnosis of a myocardial infarction is made on the basis of positive findings in two or more of:

- History
- ECG changes
- Cardiac enzyme changes

In practice the ECG is usually the diagnostic test in a patient with a suggestive history. Determination of cardiac enzymes may be used to make a retrospective diagnosis of MI.

Immediate Management

High-flow oxygen should be given
300 mg aspirin should be chewed.
Obtain Intravenous access and administer 5-10 mg diamorphine IV, 10 mg metoclopramide IV
Immediately transfer to coronary care unit.

Treatment of Choice

Aim is reperfusion. Following methods can be used:

- Pharmacological thrombolysis: Most commonly used and best validated method
- Primary coronary angioplasty: Controversial

Your notes:

Serial No. 127

Subject: Medicine

Topic: Arrhythmias

Question: A man after falling unconscious on a number of occasions was found to have a heart rate of 40 bpm.

Diagnosis: Complete Heart Block

Clinchers

- *Falling unconscious on a number of occasions:* These syncopal attacks are typical and known as Stokes Adam's attacks. The patient classically gives history of repeated syncopal attacks without any apparent reason and unrelated to any sort of posture or activity. A minority of patients with heart block may also present with life threatenting arrhythmias like VT/VF or even sudden cardiac death.
- *Heart rate of 40 bpm:* When the block is at the level of the AV node, the escape rhythm generally arises from a junctional pacemaker with a rate of 45-60 beats per minute. Such patients frequently are haemodynamically stable, and their heart rates increase in response to exercise and atropine. When the block is below the AV node, the escape rhythm arises from the His bundle or the bundle branch-Purkinje system at rates less than 45 beats per minute. These patients generally are haemodynamically unstable, and their heart rates are unresponsive to exercise and atropine.

CONFUSA

- A vasovagal syncope can also present with history of repeated falls and bradycardia(because of increased vagal tone). However, there is always a triggering factor in such cases (which is absent in complete heart block).
- The factors which can trigger vasovagal syncope can be emotion, fear and pain, heavy meals and alcohol, micturition, defaecation and coughing, prolonged upright posture, a warm environment and dehydration.
- A Tilt table test is used to differentiate between the two. A positive tilt table test (i.e. patient becoming symptomatic during the tilt and developing bradycardia or hypotension) signifies vasovagal syncope.

Investigation of Choice

- 12 lead ECG.
- 24 hour tape may be necessary if diagnosis in doubt.

Immediate Management

Give atropine to reduce vagal effect
Temporary pacing required for profound bradycardia and haemodynamic instability

Treatment of Choice

Implantation pacemakers indicated in 3rd degree heart block (even if asymptomatic).

Your notes:

Serial No. 128

Subject: Medicine

Topic: Arrhythmias

Question: A 25-year-old female with sweaty palms, tremors and weight loss. Heart rate is 140 bpm/ irregular.

Diagnosis: Atrial fibrillation (secondary to hyperthyroidism)

Clinchers

- *A 25-year-old female:*All thyroid diseases are more common in women, with Grave's Disease being 10 times more common in females than males.
- *Sweaty palms, tremors and weight loss:* Hyperactivity, irritability, altered mood, intolerance to heat, sweating, palpitations, fatigue, weakness, losing weight even with increased appetite, diarrhoea, steatorrhoea, polyuria, oligo/amenorrhoea, loss of libido are the most commonly encountered symptoms in hyperthyroidism.
- *Heart rate is 140 bpm/irregular:*This is signifying sinus tachycardia and atrial fibrillation, again commonly seen with hyperthyroidism.

CONFUSA

- Phaeochromocytoma can also present as palpitations, tachycardia, sweating, anxiety, panic attacks, tremor hyperthermia and weight loss. The patient is usually hypertensive.
- The female predominance and the absence of hypertension in the history in the given question, points more towards hyperthyroidism as the most probable cause.

Investigation of Choice

TSH can exclude primary thyrotoxicosis. Confirm diagnosis with free T4 levels.

Immediate Management

Beta blockers resolve many of the acute symptoms of hyperthyroidism, e.g. tachycardia, tremor, restlessness - within 1-2 days of starting therapy. Propanolol is the most commonly used beta blocker for the purpose.

Treatment of Choice

The treatment of choice is carbimazole in the UK. Propylthiouracil is an alternative.

Your notes:

Serial No. 129

Subject: Medicine

Topic: Arrhythmias

Question: A 32-year-old female complains of rapid palpitations and syncope. Her pulse rate is 160 bpm/ regular.

Diagnosis: Supraventricular tachycardia (SVT)

Clinchers

- *32-year-old female:* Incidence of SVT is more common in females and increases with age. However, attacks may begin in childhood or adult life. Recurrence is very common.
- *Rapid palpitations and syncope:* The patient usually complains of fast palpitations, presyncope or syncope, chest pain, fatigue, diaphoresis or polyuria. This is usually triggered by exertion or anxiety.
- *Her pulse rate is 160 bpm/regular:* The rhythm is regular and the rate is between 130 and 250 beats per minute with narrow QRS complexes and inverted P waves.

CONFUSA

- An underlying cause, which could have triggered the attack should always be searched for, once the normal rhytm is established. Not all cases are due to structural abnormalities in the heart.
- A cardiac enzyme evaluation should be ordered for patients with chest pain; patients with risk factors for myocardial infarction; and patients who are otherwise unstable and present with heart failure, hypotension, or pulmonary oedema.
- Carefully rule out ventricular tachycardia.

Investigation of Choice

ECG, to confirm the diagnosis and rule out other causes of a fast heart rate.

A transthoracic echocardiogram may be helpful if structural heart disease is suggested.

Immediate Management

- If patient compromised - DC cardioversion
- Vagal manoeuvres
- Adenosine 6 mg IV bolus into a big vein; if unsuccessful give 12 mg again twice at 2 min intervals.
- if adenosine fails, verapamil 5-10 mg IV over 2 min.

Treatment of Choice

- Patient can be maintained on long-term calcium channel blockers (Verapamil).
- Frequent attacks may require radioablation of the abnormal tract.
- Infrequent attacks with very mild symptoms may not require any treatment at all.

Your notes:

Serial No. 132

Subject: Medicine

Topic: Arrhythmias

Question: A woman with family history of coronary artery disease. She has noticed palpitations especially during the night. She describes a sensation of her heartbeat momentarily stopping, and then racing.

Diagnosis: Ventricular extrasystoles

Clinchers

- *Woman:*Ventricular extrasystoles are more common in men than women, and the incidence increases with age.
- *Family history of coronary artery disease:*A positive family history of coronary artery disease makes this woman at high risk for developing coronary artery disease and its complications for herself. Chances are that she might have had a silent myocardial infarction, the present ventricular ectopics being secondary to that.
- *Palpitations especially during the night:*Ventricular extrasystoles are more common with factors which increase the vagal tone, therby palpitations more commonly observed at night while asleep and usually gets abolished on exercising.
- *A sensation of her heartbeat momentarily stopping, and then racing:*This is the typical presentation of a ventricular extrasystole.A premature beat is followed by a compensatory pause, which is felt by the patient as 'heartbeat momentarily stopping'. This is followed by runs of normal beats.

CONFUSA

- Extrasystoles are usually normal, being common in middle age. However, patients with ventricular extrasystole are at the risk of sudden death.
- Ventricular extrasystoles are the most common arrhythmias after myocardial infarction and are associated with an increased risk of mortality.
- If ventricular ectopics coincide with the preceding T wave (R on T phenomenon) more frequently than 10 times per minute can precipitate ventricular fibrillation.

Investigation of Choice

- ECG

Rule out underlying cause which could have precipitated this, viz:

- Myocardial ischaemia—measure cardiac enzymes
- Drug history—Digitalis, tricyclics, quinine
- Hyperthyroidism—Thyroid function tests
- Hyperkalaemia and hypercalcaemia—Serum electrolytes
- Heart diseases with enlargement of the atria, e.g. mitral stenosis—ECHO
- long QT syndromes—ECG

Immediate Management

- R on T phenomenon (>10 times/minute) requires IV Lignocaine
- Maintain electrolyte balance
- Treat associated congestive heart failure or myocardial ischaemia/infarction.

Treatment of Choice

- Beta blockers may provide symptomatic relief especially for those associated with an underlying MI.
- Class I antiarrhythmic: Phenytoin (4 mg/kg IV at a maximum rate of 50 mg/min, repeated after 10 min if required); promotes AVN conduction.
- Patients deemed to be at high risk of sudden cardiac death may benefit from implantable cardioverter defibrillator (ICD) implantation.

Your notes:

Serial No. 133

Subject: Medicine

Topic: Arrhythmias

Question: A man complains of episodes of palpitations which last for few minutes and leave him dizzy. His pulse appears to be normal at the point of examination.

Diagnosis: Ventricular tachycardia (VT)

Clinchers

- *Man:* VT is more common in males than females, most common underlying cause being myocardial ischaemia, which holds good male predominance. Again, because of the similar reasons incidence increases with age, regardless of sex. VT in the young is usually related to structural heart disease like dilated cardiomyopathy and the like.
- *Episodes of palpitations which last for few minutes:* VT is typically described as any rapid rhythm, faster than 100-120 beats per minute, arising in the ventricle. It is usually non-sustained and resolves by itself.
- *Leave him dizzy:* During VT, cardiac output is reduced due to the rapid heart rate and lack of a properly timed or coordinated atrial contraction.This leaves the patient dizzy or with even frank syncope because of diminished cerebral perfusion.
- *His pulse appears to be normal at the point of examination:* Most VT are non-sustained and patient may appear apparently normal at the time of examination.

CONFUSA

- A sustained VT is the one, which lasts longer than 30 seconds. It is usually associated with various serious heart conditions including:
  - Myocardial infarction.
  - Left ventricular aneurysm
  - Cardiomyopathy (hypertrophic, alcoholic)
  - Right ventricular dysplasia.
- SVT with abberant ventricular conduction can also present with similar features. It needs to be carefully differentiated from VT.

Investigation of Choice

24 hour holter monitoring is required to know the exact nature of the arrhythmia.

Immediate Management

- High flow oxygen
- Gain IV access
- Check serum potassium; if less than 4 mmol/L - give up to 60 mmol potassium chloride at maximum rate of 30 mmol per hour.

- if hypokalaemic, assume patient also to be hypomagnesaemic: give 10 mmol magnesium sulphate over 30 minutes (5 mls of 50% solution)

Treatment of Choice

In hemodynamically unstable: DC cardioversion

In hemodynamically stable: Amiodarone 150 mg in 20 mls 5% solution over 10 minutes

[Lignocaine is only used as 2nd line drug in the UK, to treat VT- given as 50 mg over 2 minutes repeated every 5 minutes up to a maximum of 200 mg, followed by lignocaine infusion at 2 - 4 mg per minute.

Your notes:

Serial No. 159

Subject: Medicine

Topic: Falls

Question: A 70-year-old lady shopping in a supermarket fainted suddenly and sustained fracture neck of femur. Her daughter who was with her said she went pale before fainting.

Diagnosis: Vasovagal syncope

Clinchers

- *70-year-old lady:* Vasovagal syncope is more common among the elderly, perhaps due to blunted sympathethic reflexes. Its most common at the age of 60-70 years with females more commonly affected than males.
- *Shopping in a supermarket:* Certain factors which predispose an individual to vasovagal syncope are prolonged upright posture, emotion, fear and pain, heavy meals and alcohol, micturition, defaecation and coughing, a warm environment and dehydration
- *Fainted suddenly:* Patient usually feels as slight prodrome of light headedness following which there is sudden loss of consciousness and if not supported, patient sustains a fall.
- *Sustained fracture neck of femur:* Osteoporosis and the subsequent weakness of bones in post menopausal age group, makes females more vulnerable for fractures even after trivial falls.
- *Went pale before fainting:*The peripheral pooling of blood, bradycardia and hypotension are the cardiological consequences of a vasovagal attack. Hence, a witness usually reports that the patient appeared pale, cold and clammy just before the attack.

CONFUSA

Stokes Adams may closely mimic a vasovagal syncope. However, the positive history of prolonged standing makes vasovagal syncope more strong a possibility.

Note that in Stokes Adams also the patient may appear pale just before the syncopal attack, however, Stokes Adams doesn't need any predisposing factor as such to precipitate syncope. It can appear anytime anywhere, even in sleep. Previous history of recurrent unexplained falls in an elderly with severe bradycardia (<40bpm) goes in favour of a Stokes Adams attack.

Investigation of Choice

Tilt a table test - Patient is made to lie flat on the tilt-table for 30 minutes, during which time baseline values of pulse-rate and blood pressure are measured.

The tilt-table test is positive if the patient becomes symptomatic during the tilt and there is bradycardia or hypotension.

A positive tilt-table test signify neurally mediated syncope (vasovagal).

A negative test should prompt further investigations into the cause of the syncope.

Immediate Management

Reassurance;
Adopt proper posture and ensure adequate fluid and salt intake.

Treatment of Choice

Avoidance of triggering situations (e.g., prolonged standing, hot tubs),
support stockings to reduce venous pooling.
Discontinuation of offending medications (eg, nitrates) that are not necessary also may be helpful.

Your notes:

PAPER 2

Serial No. 108

Subject: Medicine

Topic: CVS

Question: A 40-year-old woman presents with malaise and low-grade fever for 2 weeks. She recently had treatment for a dental abscess. On examination she has splinter haemorrhages and an early diastolic murmur.

Diagnosis: Infective Endocarditis

Clinchers

- *A 40-year-old woman:* Infective endocarditis is three times more common in the males than the females. It can affect almost anybody of any age, however, the frequency definitely higher in adults more than 40 years.
- *Malaise and low-grade fever for 2 weeks:* The symptoms of the native valve endocarditis usually starts in very subtle fashion, with very non-specific influneza like symptoms. When the treatnent is delayed for weeks-months, then the immunological and valvular phenomenon develops.
- *She recently had treatment for a dental abscess:* In most cases of native valve endocarditis, a history of dental or other invasive procedures within 2-6 weeks of appearance of the endocarditis symptoms. Most cases of dental related endocarditis are due to *Streptococcus viridans*.

CONFUSA

- Most acute cases of IE are casued by *Staphylococcus aureus*.
- Most subacute cases of IE are caused by *Streptococcus viridans*.
- Most early cases (within 60 days) of prosthetic valve endocarditis is caused by *Staph aureus*.
- Most late cases (after 60 days) of prosthetic valve endocraditis are caused by *Streptococcous viridans*.
- Right sided endocarditis is especially common in IV drug abusers.
- Right sided endocarditis invariably affects tricuspid valve.

Investigation of Choice

Blood culture will reveal the causative organism.
ECHO will demonstrate vegetations on the affected valve.

Immediate Management
Symptomatic management under expert guidance.

Treatment of Choice
Antibiotics: Empirical treatment: IV Benzylpenicillin plus IV Gentamicin If staphylococcal endocarditis is suspected, vancomycin is substituted for penicillin.

Your notes:

Serial No. 137

Subject: Medicine

Topic: Arrhythmias

Question: A woman experiences 'thumping' in her chest associated with breathlessness, while asleep. She sits up to get symptoms resolve in few minutes time.

Diagnosis: Atrial Myxoma

Clinchers

- *A woman:* Atrial myxomas predominantly occur in females, with more than 75% sporadic cases seen females. The usual age of presentation is anywhere between 3 and 86 years, however, highest incidence is observed around 40-60 years.
- *'Thumping', with breathlessness, while asleep:* The most common symptom patients present with is dyspnoea, whether exertional, nocturnal or posture specific.
- *She sits up to get symptoms resolve in few minutes time:* This appears to be most typical of atrial myxoma, as the tumour obstructing the outflow tract of heart (usually left sided) can cause increase severity of symptoms. As soon as the patient gets up to assume an erect posture, the obstruction is relieved and the symptoms resolve out.

CONFUSA

The symptoms of atrial myxoma can vary from totally symptom free to sudden death. Patient may present with unusual palpiations or features of right/left heart failure, which usually resolve by the changing postures (until and unless the tumour is too large). It can also present with features of thromboembolism, dizziness or syncope. Constitutional symptoms like fever, weight loss, arthralgias, and Raynaud phenomenon are observed in 50% of patients.

Investigation of Choice
ECHO – Transthoracic or Transoesophageal

Immediate Management
Consult expert advice

Treatment of Choice
Surgical resection

Your notes:

Serial No. 138

Subject: Medicine

Topic: Arrhythmias

Question: A woman with family history of coronary artery disease. She has noticed palpitations especially during the night. She describes a sensation of her heartbeat momentarily stopping, and then racing.

Diagnosis: Ventricular extrasystoles

Clinchers

- *Woman:* Ventricular extrasystoles are more common in men than women, and the incidence increases with age.
- *Family history of coronary artery disease:* A positive family history of coronary artery disease makes this woman at high risk for developing coronary artery disease and its complications for herself. Chances are that she might have had a silent myocardial infarction, the present ventricular ectopics being secondary to that.
- *Palpitations especially during the night:* Ventricular extrasystoles are more common with factors which increase the vagal tone, therby palpitations more commonly observed at night while asleep and usually gets abolished on exercising.
- *A sensation of her heartbeat momentarily stopping, and then racing:* This is the typical presentation of a ventricular extrasystole. A premature beat is followed by a compensatory pause, which is felt by the patient as 'heartbeat momentarily stopping'. This is followed by runs of normal beats.

CONFUSA

- Extrasystoles are usually normal, being common in middle age. However, patients with ventricular extrasystole are at the risk of sudden death.
- Ventricular extrasystoles are the most common arrhythmias after myocardial infarction and are associated with an increased risk of mortality.
- If ventricular ectopics coincide with the preceding T wave (R on T phenomenon) more frequently than 10 times per minute can precipitate ventricular fibrillation.

Investigation of Choice

ECG

Rule out underlying cause which could have precipitated this, viz:

- Myocardial ischaemia - measure cardiac enzymes
- Drug history - Digitalis, tricyclics, quinine
- Hyperthyroidism - Thyroid function tests
- Hyperkalaemia and hypercalcaemia - Serum electrolytes
- Heart diseases with enlargement of the atria, e.g. mitral stenosis - ECHO
- long QT syndromes- ECG

Immediate Management

R on T phenomenon (>10 times/minute) requires IV Lignocaine

Maintain electrolyte balance

Treat associated congestive heart failure or myocardial ischaemia/infarction.

Treatment of Choice

- Beta-blockers may provide symptomatic relief especially for those associated with an underlying MI.
- Class I anti-arrhythmic: Phenytoin (4 mg/kg IV at a maximum rate of 50 mg/min, repeated after 10 min if required); promotes AVN conduction.
- Patients deemed to be at high risk of sudden cardiac death may benefit from implantable cardioverter defibrillator (ICD) implantation.

Your notes:

Serial No. 139

Subject: Medicine

Topic: Arrhythmias

Question: A man complains of episodes of palpitations which last for few minutes and leave him dizzy. His pulse appears to be normal at the point of examination.

Diagnosis: Ventricular tachycardia (VT)

Clinchers

- *Man:* VT is more common in males than females, most common underlying cause being myocardial ischaemia, which holds good male predominance. Again, because of the similar reasons incidence increases with age, regardless of sex. VT in the young is usually related to structural heart disease like dilated cardiomyopathy and the like.
- *Episodes of palpitations which last for few minutes:* VT is typically described as any rapid rhythm, faster than 100-120 beats per minute, arising in the ventricle. It is usually non-sustained and resolves by itself.
- *Leave him dizzy:* During VT, cardiac output is reduced due to the rapid heart rate and lack of a properly timed or coordinated atrial contraction.This leaves the patient dizzy or with even frank syncope because of diminished cerebral perfusion.
- *His pulse appears to be normal at the point of examination:* Most VT are non-sustained and patient may appear apparently normal at the time of examination.

CONFUSA

- A sustained VT is the one, which lasts longer than 30 seconds. It is usually associated with various serious heart conditions including:
  - Myocardial infarction
  - Left ventricular aneurysm
  - Cardiomyopathy (hypertrophic, alcoholic)
  - Right ventricular dysplasia.
- SVT with abberant ventricular conduction can also present with similar features. It needs to be carefully differentiated from VT.

Investigation of Choice

24 hour holter monitoring is required to know the exact nature of the arrhythmia.

Immediate Management

- High flow oxygen
- Gain IV access
- Check serum potassium; if less than 4 mmol/L - give up to 60 mmol potassium chloride at maximum rate of 30 mmol per hour
- if hypokalaemic, assume patient also to be hypomagnesaemic: give 10 mmol magnesium sulphate over 30 minutes (5 ml of 50% solution)

Treatment of Choice

In hemodynamically unstable: DC cardioversion

In hemodynamically stable: Amiodarone 150 mg in 20 ml 5% solution over 10 minutes

[Lignocaine is only used as 2nd line drug in the UK, to treat VT- given as 50 mg over 2 minutes repeated every 5 minutes up to a maximum of 200 mg, followed by lignocaine infusion at 2 - 4 mg per minute.

Your notes:

Serial No. 140

Subject: Medicine

Topic: Arrhythmias

Question: A man after falling unconscious on a number of occasions was found to have a heart rate of 40 bpm.

Diagnosis: Complete heart block

Clinchers

- *Falling unconscious on a number of occasions:* These syncopal attacks are typical and known as Stokes Adam's attacks. The patient classically gives history of repeated syncopal attacks without any apparent reason and unrelated to any sort of posture or activity. A minority of patients with heart block may also present with life threatenting arrhythmias like VT/VF or even sudden cardiac death.
- *Heart rate of 40 bpm:* When the block is at the level of the AV node, the escape rhythm generally arises from a junctional pacemaker with a rate of 45-60 beats per minute. Such patients frequently are hemodynamically stable, and their heart rates increase in response to exercise and atropine. When the block is below the AV node, the escape rhythm arises from the His bundle or the bundle branch-Purkinje system at rates less than 45 beats per minute. These patients generally are hemodynamically unstable, and their heart rates are unresponsive to exercise and atropine.

CONFUSA

- A vasovagal syncope can also present with history of repeated falls and bradycardia(because of increased vagal tone). However, there is always a triggering factor in such cases (which is absent in complete heart block).
- The factors which can trigger vasovagal syncope can be emotion, fear and pain, heavy meals and alcohol, micturition, defaecation and coughing, prolonged upright posture, a warm environment and dehydration.
- A Tilt table test is used to differentiate between the two. A positive tilt table test (i.e., patient becoming symptomatic during the tilt and developing bradycardia or hypotension) signifies vasovagal syncope.

Investigation of Choice

12 lead ECG.

24 hours tape may be necessary if diagnosis in doubt.

Immediate Management

Give atropine to reduce vagal effect

Temporary pacing required for profound bradycardia and hemodynamic instability

Treatment of Choice

Implantation pacemakers indicated in 3rd degree heart block (even if asymptomatic).

Your notes:

Serial No. 162

Subject: Medicine

Topic: Cardiology

Question: A 56-year-old male presents with severe chest pain. His JVP is normal and no positive findings on the Chest X ray. He is tachycardic with pule rate of 110 bpm and his BP is 120/80 PR 110 bpm. The ECG taken shows changes in V1, 2, 3.

Diagnosis: Myocardial infarction (Anteroseptal)

Clinchers

- *56-year-old, male:* the incidence of MI is higher in males than females, however, the incidence is almost the same among the 2 sexes when postmenopausal age is taken in view.
- *JVP normal:* JVP is usually normal in isolated cases of myocardial infarction, however, its usually raised in cases of posterior wall infarction which is usually associated with right ventricular infarction and dysfunction.
- *CXR normal:* Chest X ray is usually normal in early cases of infarction, however, it is usually taken to assess the patient's heart size and the presence or absence of decompensated CHF with or without pulmonary oedema. A CXR may also assist in ruling out concomitant disease, such as pneumonia or aortic dissection.
- *BP 120/80 PR 110 bpm:* The tachycardia is usually due to agitation caused by intense chest pain. Both hypertension and hypotension can be present in MI depending on the extent of infarct and presence of cardiac failure.
- *Slide: ECG Q waves in V1, 2, 3:* Definitive diagnosis of myocardial infarction requires the presence of Q waves in the ECG. It takes hours to weeks to develop. Pathological Q waves are defined as duration beyond 40 msec or >¼ of R-wave amplitude. Over the next few hours after infarction, the ST segments return to normal and shortly after, the T waves become inverted but Q waves remain. If occlusion of the coronary artery is incomplete infarction can occur without Q waves.

CONFUSA

- The ECG changes of myocardial infarction vary according to the site of the infarction and whether it is partial or full thickness.
- Changes in Leads I and aVR signify anterior wall involvement.
- Typical changes in leads II, III, and aVF suggest inferior wall infarction.
- The V leads will show if it is anterior-septal with early V leads(V1,2,3) affected or anterior-lateral with late V(V4,5,6) leads involved.
- If there is ST depression in V1 and 2 but no other signs always check changes in V7,8,9 to rule out a posterior infarct.

Investigation of Choice

Diagnosis of a myocardial infarction is made on the basis of positive findings in two or more of:

- History
- ECG changes
- Cardiac enzyme changes

In practise the ECG is usually the diagnostic test in a patient with a suggestive history. Determination of cardiac enzymes may be used to make a retrospective diagnosis of MI.

Immediate Management

- High-flow oxygen should be given
- 300 mg aspirin should be chewed.
- Obtain Intravenous access and administer 5-10 mg diamorphine iv, 10 mg metoclopramide IV
- Immediately transfer to coronary care unit.

Treatment of Choice

Aim is reperfusion. Following methods can be used:

- Pharmacological thrombolysis: Most commonly used and best validated method
- Primary coronary angioplasty: Controversial

Your notes:

PAPER 3

36. A 17-year-old girl with hypertension of 160/100 is found to have a femoral pulse delay.

Diagnosis: Coarctation of aorta.

Clinchers

- *17-year-old girl:* Coarctation of aorta is often asymptomatic for many years. Headaches and nose bleeds (due to hypertension) and claudication and cold legs (due to poor blood flow in lower limbs) may be present. It is associated with Turner's syndrome. Primary amenorrhoea must be present if that is the case. But it must be noted that coarctation is twice as common in males as in females.
- *Hypertension of 160/100:* Hypertension is typically present in the upper limbs. Decreased renal perfusion can lead to the development of systemic hypertension that persists even after surgical correction.
- *Femoral pulse delay:* Weak and delayed (radiofemoral delay) pulses are characteristically present in the legs.

CONFUSA

Aortic stenosis or sclerosis are basically the disease of the aortic valve and not of aorta itself. However, in 80% of cases coarctation of aorta is associated with a bicuspid (an potentially stenotic) aortic valve.

Investigation of Choice

- *Screening:* Chest X-ray.
- *Findings:* Dilated aorta indented at the site of coarctation (shaped like a figure of 3). Rib notching in adults.
- *Definitive:* Aortography.

Treatment of Choice

Surgical excision of coarctation and end-to-end anastomosis of aorta:

- *Extensive coarctation:* prosthetic vascular grafts.
- *Childhood operation:* prevents renal systemic hypertension
- *Alternative:* Balloon dilatation

Your notes:

70. A 23-year-old man is brought into the accident and emergency department from the local park, with a red swollen arm. He is found to have a blood pressure of 100/60 mmHg.

Diagnosis: Anaphylactic shock secondary to bee sting.

Clinchers

Brought from local park, with a red swollen arm: This situation is pointing towards a bee sting sustained in the park. Normally bee stings do not produce swelling and redness of the whole arm until and unless a component of anaphylaxis is there. Time to onset is variable, but symptoms usually occur within seconds to minutes of exposure to the offending antigen.

Symptoms of anaphylaxis are usually:

- *Respiratory:* Mucous membrane swelling (lips, larynx), hoarseness, stridor, wheezing.
- *CVS:* Tachycardia, hypotension (in this case BP is 100/60 mmHg)
- *Cutaneous:* Pruritus, urticaria, angioedema

Since anaphylaxis is a type I IgE mediated response, this person must have had a previous exposure to the bee sting.

CONFUSA

Anaphylactoid reactions are different from anaphylaxis as they result from direct release of mediators from inflammatory cells, without involving antibodies (anaphylaxis is IgE mediated), usually in response to a drug, e.g. N-acetylcysteine.

Investigation of Choice

Check for laryngeal oedema as it can be fatal.

Immediate Management

- Secure airway + 100% O_2
- Intubate if respiratory obstruction is imminent

Treatment of Choice

Adrenaline IM (0.5 ml of 1:1000)

Note: Adrenaline is not given IV unless the patient is severely ill, or has no pulse.

Prophylaxis can be effectuated by desensitisation to hymenoptera venom.

Your notes:

116. A tall 34-year-old man develops severe central chest pain radiating to his back. He soon develops a dense hemiplegia.

Diagnosis: Dissecting aortic aneurysm (DAA)

Clinchers

- *Tall 34-year-old man:* Peak incidence of DAA occurs in sixth and seventh decade. Men are more commonly affected. DAA in young 34-year-old man (tall) may focus our attention towards Marfan's syndrome. Marfan's sydnrome is a dominent connective tissue disease with following criterias (diagnostic, e.g. > 2 criteria with positive family history)—lens dislocation, aortic dissection/dilatation, dural ectasia and skeletal features, e.g. arachnodactyly (long spidery fingers) armspan greater than height.
- *Severe central chest pain radiating to his back:* DAA presents with suddent onset, severe and tearing chest pain which may be localised to front or back. Other causes of chest pain are
  - *Cardiovascular:*
    - Angina
    - Myocardial infarction
    - Acute aortic dissection
    - Pericarditis.
  - *Gastrointestinal*
    - Oesophageal spasm
    - Reflux oesophagitis
    - Peptic ulcer disease
  - *Pulmonary*
    - Pneumonia
    - Pulmonary embolism
    - Pneumothorax
  - *Musculoskeletal*
    - Chest wall injuries
    - Costochondritis
    - Rib secondaries
    - Herpes zoster
  - *Emotional*
    - Depression
    - De Costa's syndrome
- *Develops dense hemiplegia:* Hemiplegia and hemianesthesia both are neurological findings in DAA due to carotid artery obstruction. It may also lead to spinal cord ischaemia (paraplegia).

CONFUSA

Echocardiogram that shows no evidence of ischaemia is helpful in distinguishing aortic dissection from myocardial infarction.

Investigation of Choice

Chest X-ray/aortography or noninvasive techniques like two-dimensional echocardiography, CT scan or MRI (If haemodynamically compromised). MRI gives the best differentiation owing to high resolution.

Immediate Management

Monitor hemodynamics and urine output. Unless hypotension is there, aim at reducing cardiac contractility and systemic arterial pressure.

Treatment of Choice

For acute aortic dissection, beta-adrenergic blockers should be administered IV to achieve heart rate of about 60 beats/minute, followed by sodium nitroprusside infusion to lower systolic BP to 120 mmHg.

Long-term aim—control hypertension and reduce cardiac contractility.

Your notes:

117. An elderly gentleman suffers a sudden severe crushing central chest pain radiating to his neck

Diagnosis: Myocardial infarction (MI).

Clinchers

- *Elderly gentleman:* Myocardial infarction (MI) occurs in elderly, more common in males. Other risk factors include family history of IHD, smoking, hypertension, diabetes, hyperlipidaemia, obesity and sedentary lifestyle.
- *Sudden onset:* Chest pain in MI is of sudden onset, lasting >20 minutes which may be associated with nausea, sweatiness, dyspnoea, and palpitations.
- *Severe, central crushing chest pain radiating to neck:* Crushing, squeezing and heavy are some adjectives used by the patient to describe the pain in MI. The pain is severe involving central portion of chest and/or the epigastrium radiating to arms, back, lower jaw and neck.

CONFUSA

When the pain begins during a period of exertion, it does not usually subside with cessation of activity in contrast to angina pectoris.

Two out of three are essential for diagnosis of MI, A typical history ECG changes and cardiac enzyme rise.

Investigation of Choice

- *Screening:* ECG changes—hyperacute T wave, ST elevation or new LBBB occur within hours of acute Q wave
- *Definitive:* Cardiac enzymes - and troponin T increases.

Immediate Management

- High flow O_2 by facemask

↓

- Aspirin 300 mg chewed (unless clear contraindication)

↓

- Morphine 5-10 mg IV + metoclopromide 10 mg IV

↓

- GTN sublingually 2 puff or 1 tablet as required

↓

β-blockers

↓

thrombolysis

Your notes:

118. A middle-aged man has severe chest pain. Repeated ST elevation patterns are seen and a Pericardial rub is heard.

Diagnosis: Pericarditis.

Clinchers

- *Severe chest pain:* The pain in pericarditis is often severe. It is characteristically reterosternal of left precordial, referred to the back and the trapezius. Pain gets worse on inspiration or lying flat, relieved by sitting up and learning forward.
- *Repeated ST elevation pattern:* ECG classically shows concave (saddle-shaped) ST segment elevation, but may be normal.
- *Pericardial rub:* This is the most important physical sign of pericarditis. It may have upto three components per cardiac cycle, heard most frequently during expiration with patient in sitting position.

CONFUSA

Myocardial infarction can be confused here as with acute pericarditis, serum transaminase and creatine kinase levels rise. However, these enzyme elevations in pericarditis are quite modest, given the extensive ECG. ST segment elevation in pericarditis.

Investigation of Choice

ECG.

Immediate Management

Observe for development of pericardial effusion, and if it is there watch for tamponade. If manifestations of tamponade appear pericardiocentesis must be carried out at once.

Your notes:

179. A 69-year-old man develops crushing chest pain associated with nausea and profuse sweating radia–ting to the neck. By the time he gets to the hospital [quarter of an hour later] the pain is gone.

Diagnosis: Angina pectoris

Clinchers

Angina pectoris, the most common clinical manifes-tation of coronary artery disease, results from an imbalance between myocardial O_2 supply and demand, most commonly resulting from atherosclerotic coronary artery aneurysm.

- *69-year-old man:* Angina, like other common heart ailments, increase in incidence with age.
- *Crushing chest pain:* It may present variably as a central chest tightness or heaviness, crushing chest (more like MI). Usually it is precipitated by exertion and relieved by rest.
- *Nausea and profuse sweating:* Associated symptoms of an acute attack are: dyspnoea, nausea, vomiting, sweatiness, faintness.
- *Radiating to neck:* The pain may radiate to
  - One/both arms
  - Neck
  - Jaw
  - Teeth

CONFUSA

The main clinical criterion to differentiate between severe episode of angina and MI (myocardial infarction) is the duration of pain. If the pain is for more than 20 minutes (OHCM, 104) it qualifies as MI. All other characteristics and associations of the pain are same in both conditions.

Investigation of Choice

- ECG (usually normal, may show ST depression)
- If resting ECG normal—do exercise ECG

Immediate Management

GTN spray/sublingual tablet for an acute attack.

Treatment of Choice

Aspirin (75-150 mg/24 h)

+

According to angina guidelines in UK.

Your notes:

PAPER 4

48. Female after anterior resection of rectum com-plains of anterior chest pain radiating to her left arm.

Diagnosis: Myocardial infarction (probably).

Clinchers

- *Anterior resection of rectum:* It suggest that a rectal tumour has been resected. In any pelvic surgery there is an increased incidence of arterial or venous embolisation postoperatively which can lead to coronary artery thrombosis or pulmonary embolism.
- *Anterior chest pain radiating to left arm:* This is a typical pain presentation it is MI as angina usually require also some precipitant (e.g. exertion) and patient also give a previous history most of the times.

CONFUSA

Although pain from pulmonary embolism can present in the same way as that of MI, it is highly unlikely as an answer in this question as the presentation is not cliched. Usually GMC do not ask for such "far-sighted" diagnoses.

Investigation of Choice

12 lead ECG

Immediate Management

High flow O_2 by facemask.

Treatment of Choice

See MI protocol on page 781, OHCM, 5th edn.

Your notes:

110. A 17-year-old girl with hypertension of 160/100 is found to have a femoral pulse delay.

Diagnosis: Coarctation of aorta (CoA)

Clinchers

- *17-year-old:* The condition often remain asymptomatic for many years. Headache, epistaxis, cold extremities, and claudication with exercise may occur, and attention is usually directed to the cardiovascular system when a heart murmur or hypertension in the upper extremities and absence, marked diminution, or delayed pulsations in the femoral arteries are detected incidentally on physical examination.
- *Girl:* Although CoA is twice as common in males as in females, it association with Turner's syndrome accounts for majority of its incidence in females.
- *Hypertension of 160/110:* Blood pressure in upper limbs remains elevated in CoA. BP measurement in lower limbs should be done in order to get an idea.
- *Femoral pulse delay:* Radiofemoral delay is characteristic of the condition.

CONFUSA

When surgery for CoA is performed in childhood, hypertension usually resolves completely. However, when the operation is performed on adults the hypertension persists in 70% because of previous renal damage.

Investigation of Choice

- *Screening:* CXR ("Figure of 3" appearance)
- *Definitive:* MRI/aortography/digital vascular imaging).

Immediate Management

Screen for Turner's syndrome.

Treatment of Choice

Surgery/balloon dilatation.

Your notes:

116. Patient, 12 hours after MI presents with recurrent chest pain, breathlessness, heart rate—40/min.

Diagnosis: Heart block with haemodynamic compromise

Clinchers

- *12 hours after MI:* It means that it must be an acute complication of MI. Complication of MI in acute phase (i.e. within first two or three days following MI are—cardiac arrhythmia, cardiac failure and pericarditis. Late complications of MI are post-myocardiac infarction syndrome (Dressler's syndrome), ventricular aneurysm, and recurrent cardiac arrhythmias.
- *Recurrent chest pain and breathlessness:* These are the symptomatologies of the associated haemodynamic compromise.
- *Heart rate—40/min:* It is low as bradycardia is present.

CONFUSA

Condition of heart block in this patient may require pace maker insertion. But it may not be necessary after inferior MI if:

- QRS is narrow and reasonably stable
- And pulse $\geq$ 40-50 (as in this patient).

A more detailed evaluation is required to consider pacemaker insertion in this patient.

Investigation of Choice

ECG monitoring

Immediate Management

Atropine IV (0.5 mg initial, upto 2.0 mg total)

Treatment of Choice

Persistent bradycardia (<40 bpm) despite atropine is treated with electrical pacing.

Your notes:

117. Patient with pulmonary oedema features presents with irregular pulse, heart rate—140 bpm.

Diagnosis: Acute atrial fibrillation (AF)

Clinchers

- *Pulmonary oedema:* It is indicative of heart failure. Heart failure usually precipitates AF due to atrial irritation.
- *Irregular pulse:* The pulse in AF is characteristically irregularly irregular, the apical pulse rate is greater than radial rate and the first heart sound is of variable intensity.
- *Heart rate—140/bpm:* AF is a chaotic, irregular atrial rhythm at 300-600 bpm. But radial pulse is always lesser. It is so as the AV node responds intermittently producing an irregular ventricular rate.

CONFUSA

Atrial fibrillation is an early complication of myocardial infarction, occurring in about 10% patients. Apart from heart failure, other precipitants of AF can be
- Pericarditis
- Acute ischaemia or infarction

Investigation of Choice

ECG (absent P waves; irregular QRS complexes)

Immediate Management

IV digoxin or IV amiodarone

Treatment of Choice

Treatment of underlying pathology (in this case, heart failure).

Your notes:

119. 10 days after MI, female presents with chest pain on inspiration, persistently elevated ST segment on ECG.

Diagnosis: Acute pericarditis

Clinchers

- *10 days after MI:* Acute pericarditis is common in the first few days after MI, particularly in anterior wall infarction.
- *Chest pain on inspiration:* It is characterised by sharp chest pain, aggravated by
  - Movement
  - Respiration
  - Lying down (characteristic)
- *Persistently elevated ST segment:* ECG in acute pericarditis shows generalised ST segment elevation (concave upward) with upright, peaked T waves.

CONFUSA

Sequence of ECG changes in MI are:
1. Normal ECG
2. ST elevation
3. Appearance of Q waves
4. Normalization of ST segments
5. Inversion of T waves

So ST elevation is a normal feature in MI. However, if it remains persistently elevated, always suspect pericarditis, especially with saddle-shaped ST elevation.

Note:
- In pericarditis after MI, anticoagulation is avoided.
- In case of recurrent pericarditis, suspect Dressler's syndrome.

Investigation of Choice

ECG (already done in this patient).
Each to check effusions.

Immediate Management

Stop anticoagulation if continuing after MI.

Treatment of Choice

NSAIDs.

Your notes:

120. Patient after MI found to have a harsh pansystolic murmur at the apex.

Diagnosis: Papillary muscle rupture.

Clinchers

- *After MI:* Mitral valve papillary muscle rupture is common complication of MI.
- *Harsh pansystolic murmur at apex:* It is due to mitral regurgitation. It can also be a finding in ventricular septal perforation, more common than papillary muscle rupture, after MI. A systolic thrill may be found in both the cases.

CONFUSA

The cardiac rupture syndrome results from the mechanical weakening that occurs in necrotic and subsequently inflamed myocardium and includes:

1. *Rupture of ventricular free wall (most common)*—with haemopericardium and cardiac tamponade and usually fatal.
2. *Rupture of ventricular septum (less commonly)*—leading to a left to right shunt.
3. *Papillary muscle rupture (least common)*—resulting in acute onset of severe mitral regurgitation.

Note:

- Pansystolic murmur can be heard in (2) and (3).
- ECG is usually normal in cardiac rupture.

Investigation of Choice

Echocardiography (colour flow doppler)

Immediate Management

Lowering aortic systolic pressure

- Intraortic balloon counter pulsation
- Nitroglycerin/Nitroprusside

Treatment of Choice

Surgical repair/mitral valve repalcement.

Your notes:

121. Man with recurrent amaurosis fugax of right eye.

Diagnosis: Carotid artery stenosis.

Clinchers

- *Man:* The incidence of artherosclerosis, which is the causative factor of carotid artery stenosis is more in males.
- *Recurrent amaurosis fugax:* Amaurosis fugax is sudden transient loss of vision in one eye. A TIA causing an episode of amaurosis fugax is often the first clinical evidence of internal carotid artery stenosis, which may herald a hemiparesis. A recurrent event points more towards this pathology.

CONFUSA

Amaurosis fugax occurs as a benign event in migraine, but in that case recurrent unilateral headache will be a more predominant symptom. Vertebrobasilar insufficiency or emboli can be confused with amaurosis fugax, because many patients mistakenly ascribe symptoms to their left or right eye, when in fact they are occurring in the left or right hemifield of both eyes

In amaurosis fugax, the patient typically describes the blindness as a "sudden falling of a curtain in front of the eye". The other conditions with such a description is retinal detachment, but that is usually precede by a prodrome of photopsia and is differentiable on retinoscopy.

Other common cause for sudden uniocular blindness is multiple sclerosis but that will not be painless, (as in above two conditions) as retrobulbar pain is frequently present, and the patient will give a typical history of multiple sclerosis.

Common causes of amaurosis fugax

- Carotid TIA
- Embolisation of retinal circulation
- Papilloedema
- Giant cell arteritis
- Raynaud's disease
- Hypertensive retinopathy
- Migraine
- Venous stasis retinopathy
- As a prodromal symptom of:
  - Central retinal artery occlusion
  - Carotid artery occlusion.

Investigation of Choice

- *Screening:* Carotid artery doppler.
- *Definitive:* Carotid angiography.

Immediate Management
Aspirin 75 mg pO/d.

Treatment of Choice
Carotid endarterectomy (if the patient is good operative risk).

Your notes:

193. Female on treatment for supraventricular tachycardia complains of seeing dots and glare on driving at night, exophthalmos, no goitre.

Diagnosis: Drug induced thyrotoxicosis.

Clinchers

- *Female:* Thyroid disorders are overall more prevalent in females, however drug induced thyrotoxicosis have an equal incidence in both sexes:
- *On treatment for SVT:* Given her existing clinical profile, she must be on treatment with amiodarone. Amiodarone is used in a wide range of ventricular and supraventricular arrhythmias. However, because of its toxic potential, its use is limited to resistant VT and recurrent VF. It is also used to maintain sinus rhythm in AF when other drugs here failed. Rapid termination of ventricular and supraventricular arrhythmias can be obtained by IV injection. WPW tachyarrhythmia can be obtained by suppression of both normal and aberrant pathways. Its long duration of action make it suitable for long-term prophylactic use; but close monitoring is required.
- *Complains of seeing dots and glare on driving at night:* This is due to corneal oedema occurring due to inflammatory reaction in thyrotoxicosis. Otherwise also it can be due to corneal microdeposits occurring due to long-term use of amiodarone.
- *Exophthalmos, no goitre:* Absence of goitre excludes a primary thyroid abnormality. Exophthalmos is due to retro-orbital inflammatory and oedema characteristically seen in thyrotoxicosis.

CONFUSA

Had she not been taking drugs for SVT, this clinical profile would have qualified for a diagnosis of Graves' disease. Amiodarone is an iodine containing highly lipophilic long acting antiarrhythmic drug. It interferes with thyroid function in many ways including inhibition of peripheral conversion of T_4 to T_3.

Investigation of Choice
Serum T_4.

Immediate Management
Review SVT treatment by a cardiologist.

Treatment of Choice
Discontinue amiodarone

PAPER 5

45. Chest X-ray shows signs of left ventricular dilatation and an electrocardiograph (ECG) shows Q waves with ST elevation.

Diagnosis: Myocardial infarction

Clinchers

- *Left ventricular dilatation:* Cardiomegaly may be identified on CXR is cases of MI.
- *Q waves:* Acute Q waves signify transmural infarction. T wave inversion and the development of Q waves follow over hours to days.
- *ST elevation:* Hyperacute T waves, ST elevation or new LBBB occur with hours of acute Q waves.

CONFUSA

This complication most often occurs in older patients because of pre-existing pathology. Cholecystectomy may be adviced when the patient is young and other wise well, as symptomless stones may eventually produce the numerous problems. If the patient is elderly and unfit, symptomless stones are left untreated.

Investigation of Choice

ECG

Immediate Management

High flow O_2 + IV morphine

Treatment of Choice

Thrombolysis.

Your notes:

111. A teenage boy with dyspnoea and chest pain is brought into Accident and Emergency. He has a history of rheumatic fever. An ECG demonstrates left atrial hypertrophy and left ventricular hypertrophy. It also demonstrates Q waves and raised ST-segment.

Diagnosis: Myocardial infarction (MI)

Clinchers

- *Teenage boys:* Although the incidence of MI is increasing in younger age, an acute MI in teenage is rare. In this case suspicion should be raised for familial hypercholesterolaemia or cocaine use which can produce MI at such a young age.
- *Dyspnoea and chest pain:* The cardinal feature of AMI.
- *History of rheumatic fever:* Aortic insufficiency due to residual heart damage after rheumatic fever can cause MI as a major coronary blood supply from aorta is compromised.
- *ECG: LAH + LVH + Q waves + raised ST segment:* LAH and LVH confirms our suspicion of aortic stenosis (and hence aortic insufficiency) to be the cause of MI. Q waves signify a transmural infarct. Total occlusion of the infarct artery produces ST-segment elevation, and most such individuals ultimately evolve a Q-wave MI.

ECG progression in MI

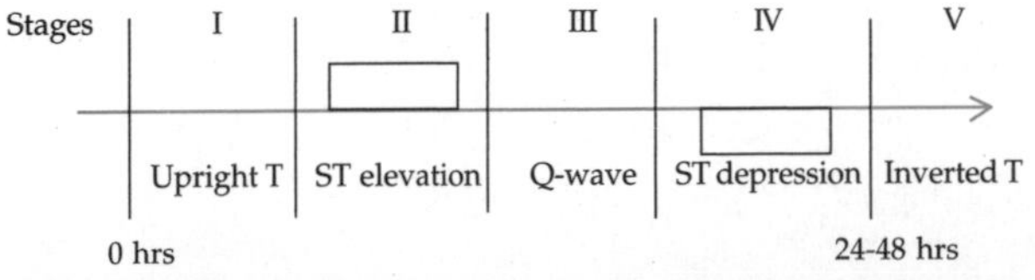

CONFUSA

ECG pathologic correlation are far from perfect and, therefore a more rational nomenclature for designating electrocardiographic infarction is now commonly in use, with the terms Q-wave and non-Q-wave infarction replacing the terms transmural and non-transmural infarction, respectively. A small population may sustain only a non-Q wave MI. When the obstructing thrombus is subtotally occlusive obstruction is transient or a rich collateral network is present, no ST-segment elevation is seen.

Investigation of Choice

12 lead ECG

Immediate Management

High flow O_2 + IV morphine

Treatment of Choice

Anticoagulation

112. An elderly woman is found unconscious at home. An ECG demonstrates sinus bradycardia. J waves, ST-depression, and flattened T waves.

Diagnosis: Hypothermia (Urban or subacute hypothermia)

Clinchers

- *Elderly woman:* Old age and no one to look after are important predisposing factors for hypothermia. The victim is usually exposed to moderate cold for days, often with several predisposing factors.
- *Unconscious at home:* The most common cause in UK of an elderly to be found unconscious at home with no obvious injuries is hypothermia. Upto 3% of medical patients admitted to UK hospitals during winter months have core temperature below 35°C.
- *ECG: sinus bradycardia + ST depression + flattened T waves:* There all suggest prolonged repolarisation, a characteristic features of hypothermia.
- *J waves:* It is characteristic notching of the S-wave (usually seen in V4). It is also called osborn wave and is present in 80% of patients with severe hypothermia.

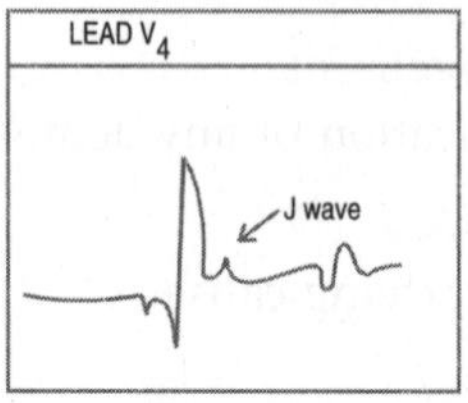

CONFUSA

- Do not assume that if vital signs seem to be absent, the patient must be dead:rewarm and re-examine
- Do not rewarm too fast, causing peripheral vasodilatation, shock and death. Thermal blankets may cause too rapid warming in old patients.
- Treat the patient gently the most common precipitant of VF hypothermia is mechanical irritation of the body.

Investigation of Choice

Core tempeature (< 35°C) +
Urgent U and E, plasma glucose and amylase, TFT + ECG (definitive if J waves present)

Immediate Management

Slowly rewarm after removal of cold stimuli (½°C increase per hour)

Treatment of Choice

Warming + treatment of complications (if any)

113. A patient's ECG shows a biphasic P-wave.

Diagnosis: Left atrial hypertrophy (LAH)

Clinchers

Left atrial overload typically produces a biphasic P-wave in V_1 with a broad negative component or a broad (≥ 120 ms), often notched P-wave in one or more leads.

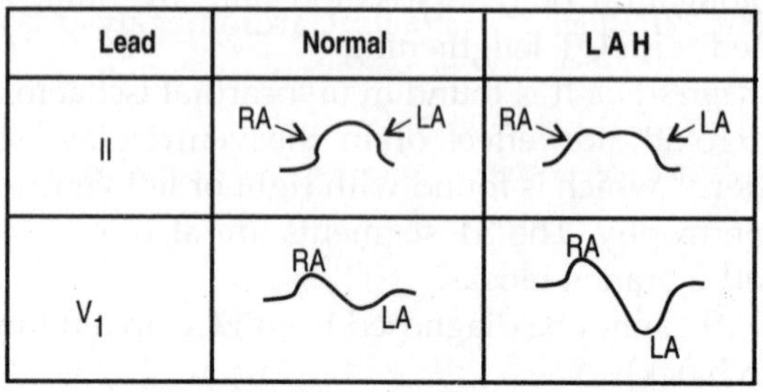

CONFUSA

Biphasic P-wave in lead V_1 is with a prominent negative component representing delayed depolarisation of the LA.

Investigation of Choice

- *Screening:* ECG
- *Definitive:* Echocardiography

Immediate Management

Specialist referral

Treatment of Choice

As per the cause of LAH.

Your notes:

114. A patient's ECG shows T-wave inversion and ST depression.

Diagnosis: Ischaemic heart disease

Clinchers

- *T-wave inversion:* It may signify previous MI. T-wave inversions due to chronic ischaemia correlate with prolongation of repolarisation and are often associated with QT lengthening.
- *ST depression:* It is found in myocardial ischaemia, as a digoxin side effect or in the ventricular "strain pattern" which is found with right or left ventricular hypertrophy. The ST segments are also inverted in bundle branch blocks.

(*Note:* MI cannot be diagnosed from ECG in left bundle branch block).

CONFUSA

Negative T waves can be sign of a sub-endocardial myocardial infarction. They are found in the resolution phase of myocardial infarction and in ischaemic heart disease without evidence of myocardial death.

Note:

- Horizontal depression of ST segment—ischaemia
- Down sloping depression of ST segment—digoxin

Investigation of Choice

ECG

Immediate Management

Specialist evaluation

Treatment of Choice

As per the cause.

Your notes:

115. A 25-year-old woman complains of tiredness and malaise. Her T waves are widespread and deep.

Diagnosis: Myocarditis

Clinchers

- *25-year-old-woman:* Although most common cause of myocarditis is infection in females autoimmune disease results in significant number of cases.
- *Tiredness and malaise*: Symptoms of myocarditis are usually fatigue, dyspnoea, chest pain and palpitations.
- *T waves widespread and deep:* This signify T waves inversion which characteristically occurs in myocardial along with other T-wave abnormalities.

CONFUSA

In myocarditis, ECG demonstrates ST and T-wave abnormalities and arrhythmias. Head blocks may be seen with diphtheric myocarditis, while Chaga's disease produces both heart block and ventricular tachyarrhythmias.

Investigation of Choice

Serology + ECG

Immediate Management

Bedrest and eradication of any acute infection

Treatment of Choice

Treatment of underlying cause

+

Supportive treatment.

Your notes:

127. An obese 45-year-old man complains of recurring chest pain which radiates to his neck lasting 20 minutes. It coincides with his weekly executive board meetings.

Diagnosis: Stable angina

Clinchers

- *Obese:* Obesity, particularly central obesity, is associated with coronary artery disease, but it is not certain which obesity itself is independently linked to the condition.
- *45-year-old:* Coronary artery disease rates increase with age.
- *Man:* Males constitutes approximately 70% of cases
- *Recurring chest pain:* Indicates angina most in this clinical profile.
- *Radiates to neck:* Angina can radiate to the left shoulder and to both arms and especially to the ulnar surfaces of the forearm and hand. It can also arise in or radiate to the back, neck, jaw, teeth or epigastrium.
- *Lasting 20 minutes:* The pain fades quickly i.e. with 1-5 minutes and never last more than 20 minutes.
- *Concides with....:* This is the precipitant (i.e. stress) and hence it is stable angina.

CONFUSA

Stable angina is one which is precipitated by exertion (e.g. exercise, hurrying or sexual activity) or emotion (e.g. stress, anger, fright or frustration) and are relieved by rest. When it occurs at rest it is called unstable angina. Occasionally the pain of stable angina disappears with continued exertion. Cardiac syndrome X refers to these patients with a good history of angina, a positive exercise test and angiographically normal coronary arteries.

Investigation of Choice
Exercise ECG (confirms the diagnosis)

Immediate Management
GTN sublingual for termination of an acute attack.

Treatment of Choice
Aspirin (75 mg daily).

Your notes:

141. A patient in her third pregnancy presents to her GP at 12 weeks gestation. She was mildly hypertensive in both of her previous pregnancies. Her BP is 150/100 mmHg. Two weeks later at the hospital antenatal clinic her BP is 150/95 mmHg.

Diagnosis: Essential hypertension (EH)

Clinchers

- *Third pregnancy:* EH is common in older multiparas, and present before pregnancy or in first trimester (in this case 12 weeks).
- *Mildly hypertensive in both of her previous pregnancies:* Those with EH are five times more likely to develop pre-eclampsia. Also increased BP is a positive risk factor for PIH.
- *BP is 150/100 mmHg, two weeks later 150/95 mmHg:* Isolated BP measurements are never reliable in pregnancy. So BP has to be recorded on at least two occasions (at least >4 hr apart) to make a diagnosis. In this case the BP is more or less the same on two occasions (two weeks apart). Also the diastolic BP is > 90 mmHg on both occasions.

CONFUSA

If the symptoms are episodic, think of phaeochromocytoma. PIH by definition does not present before 20 weeks for the first-time.

Investigation of Choice
24 hours urinary proteins (to screen for pre-eclampsia).

Immediate Management
BP monitoring (biweekly).

Treatment of Choice
Oral antihypertensive (as BP should be kept < 140/90 mmHg).

Your notes:

189. A 30-year-old man with Marfan's syndrome has sudden central chest pain going through to the back.

Diagnosis: Aortic dissection (acute).

Clinchers

- *30-year-old*: In patients with Marfan's syndrome aortic dissection tends to present in a relatively younger age.
- *Marfan's syndrome*: It increases the risk of ascending aortic dissection. In fact it is the major cause of mortality in it.
- *Sudden central chest pain going to back*: Sudden onset of pain, localised to front or back of chest, often interscapular region and typically migrates with propapation of dissection.

CONFUSA

Aortic dissection is a potentially life-threatening condition in which disruption of aortic intima allows dissection of blood into vessel wall, may involves ascending aorta (type II) descending aorta (type III), or both (type I). Alternative classification type A –ascending aortic dissection, type B—limited to descending aorta. Involvement of the ascending aorta is most lethal form.

Investigation of Choice

Screening/CXR, Definitive/CT/MRI/USG (TOE).

Immediate Management

Crossmatch and inform surgeons.

Treatment of Choice

Emegent surgical repair/always required in ascending aortic dissection.

Your notes:

190. A 57-year-old man develops crushing pain in the chest associated with nausea and profuse sweating. The pain is still present when he arrives in hospital an hour later.

Diagnosis: Acute myocardial infarction (AMI).

Clinchers

- *57-year-old*: Incidence of MI increases with age as age is a nonmodifiable risk factor.
- *Man*: Male sex is also a nonmodifiable risk factor
- *Crushing pain*: There is acute central chest pain and is classically described as crushing or heavy. Some patients say it feels like a tight band around their chest; others describe it as like someone sitting on them. It is common for the patient to clench his or her first as an aid to description.
- *Associated with nausea and profuse sweating*: Accompanying symptoms such as sweating, pallor, nausea or general malaise are almost helpful in making a diagnosis as the character of pain.
- *Still present when he arrives in hospital an hour later*: The pain usually lasts longer than 30 minutes (20 minutes according to OHCM). This feature differentiates it form angina.

CONFUSA

Be aware of the middle-aged man with 'indigestion' especially if he has no past dyspeptic history of significance. A few days of vague retrosternal pain is not a history of dyspepsia. It is much more likely to be the warning pain which often predate as MI. Recurrent belching is a sign of autonomic disturbance and as such may accompany as infarction. Even synptomatic relief from antacids should not be relived upon to relied upon to point away from the heart. Some patients present with very atypical pain, both in site and character. Examples of this would be pain localized to the abdomen or to the left shoulder or arm alone.

Investigation of Choice

ECG (hyperacute T waves, ST elevation or new LBBB)

Immediate Management

High flow O_2 + 10 mg IV morphine + anticoagulation.

Treatment of Choice

Thrombolysis.

Your notes:

PAPER 6

84. A 30-year-old man with Marfan's syndrome has sudden central chest pain going through to the back.

Diagnosis: Aortic dissection (acute).

Clinchers

- *30-year-old*: In patients with Marfan's syndrome aortic dissection tends to present in a relatively younger age.
- *Marfan's syndrome*: It increases the risk of ascending aortic dissection. In fact it is the major cause of mortality in it.
- *Sudden central chest pain going to back*: Sudden onset of pain, localised to front or back of chest, often intersapular region and typically migrates with propapation of dissection.

CONFUSA

Aortic dissection is a potentially life-threatening condition in which disruption of aortic intima allows dissection of blood into vessel wall, may involves ascending aorta (type II) descending aorta (type III), or both (type I). Alternative classification type A –ascending aortic dissection, type B—limited to descending aorta. Involvement of the ascending aorta is most lethal form.

Investigation of Choice
Screening/CXR, Definitive/CT/MRI/USG (TOE).

Immediate Management
Crossmatch and inform surgeons.

Treatment of Choice
Emegent surgical repair/always required in ascending aortic dissection.

Your notes:

85. A 57-year-old man develops crushing pain in the chest associated with nausea and profuse sweating. The pain is still present when he arrives in hospital an hour later.

Diagnosis: Acute myocardial infarction (AMI).

Clinchers

- *57-year-old*: Incidence of MI increases with age as age is a nonmodifiable risk factor.
- *Man*: Male sex is also a nonmodifiable risk factor
- *Crushing pain*: There is acute central chest pain and is classically described as crushing or heavy. Some patients say it feels like a tight band around their chest; others describe it as like someone sitting on them. It is common for the patient to clench his or her first as an aid to description.
- *Associated with nausea and profuse sweating*: Accompanying symptoms such as sweating, pallor, nausea or general malaise are almost helpful in making a diagnosis as the character of pain.
- *Still present when he arrives in hospital an hour later*: The pain usually lasts longer than 30 minutes (20 minutes according to OHCM). This feature differentiates it form angina.

CONFUSA

Be aware of the middle-aged man with 'indigestion' especially if he has no past dyspeptic history of significance. A few days of vague retrosternal pain is not a history of dyspepsia. It is much more likely to be the warning pain which often predate as MI. Recurrent belching is a sign of autonomic disturbance and as such may accompany as infarction. Even symptomatic relief from antacids should not be relived upon to point away from the heart. Some patients present with very atypicaly pain, both in site and character. Examples of this would be pain localised to the abdomen or to the left shoulder or arm alone.

Investigation of Choice
ECG (hyperacute T waves, ST elevation or new LBBB)

Immediate Management
High flow O_2 + 10 mg IV morphine + anticoagulation.

Treatment of Choice
Thrombolysis.

Your notes:

156. A 65-year-old man presents with severe, retrosternal chest pain and sweating. An ECG shows an acute anterolateral myocardial infarction.

Diagnosis: Acute myocardial infarction (MI).

Clinchers

- *65-year-old man:* The incidence and severity of almost all the risk factors of MI increases with age, hence contributing to increase the risk for MI. Male sex is a definitive risk factor for MI.
- *Severe, retrosternal chest pain:* Pain is the most common presenting complaint. In some instances, the discomfort may be severe enough to be described as the worst pain the patient has even felt. The pain is deep and visceral; adjectives commonly used to describe it are heavy, squeezing and crushing, although occasionally it is described as stabbing or burning. It is similar in character to exertional angina, but usually is more severe and lasts longer (>20 minutes). Typically the pain involves the central portion of the chest and/or the epigastrium, and an occasion it radiates to arms (most commonly), abdomen, back, lower jaw and neck.
- *Severe retrosternal chest pain:* The pain of MI may radiate as high as the occipital area but not below the umbilicus. Painless infarcts also occur especially in:
  - Diabetes mellitus
  - Elderly (present as sudden onset breathlessness, which may progress to pulmonary oedema)
- *Vomiting and sweating:* Due to intense sympathetic stimulation.
- *Anterolateral MI:* If the infarction involves both the anterior and lateral surfaces of heart, a Q wave will be present in V_3 and V_4 and in the leads that look at the lateral surface—I, VL and V_{5-6}.

Investigation of Choice
12 lead ECG.

Immediate Management
High flow O_2 by face mask (caution, if COPD).

Treatment of Choice
IV opiate (5-10 mg), repeated every 5 min.

181. Patient, 12 hours after MI presents with recurrent chest pain, breathlessness, heart rate—40/min.

Diagnosis: Heart block with haemodynamic compromise

Clinchers

- *12 hours after MI:* It means that it must be an acute complication of MI. Complication of MI in acute phase (i.e. within first two or three days following MI are—cardiac arrhythmia, cardiac failure and pericarditis. Late complications of MI are post-myocardiac infarction syndrome (Dressler's syndrome), ventricular aneurysm, and recurrent cardiac arrhythmias.
- *Recurrent chest pain and breathlessness:* These are the symptomatologies of the associated haemodynamic compromise.
- *Heart rate—40/min:* It is low as bradycardia is present.

CONFUSA

Condition of heart block in this patient may require pacemaker insertion. But it may not be necessary after inferior MI if:
- QRS is narrow and reasonably stable
- And pulse ≥ 40-50 (as in this patient).

A more detailed evaluation is required to consider pacemaker insertion in this patient.

Investigation of Choice
ECG monitoring

Immediate Management
Atropine IV (0.5 mg initial, upto 2.0 mg total)

Treatment of Choice
Persistent bradycardia (<40 bpm) despite atropine is treated with electrical pacing.

Your notes:

182. Patient with pulmonary oedema features presents with irregular pulse, heart rate—140 bpm.

Diagnosis: Acute atrial fibrillation (AF)

Clinchers

- *Pulmonary oedema:* It is indicative of heart failure. Heart failure usually precipitates AF due to atrial irritation.
- *Irregular pulse:* The pulse in AF is characteristically irregularly irregular, the apical pulse rate is greater than radial rate and the first heart sound is of variable intensity.
- *Heart rate—140/bpm:* AF is a chaotic, irregular atrial rhythm at 300-600 bpm. But radial pulse is always lesser. It is so as the AV node responds intermittently producing an irregular ventricular rate.

CONFUSA

Atrial fibrillation is an early complication of myocardial infarction, occurring in about 10% patients. Apart from heart failure, other precipitants of AF can be
- Pericarditis
- Acute ischaemia or infarction

Investigation of Choice

ECG (absent P waves; irregular QRS complexes)

Immediate Management

IV digoxin or IV amiodarone

Treatment of Choice

Treatment of underlying pathology (in this case, heart failure).

Your notes:

184. Ten days after MI, female presents with chest pain on inspiration, persistently elevated ST segment on ECG.

Diagnosis: Acute pericarditis

Clinchers

- *Ten days after MI:* Acute pericarditis is common in the first few days after MI, particularly in anterior wall infarction.
- *Chest pain on inspiration:* It is characterised by sharp chest pain, aggravated by
  - Movement
  - Respiration
  - Lying down (characteristic)
- *Persistently elevated ST segment:* ECG in acute pericarditis shows generalised ST segment elevation (concave upward) with upright, peaked T waves.

CONFUSA

Sequence of ECG changes in MI are:
1. Normal ECG
2. ST elevation
3. Appearance of Q waves
4. Normalization of ST segments
5. Inversion of T waves.

So ST elevation is a normal feature in MI. However, if it remains persistently elevated, always suspect pericarditis, especially with saddle-shaped ST elevation.

Note:
- In pericarditis after MI, anticoagulation is avoided.
- In case of recurrent pericarditis, suspect Dressler's syndrome.

Investigation of Choice

ECG (already done in this patient).
Each to check effusions.

Immediate Management

Stop anticoagulation if continuing after MI.

Treatment of Choice

NSAIDs.

Your notes:

185. Patient after MI found to have a harsh pansystolic murmur at the apex.

Diagnosis: Papillary muscle rupture.

Clinchers

- *After MI:* Mitral valve papillary muscle rupture is common complication of MI.
- *Harsh pansystolic murmur at apex:* It is due to mitral regurgitation. It can also be a finding in ventricular septal perforation, more common than papillary muscle rupture, after MI. A systolic thrill may be found in both the cases.

CONFUSA

The cardiac rupture syndrome results from the mechanical weakening that occurs in necrotic and subsequently inflamed myocardium and includes:

1. *Rupture of ventricular free wall (most common)*—with haemopericardium and cardiac tamponade and usually fatal.
2. *Rupture of ventricular septum (less commonly)*—leading to a left to right shunt.
3. *Papillary muscle rupture (least common)*—resulting in acute onset of severe mitral regurgitation.

Note:

- Pansystolic murmur can be heard in (2) and (3).
- ECG is usually normal in cardiac rupture.

Investigation of Choice

Echocardiography (colour flow doppler)

Immediate Management

Lowering aortic systolic pressure

- Intraortic balloon counter pulsation
- Nitroglycerin/Nitroprusside

Treatment of Choice

Surgical repair/mitral valve repalcement.

Your notes:

PAPER 7

16. Patient had bilateral fluffy opacities and increased interstitial markings. Had low oxygen, normal CO_2.

Diagnosis: Pulmonary oedema.

Clinchers

- *Bilateral fluffy opacities and increased intestinal markings:* These are the chest radiograph findings seen in pulmonary oedema. Other findings that may be found on CXR are:
  - Blurring of vascular outlines
  - Butterfly pattern (bat wing appearance) of distribution of alveolar oedema
  - Heart may be enlarged or normal.
- *Other features essential for diagnosis of pulmonary oedema:*
  - Acute onset or worsening of dyspnoea at rest
  - Tachycardia, cyanosis, pink frothy sputum
  - Pulmonary rales, ronchi, expiratory wheezing
  - Arterial hypoxaemia.
- *Causes of pulmonary oedema:*
  - *Cardiovascular*
    - Left ventricular failure—post MI
    - Ischaemic heart disease
    - Mitral stenosis/arrhythmias.
  - *ARDS* (lung damage and release of inflammatory mediators) increased capillary permeability cause noncardiogenic pulmonary oedema.

    CXR findings in left ventricular failure

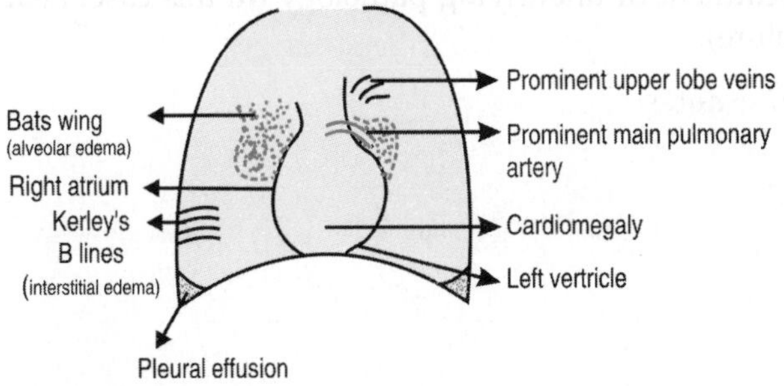

Investigation of Choice

- CxR
- EEG (may indicate cause).

Immediate Management

- Sit patient upright
- Oxygen (100% if no history of previous lung disease).

Treatment of Choice

Investigate while continuing treatment.

43. Patient with history of suggestive of atherosclerosis, now presenting with shock.

Diagnosis: Aortic aneurysm.

Clinchers

- *History suggestive of atherosclerosis:* Atheroma is the usual cause for arterial aneurysms. Other causes include:
  - Penetrating injuries
  - Infections
    - Endocarditis
    - Syphilis.
- *Shock:* Fifty percent of the patients of ruptured aortic aneurysm die from the initial rupture and never reach hospital. Those which do reach hospital are usually profoundly shocked (cold, clammy, tachycardia, hypotensive) with generalised abdominal tenderness.

CONFUSA

The ECG often shows ischaemic changes as this group of patients has generalised atherosclerosis and coronary ischaemia is worsened by hypotension. The main differential diagnosis is pancreatitis. If in doubt, assume a ruptured aneurysm. No investigation should delay the surgical referral.

Investigation of Choice
USG.

Immediate Management
Immediate surgical referral or take the patient to OT
+
Treat shock.

Treatment of Choice
Surgery (aortic clamp + Dacron graft).

Your notes:

46. A 60-year-old attends A and E and it is thought he may have aortic aneurysm.

Diagnosis: Unruptured aortic aneurysm (AA).

Clinchers

- *60-year-old:* Prevalence of AA is 3% of those above 50 years.
- *It is thought he may have aortic aneurysm:* The most common aortic aneurysms are abdominal between the renal and iliac arteries. They are usually due to atherosclerosis. The incidence increases with age, with men being affected four to five times more frequently. An ultrasound of the abdomen for evaluation of asymptomatic aneurysms will demonstrate the size of the aneurysm, the thickness of aortic wall and whether any leak has occurred.

CONFUSA

Angiography underestimates the size and extent of a true aneurysm, as it images the lumen, which is usually narrowed by thrombus. In addition, it may be dangerous, as the guide wire or cannual may perforate the aneurysm wall. It is useful in false aneurysm to identify the connection.

Investigation of Choice
Abdominal ultrasound.

Immediate Management
Evaluate for surgery.

Treatment of Choice
Prophylactic surgery for aneurysm > 5.5-6 cm.

Your notes:

47. A tall 34-year-old man develops severe central chest pain radiating to his back. He soon develops a dense hemiplegia.

Diagnosis: Dissecting aortic aneurysm (DAA)

Clinchers

- *Tall 34-year-old man:* Peak incidence of DAA occurs in sixth and seventh decade. Men are more commonly affected. DAA in young 34-year-old man (tall) may focus our attention towards Marfan's syndrome. Marfan's sydnrome is a dominent connective tissue disease with following criteria (diagnostic, e.g. > 2 criteria with positive family history)—lens dislocation, aortic dissection/dilatation, dural ectasia and skeletal features, e.g. arachnodactyly (long spidery fingers) armspan greater than height.
- *Severe central chest pain radiating to his back:* DAA presents with suddent onset, severe and tearing chest pain which may be localised to front or back. Other causes of chest pain are
  - *Cardiovascular:*
    - Angina
    - Myocardial infarction
    - Acute aortic dissection
    - Pericarditis.
  - *Gastrointestinal*
    - Oesophageal spasm
    - Reflux oesophagitis
    - Peptic ulcer disease
  - *Pulmonary*
    - Pneumonia
    - Pulmonary embolism
    - Pneumothorax
  - *Musculoskeletal*
    - Chest wall injuries
    - Costochondritis
    - Rib secondaries
    - Herpes zoster
  - *Emotional*
    - Depression
    - De Costa's syndrome
- *Develops dense hemiplegia:* Hemiplegia and hemianesthesia both are neurological findings in DAA due to carotid artery obstruction. It may also lead to spinal cord ischaemia (paraplegia).

CONFUSA
Echocardiogram that shows no evidence of ischaemia is helpful in distinguishing aortic dissection from myocardial infarction.

Investigation of Choice

Chest X-ray/aortography or noninvasive techniques like two-dimensional echocardiography, CT scan or MRI (If haemodynamically compromised). MRI gives the best differentiation owing to high resolution.

Immediate Management

Monitor haemodynamics and urine output. Unless hypotension is there, aim at reducing cardiac contractility and systemic arterial pressure.

Treatment of Choice

For acute aortic dissection, beta-adrenergic blockers should be administered IV to achieve heart rate of about 60 beats/minute, followed by sodium nitroprusside infusion to lower systolic BP to 120 mmHg.

Long-term aim—control hypertension and reduce cardiac contractility.

Your notes:

48. A patient is to have a repair of of his aortic aneurysm but also has severe myocardial ischaemia.

Diagnosis: Risk of MI during surgery.

Clinchers

Coronary artery disease is common in the population who develop aortic aneurysms. It need to be ruled out before surgery as cross clamping the aorta during surgery dramatically increases the peripheral resistance against which the heart must work, and this extra stress, coupled with the metabolic stress that occurs when the legs are reperfused, may precipitate a myocardial infarct.

CONFUSA

Preoperative assessment includes evaluating the patient's operative risk by screening for coincident cardiac disease (by ECG, echocardiography or MUGA scan to assess the ventricular ejection fraction) and for carotid arterial disease.

Investigation of Choice

Coronary angiography.

Immediate Management

Refer surgery.

Treatment of Choice

Symptomatic.

Your notes:

49. Patient with aortic aneurysm has unstable angina.

Diagnosis: Dessecting aortic aneurysm (ascending aorta)

Clinchers

- *Aortic aneurysm:* The most common pathologic condition associated with aortic aneurysm is atherosclerosis. It is controversial whether atherosclerosis itself actually causes aortic aneurysm or develops as a secondary event in the dilated aorta. Causality is implied by studies that have shown that many patients with aortic aneurysms have coexisting risk factors and atherosclerosis in other blood vessels.
- *Unstable angina.* Unstable angina may be primary, i.e. occur in the absence of an extrathoracic condition that has intensified myocardial ischaemia, or it may be precipitated by a condition extrinsic to the coronary vascular bed that has intensified myocardial ischaemia, such as anaemia, fever, infection, tachyarrhythmias, emotional stress or hypoxaemia. Unstable angina may also develop shortly after MI.

CONFUSA

An ECG could be done urgently in this case as an ECG that shows no evidence of ischaemia is helpful in distinjuishing aortic dissection from myocardial infarction. Rarely, the dissection involves the right or left coronary and causes acute myocardial infarction or unstable angina.

Investigation of Choice

ECG + Aortography + concomitant coronary angiography.

Immediate Management

Cross match > 6 units of blood + take to OT.

Treatment of Choice

Surgery.

Your notes:

50. Elderly patient suspected of having aortic dissection with complaint of abdominal pain yesterday, but is now haemodynamically stable.

Diagnosis: Aortic dissection (AD)—suspected.

Clinchers

- *Elderly:* The peak incidence of AD is in sixth and seventh decades. Men are more affected than women by a ratio of 2:1.
- *Suspected of having aortic dissection with complaint of abdominal pain:* Acute AD presents with a sudden onset of pain, which is often described as very severe and tearing and is associated with diaphoresis. The pain may be localised to the front or back of the chest, often the interscapular region, and typically migrates with preparation of dissection.
- *Now haemodynamically stable:* If hypotension is not present, therapy should be aimed at reducing cardiac contractility and systemic arterial pressure, and thereby shear stress.

CONFUSA

CT scan and MRI are each highly accurate in identifying the intimal flap and the extent of the dissection. They are useful in recognising intramural haemorrhage and penetrating ulcers. MRI also can detect blood flow which may be useful is characterising antegrade versus retrograde dissection. These noninvasive tests are now becoming the diagnostic procedures of choice. Their relative utility depends on the availability and expertise in individual institutions as well as on the haemodynamic stability of the patient, with CT and MRI obviously less suitable for more unstable patients. Still trans-oesophageal echocardiography should be the first investigation.

Investigation of Choice

Echocardiography (Trans-oesophageal).

Immediate Management

Evaluation by a specialist.

Treatment of Choice

As per the findings of echocardiography.

Your notes:

51. A patient presents with intermittent abdominal Pain for about 30 minutes after meals. Also has history of abdominal pain radiating to the back. On examination-abdominal bruit. Also has intermittent claudication.

Diagnosis: Generalised atherosclerosis.

Clinchers

- *Intermittent abdominal pain for 30 minutes after meals:* Severe abdominal pain, often colicky, following meals, is seen in acute mesenteric ischaemia. Other causes of acute abdomen are given in the confusa.
- *On examination abdominal bruit:* Abdominal bruits are often present in normal subjects. They should not necessarily be ascribed to an ischaemic bowel, on this basis alone. It occurs due to partial obstruction to flow in the vessels.
- *Intermittent claudication:* It is a sign of chronic ischaemia, almost always due to atherosclerosis.

CONFUSA

Differential diagnosis of acute abdomen—perforated viscus (especially peptic ulcer), acute cholecystitis, and biliary colic, acute intestinal obstruction, mesenteric vascular occlusion, Renal colic, myocardial infarction, dissecting aortic aneurysm.

Investigation of Choice

If we go by the options in this question, mesenteric angiogram, should be the answer.

Immediate Management

Go for tests to exclude diabetes mellitus, arteritis (ESR/CRP)

Do FBC (anaemia, infection), lipids, ECG

Arteriography.

Treatment of Choice

- Quit smoking
- Weight
- Exercise

If tests confirm any disease, treat it (e.g. treat DM, BP-, hyperlipidaemia).

Your notes:

91. A patient who developed myocardial infarction one month ago is now breathless and has basal crackles.

Diagnosis: Pulmonary oedema (post MI).

Clinchers

- *Developed MI one month ago:* Left ventricular failure is an important complication of MI. For other complications of MI refer to page 108 (OHCM) 5th edn.
- *Breathlessness and basal crackles:* These are features of presenting with acute onset of dyspnoea (with history of recent MI), and on examination pulmonary rales, ronchi, fine lung crackles, is suggestive of pulmonary oedema.

CONFUSA

Look for cardiomegaly and signs of pulmonary oedema on CXR [refer to figure in Q16 (July 2001)] and for signs of myocardial infarction on ECG to confirm the diagnosis.

Investigation of Choice

- CXR and ECG
- ABG

Immediate Management

- Sit patient upright and give oxygen.

Treatment of Choice

Most appropriate management

- *Diuretics* (furosemide 40 mg LV) produce venodilation prior to diuresis.
- *Diamorphine* given 2.5-5 mg IV slowly increases venous capacitance and relieves anxiety.
- Sublingual or IV nitrates, phlebotomy and plasma pheresis are other methods of reducing left ventricular preload.

Your notes:

92. Patient presents with one and a half hours of epigastric pain radiating to his arm. ECG shows acute inferior myocardial infarction. Oxygen + analgesia have already been given.

Diagnosis: Acute myocardial infarction.

Clinchers

- *Myocardial infarction:* Usually occurs from occlusion of coronary artery, resulting from rupture of the atheromatous plaque. It may occur due to coronary spasm, emboli or vasculitis.
- *Epigastric pain radiating to arm:* Acute prolonged (> 20 min) anterior chest discomfort, which may be associated with dyspnoea, palpitations and nausea, are the symptoms of MI. Diagnosis confirmed by ECG, and raised cardiac enzyme levels (CK, AST, LDH). In 20% cases ECG may be normal initially.

CONFUSA

Differentiate if from angina, pericarditis, aortic dissection, myocarditis, pulmonary embolism and oesophageal reflux/spasm.

Investigation of Choice

ECG and cardiac enzymes.

Immediate Management

- High flow O_2 by mask (caution if COPD).
- Aspirin in 300 mg chewed.
- Analgesia (morphine 5-10 mg IV + antiemetic e.g. metoclopramide 10 mg IV.

Next step in management

Thyrombolysis is indicated after oxygen and analgesia in this patient, since his presentation is of only one and a half hour duration.

The British Heart Foundation advices that the time from the onset of pain to thrombolysis should be < 90 minutes (< 60 min if possible). Benefits of thrombolysis (reduces mortality) are seen if given upto more than 12 hours of onset of chest pain, but some benefit upto 24 hours.

Streptokinase (SK) is the usual thrombolytic agent. Do not repeat (SK) unless it is within 4 days of first administration. Use Alteplase if the patient has previously received SK.

Your notes:

93. Patient recovering from myocardial infarction has a heart rate of 36/minute.

Diagnosis: Bradycardia/heart block.

Clinchers

- *Recovering from myocardial infarction:* Sinus bradycardia or heart block is complication of myocardial infarction. Other complications are:
  - Cardiac arrest/cardiogenic shock
  - Unstable angina
  - Tachyarrhythmias
  - Left ventricular failure
  - Right ventricular failure/infarction
  - Pericarditis, DVT, pulmonary embolism
  - Cardiac tamponade, mitral regurgitation
  - Ventricular septal defect
  - Left ventricular aneurysm
- *Heart rate of 36/minute:* May be due to sinus bradycardia of AV block. Sinus bradycardia is common in inferior infarction. First degree AV block does not require any treatment, but watch carefully as it progresses to higher degrees.

  Mobitz type I form is often transient and requires treatment only if heart rate becomes slow enough to cause symptoms. Complete A-V block occurs in upto 5% of acute inferior infractions, usually preceded by second degree block. Treatment becomes necessary because of resulting hypotension and low cardiac output.

  In anterior infarction, the site of block is distal below the AV node. Here urgent ventricular pacing is mandatory.

Investigation of Choice

ECG

Immediate Management

Atropine 0.6 to 1.2 mg IV or cardiac pacing as explained below.

Treatment of Choice

In sinus bradycardia, observation or withdrawal of offending agent is usually sufficient. If associated with signs of low cardiac output, atropine 0.6-1.2 mg IV is usually effecting. Consider temporary *cardiac pacing* if not response.

Mobitz (type I) does not require pacing, unless poorly tolerated. Mobitz (type II), should be paced, as it carries risk of complete block.

Your notes:

94. A 57-year-old man develops crushing pain in the chest associated with nausea and profuse sweating. The pain is still present when he arrives in hospital by an hour later.

Diagnosis: Myocardial infarction (MI)

Clinchers

- *Crushing pain in chest with nausea and sweating:* This is a typical presentation of myocardial infarction. The pain is acute in onset and lasts for more than 20 minutes.

  The diagnosis is supported by ECG changes and raised cardiac enzymes.
- *ECG changes in MI:* Hyper acute T wave, ST elevation or new LBBB occurs within hours of acute Q wave (transmural infarction). T wave inversion and development of Q waves follows over hour to days. In non Q wave (subendocardial) infarction, ECG findings are less specific, e.g. T wave inversion, ST depression.

Investigation of Choice

ECG and cardiac enzymes.

Immediate Management

High flow oxygen by mask and morphine (with metoclopromide).

Treatment of Choice

Already discussed in Q 92 (July 2001).

Your notes:

147. A patient's ECG shows T wave inversion and ST depression.

Diagnosis: Ischaemic heart disease

Clinchers

- *T wave inversion:* It may signify previous MI. T wave inversions due to chronic ischaemia correlate with prolongation of repolarisation and are often associated with QT lengthening.
- *ST depression:* It is found in myocardial ischaemia, as a digoxin side effect or in the ventricular "strain pattern" which is found with right or left ventricular hypertrophy. The ST segments are also inverted in bundle branch blocks.

(*Note:* MI cannot be diagnosed from ECG in left bundle branch block).

CONFUSA

Negative T waves can be sign of a sub-endocardial myocardial infarction. They are found in the resolution phase of myocardial infarction and in ischaemic heart disease without evidence of myocardial death:

Note

- Horizontal depression of ST segment—ischaemia
- Downsloping depression of ST segment—digoxin

Investigation of Choice

ECG

Immediate Management

Specialist evaluation

Treatment of Choice

As per the cause.

Your notes:

148. Three days of intravenous broad spectrum antibiotics beginning with induction of anaesthesia.

Diagnosis (Answer): Heart valve replacement

Clinchers

- The required prophylactic regimen is
  Amoxycillin 1g IV + Gentamicin 120 mg IV
  first dose is given at indcution of anaesthesia and is continued upto 3 days.

CONFUSA

Infection of valve post operating is a situation alcin to infective endocarditis of a native valve. For more detailed notes on chemoprophylaxis in various disease states refer to British national formularly or www.bnf.org.

Investigation of Choice

As per the requirements of the operation.

Immediate Management

Antimicrobial chemoprophylaxis

Treatment of Choice

Stated as the question itself.

Your notes:

4 Connective Tissue Disorders

PAPER 1

Serial No. 90

Subject: Medicine

Topic: Renal

Question: Urea 8.9 mmol/L
Creatinine 180 micromol/L
positive antinuclear antibody and
high titres of anti-dsDNA antibodies.

Diagnosis: Lupus nephritis

Clinchers

- *Urea 8.9 mmol/L; creatinine 180 micromol/L:* This signify acute renal failure; features of acute failure like hematuria, proteinuria, red cell casts and hypertension are also commonly seen. Hypertension is poor prognostic sign and requires aggressive treatment.
- *Positive antinuclear antibody:* This is diagnostic of SLE.
- *High titres of anti-dsDNA antibodies:* Active glomerulonephritis in SLE is hallmarked by high titres of anti-dsDNA antibodies and hypocomplimentaemia

CONFUSA

- Lupus nephritis is more common in females because the overall prevalence of SLE is higher in females (ie, female-to-male ratio of 9:1); however, males with SLE have an increased prevalence of clinical renal disease with a worse prognosis.
- In any young female with features of acute renal failure with rash/ arthritis, don't forget to rule out SLE as an important cause.

Investigation of Choice

- Antibodies to double stranded DNA and the antinuclear antibody anti-Sm are highly specific for SLE.
- Measure disease activity with anti-dsDNA, complement determinations (C3, C4, and CH_{50}), and erythrocyte sedimentation rate (ESR) or C-reactive protein.
- Renal function tests
- Renal biopsy should be considered for any patient with SLE who has clinical or laboratory evidence of active nephritis, especially with the first episode of nephritis.

Immediate Management

- Protein and fat restricted diet
- Hypertension- ACE inhibitors
- Osteoporosis (usually steroid induced) - calcium supplementation
- Avoid pregnancy
- Avoid nephrotoxic drugs
- Corticosteroids are mainstay of treatment for lupus nephritis. Immunosuppressive agents, especially cyclophosphamide, azathioprine, or mycophenolate mofetil, are used if the patient has aggressive proliferative renal lesions or if the patient has an inadequate response or excessive sensitivity to corticosteroids.

Treatment of Choice

Hemodialysis
Renal transplantation

Your notes:

Autoantibodies in SLE:

- antibodies to ds-DNA and the ANA anti-Sm, are highly specific for SLE but are poor "markers" because of their low prevalences, 50-70% and 7-30%
- anti-Ro and anti-La antinuclear antibodies occur in both SLE and Sjögren's syndrome
- anti-Ro is important in pregnancy since it is associated with babies born with congenital heart block
- anti U1 ribonucleoprotein, formerly, anti-RNP, is not specific for SLE
- anti-histone antibodies indicate drug induced SLE
- anti-cardiolipin is associated with thrombosis (arterial or venous), chorea, and livedo reticularis

Serial No. 153

Subject: Medicine

Topic: Headache

Question: A patient presents with unilateral temporal headache.

Diagnosis: Temporal arteritis

Clinchers

➢ *Unilateral temporal headache:* Headache, is the most universal symptom, present in with temporal arteritis and there are certain features in temporal arteritis headache which distinguishes it from other types of headaches:

- Headache most commonly tends to be unilateral, classically concentrating on the temporal region.
- Its insidious in onset typically worse at night.
- Underlying pain described as a burning or jabbing sensation may involve the surface of the scalp and face. Intracranial arteries are rarely involved.
- Scalp tenderness is typical -simple acts such as combing hair or resting the head on a pillow exacerbate pain.

CONFUSA

GMC is in the habit to provide us with such minimum information in a question that for few seconds we think in bewilderment that a unilateral temporal headache can be caused by any or all of the causes listed in the options. However, if you look carefully you can easily rule out other possibilities.

- An absence of history of injury rules out all types skull fractures as a probable cause.
- An absence of typical aura associated with migraine, rules out that possibility too.
- Again, absence of features of papilloedema or neurological deficits rules out intracranial space occupying lesion as the probable cause.
- Takayasu's arteritis typically involves main branches of aorta.

Investigation of Choice

ESR

Temopral artery biopsy

Immediate Management

Sudden loss of vision is an ophthalmological emergency and requires immediate referral to the eye emergency department (may require upto 1 mg/kg of prednisolone per day).

Treatment of Choice

In the absence of visual symptoms, giant cell arteritis is treated with 30-40 mg per day of prednisolone.

Your notes:

Serial No. 166

Subject: Medicine

Topic: Connective tissue diseases

Question: A 27-year-old female with sharp chest pain, which becomes worse on coughing or taking deep breaths. She has a red rash over her cheeks and nose.

Diagnosis: SLE

Clinchers

- *27-year-old female:* SLE is eight times more common in females affecting mainly women between 15 and 40 years of age. More common in Afro-Carribean, Asians and Chinese.
- *Sharp chest pain, chest pain which becomes worse on coughing or taking deep breaths:*This is typically describing pleurisy occurring due to inflammation of the pleura. Very common pulmonary manifestation of SLE. Lungs can also be affected in the form of pleural effusion, pericardial effusion, interstitial pneumonia and the 'small lung syndrome'.
- *Red rash over her cheeks and nose:*The 'butterfly rash' (rash over the butterfly area of face- cheeks and the nose) is the most common dermatological manifestation of SLE. However, this rash can also be present on other sun exposed areas like hands, wrists, etc.

CONFUSA

Diagnosis of SLE is based on the following criteria proposed by The American Rheumatism Association, of which at least 4 must be present:

- Malar rash
- Discoid rash
- Oral/nasopharyngeal ulcers
- Photosensitivity
- Arthritis - non-erosive
- Serositis - pleuritis or pericarditis
- Renal disease - proteinuria > 0.5 g/day or cellular casts
- Neurologic disease - seizures, psychosis
- Haemtologic disease - haemolytic anaemia, leukopenia, lymphopenia, thrombocytopenia
- Immunologic disease - anti-DNA, anti-Sm, LE, false positive serology for syphilis (> 6 months duration)
- Positive antinuclear antibodies in absence of drug induced lupus

Investigation of Choice

There is no single test; see the criteria listed above in confusa.

Immediate Management

Mild disease may respond to rest and NSAIDs

Treatment of Choice

Corticosteroid therapy

Your notes:

Serial No. 167

Subject: Medicine

Topic: Connective tissue diseases

Question: A 45-year-old male presents with chest pain and joint pains. He also complains of dry gritty eyes.

Diagnosis: Sjögren's syndrome

Clinchers

- *45-year-old male:* Sjögren's syndrome commonly affects females (9 times more than males) of 35-45 years age, but can appear anytime between 15 and 65 years of age.
- *Chest pain and joint pains:* Dry secretions in the chest may predipose individuals to variety of complications, especially infections. The musculoskeletal involvement can occur in the form of arthralgia, myalgia and fatigue.
- *Dry gritty eyes:* Dry eyes and mouth are the most common presenting symptoms and are essential for the diagnosis. It occurs due to lymphocytic infiltration of lacrimal and salivary glands respectively.

CONFUSA

- Reiters disease also present with arthralgia and 'gritty' eyes. However, the grittiness is more associated with the underlying conjunctivitis. Most patients also give the history of associated urethritis or gastroenteritis. There appears to be a strong association with HLA B27 (~75%) and other seronegative arthropathies.

Investigation of Choice

Schrimer test

Salivary gland or lip biopsy can also be undertaken.

Immediate Management

Symptomatic

Tear substitutes

saliva substitutes.

Systemic cholinergic agonists for symptomatic treatment of dryness.

NSAIDs for arthralgia

Treatment of Choice

Steroids and immunosuppressive agents

Your notes:

Serial No. 168

Subject: Medicine

Topic: Connective tissue diseases

Question: A 39-year-old lady presents with dull ache in the chest and arthritis. Chest X-ray shows bilateral enlarged hilar lymph nodes.

Diagnosis: Sarcoidosis

Clinchers

- *39-year-old lady:* Sarcoidosis affects women more than men and usually present at the age of 20-40 years. However, it can effect population of any age group.
- *Dull ache in the chest:* Lungs are the most common organ involved in sarcoidosis, affecting more than 90% patients. Pulmonary affection is usually in the form of dry cough, occasional hemoptysis and dyspnoea on exertion.
- *Arthritis:* Musculoskeletal involvement is in the form of asymmetrical arthopathy, commonly involving the knee and ankle joints.
- *Bilateral enlarged hilar lymph nodes:* This is the most important pathological finiding observed in sarcoidosis. For any adult female with features like dry cough and chest pain with systemic features of malaise, low grade fever and hilar lymphadenopathy on CXR, sarcoidosis should be ruled out.

CONFUSA

Pulmonary tuberculosis also presents with low grade fever, malaise and weight loss. Even hilar lymphadenopathy can be observed on CXR. However, the cough in tuberculosis is productive, with occasional hemoptysis. Travel history or recent migration from tuberculosis endemic regions like asia, will also provide necessary clues to make a diagnosis of tuberculosis.

Investigation of Choice

Transbronchial biopsy to demonstrate presence of non-caseating granulomas is required for definitve diagnosis.

Chest X ray for screening

Gallium scan for staging.

Immediate Management

None spontaneous remission occurs in 90% of patients with only bilateral hilar lymphadenopathy and 50% of patients with bilateral hilar lymphadenopathy and pulmonary shadowing

Treatment of Choice

Prednisolone 20-40 mg per 24 h PO for 4-6 weeks, in cases of persistent or deteriorating disease.

PAPER 2

Serial No. 11

Subject: Paediatrics

Topic: Rash

Question: A 7-year-old child with cervical lymphadenopathy, conjunctivitis and a rash on hand which started to peel after the fifth day.

Diagnosis: Kawasaki's disease

Clinchers

- *7 year old child:* Kawasaki disease is a febrile systemic vasculitis predominantly affecting children under the age of 5. The highest incidence is in Japan but is becoming increasingly recognised in the West.
- *Cervical lymphadenopathy:* Acute, non-purulent cervical lymphadenopathy is present in more than 60% and considered as one of the major features of the disease, required for the diagnosis of the condition.
- *Conjunctivitis:* This is also one of the major feature of Kawasaki's disease and present as bilateral non-purulent conjunctival congestion.
- *Rash on hand which started to peel after the fifth day:* The rash is typically polymorphous appearing from days 1 to 5 of the fever; without any vesicles or crusts

CONFUSA

Major features include:
- Fever more than 5 days
- Bilateral non-purulent conjunctival congestion
- Dry, fissured mouth and lips and a strawberry red tongue
- Acute, non-purulent cervical lymphadenopathy in more than 60%
- Polymorphous exanthema for days 1 to 5 of the fever; typically there are no vesicles or crusts

Pulmonary tuberculosis also presents with low grade fever, malaise and weight loss. Even hilar lymphadenopathy can be observed on CXR. However, the cough in tuberculosis is productive, with occasional haemoptysis. Travel history or recent migration from tuberculosis endemic regions like asia, will also provide necessary clues to make a diagnosis of tuberculosis.

Investigation of Choice

Nonspecific changes
-thrombocytosis
-raised ESR/C-reactive protein
-raised bilirubin
-raised transaminases
-raised alpha2- globulin
Follow-up- Echocardiograms

Immediate Management

Consult expert advice

Treatment of Choice

Intravenous immunoglobulin
Aspirin: 30 mg/kg/day in divided doses for 2 weeks
Plasmapheresis

Your notes:

PAPER 3

77. An 82-year-old woman complains of stiffness and muscle pain to the point where she is finding it difficult to brush her hair and get out of a chair. She now presents with sudden loss of vision in her left eye.

Diagnosis: Polymyalgia rheumatica (PMR)

Clinchers

- *82-year-old:* The patient of PMR is always over 50 years.
- *Weakness and muscle pain:* PMR causes a sudden onset of severe pain and stiffness of the shoulders and neck, and of the hips and lumbar spine (a limb girdle pattern).
- *Finding it difficult to brush her hair:* This implies a shoulder girdle weakness as she has difficulty lifting her hand overhead.
- *Difficulty getting out of chair:* This implies a hip girdle weakness.
- *Sudden loss of vision in her left eye:* PMR is associated with temporal arteritis in 25% of people (the patient may have current PMR, a history of rencet PMR, or be on treatment for PMR). Involvement of the ophthalmic arteritis in temporal arteritis causes sudden painless temporary and permanent visual loss.

CONFUSA

It is often difficult to remember the differentiating clinical features of common 'PLAB' myopathies. Here is a refreshes:
Polymyositis—proximal pain and weakness
PMR—Proximal morning stiffness and pain
Myopathy—No pain, no stiffness, only weakness

Investigation of Choice

ESR and/or CRP.

Immediate Management

Ophthalmology referral urgently.

Treatment of Choice

Prednisolone high dose IV immediately.

Your notes:

111. A middle-aged woman with a history of rheumatoid arthritis develops sudden swelling in one of her knees. This knee is swollen and hot to touch.

Diagnosis: Pseudogout.

Clinchers

- *Middle-aged:* Though pseudogout occurs more commonly in old age, no age after thirties is exempt from it.
- *Woman:* There is a slight preponderance of female incidence.
- *Sudden swelling in one of her knees:* Knee is the main joint to get involved in it. A minority will have involvement of multiple joints.
- *This knee is swollen and hot to touch:* involved joint is erythematous, swollen, warm and painful.
- *History of rheumatoid arthritis:* Any existing arthritis is a risk factor for pseudogout. Other risk factors are old age, dehydration, intercurrent illness, hyperparathyroidism, myxoedema, diabetes mellitus, phosphate decrease, magnesium deficiency, hemochromatosis, acromegaly, gout, ochronosis, surgery.

CONFUSA

Acute pseudogout is less severe and longer lasting than gout and affects different joints. Pseudogout can even be secondary to gout. It cannot be septic arthritis also as there is no preceding history of joint trauma of presence of fever.

Investigation of Choice

- *Screening:* Wrist X-ray (calcium deposition in triangular ligament or chondrocalcinosis)
- *Definitive:* Joint fluid aspiration and microscopy (positively birefringent calcium pyrophosphate crystals in plane polarised light).

Immediate Management

Analgesia.

Treatment of Choice

NSAIDs ± intra-articular injection of glucocorticoids ± colchicine.

Your notes:

112. An elderly man with recently diagnosed heart failure has been treated with diuretics. He now develops severe joint pain in his left ankle with swelling and redness.

Diagnosis: Gout (acute attack).

Clinchers

- *Diuretics:* Attacks of gout can be precipitated by:
  - Trauma
  - Surgery/some antibiotics
  - Starvation/purine rich foods (liver, offal, oily fish)
  - Infection
  - Diuretics
  - Alcohol
- *Severe joint pain in his left ankle:* Gout produces an acute inflammatory arthritis which is exquisitely painful monoarthritis (usually) but can be polyarticular also. It is often accompanied by fever. It usually affects the distal joints of the hands and feet and the knees. It particularly (and characteristically) affects the metatarso-phalangeal joints of the great toes.
- *Swelling and redness of ankle:* In acute attacks the affected joints, usually single, become severely painful, swollen, often red and impossible to move. This usually settles in less than three weeks.

CONFUSA

Gout is a chronic disease, but is characterised by acute attacks. Predisposing conditions to gout can be blood dyscrasias such as myeloid leukaemia and polycythaemia. Most common extra-articular complication of gout is recurrent renal stones. Paradoxically renal failure can be a cause for gout.

Investigation of Choice

Synovial fluid microscopy (urate crystals—negatively birefringent).

Immediate Management

Pain relief by NSAID (Ibuprofen/Naproxen)

- If NSAID contraindicated—colchicine
- If cholchicine contraindicated—streroids

Treatment of Choice

Allopurinol (but not until 3 weeks after an attack).

Note: Aspirin is absolutely contraindicated in gout.

Your notes:

113. A 78-year-old woman complains of a stiff left hip joint after walking some distance. This is most evident when she attempts to abduct the hip joint (limited abduction).

Diagnosis: Osteoarthritis (OA).

Clinchers

- *78-year-old woman:* The mean age of onset of OA is 5 years. OA is sympatomatic three times more in women.
- *Shift hip joint after walking some distance:* Typically in OA, there is pain on movement. It is usually worse at end of day. There may be some background pain at rest.
- *Limited adduction of hip joint:* There can be stiffness of the joint which limits the movements (poor range of movements). There can be associated joint instability. Joints affected in OA
  - Most commonly: DIP joints, first MCP joint, cervical and lumbar spine
  - Next most common: Hip joint
  - Other most common: Knee joint.

CONFUSA

Lets have a good look at the differentiating features of osteoarthritis and rheumatoid arthritis, the two most common arthritis of elderly females

	OA	*RA*
Joint stiffness	Late evening	Early evening
Palpable osteophytes	+	-
Skin redness	+/-	+
Swelling	+/-	+
Ligaments stretch	-	+
Age	Usually older	Usually adolescents
Arthrodesis use	Good	Poor
Fibrillation	+	-
Pannus	-	+
Bone arround joint	Sclerotic	Osteoporotic
Joint deformity	Varus	Valgus

Investigation of Choice

Joint X-ray (findings: loss of joint space, subchondral sclerosis, subchondral cysts, marginal osteophytes).

Immediate Management

Paracetamol for pain.

Treatment of Choice

Reduce weight + walking aid
  - Contralateral hand—for hip
  - Ipsilateral hand—for knee
- Joint replacement is done for end stage disease.
- If PCM does not bring relief from pain, then give
  - Day pain—NSAID
  - Night pain—TCA in low doses (tricyclic antidepressant)

114. A 34-year-old woman complains of bilateral stiff and painful joints in her hands and feet.

Diagnosis: Rheumatoid arthritis (RA)

Clinchers

- *34-year-old woman:* Although the peak onset of RA is fifth decade, no age is exempt from it. The incidence of RA is three times more in women.
- *Bilateral:* RA is a symmetrical arthropathy, i.e. affect the same joints bilaterally.
- *Stiff and painful joints in her hands and feet:* RA presents typically with swollen, painful and stiff hands and feet, especially in the morning. This gradually gets and feet, especially in the morning. This gradually gets worse and large joints become involved

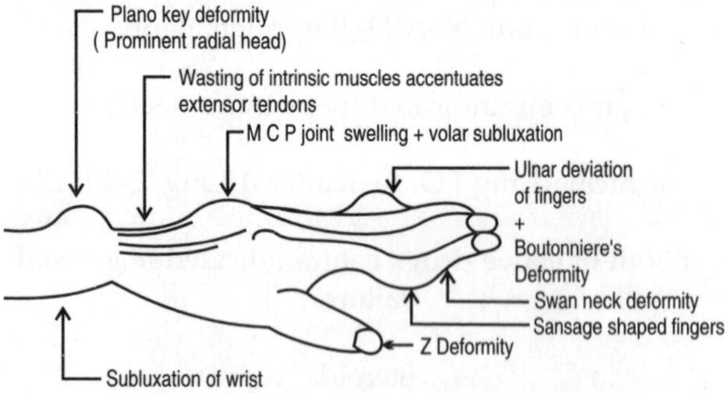

"Handy" thesaurus for signs of RA

CONFUSA

In the PLAB exams, Felty's syndrome has been indirectly asked on at least a couple of occasions. So always keep an eye open for any mention of splenomegaly in a patient of RA.
(Felty's syndrome: RA + Splenomegaly + WCC $^{-}$)

Investigation of Choice

Rheumatoid factor often negative at start, but becomes positive in 80% over the time. But note that it may be false positive in several other chronic diseases.

Immediate Management

Analgesia.

Treatment of Choice

- Naproxen/Ibuprofen
- Disease modifying drugs if:
  - 12 week trial of 3 NSAIDs do not control pain.
  - Synovitis > 2 months.

Your notes:

124. A 23-year-old woman has a history of a termination of pregancy at 12 weeks. She subsequently suffers a spontaneous miscarriage after 22 weeks of pregnancy. She has history of deep vein thrombosis (DVT).

Diagnosis: Antiphospholipid syndrome.

Clinchers

- *History of termination of pregnancy at 12 weeks and now suffer with miscarriage at 22 weeks:* Untreated < 20% of pregnancies proceed to live birth in antiphospholipid syndrome. This is due to:
  - First trimester loss
  - Placental thrombosis causing placental insufficiency leading to:
    - Intrauterine growth retardation and
    - Fetal death
- *History of DVT:* Apart from recurrent pregnancy loss history of arterial thrombosis/venous thrombosis supports the diagnosis of DVT.

Investigation of Choice

Lupus plasma marker.

Treatment of Choice

Careful regular foetal assessment (Doppler flow studies and ulstrasound for growth are required for 20 weeks). Treat affected woman from conception with aspirin 75 mg daily (heparin SC/12 h until 34 weeks improves outcome). In this question since she has suffered from prior thrombosis, she should be given Warfarin (may cause abnormal foetal cartilage development) or heparin (causes maternal osteoporosis).
Some recommend
Heparin—first trimester
Warfarin—thereafter until time of delivery.
Use one of these postpartum as risk of thrombosis is high.

Your notes:

PAPER 4

122. An elderly female with scalp tenderness on both sides of the head, complains of headache, sudden loss of vision in one eye.

Diagnosis: Giant cell arteritis (GCA)

Clinchers

- *Elderly females:* Common in elderly (rare under 55 years). More incidence in females.
- *Scalp tenderness:* Pain is felt over the inflamed superficial, temporal or occipital arteries. Touching the skin over the inflamed vessel (e.g. combing the hair) causes pain. Arterial pulsation is soon lost and the artery becomes hard, tortuous and thickened. The skin over the vessels may become red. Rarely, gangrenous patches appear on the scalp.
- *Headache:* Invariably present in GCA because of arteritis.
- *Sudden loss of vision in one eye:* Visual loss owing to inflammation and occlusion of the ciliary and/or central retinal artery occurs in 25% of cases of untreated GCA. The patient complains of sudden uniocular visual loss, either partial or complete, which is painless. Amaurosis fugax may precede total visual loss, which is usually permanent, if the transient loss of vision lasts more than an hour.

CONFUSA

Do not think that GCA is only confined to arteries of the scalp. There is always associated inflammation of other branches of the external carotid (i.e. facial, maxillary and lingual) and their involvement produces clinically important features, e.g. jaw claudication (pain worse or eating), painful opening of mouth, painful movements of tongue, etc.

Investigation of Choice

- *Screening:* ESR
- *Definitive:* Temporal artery biopsy

Immediate Management

IV steroid (since visual symptoms are present)

Treatment of Choice

Prednisolone 60-100 mg (i.e. high dose) for 2 years

Note: Headache subsides within hours of the first large dose of steroid.

Your notes:

153. Patient with hot swollen metatarsal joint, pain does not decrease with paracetamol.

Diagnosis: Acute gout

Clinchers

- *Hot swollen metatarsal joint:* Involvement of this joint is almost pathognomic of gout and is known publically as *podagra*. In acute stage there is severe pain, redness and swelling in the affected joint. Attack is due to deposition of sodium monourate crystals in joints.
- *Does not decrease with paracetamol:* Usually the pain of gout is severe and does not respond to simple analgesia. NSAIDs are often required. But note that aspirin is contraindicated as it increases serum urate.

CONFUSA

Here is the UK protocol of treatment of an episode of acute gout: NSAID (Ibuprofen, naproxen)

↓

If contraindicated (peptic ulcers, etc)

↓

Colchicine 1 mg PO, thereafter 0.5 mg/2-3 h PO

↓

If both of above drugs contraindicated (e.g. renal failure)

↓

Steroids

Investigation of Choice

Synovial fluid microscopy (negatively birefringent crystals and neutrophils with ingested crystals).

Immediate Management

Pain relief

Treatment of Choice

NSAIDs.

Your notes:

154. Pregnant woman with numbness, tingling on lateral side of hand.

Diagnosis: Carpal tunnel syndrome (CTS)

Clinchers

- *Pregnancy:* CTS is associated with
  - Pregnancy
  - Rheumatoid arthritis
  - DM
  - Hypothyroidism
  - Dialysis
  - Trauma
- *Numbness, tingling on lateral side of hand:* There is aching pain in the hand and arm (especially at night), and paraesthesiae in the thumb, index and middle fingers (lateral side of hand in anatomical position).

CONFUSA

The paraesthesiae and pain in CTS are relieved by dangling the hand over the edge of the bed and shaking it. There may be sensory loss and weakness of abductor pollicis brevis with associated wasting of thenar eminence. Light touch, two point discrimination and sweating may be impaired.

Investigation of Choice

Neurophysiology (to assess axonal degeneration and find level of brim)

Immediate Management

Phalen test or tinel test can be used on screening tests but are unreliable.

Treatment of Choice

Splinting ± Yoga (Namaste posture)

If the symptoms do not improve after pregnancy, the following may be used

- Local hydrocortisone injection
- Surgical decompression

Your notes:

PAPER 5

16. A 78-year-old man has had a painful scalp and headache for three weeks, and is generally unwell, complains of acute onset of blindness in his right eye.

Diagnosis: Temporal arteritis

Clinchers

- *Painful scalp and headache:* Interruption of blood flow to visual cortex causes sudden greying of vision, and other symptoms that mimic migraine.

  Transient mono-ocular blindness usually occurs from a retinal embolus or severe ipsilateral carotid stenosis.
- *Acute onset blindness in right eye:* Anterior ischaemic optic neuropathy (AION) is an infarction of the optic nerve head due to inadequate perfusion via the posterior ciliary arteries. Patient has sudden loss, often upon awakening, and painless swelling of the optic disc. Arteric AION is caused by *temporal arteritis.*

CONFUSA

Malignant hypertension can cause visual loss from exudates, haemorrhages, cotton wool spots (focal nerve fibre layer infarct) and optic disc oedema.

Investigation of Choice

Visual field mapping

Ophthalmoscopy

ESR

Immediate Management

Immediate glucocorticoid therapy

Treatment of Choice

Glucocorticoid therapy for at least 2 years.

Your notes:

166. A 29-year-old man with known arthritis presented with a painful red eye and a brownish rash on his feet. He has recently been treated for dysentery.

Diagnosis: Reiter's syndrome

Clinchers

- *29-year-old man:* The sex ratio following enteric infection is 1:1, but genitourinary acquired reactive arthritis is predominantly seen in young males.
- *Known arthritis + painful red eye:* Reiter's syndrome describes the triad of arthritis, conjunctivitis, and non-gonococcal urethritis or enteritis (mnemonic: cannot see, cannot pree, cannot climb a tree).
- *Brownish rash on his feet:* Mucocutaneous lesions are seen in approximately one-third of patients. These are cutaneous vesicles that become hyperkeratotic, most common on soles and palms.
- *Recently been treated for dysentery:* In individuals with appropriate genetic background (HLA-B27 positivity), reactive arthritis, *Shigella, Salmonella, Yersinia* and *Campylobacter enteritis.*

CONFUSA

Differential diagnosis is from septic arthritis (gram +/-) gonococcal arthritis, crystalline arthritis, psoriatic arthritis.

Investigation of Choice
Stool cultures.

Immediate Management
HIV screening (required in all patients).

Treatment of Choice
Symptomatic.

Your notes:

167. A 30-year-old woman presented to the family GP complaining of difficulty in lifting her arms up. She also reported having difficulty getting up and down stairs. A scaly, erythematous rash was noticed on the dorsum of the hand, and knuckles. She had earlier complained dysphagia.

Diagnosis: Dermatomyositis.

Clinchers

- *30-year-old woman:* The disease may develop at any age. Affected females outnumber males by 2:1.
- *Difficulty in lifting her arms up:* Patient first become aware of weakness of the proximal limb muscles. When shoulder girdle muscles are involved, placing an object on a high shelf or combing the hair becomes difficult.
- *Difficulty getting up and down stairs:* Hip girdle weakness causes difficulty in arising from the squatting or kneeling position and in climbing or descending stairs.
- *Scaly, erythematous rash was noticed on dorsum of hand and knuckles:* The classic iliac-coloured (heliotrope) rash is on the eyelids, bridge of nose, cheeks (butterfly distribution) forehead, chest elbows, knees and knuckles, and around the nail beds.
- *Dysphagia:* At presentation 25% of patients have dysphagia.

CONFUSA

Dermatomyositis and polymyositis are conditions of presumed autoimmune aetiology in which the skeletal muscle is damaged by a nonsuppurative inflammatory process dominated by lymphocytic infiltration. The term polymyositis is applied when the condition spares the skin, and the term dermatomyositis when polymyositis is associated with a characteristic skin rash.

Investigation of Choice

- *Screening:* Muscle enzyme (CK) levels
- *Definitive:* Muscle biopsy.

Immediate Management
Exclude retinitis (cotton wool patches).

Treatment of Choice
Rest + prednisolone.

168. A mother brought her 10-year-old son to the GP, with a history of joint pains and recurrent oral ulcers. On examination the boy had hypopyon and mild conjuctivitis.

Diagnosis: Behcet's syndrome.

Clinchers

- *10-year-old son:* It predominantly presents in adolescent males.
- *Joint pains and recurrent oral ulcers:* Behcet's syndrome represents a triad of arthritis, ocular symptoms (pain, visual loss, floaters, irits, hpopyon, retinal vein occlusion) and painful ulcers in mouth, scrotum or labia (Mnemonic: Cannot see, cannot pee, cannot eat spicy curry).
- *Hypopyon and mild conjunctivitis:* Confirms our suspicion of Behcet's syndrome.

CONFUSA

Apart from above mentioned symptoms, GIT involvement as colitis may be present. CNS manifestations can be meningoencephalitis, - IVP, brainstem signs, dementia, myelopathy, encephalopathy, cerebral vein thrombosis, etc.

Investigation of Choice

HLA-B5/51 screening.

Immediate Management

Specialist referral.

Treatment of Choice

Colchicine, steroids (topical ± oral), cyclosporin, and chlorambucil have been used.

Your notes:

170. A 30-year-old woman presented with tender, red nodules on both lower limbs and forearms. She had painful joints and was febrile. She had a month history of a productive cough and investigations revealed raised, angiotensin converting enzyme levels.

Diagnosis: Sarcoidosis.

Clinchers

- *30-year-old woman:* The peak incidence is in the third and fourth decade with a female preponderance.
- *Tender, red nodules on both lower limbs and forearms:* This is erythema nodosum of which sarcoidosis is the most common cause:
- *Painful joints:* Arthralgia is common in it and can be presenting feature.
- *Was febrile:* 4% of patients present with fever (in UK).
- *Month's history of productive cough:* Dry or productive cough (an secondary infection) with progressive dyspnoea and chest pain are the most common pulmonary manifestations.
- *Raised ACE levels:* This is characteristic and is two standard deviations above the normal mean value in over 75% of patients with untreated sarcoidosis.

CONFUSA

The Kveim test, which involved as intradermal injection of sarcoid tissue, was regularly used for confirmation of the diagnosis. It should not be used because of the risk of transmission of infection. It is less sensitive and less specific than transbronchial biopsy which has superceded it. Patients with bilateral hilar lymphadenopathy alone do not require treatment.

Investigation of Choice

- *Screening:*
  CXR
  Serum ACE levels (-)
- *Definitive:* Transbronchial biopsy.

Immediate Management

Lung function tests

Treatment of Choice

Acute sarcoidosis: Bed-rest + NSAIDs + corticosteroids.

Note: Corticosteroids should be given only if needed, i.e. in

- Parenchymal lung disease
- Uveitis
- Hypercalcaemia
- Neurological or cardiac involvement.

PAPER 6

6. A 78-year-old man has had a painful scalp and headache for three weeks, and is generally unwell, complains of acute onset of blindness in his right eye.

Diagnosis: Temporal arteritis

Clinchers

- *Painful scalp and headache:* Interruption of blood flow to visual cortex causes sudden greying of vision, and other symptoms that mimic migraine.

  Transient monoocular blindness usually occurs from a retinal embolus or severe ipsilateral carotid stenosis.
- *Acute onset blindness in right eye:* Anterior ischaemic optic neuropathy (AION) is an infarction of the optic nerve head due to inadequate perfusion via the posterior ciliary arteries. Patient has sudden loss, often upon awakening, and painless swelling of the optic disc. Arteric AION is caused by *temporal arteritis.*

CONFUSA

Malignant hypertension can cause visual loss from exudates, haemorrhages, cotton wool spots (focal nerve fibre layer infarct) and optic disc oedema.

Investigation of Choice

Visual field mapping
Ophthalmoscopy
ESR

Immediate Management

Immediate glucocorticoid therapy

Treatment of Choice

Glucocorticoid therapy for at least 2 years.

Your notes:

147. An 82-year-old woman complains of stiffness and muscle pain to the point where she is finding it difficult to brush her hair and get out of a chair. She now presents with sudden loss of vision in her left eye.

Diagnosis: Polymyalgia rheumatica (PMR)

Clinchers

- *82-year-old:* The patient of PMR is always over 50 years.
- *Weakness and muscle pain:* PMR causes a sudden onset of severe pain and stiffness of the shoulders and neck, and of the hips and lumbar spine (a limb girdle pattern).
- *Finding it difficult to brush her hair:* This implies a shoulder girdle weakness as she has difficulty lifting her hand overhead.
- *Difficulty getting out of chair:* This implies a hip girdle weakness.
- *Sudden loss of vision in her left eye:* PMR is associated with temporal arteritis in 25% of people (the patient may have current PMR, a history of rencet PMR, or be on treatment for PMR). Involvement of the ophthalmic arteritis in temporal arteritis causes sudden painless temporary and permanent visual loss.

CONFUSA

It is often difficult to remember the differentiating clinical features of common 'PLAB' myopathies. Here is a refreshes:
Polymyositis—proximal pain and weakness
PMR—Proximal morning stiffness and pain
Myopathy—No pain, no stiffness, only weakness

Investigation of Choice

ESR and/or CRP.

Immediate Management

Ophthalmology referral urgently.

Treatment of Choice

Prednisolone high dose IV immediately.

Your notes:

158. A 25-year-old woman has just been diagnosed a having rheumatoid arthritis and her rheumatologist has begun giving her gold injections. She continues to complain of joint pain and stiffness, particularly for the first two hours of each day.

Diagnosis: Rheumatoid arthritis (RA).

Clinchers

- *25-year-old:* RA presents from early childhood (rare) to late old age. The most common age of onset is between 30 and 50 years.
- *Woman:* Women before menopause are affected three times more often than men. After the menopause the frequency of onset is similar between the sexes.
- *Gold injections:* gold is a disease modifying anti-rheumatic drug (DMARD). Usually DMARDs are used after symptomatic treatment, but in seropositive patients with a poor prognosis they should be used early, before the appearance of erosions on X-rays of hands and feet. DMARDs are only prescribed by a rheumatologist in UK. DMARDs exert minimal direct nonspecific anti-inflammatory or analgesic effects, and therefore NSAIDs must be continued during their administration (except in few cases when the true remissions are induced with them).
- *Continues to complain of joint pain and stiffness:* As already explained, DMARDs have very poor analgesic action and NSAIDs have to be given with them. Moreover NSAIDs produce symptomatic improvement in morning stiffness.
- *Particularly in the first two hours of each day:* This is an indirect way to describe the pathognomonic morning stiffness.

CONFUSA

The cheapest and most safe (in terms of propensity to cause GI bleed). NSAID is ibuprofen. Naproxen is an alternative and advantageous in having only twice daily dosage and being more anti-inflammatory. Diclofenac can also be given. NSAIDs should be combined with a gastroprotection agent (proton pump inhibitor or prostaglandin analogue misoprostol) if there is—

- History of
  - peptic ulcer disease
  - dyspepsia.
- Age > 70
- Taking
  - steroids
  - aspirin.

Note: Avoid NSAIDs

- On warfarin
- Active peptic ulcer disease
- Asthma

Investigation of Choice

Rheumatoid factor (often negative initially, if positive at onset, the treatment plan differs—see above).

Immediate Management

Physiotherapy referral for exercise programmes.

Treatment of Choice

Oral NSAIDs

171. A 73-year-old complains of a severe right sided headache associated with an acute loss of right sided vision. Urgent treatment is needed to prevent left sided vision loss.

Diagnosis: Giant cell arteritis (GCA).

Clinchers
- ➢ *73-year-old:* Cranial arteritis is common after 55 years of age (60 years according to Kumar and Clark).
- ➢ *Severe right sided headache:* Headache is almost invariable in GCA. Pain is felt over the inflamed superficial, temporal or occipital arteries. Though the disease process ultimately involves arteries bilaterally, in the initial stages it is usually unilateral.
- ➢ *Associated with an acute loss of right sided vision:* Visual loss owing to inflammation and occlusion of the ciliary and/or central retinal artery occurs in 25% of cases and untreated GCA. It is characteristically sudden, painless, partial or complete, uniocular visual loss. Amaurosis fugax may precede total visual loss.
- ➢ *Urgent treatment is needed to prevent left sided vision loss:* Urgent GCA patients need to have an ESR and high dose. Oral steroids immediately. However if visual symptoms are present, give higher doses IV as it could be sight saving.

CONFUSA

Other forms of arteritis, such as SLE and PAN, can occasionally present with similar featurs (but PLAB questions on GCA are usually straight forward). Also note that GCA is closely related to polymyalgia rheumatica and these can occur in the same patient.

Investigation of Choice
- *Screening:* ESR.
- *Definitive:* Temporal artery biopsy (skip lesions occur, so repeat any negative biopsy if there are strong clinical pointers)

Immediate Management

Two things are to be done immediately
1. ESR
2. High dose oral steroids (IV if visual symptoms).

Treatment of Choice

Prednisolone, 40-60 mg/24 h, PO
- Dose is reduced as ESR falls/is increased if symptoms recurs.
- Headache subsides within hours of first large dose.
- Remission in 2 years usually.
- Steroid treatment is the main cause of death in long-term in GCA patients.

176. A middle-aged woman with a history of rheumatoid arthritis develops sudden swelling in One of her knees. This knee is swollen and hot to touch.

Diagnosis: Pseudogout.

Clinchers
- ➢ *Middle-aged:* Though pseudogout occurs more commonly in old age, no age after thirties is exempt from it.
- ➢ *Woman:* There is a slight preponderance of female incidence.
- ➢ *Sudden swelling in one of her knees:* Knee is the main joint to get involved in it. A minority will have involvement of multiple joints.
- ➢ *This knee is swollen and hot to touch:* involved joint is erythematous, swollen, warm and painful.
- ➢ *History of rheumatoid arthritis:* Any existing arthritis is a risk factor for pseudogout. Other risk factors are old age, dehydration, intercurrent illness, hyperparathyroidism, myxoedema, diabetes mellitus, phosphate decrease, magnesium deficiency, haemochromatosis, acromegaly, gout, ochronosis, surgery.

CONFUSA

Acute pseudogout is less severe and longer lasting than gout and affects different joints. Pseudogout can even be secondary to gout. It cannot be septic arthritis also as there is no preceding history of joint trauma of presence of fever.

Investigation of Choice
- *Screening:* Wrist X-ray (calcium deposition in triangular ligament or chondrocalcinosis)
- *Definitive:* Joint fluid aspiration and microscopy (positively birefringent calcium pyrophosphate crystals in plane polarised light).

Immediate Management

Analgesia.

Treatment of Choice

NSAIDs ± intra-articular injection of glucocorticoids ± colchicine.

Your notes:

177. An elderly man with recently diagnosed heart failure has been treated with diuretics. He now develops severe joint pain in his left ankle with swelling and redness.

Diagnosis: Gout (acute attack).

Clinchers

- *Diuretics:* Attacks of gout can be precipitated by:
  - Trauma
  - Surgery/some antibiotics
  - Starvation/purine rich foods (liver, offal, oily fish)
  - Infection
  - Diuretics
  - Alcohol
- *Severe joint pain in his left ankle:* Gout produces an acute inflammatory arthritis which is exquisitely painful monoarthritis (usually) but can be polyarticular also. It is often accompanied by fever. It usually affects the distal joints of the hands and feet and the knees. It particularly (and characteristically) affects the metatarsophalangeal joints of the great toes.
- *Swelling and redness of ankle:* In acute attacks the affected joints, usually single, become severely painful, swollen, often red and impossible to move. This usually settles in less than three weeks.

CONFUSA

Gout is a chronic disease, but is characterised by acute attacks. Predisposing conditions to gout can be blood dyscrasias such as myeloid leukaemia and polycythaemia. Most common extra-articular complication of gout is recurrent renal stones. Paradoxically renal failure can be a cause for gout.

Investigation of Choice

Synovial fluid microscopy (urate crystals—negatively birefringent).

Immediate Management

Pain relief by NSAID (Ibuprofen/Naproxen)

- If NSAID contraindicated—colchicine
- If cholchicine contraindicated—stereoids

Treatment of Choice

Allopurinol (but not until 3 weeks after an attack).

Note: Aspirin is absolutely contraindicated in gout.

Your notes:

178. A 78-year-old woman complains of a stiff left hip joint after walking some distance. This is most evident when she attempts to abduct the hip joint (limited abduction).

Diagnosis: Osteoarthritis (OA).

Clinchers

- *78-year-old woman:* The mean age of onset of OA is 5 years. OA is sympatomatic three times more in women.
- *Shift hip joint after walking some distance:* Typically in OA, there is pain on movement. It is usually worse at end of day. There may be some background pain at rest.
- *Limited adduction of hip joint:* There can be stiffness of the joint which limits the movements (poor range of movements). There can be associated joint instability. Joints affected in OA
  - Most commonly: DIP joints, first MCP joint, cervical and lumbar spine
  - Next most common: Hip joint
  - Other most common: Knee joint.

CONFUSA

Lets have a good look at the differentiating features of osteoarthritis and rheumatoid arthritis, the two most common arthritis of elderly females

	OA	*RA*
Joint stiffness	Late evening	Early evening
Palpable osteophytes	+	-
Skin redness	+/-	+
Swelling	+/-	+
Ligaments stretch	-	+
Age	Usually older	Usually adolescents
Arthrodesis use	Good	Poor
Fibrillation	+	-
Pannus	-	+
Bone arround joint	Sclerotic	Osteoporotic
Joint deformity	Varus	Valgus

Investigation of Choice

Joint X-ray (findings: Loss of joint space, Subchondral sclerosis, Subchondral cysts, Marginal osteophytes).

Immediate Management Paracetamol for pain.

Treatment of Choice

Reduce weight + walking aid

- Contralateral hand—for hip
- Ipsilateral hand—for knee

- Joint replacement is done for end stage disease.
- If PCM does not bring relief from pain, then give
  - Day pain—NSAID
  - Night pain—TCA in low doses (tricyclic anti-depressant)

179. A 34-year-old woman complains of bilateral stiff and painful joints in her hands and feet.

Diagnosis: Rheumatoid arthritis (RA)

Clinchers

- *34-year-old woman:* Although the peak onset of RA is fifth decade, no age is exempt from it. The incidence of RA is three times more in women.
- *Bilateral:* RA is a symmetrical arthropathy, i.e. affect the same joints bilaterally.
- *Stiff and painful joints in her hands and feet:* RA presents typically with swollen, painful and stiff hands and feet, especially in the morning. This gradually gets and feet, especially in the morning. This gradually gets worse and large joints become involved

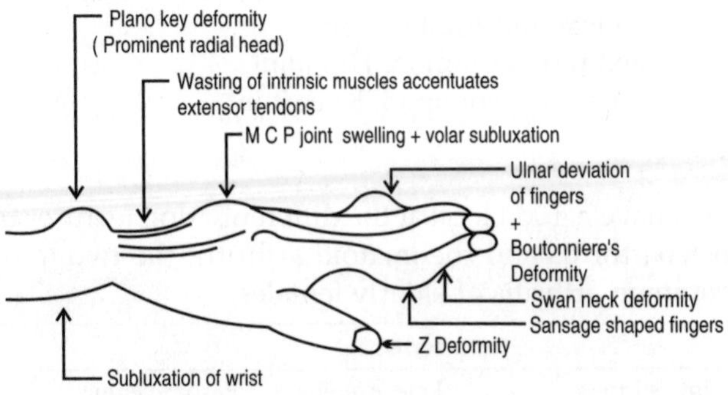

"Handy" thesaurus for signs of RA

CONFUSA

In the PLAB exams, Felty's syndrome has been indirectly asked on at least a couple of occasions. So always keep an eye open for any mention of splenomegaly in a patient of RA.
(Felty's syndrome: RA + Splenomegaly + WCC $^-$)

Investigation of Choice

Rheumatoid factor often negative at start, but becomes positive in 80% over the time. But note that it may be false positive in several other chronic diseases.

Immediate Management

Analgesia.

Treatment of Choice

- Naproxen/Ibuprofen
- Disease modifying drugs if:
  - 12 week trial of 3 NSAIDs do not control pain.
  - Synovitis > 2 months.

Your notes:

PAPER 7

70. A middle aged woman presents with recurrent nausea, weight loss and fever. She has pain, stiffness and weakness in her hips and shoulders. She does not have a rash, but the skin around the neck and shoulders appears thickened.

Diagnosis: Polymyositis

Clinchers

- *Middle-aged women:* Primary idiopathic polymyositis is twice as common in females as in males.
- *Recurrent nausea, weight loss and fever:* These are the systemic symptoms of polymyositis. These also include arthralgias and Raynaud's phenomenon.
- *Pain, stiffness and weakness in her hips and shoulders:* There is insidious, symmetrical, proximal muscle weakness which results from muscle inflammation. It is a presumed autoimmune disease in which skeletal muscle is damaged by an inflammatory process dominated by lymphocytic infiltration.
- *Skin around neck and shoulders appears thickened:* This can be scleroderma which is so frequently associated with this disease. Other associations usually are:
  - RA
  - SLE
  - MCTD
- *No rash:* This rules out dermatomyositis whose characteristics heliotrope rash usually precede muscle changes.

CONFUSA

Patients with dermatomyositis who have skin rash may not require muscle biopsy. In polymyositis, biopsy usually need to:
- Make a firm diagnosis
- Rule out other myopathies.

Investigation of Choice

- Muscle enzyme (CK) levels ($^-$)
- EMG (fibrillation potentials)
- Muscle biopsy.

Immediate Management

Refer to rheumatology.

Treatment of Choice

High dose immune globulin + rest + prednisolone.

Your notes:

136. A 70-year-old with complaint of malaise, weight loss, anorexia. Then develops sudden left-sided visual loss.

Diagnosis: Temporal arteritis (suspected)

Clinchers

- *70-year-old:* It occurs almost exclusively in individuals older than 55 years; however, well-documented cases have occured in patients 40 years old or younger.
- *Malaise, weightloss, anorexia:* The non-specific manifestations of temporal arteritis include malaise, fatigue, anorexia, weight loss, sweats and arthralgias.
- *Sudden left sided visual loss:* A well-recognised and dreaded complication of temporal arteritis, particularly in untreated patients, is ocular involvement due primarily to ischaemic optic neuritis, which may lead to serious visual symptoms, even sudden blindness in some patients.

CONFUSA

Most patients have complaints relating to the head or eyes for months before objective eye involvement. Attention to such symptoms with institution of appropriate therapy will usually avoid this complication. In patients with involvement of the temporal artery, headache is the predominant symptom and may be associated with a tender, thickened or nodular artery, which may pulsate early in the disease but become occluded later. Scalp pain and claudication of the jaw and tongue may occur.

Investigation of Choice

- *Screening:* ESR (elevated).
- *Definitive:* Temporal artery biopsy.

Immediate Management

Steroid therapy

Treatment of Choice

IV steroids immediately.

Your notes:

138. A 50-year-old woman with history of symmetrical joint pains complains of eye symptoms and Schirmer's test is positive.

Diagnosis: Sjögren's syndrome

Clinchers

- *50-year-old woman:* The disease affects predominantly middle aged women (female to male ratio 9:1), although it can be seen in all ages, including childhood.
- *History of symmetrical jiont pains:* Extraglandular (systemic) manifestations are seen in one-third of patients with Sjögren's syndrome, while they are very rare in patients with Sjögren's syndrome associated with rehumatoid arthritis. These patients complain more often to easy fatiguability, low grade fever, myalgias and arthralgias. Most patients with primary Sjögren's syndrome experience at least one episode of nonerosive arthritis during the course of their disease.
- *Eye symptoms:* Ocular involvement is a major manifestation of Sjögren's syndrome. Patient usually complains of dry eyes with a sandy or gritty feeling under the eyelids. Other symptoms include burning, accumulation of thick strands at the inter canthi, decreased tearing, redness, itching, eye fatigue and increased photosensitivity.
- *Schirmer's test is positive:* It is done by placing a strip of filter paper overlapping lower lid. Tears should soak more than 15 mm in 5 minutes normally (negative test). It is positive in dry eye syndromes (keratoconjunctivitis sicca) which includes Sjögren's syndrome.

CONFUSA

The differential diagnosis of Sjögren's syndrome includes other conditions that may cause dry mouth or eyes or parotid salivary gland enlargement. Human immunodeficiency virus (HIV) infection and sarcoidosis appear to produce a clinical picture indistinguishable from Sjögren's syndrome.

Investigation of Choice

Schirmer's test (alread done in this case)

Immediate Management

Ophthalmology referral

Treatment of Choice

Artificial tears + other symptomatic treatment + steroids.

146. A 40-year-old hypertensive male with complaint of left knee pain. Also history of similar attacks. Joint aspirate is cloudy.

Diagnosis: Gout

Clinchers

- *40-year-old-male:* Acute gout presents typically in a middle-aged made with sudden onset of agonizing pain in the joint.
- *Hypertensive:* Hypertension *per se* can impair uric acid excretion (Kumar and Clark, 483, 4th edn). This can lead to hyperuricaemia and hence gout. Otherwise this person would have been on thiazide diuretics (a first line antihypertensive) which can precipitate gout in an already hyperuricaemia state.
- *Left knee pain:* The most common joint to be involved is first MTP joint (podagra). In 25% of attacks, a joint other than the great toe is affected. Knee is frequently affected in these cases.
- *History of similar attacks:* Occasionally, individuals report a prodrome or previous episodes of milder pain lasting hours.
- *Aspirate is cloudy:* Urate crystals are precipitated in the synovial fluid only when it become supersaturated. Also neutrophils and other inflammatory residues are present in it. All this make the synovial fluid look cloudy when aspirated during an acute attack.

CONFUSA

After initial assessment and first parenteral dose of NSAIDs, the patient of acute gout should be referred back to the GP in order that he or she can:

- Assess progress
- Measure serum urate
- Exclude precipitating causes (FBC and EXR indicated)
- Consider Allopurinol therapy.

Note: Allopurinol is not given within 3 weeks of an acute attack.

Synovial fluid	*Appearance*	*Colour*	*Viscosity*
Normal	Clear	Colourless	High
Non-inflammatory	Clear	Straw	High
Haemorrhagic	Bloody	Xanthochromic	Variable
Acute inflammatory	Turbid	Yellow	Decreased
• Acute gout			
• Rheumatic fever			
• Rheumatoid arthritis			
Septic	Turbid	Yellow	Decreased
• TB			
• Gonorrhoea			
• Septic (non-gonococcal)			

Investigation of Choice

Synovial fluid microscopy.

Immediate Management

A wool and crepe bandage required to protect the joint together with non-weight-bearing crutches. The inflamed area must be rested and elevated.

Treatment of Choice

For an acute attack:

NSAID Ibuprofen/Naproxen)

- If NSAID contraindicated: Colchicine
- Decreases if both NSAID and colchicine contraindicated (e.g. renal failure)

Steroids.

Your notes:

149. A middle-aged woman with a history of rheumatoid arthritis develops sudden swelling in one of her knees. This knee is swollen and hot to touch.

Diagnosis: Pseudogout.

Clinchers

- *Middle-aged:* Though pseudogout occurs more commonly in old age, no age after thirties is exempt from it.
- *Woman:* There is a slight preponderance of female incidence.
- *Sudden swelling in one of her knees:* Knee is the main joint to get involved in it. A minority will have involvement of multiple joints.
- *This knee is swollen and hot to touch:* involved joint is erythematous, swollen, warm and painful.
- *History of rheumatoid arthritis:* Any existing arthritis is a risk factor for pseudogout. Other risk factors are old age, dehydration, intercurrent illness, hyperparathyroidism, myxoedema, diabetes mellitus, phosphate decrease, magnesium deficiency, haemochromatosis, acromegaly, gout, ochronosis, surgery.

CONFUSA

Acute pseudogout is less severe and longer lasting than gout and affects different joints. Pseudogout can even be secondary to gout. It cannot be septic arthritis also as there is no preceding history of joint trauma of presence of fever.

Investigation of Choice

- *Screening:* Wrist X-ray (calcium deposition in triangular ligament or chondrocalcinosis)
- *Definitive:* Joint fluid aspiration and microscopy (positively birefringent calcium pyrophosphate crystals in plane polarised light).

Immediate Management

Analgesia.

Treatment of Choice

NSAIDs ± intra-articular injection of glucocorticoids ± colchicine.

Your notes:

150. A 78-year-old woman complains of a stiff left hip joint after walking some distance. This is most evident when she attempts to abduct the hip joint (limited abduction).

Diagnosis: Osteoarthritis (OA).

Clinchers

- *78-year-old woman:* The mean age of onset of OA is 5 years. OA is sympatomatic three times more in women.
- *Stiff hip joint after walking some distance:* Typically in OA, there is pain on movement. It is usually worse at end of day. There may be some background pain at rest.
- *Limited adduction of hip joint:* There can be stiffness of the joint which limits the movements (poor range of movements). There can be associated joint instability.

  Joints affected in OA
  - Most commonly: DIP joints, first MCP joint, cervical and lumbar spine
  - Next most common: Hip joint
  - Other most common: Knee joint.

CONFUSA

Lets have a good look at the differentiating features of osteoarthritis and rheumatoid arthritis, the two most common arthritis of elderly females

	OA	*RA*
Joint stiffness	Late evening	Early evening
Palpable osteophytes	+	-
Skin redness	+/-	+
Swelling	+/-	+
Ligaments stretch	-	+
Age	Usually older	Usually adolescents
Arthrodesis use	Good	Poor
Fibrillation	+	-
Pannus	-	+
Bone around joint	Sclerotic	Osteoporotic
Joint deformity	Varus	Valgus

Investigation of Choice

Joint X-ray (findings: loss of joint space, subchondral sclerosis, subchondral cysts, marginal osteophytes).

Immediate Management Paracetamol for pain.

Treatment of Choice

Reduce weight + walking aid
  - Contralateral hand—for hip
  - Ipsilateral hand—for knee
- Joint replacement is done for end stage disease.
- If PCM does not bring relief from pain, then give
  - Day pain—NSAID
  - Night pain—TCA in low doses (tricyclic antidepressant)

5 Dermatology

PAPER 1

Serial No. 58

Subject: Medicine

Topic: Dermatology (Colored Slide)

Question: A-30-year old lady presents with breathlessness and perihilar shadow. On examination she had red erythematous lesions on her shins.

Diagnosis: Erythema nodosum (Sarcoidosis)

Clinchers

- *30-year-old lady:* Women are affected more often than men with erythema nodosum, with a male-to-female ratio of 1:4. It is more common in young adults aged 18-34 years.
- *Breathlessness:* This is signifying some primary lung pathology in this lady, most probably sarcoidosis as the most common association with erythema nodosum.
- *Perihilar shadow:* Hilar adenopathy may develop as part of the hypersensitivity reaction of EN. Bilateral hilar lymphadenopathy is associated with sarcoidosis, while unilateral changes may occur with infections and malignancy.
- *Red erythematous lesions on her shins:* This is the classical description of erythema nodosum; painful, palpable, dusky blue nodules or plaques. Characteristically, lesions appear on the anterior leg; however, they may appear on any surface.

CONFUSA

- In an adult female with features of arthritis, hilar lymphadenopathy and skin lesions typically on shins, always rule out sarcoidosis.
- In children, the most common cause of erythema nodosum is streptococcal throat infection.

Investigation of Choice

Investigation should be directed at finding an underlying cause:

- Careful history - especially attention to drugs (sulfonamides, OCPs)
- ESR
- Throat swab, ASO titre (Streptococcal infection)
- CXR for sarcoid, and tuberculosis
- Mantoux test - if negative, Kveim test.

Immediate Management

NSAIDs may be given for joint pain and painful skin nodules. Topical steroids are of no value.

Treatment of Choice

Treatment of the underlying condition.

Your notes:

Serial No. 59

Subject: Medicine

Topic: Dermatology (Coloured Slide)

Question: A-46-year-old man on steroids for his asthma comes with fever and chest pain. On examination he has a fine vesicular rash on his right thoracic dermatome.

Diagnosis: Herpes zoster

Clinchers

- *46-year-old man:* There appears to be no sex prediliction for herpes zoster. People of all ages can be affected, but incidence increases with age, presumably through the general decrease in immune function that occurs with aging.
- *On steroids for asthma:* patients taking high-dose corticosteroid treatment are at risk of developing shingles.
- *Fever and chest pain:* The systemic manifestations of the condition precede the onset of rash by 48-72 hr and present as malaise, myalgia, headache,fever and unusual skin sensations or pain within the affected dermatome.
- *Fine rash on his right thoracic dermatome:* Most commonly affected dermatomes are the lower thoracic region, ophthalmic division of the trigeminal nerve and occasionally motor nerves, causing paralysis (say, facial paralysis in Ramsay Hunt syndrome, or urinary retention).

CONFUSA

- Herpes zoster in persons younger than 50 years may be an indicator of an immunocompromised state. Therefore, younger patients with zoster should be assessed for evidence of immunodeficiency, including HIV.
- Patients are infectious until lesions are dried. Anyone who has not previously had varicella is at risk of acquiring this readily transmitted virus. Pregnant women and immunosuppressed patients have the highest risk of serious sequelae.
- Postherpetic neuralgia is persistent or recurring pain lasting 30 or more days after the acute infection or after all lesions have crusted.

Investigation of Choice

Its basically a clinical diagnosis in the light of a proper history.

Immediate Management

Analgesics to reduce pain

Treatment of Choice

- Oral aciclovir administration of 800 mg five times per day for 7 days (compared with placebo) has been demonstrated to reduce the duration of the rash and reduce the acute pain (those with the worst pain gain most) in immunocompetent patients treated within 48 hours of the onset of the last vesicle.
- IV Aciclovir is the preferred treatment for immunosuppressed patients or patients with ocular herpes zoster or motor shingles.

Your notes:

Serial No. 60

Subject: Medicine

Topic: Dermatology (Coloured Slide)

Question: A 42-year-old male with multiple generalised soft hyperpigmented nodules located mainly on the trunk.

Diagnosis: Neurofibromatosis Type I (NF 1, von Recklinhausen's disease or peripheral neurofibromatosis)

Clinchers

- *42-year-old male:* Its slightly more common in males than females. Its autosomal dominantly inherited and though, the change is present at birth, manifestation develop over years.
- *Multiple generalized:* This is the typical description of peripheral generalized neurofibromatosis.
- *Soft, hyperpigmented nodules:* Subcutaneous or cutaneous neurofibromas appear over time in older children, adolescents, and adults. Deep lesions may be detected only by palpation, whereas cutaneous lesions may appear initially as small papules. Puberty and pregnancy may be associated with increased numbers of neurofibromas and more rapid growth of preexisting lesions.
- *Located mainly on trunk:* Although generalised, favoured sites are trunk, extremities, scalp, or face.

CONFUSA

- Patients with the Neurofibromatosis 2 or central Neurofibromatosis demonstrate a relative paucity of cutaneous findings but have high incidence of meningioma as well as acoustic neuromas, which often are bilateral. Prognosis is worse than that of NF 1.
- NF 1 can be associated with hypertension and can be due to associated phaeochromocytoma or renal artery stenosis.

Investigation of Choice

The diagnosis of neurofibromatosis is based on the clinical findings. Cardinal features are numerous cafe au lait spots - greater than six - and skin tumours. A positive family history in antecedent and collateral members makes diagnosis even more certain.

Immediate Management

Do not excise unless there is evidence of malignancy or are cosmetically objectionable.

Treatment of Choice

Excise in case of cosmetically unsightable or producing pressure effects.

Your notes:

Serial No. 63

Subject: Medicine

Topic: Dermatology (Coloured slides)

Question: A 34-year-old woman had a pigmented lesion on her foot which has now rapidly increased in size and shows ulceration.

Diagnosis: Malignant melanoma

Clinchers

- *34-year-old woman:*Malignant melanoma is twice more common in females than males, peaking at about 35-55 years; Its rarely seen before puberty.
- *Pigmented lesion on her foot:* Lower leg is the most common site in females but in males, the trunk is most affected. Other common sites are the head and neck.
- *Now rapidly increased in size and shows ulceration:* A changing mole is the most common warning sign for melanoma. Variation in colour and/or increase in diameter, height, or asymmetry of borders of a pigmented lesion are noted by more than 80% of patients with melanoma at the time of diagnosis.

CONFUSA

7 Point Check List:

- For pigmented lesions, clinicians should be aware of and use the 7-point weighted checklist for assessment:
  - *Major features of lesions:*
    - change in size
    - irregular shape
    - irregular colour.
  - *Minor features of lesions:*
    - largest diameter 7 mm or more
    - inflammation
    - oozing
    - change in sensation

Lesions scoring 3 points or more (based on major features scoring 2 points each and minor features scoring 1 point each) in the 7-point checklist above are suspicious.

Investigation of Choice

Excision Biopsy

Immediate Management

Refer urgently patients with a lesion suspected to be melanoma. Excision in primary care should be avoided.

Treatment of Choice

Excision with a margin of 3-5 cm.

Can be combined with radiotherapy, immunotherapy or hormonal therapy.

Cytotoxic agents imidazole carboxamide - DTIC - and vindesine may be used.

Isolated limb perfusion (with melphalan) can be considered in recurrent tumours and deeply invasive ones on a limb.

Involved regional nodes are removed by block dissection. Prophylactic lymph node dissection is not practiced in UK.

Your notes:

PAPER 3

13. A 32-year-old woman has chickenpox. She scratches herself excessively and develops a blue discolouration on the abdomen. She has a history of not passing urine in the last 24 hours. She continues to scratch herself and the discolouration increases in size.

Diagnosis: Toxic epidermal necrolysis (TEN)

Clinchers

- *Chickenpox:* The most common infectious complication of varicella is secondary bacterial superinfection of the skin, which is usually caused by *Streptococcus pyogenes* or *Staphylococcus aureus.*
- *Scratches herself:* This complication mostly results from excoriation of skin lesions after scratching. About 3% of the general population harbour the toxin producing *Staphylococcus aureus* on their skin.
- *32-year-old woman:* TEN occurs predominantly in middle-aged and elderly women. More commonly it is due to drug reactions but infections causes are also prevalent.
- *Blue discolouration on abdomen:* There is erythroderma with extensive desquamation and in places blistering and erosions.
- *History of not passing urine in last 24 hours:* TEN produces rapid dehydration and sickness. The patient need to be nursed as though they had extensive burns.

CONFUSA

Staphylococcal scalded skin syndrome presents with similar symptoms but is usually a disease of newborns (In older patients the same disease is termed as TEN). Gas gangrene can be a diagnosis in this case if there had been any mention of crepitus.

Investigation of Choice

Pus or staphylococcal organisms are not present in the lesion so the diagnosis has to be totally clinical.

Immediate Management

Fluid resuscitation + systemic steroids + antibiotics (flucloxacillin).

Treatment of Choice

Debridement of nectoric tissue + flucloxacillin.

Your notes:

91. A fair 18-year-old girl has had dark black facial patches, one of which is now growing rapidly in size.

Diagnosis: Malignant melanoma (MM)—Superficial spreading type.

Clinchers

- *Fair:* It is seen in all racial types but is more common in fair-skinned caucasian types.
- *18-year-old girl:* Malignant melanoma is extremely rare before puberty but can occur at any age after that. The incidence is slightly more common in females.
- *Dark black facial patches:* Some 30% of lesions of MM develop from a pre-existing melanocytic naevus and other develop *de novo* on any part of skin surface. Benign moles may be very dark brown or black but are usually a uniform colour.
- *One of which is now growing rapidly in size:* Any change in the size, shape or colour of a pre-existing lesion should be suspected of being MM. Particular signs that are valuable in recognition of MM are irregularity in the margin, irregularity in the degree of pigmentation and erosion or cursting of skin surface.

CONFUSA

Acral lentiginous melanoma is more frequent in black skinned individuals and subjects of Japanese and Asian descent. It has particularly poor prognosis.

Investigation of Choice

Clinical examination by a dermatologist.

Immediate Management

Examine whole body to rule out other foci.

Treatment of Choice

Excision biopsy with wide margin of normal skin and subsequent pathological examination.

Your notes:

92. A 70-year-old bald gardener has had a brownish patch on his scalp which has been slowly growing for the last 30 years.

Diagnosis: Solar keratoses (actinic keratosis, senile keratosis).

Clinchers

- *70-year-old:* Usually found in elderly (hence the name senile keratosis) due to cumulative effect of sun exposure over the years.
- *Bald:* It means that his scalp is a perennially sun exposed area and hence a potential site for solar keratotis.
- *Gardener:* As he is a gardener, sun exposure is a professional hazard to him. Men seem to be at more risk than women.
- *Brownish patch on his scalp:* It appear as crumbly yellow-white crusts (may be brownish) in fair skinned people. It is a raised, scaling or warty hyperkeratotic plaque or papule.
- *Slowly growing for the last 30 years:* Solar keratoses are typically slow growing and any rapid growth in them should raise suspicious of a malignant change (SCC more common).

CONFUSA

Clinical diagnosis of solar keratosis may be quite difficult even for experienced clinicians. So a simple biopsy must be done.

Investigation of Choice
Simple biopsy.

Immediate Management
Avoid further sun exposure.

Treatment of Choice
Cautery/cryotherapy/5-FU cream.

Your notes:

93. A young HIV positive man develops raised patches in his skin and in his mouth.

Diagnosis: Kaposi's sarcoma (Idiopathic haemorrhagic sarcoma).

Clinchers

- *Young HIV positive man:* There are many cutaneous manifestations of HIV disease, due to both infectious and noninfectious conditions.
  - *Infections:* Oral candidiasis, molluscum contagiosum, HSV, varicella zoster, cryptococcosis (on face), scabies, oral hairy leukoplakia.
  - *Others:* Seborrhic dermatitis, psoriasis, eosinophilic folliculitis, drug reactions.
- *Develops raised patches in his skin and in his mouth:* Kaposi's sarcoma typically affects both skin and mucus membranes (especially oral mucosa). It presents as purpulish macules, papules, nodules and plaques affecting the feet, legs, face and oral mucosa (in fact before the advent of HIV, it was known to affect only mucosa surfaces).

CONFUSA

Lichen planus is another disease which presents as raised purple polygonal plaques on both skin and oral mucosa. However, it is not so typically associated with HIV, is itchy and characteristically differentiated by Wickham's striaes (whitish criss-cross lines). Another differential diagnosis is bacillary angiomatosis (Bartonella).

Investigation of Choice
Biopsy.

Immediate Management
Examine whole body as the disease is usually multifocal.

Treatment of Choice
- Cryotherapy
- Intralesional vincristine
- Radiotherapy
- Treatment of HIV disease

Your notes:

94. A builder has been exposed to sun for long periods of time develops an ulcerated lesion on his face.

Diagnosis: Squamous cell carcinoma (SCC).

Clinchers

- *Builder:* Sun exposure is a professional hazard for him.
- *Exposed to sun for long periods of time:* UV rays exposure is by far the most important causative factor of both actinic keratoses and SCC.
- *Develops an ulcerated lesion on his face:* SCC presents as a persistently ulcerated or crusted from irregular lesion. It is usually found on sun-exposed sites (face in this question). It may occur in pre-existing actinic keratoses which might be present because of his profession (builder).

CONFUSA

The main problem is to differentiate between a BCC and SCC.

BCC	*SCC*
• Rolled margins	• Everted margins
• Pearly	• Ulcerated
• Usually on face	• Ears, dorsa of hands, bald-scalp

Investigation of Choice

Clinical evaluation by a dermatologist.

Immediate Management

Clinical evaluation by a dermatologist.

Treatment of Choice

- Excision
- Metastases are relatively uncommon but more frequent at certain sites, e.g. ears.

Your notes:

95. An 18-year-old girl with moles on her back of different colour and sizes.

Diagnosis: Intradermal melanoma (Naevi).

Clinchers

- *18-year-old girl moles on her back:* Nearly everyone possesses one or more moles some have hundreds, although they may not become apparent until after puberty. Those moles that are entirely within the dermis remain benign, but a small percentage of the junctional naevi, so called because they are seen in the basal layer of the epidermis at its junction, with the dermis, may undergo malignant change.
- *Of different colour and sizes:* Intradermal melanoma is the most common variety of mole. The naevus may be light or dark in colour and may be flat or raised, hairy or hairless. A hairy mole is nearly always intradermal. They never undergo malignant change, and need no treatment unless the diagnosis is uncertain.

CONFUSA

Intradermal melanoma may be found in every situation except the palm of the hand, the sole of the foot or the scrotal skin.

Investigation of Choice

Histology only on suspicious of a malignant change (excision biopsy).

Immediate Management

Reassurance.

Treatment of Choice

None required.

Your notes:

PAPER 4

96. A bottle-fed baby has developed flexural eczema. His brother has the same history. Family history of asthma. Mom is presently avoiding using soap.

Diagnosis: Atopic infantile eczema.

Clinchers

- *Bottle-fed baby develops flexural eczema:* Infantile eczema is common (most children will grow out of it before the teenage years). Breastfeeding is protective.
- *Brother has same history + family history of asthma:* There is a strong genetic component often with a positive family history of atopy. IL-4 receptor mutation has been found in atopic families.
- *Mom is presently avoiding using soap:* It deinforces the finding of family history of atopy in this case (This is irritant dermatitis). If one parent has atopic disease the risk for a child of developing eczema is about 20-30%. If both parents have atopic eczema the risk is greater than 50%.

CONFUSA

Animal dander often aggravates eczema and elevated IgE RAST is typical. A proportion of atopic children have significant hood allergies, e.g. egg, fish which can exacerbate eczema. Infantile eczema gets better with time although asthma is often the next events along the line.

Immediate Management

Encourage the mother to breastfeed.

Treatment of Choice

- Hydrocortisone cream for acute flare ups (1% hydrocortisone)
- Trimeprazine for sleep, deprivation due to itching.

Your notes:

97. Young girl with eczema, treated with emollient and topical hydrocortisone, did not get better.

Diagnosis: Eczema not responding to first line drug.

Clinchers

- *Young girls:* Young children should be treated with mild and moderately patent steroids on the body.
- *Treated with emollient and topical hydrocortisone, did not get better:* Hydrocortisone is a mild steroid. Since it is not improving the condition, a trial with a higher dose is needed before changing the drug (a high potency steroid) or treatment modality.

CONFUSA

Classification of topical steroids by potency	
Very potent	Choketasol
	Diflucortolone
Potent	Betamethasone
	Fluocinolone
Moderately potent	Clobetasone
	Aldometrasone
Mild	Hydrocortisone

Investigation of Choice

Usually not required.

Immediate Management

Reassurance (as it can precipitate depression especially, in young girls)

Treatment of Choice

2.5% hydrocortisone topically.

Your notes:

98. Young girl with severe eczema,weeping vesicles, skin swab was taken, topical steroids didn't work.

Diagnosis: Severe non-responsive eczema

Clinchers

- *Young girl:* A failure to treatment can produce anxiety or depression especially in a young girl.
- *Severe eczema, weeping vesicles:* It signify a severe acute attack of eczema and should be treated on an urgent basis. Bacterial infections often exacerbate eczema to this extent.
- *Skin swab taken: Staph aureus* commonly colonies lesions and staph endotoxin is known to act as super antigen. Its elimination is a prerequisite for definitive treatment.
- *Topical steroids did not work:* It means that oral steroids will have to be given a trial.

CONFUSA

If the skin infection is by *Streptococcus*, give penicillin V (500 mg QID). Erythromycin (500 mg QID) is useful if there is already to penicillin.

Investigation of Choice
Skin swab (already taken)

Immediate Management
Topical antiseptics

Treatment of Choice
Steroids + flucloxacillin.

Your notes:

99. A 49-year-old woman complains of itchy blisters, which are occurring in groups on her knees and elbows. The itch is becoming unbearable and she is contemplating suicide. She responds to 180 mg of Dapsone within 48 hours of treatment.

Diagnosis: Coeliac disease (Gluten sensitive enteropathy).

Clinchers

- *49-year-old female:* It can present at any age. The peak incidence in adults is in the third and fourth decades with a females preponderance.
- *Itchy blisters which are occurring in group on her knees and elbows:* This is an uncommon blistering subepidermal eruption of the skin associated with gluten sensitive enteropathy. The clinical term for it is gluten sensitive enteropathy.
- *Itch is becoming unbearable and she is contemplating suicide:* This disease can produce severe depression in females and can lead to suicide.
- *Responds to 180 mg of dapsone within 48 hours of treatment:* This confirms our diagnosis.

CONFUSA

The skin condition (dermatitis herpetiformis) responds to dapsone but both the gut and the skin will improve only on a gluten free diet in this disease.

Investigation of Choice
Endomysial antibodies (IgA).

Immediate Management
Psychiatric referral (as she is contemplating suicide)

Treatment of Choice
Gluten free diet
+
Dapsone

Your notes:

100. An 18-month-old baby, red swollen lips after eating egg. Presently under treatment with emollients and topical hydrocortisone three times a day.

Diagnosis: Food allergy (egg)

Clinchers

- *18-month-old baby, red swollen lips after eating egg:* A proportion of topic children have significant food allergies, e.g. egg, fish, etc.
- *Presently under treatment with emollients and topical hydrocortisone:* Any episode of food allergy in eczema typically worsens it. So use high dose (2.5%) hydrocortisone for a few days as a prophylactic measure.

CONFUSA

Red swollen lips suggests anaphylaxis and require prompt treatment with IM epinephrine and enough interventions to prevent laryngeal oedema from developing.

Investigation of Choice
None.

Immediate Management
Follow anaphylaxis protocol

Treatment of Choice
Admission to hospital.

Your notes:

PAPER 5

107. It is a skin-to-skin contact disease.

Diagnosis: Scabies

Clinchers

Scabies is spread by prolonged close contact such as within households or institutions, and by sexual contact. It presents clinically with itchy red papules (or ocassionally vesicles and pustules) which can occur anywhere in the skin but rarely on the face, except in neonates.

CONFUSA

Crusted scabies (Norwegian scabies) is a clinical variant that occurs in immunosuppressed individuals where huge number of mites are carried in the skin. The patient is extremely infections after relatively minimal contact. Clinically this presents as hyperkeratotic crusted lesions especially on the hands and feet. Itch is often absent or minimal. Lesions may progress such that the patient has a widespread erythema with irregular crusted plaques. It can therefore mimic eczema or psoriasis.

Investigation of Choice
Microscopy (demonstration of a mite is definitive)

Immediate Management
Trace all contacts

Treatment of Choice
Topical scabicide
(malathion or 5% permerthrin to the whole body and washed off after 24 hours).

Your notes:

169. A 40-year-old sheep farmer from Kent presented to her GP complaining of muscle and joint pain with an associated chronic headache, which has been present for 3 weeks. On examination, she had an erythematous annular rash with a central clear area, on her abdomen.

Diagnosis: Lyme's disease.

Clinchers

- *40-year-old sheep farmer from kent:* It was originally described in Lyme, connecticut (USA),but is now known to occur in UK (new forest-kent). It spreads by deer or sheep ticks (bite).
- *Muscle and joint pain + headache for 3 weeks:* Headache, fever, malaise, myalgia, arthralgia and lymphadenopathy are the common accompaniments of the first stage of the disease.
- *Erythematous annular rash with a central clear area on her abdomen:* It is the characteristic rash of Lyme's disease and is known as erythema chronicum migrans. It heralds the first stage of disease as a small papule which develops into a spreading large erythematous ring with central fading. It lasts from 48 hr- 3 months and may be multiple.

CONFUSA

The 'agent' causing human granulocyte erlichiosis is also transmitted by the same ticks. It produces a similar clinical picture and can be co-transmitted.

Investigation of Choice

Clinical ± serology (if negative, PCR).

Immediate Management

Exclude CNS and CVS involvement.

Treatment of Choice

Doxycycline 100 mg/12 h PO for 10-21 days (Amoxycillin or penicillin V if < 12 years).

Your notes:

173. A Welsh farmer with malaise and arthralgia is increasingly anxious about a skin lesion which started as a papule (Diameter approx 1 mm) which has progressed to a red ring (Diameter approx 50 mm) with central fading.

Diagnosis: Borrelia burgdorferi infection (Lyme disease).

Clinchers

- *Welsh farmer:* Ticks (on deer and sheep) spreading this infection are widespread in the UK, particularly in forests, and woodlands.
- *Malaise and arthralgia:* These are nonspecific symptoms of Lyme diseases are headache, fever, malaise, myalgia, arthralgia and lymphadenopathy.
- *Skin lesion which started as a papule.... progressed to a red ring with central fading:* This is the typical description of erythema chronicum migrans which heralds this disease and is virtually pathognomic.

CONFUSA

Lyme disease is caused by Borrelia burgdorferi sensu lato. The disease is transmitted by Ixodes dammini or related ixodid ticks (Ixodes ricinus in Europe). In the UK, 300-500 cases are reported annually. Prompt removal of any tick is essential as infection is unlikely to take place until the tick begins to engorge. Ticks should be removed by grasping them with forceps near to the point of attachment to the skin and then withdrawn by gentle traction.

Investigation of Choice

Clinical ± serology (if negative, PCR).

Immediate Management

Rule out CNS and CVS involvement

Treatment of Choice

Doxycycline
(amoxycillin or penicillin V if < 12 years).

Your notes:

174. A 42-year-old woman who reports a loss in weight, presents with a shiny erythematous lesion on her shin. It's centre appear yellowish and edges are beginning to ulcerate with undermining. (Fasting blood glucose is 5.3 mmol/L).

Diagnosis: Necrobiosis lipoidica (NL).

Clinchers

- *42-year-old:* NIDDM may be present in subclinical form for years before diagnosis and the incidence increases markedly with age and degree of obesity.
- *Loss of weight:* This due to fluid depletion and the accelerated breakdown of fat and muscle secondary to insulin deficiency.
- *Shiny, erythematous lesion on her shin:*NL is a shiny plaque like lesion with erythematous margins. It is usually found over the anterior surfaces of the legs (Shins).
- *Centre appears yellowish and edges are begining to ulcerate with undermining:* This is an almost "dictionary description" of the lesion of NL.
- *Fasting blood glucose in 5.3 mmol/L":* Although skin manifestations in diabetes can occur in well-controlled but long-standing diabetes (as in this case), majority of them only present along with glycosuria and hyperglycaemia.

CONFUSA

Diabetic dermopathy ("Shin spots") is a similar but different clinical entity. Its lesions are also located over the anterior tibial surface. The lesions are small, rounded plaques with a raised border. They many crust at the edges and ulcerate centrally (opposite to what is seen in NL).

Investigation of Choice
Complete blood sugar profile

Immediate Management
Take family history of DM + rule out any malignancy.

Treatment of Choice
Strict glycaemic control if diabetes is proven.

Your notes:

PAPER 6

105. Man, slept while sunbathing comes with redness, and pain all over his body. Otherwise well.

Diagnosis: Sunburns.

Clinchers

- *Sunbathing:* It can cause sunburns if prolonged, but these are usually not serious.
- *Redness:* It is superficial erythema and is never taken into accounting when calculating the area of burn.
- *Pain:* Simple erythema is extremely painful. Even patients expected to go home after treatment may need parenteral analgesia.
- *Other wise well:* This rules out any other injury or fluid compromise. Since simple erythema do not require active treatment, he can be safely discharged home.

CONFUSA

Unprotected exposure to UV radiation can cause extremely painful, blistering, oedematous skin. In general the treatment is as for any other burn.

Investigation of Choice
None required.

Immediate Management
Oral analgesia if required.

Treatment of Choice
Reassure and discharge
+
Regular application of hydrocortisone 1% cream

Your notes:

PAPER 7

72. Patient has a large tense blister.

Diagnosis: Dermal burns

Clinchers

- *Large tense blister:* Small blisters can be left alone. Large ones can be slit open at the dependent edge to allow drainage. Alternatively they can be aspirated with a needle.

CONFUSA

Complete derooting of any blister is unnecessary and leaves a painful base. So avoid it. Blisters are absent in epidermal burns. Superficial dermal burns with blistering are usually dressed to absorb exudate, prevent desiccation, provide pain relief, encourage epithelialisation and prevent infection.

Investigation of Choice
None required.

Immediate Management
Drainage of blister/aspirate blister.

Treatment of Choice
Regular dressing.

Your notes:

75. Man, slept while sunbathing comes with redness, and pain all over his body. Otherwise well.

Diagnosis: Sunburns.

Clinchers

- *Sunbathing:* It can cause sunburns if prolonged, but these are usually not serious.
- *Redness:* It is superficial erythema and is never taken into accounting when calculating the area of burn.
- *Pain:* Simple erythema is extremely painful. Even patients expected to go home after treatment may need parenteral analgesia.
- *Other wise well:* This rules out any other injury or fluid compromise. Since simple erythema do not require active treatment, he can be safely discharged home.

CONFUSA

Unprotected exposure to UV radiation can cause extremely painful, blistering, oedematous skin. In general the treatment is as for any other burn.

Investigation of Choice
None required.

Immediate Management
Oral analgesia if required.

Treatment of Choice
Reassure and discharge
+
Regular application of hydrocortisone 1% cream

Your notes:

96. Scabies.

Diagnosis (causation): Female mite

Clinchers

Scabies is a common disorder which particularly affects children and young adults. It tends to spread within families or those living in close contact. There are markedly itchy papula eruptions affecting:

- Finger webs (esp. first)
- Wrist flexures
- Axillae
- Abdomen (esp. around umbilicus) and waist band area)
- Buttocks
- Groins
- Palms and soles (in young infants)

Note: Itchy red penile or scrotal papules are virtually diagnostic.

CONFUSA

The eruption in scabies in a skin reaction to the saliva or faeces of the female mite. Scabies mites can sometimes be extracted from burrows and can be visualised microscopically. Similarly eggs can be visualised from skin scrapings. The rash and symptom of itch will take a few weeks to settle, occasionally longer.

Investigation of Choice

The diagnosis is usually clinical. Demonstration of female mite is definitive.

Immediate Management

Crotamin cream (relieves itching till anti-scaboidals have any effect)

Treatment of Choice

Malathion/Permethrin

Note: Applied to all areas of skin, from neck down for 24 hours.

Your notes:

97. Candidial nappy rash.

Diagnosis: (causation): Immunodeficiency

Clinchers

➢ *Nappy rash:* It is usually of 4 types:
   1. Ammonia dermatitis
   2. Candida dermatitis (thrush)
   3. Seborrhoeic eczematous dermatitis.
   4. Isolated, psoriasis-like scaly plaques

➢ *Candidial:* It may be isolated from about half of all nappy rashes. Infections are red and often moist with satellite lesions.

CONFUSA

The hallmarks of candidal nappy rash are satellite spots beyond the main rash.

Investigation of Choice

Microscopy (20% KOH skin scrapings).

Immediate Management

Advise on cleliness to parents.

Treatment of Choice

Nystatin or clotrimazole cream (± 1% hydrocortisone cream).

Your notes:

98. Impetigo.

Diagnosis (causation): Close community contact (that is why it is called Impetigo contagiosa).

Clinchers

Impetigo is a common superficial bacterial infection of skin caused by

- Group A beta-haemolytic streptococci
- *Staphylococcus aureus.*

The primary lesion is a superficial pustule that rup'-tures and forms a characteristic yellow-brown "honey-coloured" crust. Lesions caused by staphylococci may be tense, clear bullae, and this less common form of the disease is called bullous impetigo. Lesions may occur on normal skin or in areas already affected by an other skin disease.

Ecthyma is a variant of impetigo that generally occurs on lower extremities and causes punched out ulcerative lesions.

Investigation of Choice

Diagnosis is usually clinical but culture from wound swab may help in confirmation

Immediate Management

Gentle debridement of adherent crusts, which is facilitated by the use of soaks and topical antibiotics

Treatment of Choice

Oral antibiotics (flucloxacillin in case of staphylococci).

Your notes:

106. Warts.

Diagnosis (transmission): Sexual contact (Most commonly).

Clinchers

Warts are caused by human papilloma virus (HPV) infection of keratinocytes. Warts can be clinically classified into four types:

1. Common warts
   - Most common in children and young adults
   - Often resolve spontaneously
   - Individual lesions can be stubbornly persistent
   - Treatment is destructive (i.e. keratolytics or cryotherapy)
2. Plantar warts
   - Large confluent lesions (mosaic warts)
   - Treatment curettage for large warts
   - Surgery contraindicated
3. Plane warts
   - Flat skin coloured or brownish lesions
   - Tend to keobnerise in scratch marks
   - Can be very resistant to treatment
4. Genital warts
   - Condylomata accuminata
   - Treatment with cryotherapy and/or podophyllin
   - Found in sexually active person.

CONFUSA

Large number of warty lesions are often seen in the immunosuppressed, e.g. transplant patients.

Investigation of Choice

Clinical diagnosis is usually sufficient.
Excision biopsy is definitive

Immediate Management

Reassume and rule out immunosuppression

Treatment of Choice

Depends upon type of wart (see clinchers)

Your notes:

6 Endocrinology

PAPER 1

Serial No. 53

Subject: Medicine

Topic: Endocrinology

Question: A heavy smoker with raised haematocrit and haemoglobin.

Diagnosis: Polycythemia (Secondary)

Clinchers

- *Heavy smoker:* Acquired polycythemia is a physiologic response to generalized or localized tissue hypoxia. In a heavy smoker, it can occur secondary to chronic obstructive pulmonary disease, due to high ventilation-to-perfusion ratios. Exposure to carbon monoxide by smoking also acts as an additive factor.
- *Raised haematocrit:* This is the primary abnormality which supports the diagnosis of polycythaemia.
- *Raised haemoglobin:* Occurs secondary to stimulation by raised levels of erythropoetin.

CONFUSA

- The main point of distinction between primary polycythemia and secondary polycythemia is the erythropoetin level. *Secondary* polycythemia occurs *secondary* to raised erythropoetin; in primary polycythemia, erythropoetin levels are low/undetectable.
- The raised hematocrit should be absolute and not due to decreased plasma volume (Gaisbock's Syndrome).

Investigation of Choice

Radioisotope measurement of red cell mass and plasma volume will confirm the diagnosis of erythrocytosis.

Immediate Management

The main fear is of thrombosis due to hyperviscosity. Phlebotomy is indicated when erythrocytosis is severe, blood is viscous and flow sluggish or prior to operative intervention.

Treatment of Choice

Treat the primary cause.

Serial No. 54

Subject: Medicine

Topic: Endocrinology

Question: A 30-year-old female presents with lethargy. Her BP is 160/100 with serum electrolytes Na^+ 149 mmol/L, K^+ 2.6 mmol/L and HCO^-_3 30 mmol/L.

Diagnosis: Conn's Syndrome

Clinchers

- *30-year-old female:* Primary hyperaldosteronism is twice as common in women as in men. Peak incidence occurs in the third to sixth decades of life.
- *Lethargy:* is attributed to hypokalemia. Patients may also present with muscle weakness, cramping, headaches, and palpitations. They can also have polydipsia and polyuria from hypokalemia-induced nephrogenic diabetes insipidus.
- *BP 160/100:* Patient may present with hypertension or one of the cardiac or neurological complications of hypertension.
- *Serum electrolytes Na^+ 149 mmol/L, K^+ 2.6 mmol/L and HCO^-_3 30 mmol/L:* The picture of mild hypernatremia with hypokalaemia in the presence of metabolic alkalosis fits perfect in the diagnosis of Conn's Syndrome.

CONFUSA

- In any case of hypokalemic hypertension in the presence of metabolic alkalosis, think of Conn's syndrome as the most probable diagnosis.
- A poorly controlled hypertensive on high doses of diuretics can also present with the same picture of hypertension, alkalosis and hypokalemia-rule out diuretics as a cause.

Investigation of Choice

- Blood electrolytes
- Plasma renin and aldosterone — low renin and high aldosterone suggests primary hyperaldosteronism
- 24 hour urinary aldosterone.

Immediate Management

Prompt treatment of hypokalemia and hypertension.

Treatment of Choice

According to the underlying cause:
- if due to adenoma — surgery after 4 to 6 weeks of spironolactone therapy (e.g. 300 mg/day)
- if due to adrenal hyperplasia — spironolactone or amiloride is generally sufficient

Your notes:

Serial No. 55

Subject: Medicine

Topic: Endocrinology

Question: A 35-year-old female presents with hypotension and lethargy. Her skin appears hyperpigmented.

Diagnosis: Addison's disease

Clinchers

- *35-year-old female:* Addison's disease is slightly more common in females. It can occur in persons of any age; however, it is most common in people aged 30-50 years.
- *Hypotension:* often marked in acute hypoadrenalism; usually postural in chronic disease with a fall in blood pressure on standing of 20 mm Hg or more after a few minutes — may cause dizziness and headache; it is due to ineffective catecholamine action.
- *Lethargy:* lassitude and muscle weakness is due to hypokalemia.
- *Hyperpigmentation:* due to high ACTH; the skin assumes a dull, grey-brown colouration.

  Exposed skin, pressure areas, palmar creases, knuckles, buccal mucosa and recent scars are the commonest sites of hyperpigmentation.

CONFUSA

In case of confusion, look for the hints at other associated autoimmnune conditions associated with Addison's Disease. Addison's disease is associated with an increased incidence of:
- Hashimoto's thyroiditis,
- Schmidt's syndrome
- Type I diabetes mellitus
- Premature ovarian failure
- Idiopathic hypoparathyroidism
- Pernicious anaemia
- Mucocutaneous candidiasis
- Vitiligo
- Alopecia
- Graves' disease
- Adrenoleukodystrophy

Investigation of Choice

ACTH levels
Synacthen Test

Immediate Management

Promptly treat patients in whom acute adrenal insufficiency is suspected — hydrocortisone 100 mg IM

Treatment of Choice

Treat cause

IV normal saline and hydrocortisone in acute situations.

In long-term replacement also add fluorocortisone with hydrocortisone.

Patients should carry a steroid card and Medic Alert bracelet.

Your notes:

Serial No. 56

Subject: Medicine

Topic: Endocrinology

Question: A 40-year-old patient complaints of lethargy, bone pain, polyuria and polydipsia. His blood glucose level is 3.0 mmol/L.

Diagnosis: Hypercalcemia

Clinchers

- *40-year-old:* Hypercalcemia in elderly usually as a part of metastatic complications of malignancy. In younger age group primary hyperparathyroidism remains the most common cause.
- *Lethargy:* increased calcium levels stimulate muscle for active contraction, which later go in for exhaustion and present as generalised lethargy and profound muscle weakness.
- *Polyuria, polydipsia:* These are among the general non specific symptoms of hypercalcemia, occurring due increased osmolality of the blood, stimulating the thirst centre of the hypothalamus.
- *Bone pain:* rapid loss of bone density leads to osteopenia, bone pains, pathological fractures and hypercalciuria.
- *Blood glucose level 3.0 mmol/L:* Normal glucose levels rules out diabetes as a cause of polyuria, polydipsia.

CONFUSA

- In a patient presenting with bone pain (or, back pain) with features of hypercalcemia along with anemia, carefully rule out Multiple Myeloma.
- In a patient who recently underwent chemotherapy for malignancy, when presenting with nonspecific symptoms of confusion, disorientation, depression with profuse thirst, think of hypercalcemia as the most probable cause.

Investigation of Choice

Serum calcium level

Serum parathormone levels

Immediate Management

- Adequate rehydration with Normal Saline
- Loop diuretics (to prevent heart failure)
- Bisphosphonates (in hypercalcemia of malignancy)
- Haemodialysis (in renal failure)
- Beta blockers (to protect against adverse cardiac effects)
- Calcitonin, Oral steroids, Mithramycin are other useful drugs.

Treatment of Choice

Treat the underlying cause

Serial No. 57

Subject: Medicine

Topic: Endocrinology

Question: A 32-year-old female presents with galactorrhoea, amenorrhoea and infertility.

Diagnosis: Hyperprolactinaema

Clinchers

- *32 year old female:* Clinical presentation in women is more obvious and occurs earlier than in men. In men, it is usually an incidental finding on brain scan -CT/ MRI or present as mass effect because of the tumor (prolactinomas).
- *Galactorrhoea:* Galactorrhoea is due to the direct physiologic effect of prolactin on breast epithelial cells.
- *Amenorrhoea, infertility:* Prolactin causes direct suppression of gonadotrophin rleasing hormones (GnRH) causing oligomenorrhoea, amenorrhoea or infertility.

CONFUSA

- Physiological hyper-prolactinaemia can occur in conditions of stress, pregnancy and lactation.
- A patient with prolactin levels which are consistently greater than 500-800 mU/L should be investigated in the absence of a pharmacological or physiological explanation.
- Prolactin levels greater than 4000 mU/L are found in patients with pathological hyperprolactinaemia.

Investigation of Choice

CT scan brain
Visual field assessment

Immediate Management

Dopamine agonists:
Bromocriptine (Drug of Choice)
Cabergoline
Quinagolide

Treatment of Choice

Transphenoidal pituitary adenomectomy

Your notes:

Serial No.122

Subject: Medicine

Topic: Endocrinology

Question: A 20-year-old girl with hypotension, hyperkalema and is mildly hyponatraemic. She has recently lost weight and her skin appears hyperpigmented.

Diagnosis: Addison's disease

Clinchers

- *A 20-year-old girl:* Addison's disease is slightly more common in females. It can occur in persons of any age; however, it is most common in people aged 30-50 years.
- *With hypotension:* often marked in acute hypoadrenalism; usually postural in chronic disease with a fall in blood pressure on standing of 20 mm Hg or more after a few minutes — may cause dizziness and headache; It is due to ineffective catecholamine action
- *Hyperkalema and is mildly hyponatremic:* hyponatraemia found in 90% of cases of primary adrenal insufficiency, hyperkalemia 65% cases, serum urea raised. Hypoglycaemia in 50% chronic cases.
- *Recently lost weight:* Weight loss is a common association with chronic adrenal insufficiency, mainly because of the loss of muscle mass. However it can be also due to associated tuberculosis.
- *Her skin appears hyperpigmented:* Hyperpigmentation is due to high ACTH; the skin assumes a dull, grey-brown colouration. Exposed skin, pressure areas, palmar creases, knuckles, buccal mucosa and recent scars are the commonest sites of hyperpigmentation.

CONFUSA

- In pregnancy, same dose of hydrocortisone can be continued, except if there is vomiting and toxaemia. Hydrocortisone 100 mg IM is given every 6 hours during labour.
- For major surgery, hydrocortisone 100 mg IM every 6 hours from premedication until oral feeds started. Twice the normal replacement is then given orally and reduced to maintenance over a few days.
- A single dose of hydrocortisone 100 mg IM is required for minimal procedures like endoscopy.

Investigation of Choice

ACTH levels
Synacthen Test

Immediate Management

Promptly treat patients in whom acute adrenal insufficiency is suspected — hydrocortisone 100 mg IM

Treatment of Choice

Treat cause

IV normal saline and hydrocortisone in acute situations.

In long term replacement also add fluorocortisone with hydrocortisone.

Patients should carry a steroid card and MedicAlert bracelet.

Your notes:

Serial No. 123

Subject: Medicine

Topic: Endocrinology

Question: A young boy with polyuria and polydipsia, has very high blood glucose levels.

Diagnosis: Type I Diabetes Mellitus (Early onset or Juvenile or Insulin Dependent Diabetes Mellitus)

Clinchers

- *A young boy:* It usually first develops in children or young adults. In the UK about 1 in 250 people develop Type 1 diabetes at some stage.
- *Polyuria and polydipsia:* This is typical presentation of IDDM; polyuria is due to the osmotic diuretic effect of glucose and ketone bodies in the urine; polydipsia is due to intracellular dehydration because of osmotic effect of high glucose levels.
- *Very high blood glucose level* :This confirms the cause of the symptoms in this young child. High glucose level in IDDM is due to insufficient insulin.

CONFUSA

- IDDM patients presenting with vomiting, abdominal pain, headache, thirst and polyuria with hyper-ventilation, drowsiness or coma-think of diabetic ketoacidosis.
- It is a medical emergency; its rapid recognition and accurate treatment are essential to prevent morbidity and mortality.
- Correcting dehydration with normal saline is a single most important step in the management of diabetic ketoacidosis.

Investigation of Choice

- Diabetes is diagnosed on the basis of history (i.e. polyuria, polydipsia and unexplained weight loss) PLUS —a random venous plasma glucose concentration >= 11.1 mmol/L.

  OR -a fasting plasma glucose concentration >= 7.0 mmol/L (whole blood >= 6.1 mmol/L).

  OR -2 hour plasma glucose concentration >= 11.1 mmol/L 2 hours after 75 g anhydrous glucose in an oral glucose tolerance test (OGTT).

Immediate Management

Refer to a Paediatric Diabetes Teams

Treatment of Choice

Acute cases like this need immediate correction of dehydration with Normal Saline.

Insulin is added to control glucose levels. Look out for signs of ketoacidosis.
Long-term insulin replacement for strict control of glucose levels is recommended.

Your notes:

Serial No. 130

Subject: Medicine

Topic: Arrhythmias

Question: An 18-year-old girl, sweaty with tremors and weight loss, says that her heart races.

Diagnosis: Hyperthyroidism

Clinchers

- *18-year-old girl:* All thyroid diseases are more common in women, with Grave's Disease being 10 times more common in females than males.
- *Sweaty with tremors and weight loss:* Hyperactivity, irritability, altered mood, intolerance to heat, sweating, palpitations, fatigue, weakness, losing weight even with increased appetite, diarrhoea, steatorrhoea, polyuria, oligo/amenorrhoea, loss of libido are the most commonly encountered symptoms in hyperthyroidism.
- *Says that her heart races:* This is signifying sinus tachycardia or atrial fibrillation, both commonly seen with hyperthyroidism.

CONFUSA

- Phaeochromocytoma can also present as palpitations, tachycardia, sweating, anxiety, panic attacks, tremor hyperthermia and weight loss. The patient is usually hypertensive.
- The female predominance and the absence of hypertension in the history in the given question, points more towards hyperthyroidism as the most probable cause.

Investigation of Choice

TSH can exclude primary thyrotoxicosis. Confirm diagnosis with free T4 levels.

Immediate Management

Beta blockers resolve many of the acute symptoms of hyperthyroidism e.g. tachycardia, tremor, restlessness — within 1-2 days of starting therapy. Propanolol is the most commonly used beta blocker for the purpose.

Treatment of Choice

The treatment of choice is carbimazole in the UK. Propylthiouracil is an alternative.

Your notes:

Serial No. 160

Subject: Medicine

Topic: Falls

Question: An elderly travelling alone was brought to Accident and Emergency from the airport in unconscious state. There are needles and a syringe in his hand baggage.

Diagnosis: Hypoglycaemia

Clinchers

- *Elderly:* Elderly, especially those more than 40 years of age are more prone for type 2 diabetes and its complications viz. hypoglycaemia, hyperglycaemia and diabeteic ketoacidosis.
- *Traveling alone:* Travelling itself puts quite a stress on the diabetic and usually a family member is advised to accompany the patient for instant recognition of symptoms of diabetic emergencies.
- *Brought to accident and emergency from the airport in unconscious state:* The most common warning symptoms of hypoglycaemia are profuse sweating, anxiety, nervousness, tremor, tachycardia, hunger, paraesthesia and patient often presents at A and E in stupor or coma. Here, the initial warning symptoms are most likely missed as the patient was traveling alone. Conditions that can lead to hypoglycaemia in people with diabetes include taking too much medication, missing or delaying a meal, eating too little food for the amount of insulin taken, exercising too strenuously, drinking too much alcohol, or any combination of these factors. The chances are high that due to his air travel, he either missed his meal or ate too little while on journey, while taking his regular dose of insulin.
- *There are needles and a syringe in his hand baggage:* This further confirms insulin, as the most likely cause of this hypoglycaemic attack.

CONFUSA

The presence of needles and a syringe in the hand baggage might have prompted you to think in the direction of opiate abuse, as heroine is also listed among the given options. However, the question typically lacks the features of opiate abuse, viz a teenage group, disheveled and dirty look, with respiratory depression, coma and pin point pupils. Morever, a drug abuser will always be in the lack of funds to support his daily needs than to afford an air travel.

Questions might look deceptively similar, but careful sorting out of facts will always lead you to the correct answer. All the hints are usually provided in the question. Your only job is to interpret them correctly.

Investigation of Choice

Plasma glucose levels

Immediate Management

50 ml of 50% glucose IV.

Glucagon 1mg IM if venous access not available.

If not recovered within 20 minutes give further injection of 25 g glucose plus 100 mg hydrocortisone.

Treatment of Choice

Strict management of glucose levels.

Your notes:

PAPER 2

Serial No. 16

Subject: Medicine

Topic: Diabetes

Question: Diabetic Ketoacidosis

Diagnosis: Diabetic Ketoacidosis

Clinchers

- Diabetic ketoacidosis occurs almost exclusively in type I diabetes.
- Patients have positive serum ketones and an arterial blood pH of less than or equal to 7.30 and/or a serum bicarbonate less than or equal to 15 mmol/l.
- The condition is stimulated by severe insulin deficiency coupled with absolute or relative increases in glucagon.
- It is a medical emergency;

CONFUSA

In diabetic ketoacidosis insulin deficiency causes excessive breakdown of adipose stores, resulting in increased levels of free fatty acids. Oxidation of such free fatty acids by the liver through acetyl CoA produces ketone bodies. Glucagon is the hormone that accelerates such fatty acid oxidation.

Investigation of Choice

Blood glucose
Ketones - urine or blood
Urea and Electrolytes
Arterial blood gases and pH

Immediate Management

Correct dehydration — Start normal saline, later change over to 5% dextrose when blood glucose is less than 15 mmol/L

Treatment of Choice

Insulin therapy
Search for and treat appropriately the precipitating factor.

Your notes:

Serial No. 17

Subject: Medicine

Topic: Diabetes

Question: Hyperosmolar non-ketotic hyperglycaemia

Diagnosis: Hyperosmolar non-ketotic hyperglycaemia

Clinchers

- Hyperosmolar non-ketotic hyperglycaemia occurs principally in patients with adult-onset diabetes.
- The condition is characterised by very high blood glucose but only a trace or +1 ketones. The plasma osmolality is very high, in the range of >350 m Osm/kg.
- It most commonly develops in patients with diabetes who have some concomitant illness that leads to a reduced fluid intake. Infection is the most common cause,
- Unlike patients with DKA, patients with hyperosmolar non ketotic hyperglycaemia do not develop ketoacidosis.
- Contributing factors include the limitation on ketogenesis by hyperosmolarity, the lower levels of free fatty acids available for ketogenesis, the availability of insulin in amounts sufficient to inhibit ketogenesis but not sufficient to prevent hyperglycaemia
- It accounts for about 10-15% of cases of diabetic decompensation (generally in elderly patients); diabetic ketoacidosis is much more common.

CONFUSA

This diagnosis of hyperosmolar non-ketotic hyperglycaemia should be considered in patients with:
-hyperglycaemia
-dehydration with marked thirst
-marked drowsiness
Hyperventilation is not present here.

Investigation of Choice

Serum Electrolytes
Serum Osmolality
Blood Glucose
Serum and Urinary Ketones

Immediate Management

Seek Expert advice

Treatment of Choice

If plasma sodium is greater than 145 mmol/L then half-normal saline is used for rehydration.
Lower doses of insulin are required because there is greater insulin sensitivity.

Serial No. 18

Subject: Medicine

Topic: Diabetes

Question: Hypoglycaemia

Diagnosis: Hypoglycaemia

Clinchers

- Hypoglycaemia in a diabetic is most often caused by over administration of oral hypoglycaemic agents or an excess dose of insulin.
- Other causes can be:
  - Injecting insulin into a scarred site — can result in delayed release of the insulin
  - Any systemic illness
  - Alcohol
  - Excess exercise and exertion.

CONFUSA

- Hypoglycaemia in presence of normal or high insulin and no elevation of ketones, consider: insulinoma, administration of insulin (no C-peptide detectable), insulin autoantibodies, administration of insulin 'sensitisers' e.g. metformin, glitazone.
- Hypoglycaemia with low insulin and no elevation of ketones, consider: a non-pancreatic neoplasma e.g. fibroma, hepatoma; anti-insulin receptor antibodies
- Hypoglycaemia with low insulin and elevation of ketones, consider:
  Addison's disease, hypopituitarism, alcohol

Investigation of Choice

Blood Glucose levels
Serum Insulin level
C-peptide

Immediate Management

Give oral sugar if patient conscious.

Treatment of Choice

If the patient is drowsy or fitting then:
Administer 50 ml of 50% glucose IV, or alternatively glucagon 1 mg IV/IM/SC Recheck the glucose by stick test after 5 mins and repeat again at 30 min.

Your notes:

Serial No. 19

Subject: Medicine

Topic: Diabetes

Question: Hyperglycaemia

Diagnosis: Hyperglycaemia

Clinchers

- Hyperglycaemia means a high blood glucose level and usually refers to a glucose level above 11 mmol/L.
- In a diabetic, hyperglycaemia perhaps suggests a poorly controlled state. It can present as simple rise in blood glucose levels or in association with diabetic ketoacidosis or non ketotic hyperosmolar hyperglycaemia.

CONFUSA

A presentation of hyperglycaemia should incite investigations for the diagnosis of diabetes in a non-diabetic and into the diagnosis of diabetic ketoacidosis or non ketotic hyperosmolar hyperglycaemia in a diabetic.

Investigation of Choice

Diabetes is diagnosed on the basis of history (i.e. polyuria, polydipsia and unexplained weight loss) PLUS
-a random venous plasma glucose concentration >= 11.1 mmol/l
OR -a fasting plasma glucose concentration >= 7.0 mmol/l (whole blood >= 6.1 mmol/l)
OR -2 hour plasma glucose concentration >= 11.1 mmol/l 2 hours after 75g anhydrous glucose in an oral glucose tolerance test (OGTT).

Immediate Management

Refer to a Diabetes Teams

Treatment of Choice

Acute cases like this need immediate correction of dehydration with Normal Saline.
Insulin is added to control glucose levels. Look out for signs of ketoacidosis.
Long term insulin replacement for strict control of glucose levels is recommended.

Your notes:

Serial No. 20

Subject: Medicine

Topic: Diabetes

Question: Syndrome X

Diagnosis: Syndrome X (also known as The metabolic syndrome, Syndrome 'X', Metabolic syndrome X, Reaven's syndrome).

Clinchers

- Syndrome X is characterised by insulin resistance, glucose intolerance with compensatory hyperinsulinaemia, hypertension and dyslipidaemia.
- Central obesity is characteristic, overt diabetes mellitus (type II); and atherosclerosis develop over time.
- It is more common in certain ethnic groups: Native or Mexican-Americans, Southern Asians.

CONFUSA

Central obesity is more highly correlated with the metabolic risk factors than body mass index (BMI) and therefore measurement of waist circumference (around the navel) is recommended to identify the body weight component of metabolic syndrome.

Investigation of Choice

The National Cholesterol Education Program (NCEP) Adult Treatment Panel (ATP) III guidelines have suggested that a diagnosis of metabolic syndrome where three or more of the following risk factors are present:
-central obesity,
-elevated triglyceride,
-low HDL,
-raised blood pressure and
-raised fasting plasma glucose

Immediate Management

None

Treatment of Choice

Directed at reducing obesity. Obesity probably leads to insulin resistance by the associated increased rate of non-esterified fatty acids causing post-receptor defects in insulin's action.
-Weight reduction
-Increased physical activity
-LDL reduction
-Treat hypertension, plus aspirin
-Treatments to reduce triglycerides and elevate HDL.
-other lifestyle factors (in addition to physical activity) must be addressed e.g. moderation in alcohol intake, and cessation of smoking and monosaturated fat in the diet.

Your notes:

Serial No. 28

Subject: Medicine

Topic: Anaemia

Question: A 28-year-old lady with history of intermittent jaundice, looks pale. Her spleen is palpable and USG abdomen shows gallstones.

Diagnosis: Congenital Spherocytosis

Clinchers

- *28-year-old lady:* Hereditary spherocytosis is an inherited disorder (autosomal dominant) of the red blood cell membrane, leading to haemolytic anaemia. It usually presents in childhood or adolescence.
- *Intermittent jaundice:* Most patients develop a partially compensated haemolytic state. Mild or intermittent jaundice is caused by rapid haemolysis of the spherocytes.
- *Looks pale:* Anaemia is invariably present, however, the severity depends upon the compensated bone marrow function.
- *Spleen is palpable:* As would be expected in any haemolytic states, splenomegaly is also a prominent feature here.
- *USG abdomen shows gallstones:* These are usually pigment stones developed due to rapid haemolysis and release of bile pigments in the circulation.

CONFUSA

Spherocytes in the peripheral blood film is also seen in cases of haemolysis and severe burns. In the absence of a definite clue in the question towards diagnosis, look for microangiopathic anaemia, e.g. DIC, TTP.

Investigation of Choice
Osmotic fragility test

Immediate Management
Folic acid supplements — 1 mg per day

Treatment of Choice
Splenectomy — eliminates the site of haemolysis.

Your notes:

Serial No. 123

Subject: Medicine

Topic: Genetics

Question: A 15-year-old girl with features of diabetes mellitus.

Diagnosis: Insulin Dependent Diabetes Mellitus (IDDM)

Clinchers

- A 15-year-old girl with features of diabetes mellitus: IDDM usually presents before 20 years of age, with both sexes being equally affected. This follows close association with HLA B8, B15, DR3 and DR4. Occasionally other autoimmune diseases like Schmidt's syndrome is present alongwith.

CONFUSA

Polygenic Inheritance: When some traits are determined by the combined effect of more than one pair of genes, it is referred to as polygenic, or continuous, traits. An example of this is human stature, colour and also IDDM. Human skin, hair, and eye colour are also polygenic traits because they are influenced by more than one allele at different loci.

Whereas, when a single gene may be responsible for a variety of traits it is called pleiotropy. The complex of symptoms that are collectively referred to as sickle-cell trait, or sickle-cell anaemia, is an example.

Investigation of Choice
Fasting plasma glucose concentration >7.0 mmol/L or 2 hr plasma glucose concentration >11.0 mmol/hr is diagnostic.

Immediate Management
Urgent referral to Diabetic Team

Treatment of Choice
Strict glycaemic control achieved by diet modifications, oral hypoglycaemics or Insulin therapy.

Your notes:

Serial No. 132

Subject: Medicine

Topic: Endocrinology

Question: A 30-year-old female presents with lethargy. Her BP is 160/100 with serum electrolytes Na^+ 149 mmol/L, K^+ 2.6 mmol/L and HCO^-_3 30 mmol/L.

Diagnosis: Conn's Syndrome

Clinchers

- *30-year-old female:* Primary hyperaldosteronism is twice as common in women as in men. Peak incidence occurs in the third to sixth decades of life.
- *Lethargy:* is attributed to hypokalemia. Patients may also present with muscle weakness, cramping, headaches, and palpitations. They can also have polydipsia and polyuria from hypokalaemia-induced nephrogenic diabetes insipidus.
- *BP 160/100:* Patient may present with hypertension or one of the cardiac or neurological complications of hypertension.
- *Serum electrolytes Na^+ 149 mmol/L, K^+ 2.6 mmol/L and HCO^-_3 30 mmol/L:* The picture of mild hypernatremia with hypokalemia in the presence of metabolic alkalosis fits perfect in the diagnosis of Conn's Syndrome.

CONFUSA

- In any case of hypokalaemic hypertension in the presence of metabolic alkalosis, think of Conn's syndrome as the most probable diagnosis.
- A poorly controlled hypertensive on high doses of diuretics can also present with the same picture of hypertension, alkalosis and hypokalaemia — rule out diuretics as a cause.

Investigation of Choice

- Blood electrolytes
- Plasma renin and aldosterone — low renin and high aldosterone suggests primary hyperaldosteronism
- 24 hour urinary aldosterone.

Immediate Management

Prompt treatment of hypokalemia and hypertension.

Treatment of Choice

According to the underlying cause:

- if due to adenoma — surgery after 4 to 6 weeks of spironolactone therapy (e.g. 300 mg/day)
- if due to adrenal hyperplasia — spironolactone or amiloride is generally sufficient.

Serial No. 133

Subject: Medicine

Topic: Endocrinology

Question: A 35-year-old female presents with hypotension and lethargy. Her skin appears hyperpigmented.

Diagnosis: Addison's disease

Clinchers

- *A 35-year-old female:* Addison's disease is slightly more common in females. It can occur in persons of any age; however, it is most common in people aged 30-50 years.
- *Hypotension:* often marked in acute hypoadrenalism; usually postural in chronic disease with a fall in blood pressure on standing of 20 mm Hg or more after a few minutes—may cause dizziness and headache; It is due to ineffective catecholamine action.
- *Lethargy:* lassitude and muscle weakness is due to hypokalemia.
- *Hyperpigmentation:* due to high ACTH; the skin assumes a dull, grey-brown colouration.
  Exposed skin, pressure areas, palmar creases, knuckles, buccal mucosa and recent scars are the commonest sites of hyperpigmentation.

CONFUSA

In case of confusion, look for the hints at other associated autoimmune conditions associated with Addison's Disease. Addison's disease is associated with an increased incidence of:

- Hashimoto's thyroiditis,
- Schmidt's syndrome
- Type I diabetes mellitus
- Premature ovarian failure
- Idiopathic hypoparathyroidism
- Pernicious anaemia
- Mucocutaneous candidiasis
- Vitiligo
- Alopecia
- Graves' disease
- Adrenoleukodystrophy

Investigation of Choice

ACTH levels
Synacthen Test

Immediate Management

Promptly treat patients in whom acute adrenal insufficiency is suspected — hydrocortisone 100 mg IM

Treatment of Choice

Treat cause

IV normal saline and hydrocortisone in acute situations.

In long-term replacement also add fluorocortisone with hydrocortisone.

Patients should carry a steroid card and MedicAlert bracelet.

Your notes:

Serial No. 134

Subject: Medicine

Topic: Endocrinology

Question: A 40-year-old patient complaints of lethargy, bone pain, polyuria and polydipsia. His blood glucose level is 3.0 mmol/L.

Diagnosis: Hypercalcaemia

Clinchers

- *40-year-old:* Hypercalcaemia in elderly usually as a part of metastatic complications of malignancy. In younger age group primary hyperparathyroidism remains the most common cause.
- *Lethargy:* increased calcium levels stimulate muscle for active contraction, which later go in for exhaustion and present as generalised lethargy and profound muscle weakness.
- *Polyuria, polydipsia:* These are among the general non specific symptoms of hypercalcaemia, occurring due increased osmolality of the blood, stimulating the thirst centre of the hypothalamus.
- *Bone pain:* rapid loss of bone density leads to osteopenia, bone pains, pathological fractures and hypercalciuria.
- *Blood glucose level 3.0 mmol/L:* Normal glucose levels rules out diabetes as a cause of polyuria, polydipsia.

CONFUSA

- In a patient presenting with bone pain (or, back pain) with features of hypercalcaemia along with anaemia, carefully rule out Multiple Myeloma.
- In a patient who recently underwent chemotherapy for malignancy, when presenting with non specific symptoms of confusion, disorientation, depression with profuse thirst, think of hypercalcaemia as the most probable cause.

Investigation of Choice

Serum calcium level

Serum parathormone levels

Immediate Management

- Adequate rehydration with Normal Saline
- Loop diuretics (to prevent heart failure)
- Bisphosphonates (in hypercalcaemia of malignancy)
- Haemodialysis (in renal failure)
- Beta blockers (to protect against adverese cardiac effects).

- Calcitonin, Oral steroids, Mithramycin are other useful drugs.

Treatment of Choice

Treat the underlying cause

Your notes:

Serial No. 135

Subject: Medicine

Topic: Endocrinology

Question: A 32-year-old female presents with galactorrhoea, amenorrhoea and infertility.

Diagnosis: Hyperprolactinaemia

Clinchers

- *A 32-year-old female:* Clinical presentation in women is more obvious and occurs earlier than in men. In men, it is usually an incidental finding on brain scan -CT/MRI or present as mass effect because of the tumor (prolactinomas).
- *Galactorrhoea:* Galactorrhea is due to the direct physiologic effect of prolactin on breast epithelial cells.
- *Amenorrhoea, infertility:* Prolactin causes direct suppression of gonadotrophin rleasing hormones (GnRH) causing oilgomenorrhoea, amenorrhoea or infertility.

CONFUSA

- Physiological hyperprolactinaemia can occur in conditions of stress, pregnancy and lactation.
- A patient with prolactin levels which are consistently greater than 500-800 mU/L should be investigated in the absence of pharmacological or physiological explanation.
- Prolactin levels greater than 4000 mU/L are found in patients with pathological hyperprolactinaemia.

Investigation of Choice

CT scan brain

Visual field assessment

Immediate Management

Dopamine agonists:

Bromocriptine (Drug of Choice)

Cabergoline

Quinagolide

Treatment of Choice

Transphenoidal pituitary adenomectomy

Your notes:

Serial No. 136

Subject: Medicine

Topic: Arrhythmias

Question: An 18-year-old girl, sweaty with tremors and weight loss, says that her heart races.

Diagnosis: Hyperthyroidism

Clinchers

- *18-year-old girl:* All thyroid diseases are more common in women, with Grave's Disease being 10 times more common in females than males.
- *Sweaty with tremors and weight loss:* Hyperactivity, irritability, altered mood, intolerance to heat, sweating, palpitations, fatigue, weakness, losing weight even with increased appetite, diarrhoea, steatorrhoea, polyuria, oligo/amenorrhoea, loss of libido are the most commonly encountered symptoms in hyperthyroidism.
- *Says that her heart races:* This is signifying sinus tachycardia or atrial fibrillation, both commonly seen with hyperthyroidism.

CONFUSA

- Phaeochromocytoma can also present as palpitations, tachycardia, sweating, anxiety, panic attacks, tremor hyperthermia and weight loss. The patient is usually hypertensive.
- The female predominance and the absence of hypertension in the history in the given question, points more towards hyperthyroidism as the most probable cause.

Investigation of Choice

TSH can exclude primary thyrotoxicosis. Confirm diagnosis with free T4 levels.

Immediate Management

Beta blockers resolve many of the acute symptoms of hyperthyroidism e.g. tachycardia, tremor, restlessness - within 1-2 days of starting therapy. Propranolol is the most commonly used beta blocker for the purpose.

Treatment of Choice

The treatment of choice is carbimazole in the UK. Propylthiouracil is an alternative.

Your notes:

Serial No. 141

Subject: Medicine

Topic: Epilepsy

Question: A 53-year-old non-alcoholic, obese man presents with sweating, tremor, drowsiness, fits and agitation.

Diagnosis: Hypoglycaemia

Clinchers

- *A 53-year-old:* Hypoglycaemia predominantly affects older individuals than the young. Females are more prone for it.
- *Non-alcoholic:* This rules out alcohol as an important cause of the presenting features in the patient. Both alcohol withdrawl and alcohol intoxication can present as agitation, tremor drowsiness and fits.
- *Obese:* This hints towards a possible undiagnosed diabetes in this patient, which is now presenting as transient reactive hypoglycaemia.
- *Sweating, tremor, drowsiness, fits and agitation:* The symptoms due to hypoglycaemia primarily occur initially due to an increase in the adrenaline activity, viz, tremor, agitation, palpitations, sweating and the like. Deficient glucose to the CNS can also lead to coma, seizures and death.

CONFUSA

Such a picture is very common in hospitalized patients and usually present in 3-5 days of admission. In most cases, the symptoms appear due to alcohol withdrawl as the patient does not gets his usual quota due to his in-hospital stay. It is always very important to rule out alcohol history and insulin therapy as the possible explanation for the condition.

Investigation of Choice

Blood glucose levels

Immediate Management

IV Dextrose or oral feeds depending on the severity of the condition.

Treatment of Choice

According to the cause identified.

Your notes:

Serial No.156

Subject: Medicine

Topic: Endocrinology

Question: A 20-year-old girl with hypotension, hyperkalaema and is mildly hyponatraemic. She has recently lost weight and her skin appears hyperpigmented.

Diagnosis: Addison's disease

Clinchers

- *A 20-year-old girl:* Addison's disease is slightly more common in females. It can occur in persons of any age; however, it is most common in people aged 30-50 years.
- *With hypotension:* often marked in acute hypoadrenalism; usually postural in chronic disease with a fall in blood pressure on standing of 20 mm Hg or more after a few minutes may cause dizziness and headache; It is due to ineffective catecholamine action
- *Hyperkalaemia and is mildly hyponatraemic:* hyponatraemia found in 90% of cases of primary adrenal insufficiency, hyperkalaemia 65% cases, serum urea raised. Hypoglycaemia in 50% chronic cases.
- *Recently lost weight:* Weight loss is a common association with chronic adrenal insufficiency, mainly because of the loss of muscle mass. However it can be also due to associated tuberculosis.
- *Her skin appears hyperpigmented:* Hyperpigmentation is due to high ACTH; the skin assumes a dull, grey-brown colouration. Exposed skin, pressure areas, palmar creases, knuckles, buccal mucosa and recent scars are the commonest sites of hyperpigmentation.

CONFUSA

- In pregnancy, same dose of hydrocortisone can be continued, except if there is vomiting and toxaemia. Hydrocortisone 100 mg IM is given every 6 hours during labour.
- For major surgery, hydrocortisone 100 mg im every 6 hours from premedication until oral feeds started. Twice the normal replacement is then given orally and reduced to maintenance over a few days.
- A single dose of hydrocortisone 100 mg im is required for minimal procedures like endoscopy.

Investigation of Choice

ACTH levels
Synacthen Test

Immediate Management

Promptly treat patients in whom acute adrenal insufficiency is suspected — hydrocortisone 100 mg IM.

Treatment of Choice

Treat cause
IV normal saline and hydrocortisone in acute situations.
In long term replacement also add fluorocortisone with hydrocortisone.
Patients should carry a steroid card and MedicAlert bracelet.

Your notes:

Serial No. 157

Subject: Medicine

Topic: Endocrinology

Question: A young boy with polyuria and polydipsia, has very high blood glucose levels.

Diagnosis: Type I Diabetes Mellitus (Early onset or Juveline or Insulin Dependent Diabetes Mellitus).

Clinchers

- *A young boy:* It usually first develops in children or young adults. In the UK about 1 in 250 people develop Type 1 diabetes at some stage.
- *Polyuria and polydipsia:*This is typical presentation of IDDM; polyuria is due to the osmotic diurectic effect of glucose and ketone bodies in the urine; polydipsia is due to intracellular dehydration because of osmotic effect of high glucose levels.
- *Very high blood glucose level:* This confirms the cause of the symptoms in this young child. High glucose level in IDDM is due to insufficient insulin.

CONFUSA

- IDDM patients presenting with vomiting, abdominal pain, headache, thirst and polyuria with hyperventilation, drowsiness or coma — think of diabetic ketoacidosis.
- It is a medical emergency; its rapid recognition and accurate treatment are essential to prevent morbidity and mortality.
- Correcting dehydration with normal saline is a single most important step in the management of diabetic ketoacidosis.

Investigation of Choice

Diabetes is diagnosed on the basis of history (i.e. polyuria, polydipsia and unexplained weight loss) PLUS

-a random venous plasma glucose concentration >= 11.1 mmol/L

OR -a fasting plasma glucose concentration >= 7.0 mmol/L (whole blood >= 6.1 mmol/L)

OR -2 hour plasma glucose concentration >= 11.1 mmol/L 2 hours after 75 g anhydrous glucose in an oral glucose tolerance test (OGTT).

Immediate Management

Refer to a Paediatric Diabetes Team

Treatment of Choice

Acute cases like this need immediate correction of dehydration with Normal Saline.

Insulin is added to control glucose levels. Look out for signs of ketoacidosis.

Long-term insulin replacement for strict control of glucose levels is recommended.

Your notes:

PAPER 3

38. A 50-year-old male complains of flushing, tremor, palpitations. He is found to have a fluctuating blood pressure of 200/120.

Diagnosis: Phaeochromocytoma.

Clinchers

- *A 50-year-old male:* Phaeochromocytomas occur at all ages but are most common in young to mild adult life. They are usually associated with MEN type II syndromes. Sometimes they are inherited (autosomal dominant).

  There is a slight female preponderance, but this fact is not proven in meta-analyses.
- *Flushing, tremor, palpitations:* Either pallor or flushing may occur during the attack paroxysmal symptoms occur which may mimic a seizure disorder or panic attack. Other symptoms can be headache, sweating, pulsatile scotomas, etc. They are precipitated by stretching, sneezing, stress, sex, smoking, surgery, parturition of cheese, alcohol or tricyclics.
- *Fluctuating blood pressure of 200/120:* Hypertension is the most common sign and is episodic (NOTE). It resonds poorly to traditional antihypertensive treatment. It might be sustained in a significant proportion of patients but even in these there are distinct crises.

CONFUSA

The main differential diagnosis is from essential hypertension with hyperadrenergic features (sweating, tachycardia, increased cardiac output), but GMC has never asked such a question. One can be confused with carcinoid syndrome which does not produce such hypertensive episodes and diarrhoea (recurrent, watery) is pathognomically present in them.

Investigation of Choice

- *Screening:* 24 h urine collection for
  - HMMA
  - VMA
  - Total/free meta-adrenalines
- *Definitive*
  - Adrenal tumor (90%)—MRI
  - Extra-adrenal (10%)—MIBG scan

Treatment of Choice

- Surgery
- Careful BP control for 2 weeks preoperative (a-blocker before b-blockers).

39. A middle-aged woman with a blood pressure of 160/110 is found to have abdominal striae and facial hirsutism.

Diagnosis: Cushing's syndrome

Clinchers

- *Middle-aged:* Peak age—30-50 years.
- *Woman:* More common in women (only for pituitary dependent adrenal hyperplasia). But the most common cause of Cushing's syndrome is iatrogenic (exogenous steroid administration).
- *Blood pressure of 160/110:* Hypertension is common (>150/90) as are other effects of glucocorticoid excess like truncal obesity, increased body weight, water retention, osteoporosis, etc.
- *Abdominal striae:* Purple abdominal striae especially on abdomen are pathognomic and occur only with ACTH dependent causes. These are secondary to weakening and rupture of collagen fibers in dermis coupled with truncal obesity.
- *Facial hirsutism:* In women, increased levels of adrenal androgens can cause acne, hirsutism, and oligomenorrhoea or amenorrhoea.

CONFUSA

Cushing's syndrome can be easily diagnosed from the clinical picture. The tough job is to differentiated between ectopic ACTH tumour or pituitary disease which is causing the syndrome. Severe hirsutism/virilization suggests an adrenal tumour. Specific diagnosis is possible only by localization tests like plasma ACTH, CRH test (Read pg. 301, OHCM, 5th edn).

Investigation of Choice

- *Screening:* Overnight dexamethasone suppression test
- *Definitive:*
  - 48 h DST
  - Cricadian rhythm of cortisol
  - Secretion (lost in Cushing's syndrome)
- *Localisation*
  - Plasma ACTH
  - High dose DST
  - CRH test
- *Others*
  - Pituitary—MRI
  - Adrenal—CT/MRI

Immediate Management

Remove source if iatrogenic

Treatment of Choice

Surgery after control of cortisol hypersecretion (Iatrogenic cases usually resolve on removal of source).

- Radiotherapy if surgery not possible.

40. A 42-year-old patient with prominent jaw and supraorbital ridges.

Diagnosis: Acromegaly

Clinchers

- *A 42-year-old:* It usually presents between the ages of 30 and 50 years. Its onset is insidious.
- *Prominent jaw and supraorbital ridges:* Most of the features of acromegaly are due to the growth of soft tissues. Main features are:
  - Large tongue
  - Prominent supraorbital ridge
  - Prognathism
  - Increased teeth spacing
  - Increased shoe size
  - Thick spade like hands

Other features are: Coarse, oily skin, deepening voice, arthralgia, kyphosis, proximal muscle weakness, paraesthesiae—due to carpal tunnel syndrome, progressive heart failure, goitre, sleep apnoea.

CONFUSA

In acromegaly, isolated growth hormone measurement may show raised secretion, but levels vary with the time of the day and other factors so random measurement are not diagnostic.

Investigation of Choice

Oral glucose tolerance test (OGTT) with growth hormone measurement is diagnostic.

Immediate Management

Obtain old photos to compare. Take new photographs of full face, torso, hands on chest.

Treatment of Choice

Transsphenoidal surgery.

Note: For older patients (or failed surgery)—external irradiation.

Your notes:

52. A young diabetic is admitted in a comatose state. His plasma glucose level is 2 mmols/L

Diagnosis: Hypoglycaemia

Clinchers

- *Young diabetic:* The most common cause of hypoglycaemia is insulin or sulfonylurea treatment in a known diabetic. It can also be due to insufficient food or change in routine of insulin (i.e. site of injection, type of insulin, new syringe size). It is more so in younger patients because there is usually no set lifestyle.
- *Comatose state:* Initially, a hypoglycaemic patient is restless and agitated but, if untreated, rapidly becomes unresponsive. There is pallor profuse sweating and a bounding pulse. Aggression can be such that the patient arrives in police custody and may be thought to be intoxicated. False neurological signs are sometimes seen.
- *His plasma glucose level is 2 mmols:* Hypoglycaemia by definition is < 2.5 mmol/L.

CONFUSA

The other two conditions which can produce comatose state in a diabetic are:

- Nonketotic (HONK) coma
- Diabetic ketoacidosis (DKA)

Investigation of Choice

- Venous blood glucose
- In case of unexplained hypoglycaemia
  - Liver function tests
  - Insulin assay
  - C peptide assay
  - Toxicology (paracetamol) screen

Immediate Management

Start treatment after taking blood sample.

Treatment of Choice

- 50 ml of 50% dextrose solution (adults)
- 2-5 ml/kg of 10% dextrose solution (child)
- If venous access is delayed:
  - Glucagon 1-2 mg IM (20 µg/kg for children)
- 50% dextrose harms veins, so follow by 0.9% saline flush.
- If there is no prompt recovery after treatment, give dexamethasone 4 mg/4h IV to combat cerebral edema after prolonged hypoglycaemia.
- Once conscious, give sugery drinks.

53. A young diabetic is admitted in a comatose state. His plasma glucose level is 17 mmols and he is dehydrated.

Diagnosis: Diabetic ketoacidosis (DKA).

Clinchers

- *Young diabetic:* DKA coma only occurs with type I diabetes, so it is more common in young diabetics (as type I diabetes usually presents in childhood).
- *Comatose state:* Apart from coma other symptoms are polyuria, polydipsia, lethargy, anorexia, hyperventilation, ketotic breath (smells like peach), dehydration, vomiting, abdominal pain, etc.
- *Plasma glucose level is 17 mmols:* Normal range of blood glucose is 3.5-5.5 mmol/L. Usually in DKA it is > 20 mmol/L. But 17 mmol/L is also a very high value.
- *Dehydrated:* Gross hyperglycaemia causes an osmotic diuresis, decreased tissue perfusion and circulatory collapse. It produces dehydration. Dehydration is more life-threatening than any hyperglycaemia—so its correction takes precedence.

CONFUSA

Some students get confused between DKA and HONK coma (hyperglycaemic hyperosmolar nonketotic coma).

DKA	*HONK*
1. Occurs only in IDDM	1. Occurs only in NIDDM
2. History of 2-3 days	2. Longer history (e.g. 1 wk)
3. Glucose usually > 20 mmol/l	3. Glucose >35 mmol/l
4. Acidosis present (pH < 7.3)	4. Acidosis absent
5. Ketotic breath present	5. No ketotic breath
6. Younger patients	6. Patient often old
7. Insulin given immediately in treatment	7. Insulin is given late, cautiously and in lower dosage

Investigation of Choice

Plasma osmolality (2[Na^+] + [urea] + [glucose])

Immediate Management

IV access and stard fluid (0.9% NS) immediately.

Treatment of Choice

Fluid replacement (0.9%NS) + 10U soluble insulin IV (if plasma glucose > 20 mmol/L).

Insulin sliding scale.

Your notes:

125. A young lady had a miscarriage in her second trimester following which she bleed profusely, needing 6 units of blood and had to be taken for surgical evacuation of her uterus. She needed medical treatment as she had milk secretion for a few days, but since she has had no periods.

Diagnosis: Sheehan's syndrome (Simmonds disease).

Clinchers

- *She bleed profusely, needing 6 units of blood:* The most common cause of Sheehan's syndrome in females is severe obstetric haemorrhage causing necrosis of pituitary (due to ischaemia).
- *Milk secretion for a few days:* This is completely normal to occur for a few days after a second trimester abortion. But eventually there will be a failure to lactate because of panhypopituitarism of Sheehan's syndrome.
- *No periods:* Amenorrhoea sets in because of failure of pituitary to secrete gonadotrophins.

CONFUSA

Galactorrhoea is milk secretion unrelated to pregnancy or postpartum period. If present it suggests pituitary function (or hyperfunction exactly) and excludes a diagnosis of Sheehan's syndrome.

Investigation of Choice

CT/MRI pituitary fossa.

Immediate Management

Refer to endocrinologist.

Treatment of Choice

Hormone therapy.

Your notes:

146. A 35-year-old female with a high blood glucose level is noted to be obese and has abdominal striae.

Diagnosis: Determination of diurnal steroid level pattern.

Clinchers

- *A 35-year-old female:* Cushings disease is more common in women with peak age between 30-50 years.
- *High blood glucose level:* One of the secondary causes of diabetes include Cushing's disease (Other endocrine diseases associated are acromegaly, pheochromocytoma, thyrotoxicosis).
- *Obese with abdominal striae:* Weight gain, menstrual irregularities, amenorrhoea, hirsutism, impotence, depression, muscle weakness are the symptoms of Cushing's disease.

Important signs include—tissue wasting, thin skin, purple abdominal striae, buffalow hump, osteoporosis water retention, etc.

Investigation of Choice

Determination of diurnal steroid level pattern.

Immediate Management

Monitor blood and urine glucose and adopt treatment accordingly.

Treatment of Choice

Manage high sugar levels and investigate for Cushing's disease. For Cushing's disease selective removal of pituitary adenoma via a transphenoidal and rarely transfrontal approach is done. Bilateral adrenalectomy is done if source cannot be located.

Your notes:

147. An elderly gentleman with frequency is found to have a raised random blood glucose level.

Diagnosis: Diabetes mellitus.

Clinchers

- *Elderly gentleman with frequency:* Signs and symptoms attributable to an osmotic diuresis (polyuria, polydipsia) supported with hyperglycaemia makes the diagnosis of diabetes mellitus unequivocal.
- *Raised random blood glucose level:* If the random blood glucose level is raised, we go for fasting venous plasma glucose. Fasting plasma glucose level $\geq$ 7 mmol/L is diagnostic. A glucose of 6-7 mmol/L implies impaired fasting glucose. If there is any doubt, the 2 hour value in oral glucose tolerance test (OGTT) should be used (diagnostic if levels >11.1 mmol/L).

Investigation of Choice

Fasting glucose level (diagnostic if $\geq$ 7 mmol/L)

Immediate Management

Monitor blood and urine glucose and adopt treatment accordingly.

Your notes:

DIABETES—treatment (NIDDM)

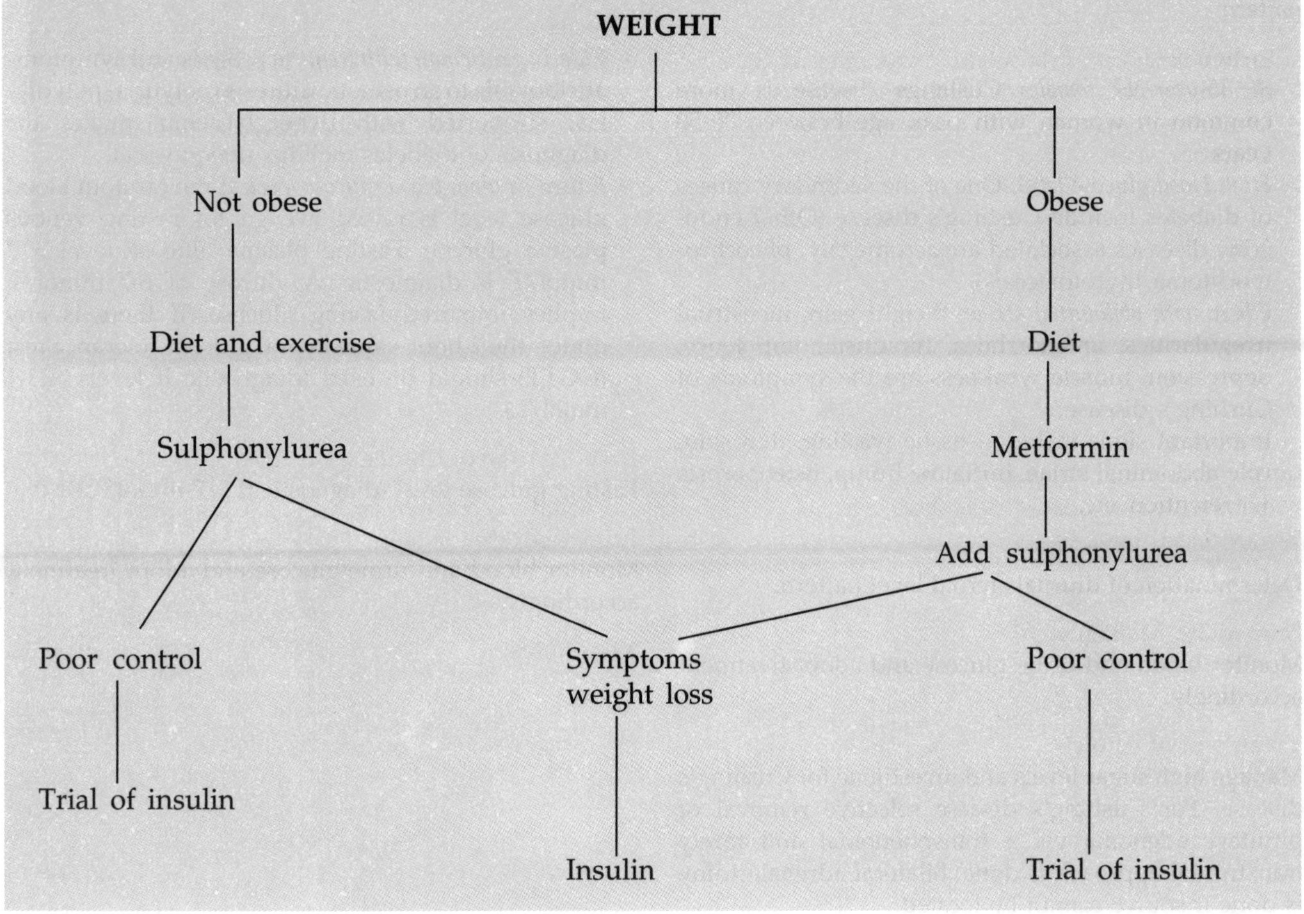

148. An elderly gentleman with polyuria is found to have a raised fasting blood glucose level.

Diagnosis: Diabetes mellitus.

Clinchers

➢ *Elderly gentleman with polyuria:* Though this question directly points towards diabetes mellitus, let us familiarise ourselves with *causes of polyuria.*

Diuretics
- Therapeutic
  - Frusemide
  - Amiloride
  - Bendrofluazide
- Osmotic
  - Hyperglycaemia
  - Hypercalcaemia
  - Mannitol
  - Urea

Diabetes insipidus
- Cranial
  - Idiopathic deficiency of ADH production
- Inherited (dominant or recessive)
  - Head injuries
  - Neurosurgery
  - Brain tumors
  - Opiates
- Nephrogenic
  - Drugs
    - Lithium
    - Demechocycline
  - Inherited (X-linked)
  - Chronic hypercalcaemia
  - Hypokalaemia
  - Chronic tubulointestinal nephritis
- Excessive fluid intake
  - Psychogenic
  - Drug induced thirst—anticholinergics
  - Hypothalamic disease

➢ *Raised fasting glucose level:* As already discussed in previous question fasting glucose (plasma) level of ≥ 7 mmol/L is diagnostic and glucose of 6-7 mmol/L implies impaired fasting glucose. We should never go for a single glucose value. In case of any trouble 2 hour value in oral glucose tolerance test (OGTT) should be used (diagnostic if value ≥ 11.1 mmol/L).

Method for performing OGTT:
- Fast overnight and give 75 gm of glucose in 300 ml under to drink.
- Venous plasma glucose before and 2 hours after drink.

Investigation of Choice: Glucose tolerance test.

Immediate Management: Go for OGTT.

149. A known diabetic on treatment has several episodes of hypoglycaemia.

Diagnosis: Improper treatment.

Clinchers

➢ *Known diabetic on treatment:* In hospital settings drugs are the most common cause of hypoglycaemia, the three drugs most frequently implicated being:
- Insulin
- Sulphonylurea
- Alcohol

➢ Here in this question we can assess glycaemic control from glycosylated haemoglobin (HbA_{1c}), the levels 8 weeks (i.e. RBC half-life). The target HbA_{1c} should be set individually. Complications increase in frequency with increasing HbA_{1c}.
In conditions interfering with HbA_{1c} measurements (e.g. some haemoglobinopathies), fructosamine (glycated plasmaprotein) levels can be assessed, this related to control over previous 1-3 weeks.

➢ Plasma HbA_{1c} values—if >7%. DM is likely and risk of microvascular complications occurs.

Investigation of Choice

Haemoglobin A_{1c} (glycosylated haemoglobin).

Immediate Management

Monitor blood and urine glucose levels and adjust the treatment accordingly.

Treatment of Choice

Educate patient—recognition and treatment of hypoglycaemia (e.g. sweets/sugar) is essential.

- Regular exercise and healthy eating habits (sugar, ⁻ saturated fat, starch-carbohydrate).

Your notes:

150. A 27-year-old woman was found to have glycosuria at a routine antenatal clinic visit. A glucose tolerance test confirmed the diagnosis of gestational diabetes. What will be your like of action.

Diagnosis: Gestational diabetes.

Clinchers

- *Gestational diabetes:* Diabetes arising for the first-time in pregnancy, is often treated with diet alone. The patient requires good education and must be encouraged to monitor blood glucose at home. A very few cases may require insulin to achieve glycaemic control. Oral hypoglycaemia should not be used in pregnancy.
- *Glycosuria:* Is common in pregnancy due to lowering of renal threshold. If glycosuria persistently present, a glucose tolerance test is performed. Some women with gestational diabetes either remain diabetic or subsequently develop diabetes.

CONFUSA

Only minority will require insulin to achieve glycaemic control.

Investigation of Choice
GTT.

Immediate Management
Dietary adjustment + monitor.

Treatment

- Women should start a simple carbohydrate restricted diet. In addition to checking her blood sugar twice a week, also test her urine for ketones.
- If simple diet does not achieve the required blood glucose levels, a twice daily regimen of medium—and short-acting insulin.
- If ketosis occurs, the diet should be relaxed and insulin started.

Your notes:

PAPER 4

106. Due to increased catecholamines.

Diagnosis: Phaeochromocytoma

Clinchers

- *Increased catecholamines:* Phaeochromocytoma is a rare catecholamine producing tumour and its clinical features are those of catecholamine excess and are frequently, but not necessarily intermittent.

  Note: These tumours are not innervated and catecholamine release does not result from neural stimulation.

Most common neurotransmitter secreted by:

- Most phaeochromocytoma—both norepinephrine and epinephrine (in ratio 80:20)
- Most extra-adrenal pheochromocytoma—only norepinephrine
- Malignant phaeochromocytoma—Dopamine and homovanillic acid

CONFUSA

Phaeochromocytoma produce some paradoxical clinical features and these should be noted, i.e. it can cause both hypertensive and hypotensive episodes (postural BP drop). Similarly it can produce both pallor and flushing. Phaeochromocytomas presents with vague episodic symptoms that the patient might be diagnosed as being depressed. This will further aggravate their problems as the tricyclic antidepressants can precipitate hypertensive episodes in them. Other precipitating factors can be:

- Stretching
- Sneezing
- Stress
- Sex
- Smoking
- Surgery
- Parturition
- Cheese
- Alcohol

Investigation of Choice

- *Screening:* 24 hour urine for HMMA, VMA
- *Definitive:* MIBG scan/clonidine suppression test

Immediate Management
Consult specialist centre for full investigations.

Treatment of Choice
Surgery after BP control

108. Increased production of aldosterone.

Diagnosis: Conn's syndrome

Clinchers

Conn's syndrome is unilateral adrenocortical adenoma and is responsible for more than 50% cases of primary hyperaldosteronism. It causes excess production of aldosterone, independent of renin-angiotensin system.

Clinical features:
- Hypertension
- Hypokalaemia   in someone not on diuretics
- Alkalosis

CONFUSA

Posture test helps in differential diagnosis of primary hyperaldosteronism. It involves measuring the effect of posture on renin, aldosterone and cortisol (measure of 9 AM lying, and at noon standing).

Interpretation

On standing	*Cortisol*	*Aldosterone*
Conn's/GRA	↓	↓
Adrenal hyperplasia	↓	↑

Investigation of Choice
- *Screening:* Posture test for renin, aldosterone and cortisol
- *Definitive:* Abdominal CT/MRI

Immediate Management

Treat hypokalaemia and alkalosis

Treatment of Choice

Surgical excision after spironolactone upto 300 mg/24h PO for 4 weeks.

CASE HISTORY

A 38-year-old overweight woman with hypertension. She has a blood pressure of 166/100 mmHg and her potassium is 3.0 mmol/L.

Diagnosis: Conn's Syndrome.

The hypokalaemic hypertension in this case suggests Conn's syndrome.

Your notes:

194. Female, swelling in the neck, tremor irritability, diarrhoea, bruit.

Diagnosis: Graves' disease

Clinchers
- *Female:* Graves' disease is more prevalent in females, especially in women aged 30-50 years (E: G » 9:1)
- *Swelling in neck:* The thyroid gland is usually smoothly enlarged but not invariably so.
- *Tremor:* Fine tremor of the outstretched hands is present and reflects the increased sympathetic activity.
- *Irritability:* It is due to the emotional lability commonly seen in hyperthyroidism. Frank psychosis may also develop.
- *Diarrhoea:* It is due to increased sympathetic activity.
- *Bruit:* The thyroid may have a bruit because of its increased vascularity in this condition.

CONFUSA

Additional signs in Graves' disease which differentiate it from other hyperthyroid conditions are:
- Bulging eyes (exophthalmos)
- Thyroid bruit
- Ophthalmoplegia
- Vitiligo
- Pretibial myxoedema
- Thyroid acropachy

Investigation of Choice

TSH receptor autoantibodies.

Immediate Management

Rule out IDDM and pernicious anaemia as these are usually associated with Graves' disease.

Treatment of Choice

Graves' disease may be treated with antithyroid drugs or radioiodine treatment; subtotal thyroidectomy is rarely indicated.

DOC—carbimazole.

Your notes:

PAPER 5

6. A 48-year-old female, insulin dependent diabetic, who has been on treatment for 20-year presents with a history of three episodes of severe hypoglycaemia. She has not changed her insulin requirement, diet or exercise pattern.

Diagnosis: Possible infection

Clinchers

- *A 48-year-old female with IDDM:* As IDDM usually have an onset at a younger age, she must be having a long history of diabetes.
- *Three episodes of severe hypoglycaemia:* Non-compliance to therapy or diet and exercise changes can induce such attacks. But since these have been specifically ruled out in this question, a possible systemic infection seems to be most probable.

CONFUSA

Infections in persons with diabetes may not occur more frequently than in nondiabetics, but they tend to be more severe, possibly because of impaired leucocyte function. In addition to common infections of the skin, urinary tract, lungs and blood stream infections like malignant external otitis, Rhinocerebral mucomycosis, emphysematous cholecystitis and emphysematous pyelonephritis, appear to have a specific relationship with diabetes.

Investigation of Choice

Blood culture

Immediate Management

Detailed history

Treatment of Choice

Treat the infection if present, with broad spectrum antibiotics

Your notes:

7. A 48-year-old female, insulin dependent diabetic, who has been on treatment for 20 years, presents with urinary frequency but no dysuria or urgency. Her blood glucose is 17.5 mmol/L.

Diagnosis: Hyperglycaemia

Clinchers

- *A 48-year-old female + IDDM:* IDDM patients prone to insulin resistance after a few years and require a greater dose of insulin else they get hyperglycaemic
- *Urinary frequency but no dysuria or urgency:* Urinary frequency alone is feature of diabetes mellitus as polyuria would be reported as increased urinary frequency.
- *17.5 mmol/L blood glucose:* Significant hyperglycaemia.

CONFUSA

Among the given list of options, the confusion can be with—Urinary tract infection, but absence of dysuria and urgency go less in its favour.

Investigation of Choice

- Blood sugar fasting.
- Urine culture and sensitivity to rule out concomitant infection since blood glucose has already been done.

Immediate Management

Increase dose of insulin.

Treatment of Choice

Better diabetic control.

Your notes:

10. A 70-year-old diabetic on treatment with metformin presents with severe epigastric pain, drowsiness and confusion.

Diagnosis: Lactic acidosis

Clinchers

- *Metformin:* Lactic acidosis is a common side effect of metformin.
- *Severe epigastric pain + drowsiness + confusion:* The usual side effects of metformin are abdominal discomfort, anorexia, nausea, metallic taste, mild diarrhoea and tiredness. Lactic acidosis is the most serious complication of metformin intake.

CONFUSA

Ketoacidosis can be a confusing option, but ketoacidosis is very uncommon in NIDDM patients Alcohol intake in a patient or metformin therapy precipitate severe lactic acidosis.

Investigation of Choice
Arterial blood gases.

Immediate Management
IV Fluids.

Treatment of Choice
$NaHCO_3$.

Your notes:

91. An overweight woman complains of having to go to the toilet more than usual. She says she does drink a lot of tea but that she is always thirsty and tired. She needs the energy.

Diagnosis: Glycosuria

Clinchers

- *Overweight:* Glycosuria can occur in diabetes mellitus or otherwise. NIDDM usually presents in overweight adults.
- *Woman:* DM is slightly more common in females because of its possible autoimmune aetiology.
- *Having to go to toilet more than usual:* This is a polyuria and occurs due to hyperglycaemia.
- *She does drink a lot of tea but that she is always thirsty:* This is polydipsia, again due to hyperglycaemia.
- *Tired + needs the energy:* Generalised weakness, feeling unwell and fatigue are the common complaints initially. Weight loss also occurs due to fluid depletion and the accelerated breakdown of fat and muscle secondary to insulin deficiency.

CONFUSA

Correlation between urine tests and simultaneous blood glucose is poor for three reasons:

- Changes in urine glucose lag behind changes in blood glucose.
- The mean renal threshold is around 10 mmol/L but the range is wide (7-13 mmol/L). The threshold also rises with age.
- Urine tests can give no guidance concerning blood glucose levels below the renal threshold.

Investigation of Choice
Blood glucose (see confusa)

Immediate Management
Dipstick test for glucose in urine

Treatment of Choice
As per the findings, but weight loss and diet control is most important.

Your notes:

103. A young diabetic is admitted in a comatose state. His plasma glucose level is 17 mmols and he is dehydrated.

Diagnosis: Diabetic ketoacidosis (DKA).

Clinchers

- *Young diabetic:* DKA coma only occurs with type I diabetes, so it is more common in young diabetics (as type I diabetes usually presents in childhood).
- *Comatose state:* Apart from coma other symptoms are polyuria, polydipsia, lethargy, anorexia, hyperventilation, ketotic breath (smells like peach), dehydration, vomiting, abdominal pain, etc.
- *Plasma glucose level is 17 mmols:* Normal range of blood glucose is 3.5-5.5 mmol/L. Usually in DKA it is > 20 mmol/L. But 17 mmol/L is also a very high value.
- *Dehydrated:* Gross hyperglycaemia causes an osmotic diuresis, decreased tissue perfusion and circulatory collapse. It produces dehydration. Dehydration is more life-threatening than any hyperglycaemia—so its correction takes precedence.

CONFUSA

Some students get confused between DKA and HONK coma (hyperglycaemic hyperosmolar nonketotic coma).

DKA	*HONK*
1. Occurs only in IDDM	1. Occurs only in NIDDM
2. History of 2-3 days	2. Longer history (e.g. 1wk)
3. Glucose usually > 20 mmol/l	3. Glucose > 35 mmol/l
4. Acidosis present (pH < 7.3)	4. Acidosis absent
5. Ketotic breath present	5. No ketotic breath
6. Younger patients	6. Patient often old
7. Insulin given immediately in treatment	7. Insulin is given late, cautiously and in lower dosage

Investigation of Choice

Plasma osmolality (2[Na^+] + [urea] + [glucose])

Immediate Management

IV access and start fluid (0.9% NS) immediately.

Treatment of Choice

Fluid replacement (0.9%NS) + 10U soluble insulin IV (if plasma glucose > 20 mmol/L).

Insulin sliding scale.

Your notes:

105. A young diabetic is admitted in a comatose state. His plasma glucose level is 2 mmols/L.

Diagnosis: Hypoglycaemia

Clinchers

- *Young diabetic:* The most common cause of hypoglycaemia is insulin or sulfonylurea treatment in a known diabetic. It can also be due to insufficient food or change in routine of insulin (i.e. site of injection, type of insulin, new syringe size). It is more so in younger patients because there is usually no set lifestyle.
- *Comatose state:* Initially, a hypoglycaemic patient is restless and agitated but, if untreated, rapidly becomes unresponsive. There is pallor profuse sweating and a bounding pulse. Aggression can be such that the patient arrives in police custody and may be thought to be intoxicated. False neurological signs are sometimes seen.
- *His plasma glucose level is 2 mmols:* Hypoglycaemia by definition is < 2.5 mmol/L.

CONFUSA

The other two conditions which can produce comatose state in a diabetic are:
- Nonketotic (HONK) coma
- Diabetic ketoacidosis (DKA)

Investigation of Choice

- Venous blood glucose
- In case of unexplained hypoglycaemia
  - Liver function tests
  - Insulin assay
  - C peptide assay
  - Toxicology (paracetamol) screen

Immediate Management

Start treatment after taking blood sample.

Treatment of Choice

- 50 ml of 50% dextrose solution (adults)
- 2-5 ml/kg of 10% dextrose solution (child)
- If venous access is delayed:
  - Glucagon 1-2 mg IM (20 µg/kg for children)
- 50% dextrose harms veins, so follow by 0.9% saline flush.
- If there is no prompt recovery after treatment, give dexamethasone 4 mg/4h IV to combat cerebral edema after prolonged hypoglycaemia.
- Once conscious, give sugary drinks.

Since in this question, blood sugar levels is already known, we should then go for urea and electrolytes, as hypoglycaemia is more common in diabetic nephropathy. Though we should remember that, most common cause of hypoglycaemia in diabetic is overdoses of hypoglycaemic drugs.

156. A 30-year-old man with AIDS presented in shock. Serum biochemistry reveals: potassium 6.7 mmol/L, bicarbonate 20 mmol/L, chloride 84 mmol/L, creatinine 160 mmol/L.

Diagnosis: Acute adrenal insufficiency

Clinchers

- *30-year-old man with AIDS:* Various endocrine abnormalities have been reported with AIDS, including reduced levels of testosterone and abnormal adrenal function. The latter may assume clinical significance in more advanced disease. When intercurrent infection superimposed upon borderline adrenal function may precipitate clear adrenal insufficiency requiring replacement doses of cortico- and mineralo-corticoid CMV is also implicated in adrenal-deficient states.
- *Presents in shock:* Acute adrenal insufficiency typically present in shock (but not always).
- *Potassium 6.7 mmol/L:* Increases as always in this condition.
- *Bicarbonate 20 mmol/L:* Mild acidosis is characteristic.
- *Chloride 84 mmol/L:* Low along with hyponatraemia.
- *Creatinine 160 μmol/L:* Slightly increased.

CONFUSA

Acute adrenal insufficiency or Addisonian crisis can occur in any one with a known Addison's disease, or someone or long-term steroids who has forgotten to take their tablets. Typically it presents with shock but an alternative presentation can be with hypoglycaemia.

Investigation of Choice

Blood for cortisol and ACTH (if possible).

Immediate Management

Start treating before biochemical results.

Treatment of Choice

Hydrocortisone sodium succinate 100 mg IV stat plasma expander followed by 0.9% saline.

175. A 32-year-old woman complains of palpitations and is found to have red oedematous swellings above both lateral malleoli, which she says are beginning to affect her feet. She is found to have digital clubbing and periorbital puffiness.

Diagnosis: Hyperthyroidism (Graves' disease).

Clinchers

- *32-year-old:* It most often occurs between ages 20 and 40 years.
- *Woman:* Hyperthyroidism affects perhaps 2-5% of all females at sometime and with a sex ratio of 5:1.
- *Red oedematous swellings above both lateral malleoli which she says are beginning to affect her feet:* This is pretibial myxoedema and is characteristic of hyperthyroidism state.
- *Palpitations:* This may be due to atrial fibrillation or other tachycardias, commonly found with hyperthyroidism.
- *Digital clubbing:* This is the rare thyroid acropachy and consists of clubbing, swollen fingers and periosteal new bone formation.
- *Periorbital puffing:* It is due to a specific immune response that causes inflammation and hence focal oedema and glycosaminoglycan deposition followed by fibrosis.

CONFUSA

The eye signs pretibial myxoedema and thyroid acropachy occur only in Graves' disease. Pretibial myxoedema is an infiltration on the skin, essential occurring only with eye disease. In Graves' disease eventually become hypothyroid.

Investigation of Choice

TSH receptor antibodies.

Immediate Management

Exclude associated disease like IDDM and pernicious anaemia.

Treatment of Choice

Carbamizole

(Side effects: drug rash; fever; arthropathy; lymphadenopathy; agranulocytosis).

Your notes:

PAPER 6

24. Patient on treatment for bipolar disorder, hypothyroidism features.

Diagnosis: Lithium side effects.

Clinchers

- *Bipolar disorder treatment:* Its first line prophylactic treatment is lithium. Majority of patients stabilizes on lithium and usually do not need alternative or second line drugs.
- *Weight gain and loss of appetite:* This suggests hypothyroidism which is in fact a prominent yet rare side effects of lithium. It is due to interference with iodination of tyrosine—decreased thyroxine synthesis.

CONFUSA

Lithium induced hypothyroidism is seen in 20% women. In men it is rare. Other main side effect of lithium on long-term usage is renal diabetes insipidus. Lithium induces granulocytosis and in-fact sometimes used to treat agranulocytosis (e.g. chemotherapy induced leukopaenia and agranulocytosis).

Investigation of Choice
TSH.

Immediate Management
Rule out primary thyroid disease.

Treatment of Choice
Thyroxine administration.

Your notes:

46. A 48-year-old female, insulin dependent diabetic, who has been on treatment for 20-year presents with a history of three episodes of severe hypoglycaemia. She has not changed her insulin requirement, diet or exercise pattern.

Diagnosis: Possible infection

Clinchers

- *48-year-old female with IDDM:* As IDDM usually have an onset at a younger age, she must be having a long history of diabetes.
- *Three episodes of severe hypoglycaemia:* Non compliance to therapy or diet and exercise changes can induce such attacks. But since these have been specifically ruled out in this question, a possible systemic infection seems to be most probable.

CONFUSA

Infections in persons with diabetes may not occur more frequently than in nondiabetics, but they tend to be more severe, possibly because of impaired leucocyte function. In addition to common infections of the skin, urinary tract, lungs and blood stream infections like malignant external otitis, Rhinocerebral mucormycosis, emphysematous cholecystitis and emphysematous pyelonephritis, appear to have a specific relationship with diabetes.

Investigation of Choice
Blood culture

Immediate Management
Detailed history

Treatment of Choice
Treat the infection if present, with broad spectrum antibiotics

Your notes:

47. A 48-year-old female, insulin dependent diabetic, who has been on treatment for 20 years, presents with urinary frequency but no dysuria or urgency. Her blood glucose is 17.5 mmol/L.

Diagnosis: Hyperglycaemia

Clinchers

- *48-year-old female + IDDM:* IDDM patients prone to insulin resistance after a few years and require a greater dose of insulin else they get hyperglycaemic
- *Urinary frequency but no dysuria or urgency:* Urinary frequency alone is a feature of diabetes mellitus as polyuria would be reported as increased urinary frequency.
- *17.5 mmol/L blood glucose:* Significant hyperglycaemia.

CONFUSA

Among the given list of options, the confusion can be with—Urinary tract infection, but absence of dysuria and urgency go less in its favour.

Investigation of Choice

- Blood sugar fasting.
- Urine culture and sensitivity to rule out concomitant infection since blood glucose has already been done.

Immediate Management

Increase dose of insulin.

Treatment of Choice

Better diabetic control.

Your notes:

49. A 68-year-old diabetic on treatment for the last 5-year presents with calf pain exacerbated by movement.

Diagnosis: Intermittent claudication

Clinchers

- *Calf pain exacerbated by movement:* This is a typical history of intermittent claudication. The pain is initially relieved by rest.
- *68-year-old diabetic:* This female has a high chances of having atherosclerosis secondary to diabetes or as a primary disease. This produces the vascular disease with diminished blood supply which cause intermittent claudication and foot ulcers.

CONFUSA

Hypertriglyceridaemia is common in diabetes and is due both to overproduction of VLDL in the liver and to a disposal defect in the periphery.

Investigation of Choice

Doppler USG lower limb (or Duplex USG)

Immediate Management

Instruction about proper foot care in an attempt to prevent ulcers.

Treatment of Choice

Maintain diabetic control properly to keep hypertriglyceridaemia under control.

+

Symptomatic management.

Your notes:

50. A 70-year-old diabetic on treatment with metformin presents with severe epigastric pain, drowsiness and confusion.

Diagnosis: Lactic acidosis

Clinchers

- *Metformin:* Lactic acidosis is a common side effect of metformin.
- *Severe epigastric pain + drowsiness + confusion:* The usual side effects of metformin are abdominal discomfort, anorexia, nausea, metallic taste, mild diarrhoea and tiredness. Lactic acidosis is the most serious complication of metformin intake.

CONFUSA

Ketoacidosis can be a confusing option, but ketoacidosis is very uncommon in NIDDM patients Alcohol intake in a patient or metformin therapy precipitates severe lactic acidosis.

Investigation of Choice

Arterial blood gases.

Immediate Management

IV Fluids.

Treatment of Choice

$NaHCO_3$.

Your notes:

52. Old lady with smooth neck swelling, bradycardia, spare coarse hair, macrocytic anaemia.

Diagnosis: Hashimoto's thyroiditis.

Clinchers

- *Old lady:* It usually occurs in women aged 60-70 years.
- *Smooth neck swelling:* The gland is usually uniformly enlarged and firm, although it may occasionally be a symmetrical and irregular.
- *Bradycardia:* It is due to hypothyroidism which may be a feature of Hashimoto's thyroiditis (although the patient is mostly euthyroid).
- *Sparse coarse hair:* The patients of hypothyroidism have a slow, deep voice and are usually overweight and apathetic, with a dry, coarse skin and thin hair, especially in the lateral third of the eyebrows.
- *Macrocytic anaemia:* Hypothyroid patients often have normochromic macrocytic anaemia.

CONFUSA

It is important to diagnose the condition correctly by demonstrating the presence of thyroid antibodies and if necessary, by biopsy, because thyroidectomy will precipitate severe hypothyroidism in these cases. Occasionally lymphoma occurs in such glands. Note that in

- Graves' disease—TSH autoantibody -
- Hashimoto's thyroiditis—thyroglobulin autoantibody increased

Investigation of Choice

Autoantibody titres (thyroglobulin)

Immediate Management

Exclude lymphoma in thyroid and other autoimmune diseases.

Treatment of Choice

T_4 replacement therapy upto 0.3 mg/day will shrink the gland and the symptoms of myxoedema should disappear.

Your notes:

53. Female on treatment for supraventricular tachycardia complains of seeing dots and glare on driving at night, exophthalmos, no goitre.

Diagnosis: Drug-induced thyrotoxicosis.

Clinchers

- *Female:* Thyroid disorders are overall more prevalent in females, however drug induced thyrotoxicosis have an equal incidence in both sexes:
- *On treatment for SVT:* Given her existing clinical profile, she must be on treatment with amiodarone. Amiodarone is used in a wide range of ventricular and supraventricular arrhythmias. However, because of its toxic potential, its use is limited to resistant VT and recurrent VF. It is also used to maintain sinus rhythm in AF when other drugs here failed. Rapid termination of ventricular and supraventricular arrhythmias can be obtained by IV injection. WPW tachyarrhythmia is obtained can be obtained by suppression of both normal and aberrant pathways. Its long duration of action make it suitable for long-term prophylactic use; but close monitoring is required.
- *Complains of seeing dots and glare on driving at night:* This is due to corneal oedema occurring due to inflammatory reaction in thyrotoxicosis. Otherwise also it can be due to corneal microdeposits occurring due to long-term use of amiodarone.
- *Exophthalmos, no goitre:* Absence of goitre excludes a primary thyroid abnormality. Exophthalmos is due to retro orbital inflammatory and oedema characteristically seen in thyrotoxicosis.

CONFUSA

Had she not been taking drugs for SVT, this clinical profile would have qualified for a diagnosis of Graves' disease. Amiodarone is an iodine containing highly lipophilic long acting antiarrhythmic drug. It interferes with thyroid function in many ways including inhibition of peripheral conversion of T_4 to T_3.

Investigation of Choice
Serum T_4.

Immediate Management
Review SVT treatment by a cardiologist.

Treatment of Choice
Discontinue amiodarone

Your notes:

54. Female, swelling in the neck, tremor irritability, diarrhoea, bruit.

Diagnosis: Graves' disease

Clinchers

- *Female:* Graves' disease is more prevalent in females, especially in women aged 30-50 years (E: G » 9:1)
- *Swelling in neck:* The thyroid gland is usually smoothly enlarged but not invariably so.
- *Tremor:* Fine tremor of the outstretched hands is present and reflects the increased sympathetic activity.
- *Irritability:* It is due to the emotional lability commonly seen in hyperthyroidism. Frank psychosis may also develop.
- *Diarrhoea:* It is due to increased sympathetic activity.
- *Bruit:* The thyroid may have a bruit because of its increased vascularity in this condition.

CONFUSA

Additional signs in Graves' disease which differentiate it from other hyperthyroid conditions are:

- Bulging eyes (exophthalmos)
- Thyroid bruit
- Ophthalmoplegia
- Vitiligo
- Pretibial myxoedema
- Thyroid acropachy

Investigation of Choice
TSH receptor autoantibodies.

Immediate Management
Rule out IDDM and pernicious anaemia as these are usually associated with Graves' disease.

Treatment of Choice
Graves' disease may be treated with antithyroid drugs or radioiodine treatment; subtotal thyroidectomy is rarely indicated.
DOC—carbimazole.

Your notes:

61. A 30-year-old man with AIDS presented in shock. Serum biochemistry reveals: potassium 6.7 mmol/L, bicarbonate 20 mmol/L, chloride 84 mmol/L, creatinine 160 mmol/L.

Diagnosis: Acute adrenal insufficiency

Clinchers

- *30-year-old man with AIDS:* Various endocrine abnormalities have been reported with AIDS, including reduced levels of testosterone and abnormal adrenal function. The latter may assume clinical significance in more advanced disease. When intercurrent infection superimposed upon borderline adrenal function may precipitate clear adrenal insufficiency requiring replacement doses of cortico- and mineralo-corticoid CMV is also implicated in adrenal-deficient states.
- *Presents in shock:* Acute adrenal insufficiency typically present in shock (but not always).
- *Potassium 6.7 mmol/L:* Increases as always in this condition.
- *Bicarbonate 20 mmol/L:* Mild acidosis is characteristic.
- *Chloride 84 mmol/L:* Low along with hyponatraemia.
- *Creatinine 160 µmol/L:* Slightly increased.

CONFUSA

Acute adrenal insufficiency or Addisonian crisis can occur in any one with a known Addison's disease, or someone or long-term steroids who has forgotten to take their tablets. Typically it presents with shock but an alternative presentation can be with hypoglycaemia.

Investigation of Choice

Blood for cortisol and ACTH (if possible).

Immediate Management

Start treating before biochemical results.

Treatment of Choice

Hydrocortisone sodium succinate 100 mg IV stat plasma expander followed by 0.9% saline.

187. Female child from Ghana, brought to the A and E with a history of nausea and vomiting, on investigations Ketone 1+, Na 148 mEq, Glucose 18 mmol/L.

Diagnosis: Diabetic ketoacidosis (DKA)

Clinchers

- *Female child from Ghana:* Although sickle cell anaemia is more prevalent in Ghana, this information is inconsequential in this question except for the fact that infections like malaria can precipitate DKA.
- *History of nausea and vomiting:* Abdominal pain, nausea and vomiting are common presenting symptoms in DKA.
- *Ketone 1+:* Ketones are usually > 2 mmol/L in DKA. Their presence almost confirms the diagnosis of DKA if blood glucose is elevated.
- *Glucose 18 mmol/L:* The cut off for DKA is glucose > 16 mmol/L.
- *Na 148 mEq:* Hypernatraemia in this case is due to severe dehydration.

CONFUSA

In case of DKA in children, dehydration may be so profound as to cause shock. DKA has a mortality rate of 9% in children. The cause of death is cerebral oedema in 50% of cases. To minimise the risk of this, metabolic abnormalities must be corrected slowly.

Investigation of Choice

ABG + serum electrolytes + blood culture + blood sugar

Immediate Management

Protect the airway and give high concentration of O_2

\+

Discuss the child with a paediatrician as soon as possible. Arrange intensive care.

Treatment of Choice

Commence a normal saline (0.9%) infusion with added potassium (20 mmol/L)

↓

Start an infusion of soluble insulin at a rate of 0.1 units/kg/hour

↓

Once blood sugar has fallen below 10 mmol/L, the IV infusion should be changed to 0.45% saline with dextrose.

↓

According to clinical improvement, can reduce insulin infusion to 0.05 units/kg/hr.

PAPER 7

69. A 40-year-old female comes with complaints of headache, bitemporal hemianopia, increase in shoe size.

Diagnosis: Acromegaly

Clinchers

- *40-year-old female:* It typically presents between the ages of 30 and 50 years. It is equally prevalent in men and women.
- *Headache and bitemporal hemianopia:* Because of the pituitary tumor (responsible for growth hormone hypersecretion). Bitemporal hemianopia is characteristic of compression of optic chiasm (most common cause of it—pituitary tumor).
- *Increase in shoe size:* GH excess results in bony and soft tissue overgrowth. The features are insidious, chronic and debilitating, i.e.
  - Increased teeth spacing
  - Increased shoe size
  - Thick spade like hands
  - Large tongue
  - Prominent supraorbital ridge
  - Prognathism.

CONFUSA

Acromegalics are said to look more like each other than their family members. Presence of bitemporal hemianopia in it clinically corroborates the presence of a pituitary tumour and that acromegaly is not due to some ectopic secretion of growth hormone.

Ectopic (other than pituitary) tumours causing acromegaly

- GnRH secreting tumours
  - Bronchial carcinoids
  - Pancreatic islet cell tumours
  - Hypothalamic gangliocytomas
  - Harmatoma
  - Gliomas
- GH secreting tumours
  - Pancreatic islet cell tumour

Investigation of Choice

MRI pituitary fossa.

Immediate Management

Obtain old photographs for comparison.

Your notes:

152. An elderly patient presents with weight gain, hypothermia and confusion.

Diagnosis: Hypothyroidism (Myxoedema coma)

Clinchers

- *Elderly:* Incidence of myxoedema coma is maximum above 65 years of age.
- *Weight gain:* In the elderly the usual symptoms are fatigue, lethargy, constipation, cold intolerance, stiffness and cramping of muscles, carpal tunnel syndrome and menorrhagia. Intellectual and motor activity slows, appetite declines and weight increases.
- *Hypothermia:* If left untreated, the patient with long standing hypothyroidism may pass into a hypothermic, stuporous state (myxoedema coma) which may be fatal.
- *Confusion:* Although very rare, severe hypothyroidism, especially in the elderly, may present with confusion or even coma.

CONFUSA

In the elderly the symptoms of hypothyroidism may be erroneously attributed to ageing itself, Parkinson's disease, depression or Alzheimer's disease. In myxoedema coma the patient may have severe cardiac failure, hypoventilation, hypoglycaemia and hyponatraemia. Occasionally with severe hypothyroidism, the elderly patient may become frankly demented or psychotic, sometimes with striking delusions (Myxoedema madness). This may occur shortly after starting T_4 replacement.

Investigation of Choice

Take

venous blood for T_3, T_4, TSH, FBC, U&E, cultures

arterial blood for PaO_2.

Immediate Management

Admit in ICU

+

High flow O_2 if cyanosed

Treatment of Choice

T_3 5-20 μg 12h/IV (slow).

Your notes:

154. A 57-year-old male comes to the A and E with his daughter, in a confused state. The daughter said that her father was started on some medication by his GP.

Diagnosis: Drug-induced (Hypoglycaemia-most probable)

Clinchers

- *57-year-old:* Mental disturbance caused by prescribed drugs is particularly common in elderly but may occur with central nervous system depressant drugs, beta blockers, digoxin and cimetidine at all ages.
- *Confused state:* Symptoms include fluctuating clouding of consciousness and restlessness with paranoid delusions and visual hallucinations in severe cases.
- *Started on some medication by his GP:* Although, drug induced psychiatric symptoms in elderly are usually a result of over dosage, there reactions may sometimes occur because of intolerance to the normal dose or after withdrawal of drug.

CONFUSA

It is often impossible to assess fully or manage a confused and distressed patient. Adequate sedation makes further therapy possible. IV diazepam or midazolam is effective and has a rapid onset of action but careful observation and monitoring are essential. Hypoglycaemia is one of the few situations where rapid diagnosis and specific therapy obviate the need for sedation.

Investigation of Choice
Blood glucose

Immediate Management
If possible, contact GP

Treatment of Choice
Symptomatic

Your notes:

161. A 39-year-old woman on thyroxine replacement comes for first check-up.

Diagnosis: Hypothyroidism (under treatment)

Clinchers

- *39-year-old:* Over replacement with thyroxine may increase the risk of atrial fibrillation in those over 60 years of age. Age of 39 years does not hold any unique significance.
- *Woman:* Overall females have a larger incidence of autoimmune diseases especially those of thyroid (most common: Hashimoto's).
- *Thyroxine replacement:* Replacement therapy with T_4 is given for life. The starting dose will depend upon the severity of the deficiency and on the age and fitness of the patient, especially cardiac performance. In the young and fit, 100 µg daily is suitable, while 50 µg daily is more appropriate for the small, old or frail. T_3 offers no significant advantage over T_4.
- *Comes for first check-up:* First review is suggested after 12 weeks of starting the treatment (6 weeks according to Kumar and Clark). It is done to assess the adequacy of replacement clinically. The aim is to restore TSH to well within the normal range. If serum TSH remain high, the dose of T_4 should be increased in 25-50 µg increments and the tests repeated six weeks later. This stepwise progression should be continued until TSH becomes normal.

CONFUSA

Thyroxine may precipitate angina especially in those with pre-existing heart disease. Osteoporosis is a theoretical risk of over replacement. The possibility of development of other autoimmune disease especially Addison's disease should be always considered in such patients. Clinical improvement on T_4 may not begin for two weeks or more, even though it is quicker on T_3, and full resolution of symptoms may take six months (although treatment is continued lifelong). During frequency about a 50 µg increase in T_4 dosage is required (due to — TIBG levels).

Investigation of Choice
TSH

Immediate Management
A detailed clinical examination

Treatment of Choice
T_4 dose adjustments according to TSH levels.

162. 40-year-old woman, euthyroid (TSH normal) complains of palpitations, weight loss and diarrhoea.

Diagnosis: Pituitary TSH tumour

Clinchers

- *40-year-old women:* Pituitary adenomas are slightly more common in middle-aged women.
- *Euthyroid (TSH normal):* In such cases TSH may be normal or increased due to overproduction by the pituitary adenoma. Otherwise is all cases of hyperthyroidism TSH is invariably decreased. T_4 should be measured to reach an accurate diagnosis.
- *Palpitations, weight loss, diarrhoea:* These are the usual symptoms of a hyperthyroid state.

CONFUSA

In any case of suspected hyperthyroidism, ask for T_3, T_4 and TSH. A minority will have elevation of only one thyroid hormone, but all will have - TSH—secretory pituitary adenoma. If TSH is normal and T_4 abnormal except for the rare phenomenon of a TSH, consider:

- Hormone binding problems, e.g. pregnancy
- Thyroid-binding globulin
- Amiodarone
- Pituitary TSH tumour

Investigation of Choice

T_3 and T_4 assay, TIG assay

Immediate Management

MRI skull

Treatment of Choice

Surgery (if possible)

Your notes:

163. 13-year-old woman, euthyroid has a soft diffuse swelling that moves with swallowing.

Diagnosis: Physiological goitre

Clinchers

- *13-year-old woman:* Incidence of thyroid disease is slightly more in females. The physiological goitre tends to occur at puberty (as in this case) and pregnancy.
- *Euthyroid:* Essentially the gland is euthyroid in this condition.
- *Soft diffuse swelling:* It is manifest as a smooth enlargement of the thyroid gland.
- *Moves with swallowing:* The characteristics of an enlarged thyroid are a mass in the neck on one or both sides of the trachea, which moves on swallowing, since it is attached to the larynx by the pretracheal fascia.

CONFUSA

This condition should be differentiated clinically from the common nodular goitre which also occurs with an euthyroid state. In it there is either a solitary nodule or multiple nodules.

Investigation of Choice

TSH and T_4 (to rule out any derangement)

Immediate Management

Rule out pregnancy

Treatment of Choice

None required

Your notes:

7 ENT

PAPER 1

Serial No. 151

Subject: Surgery

Topic: Trauma

Question: A man involved in a road traffic accident comes with CSF rhinorrhoea.

Diagnosis: Frontal bone fracture

Clinchers

- *Road traffic accident:* Most of the skull fractures are associated with high speed collision injuries typically in the setting of road traffic accidents and assaults.
- *Comes with CSF rhinorrhoea:* This CSF leakage through the nose occurs due to the fracture of cribriform plate in the anterior cranial fossa injuries. It occurs secondary to fracture of the frontal bones and is usually associated with injury to orbital bones as well.

CONFUSA

- Don't get confused with the option 'Basilar Skull Fracture' given among the listed options. Base of the skull fracture or basilar skull fracture is a broader term applied to any fracture involving the base of the skull. These include fractures of the cribiform plate, frontal, bones, sphenoid bones, temporal bone and occipital bones.

Investigation of Choice
CT Scan

Immediate Management
Primary survey including maintenance of:
Airway
Breathing
Circulation

Treatment of Choice
Most of the uncomplicated basilar skull fractures without any evidence of neurological deficits are usually managed conservatively. CSF leak usually seals off by itself by dura.

Antibiotics are administered to prevent infection, till there is CSF leak.

Serial No. 152

Subject: Surgery

Topic: Trauma

Question: A man after sustaining a fall comes with haemotympanum.

Diagnosis: Petrous temporal fracture

Clinchers

- *Man:* Skull fractures are three times more common in males than females, may be because of higher rate of road traffic accidents and assaults in males.
- *After sustaining a fall:* Most of the skull fractures are associated with high speed collision injuries typically in the setting of road traffic accidents and assaults. Falls, typically in an elderly can produce a variety if skull injuries. However, falls in children are rarely associated with fracture of skull bones, because of relative softer nature of skull bones in children.
- *Comes with haemotympanum:* The first sign of petrous temporalfracture is bleeding from external ear; it is also associated with CSF otorrhoea due to the torn tympanic membrane.

CONFUSA

- Patients with anterior cranial fossa fracture present with CSF rhinorrhea and bruising around the eyes (Raccoon eyes).
  - Patients with petrous temporal fracture present with CSF otorrhoea, haemotympanum and bruising over mastoids (Battle's Sign).
  - Temporal bone fracture is also associated with haemoptympanum, but the ossicular chain disruption (in longitudinal temporal bone fracture) typically present with conductive deafness, more than 30dB. The transverse temporal bone fracture involve the VIII cranial nerve and the labyrinth, resulting in nystagmus, ataxia, and permanent sensorineural hearing loss.

Investigation of Choice
CT Scan

Immediate Management

Primary survey including maintenance of:
Airway
Breathing
Circulation

Treatment of Choice

Most of the uncomplicated basilar skull fractures without any evidence of neurological deficits are usually managed conservatively. CSF leak usually seals off by itself by dura.

Antibiotics are administered to prevent infection, till there is CSF leak.

Your notes:

PAPER 2

Serial No. 36

Subject: ENT

Topic: Epistaxis

Question: A 50-year-old man presents with epistaxis. He has an artificial heart valve.

Diagnosis: Anticoagulant overdosage

Clinchers

- *50-year-old:* While in the young the most common cause of epistaxis is due to local trauma and the source of bleeding vessel is conveniently located anteriorly, in older people systemic causes like uncontrolled hypertension and drugs play major role.
- *Artificial heart valve:* This clearly indicates that the patient was on some sort of anticoagulant therapy which can be blamed for his present episode of epistaxis.

CONFUSA

For patients on anticoagulant therapy, the target INRs currently recommended by the British Society for Haematology are:

- INR 2–2.5 for prophylaxis of deep-vein thrombosis including surgery on high-risk patients;
- INR 2.5 for treatment of deep-vein thrombosis and pulmonary embolism, atrial fibrillation, cardioversion, dilated cardiomyopathy, mural thrombus following myocardial infarction, and rheumatic mitral valve disease;
- INR 3.5 for recurrent deep-vein thrombosis and pulmonary embolism (in patients currently receiving warfarin with INR above 2) and mechanical prosthetic heart valves.

Investigation of Choice

Check INR

Immediate Management

Assess blood loss and replace the lost amount;
Apply local pressure and ice.

Treatment of Choice

Based on the INR level found:
In cases of major bleeding

- stop warfarin;
- give phytomenadione (vitamin K1) 5 mg by slow intravenous injection;

- give prothrombin complex concentrate (factors II, VII, IX and X) 30–50 units/kg or (if no concentrate available) fresh frozen plasma 15 mL/kg.

INR more than 8.0, no bleeding or minor bleeding.
- stop warfarin,
- restart when INR less than 5.0;
- if there are other risk factors for bleeding give phytomenadione (vitamin K1) 0.5 mg by slow intravenous injection or 5 mg by mouth (for partial reversal of anticoagulation give smaller oral doses of phytomenadione e.g. 0.5–2.5 mg using the intravenous preparation orally);
- repeat dose of phytomenadione if INR still too high after 24 hours.

INR 6.0–8.0, no bleeding or minor bleeding.
- stop warfarin, restart when INR less than 5.0.

INR less than 6.0 but more than 0.5 units above target value—
- reduce dose or stop warfarin, restart when INR less than 5.0.

Unexpected bleeding at therapeutic levels—
- always investigate possibility of underlying cause e.g. unsuspected renal or gastro-intestinal tract pathology.

Your notes:

Serial No. 37

Subject: ENT

Topic: Epistaxis

Question: A 50-year-old furniture maker presents with Anaesthesia of the left check and repeated left sided episodes of epistaxis.

Diagnosis: Maxillary Carcinoma

Clinchers

- *50-year-old furniture maker:* Carcinoma of the nose and paranasal sinuses are rare and account for less than 0.1% of all cancer and only 3% of head and neck cancers. Wood dust is implicated in the development of adenocarcinoma and thus, puts those involved in the furniture industry at enhanced risk. Nickel dust is associated with the development of squamous cell carcinoma.
- *Anaesthesia of the left cheek:* the presentation of the maxillary sinus depends on the direction of the growth of the tumour and thus the compression effects produced on the path of growth. The outward growth leads to compression of branches of trigeminal nerve leading to fascial swelling, paresthesia and anaesthesia.
- *Repeated left sided episodes of epistaxis:* The growth in the medial direction usually leads to unilateral epistaxis, bloody rhinorrhoea, nasal obstruction, anosmia.

CONFUSA

Maxillary sinus cancer can produce varied symptoms:
ocular effects—proptosis, epiphora, diplopia
nasal effects—bloody rhinorrhoea, nasal obstruction, anosmia
oral effects—loose teeth, ill-fitting dentures, palatal swelling
facial effects—facial swelling or paraesthesia
metastatic lymph nodes in neck
retro-antral spread causing trismus (pterygoid invasion) or trigeminal neuralgia

Investigation of Choice

CT and/or MRI to fully delineate disease with biopsy

Immediate Management

Urgent Referral

Treatment of Choice

Most lesions will then be treated by a combination of radiotherapy and surgery.

If the ethmoids are affected, a craniofacial resection may be necessary i.e. a combined approach from below and a craniotomy from above.

Serial No. 38

Subject: ENT

Topic: Epistaxis

Question: An actor presents with repeated episodes of epistaxis as associated with whistling on breathing in through the nose.

Diagnosis: Septal Perforation

Clinchers

- *Actor:* The most common cause of nasal septal perforation is surgery, especially following submucosal resection done for deviated nasal septum. The patient in question being an actor, can be presumed to be more 'Look-conscious' and undergo such corrective surgeries.
- *Repeated episodes of epistaxis:* The injured local vessels and crusting around the perforation is responsible for repeated bleeds.
- *Whistling on breathing:* This is seen with smaller perforations and patients usually complain of whistling on breathing.

CONFUSA

In cases of septal perforation rule out the cause by definite hints in the question. A similar picture in a drug addict would be most probably due to sniffing of cocaine. Cocaine is a very strong vasoconstrictor and can cause local vasoconstriction-> ischaemia-> necrosis-> perforation. Other causes of septal perforation include repeated trauma may be due to nasal cautery when treating epistaxis, nose picking, pressure from nasal balloons, chronic infection (syphilis, tuberculosis), malignancy, cocaine addiction and inhalation of chrome salts.

Investigations

Required only if the cause is not clear;
-FBC - for exclusion of Wegener's granulomatosis
-urinalysis for haematuria
-chest radiograph
-syphilis serology
-biopsy, if still in doubt

Immediate Management

None

Treatment of Choice

A septal perforation is almost impossible to repair. Whistling is controlled by enlargement of the septal perforation.

Nasal douching with saline or bicarbonate solution will help to reduce crusting around the edge of the defect. Application of antiseptic cream will control infection.

Your notes:

Serial No. 39

Subject: ENT

Topic: Epistaxis

Question: A 45-year-old sheep farmer presents with unilateral epistaxis. Inspection reveals a bleeding polyp attached to the anterior nasal septum.

Diagnosis: Orf

Clinchers

- *45-year-old sheep farmer:* Orf is a rapidly growing cutaneous lesion caused by a pox virus. It is a condition generally seen in workers who have contact with sheep.
- *Unilateral epistaxis:* The nasal form of the disease usually presents with unilateral bleeding episodes once the lesion starts ulcerating.
- *Bleeding polyp attached to the anterior nasal septum:* This is the classical description of orf; it presents as red papules which develops rapidly within one week of exposure and develops into a polyp like structure which later ulcerates to cause bleeding.

CONFUSA

Orf is a viral disease caused by a pox virus that is widespread in sheep and goats. It can be transmitted to humans by smear infection. Orf appears as a solitary lesion or as a few lesions on the fingers, the hands, or the forearms, and it has even been reported on the face. The lesion starts as a small, firm, red-to-blue papule that grows to form a haemorrhagic, flat-topped pustule or bulla. The bulla may have a crust in its umbilicated center. The fully developed lesion is typically 2-3 cm in diameter, but it may reach 5 cm. It is often tender and may bleed easily.

Investigation of Choice

Clinical inspection in view of occupational history.

Immediate Management

Control Bleeding - apply ice, local pressure.

Treatment of Choice

None required; spontaneous recovery occurs.
If secondary bacterial infection occurs then antibiotics may be required.

Your notes:

Serial No. 40

Subject: ENT

Topic: Epistaxis

Question: An 80-year-old man presents with epistaxis of two hours duration.

Diagnosis: Hypertension

Clinchers

- *80-year-old man:* While in the young the most common cause of epistaxis is due to local trauma and the source of bleeding vessel is conveniently located anteriorly, in older people systemic causes like uncontrolled hypertension and drugs play major role.
- *Epistaxis of two hours duration:* In the absence of any other mentioned factors which can lead to epistaxis in this elderly, its safest to consider uncontrolled hypertension and arteriosclerosis as the most likely cause of the presentation.

CONFUSA

The elderly are particularly prone to suffering from shock which may be fatal. If there are signs of shock they should be admitted and transfused. Although in general those with nosebleeds are nursed sitting up to reduce venous pressure, the shocked should be nursed lying to maximize perfusion of the brain. If shocked, give high flow oxygen and ensure airway remain clear if there is heavy bleeding draining into pharynx.

Investigation of Choice

Rule out local cause, if any.
Check Pulse rate and BP

Immediate Management

Admit, Treat Shock

Treatment of Choice

Symptomatic—

- Monitor pulse and blood pressure and control as required
- Maintain sitting upright position, unless shocked
- Apply local and firm pressure over nose
- Apply ice pack over the bridge of the nose
- Nasal Packing with ribbon gauze in bismuth & iodoform paste (BIPP) if practicable

Your notes:

PAPER 3

43. A singer has a six months history of hoarseness.

Diagnosis: Vocal nodules.

Clinchers

- *Singer:* These can be two causes of hoarseness in singers that are attributable to their profession
  1. Vocal nodules
  2. Vocal cord trauma
- *Six months history of hoarseness:* A six month history rules out trauma of vocal cords as it presents acutely and there is almost always a history of prolonged rehearsals (usually happens just before a show in amateur singers). A prolonged history points towards vocal nodules.

CONFUSA

The only confusion is between nodules and trauma which can be safely distinguished by presentation and duration. However, note that it is vocal cord trauma and consequent submucosal haemorrhage that fibrose into a vocal nodule.

Investigation of Choice

Indirect laryngoscopy.

Immediate Management

Vocal rest to prevent further trauma.

Treatment of Choice

Early cases of small nodules can be managed conservatively by education of patient in proper use of voice. With this treatment many nodules in children disappear completely. But this case will require surgery because of his profession (singing). Other indications for surgery are large nodules and nodules of long standing.

CASE HISTORY

A 53-year-old woman presents with recurrent chest infections and intermittent flushing. On bronchoscopy a vascular cherry like lesion is seen in the left main bronchus.

Diagnosis: Carcinoid tumour.

- Carcinoid tumours originate from enterochromaffin cells.
- Often malignant with destructive local invasion.
- In one third cases, metastasis to regional lymph nodes and distant organs especially brain and liver in 10% cases.
- Treatment of Choice is surgical resection.

45. A 30-year-old complains of hoarseness since he came back from a football match the day before.

Diagnosis: Vocal cord trauma

Clinchers

- *30-year-old:* This is quite a young age which rules out any neoplasia in larynx or lungs. Moreover many other chronic diseases will only present symptomatically after fourth decade of life. So the cause of hoarseness has to be acute.
- *Hoarseness since he came back from a football match the day before:* The person would have been involved in persistent screaming and shouting while cheering up his side in the football match. Excessive vocal use may cause laryngeal trauma or temporary hoarseness.

CONFUSA

Other causes of traumatic hoarseness are excessive vomiting, coughing or inhaling fumes. If the hoarseness persist over one week, it suggest-some laryngeal pathology (e.g. vocal nodules) and demand immediate laryngoscopy.

Investigation of Choice

Laryngoscopy if hoarseness persists.

Immediate Management

Vocal rest.

Treatment of Choice

Symptomatic.

Your notes:

49. A nine-year-old girl has difficulty with speech. She has recently been hospitalised for a medical reason. Her speech before hospitalisation was completely normal.

Diagnosis: Meningitis.

Clinchers

- *Nine-year-old girl: Haemophilus influenzae* commonly causes meningitis in < 5 years age. Afterwards pneumococcal and meningococcal meningitis are more common.
- *Difficulty with speech:* Meningitis can produce focal neurological signs such as this. Many false localising signs may also be present because of increased intracranial tension.
- *She has recently been hospitalised for a medical reason:* Meningitis requires hospital admission.
- *Her speech before hospitalisation was completely normal:* This tell that the rise in ICT is progressive and immediate intervention is required.

CONFUSA

"Treatment for hyperthyroidism" can be a confusing option as carbamazepine (used as a first line drug) can produce agranulocytosis ® sore throat ® speech difficulty. But it can be safely excluded as hyperthyroidism per se does not warrant hospital admission and sore throat does not chiefly present as speech difficulty. Although the typical case of childhood hyperthyroidism is a prepubertal girl.

Investigation of choice

Lumbar puncture is contraindicated in the presence of focal signs. If purpura are present along with fever do blood culture, otherwise CT to find out the pressure effects of increased ICT.

Immediate Management

Benzyl penicillin after taking blood sample + high flow O_2.

Treatment of Choice

Antibiotic according to culture report.

Organism	*Antibiotic*	*Second choice*
• Unknown pyogenic	Cefotaxime	Benzyl penicillin+ Chloramphenicol
• *Meningococcus*	Benzyl penicillin	Cefotaxime
• *Pneumococcus*	Cefotaxime	Penicillin
• *Hemophilus*	Cefotaxime	Chloramphenicol

50. A four-year-old boy has delayed speech. Both his father and paternal uncle has the same problem.

Diagnosis: Familial occurrence (i.e. normal finding here).

Clinchers

- *Four-year-old boy:* Normally sequence of speech development is
  - At 1 year: Few words may be used meaningfully
  - At 1½ years: 2 word utterances ("Mommy come")
  - At 2 years: Subject-verb-object sentences
  - At 3½ years: Mastered thought, language, obstruction and elements of reason
- *Delayed speech:* If a child reaches 3 years age with < 50 words vocabulary, suspect some abnormality.
- *Both his father and paternal uncle has the same problem:* Since there are two people in the family with the same features, it is strongly suggestive of a familial occurrence.

CONFUSA

If the father and uncle now have good speech and their problem is only a delayed development of speech, then the child's parents should be reassured (after excluding deafness and other common ailments that hampers speech development).

Investigation of Choice

Evaluation by a speech therapist to classify the type of problem.

Immediate Management

Refer to speech therapist.

Treatment of Choice

Wait and watch (if no other abnormality is found).

Your notes:

86. A 7-year-old boy has right sided earache and rhinorrhoea. On examination his right sided tympanic membrane appears pink in colour.

Diagnosis: Acute suppurative otitis media (ASOM) (presuppurative stage)

Clinchers

- *7-year-old:* ASOM is more common in infants and children especially of lower socioeconomic group.
- *Right sided earache:* In presuppurative stage there is marked earache which may disturb sleep and is of throbbing nature.
- *Rhinorrchoea:* Typically ASOM follows viral infection of upper respiratory tract (hence rhinorrhoea). Most common route of spread of infection is via eustachian tube.
- *Right sided tympanic membrane appears pink in colour:* Normal tympanic membrane should be pearly grey in colour. It is abnormal (i.e. inflamed) if it looks pink. In stage of presuppurative in ASOM, because of prolonged tubal occlusion, pyogenic organisms invade tympanic cavity causing hyperemia of its lining (hence pink colour). Tympanic membrane becomes congested.

CONFUSA

This condition may be confused with sphenoidal sinusitis, whose pain refers to retroauricular region and teeth (increase on walking). But in sinusitis there will be pyogenic discharge and facial tenderness.

Investigation of Choice
Otoscopy/tympanometry.

Immediate Management
Analgesia (Paracetamol).

Treatment of Choice
Adults—IM benzylpenicillin
Less than 5 years—Amoxicillin
If resistant strain: amoxicillin + clavulinic acid.

Your notes:

87. A 4-year-old with right sided earache is examined using otoscopy. This reveals a red bulging tympanic membrane.

Diagnosis: Acute suppurative otitis media (ASOM) (suppurative stages).

Clinchers

- *4-year-old:* The most common infection causing ASOM in under 5 years age is *H. influenzae.*
- *Right sided earache:* In presuppurative stage the pain in ear becomes marked which may disturb sleep and is of throbbing nature. But in suppurative stage the pain becomes excruciating.
- *Red bulging tympanic membrane:* In suppurative stage the tympanic membrane appears red and bulging with loss of landmarks. Handle of malleus may be engulfed by the swollen and protruding tympanic membrane and may not be discernible. A yellow spot may be seen on the tympanic membrane which rupture is imminent.

CONFUSA

Pain is immediately relieved once the tympanic membrane ruptures to discharge its contents. In serous otitis media (Glue ear) the eardrum looks concave.

Investigation of Choice
Otoscopy/tympanometry.

Immediate Management
Analgesia (paracetamol).

Treatment of Choice
Myringotomy—to evacuate pus
Indications of myringotomy in ASOM
1. Bulging drum and acute pain
2. Incomplete resolution despite antibiotics
3. Persistent effusion beyond 12 weeks.

Your notes:

88. An 8-year-old boy who has been playing outside now complains of right sided earache. On inspection a green bead is seen protruding into his ear canal. The walls of the canal are red.

Diagnosis: Foreign body in ear.

Clinchers

- *8-year-old boy:* Children are prone to put inanimate foreign bodies like beads in their ear.
- *Complains of right sided earache:* Foreign bodies in ear can cause conduction deafness, discomfort usually. If they cause pain then the ear canal must be inflamed.
- *A green bead is seen protruding into his ear canal:* Beads are smooth round foreign bodies which can easily slip deeper if their removal is attempted by a inexperienced person.
- *The walls of the canal are red:* This suggests inflammation secondary to impaction of the foreign body and hence the reason for pain (as the mucosa of ear canal swells up because of inflammation).

CONFUSA

Only things that a casuality SHO should attempt to remove ear insects. They are drowned into olive oil and then syringed out. An expert should remove all other foreign bodies. Forceps should not be used for removal.

Investigation of Choice

Otoscopy.

Immediate Management

Pain relief.

Treatment of Choice

- Hooks or suction (not forceps)
- GA is often needed especially when the child is uncooperative or if inflammation is present (as in this case).

Your notes:

89. A 9-year-old girl with a history of recurrent otitis media now complains of left sided earache. On examination the right sided tympanic membrane appears scarred. On examination of the left ear, pus is seen throughout the ear canal.

Diagnosis: Recurrent acute otitis media.

Clinchers

- *9-year-old girl:* It usually occurs in infants and children.
- *History of recurrent otitis media:* It may occur 4-5 times a year. The child remain free of symptoms between the episodes. Recurrent middle ear infections may sometimes be superimposed upon an existing otitis externa.
- *Complains of left sided earache:* It can be due to otitis externa or an acute episode of otitis media in this ear.
- *Right sided tympanic membrane appears scarred:* This signifies stigmata of previous episodes of otitis media in this ear.
- *Left ear, pus is seen throughout the ear canal:* This pus can either be due to rupture of tympanic membrane (i.e. from middle ear) or due to otitis externa. But since the pain still present, we shall consider it to be from otitis externa.

CONFUSA

Chronic suppurative otitis media presents with discharge and hearing loss but no pain.

Investigation of Choice

Otoscopy.

Immediate Management

Ear toilet.

Treatment of Choice

Amoxicillin + calvulinic acid (as recurrent infections are usually resistant)
+ medicated wicks (aluminium acetate or silver nitrate).

Your notes:

90. A 54-year-old female develops mild fever, malaise and ear pain. 3 days dilater she developed multiple painful vesicles over her ear canal and external meatus.

Diagnosis: Herpes zoster

Clinchers

- *Mild fever, malaise, ear pain:* Fever, malaise signifies viral infection. Herpes zoster oticus is a viral infection involving geniculate ganglion of facial nerve. There may be anaesthesia of face, giddiness and hearing impairment due to involvement of V and VIII nerves.
- *Multiple painful vesicles;* Herpes zoster infection (oticus) is characterised by appearance of vesicles on the tympanic membrane, deep meatus, concha and reteroauticular sulcus. There may be a vesicular rash in the external auditory canal and pinna.

CONFUSA

Nose tip involvement is virtually diagnostic if present in a case of Herpes Zoster. It is known as Hutchinson's signs and means involvement of the nasociliary branch of the trigeminal nerve which also supplies the globe and makes it highly likely that the eye will be affected.

Investigation of Choice

Fluorescent antibody tests and Tzank smears (but both rarely needed as the diagnosis is clinically easy).

Immediate Management

Keeping cool may reduce the number of lesions. Tell her to avoid scratching. Give adequate analgesia.

Treatment of Choice

Aciclovir 800 mg
- five times a day
- for 7 days

Your notes:

PAPER 4

2. Man with poor physical hygiene presents with pain and deafness after taking a shower.

Diagnosis: Wax impaction.

Clinchers

- *Man with poor physical hygiene*: Wax impaction is common in people with poor hygiene.
- *Pain and deafness after shower*: During bathing and swimming if water enters the ear, it may swell the wax and this will give rise to sudden pain, sense of blocked ear and/or hearing loss.

Tinnitus and giddiness may result from impaction of wax against the drum head. Patient may also complain of reflux cough, due to stimulation of auricular branch of vagus.

Wax or cerumen is secreted by ceruminous glands (modified sweat glands) situated in cartilaginous part of meatus.

Treatment of Choice

Treatment consists of its removal by syringing or instrumental manipulation. Hard impacted mass may sometimes require prior softening with wax solvents.

Your notes:

3. Woman presents with deafness and corneal anaesthesia. On MRI, a widened internal auditory meatus is seen.

Diagnosis: Acoustic neuroma.

Clinchers

- *Woman:* No significance. Acoustic neuroma is present equally in both the sexes. It is mostly seen in age group of 40-60 years.
- *Deafness:* Progressive unilateral sensorineural hearing loss often accompanied by tinnitus is the presenting symptom of acoustic neuroma.
- *Corneal anaesthesia:* Acoustic neuroma may uninvolve V, IX, X and XI cranial nerve as it grows. The earliest cranial nerve to be involved is V cranial nerve, presenting with reduced corneal sensitivity, numbness or paraesthesia of face.
- *Widened internal auditory meatus:* Acoustic neuroma, a benign, slow growing tumour of 8th nerve expands and causes widening and erosion of the internal auditory meatus.

CONFUSA

Acoustic neuroma should be differentiated from the cochlear pathology (i.e. Meniere's disease) and other cerebellopontine angle tumours, e.g. meningioma, primary cholesteatoma and arachnoidal cyst.

Treatment of Choice

Surgical removal.

Your notes:

4. Male, 20 years, with history of head injury, bruising on the side of head complains of hearing loss.

Diagnosis: Petrous temporal bone fracture.

Clinchers

- *Head injury:* Head injury can cause hearing loss due to:
  - Ossicular disruption
  - Haemotympanum
  - CSF otorrhoea
  - VIII cranial nerve palsy

  All these can occur in fracture of petrous temporal bone which houses of the middle ear and VIII nerve.
- *Bruising on side of head:* This almost confirms our suspicion of pterous temporal bone.

CONFUSA

A complaint of reduced hearing in one ear after trauma points to a haemotympanum most commonly. Blood in the external auditory meatus after trauma is usually caused by basal fracture but is rarely secondary to temporomandibular joint injury. In such cases direct auroscopic examination of the canal should be avoided as it may introduce infection via torn meninges.

Investigation of Choice

Skull X-rays (special views).

Immediate Management

GCS + admit

Treatment of Choice

Usually conservative. For hearing loss discuss with an ENT surgeon.

Your notes:

5. A 54-year-old female develops mild fever, malaise and ear pain. 3 days later she developed multiple painful vesicles over her ear canal and external meatus.

Diagnosis: Herpes zoster

Clinchers

- *Mild fever, malaise, ear pain:* Fever, malaise signifies viral infection. Herpes zoster oticus is a viral infection involving geniculate ganglion of facial nerve. There may be anaesthesia of face, giddiness and hearing impairment due to involvement of V and VIII nerves.
- *Multiple painful vesicles;* Herpes zoster infection (oticus) is characterised by appearance of vesicles on the tympanic membrane, deep meatus, concha and reteroauricular sulcus. There may be a vesicular rash in the external auditory canal and pinna.

CONFUSA

Nose tip involvement is virtually diagnostic if present in a case of Herpes zoster. It is known as Hutchinsons signs and means involvement of the nasociliary branch of the trigeminal nerve which also supplies the globe and makes it highly likely that the eye will be affected.

Investigation of Choice

Fluoroscent antibody tests and Tzank smears (but both rarely needed as the diagnosis is clinically easy).

Immediate Management

Keeping cool may reduce the number of lesions. Tell her to avoid scratching. Give adequate analgesia.

Treatment of Choice

Aciclovir 800 mg
- five times a day
- for 7 days.

Your notes:

6. A sheep farmer with a bleeding polyp on anterior part of nasal septum.

Diagnosis: Orf

Clinchers

- *Sheep farmer:* Certain pox viruses can cause localized vesicular lesions when humans come into direct contact with infected animals. *Orf virus* is one such virus, which is known as contagious pustular dermatitis virus, caught from sheep.
- *Bleeding polyp on anterior part of nasal septum:* People who come into contact with the affected fluid from animal lesions (especially from young lambs) may develop lesions on the hands and the body parts they touch (especially face and nose).

CONFUSA

Occasionally Orf infection is transmitted from goats.

Investigation of Choice

None

Immediate Management

Tell him not to touch vesicles

Treatment of Choice

Lesions resolve spontaneously after 4-6 weeks and immunity lasts life-long.

Your notes:

7. Man working in a chrome factory presents with whistling sound on talking.

Diagnosis: Nasal perforation.

Clinchers

➢ *Working in chrome factory:* Inhalation of chrome salts is an important cause of septal perforation.
➢ *Whistling sound:* Signifies perforation.
➢ *Causes of septal perforation*
- Inhalation of chrome salts
- Postseptal surgery
- Trauma/nose picking
- Sniffing cocaine
- Rodent ulcer
- Malignancy
- Granuloma Wegners
- Infections (TB, syphilis)
- Perforations irritable, crust and bleed.

Immediate Management
Symptomatic.

Treatment of Choice
Symptomatic (closure of perforation is difficult).

Your notes:

8. Man with prosthetic heart valve presents with epistaxis.

Diagnosis: Anticoagulant overdose.

Clinchers

➢ *Prosthetic heart valve:* Patients with prosthetic heart valves are treated with anticoagulants, indefinitely.
➢ *Epistaxis:* Littles area is very prone to bleeding. Here there is convergence of the anterior ethmoidal artery, the septal branches of the sphenopalatine and the superior labial arteries and greater palatine.

Anticoagulant overdose is an important cause of bleeding tendency (e.g. Warfarin anticoagulation).

Other causes of epistaxis are degenerative arterial disease and hypertension in older people, and local causes are atrophic rhinitis, hereditary telangiectasia and tumours of the nose of sinuses.

Investigation of Choice
INR.

Immediate Management
Treat shock and replace blood if necessary.

Treatment of Choice
Titrate the dose of anticoagulant for prosthetic heart valve. For epistaxis:
- Apply firm uninterrupted pressure of nostrils f/w finger and thumb for 10 minutes, possibly with ice pack over bridge of nose.
- If still bleeding spray—2.5-10% cocaine solution over mucosa. This will anaesthetise the mucosa and reduce bleeding by constricting vessels. Cauterise any bleeding points.
- Pack the nose.
- If bleeding recurs, further packs.
- Rarely arterial ligation.
- In severe, resistant bleeds, consider embolisation of the feeding vessel.

Your notes:

9. Man who is involved in furniture making presents with recurrent epistaxis and anaesthesia of right cheek.

Diagnosis: Carcinoma of maxillary antrum.

Clinchers

- *Involved in furniture making:* People working in hardwood furniture industry, nickel refining, leather work and manufacture of mustard gas has shown higher incidence of sinunasal cancer.

  Maxillary carcinoma is common in Bantus of South Africa. They use locally made snuff, rich in nickel and chromium.
- *Recurrent epistaxis and anaesthesia of maxillary antrum:* These are the early features of maxillary antrum. Other features are nasal stiffness, blood stained discharge, facial paraesthesia or pain and epiphora.

CONFUSA

Workers of furniture industry develop adenocarcinoma of the ethmoids and upper nasal cavity, while those engaged in nickel refining get squamous cell and anaplastic carcinoma.

Investigation of Choice

Radiograph of sinuses. CT scan helps in staging the disease. Biopsy confirm the suspicion of malignancy.

Immediate Management

Embolization of feeding vessel as epistaxis of malignancy is not remediable by simple measures.

Treatment of Choice

Investigate as above for malignancy. If malignancy proved, histological nature of malignancy is important in deciding the line of treatment, e.g. in squamous cell carcinoma, combination of radiotherapy and surgery gives better result then either alone.

Your notes:

10. An 80-year-old man with history of epistaxis since 2 hours.

Diagnosis: Hypertension.

Clinchers

- *An 80-year-old man:* Since only age is specified in this question, and no other relevant history is given, we can think of only two important factor, that relate age to epistaxis. They are:
  - Hypertension and
  - Degenerative arterial disease.
- *Since 2 hours:* This further supports our diagnosis of hypertension. Since local causes of epistaxis (atrophic rhinitis, hereditary telangectasia and tumour of nose and sinuses) can be excluded.

Immediate Management

Immediate lowering of BP.

Treatment of Choice

- For epistaxis refer Q-8 (March 2002)
- For hypertension—hypertension is a major risk factor for stroke and myocardial infarction. Our aim should be for BP < 140/85, but in 130/80 in patients with diabetes.

Your notes:

PAPER 5

88. A 20-year-old man says his face hurts, especially around the eyes and cheeks. When he bends forwards it worsens and makes him cry.

Diagnosis: Sinusitis (maxillary)

Clinchers

- *20-year-old:* Sinusitis is common at all ages in adults (as the sinuses are well developed and accumulate the predisposing pathologies by the adult age).
- *Man:* Males are slightly more affected.
- *Face hurts, especially around the eyes and cheeks:* Typically it is situated over the upper jaw, but may be referred to the gums or teeth. For this reason patient may primarily consult a dentist. Pain is aggravated by stooping, coughing or chewing. Occasionally pain is referred to the ipsilateral supraorbital region and thus may simulate frontal sinus infection.
- *Makes him cry:* That signifies that the pain is severe as is the case with it.

CONFUSA

Sinusitis is an infection of the paranasal sinuses that often complicate, upper respiratory tract infections (e.g. coryza and allergic rhinitis). Acute infections are usually caused by *Streptococcus pneumoniae* and *Haemophilus influenzae*. Symptoms include frontal headache and facial pain and tenderness, usually with nasal discharge but are often difficult to differentiate from symptoms of the common cold.

Investigation of Choice

X-rays (Water's view)

Immediate Management

Steam inhalation

Treatment of Choice

Antimicrobial drugs + nasal decongestants.

Your notes:

138. Sinusitis in patient allergic to penicillin

Diagnosis: Stated as the question itself.

Clinchers

Treatment of sinusitis is always with antibiotics. Many strains of *H. influenzae* are resistant to amoxycillin so co-amoxiclav or cofactor are preferred. Erythromycin is an alternative for those with penicillin allergy.

CONFUSA

In addition, nasal treatment with decongestants such as xylometazoline or anti-inflammatory therapy with topical corticosteroids such as fluticasone proprionate nasal spray should be given to reduce swelling of the mucosa and unblock the sinus openings.

Investigation of Choice

Clinical diagnosis

Immediate Management

Rule out liver disease before starting erythromycin treatment.

Treatment of Choice

Erythromycin.

Your notes:

139. Acute otitis media.

Diagnosis: Stated as the question itself.

Clinchers

Treatment with antibacterials is indicated in all cases with fever and severe earache. As the most common organisms and *strep. pneumonia* and *H. influenzae,* the drugs which are effective in acute otitis media are ampicillin (50 mg/kg/day in 4 divided doses), amoxicillin (40 mg/kg/day) in 3 divided doses). It must be continued for a minimum of 10 days, till tympanic membrane regains normal appearance and hearing returns to normal.

CONFUSA

Those allergic to penicillins can be given cofactor, cotrimoxaole or erythromycin. In cases where beta-lactamase producing *H. influenzae* or moraxella catarrhalis are isolated antibiotics like amoxicillin-clavulnate (Augmentin), cefuroxime axetil or cefixime may be used. Early discontinuance of therapy with relief of earache and fever, or therapy given in inadequate doses may lead to secretory otitis medial and residual hearing loss.

Investigation of Choice

Bacteriology

Immediate Management

Ear toilet + analgesia

Treatment of Choice

Amoxicillin.

Your notes:

PAPER 6

121. Man treated with gentamicin for peritonitis for 10 days presents with deafness.

Diagnosis: Ototoxicity.

Clinchers

Various drugs and chemicals can damage the inner ear and cause sensorineural deafness and tinnitus.

Symptoms of ototoxicity are—hearing loss, tinnitus, and/or giddiness, may manifest during treatment or after completion of treatment.

Ototoxic drugs: *Aminoglycoside antibiotics*: Gentamicin is the most important of all. Other includes—streptomycin, tobramycin, neomycin, etc.

- *Diuretics*: Fuorosemide, ethacrinic, etc.
- *Antimalarials*: Quinine, chloroquine.
- *Cytotoxic drugs*: Nitrogen, mustard, cisplatin
- *Analgesics*: Salicylates, indomethacin, ibuprofen.
- *Chemicals*: Alcohol, tobacco, marijuana, carbon monoxide poisoning.

Investigation of Choice

Rinne test (positive), i.e. air conduction < bone conduction.

Immediate Management

Weber lateralised to better ear.

Treatment of Choice

Stop gentamicin at once.

Your notes:

122. A patient with poor hygienic condition presents with hearing loss after taking a shower.

Diagnosis: Ear wax

Clinchers

- *Poor hygiene*: Normally only small amount of wax is secreted by ceruminous glands, which dries up and is later expelled from the meatus by movement of yaw. In people with poor hygiene wax dries up and forms hard impacted mass.
- *Prevents with hearing loss*: Wax impacted patients generally present with impairment of hearing or sense of blocked ear. Tinnitus of giddiness may result from impaction of wax against the drum head.
- *After taking a shower:* It confirms our diagnosis as wax impaction usually presents in this way (as wax swells up by absorbint water).

CONFUSA

Some times the onset of symptoms may be sudden. This is when water enters the ear canal during bathing or swimming and wax smells up.

Investigation of Choice

Otoscopy.

Immediate Management

Removal of wax by syringing or instrumental manipulation.

Treatment of Choice

Remove wax by syringing or instrumental manipulation. Hard impacted mass may sometimes require prior softening with wax solvents.

Advice hygiene.

Your notes:

123. Woman presents with deafness and corneal anaesthesia. On MRI, a widened internal auditory meatus is seen.

Diagnosis: Acoustic neuroma.

Clinchers

- *Woman:* No significance. Acoustic neuroma is present equally in both the sexes. It is mostly seen in age group of 40-60 years.
- *Deafness:* Progressive unilateral sensorineural hearing loss often accompanied by tinnitus is the presenting symptom of acoustic neuroma.
- *Corneal anaesthesia:* Acoustic neuroma may uninvolve V, IX, X and XI cranial nerve as it grows. The earliest cranial nerve to be involved is V cranial nerve, presenting with reduced corneal sensitivity, numbness or paraesthesia of face.
- *Widened internal auditory meatus:* Acoustic neuroma, a benign, slow growing tumour of 8th nerve expands and causes widening and erosion of the internal auditory meatus.

CONFUSA

Acoustic neuroma should be differentiated from the cochlear pathology (i.e. Meniere's disease) and other cerebellopontine angle tumours, e.g. meningioma, primary cholesteatoma and arachnoidal cyst.

Treatment of Choice

Surgical removal.

Your notes:

124. Male, 20 years, with history of head injury, bruising on the side of head complains of hearing loss.

Diagnosis: Petrous temporal bone fracture.

Clinchers

- *Head injury:* Head injury can cause hearing loss due to:
  - Ossicular disruption
  - Haemotympanum
  - CSF otorrhoea
  - VIII cranial nerve palsy

  All these can occur in fracture of petrous temporal bone which houses the middle ear and VIII nerve.
- *Bruising on side of head:* This almost confirms our suspicion of pterous temporal bone.

CONFUSA

A complaint of reduced hearing in one ear after trauma points to a haemotympanum most commonly. Blood in the external auditory meatus after trauma is usually caused by basal fracture but is rarely secondary to temporomandibular joint injury. In such cases direct auroscopic examination of the canal should be avoided as it may introduce infection via torn meninges.

Investigation of Choice

Skull X-rays (special views).

Immediate Management

GCS + admit

Treatment of Choice

Usually conservative. For hearing loss discuss with an ENT surgeon.

Your notes:

125. A 54-year-old female develops mild fever, malaise and ear pain. 3 days later she developed multiple painful vesicles over her ear canal and external meatus.

Diagnosis: Herpes zoster

Clinchers

- *Mild fever, malaise, ear pain:* Fever, malaise signifies viral infection. Herpes zoster oticus is a viral infection involving geniculate ganglion of facial nerve. There may be anaesthesia of face, giddiness and hearing impairment due to involvement of V and VIII nerves.
- *Multiple painful vesicles:* Herpes zoster infection (oticus) is characterised by appearance of vesicles on the tympanic membrane, deep meatus, concha and reteroauricular sulcus. There may be a vesicular rash in the external auditory canal and pinna.

CONFUSA

Nose tip involvement is virtually diagnostic if present in a case of Herpes zoster. It is known as Hutchinsons signs and means involvement of the nasociliary branch of the trigeminal nerve which also supplies the globe and makes it highly likely that the eye will be affected.

Investigation of Choice

Fluoroscent antibody tests and Tzank smears (but both rarely needed as the diagnosis is clinically easy).

Immediate Management

Keeping cool may reduce the number of lesions. Tell her to avoid scratching. Give adequate analgesia.

Treatment of Choice

Aciclovir 800 mg
- five times a day
- for 7 days

Your notes:

136. There is minor bleeding from the nose, but the site of bleeding is difficult to localize.

Diagnosis: Epistaxis

Clinchers

In case of active anterior epistaxis nose is cleared of blood clots by suction, and attempt is made to localise the bleeding sites. In minor bleeds from the accessible sites cauterisation of bleeding area can be done.

When the bleeding is profuse or when site of bleeding is difficult to localise, anterior packing should be done.

CONFUSA
In profuse bleeding and/or when site of bleeding is not localised, anterior packing is the Treatment of Choice. When the bleeding point has been localised, cauterization is useful in anterior epistaxis.

Investigation of Choice

Keep a check on pulse, BP and respiration.

Immediate Management

Anterior packing.

Treatment of Choice

Investigate and treat the patient for any underlying local or general cause.

Causes of Epistaxis

Local causes:
- Trauma
- Infections
- Foreign body
- Neoplasm of nose of paranasal sinuses
- Atmospheric changes
- Deviated nasal septum

General causes:
- Cardiovascular system (e.g. HT, mitral stenosis, arteriosclerosis).
- Disorder of blood and blood vessels.
- Liver disease (prothrombin deficiency).
- Drugs (Excess salicylates and anticoagulant for heart disease)
- Mediastinal compression
- Vicarious menstruation (epistaxis occurring at time of menstruation.

Your notes:

137. A patient with nose bleeding, on examination vascular damage is found, there is still some leakage.

Diagnosis: Epistaxis

Clinchers

Most of the time bleeding occurs from littles area and can easily be controlled by pinching the nose with thumb and index finger for about 5 minutes. But in this question since on examination, vascular damage is found, this area should be anaesthetised, and bleeding point cauterised with a bead of silver nitrate or coagulated with electrocautery.

It is important to note that whenever the bleeding point is not localised, anterior packing should be done, and when bleeding point is localised, then electrocautery is the better option.

CONFUSA
Anterior packing is preferred when the bleeding point is not localised. Here cauterization is better option.

Investigation of Choice

Keep check on pulse, BP and respiration.

Immediate Management

Electrocautery

Treatment of Choice

Investigate and treat the patient for underlying local or general cause.

Causes of Epistaxis

Refer Q 136.

Your notes:

139. Man who is involved in furniture making presents with recurrent epistaxis and anaesthesia of right cheek.

Diagnosis: Carcinoma of maxillary antrum.

Clinchers

➢ *Involved in furniture making:* People working in hardwood furniture industry, nickel refining, leather work and manufacture of mustard gas has shown higher incidence of sinunasal cancer.

Maxillary carcinoma is common in Bantus of South Africa. They use locally made snuff, rich in nickel and chromium.

➢ *Recurrent epistaxis and anaesthesia of maxillary antrum:* These are the early features of maxillary antrum. Other features are nasal stiffness, blood stained discharge, facial paraesthesia or pain and epiphora.

CONFUSA

Workers of furniture industry develop adenocarcinoma of the ethmoids and upper nasal cavity, while those engaged in nickel refining get squamous cell and anaplastic carcinoma.

Investigation of Choice

Radiograph of sinuses. CT scan helps in staging the disease. Biopsy confirm the suspicion of malignancy.

Immediate Management

Embolization of feeding vessel as epistaxis of malignancy is not remediable by simple measures.

Treatment of Choice

Investigate as above for malignancy. If malignancy proved, histological nature of malignancy is important in deciding the line of treatment, e.g. in squamous cell carcinoma, combination of radiotherapy and surgery gives better result then either alone.

Your notes:

140. An 80-year-old man with history of epistaxis since 2 hours.

Diagnosis: Hypertension.

Clinchers

➢ *An 80-year-old man:* Since only age is specified in this question, and no other relevant history is given, we can think of only two important factor, that relate age to epistaxis. They are:
- Hypertension and
- Degenerative arterial disease.

➢ *Since 2 hours:* This further supports our diagnosis of hypertension. Since local causes of epistaxis (atrophic rhinitis, hereditary telangectasia and tumour of nose and sinuses) can be excluded.

Immediate Management

Immediate lowering of BP.

Treatment of Choice

- For epistaxis refer Q-8 (March 2002)
- For hypertension—hypertension is a major risk factor for stroke and myocardial infarction. Our aim should be for BP < 140/85, but in 130/80 in patients with diabetes.

Your notes:

PAPER 7

76. Otosclerosis.

Diagnosis: Bilateral conductive deafness.

Clinchers

Otosclerosis is usually bilateral. Half of the patients have a family history. Symptoms usually occur in early adult life. In this disease, vascular spongy bone replaces normal bone around the oval window to which there is adherence of the stapes footplate. This produces conductive deafness.

CONFUSA

Sometimes tinnitus and vertigo are associated with conductive deafness. In conductive deafness hearing is better in background noise. Symptoms of otosclerosis are characteristically made worse by pregnancy.

Investigation of Choice

Audiogram

Immediate Management

Hearing aid

Treatment of Choice

Replacement of stapes with an implant.

Your notes:

77. Presbycusis.

Diagnosis: Bilateral sensory neural deafness.

Clinchers

In presbycusis there is loss of acuity for high frequency sounds. It starts before 30 years of age and the rate of loss of the higher frequencies is progressive thereafter. Deafness is due to loss of hair cells (sensory-neural). It is gradual in onset.

CONFUSA

Presbycusis is senile deafness. In presbycusis the hearing defect usually go unnoticed until hearing of speech is affected. This may occur with loss of high frequency sounds e.g. consonants at (~3-4 Hz are required for speech discrimination). Hearing is most affected in the present of background noise.

Investigation of Choice

Audiogram.

Immediate Management

Curtailment of smoking and stimulants like tea and coffee (to decrease associated tinnitus).

Treatment of Choice

Hearing aids.

Your notes:

78. Otitis media with effusion.

Diagnosis: Unilateral conductive deafness.

Clinchers

- *Otitis media:* It can cause hearing loss by
  - a. Conductive deafness: Due to fluid in middle ear
  - b. Sensori-neural deafness: This is usually secondary to labyrinthitis due to ascending bacterial infection through middle ear (tympanogenic) or through CSF (meningogenic)
- *Effusion:* This indicates the deafness is most probably conductive.

CONFUSA

Otitis media with effusion is commonly referred to as glue ear and is an insidious condition characterised by accumulation of non-purulent effusion in middle ear. Hearing loss is the presenting and sometimes the only symptoms. It is insiduous in onset and rarely exceeds 40 dB. Deafness may pass unnoticed by the parents and may be accidentally discovered during audiometric screening tests.

Investigation of Choice

Impedance audiometry.

Immediate Management

Examine the other ear also.

Treatment of Choice

Myringotomy and aspiration of fluid with gommet insertion.

Note: Uncomplicated or new cases can be managed by medical treatment also.

Your notes:

79. Acoustic neuroma.

Diagnosis: Unilateral sensory deafness.

Clinchers

Acoustic neuroma is a slow growing neurofibroma. It often arises from the vestibular nerve and produces progressive ipsilateral tinnitus ± sensorineural deafness.

CONFUSA

Vertigo is rare with acoustic neuroma, giddiness is common. Big tumours may give ipsilateral above the tumour may give a facial numbness. Cranial nerves especially V, VI and VII may be affected.

Investigation of Choice

MRI

Immediate Management

Rule out - ICP

Treatment of Choice

Surgery (if possible).

Your notes:

80. Noise-induced hearing loss (NIHL).

Diagnosis: Loss is not more than 60 dB.

Clinchers

- *Noise induced:* Hearing loss follows chronic exposure to less intense sounds for prolonged periods and is mainly a hazard of noisy occupations. It can cause:
  a. Temporary threshold shift: The hearing is impaired immediately after exposure to noise but recovers after an interval of a few minutes to a few hours.
  b. Permanent threshold shift: The hearing impairment is permanent and does not recover at all.
- Hearing loss: The damage caused by raise trauma depends on several factors (usually the hearing loss is not more than 60 dB):
  - Frequency: A frequency of 2000 to 3000 Hz causes more damage than lower or higher frequencies
  - Intensity and duration: As the intensity increases, permissible time for exposure is reduced
  - Continuous vs interrupted noise: Continuous noise is more harmful
  - Susceptibility of individual
  - Pre-existing ear disease.

CONFUSA

The single most successful way of reducing deafness is to limit damaging noise (< 85 dB/8 h day) exposure at work and leisure—as indicated by finding talking difficult, ringing in the ears during exposure, or sounds appearing muffled after exposure.

Investigation of Choice

Audiogram (shows a typical notch at 4 Hz, both for air and bone conduction).

Immediate Management

Work to limit exposure.

Treatment of Choice

Ear protectors should be used where noise levels exceed 85 dB. It hearing impairment has already occurred work for rehabilitation and give hearing aids.

Your notes:

101. Male patient has nasal speech, snores at night. day time he is sleepy.

Diagnosis: Obstructive sleep apnoea

Clinchers

- *Male:* This condition occurs most often in over-weight middle-aged men and affects 1-2% of the population.
- *Nasal speech:* This signifies nasal obstruction i.e. nasal deformity, rhinitis, polyp or adenoid. It is a correctable factor and occurs in upto one-third of cases.
- *Snores at night:* Apnoeas occur when the airway at the back of the throat is sucked closed while breathing in during sleep. When awake this tendency is overcome by the action of opening muscles of upper airway which become hypotonic during sleep. Partial narrowing results in snoring, occlusion in apnoea and critical narrowing in hypoapnoeas.
- *Day time he is sleepy:* Patients are worked by the struggle to breathe against the blocked throat. The awakenings are so brief that the patient remains unaware of them but is woken thousands of times per night leading to day time sleepiness and impaired performance.

CONFUSA

It can occur in children also, particularly those with enlarged tonsils. In adults, apart from nasal obstruction, other associated correctable factors may be:

- Encroachment on pharynx—obesity, acromegaly, enlarged tonsils.
- Respiratory depressant drugs—alcohol, sedatives, strong analgesics.

Investigation of Choice

- *Screening:* Noninvasive ear or finger oximetry (best performed at home).
- *Definitive:* Polysomnographic studies.

Immediate Management

Nasal continuous positive airway pressure (CPAP) till definitive treatment is undertaken.

Treatment of Choice

Correction of treatable factors (may be surgical).

Your notes:

102. 2-year-old child has been keeping well, but now has decreased hearing. Motor function is normal.

Diagnosis: Hearing impairment.

Clinchers

- *2-year-old child decreased hearing:* Hearing loss in a child may develop from causes
  - Prenatal
    - Genetic defects
    - Maternal infections
    - Drugs during pregnancy
    - Radiation to mother in first trimester
  - Perinatal
    - Prematurity
    - Birth injuries
    - Neonatal jaundice
    - Neonatal meningitis
    - Ototoxic drugs
  - Postnatal (most likely in this case)
    - Genetic
    - Nongenetic
- *Motor function is normal:* Rules out brain lesions as cause.

CONFUSA

Viral infections (measles, mumps, varicella, influenza) and meningitis and encephalitis are the most common causes of hearing loss postnatally. Genetic deafness may also present late as in familial progressive sensorineural deafness and in association with certain syndrome, e.g. Alport's, Klippel-fiel, Hurlers's, etc.

Investigation of Choice

Hearing tests.

Immediate Management

ENT referral.

Treatment of Choice

As per the cause.

Your notes:

105. A 3-year-old with a persistent and rough voice.

Diagnosis: Respiro-laryngeal dysfunction (RLD).

Clinchers

- *3-year-old:* RLD affected child commonly present at this age as this disorder is noted after development of a good speech.
- *Loud and rough voice:* It is dysphonia from incorrect vocal fold vibration or air flow regulation.

CONFUSA

Other causes of speech disorder in a 3 years old child can be:

- Deafness
- Expressive dysphasia
- Speech dyspraxia
- Audio-premotor syndrome
- Congenital aphonia (rare)

Investigation of Choice

Laryngeal airflow measurements

Immediate Management

Exclude deafness (as child can be unduly loud in its presence) and refer to ENT.

Treatment of Choice

- Voice training
- Surgical correction (rarely)

Your notes:

8 Gastroenterology

PAPER 1

Serial No. 62

Subject: Medicine

Topic: Gastroenterology (Coloured Slide)

Question: A 48-year-old female, a chronic alcoholic with history of haematesis. Oesophagogastroscopy revealed oesophageal varices.

Diagnosis: Spider naevi (secondary to alcoholic hepatitis).

Clinchers

- *48-year-old female:* Alcoholic hepatitis although more commonly seen in males, females are far more susceptible. It can occur at any age; peaking at 20-60 years of age.
- *Chronic alcoholic:* This is the strongest clue in the question which points towards alcoholic hepatitis. Heavy alcohol use is a prerequisite for the development of alcoholic hepatitis.
- *History of haematemesis:* Haematemesis usually occur as a complication of chronic liver disease which causes a portal hypertension and subsequent engorgement of the porto-systemic anastomoses.
- *Oesophagogastroscopy revealed oesophageal varices:* This confirms that the haematemesis was due to engorged varices secondary to portal hypertension.

CONFUSA

- Spider naevi are telangiectases that consist of a large arteriole from which radiate numerous small vessels that resemble a spider's legs. They are found in the distribution of the superior vena cava i.e. on the arms, neck, and chest wall. Pressure applied with a pointed object to the central arteriole causes blanching of the whole lesion. Most frequently associated with alcoholic cirrhosis.
- Venous stars are star-like lesions that occur on the dorsum of the feet, legs, back and lower chest on sites overlying the main tributary to a large vein. They result from raised venous pressure. Blood flow is from the periphery of the lesion to its centre and is not obliterated by pressure.

Investigation of Choice

Differentiate from other common lesions like venous stars, Campbell de Morgan spots, hereditary haemorrhagic telangiectasias.

Immediate Management

None

Treatment of Choice

Treatment directed at the underlying liver condition.

Your notes:

Serial No. 109

Subject: Medicine

Topic: Dyspepsia

Question: A 56-year-old male presents with dyspeptic symptoms. Cytological brushings from stomach are positive for gram-negative spiral organisms.

Diagnosis: *Helicobacter pylori* induced dyspepsia.

Clinchers

- *56-year-old male:* Infection with *H. pylori* affects 30-50% of adults in Europe and over 80% in parts of the developing world. Although no sex predilection is confirmed, females appear to be slightly more infected.
- *Dyspeptic symptoms:* Dyspepsia usually includes symptoms such as upper abdominal pain or discomfort, bloating, nausea and vomiting, early satiety and heart burn.
- *Cytological brushings from stomach positive for gram negative spiral organisms:* This confirms infection by *Helicobacter pylori*. It is typically described as a gram negative S shaped, spiral bacillus, a Unipolar flagellate, 1 by 3 micrometres in size. It is a micro-aerophilic, and produces urease and other toxins.

CONFUSA

- In a patient with documented peptic ulcer disease test for *Helicobacter pylori* should be performed.
- If the test is positive, go for eradication therapy.
- If the test is negative and/or the patient remains symptomatic then prescribe a proton pump inhibitor, in the lowest dose possible.

Investigation of Choice

- ^{13}C urea breath tests are the most reliable for diagnosis. They are the most suitable test for assessing the success of eradication therapy (>4 weeks after end of treatment). [Stop antisecretories, bismuth and antibiotics 2 weeks prior to test]
- Endoscopy with biopsy for rapid urease test is highly reliable for both diagnosis and to confirm cure.

Immediate Management

Immediate referral is indicated for significant acute gastrointestinal bleeding.

Treatment of Choice

HP eradication therapy:

- For patients who test positive, are provided with a 7-day twice-daily course of treatment consisting of a full-dose PPI, with either metronidazole 400 mg and clarithromycin 250 mg or amoxicillin 1g and clarithromycin 500 mg.

Note: For patients requiring a second course of eradication therapy, a regimen should be chosen that does not include antibiotics given previously

Your notes:

Management of Uninvestigated Dyspepsia in Primary Care

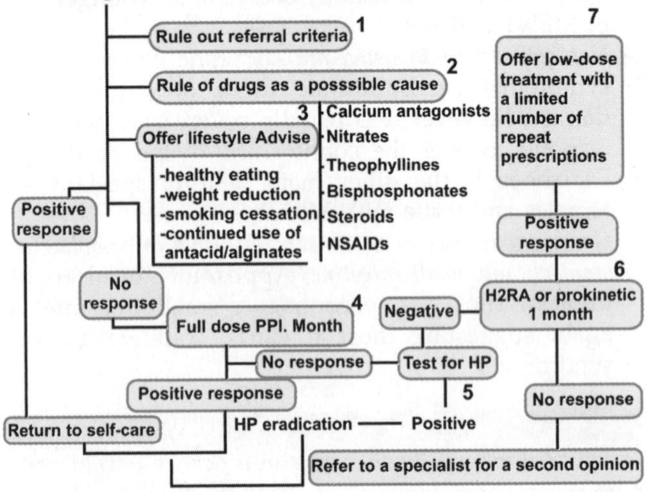

*Referral criteria:

1. Immediate referral is indicated for significant acute gastrointestinal bleeding.
2. Urgent specialist referral (with 2 weeks) for endoscopic investigation is indicated for patients of any age with dyspepsia when presenting with chronic gastrointestinal bleeding or progressive unintentional weight loss or progressive difficulty swallowing or persistent vomiting or iron deficiency anaemia or epigastric mass or suspicious barium meal.
3. Routine endoscopic investigation of patients of any age, presenting with dyspepsia and without alarm signs, is not necessary. However, for patients over 55, consider endoscopy when symptoms persist despite *Helicobacter pylori* (*H. pylori*) testing and acid suppression therapy and when patients have one or more of the following previous gastric ulcer or surgery, continuing need for NSAID treatment or raised risk of gastric cancer or anxiety about cancer. Consider managing previously investigated patients without new alarm signs according to previous endoscopic findings

Serial No. 110

Subject: Medicine

Topic: Dyspepsia

Question: A 34-year-old male with severe dyspepsia, not responding to usual anti-dyspeptic measures. Gastro-duodenoscopy shows several ulcers in oesophagus, stomach and small intestine.

Diagnosis: Zollinger Ellison Syndrome

Clinchers

- *34-year-old male:* syndrome has a slight male preponderance at about 1.3 : 1, with mean age of presentation around 40; It usually occurs at an younger age in MEN1 patients.
- *Not responding to usual anti-dyspeptic measures:* The symptoms usually mimic those of peptic ulcer disease, however it is usually severe and does not respond to over the counter anti-dyspeptic drugs. Diarrhoea is the other major feature specially in females and those with MEN1.
- *Gastroduodenoscopy shows several ulcers in oesophagus, stomach and small intestine:* Appearance of ulcers at unusual sites, viz. oesophagus, small intestine is again suggesting most towards Zollinger Ellison syndrome.

CONFUSA

- The Zollinger Ellison syndrome occurs because of excessive production of gastrin that produces excessive gastric acidity. It can occur as a component of type 1 multiple endocrine neoplasia syndrome (MEN1) or it can occur in isolation.
- MEN 1 typically affects: parathyroid gland (hyperparathyroidism), pancreatic islets (Gastrinomas) and anterior pituitary gland(Prolactinomas).
- Zollinger Ellison syndrome is the major cause of morbidity in MEN1.

Investigation of Choice

- Measurement of basal and maximal gastric acid output is mandatory to distinguish it from secondary hypergastrinaemia.

Immediate Management

Refer to specialist

Treatment of Choice

- Most patients are managed with proton pump inhibitors. Octreotide can also control acid hypersecretion in patients with Zollinger-Ellison syndrome —this treatment modality has a favourable outcome on the patients' prognosis and survival.
- Surgical resection of the primary tumour may improve prognosis and even result in a complete cure; Indicated for those without evidence of metastasis or tumours more than 2.5 cm; A single, isolated metastasis to liver can also be resected.

Your notes:

Serial No. 154

Subject: Medicine

Topic: Gastro

Question: A 37-year-old lady with chronic history of constipation, diarrhoea and passing bloody stools. Barium enema shows rose thorn ulcers.

Diagnosis: Crohn's Disease

Clinchers

- *37-year-old lady:* Women are affected with Crohn's disease more than men, with most common age of affection being 15-35 years. However, a second peak is observed at the age of 60-80 years.
- *With chronic history of constipation, diarrhoea and passing bloody stools:* The course of Crohn's disease is classically chronic and relapsing with abdominal pain, diarrhoea and weight loss as the main symptoms. Colon involvement typically presents with mucous and blood in stools.
- *Barium enema shows rose thorn ulcers:* Rose thorn ulcers typically associated with Crohn's disease, seen in large bowel involvement, are seen on double-contrast barium enema and usually deep (>3 mm). Similar but shallow ulcers seen in Ulcerative colitis are known as 'collar button ulcers'.

CONFUSA

- While large bowel involvement produces 'rose thorn ulcers' in Crohn's disease, the small bowel involvement (especially the terminal ileum) presents as Kantor String Sign. It is seen when a barium meal and follow through shows a typical stricture in the affected segment, usually the terminal ileum.
- Cobblestoning is another radiographic feature which is very characteristic of Crohn's disease, and often considered pathognomonic. Cobblestoning consists of a combination of submucosal edema and deep transverse and longitudinal fissuring which collects barium. This combination gives an appearance similar to a cobblestone street.

Investigation of Choice

Sigmoidoscopy and rectal biopsy is required to establish a diagnosis.

Immediate Management

Correct nutrition and electrolyte imbalance.

Severe fistulae may also necessitate considering total parenteral nutrition.

Treatment of Choice: Sulphasalazine

Serial No. 156

Subject: Medicine

Topic: Gastro

Question: An 18-year-old girl comes with complains of alternating diarrhoea and constipation. There is no weight loss.

Diagnosis: Irritable Bowel Syndrome.

Clinchers

- *18-year-old girl:* Irritable bowel syndrome is a functional gastrointestinal disorder which affects women twice more commonly than men. It has no age prediliction and can affect any age.
- *Alternating diarrhoea and constipation:* Abdominal discomfort associated with disordered bowel activity is the main presenting symptoms. Patients may either present with diarrhoea or constipation or both alternating. However, in females constipation is the predominant symptom.
- *No weight loss:* This rules out other serious abnormalities like inflammatory bowel disease (in young) and carcinoma colon (in the elderly).

CONFUSA

Irritable bowel syndrome can be easily confused with early stages of other organic disorders like Colonic cancer; inflammatory bowel disease, Coeliac disease, Gastroenteritis (e.g. giardiasis), ischaemic colitis, endometriosis, anxiety ± depression, somatization and panic disorders. Thus urgent referral and colonoscopy is indicated patients with suspected irritable bowel syndrome presenting with:

- Age > 50 years
- Weight loss
- Occult blood in faeces
- Family history of colorectal cancer
- Abdominal mass

Investigation of Choice

Positive diagnosis, based on symptoms can be made when there is a classical history, no alarming symptoms (see confusa above), no strong family history of GI malignancy, and the patient is young (<45) — without any investigations being necessary.

When there is diagnostic uncertainty, first line investigations are:

FBC and plasma viscosity ± stool culture, sigmoidoscopy and fecal occult blood.

TSH is done if diarrhoea is prominent.

Immediate Management
Urgent referral if alarming symptoms present.

Treatment of Choice
Reassurance and high fibre diet.
For constipation-predominant IBS - Bulk-forming agents; may also require treatment with an osmotic laxative
For diarrhoea predominant IBS - Drugs such as loperamide may be of benefit once other pathology has been excluded.

Your notes:

Table: Diagnostic criteria of IBIS

Diagnostic criteria for IBS (Rome II criteria):
At least 12 weeks, (need not be consecutive), in the preceding 12 months of abdominal discomfort or pain that has two of the three features:
- Relieved by defecation, and/or
- Associated with change of frequency of stool and/or
- Associated with change of consistency of stool.

The following cumulatively support the diagnosis of IBS:
- More than three motions per day
- Less than three motions per week
- Hard or lumpy stools
- Loose or water stools
- Straining during a bowel movement
- Urgency
- Feeling of incomplete emptying
- Passing mucus during a bowel movement
- Abdominal fullness, bloating or swelling

PAPER 2

Serial No. 41

Subject: Medicine

Topic: Gastro

Question: A patient presents with increasing constipation, and passing ribbon-like stools. He is well otherwise.

Diagnosis: Constipation (spastic)

Clinchers
- *Increasing constipation:* The history of progressively increasing constipation points towards many diagnosis such as Carcinoma colon, Carcinoma rectum, Irritable bowel disease, Inflammatory Bowel Disease, Intestinal tuberculosis as well as functional causes like diabetic neuropathy.
- *Passing ribbon-like stools:* This is suggesting narrowed colonic lumen. This narrowing can be due to any causes like a tumour or growth in the lumen or neuropathy which causes spasm of the intestinal musculature.
- *He is well otherwise:* His otherwise normal state of health rules out possibilities of carcinoma or inflammatory bowel disease. However, thorough investigations are required to rule out these possibilities with definite proofs.

CONFUSA

There are two basic kinds of constipation: atonic (lazy bowel) and spastic (narrowing of the colon, with small, ribbon-like stools). For atonic constipation, a high fibre diet and increased fluid intake is recommended. Spastic constipation may be caused by an obstruction or nervousness or anxiety. For spastic constipation it may be necessary to decrease the fibre intake until the situation is corrected.

Investigation of Choice
Barium Enema

Immediate Management
Exclude endocrine and metabolic abnormalities like hypothyroidism, hypercalcaemia, dehydration.

Treatment of Choice
According to the cause identified.

Your notes:

Serial No. 43

Subject: Medicine

Topic: Gastro

Question: A 40-year-old patient comes with two year history of epigastric pain after food and tarry stools.

Diagnosis: Peptic Ulcer

Clinchers

- *40-year-old:* Peptic ulcers is a common condition with a lifetime incidence of up to 10%, occurring four times more commonly in men than women and most common in middle age with peak at 30-50 years.
- *Two year history of epigastric pain after food:* This is the most usual symptom seen in peptic ulcers. The patient usually complains of localized epigastric pain, described as burning or gnawing, for which the patient can characteristically point to the location of maximum intensity. The pain is associated with meals. Gastric ulcers give rise to pain 15-20 minutes after meals, whereas duodenal ulceration causes pain 1-3 hours after a meal.
- *Tarry stools:* This is signifying complication of long standing peptic ulcer-gastrointestinal bleeding. It occurs in 25 to 33% of cases and accounts for 25% of ulcer deaths. Haemorrhage arises from the small blood vessels at the base of the ulcer.

CONFUSA

Peptic ulcer is a broad term including both duodenal and gastric ulcers. While duodenal ulcer is most commonly related to infection by *Helicobacter pylori*, gastric ulcer owe their existence to the factors which are related with increased serum gastrin levels and inadvertent use of NSAIDs.

Investigation of Choice
Upper GI Endoscopy with biopsy

Immediate Management
Urgent admission to hospital is required in cases of actively bleeding peptic ulcer.

Treatment of Choice
According to the cause identified:
HP eradication for duodenal ulcer
Stopping the offending drug (NSAIDs)
Proton pump inhibitors or Surgical resection for Zollinger Ellison Syndrome

Your notes:

Serial No. 44

Subject: Medicine

Topic: Gastro

Question: A 55-year-old woman presents with a six-month history of severe central abdominal pain, which comes on 30-minutes after meals. She has lost 10-kg in weight, and on examination of her abdomen there is a bruit in the epigastrium. She also suffers from intermittent claudication.

Diagnosis: Intestinal Claudication

Clinchers

- *55-year-old woman:* Atherosclerosis is the leading cause of morbidity in the Western World, accounting for more than half of all deaths. It affects nearly all adults, with a variable pattern and severity. Increases with age; more common in males than in females, particularly in younger age groups – aged 35 to 44 the prevalence in males is six times that of females, compared to just two times in 65 to 74 year olds.
- *Six-month history... after meals:* The patient typically is presenting with features suggesting of mesenteric ischaemia. Patients may present with a history of postprandial pain, typically starting 20-30 minutes after their last meal, that may last up to 60-90 minutes.
- *Lost 10-kg in weight:* Because of this typical relation of symptoms with food, they develop food fear and experience subsequent weight loss. Patients may be severely malnourished upon presentation.
- *Bruit in the epigastrium:* This is again suggesting the narrowed mesenteric artery due to probable athero-sclerosis.
- *Intermittent claudication:* Atherosclerosis of aorta and internal iliac arteries can cause intermittent claudi-cation. Presence in this patient suggests widespread atherosclerosis.

CONFUSA

Patient can also present with acute mesentric ischaemia due to embolic or thrombotic occlusion of the mesenteric artery. Look carefully for hints such as a prosthetic heart valve or atrial fibrillation which can be the source of the offending embolus. Such patients will present acutely with sudden onset of symptoms. Palpation of the abdomen would reveal no peritoneal signs and pain is usually out of proportion to examination. Auscul-tation of the abdomen may reveal a bruit.

Investigation of Choice
Mesenteric angiogram

Immediate Management
Correct dehydration

Treatment of Choice
Surgery

Your notes:

Serial No. 116

Subject: Medicine

Topic: GIT

Question: A 19-year-old female with complaint of a 1 year history of bloody diarrhoea and tenesmus. She has pale skin lesions. On examination-sigmoidoscopy shows inflammation and granulomata.

Diagnosis: Ulcerative Colitis

Clinchers

- *19 year old female:* Most cases of ulcerative colitis present between 15-30 years of age.
- *1-year history of bloody diarrhoea, tenesmus:* The onset is usually gradual and frequency of bowel is related to the severity of the disease. The stools are mixed with varying amounts of blood and mucus. The presence of tenesmus hints towards rectal involvement.
- *Has pale skin lesions:* The extra intestinal manifestations in the form of clubbing, apthous, oral ulcers, erythema nodosum, pyoderma gangrenosum, conjunctivitis, episcleritis and joint involvement, is predominantly a feature of ulcerative colitis than Crohn's disease.
- *Sigmoidoscopy shows inflammation, granulomata:* These are the classical features of ulcerative colitis.

CONFUSA

Its often difficult to differentiate between Crohn's and Ulcerative Colitis and the huge list of differences mentioned in the textbooks are of hardly of any help, especially in the stressed up environment on the exam day. Here are some useful points, which I personally found very useful for such questions.

- Young adults (<12 yrs): more likely diagnosis of Crohn's than UC.
- Extraintestinal Manifestations: More likely to be UC than Crohn's.
- Perianal fistula/fissures: More likely to be Crohn's than UC.
- Rectal involvement (tenesmus, urgency): More likely to be UC than Crohn's.
- Ileal involvement and strictures: Classical of Crohn's.
- Abnormal Sigmoidoscopy with few lesions on colonoscopy: more likely to be UC.
- Abnormal Colonoscopy with few lesions on sigmoidoscopy: more likely to be Crohn's.

Investigation of Choice
Sigmoidoscopy with rectal biopsy

Immediate Management
Specialist referral

Treatment of Choice
Mild UC(< 4 motions per day): Oral Prednisolone 20 mg + Mesalazine 500 mg
Moderate UC (4-6 motions per day): Oral Prednisolone 40 mg + Sulfasalzine 1g/12hr + twice daily steroid enemas.
Severe UC (>6 motions per day): Nil by mouth, IV hydration, IV hydrocortisone 100 mg/6h, rectal steroids

Your notes:

Serial No. 118

Subject: Medicine

Topic: GIT

Question: An 18-year-old presents with frequent diarrhoea and gaseous distention of the abdomen which is relieved by defaecation. Sigmoidoscopy is normal.

Diagnosis: Irritable Bowel Disease

Clinchers

- *18 year old:* Irritable bowel disease (IBS) is a disease of young age, highest incidence being observed among 20-40 yrs old, affecting females more commonly than the females.
- *Frequent diarrhoea, gaseous distension, relieved by defaecation:* The disease is characterise by altered bowel habits, either predominantly diarrhoea or constipation. Abdominal distension which is relieved by defaecation is almost characteristic.
- *Sigmoidoscopy is normal:* A 'pure' case of IBS doesn't have any abnormal findings on investigations, what so ever, however, rigorous investigations are indicated to rule out any organic basis of the symptoms.

CONFUSA

Be cautious in giving a diagnosis of irritable bowel if:
- Patient's age is more than 40 years,
- The history of altered habits is less than 6 months,
- There is associated anorexia or weight loss,
- There is waking at night with pain/diarrhoea,
- Associated mouth ulcers, rectal bleeding,
- Any abnormal investigations.

Investigation of Choice
Extensive investigations required to rule out any organic basis of the presenting symptoms viz. Inflammatory bowel disease, colorectal carcinoma, malabsorption or food intolerance.

Immediate Management
Careful explanation and reassurance

Treatment of Choice
Symptomatic
Constipation- Increase fibre intake
Diarrhoea- Bulking agent +/- loperamide
Tricyclic antidepressants (amitryptiline) is often useful

Your notes:

Serial No. 119

Subject: Medicine

Topic: GIT

Question: An 80-year-old with complaint of diarrhoea and urinary retention

Diagnosis: Faecal Impaction

Clinchers

- *80-year-old:* Elderly are at more risk of faecal impaction because of decreased mobility. Insufficient fibre or liquid in the diet exaggerates the problem.
- *Diarrhoea and urinary retention:* Chronic constipation can result in faecal impaction, where putty-like faeces partially obstructs the bowel. Subsequent cramping then causes the involuntary passage of liquid stools from higher up in the bowel.

CONFUSA

Faecal impaction can present with varying clinical features. It can present like:

- Chronic constipation, Diarrhoea, Urinary retention, Urinary Incontinence, Sense of fullness in the rectum; firm mass in the lower left abdomen; abdominal pain or cramps; thin, watery discharge from the rectum.
- The idea is to find out the high risk group which include elderly, or those who are immobile or on bed rest for any reason, those with back disorders that can cause nerve pressure, chronic users of laxatives or people on drugs like narcotics, antiparkinsonian drugs, atropine, phenothiazines or tricyclic anti-depressants.

Investigation of Choice

It's basically a clinical diagnosis

Immediate Management

Rule out underlying cause

Treatment of Choice

Improve diet and mobility

Correction of the underlying cause.

Your notes:

Serial No. 120

Subject: Surgery

Topic: GIT

Question: After an abdominal operation, a patient presents with subfebrile state and abdominal distention. There is associated no abdominal tenderness and constipation is present. On auscultation no bowel sounds are heard.

Diagnosis: Paralytic Ileus

Clinchers

- *After an abdominal operation:* Most common setting of paralytic ileus is post operative period, other causes being hypokalaemia, peritonitis, hypomagnesaemia, uremia, hypothyroidism and drug induced.
- *Subfebrile, abdominal distension:* Being subfebrile rules out any infectious cause of abdominal distension (viz, peritonitis). Paralytic ileus most commonly present as abdominal distension, with failure to pass flatus or faeces.
- *Associated no abdominal tenderness, constipation:* Although the patient might complain of slight abdominal pain, there is usually no abdominal tenderness. Constipation is characteristic.
- *No bowel sounds:* This adds further to our diagnosis. The bowel sounds is totally absent, apart from some occasional clicks. The patient may continue to vomit or if nasogastric tube *in situ,* would drain huge amount of fluids continuously.

CONFUSA

The above question can become quite tricky when presented like, 'A postoperative patient vomiting huge volumes of chocolate colored fluid. On auscultation, bowel sounds are absent.' Although, the picture looks quite similar to paralytic ileus, the difference in the diagnosis is made by the 'chocolate coloured fluid'. This is a typical description of Acute gastric dilatation, which occurs in postoperative period and is due to decreased vagal tone. The condition demands immediate insertion of a nasogastric tube (to regain the vagal tone) and restoration of the fluid and electrolyte loss. Re-surgery is rarely indicated.

Investigation of Choice

Clinical diagnosis.

Abdominal X-ray may show gas through out large and small bowel. However, this picture should always be supported by clinical signs.

Immediate Management

Restoration of Fluid and electrolytes.

Nil by mouth.

NG tube suction, if required.

Treatment of Choice

Rule out and correct any underlying cause (viz. electrolyte abnormality).

Colonoscopy may permit decompression of the gut, and also establishing any alternative diagnosis, if the above measures fail.

Your notes:

PAPER 3

28. An 18-year-old girl is doing her exams and is very stressed. She has missed her last period. Her pregnancy test is negative. She complains of a three months history of generalised abdominal pain and bloating.

Diagnosis: Probable irritable bowel syndrome (IBS).

Clinchers

- *18-year-old girl:* Patients are usually 20-40 years old and females are more frequently affected than males.
- *Doing her exams and is very stressed:* Symptoms of IBS are exacerbated by stress, menstruation or gastroenteritis.
- *She has missed her last period:* It might be reason for her stress in addition to her exams. On the other hand, it could also be secondary to anorexia induced by IBS.
- *Her pregnancy test is negative:* Proves that her amenorrhoea is not due to pregnancy.
- *She complains of a three month history of generalised abdominal pain and bloating:* Generalised abdominal pain and bloating are features of IBS. But IBS is diagnosed only if symptoms persist for >6 months. (The abdominal pain can also be central or lower).

CONFUSA

Coeliac disease also present with generalised abdominal pain and bloating. It could be a diagnosis in this case and should be ruled out by proper investigations. Basically IBS is a diagnosis of exclusion. But IBS < 6 months and presence of anorexia (as in this case) are usually markers of an organic disease.

Investigation of Choice

- *For young patients with a classical history:* do FBC, ESR, LFT, urinalysis, sigmoidoscopy and rectal biopsy.
- *If any marker of organic disease is present:* do either barium enema or colonoscopy.

Immediate Management

Careful explanation and reassurance.

Treatment of Choice

Symptomatic (see pg 237, OHCM, 5th edn).

Your notes:

106. A businessperson has just returned from a business trip to Asia. He now develops copious watery and bloody diarrhoea.

Diagnosis: Amoebic dysentery.

Clinchers

- *Business person:* Risk of amoebiasis in developed countries is more in travellers, recent immigrants and homosexual men.
- *Just returned from a business trip to Asia:* Highest incidence of amoebiasis is seen in developing countries in the topics, particularly Mexico, India, tropical Asia, central and south America and Africa.
- *Copious watery and bloody diarrhoea:* In amoebiasis diarrhoea develops slowly, but becomes profuse and bloody.

CONFUSA

Bacillary dysentery often has sudden onset and may cause dehydration. Stools are more watery. Acute ulcerative colitis has more gradual onset and stools are very bloody.

Investigation of Choice

Stool microscopy showing trophozoites, blood and pus cells.

Immediate Management

Correct dehydration: Oral rehydration is more beneficial than IV rehydration. In severe dehydration give 0.9% saline + 20 mmol K^+/L IVI.

Treatment of Choice

Metronidazole 800 mg/8h PO for 5 days then diloxanide furoate 500 mg/8h for 10 days to destroy gut cysts.

Your notes:

108. A young man develops bloody diarrhoea. A rigid sigmoidoscopy examination revealed granular ulceration in the sigmoid colon with proximal sparing.

Diagnosis: Crohn's involvement of the colon.

Clinchers

- *Young man:* Peak occurrence between 15 and 30 years of age and between 60 and 80 years of age, but onset may occur of any age.
- *Bloody diarrhoea:* Though bloody diarrhoea is more commonly seen in ulcerative colitis, sometimes Crohn's disease may present with bloody diarrhoea. Moreover the options include ulcerative pancolitis and not ulcerative colitis, therefore since rectal involvement is not there we can safely exclude UC.
- *Granular ulceration in the sigmoid colon with proximal sparing:* Inflammation seen in UC is continuous (no skip areas), whereas in Crohn's disease any part of GI involved, usually terminal ilium and/or colon, with linear ulcerations and submucosal thickening leading to cobblestone pattern, discontinuous skip areas are characteristic of Crohn's disease.

CONFUSA

There may be confusion with ulcerative collitis (UC) but in that case rectum involvement should be there. In UC rectal involvement is almost always seen.

Investigation of Choice

Sigmoidoscopy.

Immediate Management

Antidiarrhoeal agents, IV hydration and blood transfusion in severe cases.

Treatment of Choice

5 ASA oral or enema, metronidazole and/or ciprofloxacin.

Your notes:

109. A middle-aged woman has been on several antibiotic treatments recently because of a persistent pneumonia. She now develops a severe watery diarrhoea. Colonoscopy reveals whitish plaques scattered throughout the colon.

Diagnosis: Pseudomembranous colitis.

Clinchers

- *On several antibiotic treatments recently:* Pseudomembranes colitis is caused by overgrowth of *Clostridium difficile*, following any antibiotic therapy.
- *Severe watery diarrhoea:* Most often diarrhoea is profuse and watery, although bloody diarrhoea occurs in 5% cases.
- *Whitish plaques scattered throughout the colon:* Characteristic multiple, discrete, yellowish plaques are seen on sigmoidoscopy which on biopsy shows features of acute inflammation and ulceration with a pseudomembrane of fibrin and necrotic material.

CONFUSA

Currently, strains of *C. difficile* that produce toxins detectable in the stool the only identified cause of colitis induced by antibiotics, therefore there should be no confusion in this question.

Investigation of Choice

Sigmoidoscopy occasionally colonoscopy may be required.

Immediate Management

Should be initially directed in eradicating *C. difficile* from the stool.

Treatment of Choice

Vancomycin 125 mg/6h PO or metronidazole 400 mg/8h PO.

Your notes:

120. A 52-year-old obese man has had episodic anterior chest pain, particularly at night, for three weeks. Chest X-ray and ECG are normal.

Diagnosis: Reflux oesophagitis.

Clinchers

- *Obesity:* A risk factor for reflux oesophagitis.
- *Episodic anterior chest pain:* Refer causes of chest pain in question 116. Episodic character of chest pain is more likely to be due to angina or reflux oesophagitis.
- *At night:* Burning, retrosternal discomfort related to meals, lying down, stooping and straining is likely to be due to reflux.
- *Chest X-ray and ECG are normal:* Rules out cardiovascular + pulmonary causes of chest pain.

CONFUSA

Oesophagitis (corrosive, NSAIDs), duodenal and gastric ulcer, infections (CMV, herpes, candida).

Investigation of Choice

Investigation not required in isolated symptoms: Tests—barium swallow (shows hiatus hernia).

Immediate Management

Antacids, e.g. magnesium trisilicate mixture.

Treatment of Choice

Change in lifestyle— weight, stop smoking, alcohol intake, raise bed head, take small regular meals, avoid hot drinks, eating < 3 hours before bed.

- Upper GI endoscopy
- H_2 antagonists (ranitidine)
- Proton pump inhibitor (lansoprazole)
- Prokinetic drugs (metoclopramide)

Your notes:

181. A 35-year-old woman complains of abdominal discomfort relieved by passing flatus or defaecation. Over the last 6 months she has had episodes of diarrhoea and constipation, but denied she had lost weight. Her mother died of bowel carcinoma.

Diagnosis: Irritable bowel syndrome (IBS).

Clinchers

- *35-year-old woman:* Patients of IBS are usually between 20-40 years and females are more frequently affected.
- *Abdominal discomfort relieved by flatus or defaecation:* This is a very important point. This supports the diagnosis of IBS. Other important history is the sensation of incomplete evacuation and the passage of mucus.
- *Episode of diarrhoea and constipation:* Altered bowel habits (constipation alternating with diarrhoea) present in IBS.
- *Since last 6 months:* These symptoms must be present for atleast 3 months, before the diagnose of IBS could be established.
- *No history of weight loss:* Helps to exclude carcinoma.

Investigation of Choice

Flexible sigmoidoscopy: In over 48 years to exclude colonic neoplasm. In younger patients exclude inflammatory bowel disease.

Treatment of Choice

Though there is no treatment for IBS, focus on dietary modification with fiber supplements. Treatment should be directed to the predominant symptom.

Your notes:

PAPER 4

131. An elderly female has history of uncontrollable loose stools many times a day. On examination, packed solid faeces in rectum.

Diagnosis: Faecal impaction with overflow diarrhoea.

Clinchers

- *Elderly female:* Faecal impaction usually occurs in the elderly with constipation.
- *Loose stools many times a day:* It is faecal incontinence and is a major problem in the elderly infirm or demented patient. It is often secondary to faecal loading and impaction (overflow incontinence).

CONFUSA

Faecal incontinence in younger patients, is most commonly due to neurological disorders or childbirth trauma. Faecal impaction is rare in them.

Investigation of Choice

To find the cause for constipation so vary from patient to patient.

Immediate Management

Rule out dementia

Treatment of Choice

Manual removal of impacted faeces.

Your notes:

132. A 30-year-old female has history of alternating constipation and diarrhoea, for 7 months. She told that she is passing hard pellet like stools.

Diagnosis: Irritable bowel syndrome (IBS).

Clinchers

- *30-year-old females:* Patients are usually 20-40 years old and females are more frequently affected.
  Note: Since this disorder is chronic, patients can present at any age often teens.
- *Alternating constipation and diarrhoea:* This is the most common symptom of the altered bowel habit in IBS. Other symptoms of IBS are:
  - Central or lower abdominal pain (relieved by defaecation)
  - Abdominal bloating
  - Tenesmus
  - Mucus per rectum
- *Passing pellet like stools:* This can be due to abnormal colonic motility frequently present in IBS.
- *For 7 months:* Symptoms should be present for > 6 months for diagnosis.

CONFUSA

Half of all patients with this disorder who seek medical care have comorbid psychiatric disorders. IBS is usually a diagnosis of exclusion. There are markers of organic disease, which are usually present in this condition. These markers can represent some organic disease which will manifest itself over the time. The organic markers are:

- Age > 40 years
- History < 6 months
- Anorexia
- Weight loss
- Waking at night with pain/diarrhoea
- Mouth ulcers
- Rectal bleeding
- Abnormal investigations

Note: Presence of any of these question the diagnosis of IBS.

Investigation of Choice

Follow the following flow chart.

Any marker of organic disease?
→ Yes → Barium enema or Colonoscopy
↓ No

Diarrhoea
→ Yes → Stool culture, TSH, Faecal fats
↓ No

Constipation?
→ Yes → Plasma Ca^{2+}, TSH
↓ No

Anaemia or weight loss?
→ Yes → Endomysial antibodies (for coeliac disease)
↓ No

Immediate Management

Reassurance.

Treatment of Choice

Treatment should be directed the predominant symptom, i.e.

- Food intolerance—exclusion diets
- Constipation—high fibre diet
- Diarrhoea—bulking agent + loperamide
- Colic and bloating—antispasmodics (mebeverine, alverine citrate)
- Dyspepsia—Metoclopramide or antacids
- Psychiatric symptoms—Anxiolytics + cognitive therapy.

133. Female, 22-year-old, with bleeding and mucus per rectum, fever, loss of weight, has never been abroad.

Diagnosis: Inflammatory bowel disease (IBD)

Clinchers

- *22-year-old female:* The incidence of IBD peaks between 15 to 35 years, although it has been reported in every decade of life. Both the sexes are affected equally.
- *Bleeding and mucus per rectum:* Mucus per rectum is a symptom present both in IBD and IBS. Blood diarrhoea is more frequently seen in UC rather than CD.
- *Fever:* Fever is almost invariably present in IBD and differentiates it from IBS.
- *Loss of weight:* It is due to malabsorption in IBD.
- *Never been abroad:* This probably rules out infective causes of haemorrhagic diarrhoea i.e. *Shigella* and *E. coli*.

CONFUSA

IBD is a very frequent topic in PLAB exam and the questions are often difficult. Some students often have confusion in differentiating UC from CD. These are:

	Ulceratives colitis (UC)	*Crohn's disease (CD)*
Most common site	Colon	Ileocaecal
Rectum	Always involved	Often spared
Inflammation	Mucosa and submucosa	Transmural
Diarrhoea	Often bloody	Often not blood
Fistulas	Rare	Common
Perianal fissures	Absent	Present
Nephrolithiasis	Absent	Often present
Skin lesions	Absent	Present
Colon cancer risk	Markedly increased	Mildly increased

Investigation of Choice

- *Screening:* Colonoscopy
- *Definitive:* Biopsy

Immediate Management

Antipyretics for fever
+
Bulking agents for diarrhoea

Treatment of Choice

- Sulfasalazine
- Refractory disease: Corticosteroids
- Surgery
  - UC—curative
  - CD—if perforation likely

134. An 80-year-old woman, fever 39 degrees centigrade, acute generalised abdominal pain, diarrhoea and vomiting, slightly dehydrated.

Diagnosis: Acute gastroenteritis (GE)

Clinchers

- *80-year-old woman:* Susceptibility to infection increases in old age and debilitation.
- *Fever 39° C:* It is a common accompaniment of many GE organisms.
- *Acute generalised abdominal pain:* Crampy and diffuse abdominal pain is there in acute GI.
- *Diarrhoea and vomiting:* It is the most common symptom of GI infection seen in almost every infection. Usually it is due to activation of specific GI receptors by toxins produced by organisms.
- *Slightly dehydrated:* It is due to fluid loss in diarrhoea.

CONFUSA

Vomiting without diarrhoea is present with:
- *Clostridium botulinum*

Diarrhoea without vomiting is present with:
- *Clostridium perfringens*
- *Campylobacter* (bloody)
- *Cryptosporidium*
- *Yersinia enterocolitica*
- *Shigella* (bloody)

* Source: 558, OHCM, 5th edn.

Investigation of Choice

Stool microscopy and culture.

Immediate Management

Fluid resuscitation (oral in mild to moderate dehydration IV in severe dehydration)

Treatment of Choice

- Antibiotics (as she is systemically unwell)
- Antidiarrhoeals (as symptoms of dehydration present)
- Antiemetics (contraindicated in dysentery, but here it is not specified whether the stools are bloody).

Your notes:

150. Girl with diarrhoea and jejunal villous atrophy.

Diagnosis: Coeliac disease

Clinchers

- *Girl:* It is marginally more common in females. It can present at any age. In infancy it appears after weaning on to gluten-containing foods. The peak incidence in adults is in third and fourth decades but it is shifting towards younger ages over the years.
- *Diarrhoea:* Common GI symptoms are diarrhoea and steatorrhoea, abdominal discomfort or pain and weight loss.
- *Jejunal villous atrophy:* The mucosal appearance of a jejunal biopsy specimen in diagnostic. The mucosa of the proximal small bowel is predominantly affected, the mucosal damage decreasing in severity towards the ileum as the gluten is digested into smaller non-toxic fragments.

CONFUSA

Other causes of flat mucosa (subtotal villous atrophy)
- Zollinger-Ellison syndrome
- Hypogammaglobulinaemia

Note: The lesion in coeliac disease is subtotal villous atrophy. True atrophy of the mucosa is not present because the crypt hyperplasia compensates for villous atrophy and the total mucosal thickness is normal.

Investigation of Choice

- *Screening:* Anti-reticulin antibodies
- *Definitive:* Jejunal biopsy

Immediate Management

Compensate for malabsorption and weight loss with gluten free diets.

Treatment of Choice

Lifelong gluten-free diet.

Your notes:

165. An elderly female with past history of rectal bleeding, normal on endoscopy and enema studies done previously presents with profuse fresh rectal bleeding.

Diagnosis: Chronic intestinal ischaemia.

Clinchers

- *Elderly female:* It frequently occurs in elderlies because of increased incidence of atherosclerotic vaso-occlusive diseases in them.
- *Past history of rectal bleeding:* It suggests that there must be some definitive predisposing factor which is giving rise to recurrent emboli and hence repeated infarctions. A heart lesion (atrial fibrillation) or liver disease can be the culprits here. Other cause can be superior mesenteric artery disease.
- *Normal on endoscopy and enema studies:* Because there is no intrinsic GI pathology, there studies will always be normal.
- *Profuse fresh rectal bleeding:* It is due to ischaemic necrosis of the infarcted bowel area.

CONFUSA

Mesenteric infarction can be differentiated from other GI pains by — Hb, WCC and a moderately raised plasma amylase. There will also be a persistent metabolic acidosis. In chronic disease (as in this question) there is typical postprandial pain which is relieved by passing stools.

Investigation of Choice

Mesenteric angiogram (Barium enema if mesenteric infarction is suspected).

Immediate Management

Rule out—vasculitis/trauma/radiotherapy/strangulation.

Treatment of Choice

Surgery.

Your notes:

168. A young female with long-standing irregular bowel habit and persistent UTI.

Diagnosis: Probable Crohn's disease (CD)

Clinchers

- *Young female:* CD has peak incidence at between 20 and 40 years. It is uncommon before the age of 10 years and both sexes are equally affected.
- *Long-standing irregular bowel habit:* The major symptom of inflammatory bowel disease (including CD) is irregular bowel habit. Mainly it presents as diarrhoea, abdominal pain and weight loss.
- *Persistent UTI:* Fistula formation is common in CD and it may atypically present with symptoms of fistula rather than those of bowel. Although uncommon a persistent UTI in the setting of CD, should be suspected to be due to enterovesical fistula.

CONFUSA

Pneumaturia (air in the urine) present as bubbling while micturition and is a definitive symptom of enterovesicle fistula. Other causes of enterovesicle fistula can be malignancy and regional enteritis (chronic). Irritable bowel disease can also cause UTI (due to impaired local hygiene) but that will be recurrent rather than persistent.

Investigation of Choice
Small bowel barium enema

Immediate Management
High dose urinary antibacterials

Treatment of Choice
Surgical closure of fistula

Your notes:

187. Condition associated with gatroesophageal reflux, epithelial metaplasia, increased risk of carcinoma.

Diagnosis: Barret's oesophagus.

Clinchers

- *Gastroendophageal reflux:* The predisposing condition to Barret's is chronic reflux oesophagitis.
- *Epithelial metaplasia:* Squamous mucosa of the oesophagus shows metaplastic change and the squamocolumnar junction (ora serrata) migrates upwards in response to chronic reflux oesophagitis. The length affected may be a few can only or all of the oesophagitis.
- *Increased risk of carcinoma:* It carries a 40 fold increase in risk of adenocarcinoma.

CONFUSA

The most common carcinoma in the middle third of oesophagus is squamous cell carcinoma, whereas in the lower third it is adenocarcinoma.

Investigation of Choice
Endoscopy

Immediate Management
Exclude malignant change by biopsy.

Treatment of Choice

- *If premalignant changes are found:* Oesophageal resection (especially in younger, fit patients)
- *If no premalignant changes:* Regular endoscopy

  \+

  Intensive antireflux measures

  ±

  Epithelial laser ablation/photodynamic therapy.

Your notes:

189. Condition associated with persistent inflammation, can cause lymphoma.

Diagnosis: *Helicobacter pylori* infection.

Clinchers

- *Persistent inflammation:* Initially, *H. pylori* infection produces acute gastritis which rapidly becomes chronic active gastritis and in some peptic ulcer disease may develop. Some strains or *H. pylori* (Cag A positive strains) may be particular associated with gastroduodenal disease *H. pylori* causes tissue damage by releasing toxins—Vac A (vacuolating toxin) and Cag A (cytotoxin associated protein).
- *Can cause lymphoma:* Over 90% of patients with gastric B cell lymphomas (mucosal associated lymphoid tissue—MALT lymphoma) have *H. pylori.* Low grade tumors have been shown to regress with *H. pylori* eradication.

CONFUSA

The exact mode of transmission is unclear, but intrafamilial clustering suggests person to person spread, either oral-oral or faeco-oral. Childhood acquisition of *H. pylori* is prevalent in developing countries and its presence is also associated with lower socioeconomic status worldwide. Between one-third and two-third of the western populations have this infection and prevalence is higher in older population—presumably acquired in their childhood.

Investigation of Choice

- *Screening:* Urea breath test ^{13}C or ^{14}C (using urea as substrate)
- *Definitive:* Serological IgG antibody tests

Treatment of Choice

Triple therapy (for one week)
Omeprazole + metronidazole + clarithromycin
or
Omeprazole + metronidazole + amoxycillin.

Your notes:

PAPER 5

53. A 49-year-old lawyer complains of blood and diarrhoea. She is also suffering from abdominal pain, fever, and general ill health. On palpation you find tenderness in the lower abdomen.

Diagnosis: Severe ulcerative colitis (UC)

Clinchers

- *49-year-old lawyer (she):* The sex ratio is equal. It is uncommon before the age of 10 and most patients are between the ages of 20 and 40 at diagnosis.
- *Blood and diarrhoea:* The first symptom is watery or bloody diarrhoea. There may be a rectal discharge of mucus which is either blood-stained or purulent.
- *Abdominal pain, fever, general ill health:* Pain as an early symptom is unusual and suggest severe disease. Other indicators of severe diseases are:
  - more than four motions a day, together with
  - one or more signs of systemic illness, i.e
    - fever over 37.5°C
    - tachycardia > 90/m
    - hypoalbuminaemia < 30 g/L
    - weight loss > 3 kg
- *Tenderness in lower abdomen:* May or may not be present in UC.

CONFUSA

Diarrhoea usually implies that there is active disease proximal to the rectum. In 95 percent of cases the disease starts in the rectum and spreads proximally. Bad prognosis is indicated by:

- a severe initial attack
- disease involving whole colon
- increasing age, especially after 60 years

If the disease remains confined to the left colon, the out-look is better.

Investigation of Choice

- *Screening:* Barium enema (findings: • loss of haustrations, • granularity, • pseudopolyps)
- *Definitive:* Colonoscopy and biopsy

Immediate Management

Examine for extraintestinal manifestations i.e. arthritis/skin lesions/eye problems/liver and bile duct diseases).
+
Admit (this case is a medical emergency since this is a severe attack, 1040, Bailey, 23 edn).

Treatment of Choice

IV hydrocortisone 100-200 mg QID + rectal infusion of prednisolone + sulfasalazine maintenance/surgery.

54. A young woman presents with recurrent abdominal pain, episodic diarrhoea, malaise, and fever. Over the past few years she has felt her health to be declining. At presentation she complains of severe abdominal pain and constipation.

Diagnosis: Crohn's disease (CD)

Clinchers

- *Young woman:* It is slightly more common in females than in males but is more commonly diagnosed in young patients between the ages of 25 and 40. There does seem to be a second peak of incidence around the age of 17.
- *Recurrent abdominal pain, episodic diarrhoea, malaise, and fever:* There is often a history of mild diarrhoea extending over many months occurring in bouts accompanied by intestinal colic. Patients may complain of pain, particularly in the right iliac fossa and there may be a tender mass palpable. Intermittent fevers, secondary anaemia and weight loss are common.
- *Over the past few years she has felt her health to be declining:* It is due to generalised systemic nonspecific effects like loss of appetite, weight loss, anaemia, etc.
- *Severe abdominal pain and constipation:* This could be due to intestinal obstruction after formation of adhesions. Constipation is otherwise rare in this disease.

CONFUSA

Constipation in CD is rare and can be due to:

- After months of repeated attacks with acute inflammation of the affected area of intestine begins to narrow, with fibrosis causing abdominal pain on eating, giving rise to 'food fear' which leads to no formation of stools.
- Delay and dilatation of small intestine causing partial obstruction
- Intestinal adhesions or strictures.

Investigation of Choice

Small bowel enema

±

Technetium labelled leucocyte scan

Immediate Management

Pain relief

Treatment of Choice

Mesalazine (for acute attack like this)

55. A young woman complains of cramp-like abdominal pain, and difficulties with bowel movements. Acute abdominal pain is frequently relieved by embarrassing flatulence. Barium studies and sigmoidoscopy have proved inconclusive.

Diagnosis: Irritable bowel syndrome (IBS).

Clinchers

- *Young woman:* Symptoms of IBS typically begin young adulthood (esp. females) and the prevalence of IBS is similar in elderly and young adults.
- *Cramp like abdominal pain and difficulties with bowel movements:* Abdominal pain and altered bowel habits are non-specific symptoms found in patients with a wide variety of illnesses including IBS.
- *Acute abdominal pain is frequently relieved by embarrassing flatulence:* "Manning criteria" for IBS include abdominal pain or discomfort that is relieved by defaecation or associated with a change in stool frequency or consistency, abdominal distension, the sensation of incomplete evacuation, and the passage of mucus.
- *Barium studies and sigmoidoscopy have proved inconclusive:* A diagnosis of IBS is based on a careful history to identify characteristic symptoms (e.g. Manning criteria), physical examination, selected laboratory tests, and if necessary, further testing to exclude other disorders.

CONFUSA

Patients presenting with abdominal pain in the absence of abdominal pain may be considered to have IBS if no alternative explanation for the symptoms is found. However, patients with otherwise unexplained chronic constipation in the absence of abdominal pain are generally considered to have a distinct disorder.

Investigation of Choice

All required to exclude other diseases (but not always).

Immediate Management

Reassurance + counselling.

Treatment of Choice

Symptomatic.

Your notes:

76. A 4-year-old Irish girl looks wasted and appears short for her age. The mother reports the daughter has been vomiting on several occasions in the past, with associated diarrhoea. The SHO thinks he has an enteropathy and on serology IgA gliadin and Endomysial antibodies are found.

Diagnosis: Coeliac disease

Clinchers
- *Frequent episodes of diarrhoea with vomiting:* These are precipitated by diets containing gluten such as wheat, barley, rye.
- *Wasting:* It is failure to thrive due to malabsorption
- *a-Gliadin and anti-endomysial (IgA) antibodies:* These are almost 95% specific to coeliac disease.

CONFUSA

Other causes of malabsorption and failure to thrive such as lactose intolerance and chronic non-specific diarrhoea, which are excluded by positive anti-endomysial antibodies.

Investigation of Choice
- a-gliadin and anti-endomysial (IgA) antibodies are used for screening.
- Jejunal biopsy (villous atrophy seen) is definitive

Immediate Management

Correction of fluid and electrolyte imbalance due to malabsorption.

Treatment of Choice

Life-long gluen free diet, such as rice, maize, soya, potato, etc.

Your notes:

77. A mother brings her 5-year-old son who has been passing bloody stool associated with severe abdominal pain. On examination he is found to have mildly swollen tender wrists and red nodular tender lesions were found on his forearms.

Diagnosis: Ulcerative colitis

Clinchers
- *Bloody stools associated with abdominal pain:* This point towards a colonic pathology, most probably an inflammatory bowel disease.
- *Mildy swollen tender wrists:* since ulcerative colitis is associated with large joint arthritis.
- *Red nodular tender lesions on forearm:* These are suggestive of erythema nodosum a dermatological association of ulcerative colitis.

CONFUSA

Giardia lamblia infection is a common cause of dysentery and must be excluded. Differentiation of ulcerative colitis from colonic Crohn's disease may be particularly difficult, even when the resected colon is examined by an expert pathologist.

Investigation of Choice
- Procto-sigmoidoscopy: Inflammed friable mucosa.
- Barium enema: Loss of haustra, granular mucosa seen.

Immediate Management

Counselling of mother about taking proper care of the son.

Treatment of Choice

Initially this is medical in the uncomplicated case (Sulfasalazine and steroids), but surgery is required when medical treatment fails or when complications supervene.

Your notes:

78. An 8-year-old girl has got repeated episodes of diarrhoea. On each occasion the stool contains segments of undigested vegetables. The paediatrician recommends restricting fluids to meal times. The girls condition improves and she is thriving.

Diagnosis: Chronic non-specific diarrhoea:

Clinchers

- *Repeated episodes of diarrhoea:* It is without any associated complaints.
- *Stool containing undigested vegetables:* Suggests gastric hurrying as the cause of diarrhoea, probably due to excess fluid intake in between meals.
- *Improvement on restricting fluids to meal times:* Implies better regulation of diet.

CONFUSA

Lactose intolerance can be a confusing option which is excluded by resolution of symptomatology on restricting fluids to meal times.

Investigation of Choice

Stool microscopic examination and culture to rule out any infective pathology.

Immediate Management

Refer to a dietician

Treatment of Choice

Fluids and electrolyte management.

Your notes:

80. A 15-year-girl complains of episodic diarrhoea which typically starts in the morning with a constant urge to go to the toilet on waking, and after breakfast. She says there is associated abdominal pain in the right iliac fossa relieved by defaecation or flatus. She has had the symptoms for 3 months.

Diagnosis: Irritable Bowel Syndrome (IBS)

Clinchers

- Some characteristics of IBS are:
  - Episodic diarrhoea on walking.
- Urge of pass stool in morning, after breakfast.
  - Abdominal pain relieved by defaecation or flatus.

Since all these are present in this patient, we can safely label it as IBS, but it is better to avoid labelling as Irritable Bowel Syndrome if symptoms are present for less than 6 months.

CONFUSA

Diarrhoea of chronic disesae.

- The young age goes against colorectal carcinoma which may present similarly with diarrhoea alternating with constipation and tenesmus.
- Absence of per-rectal bleed goes against ulcerative colitis.

Investigation of Choice

Stool microscopic examination sigmoidoscopy, colonoscopy and Barium studies to exclude organic pathology.

Immediate Management

Exclusion of organic pathology

Treatment of Choice

- High fibre diet
- Psychotherapy.

Your notes:

120. A 50-year-old man is brought in by his wife who says he is always farting. He has a fresh abdominal scar. His haemoglobin is low. His mean corpuscular volume is low. His mean corpuscular haemoglobulin concentration is low. And his glucose tolerance test shows lag storage.

Diagnosis: Intestinal hurry

Clinchers

- *50-year-old man:* Occurrence of hypermotility of intestines in this age is not common without an obvious cause.
- *Always farting:* Due to malabsorption.
- *Fresh abdominal scar:* Since intestinal hurry is usually seen after postgastrectomy (dumping), postvagotomy and gastrojejunostomy, it could be due to any of these operations.
- Hb, MCV, MCHC are all low: Due to malabsorption (due to HCl deficiency) and intrinsic factor deficiency causing pernicious anaemia.
- *GTT shows lag storage:* This is characteristic of post-gastrectomy dumping syndromes and thus confirms our diagnosis.

CONFUSA

The dumping syndrome comprises attacks of fainting, vertigo and sweating after foot, rather like a hypoglycaemic attack. This is probably an osmotic effect due to gastric contents of high osmolarity passing rapidly into the jejunum, absorbing fluid into the gut lumen and producing a temporary reduction in circulating blood volume.

Investigation of Choice

GTT

Immediate Management

Bulk forming diets

Treatment of Choice

Treatment of anaemia + symptomatic

126. An obese 34-year-old man complains of epigastric pain, which seems to exacerbated by eating his favourite meal, fish and chips. He get temporary relief when hungry.

Diagnosis: Peptic ulcer (PU) disease.

Clinchers

- *Obese:* There is no *per se* relationship between obesity and PU disease. Although PU patients may gain weight due to high intake of milk to relieve symptoms.
- *34-year-old man:* In UK, ulcer rates are declining rapidly for young man and increasing rapidly for older individuals especially females DU are more common than GU in young man.
- *Epigastric pain:* The pain is typically epigastric occurs in attacks that last for days or weeks and interspersed with periods of relief. Pain that radiates into the back suggest a posterior penetrating ulcer.
- *Exacerbated by eating his favourite meal, fish and chips:* The pain is usually related to hunger, eating specific foods, or the time of the day. Often associated with heaviness, bloating or fullness after meals.
- *Get temporary relief when hungry:* The pain of duodenal ulceration is worse when hungry so this excludes it to be the cause.

CONFUSA

The relationship of the pain to food is variably and on the whole is not helpful in the diagnosis. It is a myth to say that one can differentiate between a gastric and duodenal ulcer merely on the time relationship of the pain. Peptic ulcer may come on immediately after a meal but more typically commences about 2 hours after food.

Investigation of Choice

Upper GI endoscopy

Immediate Management

Counselling (stop smoking + food advise)

Treatment of Choice

Triple therapy (for *H. pylori*)

+

Acid suppression (proton-pump inhibitor).

Your notes:

172. A 49-year-old woman complains of itchy blisters, which are occurring in groups on her knees and elbows. The itch is becoming unbearable and she is contemplating suicide. She responds to 180 mg of Dapsone within 48 hours of treatment.

Diagnosis: Coeliac disease (Gluten sensitive enteropathy).

Clinchers

- *49-year-old female:* It can present at any age. The peak incidence in adults is in the third and fourth decades with a females preponderance.
- *Itchy blisters which are occurring in group on her knees and elbows:* This is an uncommon blistering subepidermal eruption of the skin associated with gluten sensitive enteropathy. The clinical term for it is gluten sensitive enteropathy.
- *Itch is becoming unbearable and she is contemplating suicide:* This disease can produce severe depression in females and can lead to suicide.
- *Responds to 180 mg of dapsone within 48 hours of treatment:* This confirms our diagnosis.

CONFUSA

The skin condition (dermatitis herpetiformis) responds to dapsone but both the gut and the skin will improve only on a gluten free diet in this disease.

Investigation of Choice

Endomysial antibodies (IgA).

Immediate Management

Psychiatric referral (as she is contemplating suicide)

Treatment of Choice

Gluten free diet

+

Dapsone.

Your notes:

PAPER 6

28. A 49-year-old lawyer complains of blood and diarrhoea. She is also suffering from abdominal pain, fever, and general ill health. On palpation you find tenderness in the lower abdomen.

Diagnosis: Severe ulcerative colitis (UC)

Clinchers

- *49-year-old lawyer (she):* The sex ratio is equal. It is uncommon before the age of 10 and most patients are between the ages of 20 and 40 at diagnosis.
- *Blood and diarrhoea:* The first symptom is watery or bloody diarrhoea. There may be a rectal discharge of mucus which is either blood-stained or purulent.
- *Abdominal pain, fever, general ill health:* Pain as an early symptom is unusual and suggest severe disease. Other indicators of severe diseases are:
  - more than four motions a day, together with
  - one or more signs of systemic illness, i.e
    - fever over 37.5°C
    - tachycardia > 90/m
    - hypoalbuminaemia < 30 g/l
    - weight loss > 3 kg
- *Tenderness in lower abdomen:* May or may not be present in UC.

CONFUSA

Diarrhoea usually implies that there is active disease proximal to the rectum. In 95 percent of cases the disease starts in the rectum and spreads proximally. Bad prognosis is indicated by:

- a severe initial attack
- disease involving whole colon
- increasing age, especially after 60 years

If the disease remains confined to the left colon, the out look is better.

Investigation of Choice

- *Screening:* Barium enema (findings: • loss of haustrations, • granularity, • pseudopolyps)
- *Definitive:* Colonoscopy and biopsy

Immediate Management

Examine for extraintestinal manifestations i.e. arthritis/ skin lesions/eye problems/liver and bile duct diseases).

+

Admit (this case is a medical emergency since this is a severe attack, 1040, Bailey, 23 edn).

Treatment of Choice

IV hydrocortisone 100-200 mg QID + rectal infusion of prednisolone + sulfasalazine maintenance/surgery

29. A young woman presents with recurrent abdominal pain, episodic diarrhoea, malaise, and fever. Over the past few years she has felt her health to be declining. At presentation she complains of severe abdominal pain and constipation.

Diagnosis: Crohn's disease (CD)

Clinchers

- *Young woman:* It is slightly more common in females than in males but is more commonly diagnosed in young patients between the ages of 25 and 40. There does seem to be a second peak of incidence around the age of 17.
- *Recurrent abdominal pain, episodic diarrhoea, malaise, and fever:* There is often a history of mild diarrhoea extending over many months occurring in bouts accompanied by intestinal colic. Patients may complain of pain, particularly in the right iliac fossa and there may be a tender mass palpable. Intermittent fevers, secondary anaemia and weight loss are common.
- *Over the past few years she has felt her health to be declining:* It is due to generalised systemic nonspecific effects like loss of appetite, weight loss, anaemia, etc.
- *Severe abdominal pain and constipation:* This could be due to intestinal obstruction after formation of adhesions. Constipation is otherwise rare in this disease.

CONFUSA

Constipation in CD is rare and can be due to:

- After months of repeated attacks with acute inflammation of the affected area of intestine begins to narrow, with fibrosis causing abdominal pain on eating, giving rise to 'food fear' which leads to no formation of stools.
- Delay and dilatation of small intestine causing partial obstruction
- Intestinal adhesions or strictures.

Investigation of Choice

Small bowel enema

±

Technetium labelled leucocyte scan

Immediate Management

Pain relief

Treatment of Choice

Mesalazine (for acute attack like this)

30. A young woman complains of cramp-like abdominal pain, and difficulties with bowel movements. Acute abdominal pain is frequently relieved by embarrassing flatulence. Barium studies and sigmoidoscopy have proved inconclusive.

Diagnosis: Irritable bowel syndrome (IBS).

Clinchers

- *Young woman:* Symptoms of IBS typically begin young adulthood (especially females) and the prevalence of IBS is similar in elderly and young adults.
- *Cramp-like abdominal pain and difficulties with bowel movements:* Abdominal pain and altered bowel habits are non-specific symptoms found in patients with a wide variety of illnesses including IBS.
- *Acute abdominal pain is frequently relieved by embarrassing flatulence:* "Manning criteria" for IBS include abdominal pain or discomfort that is relieved by defaecation or associated with a change in stool frequency or consistency, abdominal distension, the sensation of incomplete evacuation, and the passage of mucus.
- *Barium studies and sigmoidoscopy have proved inconclusive:* A diagnosis of IBS is based on a careful history to identify characteristic symptoms (e.g. Manning criteria), physical examination, selected laboratory tests, and if necessary, further testing to exclude other disorders.

CONFUSA

Patients presenting with abdominal pain in the absence of abdominal pain may be considered to have IBS if no alternative explanation for the symptoms is found. However, patients with otherwise unexplained chronic constipation in the absence of abdominal pain are generally considered to have a distinct disorder.

Investigation of Choice

All required to exclude other diseases (but not always).

Immediate Management

Reassurance + counselling.

Treatment of Choice

Symptomatic.

Your notes:

31. A known HIV positive patient presents with pain in swallowing and some lesion in the mouth. The underlying tissue is red when the lesion is taken off.

Diagnosis: Candidiasis

Clinchers

- *Known HIV positive patient:* Let us first get familiar with complications of HIV infection. These are *Pneumocystis carinii* (this is the most common life-threatening opportunistic infection in AIDS). Infection by *M. tuberculosis, M. avium intracellulare, candidiasis, toxoplasma gondii* (a chief CNS pathogen), Cryptococcus neoformans (causes incidious meningitis). CMV retinitis, leishmaniasis, Kaposi's sarcoma.
- *Pain in swallowing:* Oesophageal involvement causes dysphagia ± retrosternal discomfort. Oropharyngeal candidiasis in an apparently fit patients suggests underlying HIV infection.
- *Some lesions in mouth:* These with oral pain and discomfort may be caused by candidiasis.
- *Underlying tissue is red when lesion is taken off:* Candidiasis causes white patches or erythema of the buccal mucosa. The patches are hard to remove and bleed if scraped.

CONFUSA

Causes of oral pain/discomfort in HIV positive patient are candidiasis, HSV or aphthous ulceration or tumours.

Investigation of Choice

Demonstration of pseudohyphae on wet smear with confirmation by culture is procedure of choice for superficial candidiasis. Deeper lesions due to Candida may be diagnosed by histologic section of biopsy specimen or by blood culture.

Treatment of Choice

- *Local treatment:* Nystatin suspension/amphotericin lozenges 4-6 times/day.
- *Systemic treatment:* Fluconazole 50-200 mg/day PO (may cause nausea, hepatitis), ketoconazole 200 mg/day PO (may cause nausea, hepatitis, rash, low platelets)

Your notes:

32. A patient comes with dysphagia for solids for 5 years and now presents with regurgitation when he eats, it relieves a few hours after meal.

Diagnosis: Achalasia

Clinchers

- *Dysphagia for solids for 5 years:* Overall course of achalasia is usually chronic, with progressive dysphagia and weight loss over months to years. Word 'solid' here signifies oesophageal cause and liquids signify pharyngeal cause.
- *Regurgitation:* Dysphagia, chest pain and regurgitation are the main symptoms of achalasia. Dysphagia occurs early, worsened by emotional stress and hurried eating.
- *Relieves a few hours after meal:* Achalasia is a motor disorder of the oesophageal smooth muscle in which the LES does not relax properly with swallowing, and the normal peristalsis of esophageal body is replaced by abnormal contractions.

CONFUSA

Achalasia associated with carcinoma is characterized by severe weight loss and a rapid down hill course if untreated.

The presence of gastroesophageal reflux argues against achalasia, and in patients with long standing heartburn, cessation of heart burn and appearance of dysphagia suggest development of achalasia in a patient with reflux oesophagitis.

Investigation of Choice

- *Chest X-ray:* Absence of gastric air bubble, air fluid level in mediastinum in upright position represents retained food in oesophagus.
- *Barium swallow:* Shows oesophageal dilatation or sigmoid shape of oesophagus in advanced cases.
- *Fluoroscopy.*

Immediate Management

Depends upon the complications (like aspiration can occur due to regurgitation therefore manage that first).

Treatment of Choice

Endoscopic balloon dilatation of Heller's Cardiomyotomy.

Your notes:

33. 65-year-old male presents with weight loss, difficulty in swallowing solid. Dysphagia is getting worse.

Diagnosis: Carcinoma oesophagus.

Clinchers

- *65-year-old male:* Risk factors for Ca oesophagus are tobacco, alcohol, achalasia, old age, Barrets oesophagus, Plummer-Vinson syndrome.
- *Weight loss:* Suspect malignancy.
- *Difficulty in swallowing solid:* Acute or progressive dysphagia requires investigation to exclude malignancy in oesophagus. If dysphagia is predominantly for solids, then suspect oesophageal cause.

Dysphagia, weight loss, retrosternal chest pain, rarely lymphadenopathy are signs of carcinoma of the oesophagus. If upper 1/3rd of oesophagus is involved it may present with hoarseness and cough.

CONFUSA

Keep in mind the differential diagnosis of dysphagia (refer to page 196, OHCM, 5th edn).

Investigation of Choice

Barium swallow, CXR

Oesophagoscopy with biopsy/brushings.

Immediate Management

Treat the complications

Treatment of Choice

Radiotherapy and surgery complete for dismal statistics (6% vs 4% 5 year survival).

Your notes:

34. A patient presents with intermittent dysphagia for both solids and liquids and chest pain. No weight loss.

Diagnosis: Diffuse oesophageal spasm

Clinchers

- *Intermittent dysphagia for both solids and liquids:* Dysphagia for both solids and liquids is seen in oesophageal spasm, correlated particularly with simultaneous-onset contractions.
- *Chest pain:* Chest pain is particularly marked in patients with oesophageal contractions of large amplitude and long duration. It usually occurs at rest, may radiate to back and arms. May mimic the pain of myocardial ischaemia.

CONFUSA

Diffuse oesophageal spasm must be differentiated from other causes of chest pain, particularly ischaemic heart disease with atypical angina. Always go for complete cardiac work up and also carefully distinguish it from reflux oesophagitis.

Investigation of Choice

Barium swallow: Shows uncoordinated simultaneous contractions, that produce the appearance of curling or multiple ripples in the wall, sacculations and pseudodiverticula—the "cork screw" oesophagus.

Your notes:

55. A 35-year-old woman who was diagnosed as having coeliac disease at the age of 12 years has had good control of her abdominal symptoms for a number of years. She presents with a recent history of weight loss, tiredness, diarrhoea and abdominal pain.

Diagnosis: Small bowel lymphoma (probable).

Clinchers

- *35-year-old:* Incidence of lymphomas peak after 30 years
- *Coeliac disease:* The risk of small bowel lymphoma is increased in patients with a prior history of:
  - Malabsorption conditions (e.g. celiac sprue)
  - Regional enteritis
  - Depressed immune function
    - Congenital immunodeficiencies
    - Prior organ transplantation
    - Autoimmune disorders
    - AIDS
- *Good control of abdominal symptoms for a number of years:* Coeliac disease symptoms are very amenable to diet control and since the symptoms are in control in this patient for many years, there is no reason that they should relapse. Considering her age and high risk, lymphoma should be ruled out.
- *Weight loss, tiredness, diarrhoea and abdominal pain:* Characteristic of any malabsorption syndrome (in this case induced by lymphoma).

CONFUSA

Primary intestinal lymphoma accounts for 20% of malignancies of small bowel. Essentially all these neoplasms are non-Hodgkin's lymphoma. Its incidence is: Ileum > jejunum > duodenum (mirrors the relative amount of normal lymphoid cells in these anatomic areas).

Investigation of Choice

- *Screening:* Contrast radiographs (infiltration and thickening of mucosal folds, mucosal nodules, ulcerations)
- *Definitive:* Surgical exploration and resection for tissue diagnosis.

Immediate Management

Rule out ethnic relation (Jews and Arabs) which produce a nonresectable immunoproliferative small intestinal disease and any non-compliance on gluten free diet.

Treatment of Choice

Surgical exploration +
Postresection radio/chemotherapy.

56. A 35-year-old woman complains of abdominal discomfort relieved by passing flatus or- defaecation. Over the last 6 months she has had episodes of diarrhoea and constipation, but denied she had lost weight. Her mother died of bowel carcinoma.

Diagnosis: Irritable bowel syndrome (IBS).

Clinchers

- *35 years old woman:* Patients of IBS are usually between 20-40 years and females are more frequently affected.
- *Abdominal discomfort relieved by flatus or defaecation:* This is a very important point. This supports the diagnosis of IBS. Other important history is the sensation of incomplete evacuation and the passage of mucus.
- *Episode of diarrhoea and constipation:* Altered bowel habits (constipation alternating with diarrhoea) present in IBS.
- *Since last 6 months:* These symptoms must be present for atleast 3 months, before the diagnose of IBS could be established.
- *No history of weight loss:* Helps to exclude carcinoma.

Investigation of Choice

Flexible sigmoidoscopy: In over 48 years to exclude colonic neoplasm. In younger patients exclude inflammatory bowel disease.

Treatment of Choice

Though there is no treatment for IBS, focus on dietary modification with fiber supplements. Treatment should be directed to the predominant symptom.

Your notes:

133. Patient has both Iron and Folate deficiency Radiology sigmoidoscopy—normal, has pale stools which are difficult to flush away.

Diagnosis: Malabsorption (pancreatic insufficiency)

Clinchers

- *Both iron and folate deficiency* Malabsorption produces the signs of following deficiencies:
  - anaemia (Fe, B_{12}, folate)
  - bleeding (vitamin K)
  - edema (protein).
- *Radiology and sigmoidoscopy normal:* This rules out other causes of malabsorption, e.g. Crohn's disease and coeliac disease.
- *Pale stools which are difficult to flush away:* This suggest pancreatic insufficiency to be the cause.

CONFUSA

Most common cause of malabsorption in UK are:
- Coeliac disease
- Crohn's disease
- Chronic pancreatitis (usually due to alcoholism).

Investigation of Choice

USG (dilated biliary tree; stones)

Immediate Management

Prescribe low fat diet + take alcohol history

Treatment of Choice

As per the causation.

159. A 50-year-old obese man with a known hiatus hernia, presents with recurrent, severe, burning retrosternal chest pain associated with acid regurgitation and increased oral flatulence.

Diagnosis: Gastro-oesophageal reflux disease (GORD)

Clinchers

- *50-year-old:* Hiatus hernia is most common in the elderly, but may occur in young fit people.
- *Obese:* Hiatus hernias probably represent a progressive weakening of the muscles of the hiatus. They occur in obese commonly.
- *Man:* Generally hiatus hernias are four times more common in females than males.
- *Known hiatus hernia:* Incompetence of cardiac sphincter is invariably present in the initial stages of hiatus hernia, but disappear as distortion of the cardia increases. This incompetence leads to GORD.
- *Recurrent, severe, burning retrosternal chest pain:* In GORD there is a burning, retrosternal discomfort that is related to:
  - Meals
  - Lying down
  - Stooping
  - Straining

It is typically relieved by antacids.

- *Acid regurgitation:* This is 'acid brash' and typical of GORD. It can also be due to bile regurgitation. Wather brash is also seen in GORD and is due to excessive salivation.
- *Increased oral flatulence:* This is due to unopposed release of intestinal gas through incomplete lower oesophageal sphincter.

CONFUSA

Gastro-oesophageal reflux occurs as a normal event, and the clinical features of GORD occurs only when the antireflux mechanisms fail sufficiently to allow gastric contents to make prolonged contact with the lower oesophageal mucosa. Hiatus hernia reduce acid clearance of oesophagus owing to trapping of acid within the hernial sac. Moreover a large hiatus hernia can impair the "pinchcork" mechanism of diaphragm. GORD can also occur with hiatus hernia.

Investigation of Choice

- *Screening:* Endoscopy ± barium swallow (show hiatus hernia)
- *Definitive:* 24 hr oesophageal pH monitoring + Oesophageal manometry.

Immediate management: Proton pump inhibitors.

Treatment of choice: Rule out gastric carcinoma (Common at this age)

163. A young female with long-standing irregular bowel habit and persistent UTI.

Diagnosis: Probable Crohn's disease (CD).

Clinchers

- *Young female:* CD has peak incidence at between 20 and 40 years. It is uncommon before the age of 10 years and both sexes are equally affected.
- *Long-standing irregular bowel habit:* The major symptom of inflammatory bowel disease (including CD) is irregular bowel habit. Mainly it presents as diarrhoea, abdominal pain and weight loss.
- *Persistent UTI:* Fistula formation is common in CD and it may atypically present with symptoms of fistula rather than those of bowel. Although uncommon a persistent UTI in the setting of CD, should be suspected to be due to enterovesical fistula.

CONFUSA

Pneumaturia (air in the urine) present as bubbling while micturition and is a definitive symptom of enterovesicle fistula. Other causes of enterovesicle fistula can be malignancy and regional enteritis (chronic). Irritable bowel disease can also cause UTI (due to impaired local hygiene) but that will be recurrent rather than persistent.

Investigation of Choice

Small bowel barium enema

Immediate Management

High dose urinary antibacterials

Treatment of Choice

Surgical closure of fistula

Your notes:

PAPER 7

15. Child with vomiting and diarrhoea. Brother had a similar problem 2 weeks ago.

Diagnosis: Gastroenteritis.

Clinchers

- *Vomiting and diarrhoea:* These are the hallmarks of gastroenterities and can be fatal as they produce dehydration ± urea and electrolyte imbalance.
- *Brother had a similar problem 2 weeks ago:* It suggests an infective etiology. 2 weeks might be the incubation period of this infection. The most common cause in Rotavirus but that has a short incubation period.

CONFUSA

Causes of secretory infective diarrhoea in children are:

- Bacteria
  - *Camphylobacter*
  - *Staphylococcus*
  - *E. coli*
  - *Salmonella*
  - *Shigella* — Where sanitation is poor
  - *Vibrio cholerae*
- Virus
  - Rotavirus
- Protozoan
  - Giardiasis
  - Amoebiasis
- Fungus
  - Cryptosporidium

Investigation of Choice

Stool for ova, cysts, parasites, and culture (electron microscopy for rotavirus).

Immediate Management

Rehydrate

Educate family about personal hygiene (as incidence of faeco-oral transmission has occurred).

Treatment of Choice

As per the cause.

Your notes:

26. A 19-year-old female with complaint of a 1 year history of bloody diarrhoea and tenesmus. Has pale skin lesions. On examination-sigmoidoscopy shows inflammation and granulomata.

Diagnosis: Ulcerative colitis (UC).

Clinchers

- *19-year-old:* It is found in any age from infancy to elderly, but the maximum incidence is between the ages of 20 and 40 years.
- *Female:* Females are more often affected than males.
- *1 year history of bloody diarrhoea and tenesmus:* The most common presentation of ulcerative colitis is diarrhoea with blood and mucus. Oedema of rectal mucosa can lead to the symptom of tenesmus.
- *Pale skin lesions:* One of the several skin manifestation seen in UC.
- *Sigmoidoscopy shows inflammation and granulomata:* Sigmoidoscopy reveals oedema of the mucosa with contact bleeding in early mild cases, proceeding to granularity of the mucosa and ten frank ulceration with pus and blood in the bowel lumen. Biopsy will give confirming histological evidence of the diagnosis.

CONFUSA

The changes in UC are confluent, with no unaffected "skip lesions" as found in Crohn's disease. Surprisingly, the inflamed colon does not become adherent to its neighbouring intra-abdominal viscera.

Investigation of Choice
Sigmoidoscopy + biopsy.

Immediate Management
Delineate family history.

Treatment of Choice
Sulphasalazine.

Your notes:

28. An 18-year-old presents with frequent diarrhoea for about 3 weeks, relieved by defaecation. Sigmoidoscopy is normal.

Diagnosis: IBS with diarrhoea (suspected).

Clinchers

- *18-year-old:* Patient is usually 20-40 years old and females are frequently affected than males.
- *Frequent diarrhoea:* Altered bowel habit i.e. constipation alternating with diarrhoea is a major feature and no cause can be found for it.
- *For 3 weeks:* Chronic symptoms, i.e. for more than 6 months are required for diagnosis of IBS (irritable bowel syndrome).
- *Relieved by defaecation:* There is central or lower abdominal pain in IBS which is characteristically relieved by defaecation.
- *Sigmoidoscopy is normal:* IBS is a diagnosis of exclusion, i.e. no pathology is found on examination and investigations.

CONFUSA

If diarrhoea is present send a stool culture and check the TSH. If the patient is young, with a classic history, check FBC, ESR, LFTs and urinalysis and perform a sigmoidoscopy and rectal biopsy.

Investigation of Choice
Stool culture + TSH.

Immediate Management
Reassurance and counselling.

Treatment of Choice
Symptomatic (see page 237, OHCM, 5th edn).

Your notes:

29. An 80-year-old with complaint of diarrhoea and urinary retention.

Diagnosis: Faecal impaction.

Clinchers

- *80-year-old:* It occurs in the elderly with constipation.
- *Diarrhoea:* It may occur paradoxically wtih the overflow of liquid colonic contents around the impacted stool.
- *Urinary retention:* Chronic constipation or impaction of faeces can result in either urinary incontinence or retention is usually acute anal discomfort.

CONFUSA

Impaction of faeces give the classical characteristic sign of indentation on PR examination. The differential diagnosis is from a rectal tumour.

Investigation of Choice

PR examination.

Immediate Management

Find the cause of constipation.

Treatment of Choice

Manual removal of impacted faeces.

Your notes:

128. Patient has both Iron and Folate deficiency Radiology sigmoidoscopy—normal, has pale stools which are difficult to flush away.

Diagnosis: Malabsorption (pancreatic insufficiency)

Clinchers

- *Both iron and folate deficiency* Malabsorption produces the signs of following deficiencies:
  - anaemia (Fe, B_{12}, folate)
  - bleeding (vitamin K)
  - edema (protein).
- *Radiology and sigmoidoscopy normal:* This rules out other causes of malabsorption, e.g. Crohn's disease and coeliac disease.
- *Pale stools which are difficult to flush away:* This suggest pancreatic insufficiency to be the cause.

CONFUSA

Most common cause of malabsorption in UK are:

- Coeliac disease
- Crohn's disease
- Chronic pancreatitis (usually due to alcoholism).

Investigation of Choice

USG (dilated biliary tree; stones)

Immediate Management

Prescribe low fat diet + take alcohol history

Treatment of Choice

As per the causation.

Your notes:

Serial No. 126

Subject: Medicine

Topic: GIT

Question: A patient presents with increasing constipation, and passing ribbon-like stools. He is well otherwise.

Diagnosis: Constipation (spastic)

Clinchers

- *Increasing constipation:* The history of progressively increasing constipation points towards many diagnosis such as Carcinoma colon, Carcinoma rectum, Irritable bowel disease, Inflammatory Bowel Disease, Intestinal tuberculosis as well as functional causes like diabetic neuropathy.
- *Passing ribbon-like stools:* This is suggesting narrowed colonic lumen. This narrowing can be due to any causes like a tumour or growth in the lumen or neuropathy which causes spasm of the intestinal musculature.
- *He is well otherwise:* His otherwise normal state of health rules out possibilities of carcinoma or inflammatory bowel disease. However, thorough investigations are required to rule out these possibilities with definite proofs.

CONFUSA

There are two basic kinds of constipation: atonic (lazy bowel) and spastic (narrowing of the colon, with small, ribbon-like stools). For atonic constipation, a high fibre diet and increased fluid intake is recommended. Spastic constipation may be caused by an obstruction or nervousness or anxiety. For spastic constipation it may be necessary to decrease the fibre intake until the situation is corrected.

Investigation of Choice

Barium Enema

Immediate Management

Exclude endocrine and metabolic abnormalities like hypothyroidism, hypercalcaemia, dehydration.

Treatment of Choice

According to the cause identified.

Your notes:

9 Haematology

PAPER 1

Serial No. 7

Subject: Medicine

Topic: Haematology

Question: An elderly man complains of bone pain and visual loss. Pathologist gives a diagnosis of multiple myeloma after bone marrow biopsy.

Diagnosis: Multiple Myeloma

Clinchers

- *An elderly man:* Multiple myeloma is the disease of elderly. The median age of patients is 68 years for men and 70 years for women. Sex incidence being equal.
- *Bone pain and visual loss:* Most common feature of myeloma is bone pain — the lumbar vertebrae are one of the most common sites of pain. Visual loss is due to hyperviscosity. Other very common feature is the presence of anaemia.
- *Pathologist gives a diagnosis of multiple myeloma after bone marrow biopsy:* In patients with myeloma, plasma cells proliferate within the bone marrow. Plasma cells are 2-3 times larger than typical lymphocytes, with eccentric smooth nuclei with clumped chromatin and have a perinuclear halo or pale zone. The cytoplasm is basophilic. Many descriptions of myeloma cells include characteristic, but not diagnostic, cytoplasmic inclusions, which include Mott cells, Russell bodies, grape cells, and morula cells.

CONFUSA

The origin of the malignant clone in myeloma is the thought to be a mutated B cell which differentiates into plasma cells. Hence all the myeloma cells are actually derived from rapid expansion of a single mutated B Cell, differentiated in the line of Plasma Cells.

The proliferating cells in myeloma occur principally in the bone marrow causing diffuse infiltration and rapid expansion (causing bone pain). These myeloma cells secrete an osteoclast stimulating factor that leads to marked bone erosion, thus causing the 'Lytic Lesions' in the bones which is so typical of multiple myeloma.

Investigation of Choice

- Serum protein electrophoresis, urine protein electrophoresis, and immunofixation are intial investigations done in cases of suspected myeloma.
- Serum protein electrophoresis is used to determine the type of each protein present and may indicate a characteristic curve (i.e. where the spike is observed; M (monoclonal) band being characteristic of the condition.)
- Urine protein electrophoresis is used to identify the presence of the Bence Jones protein in urine.
- Immunofixation is used to identify the subtype of protein (i.e. IgA lambda).
- Bone marrow biopsy may be required to confirm the diagnosis.
- Beta-2 microglobulin is very strong predictor of outcome.

Immediate Management

Supportive therapy for:

- Anemia: Blood Transfusion
- Infections: Antibiotics
- Hyperviscosity: Plasmaphoresis
- Rehydration
- Radiotherapy is used for the treatment of localised painful lesions.

Treatment of Choice

- Chemotherapy is the mainstay of treatment.
- Melphalan is the most commonly used drug for monotherapy.
- Multidrug regimens include: VAD
  - vincristine, doxorubicin (Adriamycin) and dexamethasone
  - melphalan and prednisolone.
- In younger patients autologous bone marrow transplant should be considered.

Your notes:

Serial No. 9

Subject: Medicine

Topic: Haematology

Question: A young female with lymph node enlargement and splenomegaly. Bone marrow examination confirms the diagnosis to be Acute myeloid leukaemia.

Diagnosis: Acute myeloid leukaemia (AML)

Clinchers

- *Young female:* The condition affects males and females nearly equally at all ages. AML is diagnosed in persons of all ages, from the newborns to persons advanced in age.
- *Lymph node enlargement and splenomegaly:* Splenomegaly and lymphadenopathy occur due to extramedullary infiltration of the reticuloendothelial system by the leukaemic cells.
- *Acute myeloid leukaemia:* Acute myeloid leukaemia (AML) is a group of malignant disorders characterized by the replacement of normal bone marrow with abnormal, primitive haematopoietic cells. Bone marrow aspirate and biopsy demonstrate the characteristic replacement of normal marrow elements with the monotonous sheets of leukaemic myeloblasts. The myeloblast is the first stage of the granulocytic series that is identifiable by light microscopy, the earliest recognizable cell of the neutrophil series.

CONFUSA

- Important points of difference between AML and ALL:
  - Morphological — Auer rods pathognomonic of AML
  - Histochemical stains for myeloid enzymes such as peroxidase or chloroacetate confirm AML
  - Surface markers characteristic of primitive lymphoid cells identify ALL, e.g. terminal deoxynucleotide transferase present in 95% cases of ALL
  - Primitive B lymphocyte antigens such as CALLA, B1, BA1 may help to identify ALL
  - T cell ALL diagnosed by rosette formation with sheep erythrocytes or identification of cell markers by monoclonal antibodies such as Leu-1 or Leu-9.

Investigation of Choice

- Full blood count
- Peripheral blood smear
- Bone marrow aspiration to confirm diagnosis
- Lumbar puncture—to check for meningeal leukaemia

Immediate Management

- Blood transfusion for anaemia
- Antibiotics for infections
- Hyperkalemia and hyperphosphatemia with associated hypocalcaemia result from rapid cell turnover and cell destruction. Treat elevated potassium levels promptly by using measures such as calcium gluconate, insulin and glucose regime and haemodialysis, if required.

  Maintain adequate hydration.

Treatment of Choice

Remission induction is attempted using a combination of cytotoxic agents such as cytosine arabinoside, thioguanine and daunorubicin.

Bone marrow transplantation is often undertaken either following induction of remission or after relapse.

Your notes:

Serial No. 136

Subject: Obstetrics

Topic: Prenatal Screening

Question: Pregnant lady with previous baby with severe anaemia and jaundice.

Diagnosis: Beta Thalassaemia

Clinchers

- *Previous baby with severe anaemia and jaundice:* Beta thalassaemia is an inherited disorder of haemoglobin synthesis where there is defective beta-chain production resulting in excess alpha-chain synthesis, which are unstable and precipitate in the red cell precursors causing their destruction in the bone marrow. This rapid destruction leads to two main consequences, the anemia and jaundice.
- Though an inherited disease, it usually becomes apparent after first year of life, when the fetal haemoglobin production stops.
- Patients with thalassaemia major present within the first year of life with the following features:

- Failure to thrive
- Jaundice
- Anaemia
- Hepatosplenomegaly
- Massive expansion of the marrow leads to serious bone deformities with:
  - Typical mongoloid facies
  - Frontal bossing of the skull
  - Prominent maxillae

CONFUSA

- ALL (Acute lymphatic leukaemia) can also present as severe anaemia and jaundice. However, note that ALL is not 'inherited' as thalassaemia.
- Iron deficiency anaemia also presents as hypochromic, microcytic anaemia, but with low ferritin levels. (Thalassaemia typically has raised ferritin.)
- Don't confuse this with hydrops fetalis which occurs mainly due to haemolytic disease of the newborn, where maternal antibodies are directed against fetal red blood cells to cause haemolysis. Seen in cases of Rh-incompatibility or ABO-incompatibility between the mother and the fetus.

Investigation of Choice

Prenatal diagnosis is done by foetal blood sampling or gene probe analysis of amniotic cells

Immediate Management

Counselling of the parents with proper information

Treatment of Choice

Advise against the birth of a thalassaemic child. Respect parents' decision.

Your notes:

PAPER 2

Serial No. 26

Subject: Medicine

Topic: Anaemia

Question: A 5-year-old child from South Africa is brought to the accident and emergency department deeply jaundiced. He is found to have mildly swollen, tender feet and hands. His mucosae are pale.

Diagnosis: Sickle Cell Disease

Clinchers

- *5-year-old*: The condition may present in childhood with anaemia and mild jaundice. The hand and foot syndrome due to infarcts of small bones is quite common in children and may result in digits of varying lengths.
- *South African*: The disease occurs mainly in Africans and about 25% carry the gene. It is also common in India, middle east and Southern Europe.
- *Mildly swollen*: Tender feet and hands: It is bone pain which is the most common symptom and is due to infarcts of small bones.
- *Mucosae are pale*: Due to anaemia.

CONFUSA

In a given patient the degree of anaemia is usually stable, and during a crisis Hb does not fall unless there is one or more of the following:

- Aplasia
- Acute Sequestration
- Haemolysis

Investigation of Choice

Screening: Sodium Metabisulphite test
Definitive: Hb electrophoresis (NO Hb A, 80-95% HbSS and 2-20% HbF).

Immediate Management

IV Fluids + Oxygen + Adequate analgesia

Treatment of Choice

Exchange Transfusion if severe
Penicillin prophylaxis in children
Seek advice from nearest NHS sickle Cell and Thalssaemia Counselling Centre

Your notes:

Serial No. 30

Subject: Medicine

Topic: Anaemia

Question: Following a mild viral illness, a 2-year-old child suddenly becomes severely pale. On examination there is no hepatosplenomegaly. Blood smear shows normocytic and normochromic RBCs and there are very few reticulocytes.

Diagnosis: Aplastic Anaemia

Clinchers

- *Mild viral illness:* Most cases of acquired aplastic anaemia are idiopathic. However, aplasia may develop concurrently with or following a variety of viral infections.
- *Severely pale:* The anaemia is usually severe but of slower onset than other features due to the longer survival of red cells compared to platelets and neutrophils. However, significant bleeding can lead to rapid development of severe anaemia.
- *No hepatosplenomegaly:* Hepatosplenomegaly, lymphadenopathy or bone tenderness are uncommon in aplastic anaemia but are characteristic of bone marrow failure due to leukaemia, myelofibrosis
- *Normocytic and normochromic RBCs:* The normal size and shape of red blood cells in the presence of anaemia suggest a hypoplastic bone marrow.
- *Very few reticulocytes:* This again suggests poorly reacting bone marrow in response to decreasing red blood cells.

CONFUSA

Red cells survive for around 120 days, platelets for an average 8 days and neutrophils for 1-2 days. So early problems are mainly neutropaenia and thrombocytopaenia. A 1 unit transfusion usually raises the Hb by 1-1.5 g/dl. However, transfusion may drop platelet count, so its useful to transfuse platelets before and after blood transfusion.

Investigation of Choice

Diagnosis is based upon:
A. Peripheral blood:

- neutrophils less than 0.5 x 10^9 per litre
- platelets less than 20 x 10^9 per litre
- reticulocyte count corrected for haematocrit less than 1%

B. Marrow:

- severe hypocellularity
- moderate hypocellularity with < 30% of residual cells being haematopoietic

At least two peripheral plus one marrow criteria must be satisfied.

Immediate Management

Supportive care — transfusion of red cells and platelets, and antibiotics.

Treatment of Choice

Bone marrow transplantation.

Your notes:

Serial No 121

Subject: Medicine

Topic: Genetics

Question: A 4-year-old boy gets haemarthrosis with trivial injury. He had similar episodes before maternal grandfather and uncle had a similar problem.

Diagnosis: Haemophilia A

Clinchers

- *A 4-year-old boy:* Haempohilia A is X linked recessive disease affecting 1 in 10,000 males. While the severe disease can present at birth or in utero, mild disease can be recognized on after some major trauma or surgery.
- *Gets haemarthrosis with trivial injury:* Hemarthrosis and soft tissue bleeds are common. These can occur either following injuries or even spontaneously, based on the severity of the disease.
- *Maternal grand father and uncle had a similar problem:* This clearly shows that male members of the family are affected and the disease is propagated further in family via carrier heterozygote females.

CONFUSA

While the haemophilia most commonly present as joint bleeds, soft tissue bleeds and intracranial bleeds, mucosal bleeds usually signify platelet or vessel wall abnormality and is seen in thrombocytopenia and deficient conditions like Scurvy. Keep your mind open to catch such clues, when question mentions joint bleeds or gum bleeds!
Good luck diagnosing!

Investigation of Choice

Prolonged APTT.
Pedigree analysis
Perinatal diagnosis is done by DNA analysis of the fetal tissue obtained by chorionic villus sampling.

Immediate Management

Control bleeding by infusion of Factor VIII concentrate or cryoprecipitate.

Treatment of Choice

Maintaining adequate levels of Factor VIII by regular infusions is the key.
Every effort should be made to prevent deformities arising as a consequence of joint bleeds.
Genetic counseling.

Serial No. 122

Subject: Medicine

Topic: Genetics

Question: A young girl with complaint of prolonged bleeding following dental extraction. Father had a work-up for anaemia and mother had multiple transfusions.

Diagnosis: von Willebrand's Disease

Clinchers

- *A young girl:* von Willebrand's Disease follow an autosomal dominant pattern of inheritance, affecting both sexes equally and can present at any age depending upon the severity of the disease.
- *Prolonged bleeding following dental extraction:* This is the most common mode of presentation, with most patients remaining asymptomatic and are diagnosed either following a minor procedure or during routine preoperative investigations.
- *Father had work up for anaemia:* Bleeding usually from GIT usually goes unnoticed and patients can be first brought to notice during a work up for anaemia.
- *Mother had multiple transfusions:* This again signifying the severity of disease in the mother.

CONFUSA

vWD can be classified into 3 main types, of which 70-80% are considered to be type 1.

- Type 1 vWD is most common type and is characterized by a partial quantitative decrease of qualitatively normal vWF and FVIII. This is inherited as an autosomal dominant trait; however, penetrance may vary dramatically in a single family.
- Of patients with vWD, 15-20% have type 2 disease. vWD type 2 is a variant of the disease with primarily qualitative defects of vWF. Type 2 vWD can be either autosomal dominant or recessive. Of the 5 known type 2 vWD subtypes (i.e. 2A, 2B, 2C, 2M, 2N), type 2A vWD is by far the most common (autosomal dominant).
- Type 3 is the most severe form of vWD and is inherited as an autosomal recessive trait.

Investigation of Choice

Assays of von Willebrand's Factor.

Ristocetin cofactor activity — ristocetin fails to induce platelet aggregation in von Willebrand's patients because of lack of vWF: R — a cofactor for ristocetin.

Immediate Management

Urgent referral

Treatment of Choice

Factor VIII concentrate or Cryoprecipitate are the most common replacement therapies of choice.

Your notes:

Serial No. 125

Subject: Medicine

Topic: Genetics

Question: An 18-year-old female underwent caries tooth extraction and developed profuse bleeding. On taking history she revealed menorrhagia. Her mother and her grandfather had the same disease.

Diagnosis: von Willebrand's Disease

Clinchers

- *An 18-year-old female:* von Willebrand's Disease follow an autosomal dominant pattern of inheritance, affecting both sexes equally and can present at any age depending upon the severity of the disease.
- *Tooth extraction, developed profuse bleeding:* This is the most common mode of presentation, with most patients remaining asymptomatic and are diagnosed either following a minor procedure or during routine pre operative investigations.
- *Menorrhagia:* In most cases, presentation is often of a mild haemophilia with bleeding following mild trauma or surgery. Haemarthrosis, soft tissue haematomas, epistaxis and menorrhagia may occur.
- *Mother, grandfather had the same disease:* This again relates to the familial mode of inheritance, affecting both the sexes overgeneration.

CONFUSA

vWD can be classified into 3 main types, of which 70-80% are considered to be type 1.

- Type 1 vWD is most common type and is characterized by a partial quantitative decrease of qualitatively normal vWF and FVIII. This is inherited as an autosomal dominant trait; however, penetrance may vary dramatically in a single family.
- Of patients with vWD, 15-20% have type 2 disease. vWD type 2 is a variant of the disease with primarily qualitative defects of vWF. Type 2 vWD can be either autosomal dominant or recessive. Of the 5 known type 2 vWD subtypes (i.e., 2A, 2B, 2C, 2M, 2N), type 2A vWD is by far the most common (autosomal dominant).
- Type 3 is the most severe form of vWD and is inherited as an autosomal recessive trait.

Investigation of Choice

Assays of von Willebrand's Factor.

Ristocetin cofactor activity — ristocetin fails to induce platelet aggregation in von Willebrand's patients because of lack of vWF: R — a cofactor for ristocetin.

Immediate Management

Urgent referral

Treatment of Choice

Factor VIII concentrate or Cryoprecipitate are the most common replacement therapies of choice.

Your notes:

Serial No. 131

Subject: Medicine

Topic: Endocrinology

Question: A heavy smoker with raised haematocrit and haemoglobin.

Diagnosis: Polycythaemia (Secondary)

Clinchers

- *Heavy smoker:* Acquired polycythemia is a physiologic response to generalised or localized tissue hypoxia. In a heavy smoker, it can occur secondary to chronic obstructive pulmonary disease, due to high ventilation-to-perfusion ratios. Exposure to carbon monoxide by smoking also acts as an additive factor.
- *Raised haematocrit:* This is the primary abnormality which supports the diagnosis of polycythemia.
- *Raised haemoglobin:* Occurs secondary to stimulation by raised levels of erythropoetin.

CONFUSA

- The main point of distinction between Primary polycythemia and secondary polycythemia is the erythropoetin level. ***Secondary* polycythaemia occurs *secondary* to raised erythropoetin; in primary polycythaemia, erythropoetin levels are low/undetectable.**
- The raised haematocrit should be absolute and not due to decreased plasma volume (Gaisbock's Syndrome).

Investigation of Choice

Radioisotope measurement of red cell mass and plasma volume will confirm the diagnosis of erythrocytosis.

Immediate Management

The main fear is of thrombosis due to hyperviscosity. Phlebotomy is indicated when erythrocytosis is severe, blood is viscous and flow sluggish or prior to operative intervention.

Treatment of Choice

Treat the primary cause.

Your notes:

Serial No. 132

Subject: Medicine

Topic: Endocrinology

Question: A 30-year-old female presents with lethargy. Her BP is 160/100 with serum electrolytes Na^+ 149 mmol/L, K^+ 2.6 mmol/L and HCO^-_3 30 mmol/L.

Diagnosis: Conn's Syndrome

Clinchers

- *30-year-old female:* Primary hyperaldosteronism is twice as common in women as in men. Peak incidence occurs in the third to sixth decades of life.
- *Lethargy:* is attributed to hypokalaemia. Patients may also present with muscle weakness, cramping, headaches, and palpitations. They can also have polydipsia and polyuria from hypokalaemia-induced nephrogenic diabetes insipidus.
- *BP 160/100:* Patient may present with hypertension or one of the cardiac or neurological complications of hypertension.
- *Serum electrolytes Na^+ 149 mmol/L, K^+ 2.6 mmol/L and HCO^-_3 30mmol/L:* The picture of mild hypernatremia with hypokalemia in the presence of metabolic alkalosis fits perfect in the diagnosis of Conn's Syndrome.

CONFUSA

- In any case of hypokalaemic hypertension in the presence of metabolic alkalosis, think of Conn's syndrome as the most probable diagnosis.
- A poorly controlled hypertensive on high doses of diuretics can also present with the same picture of hypertension, alkalosis and hypokalaemia—rule out diuretics as a cause.

Investigation of Choice

- Blood electrolytes
- Plasma renin and aldosterone — low renin and high aldosterone suggests primary hyperaldosteronism
- 24 hour urinary aldosterone.

Immediate Management

Prompt treatment of hypokalemia and hypertension.

Treatment of Choice

According to the underlying cause:

- if due to adenoma — surgery after 4 to 6 weeks of spironolactone therapy (e.g. 300 mg/day)
- if due to adrenal hyperplasia — spironolactone or amiloride is generally sufficient.

PAPER 3

21. A 51-year-old man is lethargic and found to be anaemic. His blood picture is found to have a granulocytic tendency with an increase in the platelet count.

Diagnosis: Myelofibrosis.

Clinchers

- *51-year-old man:* Usually it occurs in older patients.
- *Lethargic:* The disease presents insidiously with lethargy, weakness and weight loss. Patients often complains of a fullness in the upper abdomen due to splenomegaly.
- *Anaemic:* Anaemia with leucoerythroblastic features is present. Poikilocytes and red cells with characteristic tear-drop forms are seen. The WBC count may be over 100×10^9/L, and the differential WBC count may be very similar to that seen in CML; later leucopaenia may develop.
- *His blood picture is found to have a granulocytic tendency with an increase in the platelet count:* The platelet count may be very high but in later stages, thrombocytopaenia occurs. The granulocytic tendency is due to increased WBC counts (see above) with many granulocyte precursors in the peripheral blood.

CONFUSA

The major diagnostic difficulty is the differentiation of myelofibrosis from CML as in both conditions there may be marked splenomegaly and a raised WBC count with many granulocyte precursors in the peripheral blood. The main distinguishing features are the appearance of the bone marrow and the absence of the Philadelphia chromosome in myelofibrosis. Fibrosis of the marrow, often with a leucoerythroblastic anaemia, can occur secondarily to leukemia or lymphoma, tuberculosis or malignant infiltration with metastatic carcinoma, or to irradiation.

Investigation of Choice

Bone marrow trephine biopsy (show markedly increased fibrosis and megakaryocytes).

Immediate Management

Blood transfusion (as he is anaemic).

Treatment of Choice

- Support blood count + folate + analgesics + allopurinol
- Hydroxyurea/busulfan to reduce high metabolic activity and WBC and platelet levels
- Chemotherapy and radiotherapy to reduce spleen size.

22. A 5-year-old boy with generalised lymphadenopathy develops fever and neck stiffness and headache. He is found to have a lot of lymphoblasts in the blood picture.

Diagnosis: Acute lymphoblastic leukaemia (ALL).

Clinchers

- *5-year-old boy*

  cALL—2 to 4-year-old

  tALL—10 to 12-year-old

  ALL is predominantly a disease of children.
- *Generalised lymphadenopathy:* In addition the other usual signs and symptoms are bone pain, arthritis, splenomegaly, thymic enlargement and cranial nerve palsies. Marrow failure produces anaemia, infection and bleeding.
- *Fever and neck stiffness and headache:* These are the signs of leukaemic meningitis (CNS is also a potential site of relapse ALL, other such sites are testes).
- *Lot of lymphoblasts in the blood picture:* ALL manifests as a neoplastic proliferation of lymphoblasts which is evident in peripheral blood picture.

CONFUSA

Fever per se is absent in ALL (characteristically present in AML). The fever in this case may be due to secondary infections which are usually viral, but *Candida, Pneumocystis pneumonia* and bacterial septicaemia can also occur. Neck stiffness can be feature of subarachnoid haemorrhage and shigella dysentery apart from its most common cause meningitis (leukemic meningitis in this case). But beware of the fact that neck stiffness is usually absent in neonatal meningitis.

Investigation of Choice

- *Screening:* Peripheral blood smear.
- *Definitive:* Bone marrow aspiration/biopsy.

Immediate Management

- Blood and platelet transfusions
- IV antibiotics at first sign of infection
- Prophylactic neutropaenic regimen

Treatment of Choice

Chemotherapy (under UK national trials).

Your notes:

24. A 72-year-old man is having a routine examination. He is found to have a mild lymphocytosis and splenomegaly.

Diagnosis: Chronic myeloid leukaemia (CML).

Clinchers

- *72-year-old:* Though it occur most commonly in middle age, old age is no exception for it.
- *Is having a routine examination:* 10% cases of CML are detected by chance. Its symptoms are mostly chronic and insidious, e.g. weight loss, tiredness, gout, fever, sweats, bleeding or abdominal pain.
- *He is found to have a mild lymphocytosis and splenomegaly:* Splenomegaly (often massive) is characteristic of CML (Note: that AML and CML are characterised by early megaly'-spleno and/or hepato-). In the chronic phase of CML, there is only mild lymphocytosis.

CONFUSA

It might be a little difficult to rule out other conditions with such a meagre information but it is safe to diagnose CML. In CLL splenomegaly is a late presentation, i.e. even after the disease can be diagnosed from blood film but in CML the splenomegaly is positive even on presentation.

Investigation of Choice

Blood film ± bone marrow aspiration/biopsy.

Immediate Management

Hydroxyurea 0.5-2 g/24 h PO.

Treatment of Choice

- Allogenic transplantation of bone marrow
  Note: But it is attempted only if:
  - Patient < 55 years
  - Patient is in chronic phase.
- Since the age of this patient is 72 years it will not be attempted.

Your notes:

132. An 8-year-old with acute leukaemia is admitted in a comatose state. He is found to have lymphoblast depletion prevention of infectious diseases.

Diagnosis: Tumour lysis syndrome.

Clinchers

- *8-year-old:* Leukaemias are the most common type of childhood malignancies are over 95% of cases are of acute variety. In the acute series ALL accounts for 70-80% cases. The peak age of onset of ALL is 3-7 years.
- *Acute leukaemia:* As his diagnosis is known he must be on some treatment. Usually chemotherapy is given for ALL.
- *Lymphoblast depletion:* Since lymphoblasts rapidly proliferate in ALL, their depletion should raise a suspicion of any treatment with chemotherapeutic drugs. Tumour lysis syndrome is due to rapid cell death on starting chemotherapy for rapidly proliferating tumours like ALL. It results in rise in serum urate, potassium and phosphate, precipitating renal failure, which can lead to comatose condition if not treated urgently.

CONFUSA

Coma can also occurs in ALL as leukaemic blast cells can infiltrate brain to produce leukaemic meningitis.

Investigation of Choice

Serum urate level (increased).

Immediate Management

Immediate hydration.

Treatment of Choice

Haemodialysis.

Your notes:

PAPER 4

161. A middle-aged man with hepatosplenomegaly, fatigue, immature cells seen in blood film.

Diagnosis: Chronic myeloid leukaemia (CML)

Clinchers

- *Middle-aged man:* CML occurs most often in middle-age. There is a slight male predominance.
- *Hepatosplenomegaly:* In CML there is a marked splenomegaly (produces abdominal discomfort due to enlargement). Hepatomegaly is variable.
- *Fatigue:* Unlike most other leukaemias, CML present with chronic insidious and nonspecific symptoms, e.g.
  - Weight loss
  - Tiredness
  - Gout
  - Fever
  - Sweats
  - Bleeding
  - Abdominal pain
- *Immature cells:* Blood film shows raised WCC with, characteristically the whole spectrum of myeloid precursors, including a few blast cells visible on blood film.
- *Anaemia:* Hb levels are either low or normal in CML.

CONFUSA

Before causing death, CML transforms into an acute leukaemia which is rapidly fatal (within 6 months). But unlike de novo acute leukaemia, with acute phase of CML is characterised by the development of acute leukaemia which may be myeloid (60%), lymphoid (30%) or erythroid (10%) in origin. Moreover in CML this phase is refractory to treatment.

Investigation of Choice

- *Screening:* Peripheral blood smear
- *Definitive:* Bone marrow biopsy and demonstration of Ph chromosome

Immediate Management

Register for allogeneic transplantation if patient is less than < 55 years.

Treatment of Choice

Hydroxyurea (in chronic phase).

Your notes:

163. A 60-year-old man presents with fatigue and backache with localised tenderness. He also have decreased visual acuity.

Diagnosis: Myeloma

Clinchers

- *60-year-old:* Myeloma usually occurs in older age group. The peak age is 70 years.
- *Man:* Sex ratio is equal for myeloma.
- *Fatigue:* It occurs because of anaemia, renal failure or dehydration via proximal tubule dysfunction from light chain precipitation.
- *Backache with localised tenderness:* Bone pain or tenderness is the most common presentation and is often postural, e.g. back, ribs, long bones and shoulder.
- *Decreased visual acuity:* Visual acuity is decreased in myeloma (most probably due to hyperviscosity complications). On fundoscopy haemorrhages or exudates may be seen.

CONFUSA

Bone pain or tenderness in myeloma is never found in extremities. If alkaline phosphate is raised, suspect a healing pathological fracture somewhere (most common: rib). Bone scintigrams which demonstrate lesions in many other tumours are usually normal in myeloma.

Investigation of Choice

Serum/gel electrophoresis.

Immediate Management

Analgesia and transfusion as needed.

Treatment of Choice

Solitary lesions—radiotherapy
Multiple myeloma—chemotherapy

164. Old lady with Hb—3g/dl, MCV—120 fl, family history presents with fatigue, lethargy.

Diagnosis: Megaloblastic anaemia.

Clinchers

- *Old lady:* Incidence of pernicious anaemia (the most common cause of megaloblastic anaemia: which is MCV > 110 fl) increases in old age. Female to male ratio is 1.6 : 1.
- *Hb 3g/dl:* Hb is usually between 3-11 g/dl in pernicious anaemia.
- *MCV 120 fl:* MCV has to be greater than 110 fl to qualify as a megaloblastic type.
- *Family history:* Pernicious anaemia has a higher incidence in blood group A. It is secondary to atrophic gastritis and lack of gastric intrinsic factor, both of which are probably of autoimmune origin and may have a familial preponderance.
- *Fatigue, lethargy:* Most common symptom of pernicious anaemia is tiredness and weakness (seen in 90%). The second most common feature is dyspnoea (70%), sore red tongue (25%), diarrhoea and lemon tinge to skin. There may be prematurely grey hair and neuropsychiatric symptoms.

CONFUSA

A typical feature of pernicious anaemia is presence of a lemon yellow tinge to skin. This colour is produced whenever there is jaundice (mild) with a coexisting pallor (anaemia) in a fair skinned individual. One other condition producing this colour is mild haemolytic anaemia. B_{12} deficiency anaemia can be clinically differentiated from folate deficiency anaemia by the absence of neurological signs in the latter.

Investigation of Choice

Schilling test

Antibodies to intrinsic factor (most specific test)

Immediate Management

Immediate blood transfusion as Hb is 3

Treatment of Choice

Hydroxocobalamin (B_{12}) therapy

Your notes:

190. Condition associated with megaloblastic anaemia, increased risk of carcinoma.

Diagnosis: Pernicious anaemia

Clinchers

- *Megaloblastic anaemia:* Megaloblastic anaemia is caused by:
  - Vit B_{12} or folate deficiency
  - Hydroxyurea (hydroxycarbamide)

  In B_{12} deficiency, synthesis of thymidine, and hence DNA, is impaired and consequently red cell production is reduced.
- *Increased risk of carcinoma:* Since pernicious anaemia is due to malabsorption of B_{12} resulting from atrophic gastritis and lack of gastric intrinsic factor secretion, risk of carcinoma stomach increases manifold. So one should have a low threshold for endoscopy while investigating it. Since it is an autoimmune disease, risk of other autoimmune diseases also increases. Some of such classical associations are:
  - Thyroid disease
  - Vitiligo
  - Addison's disease

CONFUSA

Note that pernicious anaemia is manifestation of a disease which affects all cells of the body. Note that megaloblasts are macrocytes with MCV > 110 fl, so many conditions can lead to macrocytic anaemia (MCV > 96 fl), only a couple of them lead to megaloblastic anaemia (enumerated above). Also beware of diagnosing pernicious anaemia in those below 40 years (malabsorption more common).

Investigation of Choice

- *Screening:* Peripheral blood film
- *Definitive:* Antibodies to intrinsic factor

Immediate Management

Rule out thyroid disease (present in 25% cases of pernicious anaemia).

Treatment of Choice

- *Initial:* Hydroxocobalamin (B_{12}) 1 mg IM alternate days for weeks (or, if CNS signs, until improvement occurs)
- *Maintenance:* Hydroxocobalamin 1 mg IM every 2 month for life

PAPER 5

66. A child is brought to you with weakness, malaise, and bone pain. On physical examination you find painfully enlarged lymph nodes and hard and enlarged testicles. He has a history of sore throats and chest infections.

Diagnosis: Acute lymphoblastic leukaemia (ALL).

Clinchers

- *Child:* ALL is predominantly a disease of children.
- *Weakness, malaise and bone pain:* Apart from non-specific symptoms like weakness and malaise, there are also specific symptoms like bone pain, arthritis, splenomegaly, lymphadenopathy, thymic enlargement, CNS involvement, e.g. cranial nerve palsies.
- *Painfully enlarged lymph nodes and hard and enlarged testicles:* Patients with ALL can present with infiltration of spleen, lymph nodes, liver, skin or CNS. Involvement of testis as a foci or as an extramedullary site of relapse is not uncommon.
- *History of throats and chest infections:* This increased risk of infection occurs with absolute neutrophil counts less than 500/µl and is the leading cause of death. Infections commonly involve mucosal sites such as the pharynx and perianal area as well as the lungs and skin—particularly IV line sites.

CONFUSA

Patients with ALL present with signs and symptoms of marrow failure. These includes pallor and fatigue, bleeding and neutropaenia respectively. With platelet transfusions, haemorrhage is no longer a major cause of death, although alloimmunisation can limit optimal platelet support of patients particularly when patients have been heavily transfused.

Investigation of Choice

Peripheral blood films and bone marrow biopsy.

Immediate Management

Enrol him in national trials.

Treatment of Choice

Chemotherapy (page 654, OHCM, 5th edn).

Your notes:

67. A 51-year-old lecturer presents with lethargy, abdominal pain, fever, and weight loss. On physical examination you find a large spleen. A blood examination shows normocytic normochromic anaemia with a very high white cell count.

Diagnosis: Chronic myeloid leukaemia (CML).

Clinchers

- *51-year-old lecturer:* It occurs most often in middle age with a slight male predominance.
- *Lethargy, abdominal pain, fever, weight loss:* Characteristically CML presents with consti-tutional symptoms.
- *Large spleen:* In most patients the abnormal finding on physical examination at diagnosis is minimal to moderate splenomegaly; mild hepatomegaly is found occasionally.
- *Normocytic normochromic anaemia:* Platelet counts are almost always elevated at diagnosis and mild degree of normochromic nomocytic anaemia is present.
- *Very high white cell count:* Elevated white blood cell counts with various degrees of immaturity of the granulocytic series are observed at diagnosis.

CONFUSA

The clinical onset of the CML is generally insidious. Accordingly, some patients are diagnosed while asymptomatic, during health screening tests; other patients present with fatigue, malaise, and weight loss or have symptoms resulting from splenic enlargement, such as early satiety and LUQ pain or mass. Less common infections, thrombosis, or bleeding. Occasionally, pateints present with leucostatic manifestations due to severe leucocytosis or thrombosis such as vaso-occlusive disease, CVA, MI, venous thrombosis, priapsim, visual disturbances and pulmonary insufficiency.

Investigation of Choice

Blood film.

Immediate Management

Cytogeneic study to find Philadelphia chromosome whose absence mean poor prognosis.

Treatment of Choice

Hydroxyurea.

+

Allogenic transplantation of bone marrow (Always considered if patient is < 55 yrs).

68. An elderly man presents with backache, pallor, and shortness of breath. He has suddenly had some difficulties with his vision. Blood examination demonstrates a high ESR, and normochromic normocytic anaemia. There is rouleaux formation.

Diagnosis: Multiple myeloma.

Clinchers

- *Elderly:* Myeloma increases in incidence with age. The median age at diagnosis is 68 years. It is rare under age 40.
- *Man:* Males are slightly more commonly affected than females and Blacks have nearly twice the incidence of Whites.
- *Backache:* Bone pain is the most common symptom in myeloma. The pain usually involves the back and ribs.
- *Pallor + shortness of breath:* Due to anaemia and pneumonia respectively.
- *Difficulties with his vision:* Hyperviscosity may lead to headache, fatigue, visual disturbances and retinopathy.
- *High ESR:* Characteristic of multiple myeloma.
- *Normochromic, normocytic anaemia:* It ocucrs in about 80% of myeloma patients and is related both to the replacement of normal marrow by expanding tumour cells and to the inhibition of haematopoiesis by factors made by tumour.
- *Rouleaux formation:* Due to hyperviscosity state seen.

CONFUSA

Unlike the pain of metastatic carcinoma, which often is worse at night, the pain of myeloma is precipitated by movement. Persistent localized fracture. The bone lesions are lytic in nature and are rarely associated with osteoblastic new bone formation; therefore, radioisotope bone scanning is less useful in diagnosis than plain radiography.

Investigation of Choice

- *Screening:* ESR
- *Definitive:* Bone marrow biopsy.

Immediate Management

Analgesia + transfusion.

Treatment of Choice

Chemotherapy
(Melphalan—alone or as ABCM regimen).

132. An 8-year-old with acute leukemia is admitted in a comatose state. He is found to have lymphoblast depletion prevention of infectious diseases.

Diagnosis: Tumour lysis syndrome.

Clinchers

- *8-year-old leukaemias are the most common type of childhood:* Malignancies are over 95% of cases are of acute variety. In the acute series ALL accounts for 70-80% cases. The peak age of onset of ALL is 3-7 years.
- *Acute leukaemia:* As his diagnosis is known he must be on some treatment. Usually chemotherapy is given for ALL.
- *Lymphoblast depletion:* Since lymphoblasts rapidly proliferate in ALL, their depletion should raise a suspicion of any treatment with chemotherapeutic drugs. Tumour lysis syndrome is due to rapid cell death on starting chemotherapy for rapidly proliferating tumours like ALL. It results in rise in serum urate, potassium and phosphate, precipitating renal failure, which can lead to comatose condition if not treated urgently.

CONFUSA

Coma can also occurs in ALL as leukemic blast cells can infiltrate brain to produce leukemic meningitis.

Investigation of Choice

Serum urate level (increased).

Immediate Management

Immediate hydration.

Treatment of Choice

Haemodialysis.

Your notes:

161. A 60-year-old man presents with malaise and backpain which has been present for three months. He is found to have significant proteinuria.

Diagnosis: Multiple myeloma (MM)

Clinchers

- *Malaise and backpain:* Bone pain or tenderness is common, and often postural, e.g. back, ribs, long bones, and shoulder. Lassitude is from anaemia, renal failure or dehydration is a proximal tuble dysfunction, from light chain precipitation.
- *Significant proteinuria:* as Bence-Jones proteins are passed in urine. In MM proteinuria is not accompanied by hypertension, and the protein is nearly all light chains. Generally there is very little albumin in the urine because glomerular function is usually normal.

CONFUSA

Bone pain in multiple myeloma never occurs in the extremities. If such a symptom is present, myeloma can be safely excluded as a diagnosis.

Investigation of Choice

Serum gel electrophoresis from 'M' protein spike.

Immediate Management

Correct dehydration, if present.

Treatment of Choice

Supportive + Melphalan chemotherapy.

Also see page 306, for a case history on Multiple myeloma.

Your notes:

163. A 60-year-old man with a plethoric appearance presents with pleuritic chest pain. He has palpable splenomegaly.

Diagnosis: Polycythemia rubra vera (PCRV)

Clinchers

- *60-year-old:* It spares no age group amongst adults. Peak age is 45-60 years.
- *Man:* A slight overall male predominance has been observed.
- *Plethoric appearance:* Most often PCRV is first recognised by discovery of a high haemoglobin or haematocrit of plethoric facies.
- *Pleuritic chest pain:* It could be due to pulmonary thromboembolism—a frequent complication of PCRV. But to be sure, one needs more history.
- *Palpable splenomegaly:* Massive splenomegaly is the most common finding on clinical examination on presentation.

CONFUSA

With the exception of aquagenic pruritus (generalized itching after bathing), no symptoms can distinguish polycythaemia vera from other causes of erythrocytosis.

Investigation of Choice

Screening—PCV

Definitive—^{51}Cr studies to determine RBC mass (> 125% of predicted).

Immediate Management

PaO_2 measurement (as raised RBC mass and splenomegaly in the presence of normal PaO_2 provide a diagnosis).

+

Refer to haematologist

Treatment of Choice

IV 32p/Busulfan

(Note: The treatment is different for younger patients and is based on hydroxyurea).

Your notes:

182. A 5-year-old South African boy is brought to the accident and emergency department deeply jaundiced. He is found to have mildly swollen, tender feet and hands. His mucosae are pale.

Diagnosis: Sickle cell disease.

Clinchers

- *5-year-old:* The condition may present in childhood with anaemia and mild jaundice. The hand and food syndrome due to infarcts of small bones is quite common in children and may result in digits of varying lengths.
- *South African:* The disease occurs mainly in Africans and about 25% carry the gene. It is also common in India, Middle-east and southern Europe.
- *Mildly swollen, tender test and hands:* It is bone pain which is the most common symptom and is due to infarcts of small bones.
- *Mucosae are pale:* Due to anaemia.

CONFUSA

In a given patient the degree of anaemia is usually stable, and during a crisis Hb does not fall unless there is one or more of the following:

- Aplasia
- Acute sequestration
- Haemolysis

Investigation of Choice

- *Screening:* Sodium metabisulphite test
- *Definitive:* Hb electrophoresis (No HbA, 80-95% HbSS and 2-20% HbF).

Immediate Management

IV fluids + oxygen + adequate analgesia.

Treatment of Choice

Exchange transfusion is severe
Penicillin prophylaxis in children
Seek advice from nearest NHS sickle cell and Thalassemia counselling centre.

183. A 6-year-old Asian boy gets regular blood transfusion for his haematological abnormality. His mucosae are pale and skull is grossly bossed. Haematological investigations were done and showed; MCHC 25 g/dl, Hb 8 g/dl, MCV 74 fl.

Diagnosis: Beta thalassemia.

Clinchers

- *6-year-old:* Children affected by severe β-thalassaemia present during the first year of life.
- *Regular blood transfusion for his haematological abnormality:* Regular transfusion may be required every 4-6 weeks and are given to keep the Hb above 10 g/dL.
- *Mucosae are pale:* Because of anaemia.
- *Skull is greatly bossed:* It is due to expansion of the bone marrow due to extramedullary haematopoiesis, giving rise to characteristic thalassemic facies.
- *MCHC 25 g/dL:* It is always reduced (normal 30-36 g/dL) as is MCV and MCH.
- *Hb 8 g/dL:* It suggest β-thalassaemia major.
- *MCV 74 FL:* It is always M 75 FL in this condition.

CONFUSA

Iron overload caused by repeated transfusions (transfusion haemosiderosis) may lead to damage to the endocrine glands, liver, pancreas and the myocardium by the time patients reach adolescence. The type in question is β-thalassaemia because of severity and early age of onset. In β-thalassaemia minor, Hb is > 9 g/dl, so this is β-thalassaemia major.

Investigation of Choice

Hb electrophoresis.

Immediate Management

Transfusion to keep Hb > 9 g/dL.

Treatment of Choice

Bone marrow transplantation in young patients with HLA matched siblings.

Your notes:

184. A 10-year-old boy is brought to the accident and emergency department with a swollen right arm. His temperature is 38.5°C and is unable to move his arm due to severe pain. Blood culture confirms *Salmonella typhi* osteomyelitis. This is his second presentation this month and earlier presented with an acute onset hepatosplenomegaly associated with severe pallor. The SHO does a Sodium Metabisulphite test on the patient's blood which turns out to be positive.

Diagnosis: Sickle cell disease (SCD).

Clinchers

- *10-year-old:* The complications of sickle cell disease are common around adolescence.
- *Swollen right arm + 38.5°C + severe pain + Salmonella typhi osteomyelitis:* Osteomyelitis can occur in SCD in necrotic bone and is often due to *Salmonella.*
- *Second presentation this month:* This suggest a recurrent "crises" state which is common in SCD.
- *Sodium metabisulphite test positive:* Red cells assume their characteristic morphologic form when the haemoglobin is deoxygenated, as by treatment with a reducing agent like sodium metabisulphite.

CONFUSA

Salmonella osteomyelitis is rarely seen in normal population. Although the spleen may be enlarged in small children with sickle cell disease, repeated episodes of splenic infarction cause the spleen to be reduced to a small calcified remnant (autosplenectomy). Concurrent α-thalassaemia seems to protect on the average against the clinical manifestations of sickle disease.

Investigation of Choice
Hb electrophoresis.

Immediate Management
Transfusion to keep Hb > 9 g/dL.

Treatment of Choice
Bone marrow transplantation in young patients with HLA matched siblings.

Your notes:

PAPER 6

131. Patient with atrophic gastritis has megaloblastic anaemia.

Diagnosis: Pernicious anaemia (PA)

Clinchers

- *Atrophic gastritis:* PA is a condition in which there is atrophy of gastric mucosa with consequent failure of intrinsic factor production and vitamin B_{12} malabsorption.
- *Megaloblastic anaemia:* It is characterised by the presence in the bone marrow of erythroblasts with delayed nuclear maturation because of defective DNA synthesis (megaloblasts). Megaloblasts are large (>110 MCV) and have large immature nuclei. The nuclear chromatin is more finely dispensed than normal and has an open stippled appearance. It occurs in:
  - Vitamin B_{12} deficiency or abnormal B_{12} metabolism
  - Folic acid deficiency or abnormal metabolism
  - DNA synthesis defects, i.e.
    - Orotic aciduria
    - Drugs
      - hydroxyurea
      - azathioprine
      - AZT
  - Myelodysplasia due to dyserythropoiesis.

CONFUSA

Beware of diagnosing pernicious anaemia in those under 40 years old: look for GI malabsorption with small bowel biopsy in them. Pernicious anaemia must always be distinguished from other causes of vitamin B_{12} deficiency. Any disease involving the terminal ileum or bacter overgrowth in the small bowel can produce vitamin B_{12} deficiency. Gastrectomy can lead, in the long term, to vitamin B_{12} deficiency. A careful dietary history should be obtained.

Investigation of Choice
Schilling test (expect it to show that < 7% of an oral administered dose of labelled B_{12} is excreted—unless concurrent intrinsic factor is given).

Immediate Management
Rule out associated disease i.e.

- Thyroid disease
- Vitiligo
- Addison's disease
- Carcinoma stomach

Treatment of Choice

Hydroxycobalamin (B_{12}) IM

- 1 mg alternate days
- For 2 weeks (or, if CNS signs, until improvement stops)
- Maintenance: 1 mg IM every 2 months for life.

132. Patient who is a strict vegetarian has an MCV of 110.

Diagnosis: B_{12} deficiency anaemia.

Clinchers

- *Strict vegetarian:* Vitamin B_{12} is synthesized by certain microorganisms, and humans are ultimately dependent on animal sources. It is found in meat, fish, eggs and milk. No vegetable sources contain B_{12}. Strict vegetarians develop its deficiency if they do not even take milk or milk products.
- *MCV of 110:* This signifies a megaloblastic anaemia (criteria: MCV > 110). The peripheral blood film shows macrocytes with hypersegmented polymorphs with six or more lobes in the nucleus.

CONFUSA

Causes of vitamin B_{12} deficiency or abnormal metabolism:

I. Low dietary intake
- Vegans (as is this case)
- Alcoholics.

II. Impaired absorption

A. Stomach
- Pernicious anaemia
- Gastrectomy
- Congenital deficiency of IF.

B. Small bowel
- Ileal disease or resection
- Bacterial overgrowth
- Tropical sprue
- Fish tapeworm (*Diphyllobrothrium l..tum*).

C. Abnormal metabolism
- Congenital transcobalamin II deficiency
- Nitrous oxide (inactivates B_{12}).

Note:
- Malabsorption of B_{12} due to pancreatitis, coeliac disease or treatment with metformin is mild and does not usually result in significant vitamin B_{12} deficiency.
- Body stores of vitamin B_{12} are usually sufficient for 3 years.

Investigation of Choice

- *Screening:* Deoxyuridine suppression test or Schilling's test.
- *Definitive:* Serum vitamin B_{12} (Normal: 160 ng/L).

Immediate Management

Careful and detailed dietary history.

Treatment of Choice

Replenish stores with hydroxycobalamin (B_{12}) (Doses—see previous question).

134. Elderly patient with complaint of anaemia and has bleeding gum.

Diagnosis: Scurvy

Clinchers

- *Elderly:* Vitamin C deficiency is seen mainly in infants fed with boiled milk and in the elderly and single people who cannot be bothered to eat vegetables. It can be seen in UK among Asian countries where people prefer to eat rice and chapatis and also in food faddists.
- *Anaemia:* In scurvy the anaemia is usually hypochronic but occasionally a normochromic or megaloblastic whether iron deficiency (owing to decreased absorption or loss due to haemorrhage) or folate deficiency (folate being largely found in green vegetables) is present.
- *Bleeding gums:* Swollen, spongy gums with bleeding and superadded infection and loosening of teeth are characteristic of scurvy.

CONFUSA

Humans, along with a few other animals (e.g. primates and the guinea pigs) are unusual in not being able to synthesize ascorbic acid from glucose. Vitamin C is present in all fresh fruits and vegetables. Unfortunately, ascorbic acid is easily leached out of vegetables when they are placed in water and it is also oxidised to dehydroascorbic acid during cooking, exposure to copper or alkalis. Potatoes is a good source and many people eat a lot of them, but vitamin C is lost during storage.

Investigation of Choice

Plasma ascorbic acid level (Normal > 11μmol/L)

Immediate Management

Detailed dietary history

Treatment of Choice

Ascorbic acid

- Initial: 250 mg daily
  - Maintenance: 40 mg daily

135. Elderly patient in residential home a complaints of tiredness.

Diagnosis: Nutritional deficit (most probably)

Clinchers

- *Elderly:* Nutritional deficits in the elderly may be due to many factors such as:
  - Dental problems
  - Lack of cooking skills (particularly in widowers)
  - Depression
  - Lack of motivation
  - Disabilities.
- *Residential home stay:* This will result in vitamin D deficiency. In elderly patients who are confirmed to their houses, vitamin D supplements may be required because often these people do not go into sunlight.
- *Tiredness:* It is a common non-specific symptom of malnutrition.

CONFUSA

The daily energy requirement of elderly people (aged 60 and above, irrespective of age) has been set to approximately 1.5 × BMR. The BMR is reduced, owing to a fall in the fat-free mass, from an average of 60 kg to 50 kg in men and from 40 kg to 35 kg in women. The diet should contain the same proportions of nutrients, and essential nutrients are still required. Owing to the high prevalence of osteoporosis in elderly people, daily calcium intake should be 1-1.5 g.

Investigation of Choice

Tests for various nutritional deficiencies

Immediate Management

A detailed dietary history

Treatment of Choice

Prescribe proper diet + treatment of any deficiency.

141. A 51-year-old man is lethargic and found to be anaemic. His blood picture is found to have a granulocytic tendency with an increase in the platelet count.

Diagnosis: Myelofibrosis.

Clinchers

- *51-year-old man:* Usually it occurs in older patients.
- *Lethargic:* The disease presents insidiously with lethargy, weakness and weight loss. Patients often complains of a fullness in the upper abdomen due to splenomegaly.
- *Anaemic:* Anaemia with leucoerythroblastic features is present. Poikilocytes and red cells with characteristic tear-drop forms are seen. The WBC count may be over 100 × 10^9/L, and the differential WBC count may be very similar to that seen in CML; later leucopenia may develop.
- *His blood picture is found to have a granulocytic tendency with an increase in the platelet count:* The platelet count may be very high but in later stages, thrombocytopenia occurs. The granulocytic tendency is due to increased WBC counts (see above) with many granulocyte precursors in the peripheral blood.

CONFUSA

The major diagnostic difficulty is the differentiation of myelofibrosis from CML as in both conditions there may be marked splenomegaly and a raised WBC count with many granulocyte precursors in the peripheral blood. The main distinguishing features are the appearance of the bone marrow and the absence of the Philadelphia chromosome in myelofibrosis. Fibrosis of the marrow, often with a leucoerythroblastic anaemia, can occur secondarily to leukaemia or lymphoma, tuberculosis or malignant infiltration with metastatic carcinoma, or to irradiation.

Investigation of Choice

Bone marrow trephine biopsy (show markedly increased fibrosis and megakaryocytes).

Immediate Management

Blood transfusion (as he is anaemic).

Treatment of Choice

- Support blood count + folate + analgesics + allopurinol
- Hydroxyurea/busulfan to reduce high metabolic acitivity and WBC and platelet levels
- Chemotherapy and radiotherapy to reduce slpeen size.

142. A 5-year-old boy with generalised lymphadenopathy develops fever and neck stiffness and headache. He is found to have a lot of lymphoblasts in the blood picture.

Diagnosis: Acute lymphoblastic leukaemia (ALL)

Clinchers

- *5-year-old boy*
  cALL—2-4 yrs old
  tALL—10-12 yrs old
  ALL is predominantly a disease of children.
- *Generalised lymphadenopathy:* In addition the other usual signs and symptoms are bone pain, arthritis, splenomegaly, thymic enlargement and cranial nerve palsies. Marrow failure produces anaemia, infection and bleeding.
- *Fever and neck stiffness and headache:* These are the signs of leukemic meningitis (CNS is also a potential site of relapse ALL, other such sites are testes).
- *Lot of lymphoblasts in the blood picture:* ALL manifests as a neoplastic proliferation of lymphoblasts which is evident in peripheral blood picture.

CONFUSA

Fever per se is absent in ALL (characteristically present in AML). The fever in this case may be due to secondary infections which are usually viral, but *Candida, Pneumocystis pneumonia* and bacterial septicaemia can also occur. Neck stiffness can be feature of subarachnoid haemorrhage and *Shigella* dysentery apart from its most common cause meningitis (leukaemic meningitis in this case). But beware of the fact that neck stiffness is usually absent in neonatal meningitis.

Investigation of Choice

- *Screening:* Peripheral blood smear.
- *Definitive:* Bone marrow aspiration/biopsy.

Immediate Management

- Blood and platelet transfusions
- IV antibiotics at first sign of infection
- Prophylactic neutropenic regimen

Treatment of Choice

Chemotherapy (under UK national trials).

Your notes:

144. A 72-year-old man is having a routine examination. He is found to have a mild lymphocytosis and splenomegaly.

Diagnosis: Chronic myeloid leukaemia (CML).

Clinchers

- *72-year-old:* Though it occur most commonly in middle age, old age is no exception for it.
- *Is having a routine examination:* 10% cases of CML are detected by chance. Its symptoms are mostly chronic and insidious, e.g. weight loss, tiredness, gout, fever, sweats, bleeding or abdominal pain.
- *He is found to have a mild lymphocytosis and splenomegaly:* Splenomegaly (often massive) is characteristic of CML (Note: that AML and CML are characterised by early megaly'-spleno and/or hepato-). In the chronic phase of CML, there is only mild lymphocytosis.

CONFUSA

It might be a little difficult to rule out other conditions with such a meagre information but it is safe to diagnose CML. In CLL splenomegaly is a late presentation, i.e. even after the disease can be diagnosed from blood film but in CML the splenomegaly is positive even on presentation.

Investigation of Choice
Blood film ± bone marrow aspiration/biopsy.

Immediate Management
Hydroxyurea 0.5-2 g/24 h PO.

Treatment of Choice

- Allogenic transplantation of bone marrow
  Note: But it is attempted only if:
  - Patient < 55 years
  - Patient is in chronic phase.
- Since the age of this patient is 72 years it will not be attempted.

Your notes:

PAPER 7

37. An 8-year-old with acute leukemia is admitted in a comatose state. He is found to have lymphoblast depletion prevention of infectious diseases.

Diagnosis: Tumour lysis syndrome.

Clinchers

- *8-year-old:* Leukaemias are the most common type of childhood. Malignancies are over 95% of cases are of acute variety. In the acute series ALL accounts for 70-80% cases. The peak age of onset of ALL is 3-7 years.
- *Acute leukaemia:* As his diagnosis is known he must be on some treatment. Usually chemotherapy is given for ALL.
- *Lymphoblast depletion:* Since lymphoblasts rapidly proliferate in ALL, their depletion should raise a suspicion of any treatment with chemotherapeutic drugs. Tumour lysis syndrome is due to rapid cell death on starting chemotherapy for rapidly proliferating tumours like ALL. It results in rise in serum urate, potassium and phosphate, precipitating renal failure, which can lead to comatose condition if not treated urgently.

CONFUSA

Coma can also occurs in ALL as leukaemic blast cells can infiltrate brain to produce leukaemic meningitis.

Investigation of Choice
Serum urate level (increased).

Immediate Management
Immediate hydration.

Treatment of Choice
Haemodialysis.

Your notes:

126. Patient with atrophic gastritis has megaloblastic anaemia.

Diagnosis: Pernicious anaemia (PA)

Clinchers

- *Atrophic gastritis:* PA is a condition in which there is atrophy of gastric mucosa with consequent failure of intrinsic factor production and vitamin B_{12} malabsorption.
- *Megaloblastic anaemia:* It is characterised by the presence in the bone marrow of erythroblasts with delayed nuclear maturation because of defective DNA synthesis (megaloblasts). Megaloblasts are large (>110 MCV) and have large immature nuclei. The nuclear chromatin is more finely dispensed than normal and has an open stippled appearance. It occurs in:
  - Vitamin B_{12} deficiency or abnormal B_{12} metabolism
  - Folic acid deficiency or abnormal metabolism
  - DNA synthesis defects, i.e.
    - Orotic aciduria
    - Drugs
      - hydroxyurea
      - azathioprine
      - AZT
  - Myelodysplasia due to dyserythropoiesis.

CONFUSA

Beware of diagnosing pernicious anaemia in those under 40 years old: look for GI malabsorption with small bowel biopsy in them. Pernicious anaemia must always be distinguished from other causes of vitamin B_{12} deficiency. Any disease involving the terminal ileum or bacter overgrowth in the small bowel can produce vitamin B_{12} deficiency. Gastrectomy can lead, in the long term, to vitamin B_{12} deficiency. A careful dietary history should be obtained.

Investigation of Choice

Schilling test (expect it to show that < 7% of an oral administered dose of labelled B_{12} is excreted—unless concurrent intrinsic factor is given).

Immediate Management

Rule out associated disease i.e.

- Thyroid disease
- Vitiligo
- Addison's disease
- Carcinoma stomach

Treatment of Choice

Hydroxycobalamin (B_{12}) IM

- 1 mg alternate days
- For 2 weeks (or, if CNS signs, until improvement stops)
- Maintenance: 1 mg IM every 2 months for life.

127. Patient who is a strict vegetarian has an MCV of 110.

Diagnosis: B_{12} deficiency anaemia

Clinchers

- *Strict vegetarian:* Vitamin B_{12} is synthesized by certain micro-organisms, and humans are ultimately dependent on animal sources. It is found in meat, fish, eggs and milk. No vegetable sources contain B_{12}. Strict vegetarians develop its deficiency if they do not even take milk or milk products.
- *MCV of 110:* This signifies a megaloblastic anaemia (criteria: MCV > 110). The peripheral blood film shows macrocytes with hypersegmented polymorphs with six or more lobes in the nucleus.

CONFUSA

Causes of vitamin B_{12} deficiency or abnormal metabolism:

I. Low dietary intake
- Vegans (as is this case)
- Alcoholics.

II. Impaired absorption

A. Stomach
- Pernicious anaemia
- Gastrectomy
- Congenital deficiency of IF.

B. Small bowel
- Ileal disease or resection
- Bacterial overgrowth
- Tropical sprue
- Fish tapeworm *(Diphyllobrothrium latum).*

C. Abnormal metabolism
- Congenital transcobalamin II deficiency
- Nitrous oxide (inactivates B_{12}).

Note:
- Malabsorption of B_{12} due to pancreatitis, coeliac disease or treatment with metformin is mild and does not usually result in significant vitamin B_{12} deficiency.
- Body stores of vitamin B_{12} are usually sufficient for 3 years.

Investigation of Choice

- *Screening:* Deoxyuridine suppression test or Schilling's test.
- *Definitive:* Serum vitamin B_{12} (Normal: 160 ng/L).

Immediate Management

Careful and detailed dietary history.

Treatment of Choice

Replenish stores with hydroxycobalamin (B_{12}) (Doses—see previous question).

129. Elderly patient with complaint of anaemia and has bleeding gum.

Diagnosis: Scurvy

Clinchers

- *Elderly:* Vitamin C deficiency is seen mainly in infants fed with boiled milk and in the elderly and single people who cannot be bothered to eat vegetables. It can be seen in UK among Asian countries where people prefer to eat rice and chapatis and also in food faddists.
- *Anaemia:* In scurvy the anemia is usually hypochronic but occasionally a normochromic or megaloblastic whether iron deficiency (owing to decreased absorption or loss due to haemorrhage) or folate deficiency (folate being largely found in green vegetables) is present.
- *Bleeding gums:* Swollen, spongy gums with bleeding and superadded infection and loosening of teeth are characteristic of scurvy.

CONFUSA

Humans, along with a few other animals (e.g. primates and the guinea pigs) are unusual in not being able to synthesize ascorbic acid from glucose. Vitamin C is present in all fresh fruits and vegetables. Unfortunately, ascorbic acid is easily leached out of vegetables when they are placed in water and it is also oxidised to dehydroascorbic acid during cooking, exposure to copper or alkalis. Potatoes is a good source and many people eat a lot of them, but vitamin C is lost during storage.

Investigation of Choice

Plasma ascorbic acid level (Normal > 11μmol/L)

Immediate Management

Detailed dietary history

Treatment of Choice

Ascorbic acid

- Initial: 250 mg daily
  - Maintenance: 40 mg daily

Your notes:

130. Elderly patient in residential home a complaints of tiredness.

Diagnosis: Nutritional deficit (most probably)

Clinchers

- *Elderly:* Nutritional deficits in the elderly may be due to many factors such as:
  - Dental problems
  - Lack of cooking skills (particularly in widowers)
  - Depression
  - Lack of motivation
  - Disabilities.
- *Residential home stay:* This will result in vitamin D deficiency. In elderly patients who are confirmed to their houses, vitamin D supplements may be required because often these people do not go into sunlight.
- *Tiredness:* It is a common non-specific symptom of malnutrition.

CONFUSA

The daily energy requirement of elderly people (aged 60 and above, irrespective of age) has been set to approximately 1.5 × BMR. The BMR is reduced, owing to a fall in the fat-free mass, from an average of 60 kg to 50 kg in men and from 40 kg to 35 kg in women. The diet should contain the same proportions of nutrients, and essential nutrients are still required. Owing to the high prevalence of osteoporosis in elderly people, daily calcium intake should be 1-1.5 g.

Investigation of Choice

Tests for various nutritional deficiencies

Immediate Management

A detailed dietary history

Treatment of Choice

Prescribe proper diet + treatment of any deficiency.

Your notes:

10 Hepatobiliary System

PAPER 2

Serial No. 29

Subject: Medicine

Topic: Anaemia

Question: A man is brought in with haematemesis and melaena. He is anaemic, jaundiced, has spider naevi and gynaecomastia.

Diagnosis: Chronic Liver Disease

Clinchers

- *Haematemesis and melaena:* Raised portal hypertension in chronic liver disease leads to opening up of porto systemic anastomsis leading repeated haematemesis and malaena.
- *Anaemic:* Repeated blood loss through engorged oesophageal varices and rectal varices leads to iron deficiency anaemia, usually superimposed on anaemia of chronic disease.
- *Jaundiced:* Jaundice is a common sign in liver disease. Raised bilirubin levels are clinically detectable when the concentration exceeds 40 micromol/l.
- *Spider naevi:* Spider naevi are telangiectases that consist of a large arteriole from which radiate numerous small vessels that resemble, in the mind's eye, spider's legs. They are found in the distribution of the superior vena cava, i.e. on the arms, neck, and chest wall. Seen in liver disease and also in pregnancy.
- *Gynaecomastia:* Occurs due to altered oestradiol/testosterone ratio in chronic liver disease because of decreased inability of the liver to metabolise oestrogen.

CONFUSA

Be careful when dealing with questions like this, for the theme can be tricky and ask you to specify the cause of bleeding or the cause of anaemia. While the cause of bleeding in a case of ruptured oesophageal varices signify chronic liver disease as answer, the cause of anaemia can be either acute blood loss or due to anaemia of chronic liver disease.

Investigation of Choice

Liver Function Test

Immediate Management

Symptomatic

Treatment of Choice

Liver transplantation

Your notes:

Serial No. 32

Subject: Medicine

Topic: Drug complications

Question: A boy on treatment for generalised tonic clonic epilepsy, develops features of hepatic failure in few weeks of starting treatment.

Diagnosis: Valproate-induced liver failure

Clinchers

- *Boy on treatment for generalized tonic clonic epilepsy:* Valproate is the first drug of choice, according to NICE guidelines, in patients who have tonic-clonic seizures as part of idiopathic generalised epilepsy.
- *Features of hepatic failure:* Liver dysfunction (including fatal hepatic failure) has occurred in association with valproate, especially in children under 3 years of age.
- *Within few weeks of starting treatment:* valproate-induced liver dysfunction is usually seen in the first 6 months of therapy.

CONFUSA

Raised liver enzymes are not uncommon during valproate treatment and are usually transient. Patients should be reassessed clinically and liver function (including prothrombin time) monitored until return to normal. An abnormally prolonged prothrombin time (particularly in association with other relevant abnormalities) requires discontinuation of treatment. Any concomitant use of salicylates should be stopped.

Investigation of Choice

Liver Function Tests - Prothrombin Time

Immediate Management

Regularly monitor liver functions till it returns to normal.

In case of deterioration or abnormally prolongation of prothrombin time, discontinue valproate under coverage of 2nd line anticonvulsants.

Treatment of Choice

Discontinue valproate under coverage of 2nd line anticonvulsants.

Your notes:

PAPER 3

83. Avoidance of alcohol for six months after hepatitis A.

Diagnosis: To decrease risk of cirrhosis.

Clinchers

A small proportion of patients with hepatitis A experience relapsing hepatitis weeks to months after apparent recovery from acute hepatitis. Relapses are characterised by recurrence of symptoms, aminotransferase elevations, occasionally jaundice and faecal excretion of HAV. Rarely, liver test abnormalities persists for many months, even upto a year. So it is advisable to avoid alcohol or drugs whose metabolism is primarily through liver (especially drugs which can precipitate cholestasis), because they can induce severe liver damage in this period which can lead to cirrhosis.

CONFUSA

Kumar and Clark's textbook of medicine says that there is no reason to stop alcohol consumption other than for the few weeks when the patient is ill (pg 304, 4th edn).

Investigation of Choice

LFT (to check resolution).

Immediate Management

Symptomatic.

Treatment of Choice

Avoidance of alcohol.

Your notes:

PAPER 4

104. A chronic alcoholic presents with flapping tremors and confusion.

Diagnosis: Alcoholic liver disease.

Clinchers

- *Chronic alcoholic:* Alcohol and chronic HBV or HCV infections are the most common causes of cirrhosis.
- *Flapping tremors:* This is a coarse irregular tremor of outstretched hands better known as asterixis. It is pathognomic of chronic liver disease.
- *Confusion:* Confusion is presence hepatic disease signifies grade II of hepatic encephalopathy
  - Grade I—altered mood or behaviour
  - Grade II—increasing drowsiness, confusion, slurred speech
  - Grade III—stupor, incoherence, restlessness, significant confusion
  - Grade IV—coma.

CONFUSA

Flapping tremor can be present in
- Wilson's disease
- Haemochromatosis

Encephalopathy is suspected chronic liver disease suggests acute on chronic hepatic failure.

Investigation of Choice

- *Screening:* LFT (- bilirubin, AST > ALT-although both rise)
- *Definitive:* Liver biopsy

Immediate Management

Nurse with a 20° head up tilt in ITU

Treatment of Choice

Supportive
- 20% mannitol, slow infusion for - ICP
- 10% dextrose infusion for hypoglycemia
- Potassium and calcium supplements
- IV vitamin K for coagulopathy

Your notes:

149. Man with jaundice and ascites suddenly deteriorates.

Diagnosis: Hepatic encephalopathy.

Clinchers

- *Jaundice and ascites:* This signifies hepatic disease. Most probably it is cirrhosis of liver of which the most common cause is chronic alcoholism.
- *Suddenly deteriorates:* Sudden deterioration of the condition in the setting of chronic liver failure strongly suggests encephalopathy is failure of liver to detoxify ammonium ions into readily excretable urea, a low protein diet given prophylactically, can present it.

CONFUSA

The pathogenesis of the development of ascites in liver disease is controversial, but is probably secondary to renal sodium and water retention. Portal hypertension is also contributive as it exerts a local hydrostatic pressure and leads to increased hepatic and splanchnic production of lymph and transudation of fluid into peritoneal cavity.

Investigation of Choice

Serum albumin, bilirubin urea.

Immediate Management

Refer patient to specialised unit.

Treatment of Choice

There is no specific treatment but only support therapy, Note: Dexamethasone is of no value. Low protein, low salt diet should be given in this condition irrespective of the presence of encephalopathy.

Your notes:

179. Female 50-year-old, 5 years history of mild pruritus history of pale stools, dark urine, jaundice.

Diagnosis: Primary biliary cirrhosis (PBC).

Clinchers

- *50-year-old female:* Ninety percent of those affected are women in the age range 40-50 years. It used to be rare but now being diagnosed more frequently in its milder forms.
- *5 years history of mild pruritus:* Pruritus is often the earliest symptom, preceding jaundice by a few years.
- *Pale stools, dark urine, jaundice:* This is a characteristic picture of obstructive jaundice. It signifies a late stage of PBC—the patient is jaundiced with severe pruritus. Pigmented xanthelasma on eyelids or other deposits of cholesterol in the creases of the hands may be seen. Hepatosplenomegaly may be present.

CONFUSA

PBC is usually associated with:
- Autoimmune disorders
  - Sjögren's syndrome
  - Scleroderma
  - Rheumatoid arthritis
- Keratoconjunctivitis sicca (dry eyes and mouth) is seen in 70% of cases
- Renal tubular acidosis
- Membranous glomerulonephritis

Mitochondrial antibodies (measured routinely by ELISA—in titres more than 1: 160) are present in over 95% of patients. M2 antibody is specific. Other nonspecific antibodies (e.g. ANA and SMA) may also be present.

Investigation of Choice

- *Screening:* ELSIA for mitochondrial antibodies
- *Definitive:* Liver biopsy

Immediate Management

USG (in a jaundiced patient, extrahepatic biliary obstruction should be excluded)

Treatment of Choice

Symptomatic:
- Pruritus: colestyramine
- Diarrhoea: codeine phosphate
- Malabsorption: prophylactic fat soluble vitamin supplements
  - In case serum bilirubin > 100 μmol/L—consider liver transplantation.

180. Man with history of hemochromatosis and alcohol addiction presents with jaundice, ascites, variceal bleed. USG is unequivocal, high ferritin level.

Diagnosis: Hereditary haemochromatosis (HHC)

Clinchers

- *Mass:* Middle-aged males are more frequently and severely affected than women.
- *Haemochromatosis:* HHC is one of the most common inherited (autosomal recessive) single gene disorders in northern Europeans.
- *Alcohol addiction:* The course of the disease depends on a number of factors including sex, dietary iron intake, presence of associated hepatoxins (especially alcohol) and genotype.
- *USG unequivocal:* USG will not demonstrate anything significant. A liver biopsy is definitive (with Perl's stain).
- *High ferritin level:* Serum ferritin is elevated, usually >500 μg/L or 240 nmol/L.

CONFUSA

Haemochromatosis tend to present about 10 years later in females than males on the menstrual blood loss is protective. So while in males, its peak incidence is in middle-ages, in case of females it is usually postmenopausal. Iron overload may be present in alcoholics, but alcohol excess per se does not cause HHC. There is a history of excess alcohol intake in 25% of patients.

Investigation of Choice

- *Screening:*
  - Homozygotes
    - Serum iron (--)
    - Serum ferritin (--)
  - Heterozygotes
    - Serum ferritin (-)
    - Transferrin saturation (-)
- *Definitive*
  - Liver biopsy/MRI

Immediate Management

Manage cirrhotic symptoms

Treatment of Choice

Venesection routinely

If venesection not tolerated, chelation therapy.

PAPER 5

43. Liver function tests show raised alkaline phosphatase, raised bilirubin, normal albumin and normal hepatocellular enzymes.

Diagnosis: Stone in common bile duct (choledocholithiasis)

Clinchers

- *Liver function tests:* They are performed whenever jaundice, part or present, is a feature.
- *Raised alkaline phosphatase:* Persistently raised alkaline phosphatase is always suspicious of choledocholithiasis.
- *Raised bilirubin:* Stone in CBD is associated with jaundice in 75% cases.
- *Normal albumin and hepatocellular enzymes:* This rules out lives injury and hence suggest a CBD pathology.

CONFUSA

Differential diagnosis of stone in the CBD is as follows:
- With jaundice (75%)
  - Carcinoma pancreas or other malignant obstruction of CBD
  - Acute hepatitis
  - Other causes of jaundice
- Without jaundice (25%)
  - Renal colic
  - Intestinal obstruction or angina pectoris

Investigation of Choice
USG

Immediate Management
IV vitamin K (as depressed absorption of this fat soluble vitamin lower the serum prothrombin with consequent bleeding tendency).

Treatment of Choice
Conservative management with subsequent exploration of CBD or emergency endoscopic sphincterectomy if severe.

Your notes:

44. Ultrasound scan shows dilated common bile duct with no free intra-abdominal fluid or bowel distension.

Diagnosis: Stone in common bile duct

Clinchers

- *Dilated CBD:* USG demonstrate dilatation of the duct system suggesting distal duct obstruction and hence is an invaluable investigation in this case.
- *No free intra-abdominal fluid or bowel distention:* This rules out any biliary leakage or peritonitis. Still barium meal or upper GI endoscopy are advisable in cases of chronic cholecystitis to exclude an associated peptic ulcer or hiatus hernia.

CONFUSA

Unfortunately, USG, like CT scan, is unreliable in detecting stones in the bile ducts, especially at the lower ends.

Investigation of Choice
USG

Immediate Management
IV vitamin K (see previous Q)

Treatment of Choice
See previous Q.

Your notes:

109. It spreads by faecal-oral route.

Diagnosis: Hepatitis A virus (HAV)

Clinchers

Spread of infection is mainly by the faeco-oral route and arises from the ingestion of contaminated food or water (e.g. shellfish). Overcrowding and poor sanitation facilitate spread. There is no carrier state. In the UK it is a notifiable disease.

CONFUSA

No HAV carries state has been identified after acute type A hepatitis; perpetuation of the virus in nature depends presumably on nonepidemic, inapparent subclinical infection. Hepatitis A tends to be more symptomatic in adults. Travel to endemic areas is a common source of infection for adults from nonendemic areas. More recently recognized epidemiologic foci of HAV infection include child care centres, neonatal ICU, promiscuous homosexual men and IV drug abusers. Although HAV is rarely blood borne, several outbreaks have been recognized in recipients of clotting factor concentrates.

Investigation of Choice

Serum transaminases, IgM

Immediate Management

Notify relevant authorities

Treatment of Choice

Supportive

Rarely interferon a for fulminant hepatitis.

Your notes:

157. A 41-year-old Londoner developed a temperature of 41°C, 5 weeks after cadaveric renal transplantation. WBC is 2.1 × 1,000,000,000/L, Hb is 8.8 g/dl, creatinine 177 µmol/L. Aspartate aminotransferase (AST) 82 U/L. Alanine aminotransferase (ALT) 132 U/L.

Diagnosis: Cytomegalovirus (CMV) disease.

Clinchers

- *41-year-old Londoner:* CMV has worldwide distribution with London being no exception.
- *Temperature of 41°C:* In transplant recipients on post bone marrow transplantation, CMV present with: fever > pneumonitis > colitis > hepatitis > retinitis. In AIDS, it presents with: retinitis > colitis > CNS defects.
- *After cadavaric renal transplantation:* CMV can be acquired by direct contact, blood transfusion or organ transplantation. Transmission following organs transplantation or blood transfusion is due to silent infection in these tissues. It can well be a CMV reactivation syndrome, developed when T cell (lymphocyte) mediated immunity is compromised after organ transplantation, or in association with lymphoid neoplasms and certain acquired immunodeficiencies (in particular: HIV).
- *WBC is 2.1 × 1000,000,000/L:* Normal range is between 4-11 × 1000,000,000/L. Leukopenia is commonly seen with CMV infection in immunocompromised.
- *Aspartate transaminase (AST) of 82 IU/L:* Normal range of AST is 3-35 IU/L. This shows the LFT is deranged. Hepatitis is a common syndrome associated with CMV.
- *Alanine aminotransferase (ALT) of 132 IU/L:* Normal range of ALT is 3-35 IU/L. This shows LFT is deranged. Hepatitis is a common syndrome associated with CMV.

Variety of syndromes associated with CMV are fever, and leukopenia, hepatitis, pneumonitis, esophagitis, gastritis, colitis and retinitis.

CONFUSA

Most primary CNV infections in organ transplant recipients result from transmission of the virus in the graft itself.

Investigation of Choice

Isolation of the virus together with rise in antibody titers a fourfold and greater.

Immediate Management

Retinoscopy to exclude CMV retinitis.

Treatment of Choice Ganciclovir IV

PAPER 6

36. Man returned from trip to Asia, complains of anorexia, malaise, dark urine, pale stools.

Diagnosis: Hepatitis B (most probably)

Clinchers

- *Trip to Asia:* Hepatitis A is the most common type of viral hepatitis worldwide, often in epidemics. The disease is commonly seen in autumn and affects children and young adults. Spread of infection is mainly by the faecal-oral route and arises from the ingestion of contraminated food or water (e.g. shellfish). Overcrowding and poor sanitation facilitate spread. It is common in developing countries in Asia.
- *Anorexia malaise:* The viraemia causes the patient to feel unwell with nonspecific symptoms that includes nausea, anorexia and a distaste for cigarettes. Jaundice develops after one or two weeks.
  Note: Many recover at this stage and remain anicetric.
- *Dark urine, pale stools:* As the jaundice deepens, the urine becomes dark and stools pale owing to intrahepatic cholelithiasis.

CONFUSA

Clinically the differential diagnosis is from all other causes of jaundice—but in particular from other types of viral and drug induced hepatitis. Common causes of jaundice in travellers are:

- Viral hepatitis
- Cholangitis
- Liver abscess
- Leptospirosis
- Typhoid
- Malaria
- Dengue fever
- Yellow fever
- Haemoglobinopathies

Investigation of Choice

Viral serology and LFT

- Serum transaminases rise 22-40 days after exposure
- IgM rises from day 25 and signifies recent infection
- IgG remains detectable for life.

Immediate Management

Symptomatic and advise to avoid alcohol

Notify health authorities as it is a notifiable disease in UK

Treatment of Choice

Supportive

If fulminant hepatitis—interferon α.

37. An 80-year-old man has never been out of UK, one month history of epigastric pain, dark urine, pale stools, jaundice.

Diagnosis: Common bile duct obstruction (CBD obstruction).

Clinchers

- *80-year-old man:* The age point more towards malignancy than a stone as the cause of obstruction of CBD.
- *Never been out of UK:* Rules out infective causes like cholangitis or hepatitis.
- *One month history:* It signifies that the symptomatology is chronic and rules out infective causes and acute cholecystitis.
- *Epigastric pain:* Gallbladder pathologies produce continuous picture of any obstructive jaundice. Dark urine is due to bilirubinuria and pale stools due to decreased bile pigments.

CONFUSA

A young person is more likely to have hepatitis, so questions should be asked about drug and alcohol se, and sexual behaviour. An elderly person with gross weight loss is more likely to have a carcinoma. All patients may complain of malaise. Abdominal pain occurs in patients with biliary obstruction by gallstones and sometimes with an enlarged liver there is pain resulting from distension of the capsule.

Investigation of Choice

ERCP

Immediate Management

Heme test of stools (if positive, suspect malignancy)

Treatment of Choice

Depends on diagnosis

- Stones—cholecystectomy
- Malignancy—surgery/palliation

Your notes:

38. Female with fever, rigors, right upper quadrant pain, jaundice, USG is normal.

Diagnosis: Acute cholecystitis.

Clinchers

- *Female:* Female sex is a risk factor for cholesterol stones in gallbladder, which is the usual cause for acute cholecystitis. The disease can occur at any age.
- *Fever, rigors:* The patient is usually ill with a fever and shallow respirations.
- *Right upper quadrant (RUQ) pain:* The main symptoms are severe pain in the epigastrium and right hypochondrium. The pain is continuous, increasing in intensity over 24 hours. It can radiate to back and shoulder. It may be accompanied by nausea and vomiting. Right hypochondrium tenderness is present, being worse on inspiration (Murphy's sign). There is guarding and rebound tenderness.
- *Jaundice:* Mild jaundice occurs in 20% of cases owing to accompanying common duct stones or to surrounding oedema occluding the CBD.
- *USG is normal:* Although can accurately diagnose stones as small as 2 mm, it may be false negative in 2-4 percent of cases.

CONFUSA

A less severe case of acute pancreatitis simulates acute cholecystitis. The fever in acute cholecystitis is more marked than pancreatitis and is in range of 38-39° C with marked toxaemia and leucocytosis. Rigors are almost nerve seen in acute pancreatitis.

Investigation of Choice

Oral cholecystography (OCG)

OCG is a useful procedure for diagnosis of gallstones but has been diagnosis replaced by USG. However, OCG is still useful for

- Selection of patients for nonsurgical therapy of gallstone disease such as
  - Lithotripsy
  - Bile duct dissolution therapy
- When USG is inconclusive

Immediate Management

Nil by mouth + analgesia

Treatment of Choice

Cefuroxime 1.5 g/8 h IV

In suitable candidates do cholecystectomy (laparoscopic if no question of GB perforation).

39. Female 50-year-old, 5-year history of mild pruritus history of pale stools, dark urine, jaundice.

Diagnosis: Primary biliary cirrhosis (PBC).

Clinchers

- *50-year-old female:* Ninety percent of those affected are women in the age range 40-50 years. It used to be rare but now being diagnosed more frequently in its milder forms.
- *5 years history of mild pruritus:* Pruritus is often the earliest symptom, preceding jaundice by a few years.
- *Pale stools, dark urine, jaundice:* This is a characteristic picture of obstructive jaundice. It signifies a late stage of PBC—the patient is jaundiced with severe pruritus. Pigmented xanthelasma on eyelids or other deposits of cholesterol in the creases of the hands may be seen. Hepatosplenomegaly may be present.

CONFUSA

PBC is usually associated with:

- Autoimmune disorders
  - Sjögren's syndrome
  - Scleroderma
  - Rheumatoid arthritis
- Keratoconjunctivitis sicca (dry eyes and mouth) is seen in 70% of cases
- Renal tubular acidosis
- Membranous glomerulonephritis

Mitochondrial antibodies (measured routinely by ELISA—in titres more than 1: 160) are present in over 95% of patients. M2 antibody is specific. Other nonspecific antibodies (e.g. ANA and SMA) may also be present.

Investigation of Choice

- *Screening:* ELSIA for mitochondrial antibodies
- *Definitive:* Liver biopsy

Immediate Management

USG (in a jaundiced patient, extrahepatic biliary obstruction should be excluded)

Treatment of Choice

Symptomatic:

- Pruritus: colestyramine
- Diarrhoea: codeine phosphate
- Malabsorption: prophylactic fat soluble vitamin supplements
  - In case serum bilirubin > 100 μmol/L—consider liver transplantation.

40. Man with history of haemochromatosis and alcohol addiction presents with jaundice, ascites, variceal bleed. USG is unequivocal, high ferritin level.

Diagnosis: Hereditary haemochromatosis (HHC)

Clinchers

- *Mass:* Middle-aged males are more frequently and severely affected than women.
- *Haemochromatosis:* HHC is one of the most common inherited (autosomal recessive) single gene disorders in northern Europeans.
- *Alcohol addiction:* The course of the disease depends on a number of factors including sex, dietary iron intake, presence of associated hepatoxins (especially alcohol) and genotype.
- *USG unequivocal:* USG will not demonstrate anything significant. A liver biopsy is definitive (with Perl's stain).
- *High ferritin level:* Serum ferritin is elevated, usually >500 µg/L or 240 nmol/L.

CONFUSA

Haemochromatosis tend to present about 10 years later in females than males on the menstrual blood loss is protective. So while in males, its peak incidence is in middle-ages, in case of females it is usually postmenopausal. Iron overload may be present in alcoholics, but alcohol excess per se does not cause HHC. There is a history of excess alcohol intake in 25% of patients.

Investigation of Choice

- *Screening:*
  - Homozygotes
    - Serum iron (--)
    - Serum ferritin (--)
  - Heterozygotes
    - Serum ferritin (-)
    - Transferrin saturation (-)
- *Definitive*
  - Liver biopsy/MRI

Immediate Management

Manage cirrhotic symptoms

Treatment of Choice

Venesection routinely

If venesection not tolerated, chelation therapy.

62. A 41-year-old Londoner developed a temperature of 41°C, 5 weeks after cadaveric renal transplantation. WBC is 2.1 × 1,000,000,000/L, Hb is 8.8 g/dl, creatinine 177 µmol/L. Aspartate aminotransferase (AST) 82 U/L. Alanine aminotransferase (ALT) 132 U/L.

Diagnosis: Cytomegalovirus (CMV) disease.

Clinchers

- *41-year-old Londoner:* CMV has worldwide distribution with London being no exception.
- *Temperature of 41°C:* In transplant recipients on post bone marrow transplantation, CMV present with: fever > pneumonitis > colitis > hepatitis > retinitis. In AIDS, it presents with: retinitis > colitis > CNS defects.
- *After cadavaric renal transplantation:* CMV can be acquired by direct contact, blood transfusion or organ transplantation. Transmission following organs transplantation or blood transfusion is due to silent infection in these tissues. It can well be a CMV reactivation syndrome, developed when T cell (lymphocyte) mediated immunity is compromised after organ transplantation, or in association with lymphoid neoplasms and certain acquired immunodeficiencies (in particular: HIV).
- *WBC is 2.1 × 1000,000,000/L:* Normal range is between 4-11 × 1000,000,000/L. Leukopenia is commonly seen with CMV infection in immunocompromised.
- *Aspartate transaminase (AST) of 82 IU/L:* Normal range of AST is 3-35 IU/L. This show the LFT is deranged. Hepatitis is a common syndrome associated with CMV.
- *Alanine aminotransferase (ALT) of 132 IU/L:* Normal range of ALT is 3-35 IU/L. This shows LFT is deranged. Hepatitis is a common syndrome associated with CMV.

Variety of syndromes associated with CMV are fever, and leukopenia, hepatitis, pneumonitis, esophagitis, gastritis, colitis and retinitis.

CONFUSA

Most primary CNV infections in organ transplant recipients result from transmission of the virus in the graft itself.

Investigation of Choice

Isolation of the virus together with rise in antibody titers a fourfold and greater.

Immediate Management

Retinoscopy to exclude CMV retinitis.

Treatment of Choice Ganciclovir IV

117. Immunization of sewage workers.

Diagnosis: To decrease risk of hepatitis A.

Clinchers

Hepatitis A spreads by faecal-oral route, so sewage workers are at special risk. Active immunization against hepatitis A is available and very effective. It is made from an inactivated protein derived from hepatitis A virus.

Dose: If > 16 years, 1 IM dose (1 mL to deltoid) gives immunity for 1 year (10 years if booster is given at 6 months).

Note: Trade name of hepatitis A vaccine in UK.

- Havrix monodose.

  Passive immunization is with normal human Ig. It gives less than 3 months immunity to those at acute risk, i.e.
- Travellers
- Household contacts

CONFUSA

Sewage workers are also at risk of leptospirosis as its spread is by contact with infected rat urine. But there is no effective vaccination against it.

Investigation of Choice

IgG antibody (presence signifies previous infection).

Immediate Management

Rule out recent exposure. If present give immunoglobulin.

Treatment of Choice

Vaccination.

Your notes:

120. Immunization of hepatitis B, besides preventing hepatitis B also prevents.

Diagnosis: Reduction in risk of hepatocellular carcinoma.

Clinchers

- *Immunization of hepatitis B:* Hepatitis B vaccine (Engerix B) is given as a 1 mL dose into deltoid and is repeated at 1 and 6 months (child: 0.5 mL x 3 into anterolateral thigh). Now it is given to everyone in UK. The immunocompromised may need more boosters.
- *Besides preventing hepatitis B also prevents:* Since chronic viral hepatitis (HBV, HCV) also causes hepatocellular carcinoma in the long run, the hepatitis B vaccine is preventive against it also.

CONFUSA

Anti HBs serology advice in UK is different from rest of the world. Please note:

Anti HBs	Actions and comments
> 1000 IU/L	Retest in 4 years
100-1000 IU/L	Retest in 1 year
< 100 IU/L	Given booster and retest
< 10 IU/L	Non-responder, give booster and retest if still < 10, get consent to check hepatitis B status

Investigation of Choice

Anti HBs serology.

Immediate Management

See previous question.

Treatment of Choice

See previous question.

Your notes:

11 Infectious Diseases

PAPER 1

Serial No. 61

Subject: Medicine

Topic: Infectious Diseases (Coloured Slide)

Question: A 4-year-old boy presents with fever, photophobia and neck stiffness. He has multiple petechial lesions scatterd throughout his body.

Diagnosis: Meningococcal septicaemia

Clinchers

- *4-year-old boy:* Children younger than 4 years have the highest risk of developing meningococcal disease. Neonates are often resistant to disease because passively acquired maternal immunoglobulin G antibodies are present until approximately age 6 months.
- *Fever, photophobia, neck stiffness:* This is signifying meningitis. Meningococci are the most common cause of bacterial meningitis in UK.
- *Multiple petechial lesions:* Cutaneous manifestations of meningococcaemia are common, petechiae being the most common sign, occurring in 50-60% of patients with meningococcaemia. These are most often located on the extremities and trunk but may progress to involve any part of the body.

CONFUSA

Fatal meningococcaemia can occur even in previously immunised individuals, because immunisation is available only against strains A and C of this bacteria, however strain B is most often implicated in meningococcal meningitis.

Only close contacts (including nursery contacts) and those who had history of kissing patient's mouth are eligible for rifampicin prophylaxis.

Investigation of Choice

Lumbar Puncture (unless contraindicated).

If in doubt about raised intracranial tension, do a CT head first.

If LP cannot be done, go for blood cultures.

Immediate Management

If patient very unwell start empirical therapy immediately

Fluid resuscitation

Transfer to intensive care unit.

Treatment of Choice

Cefotaxime or ceftriaxone are 1st line drugs

2nd line: Benzylpenicillin or chloramphenicol

Your notes:

PAPER 2

Serial No 142

Subject: Medicine

Topic: Infection

Question: A 12-year-old girl is brought to Accident and Emergency department by her parents complaining of a persistent rash, photophobia, and neck pain.

Diagnosis: Meningococcal Meningitis

Clinchers

- *A 12-year-old girl:* Meningococcal meningitis is the most common form of pyogenic meningitis in the UK, usually affecting children under 5 years of age. However, no age is an exception.
- *Persistent rash, photophobia, and neck pain:* While photophobia and neck pain can occur in any CNS infections, the presence of rash is typically suggesting meningococcal meningitis, which occurs due to rapid spread of the infection into the circulation resulting in a fulminating septicemia and rash.

CONFUSA

The Glass tumbler test is one of the most commonly used test for initial diagnosis of the meningococcal meningitis. The aim is to teach mothers to identify any hemorrhagic rash on her children and thus increase the possibility of early identification and thus decreasing the mortality rates.

The basis of the test is- If a glass tumbler is pressed firmly against this haemorrhagic rash, the rash will not fade, and will remain visible through the glass.

Investigation of Choice

Lumbar puncture (rule out the signs of increased ICP before attempting Lumbar puncture).

If raised ICP, do a blood culture instead.

Immediate Management

Urgent referral

Treatment of Choice

Benzylpenicillin is the drug of choice.

The first dose should be administered by the general practitioner before transfer to hospital.

Your notes:

Serial No. 146

Subject: Surgery

Topic: Infectious Diseases

Question: A 40-year-old lady from Asia with lumps in her neck, FNAC of which revealed center of casseous material with granulomas, surrounded by fibrosis.

Diagnosis: Tuberculous lymphadenopathy

Clinchers

- *A 40-year-old lady:* Tuberculosis more commonly flares up in elderly, however, it can affect almost any age. Female: Male ratio is 2: 1 It is commoner amongst the homeless, drug addicts and alcoholics.
- *From Asia:* Countries of Asia such as India, China, Indonesia, Pakistan and Bangladesh have the largest number of cases. Recently there have been striking increases in the number of cases in the former Soviet Union and in sub-Saharan Africa also. Migration from these highly endemic area predisposes an individual for infection.
- *With lumps in her neck:* Cervical tuberculous lymphadenitis or scrofula classically presents as painless enlarging persistent mass in the neck. Associated systemic symptoms like low grade fever, weight loss and malaise can also be present.
- *FNAC of which revealed center of casseous material with graunolmas. surrounded by fibrosis:* This is the classical description of infection by tuberculosis. Caseating graulomas are almost diagnostic, however, demonstration of acid-fast bacilli (AFB) is required for a definitive diagnosis.

CONFUSA

As TB is an AIDS-defining illness, current guidelines state that it may be appropriate to offer HIV testing to patients if they are from an area or background with increased risk of HIV co-infection.

Note that lymphoma can also present as cervical lymphadenopathy, low grade fever and weight loss. Histological diagnosis would be definitive.

In the developed world, the disease is more common in some sections of society, e.g. alcoholics, undernourished, ethnic communities, the elderly, and HIV+ve individuals.

The disease is also more common in patients after gastrectomy for peptic ulcer.

Investigation of Choice

Excision biopsy

Immediate Management

- All patients should be referred for specialist advice and management usually involving a team approach including Consultant and specialist nurses.
- Disease Notification is compulsory under the Public Health Act 1984. This will trigger contact tracing and provide surveillance data. Usually this is initiated by the Specialist or doctor initiating treatment.

Treatment of Choice

Antituberculous Therapy

Your notes:

PAPER 3

30. A 27-year-old girl reliably on oral contraceptives develops a high white cell count, fever and a malodourous vaginal discharge.

Diagnosis: Staphylococcal toxic shock syndrome (TSS)

Clinchers

- *A 27-year-old girl:* Tampon use is more prevalent in 20's and 30's when active life style is more common.
- *Reliably on oral contraceptives:* OCP reduces the overall risk and incidence of PID (except monoilial vaginitis, whose risk it may increase).
- *High white cell count:* It signifies a systemic dissemination of the infection (It is absent in monoilial vaginitis until and unless the patient is immunocompromised).
- *Fever:* It also suggests a systemic dissemination of infection which is always present in TSS.
- *Malodourous vaginal discharge:* A retained tampon almost always produce an offensive discharge (In monoilial vaginitis there may be a yeasty smell).

CONFUSA

It is a somewhat tricky question and the best answer among in given options is TSS. But it could be a severe episode of simple PID also (remember OCPs reduce its incidence but not nullify it, i.e. they can occur).

Investigation of Choice

Blood culture/tampon culture.

Immediate Management

Resuscitation should be commenced immediately with oxygen and fluids.

Treatment of Choice

Antistaphylococcal therapy (flucloxacillin).

Your notes:

65. Tuberculosis.

Diagnosis: Already stated as the question.

Clinchers

GMC usually does not ask such one word questions. Most probably the person who has recapitulated these questions could not remember the clinical situations. Anyway, tuberculosis is a frequent topic and is almost invariably associated with south east asian immigrants (only in GMC questions). The other GMC 'clinchers' that appear routinely are:

- *Skin TB:* (lupus vulgaris), apple jelly nodules especially on face and neck.
- *Addison's disease:* Secondary to TB.
- *TB meningitis:* Subacute, CSF protein increase, fever
- *Bazin's disease:* Skin TB with localized areas of fat necrosis with ulceration and an indurated rash, characteristically on adolescent girl's legs.
- *Pulmonary TB:* Cough, sputum, haemoptysis, pleural effusion, chronic symptoms.

CONFUSA

Contact lens staining is an indirect and confusing side effect of antitubercular therapy. It occurs due to orange discolouration of tears (and other body fluids like sweat and urine) by rifampicin.

Investigation of Choice

- *Screening:* Mantoux test.
- *Definitive:* Sputum culture (AFB +)

Immediate Management

Rule out any immunodeficiencies (i.e. HIV, malignancy, DM, steroid treatment, debilitation).

Treatment of Choice

First 8 weeks: Rifampicin + Isoniazid + Pyrazinamide ± Ethambutol

Then for 4 months: Rifampicin + Isoniazid

- Give pyridoxine throughout treatment
- Give steroids also in meningeal and pericardial TB.

Your notes:

66. A middle-aged man has recently been operated after sustaining a perforated gallbladder. He becomes increasingly comatose and on examination is noted to have peripheral warming.

Diagnosis: Hyperdynamic (warm) septic shock

Clinchers

- *Middle-aged man:* Gallbladder perforation can be due to gallstones or trauma. Irrespective of aetiology, the thing to be ketp in mind is that bile is not a sterile fluid and contains many bacteria (Ref: Love and Bailey, 23rd edn, pg 1300).
- *Recently been operated after sustaining a perforated gall-bladder:* Peritonitis or suppurative biliary conditions predispose to serious gram-negative infections leading to hyperdynamic septic shock.
- *Becomes increasingly comatose:* Generalised capillary leakage and other fluid losses lead to severe hypovolemia with reduced cardiac output, tachycardia and vasoconstriction. The systemic infection induces cardiac depression, pulmonary hypertension, pulmonary edema and hypoxia and make him increasingly drowsy.
- *Have peripheral warming:* Initially the patient has abnormal or increased cardiac output with tachycardia and a warm, dry, skin.

CONFUSA

The patient can become cold and clammy, if severe sepsis or endotoxaemia is allowed to persist. In that case the condition may be overlooked by untrained minds.

Investigation of Choice

Blood cultures.

Immediate Management

High concentration O_2 + vigorous fluid resuscitation.

Treatment of Choice

Antibiotics IV.

Your notes:

68. A 64-year-old patient on the surgical ward has been operated on for a hernia, he presents with warm extremities and a blood pressure of 90/60 mmHg.

Diagnosis: Septic shock.

Clinchers

- *Operated on for a hernia:* Gram-negative shock is common after colonic, biliary and urological surgery and with infected severe burns.
- *Warm peripherals:* The principal effect of endotoxins is to cause vasodilatation of the peripheral circulation together with increased capillary permeability. Initially this produces warm peripheries but later on the peripheries can be cold (thereby making the differentiation difficult).
- *BP 90/60 mmHg:* Any shock results in inadequate organ perfusion. Sepsis induces hypotension usually results from a generalised maldistribution of blood flow and blood volume and from hypovolemia due to diffuse capillary leak. In septic shock the BP is < 90 mmHg systolic or 40 mmHg less than patient's normal BP and is unresponsive to fluid resuscitation.

CONFUSA

Risk factors for gram-positive bacteremia include the presence of intravascular catheters or mechanical devices, burns and IV drug use.

Investigation of Choice

Blood culture and Gram stain.

Immediate Management

Colloid/crystalloids IVI + refer to ITU for monitoring ± ionotropes (e.g. dopamine in 'renal' dose of 2-5 μg/kg/min IVI).

Treatment of Choice

This is a case of intra-abdominal sepsis. The standard treatment for it is,

Cefuroxime + metronidazole (both IV)

Your notes:

81. Immunisation of health workers who are in contact with body fluid.

Diagnosis: Risk of hepatitis B

Clinchers

- *Health workers:* Health workers should be particularly immunised against hepatitis B vaccine as its seroconversion rate after accidental exposure are dangerously high (much more than HIV). Now the protocol is to immunise everyone (and not just health workers) for hepatitis B vaccine in UK. The past strategy of vaccinating at risk gropus—health workers, IV drug abusers, homosexual, haemodialysis patients have been unsuccessful here.
- *Who are in contact with body fluid:* Body fluid can transmit many infections of which hepatitis B, hepatitis C and HIV are of not. Of these hepatitis B has maximum potential of seroconversion but because of its effective screening and immunisation, the incidence of hepatitis C is on the rise.

CONFUSA

Older age, smoking and male sex correlates to low antibody levels even after immunisation against hepatitis B vaccine. So time boosters with serology. Often there are cases of nonresponders to the vaccine. If the question is about social worker, then hepatitis A vaccine (Havrix Monodose) would have been the answer.

Investigation of Choice

Anti-HBs status (positive in vaccinated or after recovery).

Immediate Management

Universal precautions.

Treatment of Choice

Passive immunisation (specific anti-HBV immunoglobulin) may be given to nonimmune contacts after high risk exposure).

Your notes:

82. Immunisation of hepatitis B, besides preventing hepatitis B also prevents.

Diagnosis: Reduction in risk of hepatocellular carcinoma.

Clinchers

- *Immunisation of hepatitis B:* Hepatitis B vaccine (Engerix B) is given as a 1 ml dose into deltoid and is repeated at 1 and 6 months (child: 0.5 ml x 3 into anterolateral thigh). Now it is given to everyone in UK. The immunocompromised may need more boosters.
- *Besides preventing hepatitis B also prevents:* Since chronic viral hepatitis (HBV, HCV) also causes hepatocellular carcinoma in the long run, the hepatitis B vaccine is preventive against it also.

CONFUSA

Anti-HBs serology advice in UK is different from rest of the world. Please note:

Anti-HBs	Actions and comments
> 1000 IU/L	Retest in 4 years
100-1000 IU/L	Retest in 1 year
< 100 IU/L	Given booster and retest
< 10 IU/L	Non-responder, give booster and retest if still < 10, get consent to check hepatitis B status

Investigation of Choice
Anti HBs serology.

Immediate Management
See previous question.

Treatment of Choice
See previous question.

Your notes:

84. Counselling for intravenous (IV) drug users to use needle exchange facilities.

Diagnosis: To decrease risk of hepatitis B

Clinchers

IV drug user: They constitute a risk group of hepatitis B infection. Other risk groups are:

- Health workers
- Haemophiliacs
- Hemodialysis patients
- Sexually promiscuous
- Homosexual

It is endemic in:

- Far east
- Africa
- Mediterranean

Hepatitis B spread by:

- Direct contact—common in African children
- Vertical transmission—common in Asia

CONFUSA

IV drug users are also at risk for HIV and if would have been a better choice as an answer (if given in the list of options) since hepatitis B can be more effectively prevented by vaccination. Also there is controversy over the extent to which addicts should be supplied with clear needles.

Investigation of Choice
Anti-HBs (presence signifies vaccination).

Immediate Management
Notify home office (required by law in UK).

Treatment of Choice
Motivation for a proper deaddiction.

Your notes:

85. Immunisation of sewage workers.

Diagnosis: To decrease risk of hepatitis A.

Clinchers

Hepatitis A spreads by faecal-oral route, so sewage workers are at special risk. Active immunisation against hepatitis A is available and very effective. It is made from an inactivated protein derived from hepatitis A virus.

Dose: If > 16 years, 1 IM dose (1 mL to deltoid) gives immunity for 1 year (10 years if booster is given at 6 months).

Note: Trade name of hepatitis A vaccine in UK.

- Havrix monodose.

  Passive immunisation is with normal human Ig. It gives less than 3 months immunity to those at acute risk, i.e.
  - Travellers
  - Household contacts

CONFUSA

Sewage workers are also at risk of leptospirosis as its spread is by contact with infected rat urine. But there is no effective vaccination against it.

Investigation of Choice

IgG antibody (presence signifies previous infection).

Immediate Management

Rule out recent exposure. If present give immunoglobulin.

Treatment of Choice

Vaccination.

Your notes:

97. A 26-year-old heroin addict is worried because her partner has been diagnosed as having HIV infection. She is HIV negative. She does not feel able to stop using heroin currently.

Clinchers

- *Heroin addict:* Heroin is usually taken IV by drug addicts.
- *Her partner has been diagnosed as having HIV infection:* This makes her very susceptible for HIV infection because they might be sharing needles.
- *Is HIV negative:* Usually HIV antibodies do not appear in blood till three months. A PCR antigen test is required to detect early infection after exposure. So HIV negative status is dependent on the type of test she has undergone. If it was ELISA then she need another testing after three months to completely rule out the infection.
- *She does not feel able to stop using heroin currently:* It is the duty of the doctor to counsel and convince her for deaddiction. But the first priority is to eurol her in a needle exchange programme to decrease her risk of exposure to HIV, hepatitis B and C.

CONFUSA

Narcotic withdrawal is dangerous in patients with heart disease, tuberculosis or other debilitating conditions.

Investigation of Choice

ELISA for HIV after three months.

Immediate Management

Counselling.

Treatment of Choice

Enrolment in needle exchange programme.

Your notes:

133. A 14-year-old boy presents with drowsiness and generalised headache. He is recovering from a bilateral parotitits. His CT scan is normal.

Diagnosis: Viral meningitis (aseptic meningitis)

Clinchers

- *A 14-year-old boy:* Mumps is generally a childhood disease caused by RNA paramyoxovirus. Incidence of meningitis in males is three times more after mumps.
- *Drowsiness and generalised headache:* There are cardinal symptoms of increased ICP. Other symptoms can be:
  - Irritability
  - Vomiting
  - Fits
  - Bradycardia
  - BP increase
  - Impaired consciouness (confusion)
  - Coma
  - Irregular respiration
  - Papilloedema (late sign)
- *Recovering from bilateral parotitis:* Meningitis secondary to mumps usually occur in convalescent phase. Mumps is characterised by painful swelling of the parotids, unilaterally at first, becoming bilateral in 70%.
- *CT scan is normal:* Rules out any space occupying lesion in the brain or ventricular dilatation, both of which are contraindication to lumbar puncture.

CONFUSA

In aseptic meningitis, CSF has cells but is Gram stain negative and no bacteria can be cultured on standard media. Mumps infection confers life-long immunity, so a documented history of previous infection excludes this diagnosis.

Investigation of Choice

- *Screening:* Lumbar puncture, will show a picture of aseptic meningitis
- *Definitive:* Isolation of virus from CSF.

Immediate Management

Symptomatic (hospital admission usually not required).

Treatment of Choice

Bed-rest in a quiet and dark room.

Your notes:

134. An intravenous drug abuser presents with suspected meningitis. The organism is confirmed in the CSF by India ink preparation.

Diagnosis: Cryptococcal meningitis.

Clinchers

- *IV drug abuser:* He must be having an undiagnosed HIV infection resulting in immunodeficient state. Cryptococcal meningitis does not occur in immunocompetant people.
- *Suspected meningitis:* CNS infections in HIV positive people are usually by toxoplasmosis, CMV and *Cryptococcus.* Toxoplasmosis causes a SOL and CMV causes encephalitis. *Cryptococcus* is associated with meningitis usually.
- *Organism confirmed in CSF in India Ink preparation:* This is characteristic of *Cryptococcus neoformans* (a fungi) whose thick capsule resist staining and can only be demonstrated as translucencies against black background in India ink preparations.

CONFUSA

Cryptococcal meningitis have an insidious onset and is often without neck stiffness. The etiology of neck stiffness is inflammation and it is often absent in immunodeficients and neonates. Conditions (other than meningitis) which can produce neck stiffness are *Shigella* gastroenteritis and subarachnoid haemorrhage.

Investigation of Choice

India ink staining of CSF.

or

Detection of cryptococcal antigen in blood/CSF.

Immediate Management

Transfer to ITU.

Treatment of Choice

Amphotericin/fluocytosine IV

Fluconazole can be given in milder cases (better tolerated).

Your notes:

135. An anxious mother called you to say that her son's best friend in school has caught meningitis.

Diagnosis: Immediate 'contact' of meningitis.

Clinchers

Meningitis prophylaxis:

Talk to your consultant in community disease control. Offer prophylaxis is:

- Household/nurser contacts (i.e. within droplet range)
- Those who have kissed the patient's mouth.

CONFUSA

If the student suffering from meningitis is just a classmate and the best friend of her son, then there is no need of any chemoprophylaxis.

Investigation of Choice

None required except screening the skin for any nonblanching petechiae.

Immediate Management

Reassure mother

Treatment of Choice

Rifampicin prophylaxis

- 600 mg/12 h PO for 2 days
- Children > 1 yr 10 mg/kg/12 h
  < 1 yr 10 mg/kg/12 h

  or

  Ciprofloxacin
- 500 mg PO, 1 dose, adult only

Your notes:

178. A 23-year-old male prostitute develops severe chest pain. This area of chest pain corresponds to an area with an erythematous rash.

Diagnosis: Herpes Zoster (shingles)

Clinchers

- *Male prostitute:* Undiagnosed HIV infection may be present (acquired as a professional hazard) which has caused reactivation of the Herpes virus lying dormant in ganglion cells. The etiology of the primary herpes infection can also be similar.
- *Severe chest pain:* Pain heralds infection and may precede the development of vesicles by 48-72 hrs. It is severe and burning in character. Thoracic dermatomes and ophthalmic division of trigeminal are most vulnerable.
- *Pain corresponds to an area with an erythematous rash:* Herpes zoster is characterised by a unilateral vesicular eruption within a dermatome accompanied by severe local pain. Vesicles start as erythematous maculopapules.

CONFUSA

Motor nerves are rarely affected in shingles and almost all the symptoms are sensory. Other high risk group for shingles are elderly people.

Investigation of Choice

- Rarely necessary for shingles
- HIV seropositivity tests (after consent)

Immediate Management

Aciclovir (start as early as possible) + refer to pain clinic.

Treatment of Choice

- Pain—oral analgesic or low dose amitriptyline
- Virus—Aciclovir
- Post-herpetic neuralgia prophylaxis—4 week course of prednisolone.

Your notes:

PAPER 4

33. A 10-year-old boy is drowsy, febrile with a rash.

Diagnosis: Meningococcal meningitis.

Clinchers

- *A 10-year-old boy:* It is an increase in UK and is most common seen in young children. It is also the commonest cause of death from infectious disease in UK. In recent years, there has been a marked rise in incidence in young people aged 15 to 24 and the case fatality in this age group is twice as high as that in children under five.
- *Drowsy:* In meningococcal meningitis photophobia and neck stiffness are relatively unusual features; the most common symptoms are fever, malaise and drowsiness. Although meningism, if present, is associated with a worse prognosis.
- *Febrile:* It is due to bacteremia and is a very common symptom.
- *Rash:* The characteristic purpuric skin rash can be found in over 70% of cases of meningococcal septicaemia if a careful examination is made.

CONFUSA

The rash may not be purpuric in the early stages of the disease (it may be macular initially). A rapid increase in the distribution of the purpura is often associated with circulatory failure. In children, always screen for ICP increase. If raised, do not do a lumbar puncture. All children with raised ICP with require intubation and ventilation to control the $PaCO_2$.

Investigation of Choice

Lumbar puncture (after a preliminary CT to rule out ICP-).

Immediate Management

Benzyl penicillin IM (as soon as possible—before everything).

Treatment of Choice

Benzyl penicillin slow IV
Dexamethasone and mannitol if raised ICP.

Your notes:

101. Girl goes into a forest, remembers getting bitten by a tick, redness near the bite is slowly increasing in size.

Diagnosis: Erythema chronicum migraines (Lyme disease).

Clinchers

- *Forest:* Lyme's disease spreading ticks (on deer and sheep) are widespread in the UK, particularly in the forests and woodlands.
- *Bitten by tick:* Although not every person remember getting bitten by a tick, any history of tick bite in a forest should arouse suspicion of Lyme disease. It is transmitted by ixodes dammini or related ixodid ticks (Iodes ricinus in Europe).
- *Redness near the bite is slowly increasing in size:* Erythema chronicum migraine is the rash of Lyme disease, and typically manifests as singular or multiple annular plaques. It presents as an annular rash with central clearing. It gradually increases in size with central clearing. Untreated rash usually fade within 3 months but may recur. May be multiple.

CONFUSA

Lyme's disease was originally described in Lyme, connecticut, but is now known to occur in many parts of USA, Europe and in Australia. Differential features from other erythemas is as follows:

- Erythema nodosum—painful, red, raised
- Erythema marginatum—pink coalescent rings
- Erythema multiforme—target lesions.

Investigation of Choice

Serology (if negative, do PCR).

Immediate Management

Advice regarding protection from ticks.

Treatment of Choice

Doxycycline 100 mg/12 hr PO her for 10-21 days (Amoxicillin or penicillin V if < 12 years).

Your notes:

102. A policeman bite on his hand by a heroin addict while arresting him. He comes to the A and E, on examination, a deep wound seen on his hand.

Diagnosis: Human bite

Clinchers

- *Bite by heroin addict:* As the most common mode of taking heroin is intravenous, he is most probably an IV drug abuser. Such person carries highest risk for hepatitis B or HIV because of needle sharing.
- *Deep wound on hand:* A deep wound is more dangerous as infection can reach the deep space of the hand, including the bone, joint and tendons. Moreover lacerations to hand tendons can also be present which can produce functional deficits.

CONFUSA

HIV and hepatitis B virus have both been reported to be transmitted by human bite, but these instances appear to be quite rare (837, Harrisons, 14th edn). HIV serology can be done if suspicion is there (as in this case) but wound culture and Gram staining is absolutely essential in every case. Suspicious human bite wounds should provoke careful questioning regarding domestic or child abuse. Human bite infections are usually more dangerous than other animal bites (because of diverse flora or human mouth) and upto 50% infecting organisms in human bite produces β-lactamares.

Investigation of Choice

Wound swab ± hepatitis B serology ± HIV serology

Immediate Management

Bite injuries to the hand warrant consultation with a hand surgeon for the assessment of tendon, nerve and muscular damage. So get its opinion.

+

Ensure tetanus prophylaxis

Treatment of Choice

Amoxicillin

+

Clavulinic acid

Your notes:

103. A 18-month-old baby, drowsy, febrile, headache, CT normal.

Diagnosis: Meningitis

Clinchers

- *18-month-old:* This age has a significance in meningitis as neck stiffness (inability to kiss knees) is often absent if < 18-month-old.
- *Drowsy:* It is a sing of increased intracranial pressure and if found in meningitis. Other signs of increased ICP are:
  - Irritability
  - Vomiting
  - Tense fontanelle
  - Preherniation
- *Febrile:* It is a "septic sign" of meningitis and signifies bacteremia. Other septic signs can be:
  - Arthritis
  - Odd behaviour
  - Rashes
  - Cyanosis
  - DIC
  - Pulse increased
  - BP decreased
  - Tachypnoea
  - WCC increased
- *Headache:* Can be due to both ICP and - meningitis per se.

CONFUSA

Do not expect only petechiae in meningococcal disease as it can present with any rash. Rash or skin lesions in meningococcal infection signifies a bacteremia which may well be absent sometimes. Always do a CT exam to rule out inappropriately raised ICP (evident by ventriculomegaly) or a space occupying lesion first. Only then proceed to do lumbar puncture (LP). If LP carries a risk of inadvertent herniation of brain if done in setting of severely increased ICP. (But in neonates preliminary CT is incapable of showing that LP would be safe). If LP is contraindicated (i.e. focal neurological signs, DIC, increase ICP) and you are suspecting meningococcal disease (i.e. purpura is present), blood culture would be a better option.

Investigation of Choice

Lumbar puncture

Immediate Management

Give penicillin 50 mg/kg at once before anything.

Treatment of Choice

Start a broad spectrum antibiotic (i.e. cefotaxime) if CSF is cloudy. Change according to CSF culture and sensitivity report.

- Meningococcus—Benzyl penicillin
- Pneumococcus—Cefotaxime
- Hemophilus—Cefotaxime/chloramphenicol.

Your notes:

148. Man after large bowel resection and ileostomy is septicaemic.

Diagnosis: Septicaemia

Clinchers

➢ *Large bowel resection and ileostomy:* GI surgeries especially resections produce a hyperkalemic state which produces adynamic bowel for a few days post-operatively. Also after ileostomies, a few days rest to bowel are given to allow the ileostomy to "ripe".

➢ *Septicemic:* In any septicemic condition, enteral feeding is usually not given as there decreased absorption of food from GIT. This is due to decreased tissue perfusion. This produces bloating and abdominal distension.

CONFUSA

Septicemia or localised abscess formations (most common—pelvic abscess) are common after GI surgeries because of high septic load of the intestinal contents.

Investigation of Choice

Blood culture.

Immediate Management

Nasogastric tube to drain contents of stomach.

Treatment of Choice

Intravenous parenteral nutrition.

\+

Antibiotics (broad spectrum initially, thereafter depending upon culture reports).

Your notes:

162. Man returns from Ghana presents with fever with rigors

Diagnosis: Malaria

Clinchers

➢ *Ghana:* Most of the African countries are endemic for malaria. Appropriate malarial prophylaxis should be given for travel to endemic countries.

➢ *Fever with rigors:* Typical presentation of malaria is with fever, rigors, headaches, dizziness, flu like symptoms, diarrhoea and thrombocytopenia. The rule of thumb is to suspect any patient presenting with unexplained fever and rigors with a travel history should be suspected to have malaria until proven otherwise.

CONFUSA

P.ovale has been reported predominantly from east and west Africa P.vivax is the major species in temperate zones, whereas in the topics all forms of malaria are seen. But with present day ease and speed of travel, sporadic cases of malaria are being increasingly recognised. Mosquitoes may stowaway in luggage causing malaria in non-tropical areas.

Investigation of Choice

Thick and thin blood films:

- Thick film—for demonstration of parasite
- Thin film—for identification of parasite
- Two to three blood smears taken each day for three to four days and found to be negative and necessary before a patient is declared malaria free.

Immediate Management

Analgesics and antipyretics are given as necessary. IV fluids may be required to combat dehydration and shock.

Treatment of Choice

Species	*Treatment*	*Resistant to*
P. falciparum	Quinine + tetracycline	Chloroquine
P. vivax/ovale	Chloroquine + Primaquine	-

Note:

- If species unknown treat as *P. falciparum*
  If mixed species
- if doubt over resistance—treat as resistant

176. Man returned from trip to Asia, complains of anorexia, malaise, dark urine, pale stools.

Diagnosis: Hepatitis B (most probably)

Clinchers

- *Trip to Asia:* Hepatitis A is the most common type of viral hepatitis worldwide, often in epidemics. The disease is commonly seen in autumn and affects children and young adults. Spread of infection is mainly by the faecal-oral route and arises from the ingestion of contraminated food or water (e.g. shell-fish). Overcrowding and poor sanitation facilitate spread. It is common in developing countries in Asia.
- *Anorexia malaise:* The viraemia causes the patient to feel unwell with nonspecific symptoms that includes nausea, anorexia and a distaste for cigarettes. Jaundice develops after one or two weeks.
  Note: Many recover at this stage and remain anicetric.
- *Dark urine, pale stools:* As the jaundice deepens, the urine becomes dark and stools pale owing to intra-hepatic cholelithiasis.

CONFUSA

Clinically the differential diagnosis is from all other causes of jaundice—but in particular from other types of viral and drug induced hepatitis. Common cause of jaundice in travellers are:

- Viral hepatitis
- Cholangitis
- Liver abscess
- Leptospirosis
- Typhoid
- Malaria
- Dengue fever
- Yellow fever
- Haemoglobinopathies

Investigation of Choice

Viral serology and LFT

- Serum transaminases rise 22-40 days after exposure
- IgM rises from day 25 and signifies recent infection
- IgG remains detectable for life.

Immediate Management

Symptomatic and advise to avoid alcohol

Notify health authorities as it is a notifiable disease in UK

Treatment of Choice

Supportive

If fulminant hepatitis—interferon

PAPER 5

11. A 35-year-old woman presents with a four-month history of cough, productive of sputum, and recent haemoptysis. She has lost 5 kg in weight. The chest X-ray shows right upper lobe consolidation.

Diagnosis: Tuberculosis

Clinchers

- *A 35-year-old woman:* Reactivation of primary TB occurs in usually mid-adult life (usually acquired in childhood).
- *Four-month history of cough:* Any prolonged history of cough should make one suspicious of TB.
- *Productive of sputum:* Cough in TB is almost always productive and the sputum may be mucoid, purulent or blood-stained.
- *Recent haemoptysis:* It is an regular finding in pulmonary TB.
- *Lost 5 kg weight:* It is due to associated loss of appetite.
- *Right upper lobe consolidation:* The CXR typically shows patchy or nodular shadows in the upper zones, loss of volume and fibrosis with or without cavitation.

CONFUSA

An abnormal CXR is often found with no symptoms in pulmonary TB but pulmonary TB is extremely unlikely in the absence of any radiographic abnormality. The X-ray appearances alone may strongly suggest TB, but every effort must be made to obtain microbiological evidence. A single X-ray does not give an indication of the activity of the disease. Very similar CXR appearances occur in:

- Histoplasmosis
- Cryptococcosis
- Coccidioidomycosis
- Aspergillosis

Investigation of Choice

Sputum microscopy and culture

Immediate Management

Exclude HIV after consent

+

Contact tracing

Treatment of Choice

Anti-TB drug regimen

Your notes:

12. A previously well 18-year-old has had influenzae for the last two weeks. She is deteriorating and has a swinging fever. She is coughing up copious purulent sputum. Chest X-ray shows cavitating lesions.

Diagnosis: *Staphylococcus aureus*

Clinchers

- *Previously well:* Exclude any pre-existing bacterial infection.
- *A 18-year-old: S. aureus* affects all age groups.
- *Has had influenzae for the last two weeks: S. aureus* normally causes a pneumonia only after a preceding influenzae viral illness.
- *Deteriorating:* The infection starts in the bronchi, leading to patchy areas of consolidation in one or more lobes, which break down to form abscesses, and thus the condition deteriorates during the course of infection.
- *Has a swinging fever:* It is due to abscess formation.
- *Copious purulent sputum:* Characteristic of it.
- *Cavitating lesions:* It causes a bilateral cavitating bronchopneumonia.

CONFUSA

Staphylococcal pneumonia may complicate influenza infection or occur in the young, elderly, IV drug users or patients with underlying disease (e.g. leukaemia, lymphoma, cystic fibrosis). It can lead to development of septicaemia with metastatic abscesses in other organs. In IV drug abusers symptoms of septicaemia predominates over the respiratory symptoms.

Investigation of Choice
Sputum culture

Immediate Management
O_2 to maintain $PaO_2 > 8$ kPa

Treatment of Choice
Flucloxacillin

Your notes:

13. A 65-year-old man, currently undergoing chemotherapy for chronic leukemia, has felt unwell with fever and an unproductive cough for two weeks despite treatment with broad spectrum intravenous antibiotics. The chest X-ray shows an enlarging right sided, mid-zone consolidation.

Diagnosis: Fungal pneumonia

Clinchers

- *A 65-year-old man + chemotherapy + chronic leukaemia:* All these factors suggest immunocompromised state which predispose to fungal infections.
- *Felt unwell with fever:* Malaise and pyrexia are usually present.
- *Unproductive cough:* This suggest a non-bacterial cause of the pneumonia.
- *For two weeks despite treatment with broad spectrum antibiotics:* This almost confirms the suspicious of non-bacterial pneumonia.
- *CXR shows an enlarging right sided, mid-zone consolidation:* This is the lung abscess due to fungal infection.

CONFUSA

Candida and Cryptococcus cause pneumonia in the immunosuppressed. Aspergillus gives rise to a widespread invasion of lung tissue in immunocompromised patients. *Pneumocystis carinii* occurs along with AIDS. Other fungal pneumonias can be due to *Actinomyces israelii* and *Nocardia asteroides.*

Investigation of Choice

- *Screening:* CXR
- *Definitive:* Bronchoalveolar lavage (as the cough is unproductive)

Immediate Management
FBC (to evaluate status of leukaemia)

Treatment of Choice
Antifungals

Your notes:

14. A 27-year-old male prostitute has felt generally unwell for two months with some weight loss. Over the last three weeks he has noticed a dry cough with increasing breathlessness. Two courses of antibiotics from his GP has produced no improvement. The chest X-ray shows bilateral interstitial infiltrates.

Diagnosis: Pneumocystitis carinii pneumonia (PCP)

Clinchers

- *A 27-year-old male prostitute:* Strongly suspect AIDS in this patient.
- *Generally unwell for two months:* Malaise and constitutional upset is common with *P. carinii* pneumonia.
- *Weight loss:* This can be both due to AIDS and *P. carinii* infection.
- *Last three weeks:* It usually presents with a prolonged course.
- *Dry cough with increasing breathlessness:* It presents with a dry cough, exertional dyspnoea, fever and bilateral crepitations.
- *Two courses of antibiotics.... no improvement:* Rules out a bacterial course.
- *CXR shows bilateral interstitial infiltrates:* The typical radiographic appearance of PCP is of a diffuse bilateral alveolar and interstitial shadowing beginning in the perihilar regions and spreading out in a butterfly pattern.

CONFUSA

Other CXR appearance of PCP include a localized infiltrate, nodule, cavity or a pneumothorax. In patients receiving aerosolized pentamidine for prophylaxis, infiltrates may be localized to the upper zones. In early infection the CXR is normal but high-resolution CT scans of the chest can demonstrate a characteristic ground-glass appearance even then. Definitive diagnosis rests on demonstrating the organisms in the lungs via bronchoalveolar lavage. As the organism cannot be cultured in vitro it must be directly observed either with silver staining or immunofluorescent techniques.

Investigation of Choice

- *Screening:* CXR
- *Definitive:* Bronchoalveolar lavage

Immediate Management

CD4 lymphocyte count (as PCP is usually not seen until CD4 < 200)

Treatment of Choice

IV co-trimoxazole for 21 days (side effect: typical allergic rash).

15. On return to university, a 20-year-old student presented with the onset of fever, malaise and a dry cough. The student health service gave him amoxycillin. After a week he felt no better and his chest X-ray showed patchy bilateral consolidation.

Diagnosis: *Mycoplasma pneumoniae.*

Clinchers

- *A 20-year-old:* It often occurs in patients in their teens and twenties.
- *On return to university:* It is frequent amongst those living in boarding institutions.
- *Onset of fever, malaise and dry cough:* Generalised features such as headaches and malaise often precede the chest symptoms by 1-5 days. Cough may not be obvious initially and physical signs in the chest may be scanty.
- *Amoxicillin:* It responds to erythromycin or tetracycline but not to amoxycillin. Since after a week, he is not feeling any improvement, our suspicion of mycoplasma is becoming almost certain.
- *Patchy bilateral consolidation:* This is characteristic and confirms our suspicion.

CONFUSA

On CXR, usually only one of the lower lobes is involved but sometimes there may be dramatic shadowing in both lower lobes. There is frequently no correlation between the X-ray appearances and the clinical state of the patient. Complication of *Mycoplasma pneumoniae* can be skin rash (erythema multiforme), Stevens-Johnson syndrome, meningoencephalitis Guillain-Barré syndrome.

Investigation of Choice

Mycoplasma serology

Immediate Management

Rule out extrapulmonary complications

Treatment of Choice

Erythromycin 500 mg QID for 7-10 days
(Alternative: Tetracycline)

Your notes:

50. A 60-year-old with features of septicaemia (warm peripheries, low BP etc.) after an abdominal surgery.

Diagnosis: Postoperative septicaemia

Clinchers

- *A 60-year-old:* Septicaemia is a common postoperative complication among elderly and children because of incomplete immune system
- *Features of septicaemia after an abdominal surgery:* Gram negative septicaemia is particularly seen after colonic, biliary and urological surgery. The principal effect of endotoxins is to cause vasodilatation of the peripheral circulation together with increased capillary permeability. The effects are partly direct, and partly indirect due to activation of normal tissue inflammatory responses such as the complement system and mediators such as tumor necrosis factor.

CONFUSA

Septicaemia is often overlooked as:
- The temperature may not be raised
- The WBC count may be normal or low
- Blood cultures may be negative

The hallmark is impaired tissue perfusion

Investigation of Choice

Blood culture (take sample before starting antibiotics).

Immediate Management

Colloid/crystalloid IVI + refer to ITU for monitoring ± ionotropes.

Treatment of Choice

Cefuroxime 1.5 g/8h IV.

+

Metronidazole 500 mg/6h IV.

Your notes:

79. A mother and her daughter have just returned from a tropical holiday and is concerned that her daughter has an STD, since she complains of constant perianal and vulval irritation. There is no associated vaginal discharge. She has worms coming out of her bottom at night.

Diagnosis: Enterobius vermicularis infection

Clinchers

- *Returning from a tropical holiday:* Suggests improper sanitary conditions while at holiday, conducive to feco-oral transmission of pinworms.
- *Perianal and vulval irritation:* Occurs due to worms coming out of bowel to lay eggs.
- *Worms coming out of bottom at night:* To lays eggs.

CONFUSA

Acrodermatitis enteropathica is due to zinc deficiency, where a perianal rash may occur, although worms would not be seen

Investigation of Choice

Apply sticky take to the perineum and identify eggs microscopically.

Immediate Management

Anti-pruritis.

Treatment of Choice

T. Mebendazole 100 mg PO stat repeated at 2 weeks if $\geq$ 2 years of age.
- Treatment of whole family
- Sanitary hygiene.

Your notes:

86. A 53-year-old nurse complains of facial pain. A week earlier she had a red rash and blisters around her right eye. This area of her face has now become acutely painful.

Diagnosis: Herpes zoster

Clinchers

- *A 53-year-old:* The episodes of herpes zoster become increasingly common with advancing age.
- *Nurse:* This increases the chances of acquiring chickenpox which is the primary cause of herpes zoster.
- *Facial pain:* Pain heralds an acute episode. At least 50% of patients > 50 years old with zoster reports pain months after resolution of instances lesions.
- *Red rash and blisters around her right eye:* Erythematous maculopapules which rapidly evolve into vesicles in the distribution of a dermatome is characteristic of zoster.
- *Acutely painful:* This is acute neuritis which is seen with an acute episode of zoster

CONFUSA

The Tzanck preparation has a sensitivity of only ~60% and does not distinguished varicella, herpes zoster virus from herpes simplex virus infection. Serologic tests include fluorescent antibody to membrane antigen (FAMA) and ELISA. Confirmation is possible with viral isolation in tissue culture VZV takes longer to isolate than HSV.

Investigation of Choice

- *Screening:* FAMA/ELISA
- *Definitive:* Virus isolation in tissue culture

Note: Investigations are not usually required as the diagnosis is clinically easy.

Immediate Management

Analgesia (oral)

Treatment of Choice

Aciclovir for skin lesions

Low dose amitriptyline if pain relief not possible with simple analgesics.

Your notes:

106. A 45-year-old sheep farmer complains of headache, anorexia, muscle and joint pain. He has as 'undulating' fever.

Diagnosis: Brucellosis

Clinchers

- *A 45-year-old sheep farmer:* Brucellosis is a zoonosis and often occurs in workers in close contacts with animals or carcasses. Otherwise spread is largely by ingestion of raw milk from infected cattle or goats.
- *Headache, anorexia, muscle and joint pain:* The onset is insidious, with malaise, headache, weakness, generalized myalgia and night sweats.
- *Undulating fever:* The fever pattern is classically undulant, although continuous and intermittent patterns are frequent.

CONFUSA

Brucellosis has a worldwide distribution. It has been virtually eliminated from cattle in the UK. The organism does not withstand pasteurization. The organisms usually gain entry into the human body via the mouth, though less frequently they may enter via the respiratory tract, genital tract or abraded skin. The bacilli travel in the lymphatics and infect lymph nodes. This is followed by haematogenous spread with ultimate localization of the bacilli in the reticulo-endothelial system.

Investigation of Choice

Blood culture/bone marrow culture

Immediate Management

Take travel history

Treatment of Choice

Doxycycline 100 mg/12 h PO

+

Streptomycin 1 g/day IM for 2-3 weeks.

Your notes:

110. A 67-year-old man has lost 10 kg in weight, over the last 6 months. In addition he has a 5 month history of a productive cough.

Diagnosis: Tuberculosis (TB)

Clinchers

- *A 67-year-old man:* Reactivation of TB is seen in old age debility or immunosuppressed states.
- *Lost 10 kg weight over last 6 months:* It is due to the chronic disease producing a generalised ill health and loss of appetite.
- *5 month history of productive cough:* In the majority of cases, cough eventually develops—perhaps initially non-productive and subsequently accompanied by the production of purulent sputum. Blood streaking of the sputum is frequently documented.

CONFUSA

Physical findings are of limited use in pulmonary tuberculosis. Many patients have no abnormalities detectable by chest examination, while others have detectable rales in the involved areas during inspiration, especially after coughing. Occassionally, ronchi due to partial bronchial obstruction and classical amphrotic breath sounds in areas with large cavities may be heard. The most common haematological findings are mild anaemia and leukocytosis. Hyponatraemia due to SIADH has also been found.

Investigation of Choice
Sputum microscopy and culture

Immediate Management
CXR

Treatment of Choice
Anti TB drug regimen for 6 months.

Your notes:

119. A 30-year-old salesman complains of night sweats and dizziness. His ESR is high and blood sugar is low. He has a normocytic anaemia and sterile pyuria.

Diagnosis: Tuberculosis (Genitourinary)

Clinchers

- *A 30-year-old:* Reactivation of tuberculosis occurs usually in adult life.
- *Salesman:* Since the job profile includes outdoor work and intensive community contact, there is high risk of acquiring communicable diseases.
- *Night sweats and dizziness:* Early in the cause of disease, symptoms and signs are often nonspecific and insidious, consisting mainly of fever and night sweats, weight loss, anorexia, general malaise and weakness.
- *ESR high:* It is an acute phase reactant and is invariably raised (as with almost all chronic diseases).
- *Blood sugar low:* Partly due to loss of appetite and partly due to bacteremia.
- *Normocytic anaemia:* This is the typical anaemia of chronic disease and hence points towards an existing chronic symptomatology.
- *Sterile pyuria:* The documentation of culture-negative pyuria in acidic urine should invariably raise a suspicion of tuberculosis.

CONFUSA

Genitourinary TB accounts for about 15% of all extrapulmonary cases and may involve any portion of GU tract. The kidneys are mainly involved, but it is also a cause of painless, craggy swellings in the epididymis and salpingitis, tubal abscesses and infertility in females. Unlike other systems, in GU infection the local symptoms predominate. Urinary frequency, dysuria, haematuria and flank pain are common presentation although it may be asymptomatic till late in disease.

Investigation of Choice
Culture of three morning urine specimens

Immediate Management
Find out primary foci of infection (as in almost all cases GU tuberculosis is due to haematogenous spread from elsewhere)

Treatment of Choice
Anti TB drug regimen (2+4 months)

128. An obese 29-year-old woman complains of with a cough of two weeks complains of right upper quadrant pain. She is mildly febrile. There was no abdominal tenderness on examination.

Diagnosis: Tuberculosis (TB)

Clinchers

- *Obese:* These is no as such relationship.
- *A 29-year-old woman:* It can occur in any age group although and elderly (> 70 years) are more susceptible.
- *Cough of two weeks:* Prolonged cough without any major systemic manifestations is a strong indicator of TB.
- *RUQ pain:* Although classically TB involves upper lobes, in immunocompromised states it may involve any portion of lung (basilar lobe of right lung in this case).
- *Mildly febrile:* It manifests usually as a vague illness with mid evening rise of temperature.
- *No abdominal tenderness:* This rules out cholecystitis as a differential diagnosis.

CONFUSA

TB can cause disease when there is only minimal immunosuppression and thus often appears early in the course of infection. HIV related TB frequently represents reactivation of latent TB, but there is also clear evidence of newly acquired infection and nosocomial spread in HIV-infected populations. The response of tuberculosis testing is blunted in HIV-positive individuals and is unreliable. Sputum microscopy may be negative even in pulmonary infection and culture techniques are the best diagnostic tools.

Investigation of Choice

Sputum microscopy and culture

Immediate Management

HIV screening in suspected on history

Treatment of Choice

Anti TB therapy.

Your notes:

133. A 14-year-old boy presents with drowsiness and generalised headache. He is recovering from a bilateral parotitits. His CT scan is normal.

Diagnosis: Viral meningitis (aseptic meningitis)

Clinchers

- *A 14-year-old boy:* Mumps is generally a childhood disease caused by RNA paramyoxovirus. Incidence of meningitis in males is three times more after mumps.
- *Drowsiness and generalised headache:* There are cardinal symptoms of increased ICP. Other symptoms can be:
  - Irritability
  - Vomiting
  - Fits
  - Bradycardia
  - BP increase
  - Impaired consciouness (confusion)
  - Coma
  - Irregular respiration
  - papilloedema (late sign)
- *Recovering from bilateral parotitis:* Meningitis secondary to mumps usually occur in convalescent phase. Mumps is characterised by painful swelling of the parotids, unilaterally at first, becoming bilateral in 70%.
- *CT scan is normal:* Rules out any space occupying lesion in the brain or ventricular dilatation, both of which are contraindication to lumbar puncture.

CONFUSA

In aseptic meningitis, CSF has cells but is Gram stain negative and no bacteria can be cultured on standard media. Mumps infection confers life-long immunity, so a documented history of previous infection excludes this diagnosis.

Investigation of Choice

- *Screening:* Lumbar puncture, will show a picture of aseptic meningitis
- *Definitive:* Isolation of virus from CSF.

Immediate Management

Symptomatic (hospital admission usually not required).

Treatment of Choice

Bed-rest in a quiet and dark room.

Your notes:

134. An intravenous drug abuser presents with suspected meningitis. The organism is confirmed in the CSF by India ink preparation.

Diagnosis: Cryptococcal meningitis.

Clinchers

- *IV drug abuser:* He must be having an undiagnosed HIV infection resulting in immunodeficient state. Cryptococcal meningitis does not occur in immunocompetant people.
- *Suspected meningitis:* CNS infections in HIV positive people are usually by toxoplasmosis, CMV and *Cryptococcus.* Toxoplasmosis causes a SOL and CMV causes encephalitis. *Cryptococcus* is associated with meningitis usually.
- *Organism confirmed in CSF in India Ink preparation:* This is characteristic of *Cryptococcus neoformans* (a fungi) whose thick capsule resist staining and can only be demonstrated as translucencies against black background in India ink preparations.

CONFUSA

Cryptococcal meningitis have an insidious onset and is often without neck stiffness. The etiology of neck stiffness is inflammation and it is often absent in immunodeficients and neonates. Conditions (other than meningitis) which can produce neck stiffness are *Shigella* gastroenteritis and subarachnoid haemorrhage.

Investigation of Choice

India ink staining of CSF.

or

Detection of cryptococcal antigen in blood/CSF.

Immediate Management

Transfer to ITU.

Treatment of Choice

Amphotericin/fluocytosine IV

Fluconazole can be given in milder cases (better tolerated).

Your notes:

137. Pseudomembranous colitis (Patient allergic to vancomycin).

Diagnosis: Stated as the question itself

Clinchers

All suspected antibiotics should be discontinued and this alone may result in the diarrheoa stopping. Vancomycin 125 mg orally, QID for 10 days are often used but metronidazole is also effective, considerably it is less expensive and used in cases of vancomycin allergy.

CONFUSA

Relapses are common and toxic dilatation can rarely occur. There is no evidence that changing chemotherapy helps. Patients should be isolated to try to prevent spread to other susceptible individuals. Essentially any antibiotics can cause this syndrome, even metronidazole and vancomycin, which are used to treat the disease.

Investigation of Choice

Stool culture

Immediate Management

Isolation of patient in ward

Treatment of Choice

Metronidazole (Since patient is allergic to vancomycin).

Your notes:

140. Acute streptococcal sore throat (patient allergic to penicillin).

Diagnosis: Stated as the question itself

Clinchers

Streptococcal pharyngitis (Group A, beta-hemolytic) is treated with penicillin G, 200,000 to 250,000 units orally four times a day for 10 days or benzathine penicillin G 600,000 units once IM for patient less than 60 lb in weight and 1.2 million units once IM for patient > 60 lb.

CONFUSA

In penicillin-sensitive individuals, erythromycin, 20 to 40 mg/kg body weight daily in divided oral doses for 10 days is equally effective.

Investigation of Choice

Culture of throat swab

Immediate Management

Exclude liver disease before starting erythromycin treatment

+

Advise warm saline gargles

Treatment of Choice

Erythromycin.

Your notes:

152. A third-year medical student was drawing blood from a known HIV positive patient gets a needle stick injury.

Diagnosis: HIV and hepatitis B risk

Clinchers

- *Third year medical student:* Most of the needle stick injuries occur due to inexperience and faulty specimen collection techniques.
- *Known HIV positive:* HIV risk is less than 0.5% from an accidental percutaneous exposure from a known HIV positive patient.
- *Needle stick injury:* Seroconversion rate following neeld stick injury is about 0.4% for HIV and 30% for hepatitis B if HBeAg positive. The rates are comparatively higher for hollow fore needles.

CONFUSA

UK guidelines for needle stick injuries are:

- Wash well; encourage bleeding; do not suck or immerse in bleach.
- Note name, address and clinical details of 'donor'.
- Report incidence to occupational health and fill in an accident form.
- Store blood from both parties. If possible, ascertain HIV and HBsAg of both. Immunize (active + passive) against hepatitis B at once, if needed. Counsel and test recipient at 3,6 and 8 months (seroconversion may take this long).
- Give 4 weeks of drugs, if possible within 1 hour of exposure:
  - Low risk—no antiviral medication
  - Higher risk—Zidovudine 300 mg/12 h (AZT).

    +

    Lamivudine 150 mg/12 h
  - Worst episodes (i.e. deep) puncture from wide-bore needle cause bleeding)—add indinavir 800 mg/8 h.

Note:

- All drugs to be given PO
- If female, do a pregnancy test before prophylaxis
- Drug choice may change as evidence accrues

Investigation of Choice

HIV antigen testing of recipient.

Immediate Management

Sought prompt expert advise + store blood from both parties.

Treatment of Choice

Combination therapy (see confusa)

153. A healthy 20-year-old pregnant woman whose partner is a hemophiliac.

Diagnosis: Risk of HIV and haemophilia to both woman and her unborn child

Clinchers

Hemophiliacs, especially those diagnosed and treated before mid1980's, have a high-risk of having HIV infection because of the absence of HIV testing for transfusion factors

CONFUSA

It is advisable to motivate every pregnant woman to go for HIV screening as prophylactic AZT and delivery by caesarian section considerably reduce the incidence of vertical transmission from mother to child.

Investigation of Choice

HIV screening (after consent).

Immediate Management

Counselling.

Treatment of Choice

As per the test results (see confusa also).

Your notes:

154. A 28-year-old haemophiliac with a history of 20 previous blood transfusions presents with a dry cough and fever. His chest X-ray shows widespread mottling.

Diagnosis: Pneumocystitis carinii pneumonia

Clinchers

- *A 28-year-old haemophiliac with a history of 20 previous blood transfusions:* It suggests a high-risk of acquisition of HIV infection as he must have been diagnosed before 80's (he is 28 now) and must have received a few transfusions before compulsory HIV screening for transfused blood come in vogue.
- *Dry cough and fever:* Suggestive of a fungal pneunomia.
- *Widspread mottling:* In early infection the CXR is normal but the typical appearances are of bilateral perihilar interstitial infiltrates which can progress to confluent alveolar shadows throughout the lungs.

CONFUSA

After treatment of PCP, long-term secondary prophylaxis is required to prevent relapse, the usual regimen being co-trimoxazole 960 mg thrice-weekly. Patients sensitive to sulphonamide are given either dapsone and pyrimethamine or nebulized pentamidine. The latter only protects the lungs and does not penetrate the upper lobes particularly efficiently; hence if relapses occur on this regimen they may be either atypical or may be extrapulmonary.

Investigation of Choice

- *Screening:* CXR
- *Definitive:* Bronchoalveolar lavage.

Immediate Management

HIV testing

Treatment of Choice

Co-trimoxazole.

Your notes:

155. A 20-year-old sexually active woman who is going to Thailand for a holiday.

Diagnosis: Risk of HIV

Clinchers

Thailand is a country with high rates of HIV positivity. It is advisable for any sexually active traveller to carry his or her own supply of condoms whenever travelling outside the country.

CONFUSA

The practice of safe sex is the most effective way for sexually active uninfected individuals to avoid contracting HIV infection and for infected individuals to avoid spreading infection. Abstinence from sexual relations is the only absolute way to prevent sexual transmission of HIV infection, but it is not practical. Use of condoms, preferably together with the HIV-inhibiting spermicide nonoxynol-9, can markedly decrease the chance of HIV transmission. It should be remembered that condoms are not 100% effective in preventing transmission of HIV infection, and there is an approximately 10 percent failure rate of condoms used for contraceptive purposes. Latex condoms are preferable, since virus has been shown to leak through natural skin condoms. Petroleum-based gels should never be used for lubrication of the condom, since they increase the likelihood of condom rupture.

Investigation of Choice

None required

Immediate Management

Counselling

Treatment of Choice

Advice to carry condoms and practice safe sex.

Your notes:

PAPER 6

41. Man after trip to Asia presents with red, swollen scrotum.

Diagnosis: Epididymo-orchitis

Clinchers

- *Trip to Asia:* He might have caught gonococcal infection from sex workers in Thailand. Or it could be TB also but that needs a primary infection somewhere else.

  Chlamydia can also cause epididymo-orchitis in < 35 years old.
- *Red, swollen scrotum:* The patient will have a very painful swelling of the epididymis, often with a secondary hydrocele and constitutional effects (pyrexia, headaches and leucocytosis). There may be a history of dysuri suggesting a UTI, or urethral discharge suggesting a sexually transmitted organism.

CONFUSA

Examination of urine may reveal the presence of organisms and pus cells, but the urine need not be abnormal. Rectal examination of the prostate may reveal coexistent prostatitis. Always look for urethral discharge in a patient of epididymo-orchitis. A 'first-catch' is more likely to show abnormalities than MSU.

Investigation of Choice

Urethral swab for culture

Immediate Management

Rule out torsion of testis which usually presents like epididymo-orchitis

- If the patient is in his teens, torsion is more likely; if he is in his twenties and sexually active, epidymitis is more likely.
- In torsion the testes lie high in scrotum and pain is a bit worsened by lifting testes (relieved in epididymo-orchitis).

Treatment of Choice

Erythromycin for chlamydia

For others—ciprofloxacin.

Your notes:

116. Not eating sea shell products prevents.

Diagnosis: Hepatitis A

Clinchers

- Sea shell products can transmit the following infections:
  - Hepatitis A: because of unhygienic cooking methods employed. This is the most common infection due to their consumption and the cause is contamination with faecal matter.
  - Vibrio parahaemolyticus—It is a natural resident of sea foods.

CONFUSA

Prevention of hepatitis A
Passive immunization—with normal human immunoglobulin (0.02 ml/kg IM) gives < 3 months immunity to those at risk (travellers, household contacts).
Active immunization—Havrix monodose, an inactivated protein derived from hepatitis A virus.

Investigation of Choice

IgM (rises from day 25)
+
Serum transaminases
(both tests are done to diagnose recent infection)

Immediate Management

Counselling about healthy eating habits, especially for travellers.

Treatment of Choice

If infection occurs—symptomatic.

Your notes:

118. Not swimming in foreign lakes prevents.

Diagnosis: Schistosomiasis prevention (S. hematobium).

Clinchers

- *Foreign lakes:* Schistosomiasis is the most prevalent disease causes by flukes, affecting 200 million people worldwide. The snail vectors release cercariae which can penetrate the skin, e.g. during swimming/paddling, may cause on itchy papular rash ('swimmers itch'). It is not so common in UK reservoirs but is very common in sub Saharan Africa (particularly in lake Malawi), the middle east and Indian ocean.

CONFUSA

Hematospermia is a rare and interesting sign sometimes found in schistosoma hematobium infections.
- Leptospirosis (Weil's disease) is also avoidable by swimming in reservoirs but it is also common in UK and thus the question will not be specific about foreign lakes only.

Investigation of Choice

Finding egg in urine.

Immediate Management

Abdominal X-ray to look for bladder calcification characteristic of chronic infection.

Treatment of Choice

Praziquantel.

Your notes:

119. Immunization of health workers who are in contact with body fluid.

Diagnosis: Risk of hepatitis B

Clinchers

- *Health workers:* Health workers should be particularly immunised against hepatitis B vaccine as its seroconversion rate after accidental exposure are dangerously high (much more than HIV). Now the protocol is to immunise everyone (and not just health workers) for hepatitis B vaccine in UK. The past strategy of vaccinating at risk gropus—health workers, IV drug abusers, homosexual, hemodialysis patients have been unsuccessful here.
- *Who are in contact with body fluid:* Body fluid can transmit many infections of which hepatitis B, hepatitis C and HIV are of not. Of these hepatitis B has maximum potential of seroconversion but because of its effective screening and immunisation, the incidence of hepatitis C is on the rise.

CONFUSA

Older age, smoking and male sex correlates to low antibody levels even after immunisation against hepatitis B vaccine. So time boosters with serology. Often there are cases of nonresponders to the vaccine. If the the question is about social worker, then hepatitis A vaccine (Havrix Monodose) would have been the answer.

Investigation of Choice

Anti-HBs status (positive in vaccinated or after recovery).

Immediate Management

Universal precautions.

Treatment of Choice

Passive immunization (specific anti-HBV immunoglobulin) may be given to nonimmune contacts after high risk exposure).

Your notes:

PAPER 7

36. A young boy back from holiday in north Africa presents with night fever, weight loss. Began on antibiotics with minimal improvement. CSF shows: protein-960 mg/dl, glucose-2 mmol/L, cells-Lymphocytes.

Diagnosis: ZN staining

Clinchers

- *Young boy back from holiday in north Africa:* Africa especially the northern parts are endemic for tuberculosis infection.
- *Night fever and weight loss:* Tubercular meningitis commences with vague headache, low grade evening or night time pyrexia and weight loss due to loss of appetite (anorexia) and vomiting.
- *Began on antibiotics with minimal improvement:* Conventional or common antibiotics have insignificant effect on tubercle bacilli. A specific treatment (INH + Rmp) is required.
- *CSF shows protein—960 mg/dl; glucose—2 mmol/L; cells—lymphocytes:* Tuberculous meningitides have protein in CSF in range of 500-3000 mg/L; glucose < 1/3 blood glucose and 0-200/mm^3 polymorphs.

CONFUSA

Meningitic signs may take some weeks to develop in tubercular meningitis. Cryptococcal meningitis is the main differential diagnosis although syphilis, sarcoidosis and Behcet's syndrome can also cause chronic meningitis.

Investigation of Choice

LP (Now: ZN staining).

Immediate Management

CXR (to rule out pulmonary TB).

Treatment of Choice

At least nine months treatment with anti-TB drugs.

Your notes:

38. A 14-year-old boy presents with drowsiness and generalised headache. He is recovering from a bilateral parotitis. His CT scan is normal.

Diagnosis: Viral meningitis (aseptic meningitis)

Clinchers

- *A 14-year-old boy:* Mumps is generally a childhood disease caused by RNA paramyxovirus. Incidence of meningitis in males is three times more after mumps.
- *Drowsiness and generalised headache:* There are cardinal symptoms of increased ICP. Other symptoms can be:
  - Irritability
  - Vomiting
  - Fits
  - Bradycardia
  - BP increase
  - Impaired consciouness (confusion)
  - Coma
  - Irregular respiration
  - Papilloedema (late sign)
- *Recovering from bilateral parotitis:* Meningitis secondary to mumps usually occur in convalescent phase. Mumps is characterised by painful swelling of the parotids, unilaterally at first, becoming bilateral in 70%.
- *CT scan is normal:* Rules out any space occupying lesion in the brain or ventricular dilatation, both of which are contraindication to lumbar puncture.

CONFUSA

In aseptic meningitis, CSF has cells but is Gram stain negative and no bacteria can be cultured on standard media. Mumps infection confers life-long immunity, so a documented history of previous infection excludes this diagnosis.

Investigation of Choice

- *Screening:* Lumbar puncture, will show a picture of aseptic meningitis
- *Definitive:* Isolation of virus from CSF.

Immediate Management

Symptomatic (hospital admission usually not required).

Treatment of Choice

Bedrest in a quiet and dark room.

Your notes:

39. An intravenous drug abuser presents with suspected meningitis. The organism is confirmed in the CSF by India ink preparation.

Diagnosis: Cryptococcal meningitis.

Clinchers

- *IV drug abuser:* He must be having an undiagnosed HIV infection resulting in immunodeficient state. Cryptococcal meningitis does not occur in immunocompetant people.
- *Suspected meningitis:* CNS infections in HIV positive people are usually by toxoplasmosis, CMV and *Cryptococcus.* Toxoplasmosis causes a SOL and CMV causes encephalitis. *Cryptococcus* is associated with meningitis usually.
- *Organism confirmed in CSF in India Ink preparation:* This is characteristic of *Cryptococcus neoformans* (a fungi) whose thick capsule resist staining and can only be demonstrated as translucencies against black background in India ink preparations.

CONFUSA

Cryptococcal meningitis have an insidious onset and is often without neck stiffness. The etiology of neck stiffness is inflammation and it is often absent in immunodeficients and neonates. Conditions (other than meningitis) which can produce neck stiffness are *Shigella* gastroenteritis and subarachnoid haemorrhage.

Investigation of Choice

India ink staining of CSF.
or
Detection of cryptococcal antigen in blood/CSF.

Immediate Management

Transfer to ITU.

Treatment of Choice

Amphotericin/fluocytosine IV
Fluconazole can be given in milder cases (better tolerated).

Your notes:

99. **Toxoplasmosis**

Diagnosis (Causation): Animal to human

Clinchers

- The principal source of human toxoplasma infection remains uncertain. Transmission usually takes place by oral route and can be attributable to infestion of either sporulated oocysts from contaminated soil or bradyzoites from under cooked meat. During acute feline infection, a cat may excrete as many as 100 million parasites per day. These very stable sporozoite containing oocysts are highly infectious and may remain viable for many years in the soil. Human infected during a well-documented outbreak of oocyst-transmitted infection develop stage-specific antibodies to the oocyst/sporozoite.

CONFUSA

Though the actual transmission is through food or ingestion, amont the given list of options the choice "Animal to human" seem to be the most appropriate. Though "immunodeficiency" can also be a probable answer, the former choice is still a more valid answer.

Investigation of Choice

Serology.

Immediate Management

Rule out ocular toxoplasmosis by retinoscopy.

Treatment of Choice

Immunologically competant adults and older children who have only lymphadenopathy do not require specific therapy unless they have persistent and severe symptoms.

Your notes:

100. A first year university student develops headache, fever, photophobia, in the 1st week of term.

Diagnosis: Bacterial meningitis (probable)

Clinchers

- *A first year university student:* Overcrowded closed communities, schools, colleges, universities and day centres are risk factors for acquisition of infections meningitis.
- *Headache, photophobia:* These features along with stiff neck, Kernig's sign Brudzinskin's sign and ophisthotonus are constituents of "meningism".
- *Fever:* It signifies septicaemia and suggests bacterial infection. Other feature of septicaemia can be malaise, fever, arthritis, odd behaviour, rash, DIC, hypotension, tachycardia and tachypnoea.

CONFUSA

Any petechiae suggest meningococcus. If it is so, never delay treatment for any tests. This rash can be found in over 70% cases of meningococcal septicaemia if a careful examination is made. In early stages, the rash may be macular.

Investigation of Choice

Lumbar puncture.

Immediate Management

Give benzyl penicillin before anything (confirm if the GP has already given it).

Treatment of Choice

Benzyl penicillin should be given by slow IV infusion immediately after the diagnosis of bacterial meningitis or suspected meningococcal septicaemia.

Causation: **Close community contact.**

Your notes:

107. Typhoid fever.

Diagnosis (transmission): Faecal-oral

Clinchers

Typhoid is caused by *Salmonella typhi.* Its incubation period is 3-21 days. Patients usually present with malaise, headache, high fever with relative bradycardia, cough and constipation (or diarrhoea). Epistaxis, bruising, abdominal pain, and splenomegaly may occur. Complications can be osteomyelitis, DVT, GI bleed or perforation, cholecystitis, myocarditis, pyelonephritis, meningitis, abscess.

Note: Infection is said to have cleared when 6 consecutive cultures of urine and faeces are negative.

CONFUSA

CNS signs, i.e. coma, delirium or meningism in typhoid fever are serious. Diarrhoea is more common after the first week. Rose spots occur on the trunk of 40% but may be very difficult to see. High fever with relative bradycardia is a very suggestive of typhoid fever.

Investigation of Choice

- First 10 days—blood culture
- Later—urine/stool cultures.

Immediate Management

Fluid replacement and good nutrition.

Treatment of Choice

Chloramphenicol/ciprofloxacin

In encephalopathy ± shock, give dexamethasone 3 mg/kg

IV stat, then 1 mg/kg/6 h for 48 h.

Your notes:

108. Hepatitis C.

Diagnosis (transmission): Blood borne

Clinchers

It is caused by a RNA flavivirus. It spreads via:

- Blood products
- IVDU
- Sexual
- Unknown (40%).

Early infection is often mild and asymptomatic. About 85% develop chronic infection and 20-30% get cirrhosis within 20 years. It also increases the risk of hepato-cellular carcinoma.

Investigation of Choice

Anti HCV antibodies; RIBA; HCV-PCR

Liver biopsy if HCV-PCR +ve.

Treatment of Choice

Interferon a + Ribavarin.

Your notes:

109. HIV.

Diagnosis (Transmission): Sexual transmission or blood borne.

Clinchers
HIV infection is acquired by percutaneous exposure to bodily secretions, fluids and blood like semen, peritoneal fluid, pleural fluid or vaginal secretions.

CONFUSA

Tears and saliva have not been proved transmit HIV infection. Although HIV has been isolated from them but, is found in such minute quantities in them that it cannot effectuate a seroconversion reaction after exposure.

Investigation of Choice
ELISA/PCR

Immediate Management
Counselling

Treatment of Choice
Prophylactic drug cocktail till AIDS develops.

Your notes:

110. Lyme disease.

Diagnosis (Transmission): Tick borne.

Clinchers
Lyme disease is infection caused by Borrelia burgorferi. Although originally described in Lyme (connecticut) it is now widespread, e.g. New forest in UK. It is transmitted by Ixoedes tick bite.

CONFUSA

Lyme disease is a frequently asked topic in PLAB exam, so read everything about it. Another GMC favourite about Lyme disease is Erythema chronicum migrans, the cutaneous manifestation of Lyme disease.

Investigation of Choice
Clinical ± serology

Immediate Management
Travel history

Treatment of Choice
Doxycycline 100 mg/12 h PO (Amoxicillin or penicillin V if < 12 years)

Your notes:

153. Elderly patient with complaint of fever and increasing confusion.

Diagnosis: Infection toxicity

Clinchers

- *Fever:* Infection, particularly of the central nervous system can cause an acute confusional state. Elderly patients with any infection (e.g. chest or urinary tract) can present in such a way that the underlying medical condition is completely masked.
- *Increasing confusion:* The diagnosis of sepsis is easily missed, particularly in the elderly when the classical signs may not be present. Mild confusion, tachycardia and tachypnoea may be the only clues, sometimes with unexplained hypotension, a reduction in urine output, a rising plasma creatinine and glucose intolerance.

CONFUSA

The clinical signs of sepsis are not always associated with bacteremia and can occur with noninfectious processes such as pancreatitis or severe trauma. In order to avoid confusion, the term systemic inflammatory response syndrome (SIRS) has been suggested to describe the disseminated inflammation that can complicate this diverse range of disorders.

Investigation of Choice

Blood culture

Immediate Management

Refer to ITU if possible for monitoring ± ionotropes

Treatment of Choice

IV ceturoxine 1.5 g/8 h (after blood culture).

Your notes:

12 Medicolegal Issues

PAPER 3

2. A 70-year-old man is receiving treatment for Alzheimer's disease. He is looked after by a 23-year-old granddaughter. He has recently developed faecal incontinence. The SHO notices bruises on both wrists and back.

Diagnosis: Elderly abuse.

Clinchers

- *70-year-old:* Proves that he is an elderly person!
- *Alzheimer's disease:* Such patients are usually very difficult to look after and one usually requires the services of a trained nurse to care for such demented persons.
- *Faecal incontinence:* Must have compounded the problems of the young granddaughter who was looking after him.
- *Bruises on both wrists and back:* Bruises on both wrists strongly suggest towards use of handcuffs on him, (which his granddaughter might have used to prevent him from wandering aimlessly and getting lost—a frequent occurrence in dementia). The bruises on the back could result either from direct assaults or from the violent attempts of the patient to get free from the handcuffs (thereby bruising his back against wall/bed/chair).

CONFUSA

This is a straight forward question with only a mild confusion between some terminologies in the options. It can qualify as a physical abuse also, but elderly abuse is more specific and his children rather than the granddaughter are more responsible for his condition.

Investigation of Choice
Detailed history.

Immediate Management
Admission in hospital and inform social services.

Treatment of Choice
Rehabilitation.

Your notes:

3. An anxious mother brings her 6-year-old daughter who is bleeding per vaginum. Six months prior to this presentation the girl had a confirmed streptococcal sorethroat infection. She is otherwise normal.

Diagnosis: Sexual abuse.

Clinchers

- *6-year-old:* Usually such a young child cannot give a proper history of sexual abuse.
- *Bleeding per vaginum:* A common finding in children's sexual abuse. Other common finding is presence of veneral disease before puberty.
- *Confirmed streptococcal sorethroat six months back:* This is important as it can be a precipitating factor of Henoch-Schölein purpura. However, it usually does not occur after so long as six months as it is IgA mediated. It usually presents within 2-6 weeks.
- *Otherwise normal:* Rules out any systemic disease.

CONFUSA

The main differential diagnosis in this case is HSP. However, the main finding in HSP is a purpura on extensor surfaces which is excluded in this question (as the child is otherwise normal). So it is safe to answer as a childhood sexual abuse. (Also do not forget the theme is non-accidental injury).

Investigation of Choice
Forensic specimens (pubic hair, vaginal swabs) by an expert.

Immediate Management
Inform social services.

Treatment of Choice
Follow local guidelines of the region.

Your notes:

4. A 4-day-old girl is brought to casualty by the maternal grandparent who is worried about two dark bluish patches on the child's buttocks. Child's mother is white and the father is black.

Diagnosis: Battered baby.

Clinchers

- *Brought to casualty by the maternal grandparent.* Always suspect abuse if accompanying adult is not a parent.
- *Two dark bluish patches on the child's buttocks.* Injury to buttocks is one of the most common finding in battered baby syndrome.
- *Child's mother is white and the father is black.* Inter-racial marriages are often a risk factor for battered baby syndrome.

CONFUSA

The main differential diagnosis in this case is 'birth marks' or congenital nevus. But they are usually present either at birth or after seven days (Strawberry angioma). Here the socio-cultural history is also raising suspicious of battered baby syndrome.

Investigation of Choice
Detailed history from accompanying adult + complete physical examination.

Immediate Management
Inform social services.

Treatment of Choice
Follow local guidelines of region/hospital.

Your notes:

5. An 8-year-old girl is noted to have fresh bloody staining of her pants. She also suffers from eneuresis. she has recently started horse-riding lessons

Diagnosis: Accidental injury.

Clinchers

- *Fresh bloody staining of her pant:* Most probably from trauma as the history given in question does not potray any illness.
- *She also suffers from eneuresis:* Bedwetting occurs on most nights in 15% of 5-year-old, and is still a problem in upto 3% of 15-year-old (usually from delayed maturation of bladder control). So it is probably normal.
- *She has recently started horse-riding lessons:* It can be reason for trauma, most probably rupture of hymen, which is common in horse-riding training for adolescent girls.

CONFUSA

GMC has tried to mislead us by putting the history of eneuresis in this question. But eneuresis has nothing to do with bleeding anywhere. So the question is still straight enough.

Investigation of Choice
For bleeding: Local examination.
For eneuresis: Test for UTI, GU abnormality and DM.

Immediate Management
Reassurance.

Treatment of Choice
Desmopressin nasal spray.

Your notes:

PAPER 4

32. A young boy is brought to A and E by his grandparents. He is unconscious with a bruise on the temporal area.

Diagnosis: Nonaccidental injury (probably).

Clinchers

- *Brought by grandparents:* Always suspect a nonaccidental injury whenever the accompanying adult to a suspiciously injured child is not an immediate parent.
- *Unconscious:* Due to head injury, most probably cerebral contusion in this case. But injury to temporal area is a risk factor for massive extradural hematomas (due to rupture of lateral sinus).
- *Bruise on temporal area:* This necessitates a radiological investigation, CT-skull in this case as he is unconscious. Otherwise a skull X-ray would have sufficed.

CONFUSA

Diagnosis of child abuse is a complex problem. False accusations may produce great distress. In suspicious circumstances, experienced advice should be obtained before a full examination is undertaken.

Investigation of Choice

CT skull.

Immediate Management

Admit to hospital. Refer to neurosurgery if CT is abnormal. Look for the child name on the child protection register.

Treatment of Choice

As per the CT findings. If normal, admit for 24 hours and if nonaccidental injury is proven, inform social services.

Your notes:

87. Child brought to A and E, age 6 months, swollen thigh, X-ray shows transverse fracture of shaft of femur.

Diagnosis: Non-accidental injury (NAI) probable.

Clinchers

- *Age 6 months:* One-third of NAI occurs under 6 months of age (other one-third between 6 months and 3 years and next one-third after that). It is due to stress of looking after young children.
- *Transverse fracture of femoral shaft:* Any fracture in a child under 12-year-old should raised suspicious of NAI until prove otherwise.

CONFUSA

A skeletal survey—to look for occult injuries—is usually only indicated in children under 2 years of age.

Osteogenesis imperfecta can also clinically present in this way but it would have been diagnosed on the X-ray (already done in this child) because of its typical radiological characteristics:

- translucent bone
- trefoil pelvis
- wormian bones (irregular patches of ossification)

Investigation of Choice

Skeletal survey (to find out other old injuries)

Immediate Management

Look for child's name on child protection register.

Treatment of Choice

Follow local protocol.

Your notes:

88. A 9-year-old female child with itching, sore vagina, perineum is red and excoriated.

Diagnosis: Sexual abuse

Clinchers

- *9-year-old:* In UK, before the age of 16, at least one in 10 girls and one in 15 boys will have been sexually assaulted. The peak incidence of first assault is at about 8-year-old.
- *Itching and sore vagina, perineum is red and excoriated:* Most probably there are symptoms of venereal disease. Presence of venereal disease in a prepubertal, child should always be considered as sexual abuse until proven otherwise.

CONFUSA

Sexual abuse of children can occur in all socio-economic, cultural and religion groups and is associated with:

- Acute perineal injury
- Chronic perineal damage
- Genitourinary infection
- Sexually precocious behaviour
- Sexualized drawings and play
- Regressive patterns of behaviour
- Eating and sleep disorders
- Psychosomatic symptoms
- Withdrawal and depression
- Self harm
- Promiscuity
- Running away from home

Investigation of Choice
Examine under anaesthesia.

Immediate Management
Referred for consideration of the need for child protection.

Treatment of Choice
Follow local protocol after informing social services.

Your notes:

90. Child with forearm bruise, brought by teacher, Mom says she held her to prevent her from running across the road.

Diagnosis: Non-accidental injury (NAI) (probably)

Clinchers

- *Forearm bruise:* It is a common site of bruising by holding or bondage. They can occur by light grasp because of a pre-existing coagulopathy (haemophilia) or tight and violent grasp or bondage in NAI.
- *Brought by teacher:* Always suspect NAI when the accompanying adult is not one of the immediate parent.
- *Mom say she held her to prevent her from running across the road:* It can be a true explanation if the child have a coagulopathy. But then the mother would herself be bothered enough to bring her to medical attention. But since it did not happen, a NAI becomes a more probable diagnosis.

CONFUSA

Confirm the doubts of NAI by excluding coagulopathy definitely through laboratory tests. Most common coagulopathy is haemophilia.

Investigation of Choice
Coagulation profile.

Immediate Management
Informal social services if NAI is confirmed.

Treatment of Choice
Depends on investigation report. Follow local protocol if NAI.

Your notes:

PAPER 5

122. A 70-year-old man is receiving treatment for Alzheimer's disease. He is looked after by a 23-year-old granddaughter. He has recently developed faecal incontinence. The SHO notices bruises on both wrists and back.

Diagnosis: Elderly abuse.

Clinchers

- *70-year-old:* Proves that he is an elderly person!
- *Alzheimer's disease:* Such patients are usually very difficult to look after and one usually requires the services of a trained nurse to care for such demented persons.
- *Faecal incontinence:* Must have compounded the problems of the young granddaughter who was looking after him.
- *Bruises on both wrists and back:* Bruises on both wrists strongly suggest towards use of handcuffs on him, (which his granddaughter might have used to prevent him from wandering aimlessly and getting lost—a frequent occurrence in dementia). The bruises on the back could result either from direct assaults or from the violent attempts of the patient to get free from the handcuffs (thereby bruising his back against wall/bed/chair).

CONFUSA

This is a straight forward question with only a mild confusion between some terminologies in the options. It can qualify as a physical abuse alos, but elderly abuse is more specific and his children rather than the granddaughter are more responsible for his condition.

Investigation of Choice
Detailed history.

Immediate Management
Admission in hospital and inform social services.

Treatment of Choice
Rehabilitation.

Your notes:

123. An anxious mother brings her 6-year-old daughter who is bleeding per vaginum. Six months prior to this presentation the girl had a confirmed streptococcal sorethroat infection. She is otherwise normal.

Diagnosis: Sexual abuse.

Clinchers

- *6-year-old:* Usually such a young child cannot give a proper history of sexual abuse.
- *Bleeding per vaginum:* A common finding in children's sexual abuse. Other common finding is presence of veneral disease before puberty.
- *Confirmed streptococcal sorethroat six months back:* This is important as it can be a precipitating factor of Henoch-Schölein purpura. However, it usually does not occur after so long as six months as it is IgA mediated. It usually presents within 2-6 weeks.
- *Otherwise normal:* Rules out any systemic disease.

CONFUSA

The main differential diagnosis in this case is HSP. However, the main finding in HSP is a purpura on extensor surfaces which is excluded in this question (as the child is otherwise normal). So it is safe to answer as a childhood sexual abuse. (Also do not forget the theme is non-accidental injury).

Investigation of Choice
Forensic specimens (pubic hair, vaginal swabs) by an expert.

Immediate Management
Inform social services.

Treatment of Choice
Follow local guidelines of the region.

Your notes:

124. A 4-day-old girl is brought to casualty by the maternal grandparent who is worried about two dark bluish patches on the child's buttocks. Child's mother is white and the father is black.

Diagnosis: Battered baby.

Clinchers

- *Brought to casualty by the maternal grandparent.* Always suspect abuse if accompanying adult is not a parent.
- *Two dark bluish patches on the child's buttocks.* Injury to buttocks is one of the most common finding in battered baby syndrome.
- *Child's mother is white and the father is black.* Inter-racial marriages are often a risk factor for battered baby syndrome.

CONFUSA

The main differential diagnosis in this case is 'birth marks' or congenital naevus. But they are usually present either at birth or after seven days (Strawberry angioma). Here the socio-cultural history is also raising suspicious of battered baby syndrome.

Investigation of Choice

Detailed history from accompanying adult + complete physical examination.

Immediate Management

Inform social services.

Treatment of Choice

Follow local guidelines of region/hospital.

Your notes:

125. An 8-year-old girl is noted to have fresh bloody staining of her pants. She also suffers from eneuresis. she has recently started horse-riding lessons

Diagnosis: Accidental injury.

Clinchers

- *Fresh bloody staining of her pant:* Most probably from trauma as the history given in question does not potray any illness.
- *She also suffers from eneuresis:* Bedwetting occurs on most nights in 15% of 5-year-old, and is still a problem in upto 3% of 15-year-old (usually from delayed maturation of bladder control). So it is probably normal.
- *She has recently started horse-riding lessons:* It can be reason for trauma, most probably rupture of hymen, which is common in horse riding training for adolescent girls.

CONFUSA

GMC has tried to mislead us by putting the history of eneuresis in this question. But eneuresis has nothing to do with bleeding anywhere. So the question is still straight enough.

Investigation of Choice

For bleeding: Local examination.
For eneuresis: Test for UTI, GU abnormality and DM.

Immediate Management

Reassurance.

Treatment of Choice

Desmopressin nasal spray.

Your notes:

PAPER 6

92. A 70-year-old man is receiving treatment for Alzheimer's disease. He is looked after by a 23-year-old granddaughter. He has recently developed faecal incontinence. The SHO notices bruises on both wrists and back.

Diagnosis: Elderly abuse.

Clinchers

- *70-year-old:* Proves that he is an elderly person!
- *Alzheimer's disease:* Such patients are usually very difficult to look after and one usually requires the services of a trained nurse to care for such demented persons.
- *Faecal incontinence:* Must have compounded the problems of the young granddaughter who was looking after him.
- *Bruises on both wrists and back:* Bruises on both wrists strongly suggest towards use of handcuffs on him, (which his granddaughter might have used to prevent him from wandering aimlessly and getting lost—a frequent occurrence in dementia). The bruises on the back could result either from direct assaults or from the violent attempts of the patient to get free from the handcuffs (thereby bruising his back against wall/bed/chair).

CONFUSA

This is a straight forward question with only a mild confusion between some terminologies in the options. It can qualify as a physical abuse alos, but elderly abuse is more specific and his children rather than the granddaughter are more responsible for his condition.

Investigation of Choice
Detailed history.

Immediate Management
Admission in hospital and inform social services.

Treatment of Choice
Rehabilitation.

Your notes:

93. An anxious mother brings her 6-year-old daughter who is bleeding per vaginum. Six months prior to this presentation the girl had a confirmed streptococcal sorethroat infection. She is otherwise normal.

Diagnosis: Sexual abuse.

Clinchers

- *6-year-old:* Usually such a young child cannot give a proper history of sexual abuse.
- *Bleeding per vaginum:* A common finding in children's sexual abuse. Other common finding is presence of veneral disease before puberty.
- *Confirmed streptococcal sorethroat six months back:* This is important as it can be a precipitating factor of Henoch-Schölein purpura. However, it usually does not occur after so long as six months as it is IgA mediated. It usually presents within 2-6 weeks.
- *Otherwise normal:* Rules out any systemic disease.

CONFUSA

The main differential diagnosis in this case is HSP. However, the main finding in HSP is a purpura on extensor surfaces which is excluded in this question (as the child is otherwise normal). So it is safe to answer as a childhood sexual abuse. (Also do not forget the theme is non-accidental injury).

Investigation of Choice
Forensic specimens (pubic hair, vaginal swabs) by an expert.

Immediate Management
Inform social services.

Treatment of Choice
Follow local guidelines of the region.

Your notes:

94. A 4-day-old girl is brought to casualty by the maternal grandparent who is worried about two dark bluish patches on the child's buttocks. Child's mother is white and the father is black.

Diagnosis: Battered baby.

Clinchers

- *Brought to casualty by the maternal grandparent.* Always suspect abuse if accompanying adult is not a parent.
- *Two dark bluish patches on the child's buttocks.* Injury to buttocks is one of the most common finding in battered baby syndrome.
- *Child's mother is white and the father is black.* Inter-racial marriages are often a risk factor for battered baby syndrome.

CONFUSA

The main differential diagnosis in this case is 'birth marks' or congenital nevus. But they are usually present either at birth or after seven days (Strawberry angioma). Here the socio-cultural history is also raising suspicious of battered baby syndrome.

Investigation of Choice

Detailed history from accompanying adult + complete physical examination.

Immediate Management

Inform social services.

Treatment of Choice

Follow local guidelines of region/hospital.

Your notes:

PAPER 7

81. The ability of a test to detect people who does have the disease.

Answer: Sensitivity

Clinchers

Sensitivity is the percentage of the diseased people who are correctly detected or classified:

$$\text{Senstivity: } \frac{\text{number testing positive who have the disease}}{\text{total number tested who have the disease}} \times 100$$

So a test that is always positive for diseased individuals, identifying every diseased person, has a sensitivity of 100%. Therefore, a test that is insensitive leads to missed diagnosis (false negative results), whereas a sensitive test produces few false negative results.

CONFUSA

A sensitive test is obviously required in situations in which the consequence of a false negative result is serious, as in the case of a serious condition that is treatable or transmissible. High sensitivity is required of tests used to screen donated blood for HIV, or in the case of cytological screening tests for cervical cancer. Very sensitive tests are therefore used for screening or ruling out disease: if the result of a highly sensitive test is negative, it allows the disease to be ruled out with confidence.

Your notes:

82. **Measure of dispersion.**

Answer: Standard deviation

Clinchers

Standard deviation is a measure of dispersion and is used most commonly in statistical analyses. It is computed by following six steps:

1. Calculate the mean.
2. Find the difference of each observation from the mean.
3. Square the differences of observation from the mean.
4. Add the squared values to get the sum of the squares.
5. Divide this sum by the number of observations minus. One to get mean-squared deviation, called variance.
6. Find the square root of this varianace to get root-mean- squared deviation, called standard deviation.

CONFUSA

A large standard deviation shows that the measurement of the frequency distribution are widely spread out from the mean. Small standard deviation means the observations are closely spread in the neighbourhood of mean. Another measure of dispersion is mean-deviation.

Your notes:

83. **Relative risk can be obtained from these studies.**

Answer: Cohort studies

Clinchers

The estimate of disease risk associated with exposure is obtained by an index known as "Relative Risk" (RR) or risk ratio, which is defined as the ratio between the incidence of disease among exposed persons and incidence among non-exposed. It is given by formula:

$$\text{Relative risk} = \frac{\text{incidence among exposed}}{\text{incidence among non-exposed}} \times 100$$

CONFUSA

A typical case control study does not provide incidence rates from which relative risk can be calculated directly, because there is no appropriate denominator or population at risk, to calculate their rates. In general, the relative risk can be exactly determined only from a cohort study. Because relative risk is a ratio of risks, it is sometimes called the risk ratio, or morbidity ratio. In the case of outcomes involving death, rather than just disease, it may also be called the mortality ratio.

Your notes:

84. The best indicator of central value when one or more of the lowest or the highest observations are wide apart or not so evenly distributed.

Answer: Median

Clinchers

When all the observations of a variable are arranged in either ascending or descending order, the middle observation is known as median. It implies the midvalue of series.

CONFUSA

Median is sometimes a better indicator than mean, e.g. in a study of duration of stay in a hospital in general or in a specific disease ward, or disease. In such cases it is better because the stay may be unduly long in some cases.

Your notes:

85. The most frequently occurring observation in a series.

Answer: Mode

Clinchers

Mode is the most frequently occurring observation in a series, i.e. the most common or most fashionable, such as 8 mm in tuberculin test of 10 boys given below: 3, 5, 7, 8, 8, 8, 10, 11, 12

CONFUSA

Mode is rarely used in medical studies. Out of the three measures of central tendency, mean is better and utilized more often because it uses all the observations in the data and is further and in the tests of significance.

Your notes:

86. The single largest cause of death in adults in the UK.

Diagnosis: Ischaemic heart disease (IHD).

Clinchers

Coronary artery disease is the largest single cause of death in the UK. There are approximately 60 deaths per 100,000 (giving a standardised mortality rate of about 200 per 100,000).

CONFUSA

In UK, myocardial ischaemia most commonly occurs as a result of obstructive coronary disease in the form of coronary atherosclerosis. In addition to this fixed obstruction, variations in the tone of smooth muscles in the wall of a coronary artery may add an important element of dynamic or variable obstruction.

Investigation of Choice

Coronary angiography (definitive).

Immediate Management

Cardiology referral.

Treatment of Choice

As per the symptom profile.

Your notes:

87. Warfarin decreases the incidence of stroke by about 30%.

Diagnosis: Atrial fibrillation

Clinchers

There is a direct relation between the duration of anticoagulation and the risk of recurrent thrombosis. Although recommendations vary somewhat, most patients with a single uncomplicated thromboembolic event have maximal benefit after 3 to 6 months of anticoagulation. About 10% of patients on an oral anticoagulant for 1 year have a serious complication requiring medical supervision, and 0.5 to 1% have a fatal haemorrhage event despite careful medical management.

CONFUSA

Patients with paroxysmal atrial fibrillation or a porcine bioprosthetic valve, who are taking a warfarin anticoagulant as a prophylactic measure, may be protected with an INR of 1.5 to 2. In contrast, patients with lupus like anticoagulants and thromboembolism or those patients with mechanical cardiac valves require more intense anticoagulation. Satisfactory control requires an INR of 3 to 4.

Investigation of Choice

Echocardiography

Immediate Management

Evaluation by an expert

Treatment of Choice

For atrial fibrillation—anticoagulant therapy.

Your notes:

89. Probably most important public health problem in developed countries. Its ratio of frequency in women verses men increases from 0.6 to 0.7 at age 30 to 1.1 to 1.2 at age 65.

Diagnosis: Hypertension.

Clinchers

- Hypertension is the most important public health problem in the developed countries.
  It is common, asymptomatic, easily detectable, usually easily treatable, but may lead to lethal complications, if untreated.
- Increase in ratio of frequency in women with age
  In females the prevalence is closely related to age, with substantial increase occurring after age 50.
- The prevalance of hypertension depends upon the racial composition of the population studied, and criteria used to define the condition. In white-suburban population like that in the Framingham study, nearly one-fifth of individuals have BP>160/95, while almost one-half have pressures greater than 140/90. Even higher prevalence has been documented in non-white population.

Your notes:

90. Its incidence in industrialized countries of the world has defined markedly. Peak age-related incidence is between 5 and 15 years.

Diagnosis: Rheumatic fever

Clinchers

- The incidence of rheumatic fever has declined remarkably in the industrialized countries of the world, where the disease has become rare. However, in many developing countries, which account for almost two-thirds of the world's population, streptococcal infection, rheumatic fever and rheumatic heart disease remain a very significant health problem today.

CONFUSA

Epidemiology of rheumatic fever is similar to that of group-A streptococcal upper respiratory tract infection. Approximately 3 percent of individuals with untreated group A-streptococcal pharyngitis will develop rheumatic fever

Diagnosis of Rheumatic fever

- No specific laboratory tests available to establish the diagnosis of rheumatic fever. Thus diagnosis is essentially clinical, supported by clinical microbiology and clinical immunology laboratories. John's criteria's for rheumatic fever should be remembered here. There are five major and many minor criterias. Major criterias are carditis, migratory polyarthritis, Sydenham's chorea, subcutaneous nodules and erythema marginatum. Minor criterias include fever, arthralgia, elevated acute phose reactants, and prolonged PR interval.

Your notes:

13 Neurology

PAPER 1

Serial No. 38

Subject: Medicine

Topic: Epilepsy

Question: A 45-year-old lady on treatment for epilepsy develops ataxia and gum hypertrophy.

Diagnosis: Phenytoin side effect

Clinchers

- *On treatment for epilepsy:* Though once widely used antiepileptic, phenytoin is now considered only in the second line treatment of epilepsy, because of the various side effects associated with the drug.
- *Develops ataxia:* This is a dose- related side effect of phenytoin. Other dose related side effects of phenytoin include diplopia, nystagmus, dysarthria, confusion and dystonia.
- *Gum hypertrophy:* This is a long-term effect of phenytoin use. Other long-term side effects of the drug include hypertrichosis, osteomalacia, folate deficiency anaemia, polyneuropathy and aggravation of acne.

CONFUSA

- Gingival overgrowth occurs in roughly half of the patients taking phenytoin. Changes are most severe in the first year of treatment but can resolve if the drug is withdrawn. Poor oral hygiene exacerbates the effect.
- Other drugs causing gingival hypertrophy include nifedipine, cyclosporin, oral contraceptive with high oestrogen concentration.

Investigation of Choice

Ataxia signifies dose related toxicity. Check plasma levels of phenytoin

Immediate Management

Correct dose if plasma levels high.

Gum hypertrophy can be prevented with proper oral hygiene maintainence with chlohexidine.

In extreme cases, surgical excision or discontinuation of phenytoin may be essential.

Treatment of Choice

Maintain phenytoin level in therapeutic range

Proper oral hygeine.

Your notes:

Serial No. 39

Subject: Medicine

Topic: Seizures

Question: An adult with recent onset seizure. Ophthalmoscopy shows papilloedema.

Diagnosis: Intracranial Space Occupying Lesion (ICSOL)

Clinchers

- *Adult:* Idiopathic epilepsy usually presents early in childhood or adolescence. Any episode of seizure in a previously normal adult should raise the possibility of secondary causes of seizure rather than epilepsy.
- *Recent onset seizure:* This further confirms that there was no previous history of seizures in this patient.
- *Opthalmoscopy shows papilloedema:* This indicates raised intracranial tension; supporting the possibility of ICSOL.

CONFUSA

Any lesion in the form of cerebral tumour, cerebral abscess or a growing haematoma can cause structural effect and present with features of raised intracranial tension, viz papilloedema, headache, seizures, ataxia or incontinence.

Normal pressure hydrocephalus is a similar situation where typically a female presents with features of raised intracranial tensio. However, seizures is uncommon in NPH.

Investigation of Choice

CT scan is the investigation of choice.

Lumbar puncture is contraindicated in presence of features of raised intracranial tension.

Immediate Management

Maintain airway and breathing during seizures.

Control seizure with IV diazepam.

Treatment of Choice

According to the cause identified.

Your notes:

Serial No. 40

Subject: Medicine

Topic: Epilepsy

Question: A child with two episodes of jerking limb movements. Teacher says he does not concentrate in the class.

Diagnosis: Absent Seizures (Petit mal epilepsy)

Clinchers

- *Child:* Absence seizures or Petit mal is a form of primary generalised epilepsy that is seen mostly in children.
- *Two episodes of jerking limb movements:* The 'absences' can be sometimes accompanied by motor components like fluttering of eyelids, smacking movements of lips or jerking of one or more limbs.
- *He does not concentrate in the class:* These are typical 'absences' observed in the condition. The absences usually last only a few seconds but may occur many times a day. During the absence the child stops activity and stares blankly, not responding to questions, which the teacher mistakes that the child is 'not concentrating' or is 'day dreaming'. The child usually cannot recall the 'absence'.

CONFUSA

Juvenile myoclonic epilepsy (JME) is one close differential diagnosis here. JME attack is typically described as myoclonic jerky movements of limbs, usually bilateral, occurring in an adolescent, typically ocuuring in the morning shortly after awakening.

- Although 'absences' may be an associated feature in JME, occurs only very rarely. The attacks are typically precipitated by sleep deprivation or hyperventilation.
- The typical interictal EEG abnormality consists of a generalized 4- to 6-Hz spike or polyspike and slow wave discharges lasting between 1-20 seconds.

Investigation of Choice

The only diagnostic test for absence seizures is EEG. Typical absence seizures have generalized 3-Hz spike-and-wave complexes

Immediate Management

Absence seizures require emergency management only when it progresses to generalized tonic clonic form.

Treatment of Choice

Ethosuximide

Serial No. 41

Subject: Medicine

Topic: Epilepsy

Question: A 50 year old lady with jerking of thumb, followed by limb and then generalized convulsions.

Diagnosis: Simple Partial Seizure

Clinchers

- *A 50-year-old lady:* The incidence of simple partial seizure is lowest in children younger than 1 year and increases gradually up to approximately age 65 years, after which it rises exponentially. Male and females are affected equally.
- *Jerking of thumb, followed by limb and then generalized convulsions:* The sequence typically describes "Jacksonian March", so classical of simple partial seizures. The epileptinogenic foci in this patient is probably in the motor area ('Thumb area' to be specific) and it involves the adjacent areas as the epileptic potential spreads gradually.Tthe perioral area, thumb, index finger, and great toe as the areas that usually are affected first in partial seizures. These are all anatomical parts having a disproportionately large area of representation in the cortical homunculus.

CONFUSA

- In any case of simple partial seizure, imaging should be done to rule out the possibility of any structural abnormality especially in the area corresponding to the part of the body where seizure originated first (thumb, here in this case).
- This usually denotes a structural abnormality in the brain tissue which is irritating the corresponding area leading to epileptogenic potential and thus causing seizures.

Investigation of Choice

CT scan with or without contrast.

Immediate Management

If it progresses to generalized tonic clonic form, place the patient in recovery position, maintain airway and breathing. Control seizure with IV diazepam.

Treatment of Choice

Carbamazepine is the first line drug.
Individual treatment options can be tailored according to the cause identified.

Serial No. 43

Subject: Medicine

Topic: Neurology

Question: A 55 year old man with history of stroke and repeated falls, now confused and can not remember things.

Diagnosis: Vascular Dementia

Clinchers

- *A 55-year-old man:* Incidence of vascular dementia is higher in males than in females. The converse is true for Alzeihmer's. This difference probably reflects known sex differences in the incidence of cerebrovascular disease. The incidence increases with age.
- *History of stroke:* This specifies the evidence of cerebrovascualr disease in the patient the cerebravascular accidents usually precede or co incide with the occurrence of dementia.
- *Repeated falls:* Signifies transient ischemic attacks, again making the factor of cerebraovascular disease strong.
- *Now confused and can not remember things:* disorientation and step wise loss of memory is classical.

CONFUSA

Multi-infarct dementia differs from Alzheimer's disease in following aspects:

- Progress is stepwise rather than gradual
- Evidence of systemic cardiovascular disease - especially hypertension
- Focal neurological signs - pseudobulbar palsy
- Walking may be in small steps - "marche a petit pas"
- Severity of symptoms can vary throughout the day, typically being worst in the evening
- Better preservation of personality, insight and social responsiveness

Note that, a cognitively impaired patient with vascular risks factors but no history of cerebrovascular disease is most likely to have Alzeihmer's Disease.

Investigation of Choice

CT scan will show multiple cortical, and more commonly subcortical infarcts or single strokes affecting the thalamus, angular gyrus, and the territory supplied by the anterior cerebral arteries.

Immediate Management

Rule out other causes of reversible dementia (viz Vitamin B 12 deficiency, hypothyroidism).

Behaviour and psychological support.

Treatment of Choice

Aim at treating the risk factors for further strokes (viz hypertension).

Aspirin initiated to prevent further strokes.

Anticoagulants should be used very carefully keeping in mind the repititive falls.

Your notes:

Serial No. 44

Subject: Medicine

Topic: Neurology

Question: A 48-year-old man has normal memory on examination; wife complaints of him becoming aggressive lately and talking about their sexual life publicly.

Diagnosis: Frontal lobe dementia

Clinchers

- *A 48-year-old man:* can present in any age or gender. However, it closely follows cerebrovascular risk of age and sex preference, being more common in males and increasing with age.
- *Normal memory on examination:* Cognitive function and behaviour may seem entirely normal.
- *Becoming aggressive lately:* Frontal lobe syndrome usually presents with alteration in personality and social conduct. Patients usually lose sensitivity to the effects of their behaviours on others.
- *Talking about their sexual life publicly:* This is disinhibition, the most charactersitic of frontal lobe pathology. Other frontal lobe behavioural abnormalities include hyperorality, utilization behaviour (ie, picking up and manipulating any object in the environment, appropriate or not), and inappropriate sexuality.

CONFUSA

- Patients with frontal lobe dementia usually have preserved memory and visuospatial functions, while those with Alzheimer's have nearly universal involvement of these functions.
- Frontal lobe patients perform worse than Alzheimer's Disease patients on syntactic and speech fluency tasks and have more severe impairment of attention (eg, digit span).
- These differences between Frontal lobe dementia and Alzheimer's reflect the pathologic involvement of the frontal and temporal lobes, particularly in the left hemisphere, as compared to the early involvement in Alzheimer's of the hippocampi and parietal lobes.

Investigation of Choice

CT scan shows cerebral atrophy, usually of the frontal lobe and helps to rule out causes like stroke or any space occupying lesions.

Neuropsychological testing and evaluation by a speech/language pathologist with standardized language batteries is diagnostic.

Immediate Management
Identify any treatable causes of dementia.

Treatment of Choice
Symptomatic drug treatment.
Behaviour Therapy
Treat any associated depression

Your notes:

Serial No. 45

Subject: Medicine

Topic: Neurology

Question: A 65 year old lady with no medical complaints is found entering a shop at odd hours of early morning.

Diagnosis: Alzeihmer's Disease (AD)

Clinchers

- *65-year-old lady*: The risk of AD is significantly higher in women than in men. AD is most prevalent in individuals older than 60 years
- *With nomedical complaints:* This rules out any possibility of vascular dementia which can closely resembles AD.
- *Found entering a shop at odd hours of early morning:* She is showing visualspatial disorientation, characteristic of AD; there may also be an impairment of topographical memory and patients may become disoriented and get lost easily.

CONFUSA

Lewy Body dementia may appear same as AD, but differs in following aspects:

- Memory loss: Memory may be relatively normal in the early stages of Lewy body dementia, however its usually the presenting feature in AD.
- There is marked fluctuations of memory in patients with Lewy Body dementia and patient may appear severely demented and totally normal in different times of the same day. In AD, course is usually progressive; no fluctuations observed.
- Parkinsonism is an early feature of Lewy Body dementia; observed late in AD.
- Hallucinations is a major feature in Lewy body, not seen in AD.

Investigation of Choice
Apart from histology there are no specific tests for the diagnosis of Alzheimer's disease. Therefore, the principle is to rule out the differential diagnoses, and to diagnose Alzheimer's by exclusion.

Immediate Management
Avoid alcohol and drugs and treat any other disease which may exacerbate confusion.
Social and community support.

Treatment of Choice

- Cholinesterase inhibitors: Donepezil, rivastigmine, galantamine and tacrine .These drugs are available for the treatment of mild to moderate AD. There may be a slowing or even arrest of cognitive decline for about 8-9 months ; however the underlying disease process is not halted.
- Memantine is the first N-methyl-D-aspartate receptor antagonist to be licensed for the treatment of patients with moderately severe to severe Alzheimer's disease.

Your notes:

Serial No. 105

Subject: Medicine

Topic: Neurology

Question: A 60-year-old man with transient loss of vision and dysphasia which improved completely without any residual neurological deficits.

Diagnosis: Transient Ischemic Attack (Carotid Arery Territory)

Clinchers

- *60-year-old man:* Transient ischemic attacks, TIA are more commonly seen in elderly because of the associated comorbid conditions which enhance the affect of atherosclerosis, viz, diabetes, hypertension, hypercholesterolemia.
- *Transient loss of vision:* This is classical of compensated carotid artery circulation; more commonly known as amarousis fugax and presents as an attack of transient and painless loss of vision in one eye. It indicative of transient retinal ischaemia usually associated with stenosis of the ipsilateral carotid artery.
- *Dysphasia:* Patient has problem recognising or producing the right word due to involvment of Broca's or Wernicke's area.
- *Improved completely without any residual neurological deficits:* As the name suggests, TIA are typically 'transient' with symptoms reaching their maximal manifestation in fewer than 5 minutes. Manifestations are of variable duration and typically last 2-15 minutes (rarely as long as 24 h). Most TIA durations are less than 1 hour; median duration is 14 minutes in the carotid distribution and 8 minutes in vertebrobasilar ischaemia.

CONFUSA

- Transient loss of vision can present both due to monocular blindness or haemianopia. Both these can be reported as a problem in one eye. In haemianopia, patient should still be able to see through the other eye, when the affected eye is covered but in monocular blindness, covering good eye will cause complete blindness.
- Monocular attacks are associated with lesions in internal carotid artery in the neck and haemianopia usually due to a disorder in posterior circulation.

Investigation of Choice
Carotid Doppler Scanning
Carotid Angiography
CT scan

Immediate Management
Needs urgent referral.
Reduce modifiable risk factors, especially hypertension, smoking and hypercholesterolemia.

Treatment of Choice
- Antiplatelet therapy is most effective in patients in sinus rhythm;Aspirin 75 mg daily is the first choice. Dipyridamole can be considered if aspirin is not tolerated.
- Anticoagulant therapy is most effective in patients in atrial fibrillation
- Carotid endarterectomy—highly beneficial in symptomatic patients with 70-99% stenosis of the internal carotid
- ACE inhibitition—using a combination of long-acting ACE inhibitor (e.g. perindopril or ramipril) and a thiazide diuretic (e.g.indapamide) has been suggested in the National Clinical Guidelines for Stroke. London, UK.

Your notes:

Serial No. 161

Subject: Surgery

Topic: Trauma

Question: A 52-year-old chronic alcoholic comes in a state of confusion. Wife gives history of repeated falls over last few months.

Diagnosis: Subdural haematoma

Clinchers
- *52-year-old:* Most subdural haemorrhage occur in elderly, over 60 years of age because the bridging veins in the elderly are more easily torn owing to the stretching effect produced by the cerebral atrophy.
- *Chronic alcoholic:* Alcoholism is another important risk factor for the development of subdural haemorrhage because of their increased risk for blunt head trauma and also accompanying thrombocytopenia. Other risk factors for the development of subdural haemorrhage are anticoagulation therapy, haemophilia and patients on intracranial shunts which cause low CSF pressure and stretching of bridging veins.
- *State of confusion:* Fluctuating levels of consciousness, headache, dementia, personality change and even focal neurological deficits can be the presenting feature of subdural haematoma.
- *History of repeated falls over last few months:* The history confirms the mode of injury and interval of months between injury and presenting symptoms again suggest subdural haemorrhage as the most likely cause.

CONFUSA

Do not confuse lucid interval with delayed presentation of symptoms. Lucid interval in a transient gain of consciousness, after an initial period of unconsciousness. This is later followed by rapid deterioration of conscious level. All these occur within seconds to minutes following the injury to head. It characteristically denotes extradural haemorrhage.

Investigation of Choice: CT scan head

Immediate Management
Fluids to maintain systolic BP > 90 mmHg, O_2.
Consider hyperventilation to reduce CO_2 but NOT below 25-30 mmHg.
Mannitol to reduce ICP whilst awaiting surgery.

Treatment of Choice
Craniotomy to evacuate haematoma

Serial No. 165

Subject: Surgery

Topic: Trauma

Question: A man involved in an RTA, presents with headache and loss of consciousness after admission.

Diagnosis: Extradural haemorrhage

Clinchers

- *Involved in an RTA:* The most common setting of extradural haemorrhage is an adult involved in an RTA sustaining temporal or pariteal bone fracture and therby injuring middle meningeal vessels leading to torrential bleed between the skull and the dura.
- *Presents with headache:* Headache is the most common symptom due to cerebral concussion or vasogenic oedema.
- *Loss of consciousness after admission:* This is the most important clincher here, showing that patients' level of consciousness was normal at the time of admission and deteriorated later. This is signifying lucid interval- concussion followed by temporary recovery of consciousness for minutes or hours before the onset of drowsiness and possibly coma. This is most characteristic of extradural haemorrhage.

CONFUSA

The option 'intracerebral bleed' can be a cause of real confusion here. However, note that most common presentation of intracerebral bleed is in the setting of uncontrolled hypertension or in an elderly with atherosclerosis or amyloid angiopathy. Trauma can also rarely cause intracerebral bleed, but the presentation will always have definite neurological deficits to signify the site of bleeding. In the absence of any positive history (like hypertension) or neurological deficits, intracerebral bleed is an unlikely diagnosis here. Moreover, the setting of trauma and loss of consciousness after admission, points more in favour of extradural haemorrhage.

Investigation of Choice

CT scan head

Immediate Management

Immediate neurosurgery referral

Treatment of Choice

Burr holes or ideally craniotomy to evacuate haematoma.

PAPER 2

Serial No. 3

Subject: Surgery

Topic: Breast

Question: A 45-year-old women treated 3-year ago for breast carcinoma presented with back pain and lack of sensation in legs. She says that even after evacuation she feels that her bladder is full. She has been constipated for last 24-hrs.

Diagnosis: Spinal Cord Compression

Clinchers

- *A 45-year-old women treated 3-year ago for breast carcinoma:* Any positive history of breast cancer should raise suspicion of a recurrence or metastases if there are unexplained or new neurological symptoms.
- *Back pain and lack of sensation in legs:* Back pain suggests vertebral metastasis. The vertebral metastasis can impinge upon the spinal cord producing compression effects, which the patients observes as lack of sensation in the lower limbs. A definite sensory level is usually present.
- *Bladder is full, constipated for last 24-hrs:* Bowel and bladder dysfunction are pathognomic of spinal cord compression if there is associated history of weakness in lower limbs.

CONFUSA

Causes of cord compression in a metastatic disease are usually:

- Extension of tumour from a vertebral body
- Direct extension of tumour
- Crush fracture

Investigation of Choice

Screening: X-ray spine
Definitive: Myelogram

Immediate Management

Discuss with neurosurgeon and clinical oncologist immediately.

Treatment of Choice

Dexamethasone—8-16 mg IV, then 4 mg/ 6h PO
surgical decompression

Your notes:

Serial No. 4

Subject: Surgery

Topic: Breast

Question: A 43-year-old woman treated 2-years ago for grade 3 axillary node positive breast carcinoma, present with confusion, headache and vomiting. On examination she is drowsy but has no focal neurological signs. She has diplopia and O/E, papilloedema is present.

Diagnosis: Cerebral metastases

Clinchers

- *A 43-year-old woman treated...breast carcinoma:* Presence of axillary lymphnode metastasis in breast carcinoma is a poor prognostic factor. It signifies a high risk of recurrence of the carcinoma even if a block dissection of lymph nodes in axilla is done.
- *Confusion, headache and vomiting:* These all are symptoms of increased ICT and suggests the presence of a space occupying lesion in brain.
- *She is drowsy:* Due to increased ICT
- *No focal neurological signs:* So any focal pathology of brain is excluded.
- *Diplopia, papillaedema:* This again signify raised ICT.

CONFUSA

Although brain is a comparatively rare site of breast metastases, the presence of such symptoms with a positive history of breast carcinoma commands an intensive evaluation of the recurrence.

Investigation of Choice
CT skull

Immediate Management
Mannitol IV

Treatment of Choice
Chemotherapy+ Radiotherapy

Your notes:

Serial No. 31

Subject: Medicine

Topic: Drug Complications

Question: An epileptic patient on treatment develops nausea vomiting with oliguria and raised levels of urea and creatinine.

Diagnosis: Carbamazepine side effect

Clinchers

- *Epileptic on treatment:* Carbamazepine is an anti-convulsant and analgesic drug that is used in the treatment of pain associated with trigeminal neuralgia and in epilepsy, especially in partial seizures, particularly of the temporal lobe type, and in major tonic-clonic epilepsy.
- *Nausea and vomiting:* Carbamazepine is associated with acute renal failure. Nausea, vomiting and anorexia being non specific signs of uraemia, occurs due to nitrogenous substances irritating chemoreceptor trigger zone (CTZ).
- *Oliguria:* Acute renal failure should be immediately suspected on any patient on carbamazepine, developing oliguria or anuria.
- *Raised levels of urea and creatinine:* confirms the diagnosis of acute renal failure.

CONFUSA

Diagnosis of acute renal failure due to carbamazepine should always be supported by laboratory evidence as the anuria can also be due to anticholinergic side effect of carbamazepine. In a patient on antiepileptics developing renal dysfunction, hepatic impairment, agranulocytosis or water intoxication/hyponatraemia, always think of the possibility of carbamazepine toxicity.

Investigation of Choice
BUN and other renal function tests.
Serum levels of carbamazepine.

Immediate Management
Supportive

Treatment of Choice
Withdraw drug under coverage of another antiepileptic and diazepam.

Your Notes

Serial No. 33

Subject: Medicine

Topic: Drug Complications

Question: A 45-year-old lady on treatment for epilepsy develops ataxia and gum hypertrophy.

Diagnosis: Phenytoin side effect

Clinchers

- *On treatment for epilepsy:* Though once widely used antiepileptic, phenytoin is now considered only in the second line treatment of epilepsy, because of the various side effects associated with the drug.
- *Develops ataxia:* This is a dose- related side effect of phenytoin. Other dose related side effects of phenytoin include diplopia, nystagmus, dysarthria, confusion and dystonia.
- *Gum hypertrophy:* This is a long term effect of phenytoin use. Other long term side effects of the drug include hypertrichosis, osteomalacia, folate deficiency anaemia, polyneuropathy and aggravation of acne.

CONFUSA

Gingival overgrowth occurs in roughly half of the patients taking phenytoin. Changes are most severe in the first year of treatment but can resolve if the drug is withdrawn. Poor oral hygiene exacerbates the effect. Other drugs causing gingival hypertrophy include nifedipine, cyclosporin, oral contraceptive with high oestrogen concentration.

Investigation of Choice

Ataxia signifies dose related toxicity. Check plasma levels of phenytoin

Immediate Management

Correct dose if plasma levels high.
Gum hypertrophy can be prevented with proper oral hygiene maintenance with chlorhexidine.
In extreme cases, surgical excision or discontinuation of phenytoin may be essential.

Treatment of Choice

Maintain phenytoin level in therapeutic range.
Proper oral hygiene.

Your notes:

Serial No. 34

Subject: Medicine

Topic: Drug Complications

Question: A 12-year-old boy is started on antiepileptic for his absence seizures. After few days he develops fever, sore throat and ataxia.

Diagnosis: Ethosuximide Side effect

Clinchers

- *A 12-year-old boy:* Absence seizures usually occur in children and adolescents. Most patients usually grow out of it by the time they are adults.
- *Started on antiepileptic for his absence seizures:* Ehtosuximide is usually the first line of drug used for the treatment of absence seizures.
- *Develops fever, sore throat:* This may signify agranulocytosis, a rare but fatal complication associated with ethosuximide. Any patient on ethosuximide with fever, sore throat, mouth ulcers or easy bruising should be investigated thoroughly for agranulocytosis.
- *Ataxia:* The neurological side effects associated with ethosuximide use include drowsiness, headache, dizziness, euphoria, hiccups, irritability, hyperactivity, lethargy, fatigue, and ataxia. Psychiatric or psychological aberrations associated with ethosuximide administration have included disturbances of sleep, night terrors, inability to concentrate, and aggressiveness. These effects may be noted particularly in patients who have previously exhibited psychological abnormalities. There have been rare reports of paranoid psychosis, increased libido, and increased state of depression with overt suicidal intentions.

CONFUSA

While in absence seizures associated with both tonic or myoclonic component, sodium valproate is most useful; ethosuximide is effecting in controlling mainly the myoclonic seizures; Lamotrigine can control all seizure types. Note that phenytoin, carbamazepine and vigabatrin may exacerbate absences, especially if associated with myoclonus, and so should be avoided.

Investigation of Choice

White blood cell count
Serum Ethosuximide levels

Immediate Management

Gradual with drawl of the offending drug.
Start broad spectrum antibiotics.

Treatment of Choice

Replace gradually with valproate or lamotrigine. Avoid abrupt stopping of drug.

Your notes:

Serial No. 35

Subject: Medicine

Topic: Drug Complications

Question: A known epileptic on treatment, is started on some antibiotic for upper respiratory tract infections. She is now extremely drowsy and develops a bout of seizure. Her plasma sodium level is found to be very low.

Diagnosis:

Clinchers

- *Known epileptic on treatment, is started on some antibiotic:* Most of the known antiepileptics share the cytochrome P450 pathway for metabolism, and any antibiotic sharing the same pathway can be the cause of increased or decreased levels of the drug in the serum because of decreased or increased metabolism respectively.
- *She is now extremely drowsy:* This is signifying developing toxicity of the antiepileptic drug. (most antiepileptics are CNS depressants).
- *A bout of seizure, plasma sodium level is found to be very low:* This is signifying water intoxication, characteristically associated with carbamazepine. This can occur with high plasma levels of carbamazepine and may cause hyponatraemia, confusion and exacerbation of seizures. The disturbance in the antiepileptic level was most probably induced by the antibiotic started for her infection.

CONFUSA

Certain macrolides (e.g. clarithromycin or erythromycin) are known to interact with the carbamazepine antiepileptic drug. Carbamazepine-macrolide interaction leads to an increase in the level of carbamazepine in the blood, so inducing carbamazepine toxicity. Erythromycin, and to a lesser extent, clarithromycin may induce carbamazepine toxicity in clinical practice. Recall that erythromycin and clarithromycin are known to induce life threatening arrythmias when used concurrently with astemizole, terfenidine or cisapride.

Investigation of Choice

Check carbamazepine levels to confirm toxicity.

Immediate Management

Control seizure with diazepam

Treatment of Choice

Change the offending antibiotic

Serial No. 51

Subject: Medicine

Topic: Neurology

Question: A 61-year-old man presents with sudden onset dysarthria, headache, vertigo and dysphagia. He gives history of myocardial infarction 8 months back.

Diagnosis: Vertebrobasilar Stroke

Clinchers

- *A 61-year-old man:* Stroke or cerebrovascular accidents are most commonly seen in men than women and the incidence usually increases with age. After menopause, incidence is similar for both sexes.
- *Sudden onset:* Most patients with thromobotic occlusion of vertebral artery typically have a waxing and waning course of symptoms, with as many as 50% experiencing transient ischaemic attacks for several days to weeks prior to the occlusion. In contrast, embolic events are sudden, without prodrome or warning, with acute and dramatic presentation.
- *Dysarthria, headache, vertigo and dysphagia:* The common features associated with vertebrobasilar stroke include vertigo, diplopia, dysarthria, and weakness or sensory disturbance affecting one or other, or both, limbs. It can also cause impairment of vision, dysphagia, transient global amnaesia, confusion, transient unconsciousness and hearing impairment
- *History of myocardial infarction 8 months back:* This points out that the cause of the stroke was atherosclerosis.

CONFUSA

Its easy to confuse vertebrobasilar stroke with carotid artery stroke. Remember that carotid artery insufficiency would most likely produce symptoms corresponding to anterior circulation compromise viz, confusion, homonymous haemianopia, dysphasia. This man is presenting with symptoms which is more characteristic of a posterior circulation compromise.

Investigation of Choice

CT scan is the first Investigation of Choice
Doppler and angiography can be considered.

Immediate Management

Urgent referral.

Treatment of Choice

Thrombolysis—This is becoming an accepted treatment for ischaemic stroke provided that treatment is commenced within three hours of onset and that there is no sign of haemorrhage on the CT or angiogram—this treatment option is licensed in the US and it has now been licensed in the UK (only can be initiated by a specialist with necessary training).
-Antithrombotic and antiplatelet drugs, e.g. aspirin
-Neuroprotective agents

Your notes:

Serial No. 52

Subject: Medicine

Topic: Neurology

Question: A 20-year-old male with few days history of hoarseness and dysphagia, now develops paresis of both lower limbs.

Diagnosis: Motor Neurone Disease (MND)

Clinchers

- *A 20-year-old male:* The incidence of MND is of the order of 1-2 per 10,000. Typically it affects middle aged to older people with a peak age of incidence of 65-85 years, although the range may vary from 16-77 years. Males are twice more commonly affected.
- *With few days history of hoarseness and dysphagia:* This signify bulbar palsy, Dysarthria and dysphonia result from paresis of the lips, tongue and palate; nasal speech is typical. Dysphagia occurs due to involvment of pharyngeal muscles.
- *Now develops paresis of both lower limbs:* Atrophy and weakness of the muscles are characteristic. This occurs with prominent fasciculations of the muscles involved. The hand is often affected first. The patient may become aware of stiffness and difficulty in performing fine movement. The forearms tend to be affected next, the flexors before the extensors. The lower limbs are rarely affected early. Bilateral foot drop may occur. Weakness of the muscles of the trunk and of respiration are a late feature.

CONFUSA

Poliomyelitis can also present with features of bulbar palsy and lower limb paresis; however, there is often a prodrome marked by fever, sore throat and vomiting. The CNS involvement is often preceded by meningismal features like headache, neck and back stiffness. Carefully rule out from history, travel to and from endemic areas.

Investigation of Choice
Electromyography

Immediate Management
Refer to a specialist

Treatment of Choice
There is no cure for the disease.
Riluzole is the only drug currently licensed for the treatment of MND. It is a disease modifying agent, which does not control symptoms and does not prevent death. NICE have recently issued guidelines which recommends the use of Riluzole for MND, under specialist guidance.

Symptomatic treatment includes:
Dysarthria—Speech assessment and communication aids
Dysphagia—Feeding gastrostomy; cricopharyngeal myotomy; Dysphonia - speech therapists can give expert advice on speech and swallowing difficulties
Drooling—anticholinergics, e.g. benztropine
Muscle weakness—physiotherapy, walking aids, splints
Spasticity—baclofen (20-60 mg/d) or low dose diazepam
Respiratory failure—tracheostomy and artificial ventilation may prolong life
Mood—The Motor Neurone Disease Association gives valuable help to patients and relatives

Your notes:

Serial No. 53

Subject: Medicine

Topic: Neurology

Question: A 32-year-old lady had been confined to the wheelchairs because of paraplegia for now almost 2 years. She now develops blurred vision leading to blindness.

Diagnosis: Multiple Sclerosis(MS)

Clinchers

- *A 32-year-old lady:* MS is more common in females than males and onset is usually between 16-50 years with a peak at 20-40 years.
- *Confined to the wheelchairs because of paraplegia:* This is signifying spinal cord involvement by the disease process leading to paralysis of both lower limbs. The spinal cord involvement also commonly affects the bladder functions.
- *Develops blurred vision leading to blindness:* Though the natural progress of the disease is characterised by multiple neurological deficits, optic neuritis is one most consistent finding in most patients. It presents as retrobulbar pain and patchy loss of vision. In most cases the visual loss is completely reversible.

CONFUSA

A young lady with neurological deficits that typically relapse and remit all go in favor of multiple sclerosis. In addition to this the features of optic neuritis again makes the diagnosis strong. However, in the questions dealing with paraplegia, do consider other causes viz, disc prolapse, trauma or even poliomyelitis.

Investigation of Choice

Confirm multiple sclerosis by CSF examination (typical oligoclonal bands).

MRI will shows areas of patchy demyelination.

Immediate Management

Corticosteroids are the mainstay of management of the acute relapse.

The preferred regimen is intravenous methylprednisolone, 1 g for three days. If oral treatment is preferred an initial dose of 60 mg prednisolone per day is given for a week and then reduced over three weeks.

Treatment of Choice

Disease modifying agents (beta interferon, glatiramer acetate and azathioprine) - aim at reducing the number of relapses.

Urinary frequency and incontinence treated by anticholinergics (oxybutynin) and tricyclic antidepressants (amitriptyline)

Urinary retention: offer intermittent self-catheterisation

Your notes:

Serial No. 54

Subject: Medicine

Topic: Neurology

Question: A 72-year-old patient is now totally confined to the bed. He is getting increasingly forgetful within the last a few years.

Diagnosis: Alzheimer's Disease

Clinchers

- *A 72-year-old:* The risk of AD is significantly higher in women than in men. AD is most prevalent in individuals older than 60 years. AD is the most common form of dementia seen in UK. Senile type of AD usually starts after 70 years of age.
- *Now totally confined to the bed:* This occurs in the late stage of AD; The patients become increasingly physically frail. They may start to shuffle or walk unsteadily, eventually becoming confined to bed or a wheelchair.
- *Increasingly forgetful within the last a few years:* Perhaps the most common symptom of AD is loss of memory. While in the early stages, loss of short-term memory is common and patients may forget about recent conversations or events, in the late stages, loss of memory is almost complete, with the person unable to recognise familiar objects or surroundings needing reminders even for daily routines like eating, dressing, etc.

CONFUSA

Lewy Body dementia may appear same as AD, but differs in following aspects:

- Memory loss: memory may be relatively normal in the early stages of Lewy body dementia, however its usually the presenting feature in AD.
- There is marked fluctuations of memory in patients with Lewy Body dementia and patient may appear severely demented and totally normal in different times of the same day. In AD, course is usually progressive; no fluctuations observed.
- Parkinsonism is an early feature of Lewy Body dementia; observed late in AD.
- Hallucinations is a major feature in Lewy body, not seen in AD.

Investigation of Choice

Apart from histology there are no specific tests for the diagnosis of Alzheimer's disease. Therefore, the principle is to rule out the differential diagnoses, and to diagnose Alzheimer's by exclusion.

Immediate Management

Avoid alcohol and drugs and treat any other disease which may exacerbate confusion.

Social and community support

Treatment of Choice

Cholinesterase inhibitors: Donepezil, rivastigmine, galantamine and tacrine .These drugs are available for the treatment of mild to moderate AD. There may be a slowing or even arrest of cognitive decline for about 8-9 months ; however the underlying disease process is not halted

Memantine is the first N-methyl-D-aspartate receptor antagonist to be licensed for the treatment of patients with moderately severe to severe Alzheimer's disease

Your notes:

Serial No. 55

Subject: Medicine

Topic: Neurology

Question: A 65-year-old man had a transient loss of consciousness and weakness of left hand, from which he recovered completely. However, now he appears to always look towards right side while walking. His left eye vision is normal on testing.

Diagnosis: Parietal Lobe Stroke

Clinchers

- *A 65-year-old man:* Stroke or cerebrovascular accidents are most commonly seen in men than women and the incidence usually increases with age. After menopause, incidence is similar for both sexes.
- *Transient loss of consciousness, weakness of left arm:* Loss of consciousness with neurological deficits (weakness arm) signify stroke or transient ischaemic attack. The weakness of the left arm signify the involvement of right or the nondominant cerebral hemisphere.
- *Appears to always look towards right side while walking:* this is signifying sensory or visuospatial inattention, where the patient tends to neglect one side of field or his own body. usually involves the contralateral side of affection and is typical of nondominant parietal lobe involvement.
- *Left eye vision is normal:* This rules out the visual defects which might have forced the patient to prefer one side of the visual field.

CONFUSA

The involvement of occipital lobe typically causes visual filed defects and cortical blindness on the opposite side. The cortically blind patient may have no vision but pupillary responses are intact, normal fundoscopy with normal visual imagination and dreaming. However the visual evoked occipital potentials are typically absent.

Investigation of Choice

CT scan is the first Investigation of Choice
Doppler and angiography can be considered.

Immediate Management
Urgent referral.

Treatment of Choice
Thrombolysis - this is becoming an accepted treatment for ischaemic stroke provided that treatment is commenced within three hours of onset and that there is no sign of haemorrhage on the CT or angiogram - this treatment option is licensed in the US and it has now been licensed in the UK (only can be initiated by a specialist with necessary training).
-Antithrombotic and antiplatelet drugs, e.g. aspirin
-Neuroprotective agents

Your notes:

Serial No. 56

Subject: Psychiatry

Topic: Dementia

Question: A 40-year-old lady comes with gradual loss of memory. She has right handed involuntary writhing movement. Her father and uncle had similar problems.

Diagnosis: Huntington's Chorea

Clinchers

- *A 40-year-old lady:* The average age of onset of Huntington's disease is around 35-42 years, with mean age at death being 50-56 years. However, it can occur at any age, with around 8% occurring before 20 years(Juvenile Onset Huntington's Chorea) and 28% occurring later than 50 years(Late Onset Huntington's Disease).
- *Gradual loss of memory:* The classical description of Huntington's Disease is progressive degenerative neurological disorder with movement abnormalities (chorea) and dementia. Dementia is a late feature, with a strong insight, which can lead to depression and suicidal tendencies.
- *Right handed involuntary writhing movement:* The first physical sign is often the development of chorea, and disturbance of eye movement with gaze impersistence, distractibility and initiation defects with head thrusts. This can progress through increased saccadic latency to a supranuclear gaze palsy. Early signs may be personality change, self neglect, apathy with clumsiness, fidgets with fleeting facial grimaces.
- *Father and uncle had similar problems:* Family history is a strong point in favour of the disease, as it is inherited in autosomal dominant fashion with complete penetrance.

CONFUSA

For any case of dementia with movement abnormalities, even in the absence of family history, Huntington's chorea should be considered, as most often the family history is concealed. Moreover, there is no upper limit of age at which the disease can present itself. So, a child (with juvenile onset Huntington's chorea) can be very well affected, even if the father does not show any signs of the disease (with late onset Huntington's chorea).

Also, in questions with dementia and movement disorders, look out for Kayser-Fleischer Ring to come to a diagnosis of Wilson's Disease.

Investigation of Choice

Genetic testing for CAG trinucleotide expanded repeats on chromosome 4.

Immediate Management

Consult expert advice

Treatment of Choice

No treatment arrests the advance of the disease.

Tetrabenazine is used widely to suppress chorea:

Phenothiazines: Induces Parkinsonian syndrome to reduce the chorea.

Antidepressants is also be prescribed in cases of depression.

Your notes:

Serial No. 57

Subject: Psychiatry

Topic: Dementia

Question: A 55-year-old, otherwise healthy, man is brought to A and E by his wife who says that he has become progressively more forgetful. He also tends to lose his temper more often and is emotionally labile.

Diagnosis: Alzheimer's Disease (AD)

Clinchers

- *A 55-year-old, man:* The risk of AD is significantly higher in women than in men. AD is most prevalent in individuals older than 60 years. AD is the most common form of dementia seen in UK.
- *Otherwise healthy:* This rules out any possibility of vascular dementia which can closely resembles AD.
- *Progressively more forgetful:* The memory loss in AD is classically progressive and step-wise (recall, Lewy Body dementia, where the memory loss fluctuates). In AD the autobiographical memory and memory of everyday events is lost early in the disease, whilst short term memory is initially preserved.
- *Tends to lose his temper more often and is emotionally labile:* More than 40% patients of AD also present with noncognitive changes, which mainly includes a change in personality, aggressiveness, disinhibition and other behavioural changes.

CONFUSA

Lewy Body dementia may appear same as AD, but differs in following aspects:

- Memory loss: memory may be relatively normal in the early stages of Lewy body dementia, however its usually the presenting feature in AD.
- There is marked fluctuations of memory in patients with Lewy Body dementia and patient may appear severely demented and totally normal in different times of the same day. In AD, course is usually progressive; no fluctuations observed.
- Parkinsonism is an early feature of Lewy Body dementia; observed late in AD.
- Hallucinations is a major feature in Lewy body, not seen in AD.

Investigation of Choice

Apart from histology there are no specific tests for the diagnosis of Alzheimer's disease. Therefore, the principle is to rule out the differential diagnoses, and to diagnose Alzheimer's by exclusion.

Immediate Management

Avoid alcohol and drugs and treat any other disease which may exacerbate confusion.
Social and community support

Treatment of Choice

Cholinesterase inhibitors: Donepezil, rivastigmine, galantamine and tacrine .These drugs are available for the treatment of mild to moderate AD. There may be a slowing or even arrest of cognitive decline for about 8-9 months ; however the underlying disease process is not halted
Memantine is the first N-methyl-D-aspartate receptor antagonist to be licensed for the treatment of patients with moderately severe to severe Alzheimer's disease

Your notes:

Serial No. 58

Subject: Psychiatry

Topic: Dementia

Question: A 77-year-old man with weakness in his arm and leg, from which he recovered within few days. He now presents with short term memory loss. On examination he has extensor plantar response.He had similar episodes 2 years ago and became unable to identify objects and make proper judgements.

Diagnosis: Multi-infarct Dementia (Vascular Dementia)

Clinchers

- *A 77-year-old man:* Incidence of vascular dementia is higher in males than in females. The converse is true for Alzheimer's. This difference probably reflects known sex differences in the incidence of cerebrovascular disease. The incidence increases with age.
- *Weakness in his arm and leg, from which he recovered within few days:* The patient probably suffered from a mild stroke, from which he recovered gradually. This specifies the evidence of cerebrovascualr disease in the patient the cerebravascular accidents usually precede or co incide with the occurrence of dementia.
- *Short term memory loss, unable to identify objects and make proper judgements:* Problems with short-term memory typically show up first. There may be general forgetfulness, or a tendency to misplace household items. But over time, the memory lapses become more severe, and the dementia begins to take a debilitating toll on thinking, judgment, communication, and emotional stability.
- *Extensor plantar:* This again further confirms the cerebraovascular accident which has preceded the onset of symptoms.
- *Similar episodes in past:* The history is typical; multiple strokes over time gradually accumulate and cause extensive cerebral damage and the resulting dementia, hence the name, Multi-infarct Dementia.

CONFUSA

Multi-infarct dementia differs from Alzheimer's disease in following aspects:

- Progress is stepwise rather than gradual
- Evidence of systemic cardiovascular disease - especially hypertension.
- Focal neurological signs - pseudobulbar palsy
- Walking may be in small steps - "marche a petit pas"
- Severity of symptoms can vary throughout the day, typically being worst in the evening
- Better preservation of personality, insight and social responsiveness

Note that, a cognitively impaired patient with vascular risks factors but no history of cerebrovascular disease is most likely to have Alzheimer's Disease.

Investigation of Choice

CT scan will show multiple cortical, and more commonly subcortical infarcts or single strokes affecting the thalamus, angular gyrus, and the territory supplied by the anterior cerebral arteries.

Immediate Management

Rule out other causes of reversible dementia (viz Vitamin B 12 deficiency, hypothyroidism).

Behaviour and psychological support.

Treatment of Choice

Aim at treating the risk factors for further strokes (viz hypertension).

Aspirin initiated to prevent further strokes.

Anticoagulants should be used very carefully keeping in mind the repetitive falls.

Your notes:

Serial No. 59

Subject: Psychiatry

Topic: Dementia

Question: A 59-year-old man with early loss of speech and memory with visuospatial orientation preserved.

Diagnosis: Fronto Temporal Dementia(FTD)

Clinchers

- *A 59-year-old man:* Fronto-temporal dementia is a rare form of dementia, occurring far less frequently than Alzheimer's disease. Younger people, specifically those under the age of 65, are more likely to be affected. Men and women are equally likely to develop the condition.
- *Early loss of speech and memory:* FTD, is caused by damage to the frontal lobe and/or the temporal parts of the brain. These areas are responsible for our behaviour, emotional responses and language skills. Typically, during the initial stages of fronto-temporal dementia, memory is still intact, but the personality and behaviour of the person changes.
- *Visuospatial orientation preserved:* Visuospatial orientation are preserved till late in the disease. Recall, Alzheimer's disease, where visuospatial orientation is lost early.

CONFUSA

Frontal Lobe dementia and fronto temporal dementia are easily confused as most symptoms do overlap. However, if the question mentions only about disinhibition viz, increased aggressiveness, hyperorality, utilization behaviour (i.e., picking up and manipulating any object in the environment, appropriate or not), and inappropriate sexuality, the diagnosis of frontal Lobe dementia should be sought for. If the loss of speech is also mentioned in addition to frontal lobe features, the diagnosis of fronto temporal dementia is more likely.

Investigation of Choice

Neuropsychological testing and evaluation by a speech/language pathologist with standardized language batteries is diagnostic.

CT scan shows cerebral atrophy, usually of the frontal and temporal lobe and helps to rule out causes like stroke or any space occupying lesions.

Immediate Management

Identify any treatable causes of dementia.

Treatment of Choice

Symptomatic drug treatment.

Behaviour Therapy

Treat any associated depression

Your notes:

Serial No. 76

Subject: Surgery

Topic: Trauma

Question: A man involved in an RTA, presents with headache and loss of consciousness after admission.

Diagnosis: Extradural haemorrhage

Clinchers

- *Involved in an RTA:* The most common setting of extradural haemorrhage is an adult involved in an RTA sustaining temporal or parietal bone fracture and thereby injuring middle meningeal vessels leading to torrential bleed between the skull and the dura.
- *Presents with headache:* Headache is the most common symptom due to cerebral concussion or vasogenic oedema.
- *Loss of consciousness after admission:* This is the most important clincher here, showing that patients' level of consciousness was normal at the time of admission and deteriorated later. This is signifying lucid interval-concussion followed by temporary recovery of consciousness for minutes or hours before the onset of drowsiness and possibly coma. This is most characteristic of extradural haemorrhage.

CONFUSA

Intracerebral bleed can be a cause of real confusion here. However, note that most common presentation of intracerebral bleed is in the setting of uncontrolled hypertension or in an elderly with atherosclerosis or amyloid angiopathy. Trauma can also rarely cause intracerebral bleed, but the presentation will always have definite neurological deficits to signify the site of bleeding. In the absence of any positive history (like hypertension) or neurological deficits, intracerebral bleed is an unlikely diagnosis here. Moreover, the setting of trauma and loss of consciousness after admission, points more in favour of extradural haemorrhage.

Investigation of Choice

CT scan head

Immediate Management

Immediate neurosurgery referral

Treatment of Choice

Burr holes or ideally craniotomy to evacuate haematoma.

Serial No. 77

Subject: Medicine

Topic: Headache

Question: A 45-year-old man presents with unilateral temporal headache.

Diagnosis: Temporal Arteritis

Clinchers

- *Unilateral temporal headache:* Headache, is the most universal symptom, present in with temporal arteritis and there are certain features in temporal arteritis headache which distinguishes it from other types of headaches:
  - Headache most commonly tends to be unilateral, classically concentrating on the temporal region.
  - Its insidious in onset typically worse at night.
  - Underlying pain described as a burning or jabbing sensation may involve the surface of the scalp and face. Intracranial arteries are rarely involved.
  - Scalp tenderness is typical -simple acts such as combing hair or resting the head on a pillow exacerbate pain.

CONFUSA

GMC is in the habit to provide us with such minimum information in a question that for few seconds we think in bewilderment that a unilateral temporal headache can be caused by any or all of the causes listed in the options. However, if you look carefully you can easily rule out other possibilities.

- An absence of history of injury rules out all types skull fractures as a probable cause.
- An absence of typical aura associated with migraine, rules out that possibility too.
- Again, absence of features of papilloedema or neurological deficits rules out intracranial space occupying lesion as the probable cause.
- Takayasu's arteritis typically involves main branches of aorta.

Investigation of Choice

ESR

Temopral artery biopsy

Immediate Management

Sudden loss of vision is an ophthalmological emergency and requires immediate referral to the eye emergency department (may require upto 1mg/kg of prednisolone per day).

Treatment of Choice

In the absence of visual symptoms, giant cell arteritis is treated with 30-40mg per day of prednisolone.

Your notes:

Serial No. 78

Subject: Medicine

Topic: Headache

Question: A 27-year-old female with recurrent unilateral headache and transient visual disturbances.

Diagnosis: Classical Migraine

Clinchers

- *A 27-year-old female:* Migraine commonly affects females more than males with maximum cases presenting before 30 years of age.
- *Recurrent unilateral headache:* The headache of migraine is typically frontotemporal, unilateral and pulsatile. Each episode lasts for 4-72 hrs and the diagnosis of migraine requires the headache to be recurrent, being precipitated by triggering factors, like stress, menstruation, exercise, or the like.
- *Transient visual disturbances:* Visual aura are the most common aura known to be associated with migraine. Visual aura can be in the form of fortification spectra, which are often 'C'-shaped (most common type), scotoma, objects may rotate, oscillate, or 'boil' simple flashes, specks, and shimmerings. Paresthesia are the second most common type of aura and the patient may present with attacks of numbness which subsides without any deficits, but recurs again with the next attack.

CONFUSA

While the unilateral temporal headache in an elderly, associated with visual disturbance points towards, temporal arteritis, in an young female, it points towards migraine. Note that the blindness associated with temporal arteritis is not 'transient' , is an ocular emergency and requires immediate high dose steroids, to save the other eye.

Investigation of Choice

None. Migraine is a clinical diagnosis.

Immediate Management

1st line drugs in acute attack—Soluble aspirin 600-900 mg stat in adults.

If patient vomiting—Consider Diclofenac suppositories 100 mg plus domperidone suppositories 30 mg.

If these fail a triptan (sumatriptan 100 mg) is the next line. Triptans should be considered if first-line treatment has proved ineffective or is poorly tolerated.

Treatment of Choice

Aimed at preventing further attacks. Migraine recurring four or more times per month should be treated prophylactically.

Beta blockers (Propranolol) is often used as first choice, especially when hypertension coexists.

Amitriptyline 10-150 mg daily if migraine coexists with depression.

Your notes:

Serial No. 79

Subject: Medicine

Topic: Headache

Question: A 32-year-old man presents with bouts of intense headache everyday as soon as he wakes up. He is well otherwise.

Diagnosis: Cluster Headache

Clinchers

- *A 32-year-old man:* Cluster headache most commonly affects male than females with peak attacks at around 30-40 years.
- *Bouts of intense headache:* The attacks typically come rapidly without an aura, peaking within 10 minutes. The pain is extremely intense and may be associated with lacrimation, lid swelling, red eye and rhinorrhoea. The character of the pain is usually non pulsatile and is focused around one eye or temple (usually the same side each attack).
- *As soon as he wakes up:* Attacks often cluster around the same time of the day, (hence- 'Cluster Headache') lasting an average of 45 minutes.
- *He is well otherwise:* This rules out any other serious abnormality which can be associated with similar presentations. The attacks come in "clusters" of 1-3 per day usually over approximately an eight week period. Patient is well in between these 'clusters'.

CONFUSA

The headache due to an intracranial space occupying lesion (ICSOL) is also intense, and usually wakes up the patient from sleep. However, in such questions, look carefully for the hints at associated vomiting, papilloedema or ataxia which signify raised intracranial tension. Associated neurological findings again goes strong with the diagnosis of ICSOL.

Investigation of Choice

None - its a clinical diagnosis.

Immediate Management

Consult expert advice

Treatment of Choice

- For acute attack:
  ~Inhalation of 100% oxygen
  ~Sumatriptan
  ~Intranasal lignocaine

- For Prophylaxis:
  - ~ Verapamil has been shown to reduce the attack frequency.
  - ~ Alternatives: Ergotamine, Sodium valproate

Your notes:

Serial No. 80

Subject: Medicine

Topic: Headache

Question: A 22-year-old man complains of dull headache which is worst upon awakening. He also complains of defective vision left side and vomiting.

Diagnosis: Intracranial Space Occupying Lesion (ICSOL)

Clinchers

- *Dull headache:* The headache associated with ICSOL are generally dull and generalised over the entire cranium.
- *Worst upon awakening:* The hypoventilation during sleeping, typically deprives the brain of adequate oxygen making the headache worst during early hours of morning. This again is very characteristic of ICSOL; it may even cause severe headache during sleep to wake up the patient.
- *Defective vision left side:* Neurological deficits again signify some intracranial pathology behind this headache. Visual defects can occur either due to raised intracranial tension or due to the mass directly impinging on the visual pathway.
- *Vomiting:* associated nausea, vomiting, ataxia and papilloedema are the manifestations of raised intra-cranial pressure.

CONFUSA

If the headache is present on waking, classically worsened by exercise, coughing/sneezing, straining, stooping, coitus, or influenced by posture (worse on lying or bending down), consider rising intracranial pressure. If accompanied by other signs of raised ICP such as vomiting, papilloedema, epilepsy, progressive focal neurology, or mental change. Frontal or maxillary headache, worst on stooping forward may also signify maxillary or frontal sinusitis. Always, look carefully for associated hints in the question to come to correct diagnosis.

Investigation of Choice

Admit urgently for diagnostic imaging - CT scan
LP is contraindicated

Immediate Management

Neurological Referral

Treatment of Choice

According to the cause identified.

Serial No. 83

Subject: Urogenital

Topic: Urine Retention

Question: An 18-year-old girl comes with acute pain lower abdomen and difficulty in walking. She has not passed urine since 48 hrs. She gives history of visual loss few years back, which has now resolved completely.

Diagnosis: Multiple Sclerosis (MS)

Clinchers

- *A 18-year-old girl:* MS is more common in females than males and onset is usually between 16-50 years with a peak at 20-40 years.
- *Acute pain lower abdomen, not passed urine since 48 hrs:* She is presenting with acute retention of urine. Both incontinence and retention are commonly seen in bladder dysfunction associated with multiple sclerosis.
- *Difficulty in walking:* This is signifying spinal cord involvement by the disease process, which is causing paraparesis.
- *History of visual loss few years back, which has now resolved completely:* Though the natural progress of the disease is characterised by multiple neurological deficits, optic neuritis is one most consistent finding in most patients. It presents as retrobulbar pain and patchy loss of vision.

CONFUSA

Bladder dysfunction associated with multiple sclerosis can take various forms:

- Disinhibition of detrusor muscle - produces a combination of urgency and incontinence.
- Complete urinary retention
- Retention associated with urinary tract infection - the resulting cystitis exacerbates the urgency and incontinence, and so a vicious cycle occurs.
- Also note that, spinal cord lesions may necessitate prolonged catheterization and cause urethral stricture in the long run.

Investigation of Choice

Confirm multiple sclerosis by CSF examination (typical oligoclonal bands).

MRI will shows areas of patchy demyelination.

Immediate Management

Catheterize

Treatment of Choice

Disease modifying agents (beta interferon, glatiramer acetate and azathioprine).

Urinary frequency and incontinence treated by anti-cholinergics (oxybutynin) and tricyclic antidepressants (amitriptyline)

Urinary retention: offer intermittent self-catheterisation

Your notes:

Serial No. 93

Subject: Urogenital

Topic: Incontinence Urine

Question: A young girl with history of visual loss and bilateral lower limb weakness, complains of not able to pass urine at all.

Diagnosis: Multiple Sclerosis (MS)

Clinchers

- *Young girl:* MS is more common in females than males and onset is usually between 16-50 years with a peak at 20-40 years.
- *History of visual loss:* Though the natural progress of the disease is characterised by multiple neurological deficits, optic neuritis is one most consistent finding in most patients. It presents as retrobulbar pain and patchy loss of vision.
- *Bilateral lower limb weakness:* This is signifying spinal cord involvement by the disease process.
- *Not able to pass urine at all:* She is presenting with acute retention of urine. Both incontinence and retention are commonly seen in bladder dysfunction associated with multiple sclerosis.

CONFUSA

Bladder dysfunction associated with multiple sclerosis can take various forms:

- Disinhibition of detrusor muscle - produces a combination of urgency and incontinence.
- Complete urinary retention
- Retention associated with urinary tract infection - the resulting cystitis exacerbates the urgency and incontinence, and so a vicious cycle occurs.
- Also note that, spinal cord lesions may necessitate prolonged catheterization and cause urethral stricture in the long run.

Investigation of Choice

Confirm multiple sclerosis by CSF examination (typical oligoclonal bands).

MRI will shows areas of patchy demyelination.

Immediate Management

Catheterize

Treatment of Choice

Disease modifying agents (beta interferon, glatiramer acetate and azathioprine).

Urinary frequency and incontinence treated by anti-cholinergics (oxybutynin) and tricyclic antidepressants (amitriptyline)

Urinary retention: Offer intermittent self-catheterisation

Your notes:

Serial No. 100

Subject: Urogenital

Topic: Retention Urine

Question: A 39-year-old female presents with weakness of both legs, difficulty walking and urinary retention.

Diagnosis: Spinal Cord Lesion

Clinchers

- *A 39-year-old female:* A spinal cord lesion in an young female in the absence of an obvious cause (like trauma),should always raise the possibility of multiple sclerosis, especially when there is a co-existent visual abnormality(optic neuritis).
- *Weakness of both legs, difficulty walking:* These denote motor abnormality associated with spinal cord lesions due to the involvement of the long tracts.Bilateral leg weakness (paraparesis) is the commonest presentation of spinal cord dysfunction, but quadriparesis, monoparesis or any combination of limb weakness can be seen. The associated spasiticity makes walking difficult.
- *Urinary retention:* This occurs due to involvement of the autonomic fibres. Loss of descending inhibition of segmental reflex control leads to urinary urgency and incontinence. In acute cases, however, lesions may be associated with a flaccid bladder and urinary retention.

CONFUSA

Spinal cord lesions are suspected when there are long tract signs below a certain spinal level, with or without segmental signs at that level. Segmental signs include motor weakness and atrophy in a myotomal pattern, sensory loss in a dermatomal distribution and loss of tendon reflexes at the level of the lesion. Long tract signs include upper motor neuron dysfunction (weakness, spasticity, increased tendon reflexes, and Babinski responses), bilateral sensory loss below the level of the lesion and loss of bladder control.

Investigation of Choice

Extensive investigation so as to find the probable cause for the spinal cord lesion viz, multiple sclerosis, disc prolapse, stroke, Gullian Barre Syndrome or spinal tumours.

Immediate Management

Retention can be managed by catheterizing

Treatment of Choice

According to the cause identified.

Serial No. 124

Subject: Medicine

Topic: Genetics

Question: An 11-year-old boy presents with increasing difficulty walking, tremour and instability. Father died in his 40's with same disease.

Diagnosis: Huntington's Chorea

Clinchers

- *An 11-year-old boy:* Most cases of Huntington's Chorea occur between 30-50 years of age. Only a minority of cases present as Juvenile Huntington's Disease.
- *Increasing difficulty walking, tremour and instability:* The disease often first presents with the development of chorea, which gradually worsens as the disease progresses to affect walking and speech. Patient gradually develops dementia and eventually patients develop akinesia and rigidity.
- *Father died in his 40's with same disease:* Family history of the disease is characteristic. Death usually follows within 15 years of diagnosis.

CONFUSA

Huntington's Chorea has a prevalence of about 1 in 20,000 in the UK. It is inherited as an autosomal dominant trait with full penetrance. The family history of the disease is often present, even if not clearly elicited in history. The genetic basis of the disease lies in the trinucleotide repeats –CAG. The larger the number of CAG repeats, the earlier the onset of HD. Early-onset HD is associated with paternal inheritance of the HD gene. It may be that the trinucleotide repeats are more prone to expansion during spermatogenesis than oogenesis.

Investigation of Choice

Diagnosis is based on a thorough personal and family medical history and physical examination.

Genetic testing involves taking a blood sample for DNA analysis to determine whether the distinct mutation for Huntington's disease has occurred in gene IT-15.

Immediate Management

Consult expert advice

Treatment of Choice

Tertrabenzine and phenothiazines- reduce chorea

Antidepressants

Serial No. 143

Subject: Medicine

Topic: Epilepsy

Question: A 35-year-old mechanic has recurrent epileptiform attacks. He has no history of trauma.

Clinchers

- *A 35-year-old:* Although there is no specific at which epilepsy can be diagnosed, the earlier the onset is, the better is the prognosis.
- *Mechanic:* His being a mechanic by profession poses enough social and employment stigma, as far as the diagnosis of epilepsy is concerned, because handling of machines can pose a dangerous risk and he would need to discontinue his present profession and opt for an alternative. Thus, every effort should be made to rule a possible alternative, especially if one is treatable.
- *Recurrent epileptiform attacks, no history of trauma:* Epilepsy is defined as the recurrent paroxysmal transient disturbance of brain function due to disturbance of electrical activity in the brain, where the disturbance is unrelated to infection or acute cerebral insult.

CONFUSA

A person who has suffered an epileptic attack whilst awake must refrain from driving for one year from the date of the attack, or a person who has suffered an attack whilst asleep must also refrain from driving for one year from the date of the attack.
A diagnosed epileptic patient can start driving if he has been free from epileptic seizures for 10 years or, have not taken any medication for 10 years

Investigation of Choice
EEG

Immediate Management
Specialist referral

Treatment of Choice
Antiepileptic drug therapy based on the specific condition identified

Your notes:

Serial No. 144

Subject: Medicine

Topic: Trauma

Question: An 18-year-old student is brought to the Accident and Emergency department by ambulance having been flung off his bicycle in a road traffic accident upon arrival, he is noted to have deterioration in consciousness.

Diagnosis: Head Injury

Clinchers

- *An 18-year-old student:* Road traffic accidents are by far more common in males from 15-35 years of age perhaps due to indulgence in more outdoor activities.
- *Flung off his bicycle in a road traffic accident:* The mode shows the enormous impact of the injury.
- *Deterioration in consciousness:* A sudden increase in intracranial pressure, either due to intracranial bleed or due to vasogenic/reactive oedema, can cause deteoriation in consciousness.

CONFUSA

The extent of recovery is often correlated with the duration of post-traumatic amnaesia. As a guide, post-traumatic amnaesia of more than 28 days is rarely associated with a return to work. Post-traumatic amnaesia of more than one week is likely to impair higher intellectual activity. That of less than one day should allow a return to previous activity after several months. The prognosis is better for younger patients, worse for older ones.

Investigation of Choice
CT scan head (noncontrast)

Immediate Management
Urgent referral

Treatment of Choice
Depending on the cause identified on the CT for a raised ICP.

Your notes:

Serial No. 145

Topic: Medicine

Subject: Trauma

Question: A 32-year-old boxer presents with headache, drowsiness, seizures, and a rising blood pressure.

Diagnosis: Subdural haematoma

Clinchers

- *A 32-year-old boxer:* Chronic subdural haematoma are seen in people who are predisposed to recurrent injuries due to one reason or the other, as commonly encountered in the alcoholics and the boxers. Repeated injuries cause rupture of the subcortical bridgibng veins which gradually extend over time to form an organized haematoma and cause pressure effects.
- *Headache, drowsiness, seizures, a rising blood pressure:* This occurs to the pressure effect created by the haematoma. Fluctuating consciousness is almost characteristic.

CONFUSA

A similar mechanism occur in the elderly whose brain size gradually shrink with time. This shrinkage causes the brain to be suspended in the cranium on the support of the bridging subcortical veins. Thus, even minor trauma in these elderly individuals can cause rupture of the subcortical veins and lead to acute or chronic subdural haematoma.

Investigation of Choice
Noncontrast CT scan

Immediate Management
Urgent Neurosurgery referral

Treatment of Choice
Evacuate haematoma

Your notes:

Serial No. 166

Subject: Medicine

Topic: Neurology

Question: A 55-year-old man with history of stroke and repeated falls, now confused and can not remember things.

Diagnosis: Vascular Dementia

Clinchers

- *A 55-year-old man:* Incidence of vascular dementia is higher in males than in females. The converse is true for Alzeihmer's. This difference probably reflects known sex differences in the incidence of cerebrovascular disease. The incidence increases with age.
- *History of stroke:* This specifies the evidence of cerebrovascualr disease in the patient the cerebravascular accidents usually precede or co incide with the occurrence of dementia.
- *Repeated falls:* Signifies transient ischaemic attacks, again making the factor of cerebraovascular disease strong.
- *Now confused and can not remember things:* disorientation and step wise loss of memory is classical.

CONFUSA

Multi-infarct dementia differs from Alzheimer's disease in following aspects:

- Progress is stepwise rather than gradual
- Evidence of systemic cardiovascular disease - especially hypertension
- Focal neurological signs - pseudobulbar palsy
- Walking may be in small steps - "marche a petit pas"
- Severity of symptoms can vary throughout the day, typically being worst in the evening
- Better preservation of personality, insight and social responsiveness

Note that, a cognitively impaired patient with vascular risks factors but no history of cerebrovascular disease is most likely to have Alzeihmer's Disease.

Investigation of Choice
CT scan will show multiple cortical, and more commonly subcortical infarcts or single strokes affecting the thalamus, angular gyrus, and the territory supplied by the anterior cerebral arteries.

Immediate Management

Rule out other causes of reversible dementia (viz Vitamin B 12 deficiency, hypothyroidism).

Behaviour and psychological support.

Treatment of Choice

Aim at treating the risk factors for further strokes (viz hypertension).

Aspirin initiated to prevent further strokes.

Anticoagulants should be used very carefully keeping in mind the repitive falls.

Your notes:

PAPER 3

6. A 73-year-old complains of a severe right sided headache associated with an acute loss of right sided vision. Urgent treatment is needed to prevent left sided vision loss

Diagnosis: Giant cell arteritis (GCA).

Clinchers

- *A 73-year-old:* Cranial arteritis is common after 55 years of age (60 years according to Kumar and Clark).
- *Severe right sided headache:* Headache is almost invariable in GCA. Pain is felt over the inflamed superficial, temporal or occipital arteries. Though the disease process ultimately involves arteries bilaterally, in the initial stages it is usually unilateral.
- *Associated with an acute loss of right sided vision:* Visual loss owing to inflammation and occlusion of the ciliary and/or central retinal artery occurs in 25% of cases and untreated GCA. It is characteristically sudden, painless, partial or complete, uniocular visual loss. Amaurosis fugax may precede total visual loss.
- *Urgent treatment is needed to prevent left sided vision loss:* Urgent GCA patients need to have an ESR and high dose oral steroids immediately. However if visual symptoms are present, give higher doses IV as it could be sight saving.

CONFUSA

Other forms of arteritis, such as SLE and PAN, can occasionally present with similar featurs (but PLAB questions on GCA are usually straight forward). Also note that GCA is closely related to polymyalgia rheumatica and these can occur in the same patient.

Investigation of Choice

- *Screening:* ESR.
- *Definitive:* Temporal artery biopsy (skip lesions occur, so repeat any negative biopsy if there are strong clinical pointers)

Immediate Management

Two things are to be done immediately"

1. ESR
2. High dose oral steroids (IV if visual symptoms).

Treatment of Choice

Prednisolone, 40-60 mg/24h, PO

- Dose is reduced as ESR falls/is increased if symptoms recurs.
- Headache subsides within hours of first large dose.
- Remission in 2 years usually.
- Steroid treatment is the main cause of death in long-term in GCA patients.

16. A 16-year-old girl collapses after standing for a while. Her limbs are flaccid and she is not incontinent. Following 30 seconds she recovers fully.

Diagnosis: Vasovagal syncope.

Clinchers

- *A 16-year-old girl:* Vasovagal syncope is the simple faint which the majority of the population suffer at some time, particularly in childhood, in youth or in pregnancy.
- *Collapses after standing for a while:* Prolonged standing, fear, pain, or venesection are common precipitation.
- *Her limbs are flaccid:* This differentiation it from epilepsy though some jerky movements can occur in vasovagal attacks, the limbs are never tonic-clonic.
- *She is not incontinent:* Incontinence of urine is rare and there is never incontinence of faeces in a vasovagal syncope.
- *Following 30 seconds she recovers fully:* In vasovagal syncope, the subject fallts to ground and is unconscious for less than two minutes. Recovery is rapid and there is no postictal confusion or amnaesia.

CONFUSA

The main points to differentiate between syncope and pathological causes of loss of consciouness in the presence and absence of postictal confusion and duration of the episode.

Investigation of Choice

Syncope can usually be distinguished on the basis of clinical history alone. Investigate fully if in doubt.

Immediate Management

Lie flat + elevate lower limbs + record pulse.

Treatment of Choice

Vasovagal syncope do not require any specific treatment except prophylactic avoidance of precipitants.

Common causes of sudden collapse with coma:

- Subarachnoid haemorrhage
- Brainstem CVA
- Hypoglycaemia
- Poisoning (tricyclics)
- **Head injury**

Your notes:

17. An 82-year-old has 5 episodes of loss of consciousness with no convulsions in a single day.

Diagnosis: Stokes-Adams attacks.

Clinchers

- *A 82-year-old:* Stokes-Adams attacks are important causes of recurrent episodes of loss of consciousness, particularly in the elderly.
- *5 episodes of loss of consciousness:* Attacks may happen several times a day and in any posture.
- *With no convulsions:* Convulsions are typically absent in Stokes-Adams attacks. A few clonic jerks may occur if an attack is prolonged.

CONFUSA

The question does not provide a specific picture of Stokes-Adams attacks which is palpitations ® collapse + paleness + flushing ® recovery (within seconds). However, other conditions can be easily excluded by age and recurrence.

Investigation of Choice

ECG (24 hours Holter monitoring).

Immediate Management

Lie flat + elevate lower limbs + record pulse.

Treatment of Choice

Permanent pacemaker (even when asymptomatic)

CASE HISTORY: STROKE

A 68-year-old man presents with a history of right sided weakness in arm, leg and face with loss of speech for four hours.

He is mildly confused but has no headache. He has history of ischaemic heart disease. On examination there is global dysphasia, full visual fields, UMN distribution right facial weakness and dense weakness of right side (UMN distribution) with absent reflexes and upgoing plantar response on that side.

Clinical diagnosis: Left middle cerebral artery ischaemic stroke.

Immediate Management

- O_2 by mask
- Hb, U and E, WCC, glucose, ESR
- CT scan (check haemorrhage)

18. A 50-year-old male wakes up with a tingling and numbness in his right hand. This is accompanies by slurring of speech which recovers following about four hours complications and associations of blood dyscrasias.

Diagnosis: Transient ischaemic attack (TIA) in carotid territory.

Clinchers

- *A 50-year-old male:* TIA is more common after the age of 40 as the incidence of its predisposing diseases is more after this age.
- *Wakes up with a tingling and numbness in his right hand:* Contralateral weakness/numbness is characteristic of carotid territory ischaemia. On the other hand, in vertebrobasilar territory ischaemia haemiparesis and Haemisensory loss, bilateral weakness or sensory loss are features.
- *This is accompanied by slurring of speech:* Dysarthria is a feature of both carotid and vertebrobasilar territory ischaemia but dysphasia is present in only carotid territory ischaemia.
- *Which recovers following about four hours complications:* By definition, a TIA has to fully resolve within 24 hours.
- *Associations of blood dyscrasias:* Haematological disease (polycythaemia, sickle cell, multiple myeloma) can cause TIA (though emboli from heart are the most common).

CONFUSA

Always keep in mind the differential diagnosis of TIA, which are:

- *Migraine:* Symptoms spread and intensify over minutes, often with visual scintillations before headache (headache is rare in TIA)
- *Focal epilepsy:* Symptoms spread over seconds and often include twitching and jerking

Investigation of Choice

Carotid Doppler.

Immediate Management

Antiplatelet drug (aspirin if no peptic ulcer).

Treatment of Choice

Carotid endarterectomy.

Present UK guidelines do *not* indicate thrombolysis—even if a stroke is diagnosed within four hours with normal CT (i.e. a haemorrhagic shock).

19. A 34-year-old woman has 6 month history of on and off haemiparesis which resolves with no neurological deficits.

Diagnosis: Multiple sclerosis (MS).

Clinchers

- *A 34-year-old woman:* MS has a female preponderence with mean age of onset as 30 years.
- *6 months history of on and off haemiparesis which resolves with no neurological deficits:* First presentations of MS are usually monosymptomatic: unilateral optic neuritis (pain on eye movement and rapid deterioration in central vision) numbness or tingling in the limbs, leg weakness or brainstem or cerebellar symptoms such as diplopia or ataxia. Less often there may be more than one symptom. Symptoms may be worsened by heat (e.g. a hot bath) or exercise. The early picture is usually one of relapses followed by remissions with full functional recovery. With time, remissions, become incomplete and cause accumulation of progressive disability.

CONFUSA

Isolated neurological deficits are never diagnostic, but may become so if a careful history is taken to reveal previous episodies. Nevertheless the diagnosis of MS is always clinical, requiring demonstration of lesions disseminated in time and space, unattributable to other causes.

Investigation of Choice

- None is pathognomic.
- MRI for plaque demonstration in occipital lobe.

Immediate Management

Methylprednisolone (shortens relapses)

Treatment of Choice

b-interferon 16.

CASE HISTORY: MULTIPLE SCLEROSIS (MS)

A 26-year-old man presents with several days of pain and progressive loss of vision in left eye. On examination there is loss of colour vision, acuity of 6/36 and disc swelling. He has previously had an episode of gait and bladder disturbances that recovered fully after several weeks.

Clinical Diagnosis

Optic neuritis (common first presentation of MS), along with previous episode of transverse myelitis, strongly suggests diagnosis of multiple sclerosis.

Investigation
MRI to look for demyelinating lesions of MS.
CSF: Oligoclonal bands.
Rx: IV Methyl prednisolone.

23. A 55-year-old man with history of hypertension untreated presents with haemiparesis.

Diagnosis: Intracerebral haemorrhage.

Clinchers
- *A 55-year-old man:* Elderly person are more prone to hypertensive complications especially if it is left-untreated. Incidence of hypertension in males is more.
- *History of hypertension untreated:* Intracerebral haemorrhage occurs typically in patients with untreated hypertension. SAH is also associated with hypertension but its association is not so typical and usually present with severe headache and neck stiffness.
- *Presents with haemiparesis:* Focal neurological deficits are more common with intracerebral bleeds (cf SAH) which occurs at well-defined sites (basal ganglia, pons, cerebellum and subcortical white matter) due to rupture of Charcot-Bouchard aneurysms.

CONFUSA

- Haemiplegia/haemiparesis
  - Early—suggests formation of an intracerebral haematoma
  - Late—suggests vasospasm and ischaemia
- Clinically thre is no entirely reliable way of distinguishing between intracerebral haemorrhage and thromboembolic infarction, as both produce a sudden focal deficit. Intracerebral haemorrhage, however, tends to be dramatic and accompanied by a severe headache (but still less severe than that of SAH).

Investigation of Choice
Visualized reliably by immediate CT (contrast from infarction).

Immediate Management
Urgent neurosurgical evacuation of the clot should be considered when an intracerebral haematoma behaves as an expanding mass, causing deepening coma and coning.

Treatment of Choice
Unlike thromboembolism antiplatelet drugs are contraindicated. Surgery is indicated if conservative measures fail.

Your notes:

25. A 38-year-old woman presents with cervical lymphaedenopathy. Mature lymphoblasts are seen on the blood film. Examination reveals a mild splenomegaly. She is on phenytoin for epilepsy.

Diagnosis: Phenytoin side effects.

Clinchers

- *Cervical lymphadenopathy:* It can occur as a syndrome of hypersensitivity to phenytoin. It includes rashes, DLE and neutropenia. It is rare but requires discontinuation of therapy.
- *Mature lymphoblasts.* It is also a component of the above mentioned hypersensitivity syndrome. It manifest as leukocytosis often with atypical lymphocytes and eosinophils.
- *Mild splenomegaly:* Can occur in phenytoin treatment as a response to various blood dyscrasias phenytoin causes as side effects.

CONFUSA

Acute myeloid leukaemia can be excluded as the presenting cells are not myeloblasts. Plus it need bone marrow biopsy for definitive diagnosis. Nevertheless, gum hyperplasia can occur in this condition also in addition to phenytoin therapy. (So even if you are confused, you would not be wrong). Acute lymphoblastic leukaemia is characterised by immature lymphoblasts and not mature lymphoblasts (as in this case).

Note: Cyclosporin also causes gum hypertrophy.

Investigation of Choice

Phenytoin blood levels (Normal: 40-80 µmol/L).

Immediate Management

Systemic steroids to reduce symptoms.

Treatment of Choice

Discontinue phenytoin.

Your notes:

54. A 37-year-old alcoholic is found wandering in a park. His partner says he has had a number of falls recently and in the A and E the patient is confused. The blood sugar level is normal.

Diagnosis: Head injury (probable).

Clinchers

- *Alcoholic:* Subdural haematomas are commonly seen in alcoholics. There may be no apparent injury. The first sign may be a failure to wake up after an episode of heavy drinking.
- *History of number of falls recently:* Frequent falls weaken the bridging veins which traverse the subdural space. They can bleed to give rise to subdural haematomas. This mechanism is responsible for their frequent incidence in alcoholics. Subdural haematomas are also common among elderly and HIV patients. But in them the pathogenesis is cerebral atropy ® shrinkage of brain ® stretching of bridging veins ® rupture ® haematoma.
- *Confused:* A CT scan is indicated in all cases of clouding on consciousness or low GCS in an alcoholic, as the clinical assessment is difficult in an intoxicated patient.

CONFUSA

A normal blood sugar rules out hypoglycaemia which is a more common cause of confusion in an alcoholic. On the other hand this patient could be plainly showing only the features of intoxication, but CT scan is still essential from medicolegal point of view in UK.

Investigation of Choice

CT scan (subdural haematoma—inner concave border).

Immediate Management

Admit in hospital (at least overnight).

Treatment of Choice

Depends on CT findings.

Your notes:

71. Following an alcoholic binge a 36-year-old male falls and comes to casualty with a cut in his temporal region his Glasgow Coma Scale is normal and his neck is cleared by the orthopaedic SHO.

Diagnosis: Superficial head injury.

Clinchers

- *Following an alcoholic binge*: Alcoholics warrants overnight admission in the hospital as they cannot be assessed properly on presentation for head injury. This is applicable even if the GCS is normal. Other patients warranting admission in spite of normal GCS are children and postictal (confused) patients.
- *Falls:* Most probably it is the reason for the cut in the temporal region. Note that alcoholics are more prone to develop subdural haematomas due to weakening of bridging veins because of repeated falls.
- *A cut in his temporal region:* It must be a simple laceration if there is no associated fracture of temporal bone. It requires prompt suturing to maintain haemostasis.
- *Glasgow Coma Scale is normal:* Rules out any immediate brain damage/haematoma. But not that it is difficult or even misleading in an alcoholic.
- *His neck is cleared by the orthopedic SHO:* It rules out any spinal injury.

CONFUSA

The main confusion is about whom to admit or discharge in a case of head injury. The criteria are:
Criteria for admission in a case of head injury

- Difficult to assess
  - *Child*
  - *Postictal*
  - *Alcohol intoxication*
- CNS signs
- Severe headache or vomiting
- Fracture
- Smelling of alcohol with GCS < 15

Criteria for discharge with written advise (all criteria must be fulfilled)

- Fully conscious on presentation
- No abnormal neurological signs
- Loss of consciousness < 5 min
- Post-traumatic amnaesia < 5 min
- No severe headache
- No vomiting
- No skull fracture
- No bleeding disorder
- Good home conditions

Note: Get an X-ray skull in all suspected medicolegal cases (like this one) even if you suspect no bony injury Other main confusion is about anterograde and retrograde amnaesia. Note the only the extent of anterograte amnaesia correlates with severity of injury (admit if > 5 min). Retrograde amnaesia does not correlate well with severity. Also retrograde amnaesia never occurs without anterograde amnaesia. Anterograde amnaesia (also known as post-traumatic amnaesia—PTA) if under one hour, means mild injury whereas > 24 years denotes severe injury. OHCM has stated on the contrary and thus created this confusion. But refer Kumar and Clark, pg 1084, 4th edn and lecture notes in emergency medicine, pg 36 second edition.

Investigation of Choice

X-ray skull (CT in an alcoholic is only indicated if GCS falls).

Immediate Management

Suturing of laceration.

Treatment of Choice

Monitoring and discharge with written advise after a time period.

Your notes:

72. An 8-year-old boy falls off a swing at his school. He is brought to Casualty by one of his teachers. He has a bruise over his right eye but the examination is otherwise normal. He is fully conscious with no history of blackouts since the accident. A skull X-ray is performed, which is normal.

Diagnosis: Insignificant head injury.

Clinchers

- *8-year-old boy:* Children are difficult to assess for head injury and their admission for monitoring is indicated.
- *Falls off a swing at his school:* A common mode of injury to a school going child. But the most common head injury is by RTA.
- *Brought to casualty by one of his teachers:* That means that no adult member of family is with him—a contraindication for discharge.
- *Bruise over his right eye:* Usually children do not suffer from fracture of skull bones as these are more pliable.
- *Examination is otherwise normal:* Rules out any cerebral injury GCS scoring should be done on adult scale and children. GCS if for < 5 years.
- *Fully conscious:* Also in favour of any cerebral injury but not that young children lose consciousness less readily that adults. Significant brain injury can occur without a history of loss of consciousness.
- *No history of blackouts since the accident:* Also a good prognostic sign.
- *Skull X-ray is normal:* Rules out any fracture which commands admission. But one should be aware of suture lines and normal anatomical variants while interpreting the X-rays.

CONFUSA

Assessment of consciousness in a child can be difficult. The best judge for minor alteration in consciousness in children are their parents.

Investigation of Choice

Skull X-ray (already done in this case).

Immediate Management

Antiseptic dressing of the bruise.

Treatment of Choice

Admit and monitor.

Your notes:

73. A young woman is involved in an RTA and is brought in with a Glasgow Coma Scale of 6 . A CT scan shows evidence of diffuse cerebral oedema but no evidence of haemorrhage. She has bilateral papilloedema.

Diagnosis: Vasogenic cerebral oedema

Clinchers

- *Involved in an RTA:* RTA usually produces vasogenic cerebral oedema (i.e. increased capillary permeability).
- *Glasgow Coma Scale of 6:* Because cranium defines a fixed volume, brain swelling quickly results in increased ICP which may produce a sudden clinical deterioration. If untreated the GCS may fall further and the patient may be in a risk of brain herniation.
- *CT scan shows evidence of diffuse cerebral oedema but no evidence of haemorrhage:* This rules out any focal pathology which might be responsible for increased ICT and hence rules out any surgical intervention (craniotomy/burr hole).
- *Bilateral papilloedema:* It signifies raised ICT.

CONFUSA

Papilloedema is an unreliable sign, but venous pulsation at the disc may be absent (Note: it is absent in about 50% of normal people, but loss of it is a useful sign).

Investigation of Choice

ICT monitoring (as cerebral oedema peaks in two-three days).

Immediate Management

IV dexamethasone (controversial).

Treatment of Choice

IV mannitol + restriction of free water.

Your notes:

74. A young man is involved in a fight and suffers a blow to the back of the head. A skull X-ray reveals a depressed fracture of the occiput. His Glasgow Coma Scale on admission is 14 but falls rapidly within an hour.

Diagnosis: Subdural haematoma.

Clinchers

- *Is involved in a fight:* This makes it a medicolegal case and thereby warrant at least a skull X-ray (in UK).
- *Suffers a blow to the back of the head:* A blow to the back of head, if strong enough to produce a fracture in skull, will be invariably associated with neck injury. So exclude any cervical spine injury.
- *Skull X-ray reveals a depressed fracture of the occiput:* The principle local complications of skull fractures are:
  - Meningeal artery rupture, causing an extradural haematoma
  - Dural vein tears, leading to subdural haematoma.
- *Glasgow Coma Scale on admission is 14 but falls rapidly within an hour:* Since there is no lucid interval, the suspicion is more towards a subdural haematoma (Note: *Subdural* haematomas often have *subdued* onset, i.e. after sometime—hours to days).

CONFUSA

Linear skull fractures usually do not need any surgical intervention but depressed fractures almost always need surgical elevation and debridement. Cerebral contusions may result in a similar clinical picture to subdural haematoma, with a delayed recovery from trauma.

Investigation of Choice
CT scan (since GCS is falling).

Immediate Management
Inform neurosurgery after starting resuscitation.

Treatment of Choice
Surgical elevation of fracture and evacuation of clot.

Your notes:

75. A 24-year-old patient presents with RTA. The pupil on the left side is dilated and the patient is obtunded. CT scan of the head reveals a binconvex hyperdense lesion on the temporal region.

Diagnosis: Extradural haemorrhage.

Clinchers

- *History of RTA:* Road traffic accidents produces maximum mortality due to head injuries.
- *Pupil on left side is dilated:* In cases of intracranial haematomas localising neurological symptoms (e.g. ipsilateral pupil dilatation, haemiparesis) occurs late (average 63 days in case of subdural haematoma). So the patient is in a critical stage warranting urgent surgical decompression).
- *Obtunded:* Deteriorating level of consciousness is caused by a rising ICP (due to the expanding haematoma).
- *Biconvex hyperdense lesion on the temporal region:* Fresh bleed on CT appears hyperdense. A binconvex haematoma is characterisitc of an extradural haematoma (lens-shaped). Its most common site is temporal region.

CONFUSA

In subdural haematoma, the CT appearance is usually concave on the inner side, most commonly in parietal region. Midline shift may be present.

Investigation of Choice
CT scan (already done in this patient).

Immediate Management
Urgent evacuation of the clot through multiple burr holes (as the patient is very critical and there is no spare time for transfer to a neurosurgical unit/centre).

Treatment of Choice
Identification and ligation of the bleeding vessel (usually middle meningeal vessels).

Your notes:

76. A 27-year-old woman has a long-standing history of headaches associated with nausea and vomiting. On this occasion she present with sudden loss of vision in the right half of the visual field. By the time you see her it has improved considerably.

Diagnosis: Migraine

Clinchers

- *A 27-year-old woman has a long-standing history of headaches:* Onset of migraine is usually in childhood, adolescence or early adulthood; however, initial attack may occur at any age. It is more frequent in women, family history is often positive.
- *Headaches associated with nausea and vomiting:* Classic triad of migraine is:
  1. Premonitoring visual (scotoma or scintillations), sensory or motor symptoms
  2. Unilateral throbbing headache
  3. Nausea and vomiting
- *Sudden loss of vision in the right half of visual field:* Visual symptoms of migraine can be visual chaos (cascading, distortion, melting and jumbling of print lines, dots, spots, zig-zag fortification specta) and haemianopia.
- *By the time you see her it has improved considerably:* Visual symptoms in migraine last for about 15 minutes and then improved. It is generally followed by the headache within one hour.

CONFUSA

TIAs can mimic migraines visual symptoms of migraine.

Investigation of Choice

Carotid doppler to rule out TIA.

Immediate Management

Dispersible high dose aspirin.

Treatment of Choice

Migraine prophylaxis (if attacks > twice/month) with pizotifen.

Note:

- Premenstrual migraine may respond to diuretics or depot oestrogens.
- Contraceptive pill need not be discontinued if migraine is causing no focal pathology.

Your notes:

78. A woman previously in good health, presents with sudden onset of severe occipital headache and vomiting. Her only physical sign on examination is a shift neck.

Diagnosis: Subarachnoid haemorrhage (SAH)

Clinchers

- *Woman:* Females have a slightly higher incidence of SAH. Lack of estrogen in the postmenopausal females has been cited as a reason.
- *Previously in good health:* Rules out any other medical disorder. Also most of the patient of SAH present with a sudden and spontaneous occurrence with no preceeding disorder. The typical age for SAH is 35-65 years.
- *Sudden onset:* It's onset is sudden (within a few seconds). Some patient may earlier experience a sentinal headache due to small warning leaks from the offending aneurysm.
- *Severe occipital headache:* SAH presents with a devastating headache which the patients usually describe as "the worst headache of my life" or "I thought I had been kicked in the head". It is most commonly occipital. Vomiting may accompany.
- *Stiff neck:* (Kernig's positive). It is a feature of SAH but takes six hours to develop.

CONFUSA

Other differential diagnoses for stiff neck are—Shigella gastroenteritis and meningitis.

- Focal neurology (i.e. haemiplegia) in SAH may give diagnostic clues, e.g.
  - *Early development*—suggests intracerebral hematoma
  - *Late development*—suggests vasospasm and ischaemia

Investigation of Choice

Early CT (shows subarachnoid or ventricular blood).

Immediate Management

Immediate neurosurgical opinion if

- Consciousness decrease
- Progressive focal deficit
- Suspected cerebellar haematoma

Treatment of Choice

Surgical clipping of aneurysms/guglielmi coils

+

Control hypertension

79. A 74-year-old woman had a fall two weeks ago. She is brought into the A and E department with slowly increasing drowsiness. On examination you find mild haemiparesis and unequal pupils.

Diagnosis: Subdural haematoma.

Clinchers

- *74-year-old:* Bridging veins in the skull becomes more prone to rupture in old age. It is due to cortical atrophy producing gradual shrinkage of brain and thereby producing more traction on the veins.
- *Slowly increasing drowsiness:* It means that the haematoma which is now behaving like a SOL (space occupying lesion) is still expanding and there is danger if it is not evacuated urgently.
- *Two weeks ago:* Remember subdural haematomas are usually subdued in appearance, i.e. they can occur weeks to months after the initial injury (as the bleeding is from very small veins).
- *Mild haemiparesis and unequal pupils:* Ipsilateral pupillary dilatation is a lagte sign. Focal neurological signs are an indication for urgent intervention.

CONFUSA

Do not rely on absence of ipsilateral pupillary dilatation as it is a late sign. Alteration in the conscious level is the cardinal feature; lateralising signs may be absent or minimal.

Investigation of Choice

CT scan is diagnostic, showing a collection with an inner concave border (extradural—binconvex).

Immediate Management

Urgent neurological opinion.

Treatment of Choice

Surgical evacuation of the haematoma.

Your notes:

80. A 73-year-old man presents with haemianopia, haemisensory loss, haemiparesis and aphaesia of 16 hours duration.

Diagnosis: TIA involving the carotids.

Clinchers

- *73-year-old man:* Incidence of TIA increases with age. Most common cause is atherosclerosis.
- *Haemianopia:* Homonymous haemianopia is typical of a carotid territory ischaemia.
- *Haemisensory loss:* Contralateral weakness/numbness is present in *haemiparesis* carotid territory ischaemia.
- *Aphaesia:* Dysphasia, aphaesia and dysarthria are characteristic pointers for carotid territory ischaemia.
- *Of 16 hours duration:* The sudden onset of focal CNS signs or symptoms due to temporary occlusion, usually by emboli, of part of the cerebral circulation is termed a TIA if symptoms are present for less than 24 hours and fully resolve within this period.

CONFUSA

80% of the TIA are in the carotid territory. Suspect then whenever there is:

- Unilateral paresis
- Unilateral sensory loss
- Aphaesia
- Monocular visual loss.

Investigation of Choice

CT is usually not indicated in patients over 55 years. Do a routine screen (FBC, ESR, U and E, glucose, ECG, CXR).

Immediate Management

Give O_2 + monitor vital signs.

Treatment of Choice

Oral aspirin (300 mg) unless contraindicated thereafter 150 mg daily.

CASE HISTORY: AMAUROSIS FUGAX

A 50-year-old man complains of transient painless visual loss. He describes it as 'curtain falling down' over his eyes. On auscultation carotid bruit is heard.

Diagnosis: Amaurosis fugax.

This is seen in *Central retinal artery occlusion* and *giant cell* arteritis. This may precede permanent vision loss.

131. An HIV patient develops a severe headache and confusion. She is discovered to have bilateral papilloedema.

Diagnosis: Cerebral toxoplasmosis.

Clinchers

- *HIV patient:* The most common CNS infections in a HIV poistive patient are cerebral toxoplasmosis and cryptococcal meningitis.
- *Severe headache:* The clinical presentation of cerebral toxoplasmosis is of focal neurological features, convulsions, fever, headache and possible confusion.
- *Bilateral papilloedema:* It may be positive due to increased intracranial tensions as toxoplasmosis behave like a space occupying lesion.

CONFUSA

In addition to classic presentation as a CNS mass lesion, *T. gondii* has been reported to cause a variety of other clinical problems in HIV infected patients, including a CNS presentation more characteristic of herpes simplex with a negative CT scan, chorioretinitis, pneumonia, peritonitis with ascites, gastrointestinal tract involvement, cystitis and orchitis.

Investigation of Choice

- *Screening:* CT scan—multiple ring enhancing lesions.
  Note:
  - A single lesion on CT may be found to be one of several on MRI
  - A solitary lesion on MRI mitigates against toxoplasmosis
- *Definitive:*
  Brain biopsy.

Immediate Management

Medical management of raised ICT.

Treatment of Choice

Pyrimethamine + Sulfadiazine
(side effects: Renal stones)

Your notes:

166. A 33-year-old boxer who complains of left sided weakness 24 hours after a boxing match.

Diagnosis: Subdural haematoma.

Clinchers

- *Boxer:* Bridging veins in the cranium weakens in boxers because they sustain regular blows to the head. This increases the risk of their rupture and hence the formation of a subdural haematoma.
- *24 hours after a boxing match:* Subdural haematomas usually have an insiduous and delayed presenation (subdural is subdned) because the bleeding is venous and through very small vessels. They can present even weeks or months later.
- *Left sided weakness:* Focal neurological signs appear once the haematoma short behaving like a space occupying lesion in brain.

CONFUSA

Other risk groups for subdural haematoma are:
- Alcoholics (due to recurrent falls)
- Elderly (due to cortical shrinkage)

Investigation of Choice

CT skull ("concave inside" lesion).

Immediate Management

A complete neurological assessment + decrease ICT.

Treatment of Choice

Evacuation (sugical) of haematoma.

Your notes:

168. A 48-year-old woman complains of left shoulder and neck pain after having fallen off her bicycle. She has a graze on her forehead and also complains of tingling in her left ring and little fingers [digits IV and V].

Diagnosis: Cervical spine injury.

Clinchers

- *Fallen off her bicycle:* Cervical spine injury is more likely if the mobile head hits a fixed object (deceleration accleration) that if a mobile object hits the fixed head (assault).
- *Left shoulder and neck pain:* It might be due to soft tissue injury she had sustained during the fall. Neck pain as such after trauma always require cervical spine injury to be excluded.
- *Graze on her forehead:* If it is anterior, suspect cervical joint dislocation/instability. If it is near the top of skull, suspect axial compression injury.
- *Tingling in her left ring and little fingers:* These indicated a lesion in the domain of ulnar nerve. Either an imminent cervical cord compression or injury to posterior root of ulnar nerve might be responsible.

CONFUSA

A normal neurological examination does not exclude cervical spine injury. Moreover, conscious patients with other painful injuries may not always complain of neck discomfort. So neck injury must be assumed to have occurred in all patients who have sustained polytrauma until clinical examination and good quality radiographs prove otherwise. So in a major trauma the first X-ray to be performed after resuscitation is a cross-table lateral of the cervical spine. All seven cervical vertebrae, including C8-T1 junction, must be seen.

Investigation of Choice

Cervical spine X-ray

There are three standard views of the cervical spine in UK practice:

- Lateral view (90% sensitivity)
- Upper AP (open mouth or peg) view
- Lower AP view

Supplementation oblique views are used to visualize the apophyseal joints, looking for facet joint dislocation.

Immediate Management

Neck immobilization immediately with a well-fitting hard collar and a purpose-build head holder (except in situations where the patient struggles violently—a collar above will do here).

Treatment of Choice

Skull traction × 6 weeks.

169. A 28-year-old motorcyclist has been involved in an accident and complains of loss of sensation below the umbilicus and paralysis of both legs. His BP is 80/50 mm Hg with a pulse rate of 72/min.

Diagnosis: Neurogenic shock (spinal shock)

Clinchers

- *Motor cyclist:* Most serious injuries in RTAs are sustained by motrocyclists. Injuries of head, thorax and legs are more frequent in them.
- *Loss of sensation below the umbilicus and paralysis of both legs:* This suggest cord compression at T_{10} level (as umbilicus is supplied by T_{10} dermatome). There is complete anaesthesia and flaccid paralysis of all segments and muscles innervated below the level affected. Tendon reflexes are absent and there is retention of urine.
- *BP is 80/150 mmHg:* Hypotension in neurogenic shock is not due to hypovolaemia but due to sympathetic interruption below the lesion.
- *Pulse rate at 72/min:* Pulse rate is always normal in neurogenic shock.

CONFUSA

Neurogenic shock is the only "shock" in which tachycardia is absent. The thoracic spine lesions are more likely to be complete than cervical and lumbar lesions because of least free space between cord and canal. Also it has the poorest blood supply. Ischaemic injury often spreads below the level of mechanical injury.

Investigation of Choice

MRI spine (around T_{10} level)

Immediate Management

Arrange early and expert transfer to a spinal injuries unit after proper immobilization (in semiprone position).

Treatment of Choice

Surgical decompression

+

Methylprednisolone

(started within 8 hours of trauma).

Your notes:

PAPER 4

26. A chronic alcoholic with history of recurrent falls comes to A and E with complains of ataxia. Blood glucose is 7.

Diagnosis: Subdural haematoma.

Clinchers

- *Chronic alcoholic:* Chronic alcoholics are more prone for subdural haematomas because of recurrent falls weakens the bridging veins.
- *No recurrent falls:* This substantiates the above argument.
- *Complains of ataxia:* Unsteadiness, sleepiness, headache and personality changes are frequent symptoms in an evolving subdural haematoma.
- *Blood glucose is 7:* This rules out hypoglycemia to be a cause for all of the above symptoms.

CONFUSA

Drunkenness increases the risk of sustaining a head injury and of that injury causing brain damage. Nevertheless, changes in conscious level must not be attributed to alcohol or other drugs except by exclusion and in retrospect. The plasma osmolality may be a useful investigation in this circumstance.

Investigation of Choice
CT skull.

Immediate Management
ICP lowering.

Treatment of Choice
Evacuation of haematoma via surgery or burr holes.

Your notes:

27. A 17-year-old rugby player becomes unconscious after a fall. After sometime,he recovers,gives his name and address to the people in the ambulance. Later condition deteriorates.

Diagnosis: Extradural haematoma.

Clinchers

- *Becomes unconscious after a fall:* Initial loss of consciousness is due to cerebral contusion (because of the severity of attack). It resolves in sometime usually.
- *He recovers, gives his name and address to the people in the ambulance:* This is the characteristic lucid interval, between initial trauma and onset or return of depressed consciousness. It is typical for extradural haematoma.
- *Later condition deteriorates:* Now, the impairment is due to local pressure effects and increasing ICP.

CONFUSA

The lucid interval is said to be characteristic for extradural haematoma but is by no means inevitable. Extradural collections are typically seen on CT scanning as binconvex, whereas subdural collections have inner concave borders. The classical unilateral, fixed, dilated, pupil is a very late sign in extradural bleeds (it occurs as a result of a ipsilateral third nerve palsy which is caused by cerebral herniation). An impaired level of consciousness is the first feature. Limb weakness, from direct pressure on the motor cortex, is usually found on the contralateral side. Lateralizing signs may be preterminal.

Investigation of Choice
CT skull.

Immediate Management
ICP lowering.

Treatment of Choice
Surgical evacuation or multiple burr holes.

Your notes:

28. A child becomes unconscious after falling off his bicycle, later he is better and active. Only complaint is headache.

Diagnosis: Mild injury.

Clinchers
- *Unconscious:* This is due to cerebral contusion that can produce unconsciousness immediately after injury.
- *Better and acting now:* This rules out any immediate neurological impairment or injury. However, a watch should be kept as extradural haematoma can still develop.
- *Only complaint in headache:* It is due to local pain and resolving cerebral contusion.

CONFUSA

An extradural haematoma cannot be ruled out till it develops. But among the given options, mild injury is the most suitable answer. However, a more correct and definitive criterion of mild head injury is GCS 13-15.

Investigation of Choice
X-ray skull (to rule out any fracture).

Immediate Management
A complete neurological evaluation.

Treatment of Choice
Discharge with written advise (only if some responsible adult is accompanying him) and analgaesia.

Your notes:

29. Man with head trauma—GCS found to be 12.

Diagnosis: Moderate injury

Clinchers
- *Glasgow Coma Scale (GCS)*
  - Maximum possible score = 15 (not necessarily equivalent to alert and oriented)
  - Minimum possible score = 3 (even if dead)
  - Coma = GCS ≤ 8
  - Minor/mild injury = GSS 13-15
  - Mild injury = GCS 9-12
  - Severe injury = GCS ≤ 8
- *TIP:* Mnaemonic to remember best motor response scoring in GCS

See = C	obeys Commands	6
Low = Lo	Localises pain	5
Wit	Withdraws from pain	4
Flex Fl	abnormal flexion	3
ex	extension to pain	2
None	None	1

CONFUSA

Some centre in UK score GCS and of 14, not 15, omitting 'withdrawal to pain' in the best motor response category.

Investigation of Choice
Skull X-ray.

Immediate Management
Rule out cervical spine injury.

Treatment of Choice
Monitoring for any complication or neurological impairment.

Your notes:

30. Man with GCS=5, haemotympanum.

Diagnosis: Fracture base of skull.

Clinchers

➢ *GCS 5:* The implies a severe brain injury as GCS ≤ 8 is coma.

➢ *Haemotympanum:* It is a characteristic finding after fracture base of skull. It may produce reduced hearing so a complaint of reduced hearing in one ear after head injury moments an urgent otoscopy. Other pointers for fracture base of skull are:
- Bleeding from ear canal
- Bleeding from nose in absence of direct injury
- Nasopharyngeal bleeding (this may be torsential and even severe enough to compromise the airway)
- Cerebrospinal fluid leakage from the nose or ear
- Subconjunctival haemorrhage without a posterior edge
- Retro-orbital haematoma
- Bilateral periorbital haematomas (*racoon or panda eyes)*
- Bruising around the mastoid area (*Battle's sign*)

CONFUSA

Blood in the external auditory meatus after trauma is usually caused by basal fracture but is rarely secondary to temporomandibular joint injury. Deep auroscopic examination of the canal should be avoided as it may introduce infection via torn meninges. These are usually no radiographic signs of a basal skull fracture. However, there may be:
- Blood in the sphenoid sinus (look for a fluid level)
- A fracture line which appears to continue towards the base of the skull

Investigation of Choice
- *Screening:* Skull X-ray.
- *Definitive:* CT scan.

Immediate Management

Admission for observation for 48 hours + get neuro-surgeon's opinion.

Treatment of Choice

Surgical repair if appropriate, otherwise symptomatic.

Your notes:

34. A old lady fell and broke her hand one week back. After that slowly increasing confusion. Today her relatives could not wake her up from sleep.

Diagnosis: Subdural haematoma.

Clinchers

➢ *Broke her hand one week back:* Since she fall and the injury was severe enough to break hand, she might have suthered head injury also (common in injuries due to fall). At that time it might have been ignored because of masking by severe pain in the hand.

➢ *Slowly increasing confusion since one week:* Development of subdural haemorrhage may be insidious and fluctuating level of consciousness if often present as a preceding symptom.

➢ *Today her relatives could not wake her up from sleep:* It could be because of unconscious produced by increased ICP and local pressure effects of the subdural haematoma.

CONFUSA

The elderly are more susceptible to subdural haematoma formation after trivial injuries, as brain shrinkage makes bridging veins more vulnerable. Other at risk are those prone to falls (epileptics, alcoholics) and those on long-term anticoagulation. Midline shift is often visible on CT scan except in bilateral isodense clots.

Investigation of Choice

CT skull (Clot ± midline shift)

Immediate Management

ICP lowering.

Treatment of Choice

Evacuation of haematoma via surgery/burr holes.

Your notes:

60. An elderly hypertensive with recurrent faints presents with deteriorating mental functions.

Diagnosis: Multi-infarct dementia (MID)

Clinchers

- *Hypertensive:* Hypertension is a risk factor for CVA which in turn is a cause for MID.
- *Recurrent faints:* There is usually a history of transient ischaemic attacks with brief impairment of consciousness, fleeting pareses or visual loss. The dementia may follow a succession of acute CVA or less commonly, a single major stroke. Vessel occlusion is the most common cause of vascular dementia, and this may produce a variety of cognitive defects depending on the site of the ischaemic damage.

Note: MID results from involvement of several vessels supplying the cerebral cortex and subcortical structures and is typically associated with signs of cortical dysfunction.

CONFUSA

MID is the second most common cause of dementia in UK and is distinguished from Alzheimer's disease by its history of onset, clinical features and subsequent course. MID is also known as vascular dementia, so do not get confused between them!

Investigation of Choice

CT/MRI.

Immediate Management

Usually nonrequired.

Treatment of Choice

Symptomatic.

Your notes:

68. Female brings her husband to A and E, says he talks about their sex life in public. There is loss of inhibition (intellect normal) in him.

Diagnosis: Frontal lobe dementia (FLD).

Clinchers

- *Talks about sex life in public:* In FLD, the patient typically have loss of inhibitions (indiscreet, indolent, indecent). In fact this feature differentiates FLD from other dementias.
- *Normal intellect:* FLD patients may do better than those with Alzheimer's dementia on construction and calculation tasks.

CONFUSA

FLD is not a specific entity (not even regarded as such by some authors) and the designation usually includes Pick's disease. In FLD, in addition to progressive memory loss and confusion, the patients are often irritable.

Investigation of Choice

Neuroimaging (atrophy confined to frontal or frontal and temporal lobes)

Immediate Management

Counselling of the wife on how to take care of him.

Treatment of Choice

Symptomatic.

Your notes:

69. Man has cough and fever since 2 days. Wife notices he has disorientation in time and place, decreased concentration and confused. He was mentally OK 1 day back.

Diagnosis: Delirium.

Clinchers

- *Cough and fever since 2 days:* Medical conditions which can cause delirium are:
  - Febrile illness
  - Septicaemia
  - Organ failure (cardiac, renal, hepatic)
  - Hypoglycaemia
  - Postoperative hypoxia

  Or it can occur because of prescribed drugs in illness, i.e.
  - Any drug with anticholinergic properties (highly likely in this case)
  - Sedatives including opiates
  - Digoxin
  - Diuretics
  - Lithium
  - Steroids
- *Disorientation in time and place:* This is typical of delirium. Orientation in "person" is usually normal.
- *Decreased concentration and confused:* Impaired concentration and memory is a feature of delirium. Confusion is so prominent that delirium is also known as acute confusional state.
- *Mentally OK 1 day back:* It proves that the condition is acute in onset. Note that delirium is always acute in onset.

CONFUSA

In delirium there is usually no disorientation in "person" element, only disorientation in time and place are found. Clouding of consciousness is the most important diagnostic sign. It is manifested as drowsiness, decreased awareness of surroundings, disorientation and distractibility. At its most severe the patient may be unresponsive, but more commonly the impaired consciousness is quite subtle. Often the first clue to the presence of delirium is one of its features other than delirium.

Investigation of Choice
Neuroimaging to rule out SOL or encephalitis.

Immediate Management
Take psychiatric opinion.

Treatment of Choice
Symptomatic + treat the cause.

76. Fracture of anterior cranial fossa, rhinorrhoea, anosmia.

Diagnosis: Olfactory (I cranial nerve)

Clinchers

- *Fracture of anterior cranial fossa:* Palsy of first cranial nerve is often followed by head trauma especially the fracture of anterior cranial fossa due to local trauma to the nerve.
- *Rhinorrhoea:* This must be CSF leakage from the fracture of cribriform plate of ethmoid. It must be confirmed to be CSF by glucose dipstick testing.
- *Anosmia:* Sense of olfaction is definitely lost. To examine occlude each nostril sequentially. Use a mild test stimulus such as soap, toothpaste, coffee or lemon oil. With the eyes closed, the patient sniffs and try to identify the stimulus.

CONFUSA

Anosmia may also be produced by
- tumours of the olfactory groove
  - meningioma
  - frontal glioma
- meningitis

The sense of smell is often lost, sometimes permanently, after upper respiratory viral infections. It is diminished in nasal obstruction.

Investigation of Choice
Glucose dipstick test for CSF rhinorrhoea.

Immediate Management
Neurosurgery opinion.

Treatment of Choice
Conservative/surgical repair.

Your notes:

77. Cavernous sinus affected, pupil not responding to light and accommodation ,ptosis present.

Diagnosis: Oculomotor (III cranial nerve)

Clinchers

- *Cavernous sinus affected:* Cavernous sinus carries in its lateral wall the third and fourth cranial nerves and the ophthalmic and maxillary divisions of the fifth nerve. Hence in its pathology, any of these can be affected.
- *Pupil not responding to light:* A fixed and dilated pupil is characteristics of III nerve palsy and signify a complete palsy.
- *Ptosis present:* Total palsy of the oculomotor nerve lesions causes:
  - Ptosis (as it supplies, levator palpebrae superioris), which is unilateral and complete
  - The eye facing down and out
  - A fixed and dilated pupil.

An early or partial oculomotor palsy can present in any combination of the above features.

CONFUSA

Early dilatation of pupil implies a compressive lesion. Third nerve palsies without a dilated pupil are due to:
- diabetes mellitus
- other vascular causes (aneurysm)

Sparing of the pupil means that parasympathetic fibres which run in a discrete busidle on the superior surface of the nerve remain undamaged, and so the pupil is of normal size and reacts normally.

Investigation of Choice
IV antibiotics.

Immediate Management
Thrombolysis (as cavernous sinus thrombosis is the most usual pathology).

Treatment of Choice
IV antibiotics.

Your notes:

78. After head trauma, patient cannot shrug his shoulder.

Diagnosis: Spinal accessory (XI cranial nerve)

Clinchers

- *Head trauma:* This motor nerve to the trapezius and sternomastoid muscles arises in the medulla and leaves the skull through the jugular foramen with the ninth and tenth nerves. It is commonly injured in fracture base of skull.
- *Cannot string his shoulder:* A lesion of the eleventh nerve causes:
  - Weakness of the sternomastoid—rotation of the head and neck of the opposite side.
  - Weakness of trapezium—should shrugging lost.

CONFUSA

Causes of XI cranial nerve palsies are:
- Polio
- Syringomyelia
- Tumours near jugular foramen
- Stroke
- Bulbar palsy
- Trauma
- TB

Over all XI nerve palsy is a rare occurrence.

Investigation of Choice
CT skull.

Immediate Management
Refer to neurosurgery unit.

Treatment of Choice
Conservative ± surgical repair of fracture base of skull.

Your notes:

79. Forehead sparing, lower face no voluntary movements. Involuntary movements possible.

Diagnosis: Facial nerve palsy (VII cranial nerve)—UMN type.

Clinchers

- *Forehead sparing:* This is characteristic of facial nerve palsy of upper motor neurone (UMN) origin. The frontalis muscle is spared; the normal furrowing of the brow is preserved, and eye closure and blinking are not affect.
- *Lowerface—no voluntary movements:* UMN lesions cause weakness of the lower part only of the face on the side opposite the lesion. The earliest sign is simply slowing of one side of the face, for example on baring the teeth. Later on, voluntary movement is preserved.
- *Involuntary movement possible:* In UMN lesions, there is sometimes relative preservation of spontaneous emotion movement (e.g., similing) compared with voluntary movement.

CONFUSA

Differences between

	LMN	*UMN*
Weakness	All muscle of face	Forehead sparing
Eye closure	Weakness	Normal
Frontalis	Involved	Spared
Side of lesion	Same	Opposite

Investigation of Choice
CT skull/MRI (cerebral infarction or tumour).

Immediate Management
Admit and take neurosurgical opinion.

Treatment of Choice
Conservative if stroke; surgery if SOL.

Your notes:

80. Fracture of base of skull, loss of taste in anterior two-thirds of tongue, deviation of angle of mouth.

Diagnosis: Facial nerve (VII cranial nerve)—LMN type.

Clinchers

- *Fracture base of skull:* Facial nerve leaves skull through the stylomastoid foramen and can be injured here in head trauma such as fracture base of skull. This will be a lower motor neurone (LMN) lesion then.
- *Loss of taste in anterior two-thirds of tongue:* Facial nerve carries taste fibers from the anterior two-thirds of the tongue via the chorda-tympani, hence this finding confirms the suspicion of a facial nerve LMN palsy.
- *Deviation of angle of mouth:* The face, especially the angle of the mouth, falls, and dribbling occurs from the corner of the mouth.

CONFUSA

Lesions of the facial nerve within the petrous temporal bone cause the combination of:

- Loss of taste on the anterior two-third of the tongue
- Hyperacusis (unpleasantly loud distortion of noise) owing to paralysis of stapedius muscle

Investigation of Choice
CT scan

Immediate Management
Admit and urgent neurosurgery referral.

Treatment of Choice
Surgical decompression (urgent).

Your notes:

89. 18-year-old female brings her baby unconscious to A and E, cyanosed, dilated fixed left pupil.

Diagnosis: Head injury

Clinchers

- *18-year-old female:* Child abuse causing NAI is more common in babies of teenaged mother as they are more prove to breakdown under stress of looking after the child. Suspect this always in an unexplained head injury. Also note that child abuse is the most common cause of a skull fracture in an infant.
- *Unconscious; cyanosed, dilated fixed pupil:* All these features point to a unilateral intracranial haematoma.

CONFUSA

Children are unique in invariably having a carer with them. This means that most can go home with their parents and a set of head injury instructions. They often sleep after trauma and should not be kept awake. Instead, they should be examined by their parents two or three times during the night. Parents are much better judges of their children's night-time behaviour than hospital doctors or nurses.

Investigation of Choice
CT skull.

Immediate Management
Immediately neurosurgery referral.

Treatment of Choice
Surgical evacuation of haematoma.

Your notes:

94. Boy brought by his friend to the A and E. History of suddenly falling to the ground, jerky movements, urine incontinence. He is confused now but neurological examination is normal.

Diagnosis: Generalised tonic clonic seizure (GTCS)

Clinchers

- *Brought by his friend:* Since after a GTCS, the patient is in postictal confusion, he is incapable of reporting himself to hospital. Usually such patients are accompanied by someone who has witnessed the seizure.
- *Suddenly falling to ground; jerky movements and urine incontinence:* A typical description of GTCS is following a vague warning, the tonic phase of the seizure commences. The body becomes rigid, for upto a minute. The patient utters a cry and falls, sometimes suffering injury. The tongue is usually bitten. There may be incontinence of urine or faeces.
- *Confused now but neurological examination is normal:* After a generalised seizure the patient may feel awful with headache, myalgia, confusion and a sore tongue. This postictal confusion is characteristic and differentiates from other causes of loss of consciousness (e.g. vagovagal). It may lost upto 24 hours.

CONFUSA

A GTCS can be mistakenly referred to a psychiatrist if no body has witnessed the seizure and the person is found wandering in a postictal delirium GTCS is a classical grand mal seizure. An atypical generalized seizure is myoclonic jerk in which also the patient falls to the ground because of violently disobedient lower limb.
Note: TV-induced seizures are almost always generalised.

Investigation of Choice
EEG (a normal EEG between seizures does not exclude epilepsy).

Immediate Management
Admission for 24 hours for investigations and observations.

Treatment of Choice
Sodium valproate (but may be unacceptable in prepubertal child because of facial coarsening effects—replace with carbamazepine then).

Your notes:

123. A 40-year-old female comes with complaints of headache, bitemporal haemianopia, increase in shoe size.

Diagnosis: Acromegaly

Clinchers

- *40-year-old female:* It typically presents between the ages of 30 and 50 years. It is equally prevalent in men and women.
- *Headache and bitemporal haemianopia:* Because of the pituitary tumour (responsible for growth hormone hypersecretion). Bitemporal haemianopia is characteristic of compression of optic chiasm (most common cause of it—pituitary tumour).
- *Increase in shoe size:* GH excess results in bony and soft tissue overgrowth. The features are insidious, chronic and debilitating, i.e.
  - Increased teeth spacing
  - Increased shoe size
  - Thick spade like hands
  - Large tongue
  - Prominent supraorbital ridge
  - Prognathism.

CONFUSA

Acromegalics are said to look more like each other than their family members. Presence of bitemporal haemianopia in it clinically corroborates the presence of a pituitary tumour and that acromegaly is not due to some ectopic secretion of growth hormone.

Ectopic (other than pituitary) tumours causing acromegaly

- GnRH secreting tumours
  - Bronchial carcinoids
  - Pancreatic islet cell tumours
  - Hypothalamic gangliocytomas
  - Harmatoma
  - Gliomas
- GH secreting tumours
  - Pancreatic islet cell tumour

Investigation of Choice

MRI pituitary fossa.

Immediate Management

Obtain old photographs for comparison.

Your notes:

124. Patient with attacks of numbness in left hand and right-sided headache.

Diagnosis: Space occupying lesion (SOL)

Clinchers

- *Attacks of numbness in left hand:* This suggests an evolving focal neurology. Usually focal neurology depends upon site of the tumour but the information provided in the question is insufficient to diagnose the site of SOL. Most probably it is a parietal lobe tumour (Haemisonsory loss, decreased two-point discrimination).
- *Right-sided headache:* It is a sign of increased ICP signs to space occupying property of the tumour. Other signs of - ICP can be:
  - Vomiting
  - Papilloedema (only in 50% of tumours)
  - Altered consciousness.

CONFUSA

Evolving focal neurology must be differentiated from false localising signs which are produced by raised ICP. VI nerve palsy is the most common due to its long intracranial course.

Investigation of Choice

CT (MRI is good for posterior fossa tumours).

Immediate Management

Refer to neurology.

Treatment of Choice

Complete removal if possible.

Your notes:

139. A 12-year-old girl, one episode of grand mal-seizure of 3 min duration in her sleep.

Diagnosis: Probable epileptic seizure.

Clinchers

- *A 12-year-old girl:* Epilepsy commonly has its onset in adolescence. The incidence is slightly more in girls.
- *One episode:* Most probably this is her first episode. Thus it warrants admission for 24 hrs for investigations and observation. But the available text is unclear about admission criteria for seizures occurring in sleep.
- *Grand mal seizures:* These are tonic clonic seizures which cannot be referred to any part of cerebral hemispheres. Limbs stiffen (the tonic phase) and then jerk forcefully (clonic phase), with loss of consciousness. There is a definitive postictal phase (with drowsiness and confusion). They are usually of 1-5 minute duration.
- *In her sleep:* Generally seizures in sleep are virtually diagnostic of epilepsy.

CONFUSA

Epilepsy is always investigated by EEG (done by an expert). CT is done only if there are:
- Infantile spasms
- Unusual features
- CNS signs
- Partial or intractable epilepsy

MRI may be more sensitive, but is not so available and may require anaesthesia or sedation.

Investigation of Choice

EEG (shows generalized burst of spikes and irregular 4-6 Hz spike-wave complexes)

Immediate Management

Check blood glucose and protect child from immediate harm if there is a convulsion.

Treatment of Choice

Carbamazepine if epilepsy is diagnosed
(phenobarbitone if child < 1 year age)

Your notes:

140. A 14-year-old girl has had been academically brilliant, lately has had difficulty with her school work. She has be caught day dreaming in class on a number of occasions.

Diagnosis: Petit mal epilepsy (absence seizures)

Clinchers

- *A 14-year-old:* It almost invariably begins in childhood.
- *Academically brilliant:* This rules out her being not interested in studies and voluntarily indulging in day dreaming.
- *Lately has had difficulty with her school work:* This suggests a problem of recent origin.
- *Day dreaming:* In petit mal, the child ceases activity, stares and pales slightly. An attack lasts a few seconds. The eyelids twitch; a few muscle jerks may occur. After an attack, the child resumes normal activity. As these seizures generally do not produce much external effects, they can pass unrecognised or mistakenly taken as "day dreaming", a decline in school performance recognised by a teacher.

CONFUSA

Children with typical absence attacks may in adult life developed generalized seizures. Typical absence attacks are never due to acquired lesions such as tumours. They are a developmental abnormality of neuronal control. Petit mal describes only 3 Hz seizures, rather than clinically similarly absence attacks which are partial attacks.

Investigation of Choice

EEG (3 Hz spike and wave EEG).

Immediate Management

Rule out any focal signs or symptoms to differentiate from atypical absence seizures (partial seizures).

Treatment of Choice

Ethosuximide

Side effects

- Ataxia
- Lethargy
- Headache
- Skin rash
- GI irritation
- Bone marrow suppression

Your notes:

146. Patient with long-standing Parkinson's disease with intractable dysphagia.

Diagnosis: Intractable dysphagia

Clinchers

- *Long-standing Parkinson's disease:* The patient now must be having severe impairment of mental foulties so as to compound the already existing dysphagia in Parkinsons's disease.
- *Intractable dysphagia:* GI symptoms in parkinsons' disease are usually:
  - Heart burn
  - Dysphagia
  - Constipation
  - Weight loss

Since malnutrition and weight loss can severely affect the quality of life of a demented elderly patient, it need some definitive management, i.e. parenteral nutrition. Any patient requiring enteral nutrition for long periods should have a gastrostomy done and feeding is done with liquid diet through PEG tube.

CONFUSA

Examine for the state of hydration also, as dehydration and malnutrition go hand-in-hand. Overhydration can mask the appearance of malnutrition, so keep this fact in mind. Usually any patient requiring enteral nutrition in excess of one day should be feeded with a nasogastric tube and in excess of two weeks should be considered for PEG tube feeding.

Investigation of Choice

Endoscopy to rule out any obstruction to esophagus.

Treatment of Choice

PEG tube feeding (gastrostomy).

Your notes:

198. Presents with weakness of both legs, difficulty walking, urine retention.

Diagnosis: Vertebral compression fracture due to metastases.

Clinchers

- *Breast carcinoma:* Bone is a common site for the disposition of secondary tumours usually of epithelial origin. Breast metastases are common in
  - Ribs
  - Thoracic vertebrae
  - Clavicles
- *Weakness of both legs:* Vertebral fractures involving the cord may entrap cord to produce paraplegia below the level of the fracture. Usually legs are involved in fracture of thoracic vertebrae. Upper limbs are also involved if there is cervical vertebral fracture.
- *Difficulty walking:* Due to paraplegia.
- *Urinary retention:* Bladder tone is lost immediately after cord injury. Distension leads to ureteric reflux and renal damage. Later on the bladder may become automatic or neurogenic bladder. Bowel dysfunction will also be present.

CONFUSA

Causes of spinal cord compression can be either extension of tumour from vertebral body (osteoblastic metastases) or crush fracture (osteoclastic metastases). Breast carcinoma commonly produces osteoclastic metastases though it can produce osteoblastic metastases too. Prostatic carcinoma produces osteoblastic metastases.

Investigation of Choice

- *Screening:* Urgent plain X-ray spine
- *Definitive:* MRI/myelogram

Immediate Management

Get neurosurgery and clinical oncology opinions.

Treatment of Choice

Dexamethasone 8-16 mg IV then 4 mg/6h PO
Surgical decompression is the definitive treatment.

Your notes:

199. Presents with headache, confusion. On examination, papilloedema present.

Diagnosis: Raised intracranial pressure (ICP) due to cerebral metastases.

Clinchers

- *Headache:* It is the most common symptom of raised intracranial pressure. It is often worse in the morning and is accompanied by nausea and vomiting. Fits or focal neurological signs may appear as the ICP rises.
- *Confusion:* It is due to cerebral oedema secondary to brain metastases.
- *Papilloedema:* It is due to oedema of retinal nerve layer and a common finding on fundoscopy (in both the eyes) in increased ICP.

CONFUSA

Breast carcinoma commonly metastasizes to brain, bone and liver. Brain metastases are usually solitary and produce reactive cerebral oedema.

Investigation of Choice
CT scan

Immediate Management
Ventilatory support.

Treatment of Choice
Dexamethasone 4 mg/6h PO
Radiotherapy/surgery for isolated metastases.

Your notes:

PAPER 5

8. A 30-year-old female, insulin-dependent diabetic, presents with failure to pass urine.

Diagnosis: Autonomic neuropathy

Clinchers

- *IDDM patient:* Such patients are more prone to autonomic neuropathy.
- *Failure to pass urine:* Retention of urine is suggestive of autonomic involvement of the bladder. That occurs with a long-standing history of diabetes. Since the patient is now 30-year-old and IDDM usually have a juvenile onset, one must be having a long history to substantiate our diagnosis.

CONFUSA

Diabetic neuropathy may affect every part of the nervous system, with the possibel exception of brain. While rarely a direct cause of death, neuropathy is a major cause of morbidity. Most common picture is that of a peripheral polyneuropathy.

Investigation of Choice
Pelvic USG.

Immediate Management
Urinary catheterisation.

Treatment of Choice
Chronic catheter drainage.

Your notes:

9. A 68-year-old diabetic on treatment for the last 5-year presents with calf pain exacerbated by movement.

Diagnosis: Intermittent claudication

Clinchers

- *Calf pain exacerbated by movement:* This is a typical history of intermittent claudication. The pain is initially relieved by rest.
- *A 68-year-old diabetic:* this female has a high chances of having atherosclerosis secondary to diabetes or as a primary disease. This produces the vascular disease with diminished blood supply which cause intermittent claudication and foot ulcers.

CONFUSA

Hypertriglyceridaemia is common in diabetes and is due both to overproduction of VLDL in the liver and to a disposal defect in the periphery.

Investigation of Choice

Doppler USG lower limb (or Duplex USG)

Immediate Management

Instruction about proper foot care in an attempt to prevent ulcers.

Treatment of Choice

Maintain diabetic control properly to keep hypertriglyceridaemia under control

+

Symptomatic management.

Your notes:

18. An 84-year-old woman notices sudden increased visual impairment. She is found to have homonymous haemianopia.

Diagnosis: Cerebral haemorrhage

Clinchers

- *A 84-year-old woman:* Incidence of rupture of cerebral vessel aneurysms increases with age. These aneurysms are common in females.
- *Sudden increased visual impairment:* Since the defect is of sudden onset, it rules out tumours or other chronic disease processes as a causation. There is no given history of trauma cerebral embolism can be ruled out as it usually do not produce permanent changes.
- *Homonymous haemianopia:* Most commonly it results from lesions in optic tract (tumours pressing it), geniculate body and optic radiations (cerebral haemorrhage). Since we have ruled out tumours to be cause, cerebral haemorrhage is a safe answer.

CONFUSA

Haemianopia denotes loss of half of the field of vision. The most common clinical form is homonymous haemianopia, in which the right of left half of the binocular field of vision is lost, owing to loss of the temporal half of one field and the nasal half of the other, a condition due to a lesion situated in any part of the visual paths from the chiasma to the occipital lobe. Right haemianopia is more quickly discovered than left owing to the fact that reading is impossible; left haemianopia is often discovered when the patient does not see food on the left side of the plate.

Investigation of Choice

MRI/CT

Immediate Management

Admit and specialist evaluation

Treatment of Choice

Symptomatic + as per radiological findings.

Your notes:

22. A 74-year-old man presents with weakness in his arm and leg (from which he recovered within a few days) and short term memory loss. He has an extensor plantar response. He had a similar episode two years ago and became unable to identify objects and to make proper judgements.

Diagnosis: Vascular dementia (multi-infarct dementia)

Clinchers

- *74-year-old:* Prevalence and severity of vascular dementia increases with age as the incidence of cerebrovascular accidents (which predispose to it). increases.
- *Man:* Male have more prevalence of vascular diseases.
- *Weakness in his arm and leg (from which he recovered within a few days):* This represents a stroke which is the predisposing factor for vascular dementia.
- *Short-term memory loss:* This signifies dementia which is most probably of new onset.
- *Extensor plantar:* It signify a pyramidal lesion as the normal flexor plantar has become extensor.
- *Similar episode two years ago..... judgements:* There is usually a history of TIAs with brief impairment of consciousness, fleeting paresis or visual loss. The dementia may follow a succession of acute CVAs or less commonly a single major stroke.

CONFUSA

Vascular dementia is the second most common cause of dementia is distinguished from Alzheimer's disease by its history of onset, clinical features and subsequent course. Vessel occlusion is the most common cause of vascular dementia, and this may produce a variety of cognitive deficits depending on the site of the ischaemic damage. It is typically associated with signs of cortical dysfunction.

Investigation of Choice
Clinical ± MRI + Psychometric testing (e.g. Wechsler scale)

Immediate Management
Counselling of family

Treatment of Choice
None

Your notes:

23. A 38-year-old haemophiliac who received several blood transfusions a few years ago presents with irritability and increasing memory deficit. He is unable to speak properly. He is on antitubercular treatment.

Diagnosis: HIV (AIDS-dementia complex)

Clinchers

- *38-year-old haemophiliac:* Prevalence of AIDS and HIV is more in older haemophiliacs who have been treated with transfusions before mid 80's (i.e. before the advent of HIV testing).
- *Irritability and increasing deficit + unable to speak properly:* This is a diffuse, progressive usually fatal HIV-related dementia, sometimes associated with a cerebellar syndrome. It is thought to be due cerebral HIV infection.
- *He is on anti TB treatment:* TB is frequently associated with AIDS that represents symptomatic state of HIV infection.

CONFUSA

AIDS dementia complex (ADC) has varying degrees of severity, ranging from mild memory impairment and poor concentration through to severe cognitive deficit, personality change and psychomotor slowing. Changes in effect are common and depressive or psychotic features may be present. The spinal cord may show vacuolar myelopathy. In severe cases brain CT scan shows atrophic changes. MRI changes consists of lesions in white matter (T_2 section). EEG may show nonspecific changes consistent with encephalopathy. CSF neopterin concentration may be raised.

Investigation of Choice
CT scan/MRI

Immediate Management
Rule out distal sensory polyneuropathy which is frequently associated with ADC.

Treatment of Choice
Zidovudine has a beneficial effect on HIV neurological disease, with startling improvement in cognitive function in many patients with ADC.

Your notes:

24. A 34-year-old woman presents with memory loss, poor concentration and inability to recognize household objects. On examination she has a right handed involuntary writhing movement. There is a strong family history of similar complaints.

Diagnosis: Huntington's chorea (HC)

Clinchers

- *A 34-year-old:* The onset is usually in middle age. Death usually occurs between 10 and 20 years after the onset.
- *Woman:* Both sexes have equal incidence as it is an autosomal dominant trait.
- *Presents with memory loss, poor concentration and inability to recognize household objects:* This is dementia.
- *Right handed involuntary writhing movements:* This is chorea. Relentlessly progressive chorea and dementia in middle life are the hallmarks of this inherited disease.
- *Strong family history of similar complaints:* Inheritance of HC is an autosomal dominant trait with full penetrance, the children of an affected parent have a 50% chance of inheriting the disease.

CONFUSA

The family history of the disease in previous generations is often concealed, either by design or default. There is steady progression, of both the dementia and chorea. No treatment arrests the disease, although Phenothaizines (e.g. sulpiride) may reduce the chorea, by causing drug induced Parkinsonism. Tetrabenazine helps to control the movements. Mutation analysis, which is accurate and specific, is available for presymptomatic testing of family members.

Investigation of Choice

Neuroimaging (if possible with the chorea, will show atropy of caudate nucleus).

Immediate Management

Patient and family counselling.

Treatment of Choice

Phenothiazines +/or tetrabenazine.

Your notes:

25. A 62-year-old patient with chronic schizophrenia presents with mask-like face and involuntary pill rolling movement in both hands. He complains of chronic cough and forgetfulness.

Diagnosis: Parkinsonism (drug induced)

Clinchers

- *A 62-year-old:* The disease is common and worldwide, with prevalence increasing sharply with age to about 1 in 200 in those above 70 years.
- *Chronic schizophrenia:* This suggests a chronic use of antipsychotics which can induce parkinsonism as a long-term side effects.
- *Mask like face:* This is the impassive facial expression which is typical of parkinsonism.
- *Involuntary pill rolling movement in both hands:* This athetosis and characteristically seen in parkinsonism (between thumb and forefingers).
- *Chronic cough:* This is due to anticholinergic side effects of antipsychotics (laryngeal dryness causes cough).
- *Forgetfulness:* Dementia usually accompanies it (but not present as such in parkinsonism).

CONFUSA

In Parkinson's disease a stoop is characteristic and the gait is shuffling and festinant and with poor arm swinging. The posture is sometimes called 'simian' to describe the ape-like forward flexion, immobility of the arms and lack of facial expression.

Investigation of Choice

There is no laboratory test for the disease. The diagnosis is made by recognising the clinical pattern.

Immediate Management

Rule out other brain diseases

Treatment of Choice

Levodopa

Your notes:

31. A 43-year-old man is brought to the Accident and Emergency Department delirious, following and injury at a rugby match. His Glasgow Coma Scale (GCS) at the scene of injury is 13. On examination, his right pupil is fixed and dilated and GCS is now 7. Initial resuscitation has been done. The neurosurgeon is 30 minutes away.

Diagnosis: Extradural haemorrhage (EDH).

Clinchers

- *Following injury:* EDH is common after direct head injuries, although subdural haematoma may also occur.
- *A lucid interval, where GCS is initially 13 and later 7:* This is a hallmark of a significant EDH.
- *Right pupil fixed and dilated:* Since ipsilateral pupillary dilatation occurs but it is a late sign.
- *Initial resuscitation has been done:* It means that now secondary management is required which in this case is management of EDH.
- *Neurosurgeon is 30 minutes away:* Since he will take time to come and evaluate this patient, immediate drilling of burr-holes should be the urgent step.

CONFUSA

CT brain scan can be definitive in forming a diagnosis but no time should be lost in conducting the investigation since GCS is rapidly decreasing.

Investigation of Choice

CT—Head.

Immediate Management

Drilling of burr holes.

Treatment of Choice

Drilling of burr holes followed by neurosurgical ligation of bleeding vessels.

Your notes:

65. A 23-year-old woman has a history of recurrent attacks of blurring of vision associated with redness, pain and photophobia. Both eyes have been affected in the past. She is currently being investigated for bowel disease and a severe backache.

Diagnosis: Multiple sclerosis

Most appropriate management: 0.5% prednisolone drops 2 hrly and cyclopentolate drops

Clinchers

- *A 23-year-old man:* Multiple sclerosis has female preponderance. Mean age of onset is 30 years.
- *Recurrent attacks of blurring of vision:* Early picture of multiple sclerosis is usually one of relapses followed by remissions become incomplete. In multiple sclerosis, plaques of demyelination are seen at the sites through at the CNS.
- *Bowel disease of severe backache:* Bowel (constipation), fatigue, motor weakness, optic neuritis, incontinence, numbness, tingling in limbs, cerebellar symptoms may be seen in multiple sclerosis.

CONFUSA

Isolated neurological deficits are never diagnostic, but may become so, if a careful history reveals previous episodes.

Investigation of Choice

MRI is sensitive

Immediate Management

Treat the complication

Treatment of Choice

No cure but following may help

- Methylprednisolone (shortens relapses), use sparingly. It does no alter overall prognosis.
- b-*interferon:* ¯ relapse rate by 1/3.

Your notes:

87. A 31-year-old man complains of facial pain between the eyes and on one side of the face. His nose and the affected eye are congested. He says the pain is severe.

Diagnosis: Trigeminal neuralgia

Clinchers (Note: See Q 90 of this theme also)

- *A 31 years old man:* It is chiefly a condition of those over 50 years old. Male to female ratio is >1.
- *Facial pain between the eyes and on one side of face:* The pain is unilateral affecting the mandibular and maxillary divisions most often and the ophthalmic division only rarely.
- *His nose and the affected eyes are congested:* It is due to vasodilatation seen along with pain.
- *Pain is severe:* There are severe paroxysms of knife like or electric-shock-like pain, lasting seconds. The face may screw up with pain (hence tic douloureux).

CONFUSA

The pain of trigeminal neuralgia characteristically does not occur at right (Reference: Kumar and Clark, 1021, 5th edn). There is controversy on this point as OHCM mentions it on the contrary (page 333, OHCM, 5th edn). The recurrence are inevitable although spontaneous remissions last for months or years. Secondary trigeminal neuralgia occurs due to multiple sclerosis (especially in young). Vascular malformation, or a cerebello-pontine angle tumours.

Investigation of Choice

Clinical diagnosis

Immediate Management

High dose analgesia for pain relief

Treatment of Choice

Carbamazepine

If drugs fail, surgery.

Your notes:

89. A 57-year-old teacher says she has facial pain, especially in the temples at night. On the right side of her face it throbs. For the past three weeks she has felt unwell and had to miss classes. Also, combing her hair has become painful.

Diagnosis: Temporal arteritis (TA)

Clinchers

- *A 57-year-old:* It is common in elderly, it is rare under 55 years.
- *Facial pain, especially in the temples at night:* Pain in invariable and is felt over the inflamed superficial temporal or occipital arteries. Touching the skin over the inflamed vessel (e.g. combing the hair) causes pain.
- *On right side of her face it throbs:* Arterial pulsation is felt initially but is soon last and the artery becomes hard, tortuous and thickened.
- *For three weeks:* It signifies a chronic condition that it is.
- *Combing her hair has become painful:* See above.

CONFUSA

Generalised muscle pains, proximal limb girdle pain and tenderness, without joint effusion, i.e. polymyalgia rheumatica occur in under half the patients. Rare complications of TA can be brainstem ischaemia, cortical blindness, ischaemic neuropathy of peripheral or cranial nerves, and involvement of the aorta, coronary, renal and mesenteric arteries are sometimes seen.

Investigation of Choice

- *Screening:* ESR (60-100 mm/h)
- *Definitive:* Biopsy of temporal artery

Immediate Management

Oral steroids (immediately)

Treatment of Choice

Steroid maintenance therapy (for at least 2 years).

Your notes:

90. **A 43-year-old mechanic complains of left sided facial pain. The pain is stabbing and runs up and down his face, especially at meal times. He has been to the dentist, but the dentist has found his teeth to be in good order.**

Diagnosis: Trigeminal neuralgia (TN)

Clinchers (Note: See Q 87 of this theme also)

- *A 43 years old:* It appears in middle or old age.
- *Left sided facial pain:* It is almost always unilateral.
- *Stabbing pain:* Severe paroxysm of knife-life or electric shock like pain, lasting seconds occur in the distribution of the fifth nerve.
- *Especially at meal times:* Each paroxysm is stereotyped, brought on by stimulation of a specific and often tiny trigger zone in the face. Washing, shaving, a cold wind or eating are examples of the trivial stimuli and provoke the intense pain.
- *He has been to dentist....:* This excludes dental causes. Very often the patient presents to dentists as they mistook the pain to be dental in origin.

CONFUSA

Onset in young adulthood raises the possibility of multiple sclerosis. Carbamazepine is effective in 75% of cases of TN or nonresponders, phenytoin or baclofen can be tried. When medications fail, surgical gangliolysis or suboccipital craniectomy for decompression of trigeminal nerve are options. Microvascular decompression is recommended (where available) if a tortuous or redundant blood vessels is found in the posterior fossa near the trigeminal nerve.

Investigation of Choice
Clinical diagnosis

Immediate Management
High dose analgesia for pain relief

Treatment of Choice
Carbamazepine (see confusa also).

Your notes:

101. **A 25-year-old found deeply unconscious is brought to the Accident and Emergency Department. He has an abrasion over his left temple and puncture marks on his left forearm.**

Diagnosis: Suspected head injury after IV drug abuse

Clinchers

- *A 25-year-old:* Incidence of drug abuse is highest in teens and twenties.
- *Deeply unconscious:* This can be either due to head injury or due to opiate overdose.
- *Abrasion over his left temple:* This raises the suspicion of a head injury. Since the patient is unconscious and thus cannot be evaluated clinically properly, it necessiates an urgent CT scan to rule out brain injury.
- *Puncture marks on left forearm:* These are highly likely to be needle marks from IV drug abuse. The suspicion is increased by the fact that the marks are on left arm (as majority of population is right handed and thus use it to self inject on the other arm).

CONFUSA

A drug addict can sustain physical injuries from falls, burns or other trauma because of altered state of consciousness. Also there is an increased possibility of them being assaulted because of a high crime rate in their community.

Investigation of Choice
CT scan skull

Immediate Management
IV naloxone (to rule out opiate intoxication)

Treatment of Choice
As per the diagnosis.

Your notes:

102. A 37-year-old alcoholic is found wandering in a park. His partner says he has had a number of falls recently and in the Accident and Emergency the patient is confused. The blood sugar level is normal.

Diagnosis: Head injury (probable).

Clinchers

- *Alcoholic:* Subdural haematomas are commonly seen in alcoholics. There may be no apparent injury. The first sign may be a failure to wake up after an episode of heavy drinking.
- *History of number of falls recently:* Frequent falls weakne the bridging veins which traverse the subdural space. They can bleed to give rise to subdural haematomas. This mechanism is responsible for their frequent incidence in alcoholics. Subdural haematomas are also common among elderly and HIV patients. But in them the pathogenesis is cerebral atropy ® shrinkage of brain ® stretching of bridging veins ® rupture ® haematoma.
- *Confused:* A CT scan is indicated in all cases of clouding on consciousness or low GCS in an alcoholic, as the clinical assessment is difficult in an intoxicated patient.

CONFUSA

A normal blood sugar rules out hypoglycemia which is a more common cause of confusion in an alcoholic. On the other hand this patient could be plainly showing only the features of intoxication, but CT scan is still essential from medicolegal point of view in UK.

Investigation of Choice

CT scan (subdural haematoma—inner concave border).

Immediate Management

Admit in hospital (at least overnight).

Treatment of Choice

Depends on CT findings.

Your notes:

131. An HIV patient develops a severe headache and confusion. She is discovered to have bilateral papillodema.

Diagnosis: Cerebral toxoplasmosis.

Clinchers

- *HIV patient:* The most common CNS infections in a HIV poistive patient are cerebral toxoplasmosis and cryptococcal meningitis.
- *Severe headache:* The clinical presentation of cerebral toxoplasmosis is of focal neurological features, convulsions, fever, headache and possible confusion.
- *Bilateral papilloedema:* It may be positive due to increased intracranial tensions as toxoplasmosis behave like a space occupying lesion.

CONFUSA

In addition to classic presentation as a CNS mass lesion, *T. gondii* has been reported to cause a variety of other clinical problems in HIV infected patients, including a CNS presentation more characteristic of herpes simplex with a negative CT scan, chorioretinitis, pneumonia, peritonitis with ascites, gastrointestinal tract involvement, cystitis and orchitis.

Investigation of Choice

- *Screening:* CT scan—multiple ring enhancing lesions.
  Note:
  - A single lesion on CT may be found to be one of several on MRI
  - A solitary lesion on MRI mitigates against toxoplasmosis
- *Definitive:*
  Brain biopsy.

Immediate Management

Medical management of raised ICT.

Treatment of Choice

Pyrimethamine + Sulfadiazine
(side effects: Renal stones)

Your notes:

150. A 65-year-old woman presents with constipation, and reports difficulty in starting or stopping to walk. She has dysarthria and dribbling.

Diagnosis: Parkinsonism (Shy-Drager syndrome)

Clinchers

- *A 65-year-old woman:* It generally commences in middle or late life and leads to progressive disability with time. The disease occurs in all ethnic groups, has an equal sex distribution and is common, with a prevalence of 1 to 2 per 1000 of general population and 1 per 100 among people older than 64 years.
- *Constipation + drabbling:* Disturbances of bladder and bowel control characteristic shy-drager syndrome.
- *Difficult in starting or stopping to walk:* Walking is often difficult to initiate and patients may have to lean forward increasingly until they can advance. They walk with small, shuffling steps, have no arm swing and they are unsteady (especially on tuning) and may have difficulty in stopping.
- *Dysarthria:* The voice is hypophasic and poorly modulated.

CONFUSA

Shy-Drager syndrome is a well-characterized severe form of multisystem atrophy that is accompanied by autonomic failure. Most patients present with autonomic dysfunction alone and other neurologic manifestations usually develop within 5 years. Patients with the stiatonigral variant exhibit a form of Parkinsonism in which bradykinesia and rigidity are more prominent that tremour.

Investigation of Choice

Clinical diagnosis

Immediate Management

Exclude other similar disease + specialist evaluation

Treatment of Choice

Levodopa
+
Speech therapy.

185. A 39-year-old male is getting progressively forgetful and is later found to have Alzheimer's disease. He has small ears and an IQ score of 67.

Diagnosis: Down's syndrome

Clinchers

- *A 39-year old male Alzheimer's disease:* Alzheimer's dementia usually manifest in late forties or in fifties. Early onset of it is commonly seen in Down's syndrome which predisposes one to it.
- *Small ears:* Facial profile of Down's syndrome is flat with oblique palpebral fissures and epicanthic folds with small ears.
- *IQ score of 67:* Severe mental retardation is a characteristic feature of Down's syndrome.

CONFUSA

Trisomy 21 (Down's syndrome) is observed with a frequency of 1 in 700 like births regardless of geography or ethnic background. Apart from Alzheimer's dementia it predisposes one to all. (Mnemonic: we all will go down together)

Investigation of Choice

Karyotyping.

Immediate Management

Genetic counselling.

Treatment of Choice

Rehabilitation.

Your notes:

PAPER 6

11. Following an alcoholic binge a 36-year-old male falls and comes to casualty with a cut in his temporal region his Glasgow Coma Scale is normal and his neck is cleared by the orthopedic SHO.

Diagnosis: Superficial head injury.

Clinchers

- *Following an alcoholic binge*: Alcoholics warrants overnight admission in the hospital as they cannot be assessed properly on presentation for head injury. This is applicable even if the GCS is normal. Other patients warranting admission in spite of normal GCS are children and postictal (confused) patients.
- *Falls:* Most probably it is the reason for the cut in the temporal region. Note that alcoholics are more prone to develop subdural haematomas due to weakening of bridging veins because of repeated falls.
- *A cut in his temporal region:* It must be a simple laceration if there is no associated fracture of temporal bone. It requires prompt suturing to maintain haemostasis.
- *Glasgow Coma Scale is normal:* Rules out any immediate brain damage/haematoma. But not that it is difficult or even misleading in an alcoholic.
- *His neck is cleared by the orthopedic SHO:* It rules out any spinal injury.

CONFUSA

The main confusion is about whom to admit or discharge in a case of head injury. The criteria are:

Criteria for admission in a case of head injury

- Difficult to assess
  - *Child*
  - *Postictal*
  - *Alcohol intoxication*
- CNS signs
- Severe headache or vomiting
- Fracture
- Smelling of alcohol with GCS < 15

Criteria for discharge with written advise (all criteria must be fulfilled)

- Fully conscious on presentation
- No abnormal neurological signs
- Loss of consciousness < 5 min
- Post-traumatic amnaesia < 5 min
- No severe headache
- No vomiting
- No skull fracture
- No bleeding disorder
- Good home conditions

Note: Get an X-ray skull in all suspected medicolegal cases (like this one) even if you suspect no bony injury.

Other main confusion is about anterograde and retrograde amnaesia. Note the only the extent of anterograte amnaesia correlates with severity of injury (admit if > 5 min). Retrograde amnaesia does not correlate well with severity. Also retrograde amnaesia never occurs without anterograde amnaesia. Anterograde amnaesia (also known as post-traumatic amnaesia—PTA) if under one hour, means mild injury whereas > 24 years denotes severe injury. OHCM has stated on the contrary and thus created this confusion. But refer Kumar and Clark, pg 1084, 4th Edn. and lecture notes in emergency medicine, pg 36 second edition.

Investigation of Choice

X-ray skull (CT in an alcoholic is only indicated if GCS falls).

Immediate Management

Suturing of laceration.

Treatment of Choice

Monitoring and discharge with written advise after a time period.

Your notes:

12. An 8-year-old boy falls off a swing at his school. He is brought to Casualty by one of his teachers. He has a bruise over his right eye but the examination is otherwise normal. He is fully conscious with no history of blackouts since the accident. A skull X-ray is performed, which is normal.

Diagnosis: Insignificant head injury.

Clinchers

- *A 8-year-old boy:* Children are difficult to assess for head injury and their admission for monitoring is indicated.
- *Falls off a swing at his school:* A common mode of injury to a school going child. But the most common head injury is by RTA.
- *Brought to casualty by one of his teachers:* That means that no adult member of family is with him—a contraindication for discharge.
- *Bruise over his right eye:* Usually children do not suffer from fracture of skull bones as these are more pliable.
- *Examination is otherwise normal:* Rules out any cerebral injury GCS scoring should be done on adult scale and children. GCS if for < 5 years.
- *Fully conscious:* Also in favour of any cerebral injury but not that young children lose consciousness less readily that adults. Significant brain injury can occur without a history of loss of consciousness.
- *No history of blackouts since the accident:* Also a good prognostic sign.
- *Skull X-ray is normal:* Rules out any fracture which commands admission. But one should be aware of suture lines and normal anatomical variants while interpreting the X-rays.

CONFUSA

Assessment of consciousness in a child can be difficult. The best judge for minor alteration in consciousness in children are their parents.

Investigation of Choice

Skull X-ray (already done in this case).

Immediate Management

Antiseptic dressing of the bruise.

Treatment of Choice

Admit and monitor.

Your notes:

13. A young woman is involved in an RTA and is brought in with a Glasgow Coma Scale of 6 . A CT scan shows evidence of diffuse cerebral oedema but no evidence of haemorrhage. She has bilateral papilledema.

Diagnosis: Vasogenic cerebral oedema

Clinchers

- *Involved in an RTA:* RTA usually produces vasogenic cerebral oedema (i.e. increased capillary permeability).
- *Glasgow Coma Scale of 6:* Because cranium defines a fixed volume, brain swelling quickly results in increased ICP which may produce a sudden clinical deterioration. If untreated the GCS may fall further and the patient may be in a risk of brain herniation.
- *CT scan shows evidence of diffuse cerebral oedema but no evidence of haemorrhage:* This rules out any focal pathology which might be responsible for increased ICT and hence rules out any surgical intervention (craniotomy/burr hole).
- *Bilateral papilloedema:* It signifies raised ICT.

CONFUSA

Papilloedema is an unreliable sign, but venous pulsation at the disc may be absent (Note: it is absent in about 50% of normal people, but loss of it is a useful sign).

Investigation of Choice

ICT monitoring (as cerebral oedema peaks in two-three days).

Immediate Management

IV dexamethasone (controversial).

Treatment of Choice

IV mannitol + restriction of free water.

Your notes:

14. A young man is involved in a fight and suffers a blow to the back of the head. A skull X-ray reveals a depressed fracture of the occiput. His Glasgow Coma Scale on admission is 14 but falls rapidly within an hour.

Diagnosis: Subdural haematoma.

Clinchers

- *Is involved in a fight:* This makes it a medicolegal case and thereby warrant at least a skull X-ray (in UK).
- *Suffers a blow to the back of the head:* A blow to the back of head, if strong enough to produce a fracture in skull, will be invariably associated with neck injury. So exclude any cervical spine injury.
- *Skull X-ray reveals a depressed fracture of the occiput:* The principle local complications of skull fractures are:
  - Meningeal artery rupture, causing an extradural haematoma.
  - Dural vein tears, leading to subdural haematoma.
- *Glasgow Coma Scale on admission is 14 but falls rapidly within an hour:* Since there is no lucid interval, the suspicion is more towards a subdural haematoma (Note: *Subdural* haematomas often have *subdued* onset, i.e. after sometime—hours to days).

CONFUSA

Linear skull fractures usually do not need any surgical intervention but depressed fractures almost always need surgical elevation and debridement. Cerebral contusions may result in a similar clinical picture to subdural haematoma, with a delayed recovery from trauma.

Investigation of Choice
CT scan (since GCS is falling).

Immediate Management
Inform neurosurgery after starting resuscitation.

Treatment of Choice
Surgical elevation of fracture and evacuation of clot.

Your notes:

15. A 24-year-old patient presents with RTA. The pupil on the left side is dilated and the patient is obtunded. CT scan of the head reveals a binconvex hyperdense lesion on the temporal region.

Diagnosis: Extradural haemorrhage.

Clinchers

- *History of RTA:* Road traffic accidents produces maximum mortality due to head injuries.
- *Pupil on left side is dilated:* In cases of intracranial haematomas localising neurological symptoms (e.g. ipsilateral pupil dilatation, haemiparesis) occurs late (average 63 days in case of subdural haematoma). So the patient is in a critical stage warranting urgent surgical decompression).
- *Obtunded:* Deteriorating level of consciousness is caused by a rising ICP (due to the expanding haematoma).
- *Biconvex hyperdense lesion on the temporal region:* Fresh bleed on CT appears hyperdense. A binconvex haematoma is characterisitc of an extradural haematoma (lens-shaped). Its most common site is temporal region.

CONFUSA

In subdural haematoma, the CT appearance is usually concave on the inner side, most commonly in parietal region. Midline shift may be present.

Investigation of Choice
CT scan (already done in this patient).

Immediate Management
Urgent evacuation of the clot through multiple burr holes (as the patient is very critical and there is no spare time for transfer to a neurosurgical unit/centre).

Treatment of Choice
Identification and ligation of the bleeding vessel (usually middle meningeal vessels).

Your notes:

89. Presents with headache, confusion. On examination, papilledoema present.

Diagnosis: Raised intracranial pressure (ICP) due to cerebral metastases.

Clinchers

- *Headache:* It is the most common symptom of raised intracranial pressure. It is often worse in the morning and is accompanied by nausea and vomiting. Fits or focal neurological signs may appear as the ICP rises.
- *Confusion:* It is due to cerebral oedema secondary to brain metastases.
- *Papilloedema:* It is due to oedema of retinal nerve layer and a common finding on fundoscopy (in both the eyes) in increased ICP.

CONFUSA

Breast carcinoma commonly metastasises to brain, bone and liver. Brain metastases are usually solitary and produce reactive cerebral oedema.

Investigation of Choice

CT scan

Immediate Management

Ventilatory support.

Treatment of Choice

Dexamethasone 4 mg/6h PO

Radiotherapy/surgery for isolated metastases.

Your notes:

111. Known patient of multiple sclerosis now with complaint of urinary incontinence, weakness in all 4 limbs and difficulty walking.

Diagnosis (of anatomical site): Cervical spinal cord.

Clinchers

- *Known patient of multiple sclerosis:* Multiple sclerosis is characterised by chronic inflammation, and selective destruction of CNS myelin: sparing the peripheral nervous system. It presents a recurrent attacks of focal neurologic dysfunction.
- *Difficult walking:* The symptoms of multiple sclerosis often worsen with fatigue, stress, exercise or left.
- *Urinary incontinence:* Sensory system involves urinary urgency or frequency, visual difficulties, abnormalities of gate and coordination.

  Motor involvement presents as heavy, stiff, weak or clumsy limb.
- Difficulty in walking, Lhermitte's sign (paraesthesia in limbs on flexing legs) and urinary symptoms are common in spinal and lesion.
- Paraparesis (weakness of both lower limbs) is characteristically diagnostic (not always) of spinal cord lesion.

CONFUSA

Initial individual plaques of MS (e.g. in optic nerve, brainstem or cord) must be distinguished from compressive, inflammatory, mass or vascular lesions. Other conditions that mimic the pattern of relapsing MS are CNS sarcoidosis, SLE and Behcet's syndrome.

Investigation of Choice

MRI of the brain and spinal cord is the first line of investigation.

Immediate Management

Refer to neurology.

Treatment of Choice

When diagnosed, inform the patient of the diagnosis. There is no cure.

- *Polyunsaturated fats*—may help.
- *Methylprednisolone*—shortens relapses
- b-interferon 1b
  - ¯ relapse rate by 1/3
  - ¯ lesion accumulation on MRI
  - Slow accumulation of disability

112. Patient has nystagmus, diplopia, and positive past pointing.

Diagnosis (of anatomical site): Brainstem and its cerebellar connections

Clinchers

- *Nystagmus:* A rhythmic oscillation of the eye is a sign of disease of either the ocular or the vestibular system and its connection. In the lesions of brainstem and the cerebellum, long lasting horizontal or rotatory jerk and nystagmus are present.
- *Diplopia:* Diplopia in multiple sclerosis is the result of many different lesions—a sixth nerve lesion and the internuclear ophthalmoplegia (INO) are true examples.
- *Positive past pointing:* It is a sign of cerebellar lesion. Others include positive and gate disturbances, nystagmus, dysarthmia, etc.

CONFUSA

A typical picture of sole brainstem demyelination is sudden diplopics and vertigo with nystagmus, but without tinnitus or deafness.

Investigation of Choice

MRI (magnetic resonance imaging).

Immediate Management

Refer to neurology.

Treatment of Choice

When diagnosed, inform the patient of the diagnosis. There is no cure.

- *Polyunsatured fats*—may help
- *Methylprednisolone*—shortens relapses
- b-interferon 1b
  - ⁻ relapse rate by 1/3
  - ⁻ lesion accumulation on MRI
  - Slow accumulation of disability.

115. A known patient of multiple sclerosis with unilateral facial paralysis with no loss of taste.

Diagnosis (of anatomical site): Facial nerve

Clinchers

- *Patient of multiple sclerosis with unilateral facial paralysis:* Facial paralysis, resembling idiopathic. Bell's palsy may be due to MS. It is a unilateral weakness of all the muscles of facial expression on the same site.
- *No loss of taste:* In MS, facial palsy is usually not associated with:
  - Ipsilateral loss of taste sensation
  - Retroaural pain at onset

Which are clinical characteristics of Bell's palsy.

CONFUSA

Chronic flickering contractions of the facial musculature, termed *facial myokymia,* is common in MS; it is thought to arise from involvement of corticobulbar tracts that deafferentation of the facial nucleus.

Investigation of Choice

MRI

Immediate Management

Refer to neurology

Treatment of Choice

When diagnosed, inform the patient of the diagnosis. There is no cure.

- *Polyunsatured fats*—may help
- *Methylprednisolone*—shortens relapses
- b-interferon 1b
  - ⁻ relapse rate by 1/3
  - ⁻ lesion accumulation on MRI
  - Slow accumulation of disability.

143. A 55-year-old man with history of hypertension untreated presents with haemiparesis

Diagnosis: Intracerebral haemorrhage.

Clinchers

- *55-year-old man:* Elderly person are more prone to hypertensive complications especially if it is left-untreated. Incidence of hypertension in males is more.
- *History of hypertension untreated:* Intracerebral haemorrhage occurs typically in patients with untreated hypertension. SAH is also associated with hypertension but its association is not so typical and usually present with severe headache and neck stiffness.
- *Presents with haemiparesis:* Focal neurological deficits are more common with intracerebral bleeds (cf SAH) which occurs at well-defined sites (basal ganglia, pons, cerebellum and subcortical white matter) due to rupture of Charcot-Bouchard aneurysms.

CONFUSA

- Hemiplegia/haemiparesis
  - Early—suggests formation of an intracerebral haematoma
  - Late—suggests vasospasm and ischaemia
- Clinically thre is no entirely reliable way of distinguishing between intracerebral haemorrhage and thromboembolic infarction, as both produce a sudden focal deficit. Intracerebral haemorrhage, however, tends to be dramatic and accompanied by a severe headache (but still less severe than that of SAH).

Investigation of Choice

Visualized reliably by immediate CT (cf. infarction).

Immediate Management

Urgent neurosurgical evacuation of the clot should be considered when an intracerebral haematoma behaves as an expanding mass, causing deepening coma and coning.

Treatment of Choice

Unlike thromboembolism antiplatelet drugs are contraindicated. Surgery is indicated if conservative measures fail.

Your notes:

146. A 27-year-old woman has a long-standing history of headaches associated with nausea and vomiting. On this occasion she present with sudden loss of vision in the right half of the visual field. By the time you see her it has improved considerably.

Diagnosis: Migraine

Clinchers

- *27-year-old woman has a long-standing history of headaches:* Onset of migraine is usually in childhood, adolescence or early adulthood; however, initial attack may occur at any age. It is more frequent in women, family history is often positive.
- *Headaches associated with nausea and vomiting:* Classic triad of migraine is:
  1. Premonitoring visual (scotoma or scintillations), sensory or motor symptoms
  2. Unilateral throbbing headache
  3. Nausea and vomiting
- *Sudden loss of vision in the right half of visual field:* Visual symptoms of migraine can be visual chaos (cascading, distortion, melting and jumbling of print lines, dots, spots, zig-zag fortification specta) and haemianopia.
- *By the time you see her it has improved considerably:* Visual symptoms in migraine last for about 15 minutes and then improved. It is generally followed by the headache within one hour.

CONFUSA

TIAs can mimic migraines visual symptoms of migraine.

Investigation of Choice

Carotid doppler to rule out TIA.

Immediate Management

Dispersible high dose aspirin.

Treatment of Choice

Migraine prophylaxis (if attacks > twice/month) with pizotifen.

Note:

- Premenstrual migraine may respond to diuretics or depot oestrogens.
- Contraceptive pill need not be discontinued if migraine is causing no focal pathology.

Your notes:

148. A woman previously in good health, presents with sudden onset of severe occipital headache and vomiting. Her only physical sign on examination is a shift neck.

Diagnosis: Subarachnoid haemorrhage (SAH)

Clinchers

- *Woman:* Females have a slightly higher incidence of SAH. Lack of estrogen in the postmenopausal females has been cited as a reason.
- *Previously in good health:* Rules out any other medical disorder. Also most of the patient of SAH present with a sudden and spontaneous occurrence with no preceeding disorder. The typical age for SAH is 35-65 years.
- *Sudden onset:* It's onset is sudden (within a few seconds). Some patient may earlier experience a sentinal headache due to small warning leaks from the offending aneurysm.
- *Severe occipital headache:* SAH presents with a devastating headache which the patients usually describe as "the worst headache of my life" or "I thought I had been kicked in the head". It is most commonly occipital. Vomiting may accompany.
- *Stiff neck:* (Kernig's positive). It is a feature of SAH but takes six hours to develop.

CONFUSA

Other differential diagnoses for stiff neck are—Shigella gastroenteritis and meningitis.

- Focal neurology (i.e. hemiplegia) in SAH may give diagnostic clues, e.g.
  - *Early development*—suggests intracerebral hematoma
  - *Late development*—suggests vasospasm and ischaemia

Investigation of Choice

Early CT (shows subarachnoid or ventricular blood).

Immediate Management

Immediate neurosurgical opinion if

- Consciousness decrease
- Progressive focal deficit
- Suspected cerebellar haematoma

Treatment of Choice

Surgical clipping of aneurysms/guglielmi coils
+
Control hypertension

149. A 74-year-old woman had a fall two weeks ago. She is brought into the A and E department with slowly increasing drowsiness. On examination you find mild haemiparesis and unequal pupils.

Diagnosis: Subdural haematoma.

Clinchers

- *74-year-old:* Bridging veins in the skull becomes more prone to rupture in old age. It is due to cortical atrophy producing gradual shrinkage of brain and thereby producing more traction on the veins.
- *Slowly increasing drowsiness:* It means that the haematoma which is now behaving like a SOL (space occupying lesion) is still expanding and there is danger if it is not evacuated urgently.
- *Two weeks ago:* Remember subdural haematomas are usually subdued in appearance i.e. they can occur weeks to months after the initial injury (as the bleeding is from very small veins).
- *Mild haemiparesis and unequal pupils:* Ipsilateral pupillary dilatation is a lagte sign. Focal neurological signs are an indication for urgent intervention.

CONFUSA

Do not rely on absence of ipsilateral pupillary dilatation as it is a late sign. Alteration in the conscious level is the cardinal feature; lateralising signs may be absent or minimal.

Investigation of Choice

CT scan is diagnostic, showing a collection with an inner concave border (extradural—binconvex).

Immediate Management

Urgent neurological opinion.

Treatment of Choice

Surgical evacuation of the haematoma.

Your notes:

150. A 73-year-old man presents with haemianopia, haemisensory loss, haemiparesis and aphaesia of 16 hours duration.

Diagnosis: TIA involving the carotids.

Clinchers

- *73-year-old man:* Incidence of TIA increases with age. Most common cause is atherosclerosis.
- *Haemianopia:* Homonymous haemianopia is typical of a carotid territory ischaemia.
- *Haemisensory loss:* Contralateral weakness/numbness is present in *haemiparesis* carotid territory ischaemia.
- *Aphaesia:* Dysphasia, aphaesia and dysarthria are characteristic pointers for carotid territory ischaemia.
- *Of 16 hours duration:* The sudden onset of focal CNS signs or symptoms due to temporary occlusion, usually by emboli, of part of the cerebral circulation is termed a TIA if symptoms are present for less than 24 hours and fully resolve within this period.

CONFUSA

80% of the TIA are in the carotid territory. Suspect then whenever there is:
- Unilateral paresis
- Unilateral sensory loss
- Aphaesia
- Monocular visual loss.

Investigation of Choice

Aim to find the cause and define vascular risk. Go for carotid angiography. CT is usually not indicated in patients over 55 years. Do a routine screen (FBC, ESR, U and E, glucose, ECG, CRX).

Immediate Management

Give O_2 + monitor vital signs.

Treatment of Choice

Oral aspirin (300 mg) unless contraindicated thereafter 150 mg daily.

Your notes:

160. A-67-year old woman reports severe paroxysms of knife-like or electric shock-like pain, lasting seconds in the lower part of the right side of her face.

Diagnosis: Trigeminal neuralgia (dic douloureux)

Clinchers

- *67 year old:* It is chiefly a condition of those over 50 years old.
- *Woman:* G/E > 1
- *Severe paroxysms of knife like or electric shock like pain lasting seconds:* The patient suffers paroxysms of intense, stabbing pain, lasting only seconds in the trigeminal nerve distribution.
- *In the lower part of the right side of her face:* Pain is unilateral, affecting the mandibular and maxillary divisions most often, and the ophthalmic division only rarely. The face may screw up with pain (hence tic doloureux). Pain may recur many times in a day and can often by precipitated by
  - touching the skin of affected area
  - washing
  - shaving
  - eating
  - talking
  - cold wind

CONFUSA

The pain characteristically do not occur at night (contraindication! OHCM, page 335, 5th edn , says it do occur at night—333, 5th edn; Kumar and Clark page 1021, 4th Edn. on the contrary—1021, 4th Edn). Spontaneous remissions last for months or years before recurrence, which is almost inevitable)

Investigation of Choice

Diagnosis is on clinical grounds alone.

Immediate Management

Exclude structural causes i.e.
- Multiple sclerosis (suspect when it present in young age)
- Vascular malformation
- Cerebellopontine angle tumours

Treatment of Choice

- Drugs:
  - Carbamazepine
  - Alternatives: Phenytoin, clonazepam
- Surgical: Used when drug therapy fails
  - Radiofrequency ablation of ganglion
  - Neurovascular decompression
  - Sectioning of sensory root
  - Alcohol injection

PAPER 7

35. A 39-year-old female presents with weakness of both legs, difficulty walking and urinary retention.

Diagnosis: Spinal cord lesion

Clinchers

- Bladder tone is lost immediately after spinal transection
- Distention leads to ureteric reflux and renal damage. Motor and sensory loss further support diagnosis of spinal cord lesion.

CONFUSA

Impairment of descending sympathetic pathways in the spinal cord leads to relative hypovolaemia and cardia. Any reduction of blood supply to the damaged cord will further impair its function. Bradycardia often responds to atropine.

Investigation of Choice

MRI spine.

Immediate Management

Intermittent catheterization may be the Treatment of Choice in the spinal unit but it is preferable to insert and retain a fairly thin catheter during the initial period of resuscitation and inter-hospital transfer. Catheterisation must be performed by an experienced member of staff using an aseptic technique.

Your notes:

61. Known patient of multiple sclerosis now with complaint of urinary incontinence, weakness in all 4 limbs and difficulty walking.

Diagnosis (of anatomical site): Cervical spinal cord.

Clinchers

- *Known patient of multiple sclerosis:* Multiple sclerosis is characterised by chronic inflammation, and selective destruction of CNS myelin: sparing the peripheral nervous system. It presents a recurrent attacks of focal neurologic dysfunction.
- *Difficult walking:* The symptoms of multiple sclerosis often worsen with fatigue, stress, exercise or left.
- *Urinary incontinence:* Sensory system involves urinary urgency or frequency, visual difficulties, abnormalities of gate and coordination.

  Motor involvement presents as heavy, stiff, weak or clumsy limb.
- Difficulty in walking, Lhermitte's sign (paraesthesia in limbs on flexing legs) and urinary symptoms are common in spinal cord lesion.
- Paraparesis (weakness of both lower limbs) is characteristically diagnostic (not always) of spinal cord lesion.

CONFUSA

Initial individual plaques of MS (e.g. in optic nerve, brainstem or cord) must be distinguished from compressive, inflammatory, mass or vascular lesions. Other conditions that mimic the pattern of relapsing MS are CNS sarcoidosis, SLE and Behcet's syndrome.

Investigation of Choice

MRI of the brain and spinal cord is the first line of investigation.

Immediate Management

Refer to neurology.

Treatment of Choice

When diagnosed, inform the patient of the diagnosis. There is no cure.

- *Polyunsaturated fats*—may help.
- *Methylprednisolone*—shortens relapses
- b-interferon 1b
  - ¯ relapse rate by 1/3
  - ¯ lesion accumulation on MRI
  - Slow accumulation of disability.

Your notes:

62. Patient has nystagmus, diplopia, and positive past pointing.

Diagnosis (of anatomical site): Brainstem and its cerebellar connections

Clinchers

- *Nystagmus:* A rhythmic oscillation of the eye is a sign of disease of either the ocular or the vestibular system and its connection. In the lesions of brainstem and the cerebellum, long lasting horizontal or rotatory jerk and nystagmus are present.
- *Diplopia:* Diplopia in multiple sclerosis is the result of many different lesions—a sixth nerve lesion and the internuclear ophthalmoplegia (INO) are true examples.
- *Positive past pointing:* It is a sign of cerebellar lesion. Others include positive gait disturbances, nystagmus, dysarthria, etc.

CONFUSA

A typical picture of sole brainstem demyelination is sudden diplopia and vertigo with nystagmus, but without tinnitus or deafness.

Investigation of Choice
MRI (magnetic resonance imaging).

Immediate Management
Refer to neurology.

Treatment of Choice
When diagnosed, inform the patient of the diagnosis. There is no cure.

- *Polyunsatured fats*—may help
- *Methylprednisolone*—shortens relapses
- b-interferon 1b
  - ¯ relapse rate by 1/3
  - ¯ lesion accumulation on MRI
  - Slow accumulation of disability.

Your notes:

63. Patient has repeated attacks of multiple sclerosis, and now has pale temporal disc

Diagnosis (of anatomical site): Optic nerve

Clinchers

- *Pale temporal disc:* Disc pallor following an attack of multiple sclerosis is a sign of optic atrophy. It is first seen in temporal region.

  The optic disc appearance depends upon the site of the plaque of multiple sclerosis, within the optic nerve. If the lesion is in the nerve head, there is disc swelling (optic neuritis). If the lesion is several millimeters behind the disc, there is generally no ophthalmoscopic feature. Here the doctor sees nothing and the patient sees nothing.

  After the attack subsides, usually there is no residual symptom, but small scotoma or defects in colour vision can be demonstrated. Disc pallor is a late sequelae of multiple sclerosis and a sign of optic atrophy.

CONFUSA

Disc swelling from optic neuritis causes early and measurably visual acuity loss, thus distinguishing it from disc swelling from raised intracranial pressure.

Investigation of Choice
MRI (magnetic resonance imaging)

Immediate Management
Refer to neurology

Treatment of Choice
When diagnosed, inform the patient of the diagnosis. There is no cure.

- *Polyunsatured fats*—may help.
- *Methylprednisolone*—shortens relapses
- b-interferon 1b
  - relapse rate by 1/3
  - lesion accumulation on MRI
  - Slow accumulation of disability.

Your notes:

64. Patient with complaint of blurring of vision, papilloedema and pain in eye.

Diagnosis (of anatomical site): Optic nerve

Clinchers

- *Blurring of vision:* Optic neuritis produces variable loss. It usually begins as blurring of the central visual field, which may remain mild or progress to severe visual loss, or rarely, to complete loss of light perception. In mild cases, the patient may complain only of a subjective loss of brightness in the affected eye. Symptoms are generally monocular, but attacks may be bilateral.
- *Papillodema:* This is due to optic neuritis fundoscopic examination in it may be normal or with swelling of optic disc.
- *Pain in eye:* Pain, localized to the orbit or supraorbital area is frequently present and may precede visual loss. The pain typically worsens with eye movement.

CONFUSA

Visual blurring in MS may result from optic neuritis or diplopia. They are distinguished by asking the patient to cover each eye sequentially and observing whether the visual difficulty clears. Diplopia in MS is often due to an internuclear ophthalmoplegia (INO) or to a sixth nerve palsy; ocular muscle palsies due to involvement of the third or fourth cranial nerve are rare.

Investigation of Choice
MRI

Immediate Management
Refer to neurology

Treatment of Choice
When diagnosed, inform the patient of the diagnosis. There is no cure.

- *Polyunsatured fats*—may help
- *Methylprednisolone*—shortens relapses
- b-interferon 1b
  - ¯ relapse rate by 1/3
  - ¯ lesion accumulation on MRI
  - Slow accumulation of disability.

Your notes:

65. A known patient of multiple sclerosis with unilateral facial paralysis with no loss of taste.

Diagnosis (of anatomical site): Facial nerve

Clinchers

- *Patient of multiple sclerosis with unilateral facial paralysis:* Facial paralysis, resembling idiopathic. Bell's palsy may be due to MS. It is a unilateral weakness of all the muscles of facial expression on the same site.
- *No loss of taste:* In MS, facial palsy is usually not associated with:
  - Ipsilateral loss of taste sensation
  - Retroaural pain at onset

Which are clinical characteristics of Bell's palsy.

CONFUSA

Chronic flickering contractions of the facial musculature, termed *facial myokymia,* is common in MS; it is thought to arise from involvement of corticobulbar tracts that deafferentation of the facial nucleus.

Investigation of Choice
MRI

Immediate Management
Refer to neurology

Treatment of Choice
When diagnosed, inform the patient of the diagnosis. There is no cure.

- *Polyunsatured fats*—may help
- *Methylprednisolone*—shortens relapses
- b-interferon 1b
  - relapse rate by 1/3
  - lesion accumulation on MRI
  - Slow accumulation of disability

Your notes:

66. Patient gets diplopia when he works very hard.

Diagnosis: Myasthenia gravis (MG)

Clinchers

➢ *Gets diplopia when he works very hard:* Fatiguability is the single most important feature of MG. Muscles are not commonly affected in the early stages:
- Proximal limb muscles
- Extraocular muscles
- Muscles of mastication, speech and facial expression.

Complex extraocular palsies, ptosis and a typical fluctuating proximal weakness are found.

CONFUSA

The reflexes are initially preserved in MG but may be fatiguable. Muscle wasting is sometimes seen late in the disease. The clinical picture of fluctuating weakness may be diagnostic. Early symptoms of weakness and fatigue are frequently dismissed by attending doctors.

Investigation of Choice

Tensilon test (only do if resuscitation facilities available)

Immediate Management

Rule out
- Thymic tumour
- Hyperthyroidism
- Rheumatoid arthritis
- SLE

Treatment of Choice

Pyridostigmine + prednisolone.

Your notes:

67. Patient with attacks of numbness in left hand and right-sided headache.

Diagnosis: Space occupying lesion (SOL)

Clinchers

➢ *Attacks of numbness in left hand:* This suggests an evolving focal neurology. Usually focal neurology depends upon site of the tumour but the information provided in the question is insufficient to diagnose the site of SOL. Most probably it is a parietal lobe tumour (Haemisonsory loss, decreased two-point discrimination).

➢ *Right-sided headache:* It is a sign of increased ICP signs to space occupying property of the tumour. Other signs of - ICP can be:
- Vomiting
- Papilloedema (only in 50% of tumours)
- Altered consciousness.

CONFUSA

Evolving focal neurology must be differentiated from false localising signs which are produced by raised ICP. VI nerve palsy is the most common due to its long intracranial course.

Investigation of Choice

CT (MRI is good for posterior fossa tumours).

Immediate Management

Refer to neurology.

Treatment of Choice

Complete removal if possible.

Your notes:

68. This disease is characterised by neurofibrillary tangels and senile plaques.

Diagnosis: Alzheimer's dementia (AD)

Clinchers

- *Neurofibrillary tangles:* These are characteristic of AD and are composed of abnormally phosphorylated tan protein.
- *Senile plaques:* These are neuritic plaques composed of AB amyloid and other proteins.

CONFUSA

Risk factors for AD are old age, positive family history. The apolipoprotein E (apoE) gene (Chromosome 21) has a role in pathogenesis. Rare genetic causes of AD are:

- Down's syndrome (trisomy 21)
- Amyloid precursor protein (APP)
- Gene mutations (chromosome 21)
- ALL.

Investigation of Choice

Neuroimaging (will help rule out frontal lobe dementia; Lewy body dementia and Picks's disease).

Immediate Management

Counsel the relatives about taking care.

Treatment of Choice

Donepezil.

Your notes:

104. A 50-year-old male wakes up with a tingling and numbness in his right hand. This is accompanied by slurring of speech which recovers following about four hours.

Diagnosis: Transient ischaemic attack (TIA) (left sided)

Clinchers

- *50-year-old:* Incidence of TIA increases with age as it is usually secondary to vascular diseases like atherosclerosis which are more prevalent in older age groups.
- *Wakes up with a tingling and numbness in his right hand:* Contralateral weakness and numbness is common carotid territory ischaemia. It means that TIA has occurred in left side of cerebrum (hence carotid source is implicated)
- *Slurring of speech:* Dysphagia is typical of carotid territory ischaemia. Dysarthria can occur in both carotid and vertebrobasilary territory ischaemia.
- *Recovers in 4 hours:* By definition a TIA has no CNS signs after 24 hours.

CONFUSA

Presence of carotid bruits suggests a carotid source of emboli. Their absence does not rule it out. Tight stenosis often have no bruit.

Investigation of Choice

Carotid Doppler

Immediate Management

Aspirin (if not peptic ulcer)

Treatment of Choice

Carotid endarterectomy (if carotid stenoses is present).

Your notes:

139. Woman, 30-year-old with complaint of blurred vision. CT is normal but she has bilateral papilledema.

Diagnosis: Pseudotumour cerebri (suspected)

Clinchers

- *Woman, 30-year-old:* Majority of its patients are young, obese, females.
- *Complaint of blurred vision:* Visual acuity is not affected by papilloedema, unless the papilloedema is severe, long-standing or accompanied by macular oedema or haemorrhage. So suspect there in this patient.
- *CT is normal:* Evaluation of papilloedema requires CT or MRI to exlcude a brain tumour. If none is found, MR angiography is appropriate in selected cases to investigate the possibility of a dural venous sinus occlusion or an arteriovenous shunt. If neuroradiologic studies are normal, the subarachnoid opening pressure should be measured by lumbar puncture to confirm that it is elevated. It if is elevated, without explanation, the diagnosis of pseudotumour cerebri is made by exclusion.
- *Bilateral papilloedema:* It connotes bilateral optic disc swelling from raised ICT.

CONFUSA

All forms of optic disc swelling, other than due to raised ICT is 'optic disc oedema'. This convention is arbitrary but serves to avoid confusion. Pseudotumour cerebri is also known as benign intracranial hypertension.

Investigation of Choice

Lumbar puncture (opening pressure)

Immediate Management

Ophthalmology referral

Treatment of Choice

Acetazolamide

Your notes:

141. A 2-year-old boy ran and hit his forehead on the door. No history of loss of consciousness , and since then is playing well. No neurological signs.

Diagnosis: Head injury (minor)

Clinchers

- *2-year-old boy:* In young children minor head injuries are also important, even if they do not produce immediate major complications as repeated minor head trauma in children has been linked to lower IQ.
- *Hit his forehead on the door:* In the preschool are group the most common injuries are those which are sustained while playing or via household accidents. Nonaccidental injuries are also significant in this age group. In the school-going child the most common cause of death is a brain injury from a RTA.
- *No history of loss of consciousness:* Young children lose consciousness lesser readily than adults. Significant brain injury may thus occur without a history of unconsciousness.
- *Since then is playing well and no neurological signs:* These rule out any grave injury and the situation do not warrant a stay in hospital.

CONFUSA

Children are unique in invariably having a carer with them. This means that most can go home with their parents and a set of head injury instructions. They often sleep after trauma and should not be kept awake. Instead, they should be examined by their parents two or three times during the night. All that is required is for the parents to be confident that their child has a normal response to mild stimulation (verbal or tactile). Parents are much better judges of their children's night-time behaviour than hospital doctors or nurses.

Investigation of Choice

Skull X-ray is unnecessary if all of the following apply:

- No LOC
- Occipital or frontal injury
- Low speed imapct or injuring agent flat and soft
- Normal neurological status at time of examination
- No scalp damage or laceration with no associated significant swelling.

So, No investigations are required in this case as it meet all of the above criterias.

Immediate Management

Give a set of head injury instructions and explain (to parents)

Treatment of Choice Discharge with advise.

142. An 8-year-old boy falls off a swing at his school. He is brought to Casualty by one of his teachers. He has a bruise over his right eye but the examination is otherwise normal. He is fully conscious with no history of blackouts since the accident. A skull X-ray is performed, which is normal.

Diagnosis: Insignificant head injury.

Clinchers

- *8-year-old boy:* Children are difficult to assess for head injury and their admission for monitoring is indicated.
- *Falls off a swing at his school:* A common mode of injury to a school going child. But the most common head injury is by RTA.
- *Brought to casualty by one of his teachers:* That means that no adult member of family is with him—a contraindication for discharge.
- *Bruise over his right eye:* Usually children do not suffer from fracture of skull bones as these are more pliable.
- *Examination is otherwise normal:* Rules out any cerebral injury GCS scoring should be done on adult scale and children. GCS if for < 5 years.
- *Fully conscious:* Also in favour of any cerebral injury but not that young children lose consciousness less readily that adults. Significant brain injury can occur without a history of loss of consciousness.
- *No history of blackouts since the accident:* Also a good prognostic sign.
- *Skull X-ray is normal:* Rules out any fracture which commands admission. But one should be aware of suture lines and normal anatomical variants while interpreting the X-rays.

CONFUSA

Assessment of consciousness in a child can be difficult. The best judge for minor alteration in consciousness in children are their parents.

Investigation of Choice

Skull X-ray (already done in this case).

Immediate Management

Antiseptic dressing of the bruise.

Treatment of Choice

Admit and monitor.

Your notes:

143. A 19-year-old met with a road traffic accident (RTA). He is talking, responding and smells of alcohol.

Diagnosis: Suspected head injury.

Clinchers

- *19-year-old:* Head injury is a major cause of death in children and young adults.
- *Road traffic accident:* RTA is a leading cause of death through head injury and was responsible for 39% deaths from trauma in the UK in 1992.
- *He is talking, responding and smells of alcohol:* Although the patient might look normal at the time of assessment, he or she might have been unconscious or concurred at the time of injury. This is difficult to assess in an intoxicated person and require admission to hospital for proper assessment. A radiological investigation (at least a skull X-ray) is required in alcoholic cases for MLC purposes as such person might have been assaulted.

CONFUSA

Drunkenness increases the risk of sustaining a head injury and of that injury causing brain damage. Nevertheless, changes in conscious level must not be attributed to alcohol or other drugs except by exclusion and in retrospect. The plasma osmolality may be a useful investigation in this circumstance.

Investigation of Choice

Skull X-ray

Immediate Management

Admit to hospital

Treatment of Choice

As per the X-ray findings.

Your notes:

144. A 74-year-old woman had a fall two weeks ago. She is brought into the A and E department with slowly increasing drowsiness. On examination you find mild haemiparesis and unequal pupils.

Diagnosis: Subdural haematoma.

Clinchers

- *74-year-old:* Bridging veins in the skull becomes more prone to rupture in old age. It is due to cortical atrophy producing gradual shrinkage of brain and thereby producing more traction on the veins.
- *Slowly increasing drowsiness:* It means that the haematoma which is now behaving like a SOL (space occupying lesion) is still expanding and there is danger if it is not evacuated urgently.
- *Two weeks ago:* Remember subdural haematomas are usually subdued in appearance i.e. they can occur weeks to months after the initial injury (as the bleeding is from very small veins).
- *Mild haemiparesis and unequal pupils:* Ipsilateral pupillary dilatation is a lagte sign. Focal neurological signs are an indication for urgent intervention.

CONFUSA

Do not rely on absence of ipsilateral pupillary dilatation as it is a late sign. Alteration in the conscious level is the cardinal feature; lateralising signs may be absent or minimal.

Investigation of Choice

CT scan is diagnostic, showing a collection with an inner concave border (extradural—binconvex).

Immediate Management

Urgent neurological opinion.

Treatment of Choice

Surgical evacuation of the haematoma.

Your notes:

145. A 24-year-old patient presents with RTA. The pupil on the left side is dilated and the patient is obtunded. CT scan of the head reveals a binconvex hyperdense lesion on the temporal region.

Diagnosis: Extradural haemorrhage.

Clinchers

- *History of RTA:* Road traffic accidents produces maximum mortality due to head injuries.
- *Pupil on left side is dilated:* In cases of intracranial haematomas localising neurological symptoms (e.g. ipsilateral pupil dilatation, haemiparesis) occurs late (average 63 days in case of subdural haematoma). So the patient is in a critical stage warranting urgent surgical decompression).
- *Obtunded:* Deteriorating level of consciousness is caused by a rising ICP (due to the expanding haematoma).
- *Biconvex hyperdense lesion on the temporal region:* Fresh bleed on CT appears hyperdense. A binconvex haematoma is characterisitc of an extradural haematoma (lens-shaped). Its most common site is temporal region.

CONFUSA

In subdural haematoma, the CT appearance is usually concave on the inner side, most commonly in parietal region. Midline shift may be present.

Investigation of Choice

CT scan (already done in this patient).

Immediate Management

Urgent evacuation of the clot through multiple burr holes (as the patient is very critical and there is no spare time for transfer to a neurosurgical unit/centre).

Treatment of Choice

Identification and ligation of the bleeding vessel (usually middle meningeal vessels).

Your notes:

151. A chronic alcoholic presents with increasing confusion and confabulation.

Diagnosis: Wernicke's-Korsakoff's syndrome (WKS)

Clinchers

- *Chronic alcoholic:* WKS can develop in heavy drinkers. The cause is severe, untreated, thiamine deficiency secondary to chronic alcohol use.
- *Increasing confusion:* The patient may be disoriented in WKS and is due to Wernicke's encephalopathy. Its patients are profoundly disoriented, indifferent, and inattentive, although rarely they have an agitated delirium related to ethanol withdrawal. If the disease is not treated stupor, coma and death may ensue.
- *Confabulation:* It is the component of Korsakoff's (or Korsakov's) psychosis in WKS. Severe loss of short term memory causes the patient to invent his or her immediate past and is called confabulation.

CONFUSA

The characteristic clinical trial of Wernicke's disease is that of ophthalmoplegia, ataxia and global confusion. However, only one third of patients with acute Wernicke's encephalopathy present with the classical clinical triad. As Korsakoff's psychosis often follows Wernicke's encephalopathy, these are together referred to as Wernicke's-Korsakoff's syndrome.

Investigation of Choice

Red cell transketolase (↓)
Plasma pyruvate (↑)

Immediate Management

Admit as it is a medical emergency

Treatment of Choice

Urgent thiamine amine

- 200-300 mg/24 h PO
  But this case is showing symptoms of Korsakoff's psychosis also, so give:
  Pabrinex (High potency ampoules of thiamine)
- 2-3 pairs of ampoules/8 h IV over 10 minutes for ≤ 2 days, then daily for 5-7 days.

Your notes:

14 Obstetrics and Gynaecology

PAPER 1

Serial No. 84

Subject: Obstetrics

Topic: PPH

Question: A primipara after instrumental delivery, lost 800 ml blood. Uterus is well contracted.

Diagnosis: Traumatic post partum haemorrhage

Clinchers

- *Primipara:* while atonic PPH is more commonly associated cause for PPH in multipara, traumatic PPH is more common in primiparous because of increased incidence of instrumental intervention.
- *Instrumental delivery:* Increases the chance of PPH.
- *800 ml blood loss:* any blood loss in excess of 500 ml is considered as PPH.
- *Uterus well contracted:* a well contracted uterus rules out atonicity as the probable cause.

CONFUSA

- PPH was defined as blood loss greater than 500 ml in an vaginal delivery and greater than 1,000 ml in a caesarean delivery.
- Early or primary PPH occurs within 24 hours after delivery and late or secondary PPH occurs 24 hours to 6 weeks after delivery.
- Don't rely completely on clinic parameters for assessment of the severity of blood loss, because in some situations clinical parameters may be unreliable; apparent normotension can be due to pre-eclampsia combined with blood loss.
- Again, think of occult PPH when you get unstable haemodynamic findings without evidence of excessive blood loss.

Investigation of Choice

Local examination to rule out cervical and vaginal lacerations.

Immediate Management

IV fluids; Blood Transfusion

Treatment of Choice

Repair of any soft tissue lacerations brought about by instrumentation.

Serial No. 85

Subject: Obstetrics

Topic: PPH

Question: A multipara with history of two previous PPH.

Diagnosis: High risk for PPH

Clinchers

- *Multipara:* multipara are at 20 times more risk for PPH.
- *History of two previous PPH:* Previous history of PPH is again a risk factor for PPH in present pregnancy.

Risk factors for PPH include:

- Prolonged third stage of labor
- Preeclampsia
- Mediolateral episiotomy
- Previous PPH
- Multiple gestation
- Arrest of descent
- Maternal hypotension
- Coagulation abnormalities
- Lacerations of the cervix, vagina, or perineum
- Asian or Hispanic ethnicity
- Delivery with forceps or vacuum
- Augmented labour
- Nulliparity, multiparity (20-fold increase in risk), and polyhydramnios

CONFUSA

- Multipara as well as primipara are at higher risk for PPH than the general ladies population.
- 80% cases of primary PPH are due to atonic uterus or retention of placental remnants.
- Retained placental products can cause both primary and secondary PPH.

Investigation of Choice

None

Immediate Management

Be vigilant to look into signs for any PPH

Treatment of Choice

In at risk cases, prophylactic oxytocics are administered Avoid 'fundal fiddling' in third stage of labour.

Serial No.86

Subject: Obstetrics

Topic: PPH

Question: A lady on 10th day post LSCS, brought with bleeding per vaginum lasting for 24 hours. She has suprapubic tenderness.

Diagnosis: Secondary PPH

Clinchers

- *10th day post LSCS:* 10 day post LSCS rules out the possibility of wound dehisence or slipping of ligatures as a cause for this presentation. However, the possibilty of infection cannot be ruled out. However, don't forget that blood stained lochia is usually seen upto 5 days post delivery and should not be confused as bleeding PV.
- *Bleeding for 24 hours:* Apparently continuous bleed signifies either retained bits of placenta or membranes or infection (endometritis).
- *Suprapubic tenderness:* This is denoting scar tenderness, which again in the view of the presentation, goes in favour of infection.

CONFUSA

The main area of confusion remains whether this presentation is one of infection as nothing is mentioned about pyrexia. However, in the view of scar tenderness and bleeding per vaginum, there appears to be very unlikely chance of any other possibility. Considering bladder injury in view of the suprapubic tenderness, is again unlikely when we look at the duration between the surgery and the presentation (10 days). Bladder injury would usually present in the immediate postoperative period.

Investigation of Choice
Exploration of uetrine cavity under general anaesthesia

Immediate Management
IV antibiotics

Treatment of Choice
IV antibiotics

Your notes:

Serial No. 87

Subject: Obstetrics

Topic: PPH

Question: A primipara after normal vaginal delivery bled 600 ml after removal of placenta.

Diagnosis: True PPH

Clinchers

- *Primipara:* Primipara are at higher risk for PPH.
- *Normal vaginal delivery:* This rules out trauma from instrumental delivery and subsequent soft tissue laceration as the cause for bleeding.
- *Bled 600 ml:* any amount of bleeding, more than 500 ml in a vaginal delivery and more than 1000 ml in caesarean section is considered as post partum haemorrhage.
- *After removal of placenta:* Bleeding occuring after extraction of placenta is considered as true postpartum Haemorrhage. The main cause being the open placental sinuses which continue to bleed if the uterus fails to contract. Retained placenta can also produce a similar picture.

CONFUSA

Third stage bleeding can occur in 2 forms:

- *With placenta in uterus:* Here, the aim is to deliver the placenta; Exploration under general anaesthesia may become necessary. Also look for soft tissue lacerations, especially if delivery was difficult or precipitate labour.
- *After placenta separates:* Its due to continued bleeding from open sinuses; While massaging uterus, check for completeness of placenta.

Note: Even if the placenta is complete, don't forget about the possibility of succenturiate lobe.

Investigation of Choice
Check placenta for completeness
Monitor vitals

Immediate Management
Massage uterus with slow, rotary motion

Treatment of Choice
Set up Hartmann's infusion,
Give 0.25 mg ergometrine IV or syntocin by infusion.
Alternatively, syntometrine or misoprostol (misoprostol preferred in hypertension)
If still bleeding despite firm uterine contractions inspect genital tract for lacerations, explore uterine cavity for retained placental products.

Serial No. 97

Subject: Gynaecology

Topic: Pelvic Inflammatory Diseases

Question: A 26-year-old female with sore vagina and whitish discharge; smear shows mycelia.

Diagnosis: Vaginal candidiasis

Clinchers

- *26-year-old:* All age groups can be affected. However, highest incidence is noted among young, sexually active women. Risk factors include oral contraceptive use, IUD use, early intercourse, increased frequency of intercourse, receptive cunnilingus, diabetes, HIV or other immunocompromised states, chronic antibiotic use, and pregnancy.
- *Sore vagina:* Pruritus is the most common symptom of vaginal candidiasis. Erythema and swelling of the labia and vulva with satellite lesions are present. Vagina is usually reddened with adherent thick, cottage cheese–like vaginal discharge. Cervix appears normal.
- *Whitish discharge:* Discharge associated with vaginal candidiasis is typically described as thick, odorless white and scanty, with an appearance similar to cottage cheese.
- *Smear shows mycelia:* This is diagnostic of candidiasis. Exudate collected from the lateral vaginal walls and Gram stained, microscopically show hyphae and budding yeasts.

CONFUSA

- Vaginal candidiasis is not a sexually transmitted infection. Candida is a normal commensal of the skin and vagina.
- Male sexual partners do not need treatment unless they have symptoms of thrush on their penis. Symptoms in men include redness, itch, and soreness of the foreskin and the glans of the penis.
- Women do not 'catch' thrush from men who have no symptoms.

Investigation of Choice

Exudate is collected from the lateral vaginal walls and Gram stained and examined microscopically for yeast forms.

Cultured on Sabouraud's dextrose agar medium

Urine is tested for sugar

Immediate Management

Maintain local hygiene

Avoid re-infection from sexual partner; sexual intercourse should be avoided until cure is complete.

Removal any local 'foreign bodies' like IUCD or vaginal diaphragms; Barrier contraceptive in the form of male condoms are the most useful contraceptive during infection.

Treatment of Choice

Intravaginal pessaries or cream inserted high into the vagina at night. Either of the following can be used:

- clotrimazole 200 mg pessary, 1 at night, for 3 nights
- clotrimazole 500 mg pessary, single dose
- miconazole 100 mg pessary, two, for 7 nights
- miconazole ovule 1.2 g, single dose at night

Alternatively a single oral dose of fluconazole can be used. (Avoid in pregnant and lactating mothers).

Your notes:

Serial No. 98

Subject: Gynaecology

Topic: Pelvic inflammatory diseases

Question: A-27-year-old sexually active female on oral contraceptives for two years, complains of mucoid discharge per vaginum.

Diagnosis: Cervical ectropion

Clinchers

- *27-year-old:* Cervical ectropion or erosion most commonly occurs in women of reproductive age group. However, it can be also seen in neonates, who are exposed high maternal oestrogen.
- *Sexually active:* Being sexually active does not prediposes one to cervical erosion directly, but use of oral contraceptives, or even high estrogen levels during pregnancy provides good enviornment for the squamous lining of the cervix to change to columnar.
- *On oral contraceptives for two years:* This is the most common cause of exogenous source of oestrogen causing change of cervical epithelium.
- *Mucoid discharge per vaginum:* most patients are asymptomatic except for some mucoid discharge. An erosion is not painful and does not cause dyspareunia; however a patient may sometimes present with bleeding or infection.

CONFUSA

Erosions are thought to be oestrogen dependent. They are seen most commonly in women taking combined oral contraceptives pills and resolve when the pill is stopped. It also frequently develops during pregnancy and resolve after delivery.

An erosion may also occur in newborn infants and may persist into childhood. This congenital erosion is not abnormal, and is due to exposure to high maternal oestrogens. Sometimes, it may also be seen during puberty.

Investigation of Choice

Speculum examination: shows a red ring around the os. The 'red ring' is actually the migrated endocervical mucous columnar epithelium over the ectocervix.

Immediate Management

A cervical smear is mandatory. It should be followed by colposcopy and cervical biopsy if the result is unsatisfactory.

Treatment of Choice

None required;

A troublesome erosion may be treated by thermal cautery with diathermy, cyrosurgery or laser treatment.

Your notes:

Serial No. 99

Subject: Gynaecology

Topic: Pelvic inflammatory diseases

Question: A 18-year-old girl with recently developed dysmenrrorhoea and deep dyspareunia. Speculum examination reveals purulent discharge from cervical os. Tested negative for gonorrhoea.

Diagnosis: Chlamydia cervicitis

Clinchers

- *18 year-old-girl:* Young age, multiple sexual partners, low socioeconomic group are important risk factors for developing PID. Insertion of intrauterine contraceptive device increases the risk by 6 times, during first 3 weeks following insertion. Most cases of PID occur in sexually active women of age 15-24 years.
- *Recently developed dysmenrrorhoea:* PID usually presents with non specific symptoms, of which dysmenrrorhoea is one of the common one.The recent onset of dysmenrrorhoea may be linked to the PID she developed after some recent 'infected' intercourse
- *Deep dyspareunia:* specific for PID and occurs due touching of inflammed cervix during intercourse which elicits severe pain.
- *Purulent discharge from cervical os:* Mucopurulent cervical discharge and cervicitis, cervical motion tenderness and adnexal tenderness are all very strong points in favour of PID.
- *Tested negative for gonorrhoea:* Gonorrhoea and chlamydia are two most common cause of PID; however, in UK maximum cases (52%) are due to Chlamydia; only 14% occur due to gonorrhoea.

CONFUSA

Dyspareunia in females is related to varied causes and should be dealt in the light of other features present. For this case, deep dyspareunia with mucopurulent discharge points directly to PID. However, other causes of deep dyspareunia should be kept in mind, viz, endometriosis (especially when deposits are present in the pouch of Douglas, uterosacral ligaments, posterior vaginal fornix), adenomyosis, prolapsed ovaries in the pouch of Douglas, retroverted and retroflexed uterus - (unlikely to cause significant dyspareunia unless associated pathology e.g. endometriosis), changed partner - changed shape / size of penis.

Investigation of Choice

Urethral and cervical swabs for chlamydia

Immediate Management

Advise abstinence from sexual intercourse until women and her partner have both completed a course of treatment. Consider empirical treatment of partner if he/she refuses screening.
Advise on use of condoms (antibiotics reduce efficacy of OCP).
Remove IUCDs, if any.
Advise against tampons.
Contact tracing and treatment (all sexual partners in previous 6 months need to be contacted and tested)

Treatment of Choice

Blind antibiotic therapy (covers *C. trachomatis*, *N. gonorrhoeae* and anaerobic infection)

- oral ofloxacin 400 mg twice a day plus oral metronidazole 400 mg twice a day for 14 days, OR,
- intramuscular ceftriaxone 250 mg immediately or intramuscular cefoxitin 2 g immediately with oral probenecid 1 g, followed by oral doxycycline 100 mg twice a day plus metronidazole 400 mg twice a day for 14 days

If pregnant, a suggested antibiotic treatment regime is: erythromycin 500 mg four times daily for 14 days and metronidazole 400 mg twice daily for seven days
Start treatment as soon as the diagnosis is suspected, don't wait for swab results.

Your notes:

Serial No. 100

Subject: Gynaecology

Topic: PID

Question: A 37-year-old lady with multiple painful, vesicular lesions at the introitus with scanty offensive discharge.

Diagnosis: Herpes genitalis

Clinchers

- *37-year-old lady:* The prevalence of HSV antibodies is slightly higher in females. However, women are more likely than men to be protected from genital HSV infection by the use of barrier methods.The rate of genital herpes is highest in sexually active ladies.
- *Multiple painful, vesicular lesions at the introitus:* Groups of small, painful blisters then appear around the genitals and/or anus, which tend to erupt in crops over 1-2 weeks. The blisters later evolve into shallow, sore ulcers. There can be inguinal lymphadenopathy and dysuria. The ulcers and blisters last up to 10-14 days, and then gradually heal and go without scarring.
- *Scanty offensive discharge:* Scanty serous vaginal discharge usually accompany which can later turn purulent due to secondary bacterial infections.

CONFUSA

Genital herpes infection in pregnancy:

- If herpes infection is apparent at the onset of labour then a caesarean section is indicated.
- In case of primary infection, aciclovir 200 mg orally five times daily is give to the mother, (usually for five days) or topical application of 5 per cent cream five times a day for 5-10 days, starting at the first sign of attack.
- Neonatal infection is uncommon in cases of recurrent genital herpes. This is because of relatively lower concentration and shedding of the virus and also, the passive immunity acquired by the foetus from the mother.

Investigation of Choice

Clinical diagnosis.

The gold standard of diagnosis is viral culture.

Immediate Management

Symptomatic measures:

- analgesia (paracetamol)
- saline baths

Advise male condom use to prevent sexual transmission from infected men to uninfected sexual partners.

Advise antiviral treatment of infected sexual partner.

Treatment of Choice

Acyclovir, 200 mg, 5 times a day for 5 days.

Alternatives to acyclovir therapy are famciclovir and valaciclovir.

Recurrent episodes may require continous acyclovir

Your notes:

Serial No. 101

Subject: Gynaecology

Topic: PID

Question: A 34-year-old lady comes with discharge per vaginum. Wet mount shows clue cells.

Diagnosis: Bacterial vaginosis

Clinchers

- *34-year-old lady:* Bacterial vaginosis most commonly occurs in sexually active females. Infection is rare in males.
- *Discharge per vaginum:* Most common and predominant symptom. In fact, bacterial vaginosis is the most common cause of vaginal discharge in women of childbearing age. The discharge is often white-grey, and fishy smelling. It tends to be heaviest just after a period, and after having sex.
- *Wet mounts show clue cells:* Clue cells are the most specific criterion for diagnosing bacterial vaginosis. Clue cells are vaginal epithelial cells that have bacteria adherent to their surfaces. The edges of the squamous epithelial cells, which normally have a sharply defined cell border, become studded with bacteria. The epithelial cells appear to be peppered with coccobacilli.

CONFUSA

- Bacterial Vaginosis is not caused by poor hygiene. In fact, excessive washing of the vagina may alter the normal balance of bacteria in the vagina, which may make Bacterial vaginosis more likely to develop.
- Bacterial vaginosis is not caused by a single bacterium. In Bacterial vaginosis, an 'overgrowth' of various bacteria occurs in the vagina. Most common bacteria present in most cases are *Gardnerella vaginalis* and *Prevotella*. In 50-60% *Mobiluncus* species may be present.
- Bacterial Vaginosis is not a sexually transmitted disease. However, it may develop after a change in sexual partner, as a change in sexual partner may affect the balance of normal bacteria in the vagina.

Investigation of Choice

Microscopy for "clue cells"

Positive amine test (Whiff Test) - a fishy ammoniacal smell when the discharge is mixed with 10% potassium hydroxide

Immediate Management

It is recommended that the male partner is treated with metronidazole at the same time because it has been found that the majority of male partners of infected partners harbour the organism in their urethras.

Treatment of Choice

Metronidazole 400-500 mg twice daily for seven days .

During pregnancy: standard treatment in the UK is oral metronidazole 400 mg twice a day for five days (Avoid metronidazole in 1st trimester).

Your notes:

Serial No. 139

Subject: Gynaecology

Topic: Pelvic inflammatory diseases

Question: A 24-year-old lady with pelvic pain and offensive vaginal discharge.

Diagnosis: Pelvic inflammatory disease

Clinchers

- *24-year-old lady:* Young age, multiple sexual partners, low socioeconomic group are important risk factors for developing PID. Insertion of intrauterine contraceptive device increases the risk by 6 times, during first 3 weeks following insertion. Most cases of PID occur in sexually active women of age 15-24 years.
- *Pelvic pain:* Pelvic pain is the most common symptom reported. However, majority of patients may be asymptomatic. Other symptoms observed are dyspareunia, abnormal vaginal discharge, menstrual irregularities.
- *Offensive vaginal discharge:* Mucopurulent vaginal discharge is the commonly observed sign in PID; it can be associated with cervical motion tenderness, adnexal tenderness or fever.

CONFUSA

- In UK, chlamydia trachomatis is the most important cause of PID, being responsible for at least 50% of identified cases
- *Neisseria gonorrhoea* ranks 2nd with 14 % cases.
- Mixed infection is seen in 8% cases(most common mixture being Chlamydia + Gonorrhoea).
- Insertion of IUCD is associated with Actinomyces israelii infection.

Investigation of Choice

Endocervical swab

Immediate Management

Advise abstinence from sexual intercourse until women and her partner have both completed a course of treatment. Consider empirical treatment of partner if he/she refuses screening.

Advise on use of condoms (antibiotics reduce efficacy of OCP).

Remove IUCDs, if any.

Advise against tampons.

Contact tracing and treatment (all sexual partners in previous 6 months need to be contacted and tested)

Treatment of Choice

Blind antibiotic therapy (covers *C. trachomatis, N. gonorrhoeae* and anaerobic infection)

- Oral ofloxacin 400 mg twice a day plus oral metronidazole 400 mg twice a day for 14 days, OR,
- Intramuscular ceftriaxone 250 mg immediately or intramuscular cefoxitin 2 g immediately with oral probenecid 1 g, followed by oral doxycycline 100 mg twice a day plus metronidazole 400 mg twice a day for 14 days

If pregnant, a suggested antibiotic treatment regime is: **Erythromycin 500 mg four times daily for 14 days and metronidazole 400 mg twice daily for seven days**

Start treatment as soon as the diagnosis is suspected, don't wait for swab results.

Your notes:

Serial No. 140

Subject: Gynaecology

Topic: Pelvic inflammatory disease

Question: An asymptomatic 25-year-old lady says her husband had a purulent urethral discharge and does not wants to talk about it.

Diagnosis: Pelvic inflammatory disease (suspected)

Clinchers

- *25-year-old lady:* Young age, multiple sexual partners, low socioeconomic group are important risk factors for developing PID. Insertion of intrauterine contraceptive device increases the risk by 6 times, during first 3 weeks following insertion. Most cases of PID occur in sexually active women of age 15-24 years.
- *Asymptomatic:* Most cases of PID are asymptomatic and present at a later date as ectopic pregnancy or infertility.
- *Her husband had a purulent urethral discharge:* This denotes some kind of sexually transmitted disease he acquired following unprotected sexual exposure.
- *Does not wants to talk about it:* He needs to be convinced for a urethral swab to be tested for chlamydia and *N. gonorrhoeae* infection.If he refuses screening, start the empirical treatment.

CONFUSA

Empirical treatment of undiagnosed urethritis in a male

Ideally management should be via a GUM clinic; however if a man is unlikely or unable to attend follow-up then empirical antibiotic treatment should be considered.

- If the infection is gathered locally (less chances for high resistance strains) the first-choice therapeutic option is: ofloxacin 200 mg twice a day (or 400 mg once a day) for 7 days.
- If the infection contracted from abroad, viz after an international travel, consider - ceftriaxone 250 mg (or cefotaxime 500 mg)by intramuscular injection (single dose), followed by Doxycycline 100 mg twice a day for 7 days.

Investigation of Choice

Contact tracing - all sexual partners in previous 6 months need to be contacted and tested for Chlamydial infections.

Immediate Management

Refer to a genitourinary clinic

Treatment of Choice

All sexual partners of chlamydia positive patients should be treated for chlamydia even if not identified on testing. Consider empirical treatment if partner refuses screening.

Your notes:

Serial No. 141

Subject: Gynaecology

Topic: Post menopausal bleeding

Question: A 67-year-old lady with bleeding per vaginum. USG shows thickened endometrium.

Diagnosis: Carcinoma endometrium

Clinchers

- *67-year-old lady:* Endometrial carcinoma is a disease manifesting in post menopausal women, the peak incidence being at the age 61 years.
- *Bleeding per vaginum:* Post menopausal bleeding is the classical presentation of endometrial carcinoma.Seen in 90% cases. This is usually slight and intermittent at first, and separated by long intervals. It later may become continuous and heavy.
- *USG shows thickened endometrium:* A thickened endometrium as seen on a transvaginal ultrasound, of more than 4 mm , in a post menopausal woman is suggestive of endometrial carcinoma.

CONFUSA

- Post menopausal bleeding is defined as bleeding from the vagina 6 months after the last period.
- Any post-menopausal bleeding should be assumed to be to endometrial carcinoma until proved otherwise.
- Other important causes of post menopausal bleeding are—exogenous oestrogens(in the form of hormone replacement therapy), atrophic endometritis/vaginitis, endometrial or cervical polyps, endometrial hyperplasia, cervical carcinoma, ring pessary or ovarian oestrogen secreting tumour.

Investigation of Choice

Primary assessment is by a Transvaginal Ultrasound. If endometrial thickening, as observed on transvaginal ultrasound is more than 4 mm, an endometrial biopsy is indicated.

In outpatient settings, hysteroscopy with/without biopsy is more practical.

Immediate Management

Refer to a cancer unit, or gynaecological oncologist in the cancer centre.

Treatment of Choice

Stage I (low risk): Total abdominal hysterectomy with bilateral salpingo-oophorectomy

Stage I (high risk): above plus post-operative radiotherapy.

Stage II: managed as Stage I high risk

Stages III and IV: Progestogen therapy may be helpful. Chemotherapy may occasionally be used in metastatic disease.

Your notes:

PAPER 2

Serial No. 62

Subject: Obstetrics

Topic: Prenatal Diagnosis

Question: A pregnant lady with high alpha feto protein.

Diagnosis: Spina bifida

Clinchers

- *A pregnant lady with high alpha feto protein:* High AFP can occur due a variety of causes like open neural tube defects, gastroschisis and anterior abdominal wall defects, renal defects, antepartum haemorrhage, intrauterine death, twin pregnancy or wrong dates.
- The most common neural tube defects associated with high AFP are anencephaly and spina bifida.
- For AFP screening, the maternal blood is taken at 14-16 weeks gestation. The outcome of the test is to prompt further investigations if positive - i.e. it is not diagnostic

CONFUSA

For pregnant ladies or those planning pregnancy, 400 mcg folic acid daily is prescribed in the peri-conceptional period and during first 12 weeks of pregnancy. For those with already one previous child with neural tube defects, folic acid is prescribed in higher dose: 4-5 mg/day folic acid. For those on antifolates, pregnancy should be avoided as far as possibles or the drug regimen should be re considered to exclude anti-folate drugs.

Investigation of Choice

Screening- AFP at 14-16 weeks
Definitive- 2nd trimester USG (Can detect anencephaly from 12th week and spina bifida from 16-20 weeks).

Immediate Management

Counsel and inform parents; advise termination of pregnancy.

Treatment of Choice

According to parent's decision.

Your notes:

Serial No. 64

Subject: Obstetrics

Topic: Prenatal diagnosis

Question: A pregnant lady is advised to take folate prior to conception and during pregnancy to prevent this condition.

Diagnosis: Spina bifida

Clinchers

- *To take folate prior to conception and during pregnancy to prevent this condition:* For pregnant ladies or those planning pregnancy, 400 mcg folic acid daily is prescribed in the peri-conceptional period and during first 12 weeks of pregnancy.
- *For those with already one previous child with neural tube defects, folic acid is prescribed in higher dose:* 4-5 mg/day folic acid.
- For those on antifolates, pregnancy should be avoided as far as possibles or the drug regimen should be re considered to exclude anti-folate drugs.

CONFUSA

Neural tube defects are associated with very high AFP levels in maternal serum. This forms the basis for screening test for high risk women (those on anticonvulsants/ chemotherapy or a previous child with neural tube defect). For AFP screening, the maternal blood is taken at 14-16 weeks gestation. The outcome of the test is to prompt further investigations if positive - i.e. it is not diagnostic. USG is required to confirm the diagnosis.

Investigation of Choice

Screening- AFP at 14-16 weeks
Definitive- 2nd trimester USG (Can detect anencephaly from 12th week and spina bifida from 16-20 weeks).

Immediate Management

Counsel and inform parents; advise termination of pregnancy.

Treatment of Choice

According to parent's decision.

Your notes:

Serial No. 66

Subject: Obstetrics

Topic: Prenatal Diagnosis

Question: A 30-year-old second gravida with previous child diagnosed with Duchenne's Muscular Dystrophy.

Diagnosis: Duchenne's muscular dystrophy (DMD)

Clinchers

- *Previous child diagnosed with Duchenne's Muscular Dystrophy:* DMD is inherited an X-linked manner, severely affecting males while female carriers only show mild myopathy features.
- The gene for Duchenne muscular dystrophy is the dystrophin locus at Xp21.
- The disease typically manifests by 5 years of age and the affected child presents with features of gradually worsening muscle power, psuedohypertrophy of calf muscles, cardiomyopathy and scoliosis.

CONFUSA

Genetic counselling is an important aspect of dealing with families with a child diagnosed with DMD. Here, the female relatives are tested to see if they are carriers. However, note that 10-20% cases of DMD occur due to spontaneous mutation and is not inherited. So, even if the mother (with already one child diagnosed with DMD) is not a carrier of dystrophin mutation, there is still a high possibility of the second child to be affected because of other eggs carrying the same mutation.

Investigation of Choice

Screening: Serum creatinine kinase
Definitive: Muscle biopsy
Prenatal diagnosis: Chorionic villous sampling and looking for dystrophin mutation.

Immediate Management

None

Treatment of Choice

Genetic counselling

Your notes:

Serial No. 67

Subject: Obstetrics

Topic: Prenatal diagnosis

Question: A 35-year-old pregnant at 16 weeks gestation was found to have a high hCG, low AFP and low oestriol.

Diagnosis: Down's syndrome

Clinchers

- *35-year-old:* The risk of having a baby with Down's syndrome is related to the age of the mother, at 35 years, risk is 1 in 400; at 37.5 years, risk is 1 in 200; at 40 years, risk is 1 in 100; at 43 years, risk is 1 in 50.
- *16 weeks gestation:* Definitive diagnosis of requires karyotyping. Cells can be obtained by either amniocentesis or chorionic villous sampling. However, at 14-16 weeks of gestation amniocentesis is more sensitive and safe for the prenatal diagnosis.
- *high hCG, low AFP and low oestriol:* This is the Triple Test, particularly offered to at risk mothers, in the antenatal period. The test measures alpha fetoprotein, human chorionic gondaotrophin and unconjugated oestriol. Low maternal serum alpha-fetoprotein (MSAFP), elevated human chorionic gonadotropin (hCG) and low unconjugated oestriol are markers for Down's syndrome.

CONFUSA

Although it is widely known that the incidence of Down's syndrome, increases with maternal age, always remember that mothers of any age can have infants with Down's syndrome and, because fewer women over the age of 40 years have babies, the majority of Down's syndrome babies are born to younger mothers.
Also note that, for definitive diagnosis, karyotyping is a must; rest all tests are only suggestive of Down's Syndrome.

Investigation of Choice

Amniocentesis with karyotyping

Immediate Management

Necessary counselling and information to the parents.

Treatment of Choice

Genetic counselling; discuss the risk with subsequent pregnancies.

Serial No. 68

Subject: Obstetrics

Topic: Prenatal diagnosis

Question: A 27-year-old epileptic at 14 weeks gestation was found to have very high AFP.

Diagnosis: Neural tube defects

Clinchers

- *27-year-old epileptic:* Maternal age is not a contributing factor for the development of neural tube defects; the main factor is folic acid deficiency and this lady presumed to be on antiepileptics, puts her baby at higher risk for developing neural tube defects. Other drugs commonly associated are chemotherapeutic agents, trimethoprim and valproate.
- *14 weeks gestation:* For AFP screening, the maternal blood is taken at 14-16 weeks gestation. The outcome of the test is to prompt further investigations if positive - i.e. it is not diagnostic.
- *Very high AFP:* High AFP can occur due a variety of causes like open neural tube defects, gastroschisis and anterior abdominal wall defects, renal defects, antepartum haemorrhage, intrauterine death,twin pregnancy or wrong dates.

CONFUSA

For pregnant ladies or those planning pregnancy, 400 mcg folic acid daily is prescribed in the periconceptional period and during first 12 weeks of pregnancy. For those with already one previous child with neural tube defects, folic acid is prescribed in higher dose: 4-5 mg/day folic acid. For those on antifolates, pregnancy should be avoided as far as possibles or the drug regimen should be re considered to exclude anti-folate drugs.

Investigation of Choice

Screening- AFP at 14-16 weeks

Definitive- 2nd trimester USG (Can detect anencephaly from 12th week and spina bifida from 16-20 weeks).

Immediate Management

Counsel and inform parents; advise termination of pregnancy.

Treatment of Choice

According to parent's decision.

Your notes:

Serial No. 69

Subject: Obstetrics

Topic: Prenatal Diagnosis

Question: A 32-year-old hypertensive with severe oilgohydramnios.

Diagnosis: Renal agenesis

Clinchers

- *Hypertensive:* Maternal usage of ACE-inhibitors are related to bilateral renal agensis in babies leading to severe oligohydramnios. Also beta blockers can cause placental insufficiency leading to oligohydramnios, but oligohydramnios associated with beta blockers is mild-moderate.
- *Severe oilgohydramnios:* It is defined clinically as the absence of fluid surrounding the foetus. On ultrasound scanning it is defined as a pool depth of amniotic fluid of less than 2 cm - the normal range is from 2 to 10 cm.

CONFUSA

Common causes leading to oligohydramnios include premature rupture of the membranes, chronic amniotic leakage, maternal NSAID or ACE inhibitor usage, postmaturity (>42 weeks gestation), placental insufficiency, congenital abnormalities of the urinary tract or twin-twin transfusion (in the donor twin).

Investigation of Choice

Ultrasound examination of the foetal kidneys and urogenital system.

Immediate Management

Bed rest with mother drinking 2l water/day (raises AFI by 30%).

Treatment of Choice

Conservative;

Fetal renal abnormality can be dealt with once born.

Amnioinfusion - saline or Ringer's lactate through the cervix if membranes ruptured or trans-abdominally if membranes intact

Your notes:

Serial No. 70

Subject: Gynaecology

Topic: Prenatal diagnosis

Question: A-28-year old pregnant lady with previous child diagnosed with congenital adrenal hyperplasia.

Diagnosis: Congenital adrenal hyperplasia

Clinchers

- *previous child diagnosed with congenital adrenal hyperplasia:* Congenital adrenal hyperplasia is a metabolic disorder related to enzymatic defects in the biosynthesis of cortical steroids.
- Typically the defects are inherited in an autosomal recessive manner, and within a particular family all inherit the same enzyme deficiency.

CONFUSA

For the prenatal diagnosis of congenital adrenal hyperplasia, elevated level of 17-hydroxyprogesterone can be demonstrated in amniotic fluid in the second trimester. However, in the presence of previously affected child, DNA analysis techniques or comparison of amniotic fluid cells with the HLA analysis, of the affected child and his/her parents can be used to predict the disease status of a foetus. Chorionic villous sampling can be performed at 8-11 weeks gestation.

Investigation of Choice
17-hydroxyprogesterone levels in the amniotic fluid in the second trimester.

Immediate Management
Counsel and inform parents

Treatment of Choice
Aim is to provide life-long replacement hydrocortisone and a salt-retaining steroid such as fludrocortisone beginning as early as possible, to allow for the normal growth and development of the foetus.

Your notes:

Serial No.71

Subject: Gynaecology

Topic: STDs

Question: A-25-year old sexually active female comes with mucopurulent discharge per vaginum. She is febrile and noted to have a diffuse pustular erythematous rash.

Diagnosis: Gonorrhoea

Clinchers

- *25-year-old sexually active female:* Gonorrhoea is primarily a disease of sexually active individuals, with most females remaining asymptomatic for long, while most males present with purulent urethritis within 3-5 days, following exposure.
- *Mucopurulent discharge per vaginum:* Symptomatic females present with purulent vaginal discharge, frequency of micturition and anorectal discomfort. There may be bartholinitis.
- *Febrile:* this signify dissemination of infection; it is assocaited with systemic features like fever, malaise, myalgia and even monoarticular arthritis.
- *Diffuse pustular eythematous rash:* This again confirms the disseminated gonococcal infection; the rash associated is typically diffuse, pustular and erythematous.

CONFUSA

Note that secondary syphilis can also present with features of fever, malaise, joint pains and rash. However, note that syphilitic rash is never pustular (always, maculopapular). The genital infection usually does not manifests itself in secondary syphilis (genital infection is more characteristically seen in primary syphilis as chancre).

Investigation of Choice
Urethral and cervical swabs for gonococci

Immediate Management
Referral to Genitourinary (GUM) clinic

Treatment of Choice
Cefixime as a 400 mg single oral dose
OR ceftriaxone 250 mg single IM dose
OR cefotaxime 500 mg single IM dose
In all cases contacts must be traced and patients rescreened around three days after treatment to confirm cure.

Serial No. 72

Subject: Gynaecology

Topic: STDs

Question: A 32-year-old female complains of offensive white, fishy odor vaginal discharge. She has recently changed her partner.

Diagnosis: Bacterial vaginosis

Clinchers

- *32-year-old female:* Bacterial vaginosis most commonly occurs in sexually active females. Infection is rare in males.
- *offensive white, fishy odor vaginal discharge:* The fishy odor vaginal discharge is characteristic of bacterial vaginosis. The discharge is often white-grey, and fishy smelling. It tends to be heaviest just after a period, and after having sex. Recall that, bacterial vaginosis is the most common cause of vaginal discharge in women of childbearing age.
- *She has recently changed her partner:* Bacterial vaginosis is caused by altered normal balance of bacteria in the vagina. It is not infective, so as to be 'caught' by the new partner. However, it may develop after a change in sexual partner, as a change in sexual partner may affect the balance of normal bacteria in the vagina.

CONFUSA

- Bacterial Vaginosis is not caused by poor hygiene. In fact, excessive washing of the vagina may alter the normal balance of bacteria in the vagina, which may make Bacterial Vaginosis more likely to develop.
- Bacterial Vaginosis is not caused by a single bacterium. In Bacterial Vaginosis, an 'overgrowth' of various bacteria occurs in the vagina. Most common bacteria present in most cases are Gardnerella vaginalis and Prevotella. In 50-60% Mobiluncus species may be present.

Investigation of Choice

Microscopy for "clue cells"

Positive amine test (Whiff Test) - a fishy ammoniacal smell when the discharge is mixed with 10% potassium hydroxide

Immediate Management

It is recommended that the male partner is treated with metronidazole at the same time because it has been found that the majority of male partners of infected partners harbour the organism in their urethras.

Treatment of Choice

Metronidazole 400-500 mg twice daily for seven days . During pregnancy: standard treatment in the UK is oral metronidazole 400 mg twice a day for five days (Avoid metronidazole in 1st trimester).

Your notes:

Serial No. 73

Subject: Gynaecology

Topic: STDs

Question: A 23-year-old female comes with complains of dysuria. Bacterial culture of urine yields no growth. Cervical tenderness is elicited on per vaginum examination.

Diagnosis: Chlamydia cervicitis

Clinchers

- *23-year-old female:* Chlamydia is the most prevalent STD in the western world, found predominantly in sexually active women. More than half cases of cervicitis and >60% cases of pelvic inflammatory diseases in females are caused due to chlamydia.
- *Dysuria, bacterial culture of urine yields no growth:* Most cases of chalmydial infections are asymptomatic or present with vague symtomps like pyuria, dysuria or vaginal discharge. The urine culture characteristically yields no growth.
- *Cervical tenderness:* Mucopurulent cervical discharge and cervicitis, cervical motion tenderness and adnexal tenderness are all very strong points in favour of cervicitis or developing PID.

CONFUSA

- Dysuria in a young woman can be an inidcation of acute cystitis; acute urethritis; or vaginitis. Cystitis is usually due to E. Coli and associated with urgency and suparpubic pain; urine culture will yield $>10^5$ colony forming units per millimetre.
- Urethritis is usually due to chalmydia or gonorrhea and is gradual in onset, associated with vaginal discharge or bleeding and lower abdominal pain. There may be a history of a new sexual partner. Look for hints of involvement of the cervix. Urine culture is negative or less than 10^2 organisms.
- Vaginits is characterized by vaginal odour and/or discharge along with pruritus, dyspareunia, 'external' dysuria. There is no urgency or increased frequency. 'External' dysuria is described as the burning sensation felt due to urine irritating already sore vagina during micturition. Its not true dysuria.

Investigation of Choice

Urethral and cervical swabs for chlamydia

Immediate Management

Advise abstinence from sexual intercourse until women and her partner have both completed a course of treatment. Consider empirical treatment of partner if he/ she refuses screening.
Advise on use of condoms (antibiotics reduce efficacy of OCP).
Remove IUCDs, if any.
Advise against tampons.
Contact tracing and treatment (all sexual partners in previous 6 months need to be contacted and tested).

Treatment of Choice

Blind antibiotic therapy (covers *C. trachomatis, N. gonorrhoeae* and anaerobic infection)
-oral ofloxacin 400 mg twice a day plus oral metronidazole 400 mg twice a day for 14 days, OR,
-intramuscular ceftriaxone 250 mg immediately or intramuscular cefoxitin 2 g immediately with oral probenecid 1 g, followed by oral doxycycline 100 mg twice a day plus metronidazole 400 mg twice a day for 14 days
If pregnant, a suggested antibiotic treatment regime is: erythromycin 500 mg four times daily for 14 days and metronidazole 400 mg twice daily for seven days
Start treatment as soon as the diagnosis is suspected, don't wait for swab results.

Your notes:

Serial No. 74

Subject: Gynaecology

Topic: STDs

Question: An-18-year old girl on OCPs, with severe vaginal itching and cheese like discharge per vaginum.

Diagnosis: Vaginal Candidiasis

Clinchers

- *18-year-old girl on OCPs:* All age groups can be affected. However, highest incidence is noted among young, sexually active women. Risk factors include oral contraceptive use, IUD use, early intercourse, increased frequency of intercourse, receptive cunnilingus, diabetes, HIV or other immunocompromised states, chronic antibiotic use, and pregnancy
- *Severe vaginal itiching:* Pruritus is the most common symptom of vaginal candidiasis. Erythema and swelling of the labia and vulva with satellite lesions are present. Vagina is usually reddened with adherent thick, cottage cheese–like vaginal discharge. Cervix appears normal.
- *Cheese like discharge:* Discharge associated with vaginal candidiasis is typically described as thick, odorless white and scanty, with an appearance similar to cottage cheese.

CONFUSA

Vaginal candidiasis is not a sexually transmitted infection. Candida is a normal commensal of the skin and vagina. Male sexual partners do not need treatment unless they have symptoms of thrush on their penis. Symptoms in men include redness, itch, and soreness of the foreskin and the glans of the penis. Women do not 'catch' thrush from men who have no symptoms.

Investigation of Choice

Exudate is collected from the lateral vaginal walls and Gram stained and examined microscopically for yeast forms.
Cultured on Sabouraud's dextrose agar medium
Urine is tested for sugar

Immediate Management

Maintain local hygiene
Avoid re-infection from sexual partner; sexual intercourse should be avoided until cure is complete
Removal any local 'foreign bodies' like IUCD or vaginal diaphragms; Barrier contraceptive in the form of male condoms are the most useful contraceptive during infection.

Treatment of Choice

Intravaginal pessaries or cream inserted high into the vagina at night. Clotrimazole and miconazole are the commonly used pessaries.
Alternatively a single oral dose of fluconazole can be used. (Avoid in pregnant and lactating mothers.)

Your notes:

Serial No. 75

Subject: Gynaecology

Topic: STDs

Question: A-27-year old sexually active female on oral contraceptives for two years, with mucoid discharge per vaginum.

Diagnosis: Cervical ectropion

Clinchers

- *27-year-old:* Cervical ectropion or erosion most commonly occurs in women of reproductive age group. However, it can be also seen in neonates, who are exposed high maternal oestrogen.
- *Sexually active:* Being sexually active does not predisposes one to cervical erosion directly, but use of oral contraceptives, or even high oestrogen levels during pregnancy provides good environment for the squamous lining of the cervix to change to columnar.
- *On oral contraceptives for two years:* This is the most common cause of exogenous source of oestrogen causing change of cervical epithelium.
- *Mucoid discharge per vaginum:* most patients are asymptomatic except for some mucoid discharge. An erosion is not painful and does not cause dyspareunia; however a patient may sometimes present with bleeding or infection.

CONFUSA

- Erosions are thought to be oestrogen dependent. They are seen most commonly in women taking combined oral contraceptives pills and resolve when the pill is stopped. It also frequently develops during pregnancy and resolve after delivery.
- An erosion may also occur in newborn infants and may persist into childhood. This congenital erosion is not abnormal, and is due to exposure to high maternal oestrogens. Sometimes, it may also be seen during puberty.

Investigation of Choice

Speculum examination: shows a red ring around the os. The 'red ring' is actually the migrated endocervical mucous columnar epithelium over the ectocervix.

Immediate Management

A cervical smear is mandatory. It should be followed by colposcopy and cervical biopsy if the result is unsatisfactory.

Treatment of Choice

None required;

A troublesome erosion may be treated by thermal cautery with diathermy, cyrosurgery or laser treatment.

Your notes:

Serial No.101

Subject: Gynaecology

Topic: PID

Question: A 24-year-old lady with pelvic pain and offensive vaginal discharge.

Diagnosis: Pelvic inflammatory disease

Clinchers

- *24-year-old lady:* Young age, multiple sexual partners, low socioeconomic group are important risk factors for developing PID. Insertion of intrauterine contraceptive device increases the risk by 6 times, during first 3 weeks following insertion. Most cases of PID occur in sexually active women of age 15-24 years.
- *Pelvic pain:* Pelvic pain is the most common symptom reported. However, majority of patients may be asymptomatic. Other symptoms observed are dyspareunia, abnormal vaginal discharge, menstrual irregularities.
- *Offensive vaginal discharge:* Mucopurulent vaginal discharge is the commonly observed sign in PID; it can be associated with cervical motion tenderness, adnexal tenderness or fever.

CONFUSA

In UK, *Chlamydia trachomatis* is the most important cause of PID, being responsible for at least 50% of identified cases. Neisseria gonorrhoea ranks 2nd with 14% cases. Mixed infection is seen in 8% cases(most common mixture being Chlamydia + Gonorrhoea).

Insertion of IUCD is associated with *Actinomyces israelii infection.*

Investigation of Choice

Endocervical swab

Immediate Management

Advise abstinence from sexual intercourse until women and her partner have both completed a course of treatment. Consider empirical treatment of partner if he/she refuses screening.

Advise on use of condoms (antibiotics reduce efficacy of OCP).

Remove IUCDs, if any.

Advise against tampons.

Contact tracing and treatment (all sexual partners in previous 6 months need to be contacted and tested)

Treatment of Choice

Blind antibiotic therapy (covers *C. trachomatis, N. gonorrhoeae* and anaerobic infection)

- oral ofloxacin 400 mg twice a day plus oral metronidazole 400 mg twice a day for 14 days, OR,
- intramuscular ceftriaxone 250 mg immediately or intramuscular cefoxitin 2 g immediately with oral probenecid 1 g, followed by oral doxycycline 100 mg twice a day plus metronidazole 400 mg twice a day for 14 days

If pregnant, a suggested antibiotic treatnent regime is: Erythromycin 500 mg four times daily for 14 days and metronidazole 400 mg twice daily for seven days

Start treatment as soon as the diagnosis is suspected, don't wait for swab results.

Your notes:

Serial No. 102

Subject: Gynaecology

Topic: PID

Question: An asymptomatic 25-year-old lady says her husband had a purulent urethral discharge and does not wants to talk about it.

Diagnosis: Pelvic inflammatory disease (suspected)

Clinchers

- *25-year-old lady:* Young age, multiple sexual partners, low socioeconomic group are important risk factors for developing PID. Insertion of intrauterine contraceptive device increases the risk by 6 times, during first 3 weeks following insertion. Most cases of PID occur in sexually active women of age 15-24 years.
- *Asymptomatic:* Most cases of PID are asymptomatic and present at a later date as ectopic pregnancy or infertility.
- *Her husband had a purulent urethral discharge:* This denotes some kind of sexually transmitted disease he acquired following unprotected sexual exposure.
- *Does not wants to talk about it:* He needs to be convinced for a urethral swab to be tested for chlamydia and N. gonorrhoea infection. If he refuses screening, start the empirical treatment.

CONFUSA

Empirical treatment of undiagnosed urethritis in a male

Ideally management should be via a GUM clinic; however if a man is unlikely or unable to attend follow-up then empirical antibiotic treatment should be considered.

- If the infection is gathered locally (less chances for high resistance strains) the first-choice therapeutic option is: ofloxacin 200 mg twice a day (or 400 mg once a day) for 7 days.
- -If the infection contracted from abroad, viz after an international travel, consider - ceftriaxone 250 mg (or cefotaxime 500 mg)by intramuscular injection (single dose), followed by Doxycycline 100 mg twice a day for 7 days .

Investigation of Choice

Contact tracing - all sexual partners in previous 6 months need to be contacted and tested for Chlamydial infections.

Immediate Management

Refer to a Genitourinary clinic (GUM clinic).

Treatment of Choice

All sexual partners of chlamydia positive patients should be treated for chlamydia even if not identified on testing. Consider empirical treatment if partner refuses screening.

Your notes:

Serial No. 103

Subject: Gynaecology

Topic: Oncology

Question: A 67-year-old lady with bleeding per vaginum. USG shows thickened endometrium.

Diagnosis: Carcinoma endometrium

Clinchers

- *67-year-old lady:* Endometrial carcinoma is a disease manifesting in post menopausal women, the peak incidence being at the age 61 years.
- *bleeding per vaginum:* Post menopausal bleeding is the classical presentation of endometrial carcinoma. Seen in 90% cases. This is usually slight and intermittent at first, and separated by long intervals. It later may become continuous and heavy.
- *USG shows thickened endometrium:* A thickened endometrium as seen on a transvaginal ultrasound, of more than 4 mm , in a postmenopausal woman is suggestive of endometrial carcinoma.

CONFUSA

Postmenopausal bleeding is defined as bleeding from the vagina 6 months after the last period. Any post-menopausal bleeding should be assumed to be to endometrial carcinoma until proved otherwise.

Other important causes of postmenopausal bleeding are - exogenous oestrogens(in the form of hormone replacement therapy), atrophic endometritis/vaginitis, endometrial or cervical polyps, endometrial hyperplasia, cervical carcinoma, ring pessary or ovarian oestrogen secreting tumour.

Investigation of Choice

Primary assessment is by a Transvaginal Ultrasound. If endometrial thickening, as observed on transvaginal ultrasound is more than 4 mm, an endometrial biopsy is indicated.

In outpatient settings, hysteroscopy with/without biopsy is more practical.

Immediate Management

Refer to a cancer unit, or gynaecological oncologist in the cancer center.

Treatment of Choice

Stage I (low risk): Total abdominal hysterectomy with bilateral salpingo-oophorectomy

Stage I (high risk): above plus post-operative radiotherapy.

Stage II: managed as Stage I high risk

Stages III and IV: Progestogen therapy may be helpful. Chemotherapy may occasionally be used in metastatic disease.

Your notes:

Serial No. 105

Subject: Gynaecology

Topic: PID

Question: A-34-year old lady comes with discharge per vaginum. Wet mount shows clue cells.

Diagnosis: Bacterial vaginosis

Clinchers

- *34-year-old lady:* Bacterial vaginosis most commonly occurs in sexually active females. Infection is rare in males.
- *Discharge per vaginum:* Most common and predominant symptom. In fact, bacterial vaginosis is the most common cause of vaginal discharge in women of childbearing age. The discharge is often white-grey, and fishy smelling. It tends to be heaviest just after a period, and after having sex.
- *Wet mounts show clue cells:* Clue cells are the most specific criterion for diagnosing bacterial vaginosis. Clue cells are vaginal epithelial cells that have bacteria adherent to their surfaces. The edges of the squamous epithelial cells, which normally have a sharply defined cell border, become studded with bacteria. The epithelial cells appear to be peppered with coccobacilli.

CONFUSA

- Bacterial Vaginosis is not caused by poor hygiene. In fact, excessive washing of the vagina may alter the normal balance of bacteria in the vagina, which may make Bacterial Vaginosis more likely to develop.
- Bacterial Vaginosis is not caused by a single bacterium. In Bacterial Vaginosis, an 'overgrowth' of various bacteria occurs in the vagina. Most common bacteria present in most cases are Gardnerella vaginalis and Prevotella. In 50-60% Mobiluncus species may be present.
- Bacterial Vaginosis is not a sexually transmitted disease. However, it may develop after a change in sexual partner, as a change in sexual partner may affect the balance of normal bacteria in the vagina.

Investigation of Choice

Microscopy for "clue cells"

Positive amine test (Whiff Test) - a fishy ammoniacal smell when the discharge is mixed with 10% potassium hydroxide

Immediate Management

It is recommended that the male partner is treated with metronidazole at the same time because it has been found that the majority of male partners of infected partners harbour the organism in their urethras.

Treatment of Choice

Metronidazole 400-500 mg twice daily for seven days .
During pregnancy: standard treatment in the UK is oral metronidazole 400 mg twice a day for five days (Avoid metronidazole in 1st trimester).

Your notes:

Serial No. 151

Subject: Gynaecology

Topic: Pelvic inflammatory diseases

Question: A 26-year-old female with sore vagina and whitish discharge; smear shows mycelia.

Diagnosis: Vaginal candidiasis

Clinchers

- *26-year-old:* All age groups can be affected. However, highest incidence is noted among young, sexually active women. Risk factors include oral contraceptive use, IUD use, early intercourse, increased frequency of intercourse, receptive cunnilingus, diabetes, HIV or other immunocompromised states, chronic antibiotic use, and pregnancy.
- *Sore vagina:* Pruritus is the most common symptom of vaginal candidiasis. Erythema and swelling of the labia and vulva with satellite lesions are present. Vagina is usually reddened with adherent thick, cottage cheese–like vaginal discharge. Cervix appears normal.
- *Whitish discharge:* Discharge associated with vaginal candidiasis is typically described as thick, odorless white and scanty, with an appearance similar to cottage cheese.
- *Smear shows mycelia:* This is diagnostic of candidiasis. Exudate collected from the lateral vaginal walls and Gram stained, microscopically show hyphae and budding yeasts.

CONFUSA

- Vaginal candidiasis is not a sexually transmitted infection. Candida is a normal commensal of the skin and vagina.
- Male sexual partners do not need treatment unless they have symptoms of thrush on their penis. Symptoms in men include redness, itch, and soreness of the foreskin and the glans of the penis.
- Women do not 'catch' thrush from men who have no symptoms.

Investigation of Choice

Exudate is collected from the lateral vaginal walls and Gram stained and examined microscopically for yeast forms.
Cultured on Sabouraud's dextrose agar medium
Urine is tested for sugar

Immediate Management

Maintain local hygiene
Avoid re-infection from sexual partner; sexual intercourse should be avoided until cure is complete
Removal any local 'foreign bodies' like IUCD or vaginal diaphragms; Barrier contraceptive in the form of male condoms are the most useful contraceptive during infection.

Treatment of Choice

Intravaginal pessaries or cream inserted high into the vagina at night. Either of the following can be used:

- clotrimazole 200 mg pessary, 1 at night, for 3 nights
- clotrimazole 500 mg pessary, single dose
- miconazole 100 mg pessary, two, for 7 nights
- miconazole ovule 1.2 g, single dose at night

Alternatively a single oral dose of fluconazole can be used. (Avoid in pregnant and lactating mothers.

Your notes:

Serial No. 152

Subject: Gynaecology

Topic: Pelvic inflammatory diseases

Question: A 27-year-old sexually active female on oral contraceptives for two years, complains of mucoid discharge per vaginum.

Diagnosis: Cervical ectropion

Clinchers

- *27-year-old:* Cervical ectropion or erosion most commonly occurs in women of reproductive age group. However, it can be also seen in neonates, who are exposed high maternal oestrogen.
- *Sexually active:* Being sexually active does not prediposes one to cervical erosion directly, but use of oral contraceptives, or even high estrogen levels during pregnancy provides good environment for the squamous lining of the cervix to change to columnar.
- *On oral contraceptives for two years:* This is the most common cause of exogenous source of oestrogen causing change of cervical epithelium.
- *Mucoid discharge per vaginum:* Most patients are asymptomatic except for some mucoid discharge. An erosion is not painful and does not cause dyspareunia; however a patient may sometimes present with bleeding or infection.

CONFUSA

Erosions are thought to be oestrogen dependent. They are seen most commonly in women taking combined oral contraceptives pills and resolve when the pill is stopped. It also frequently develops during pregnancy and resolve after delivery.
An erosion may also occur in newborn infants and may persist into childhood. This congenital erosion is not abnormal, and is due to exposure to high maternal oestrogens. Sometimes, it may also be seen during puberty.

Investigation of Choice

Speculum examination: shows a red ring around the os. The 'red ring' is actually the migrated endocervical mucous columnar epithelium over the ectocervix.

Immediate Management

A cervical smear is mandatory. It should be followed by colposcopy and cervical biopsy if the result is unsatisfactory.

Treatment of Choice

None required;
A troublesome erosion may be treated by thermal cautery with diathermy, cryosurgery or laser treatment.

Your notes:

Serial No. 153

Subject: Gynaecology

Topic: Pelvic inflammatory diseases

Question: A 18-year-old girl with recently developed dysmennorhoea and deep dyspareunia. Speculum examination reveals purulent discharge from cervical os. Tested negative for gonorrhoea.

Diagnosis: Chlamydia cervicitis

Clinchers

- *18-year-old girl:* Young age, multiple sexual partners, low socioeconomic group are important risk factors for developing PID. Insertion of intrauterine contraceptive device increases the risk by 6 times, during first 3 weeks following insertion. Most cases of PID occur in sexually active women of age 15-24 years.
- *Recently developed dysmennorhoea:* PID usually presents with non specific symptoms, of which dysmennorhea is one of the common one. The recent onset of dysmenorrhoea may be linked to the PID she developed after some recent 'infected' intercourse
- *Deep dyspareunia:* specific for PID and occurs due touching of inflammed cervix during intercourse which elicits severe pain.
- *Purulent discharge from cervical os:* Mucopurulent cervical discharge and cervicitis, cervical motion tenderness and adnexal tenderness are all very strong points in favour of PID.
- *Tested negative for gonorrhoea:* Gonorrhoea and chlamydia are two most common cause of PID; however, in UK maximum cases (52%) are due to Chlamydia; only 14% occur due to gonorrhoea.

CONFUSA

Dyspareunia in females is related to varied causes and should be dealt in the light of other features present. For this case, deep dyspareunia with mucopurulent discharge points directly to PID. However, other causes of deep dyspareunia should be kept in mind, viz, endometriosis (especially when deposits are present in the pouch of Douglas, uterosacral ligaments, posterior vaginal fornix), adenomyosis, prolapsed ovaries in the pouch of Douglas, retroverted and retroflexed uterus - (unlikely to cause significant dyspareunia unless associated pathology e.g. endometriosis), changed partner - changed shape / size of penis.

Investigation of Choice

Urethral and cervical swabs for chlamydia

Immediate Management

Advise abstinence from sexual intercourse until women and her partner have both completed a course of treatment. Consider empirical treatment of partner if he/she refuses screening.

Advise on use of condoms (antibiotics reduce efficacy of OCP).

Remove IUCDs, if any.

Advise against tampons.

Contact tracing and treatment (all sexual partners in previous 6 months need to be contacted and tested)

Treatment of Choice

Blind antibiotic therapy (covers *C. trachomatis, N. gonorrhoeae* and anaerobic infection)

- oral ofloxacin 400 mg twice a day plus oral metronidazole 400 mg twice a day for 14 days, OR,
- intramuscular ceftriaxone 250 mg immediately or intramuscular cefoxitin 2 g immediately with oral probenecid 1 g, followed by oral doxycycline 100 mg twice a day plus metronidazole 400 mg twice a day for 14 days

If pregnant, a suggested antibiotic treatment regime is: **erythromycin 500 mg four times daily for 14 days and metronidazole 400 mg twice daily for seven days**

Start treatment as soon as the diagnosis is suspected, don't wait for swab results.

Your notes:

Serial No. 154

Subject: Gynaecology

Topic: PID

Question: A 37-year-old lady with multiple painful, vesicular lesions at the introitus with scanty offensive discharge.

Diagnosis: Herpes genitalis

Clinchers

- *37-year-old lady:* The prevalence of HSV antibodies is slightly higher in females. However, women are more likely than men to be protected from genital HSV infection by the use of barrier methods.The rate of genital herpes is highest in sexually active ladies.
- *Multiple painful, vesicular lesions at the introitus:* Groups of small, painful blisters then appear around the genitals and/or anus, which tend to erupt in crops over 1-2 weeks. The blisters later evolve into shallow, sore ulcers. There can be inguinal lymphadenopathy and dysuria. The ulcers and blisters last up to 10-14 days, and then gradually heal and go without scarring.
- *Scanty offensive discharge:* scanty serous vaginal discharge usually accompany which can later turn purulent due to secondary bacterial infections.

CONFUSA

Genital herpes infection in pregnancy:

- If herpes infection is apparent at the onset of labour then a caesarean section is indicated.
- In case of primary infection, acyclovir 200 mg orally five times daily is given to the mother (usually for five days) or topical application of 5 per cent cream five times a day for 5-10 days, starting at the first sign of attack.
- Neonatal infection is uncommon in cases of recurrent genital herpes. This is because of relatively lower concentration and shedding of the virus and also, the passive immunity acquired by the foetus from the mother.

Investigation of Choice

Clinical diagnosis.

The gold standard of diagnosis is viral culture.

Immediate Management

Symptomatic measures:

- analgesia (paracetamol)
- saline baths

Advise male condom use to prevent sexual transmission from infected men to uninfected sexual partners.

Advise antiviral treatment of infected sexual partner.

Treatment of Choice

Acyclovir, 200 mg, 5 times a day for 5 days.

Alternatives to acyclovir therapy are famciclovir and valaciclovir.

Recurrent episodes may require continuous acyclovir.

Your notes:

Serial No. 155

Subject: Gynaecology

Topic: PID

Question: A 34-year-old lady comes with discharge per vaginum. Wet mount shows clue cells.

Diagnosis: Bacterial vaginosis

Clinchers

- *34-year-old lady:* Bacterial vaginosis most commonly occurs in sexually active females. Infection is rare in males.
- *Discharge per vaginum:* Most common and predominant symptom. In fact, bacterial vaginosis is the most common cause of vaginal discharge in women of childbearing age. The discharge is often white-grey, and fishy smelling. It tends to be heaviest just after a period, and after having sex.
- *Wet mounts show clue cells:* Clue cells are the most specific criterion for diagnosing bacterial vaginosis. Clue cells are vaginal epithelial cells that have bacteria adherent to their surfaces. The edges of the squamous epithelial cells, which normally have a sharply defined cell border, become studded with bacteria. The epithelial cells appear to be peppered with coccobacilli.

CONFUSA

- Bacterial vaginosis is not caused by poor hygiene. In fact, excessive washing of the vagina may alter the normal balance of bacteria in the vagina, which may make bacterial vaginosis more likely to develop.
- Bacterial Vaginosis is not caused by a single bacterium. In bacterial vaginosis, an 'overgrowth' of various bacteria occurs in the vagina. Most common bacteria present in most cases are Gardnerella vaginalis and Prevotella. In 50-60% Mobiluncus species may be present.
- Bacterial vaginosis is not a sexually transmitted disease. However, it may develop after a change in sexual partner, as a change in sexual partner may affect the balance of normal bacteria in the vagina.

Investigation of Choice

Microscopy for "clue cells"

Positive amine test (Whiff Test) - a fishy ammoniacal smell when the discharge is mixed with 10% potassium hydroxide.

Immediate Management

It is recommended that the male partner is treated with metronidazole at the same time because it has been found that the majority of male partners of infected partners harbour the organism in their urethras.

Treatment of Choice

Metronidazole 400-500 mg twice daily for seven days .

During pregnancy: standard treatment in the UK is oral metronidazole 400 mg twice a day for five days (Avoid metronidazole in 1st trimester).

Your notes:

PAPER 3

26. A pregnant woman with an LMP of 9 weeks and a positive home pregnancy test presents with an enlarged tender uterus and bright red bleeding per vaginum. On examination her cervical os is fully open.

Diagnosis: Inevitable abortion.

Clinchers

- *Pregnant woman with an LMP of 9 weeks:* Inevitable abortion in first trimester presents with bleeding. In second trimester, however, it may start with rupture of membranes or intermittent lower abdominal pain (mini labour).
- *Positive home pregnancy test:* Proves that her amenorrhoea is due to pregnancy only. This rules out other causes of vaginal bleeding.
- *Presents with an enlarged tender uterus:* Pain appears usually following haemorrhage (bleeding is usually painless). Most common presentation is with painful (colicky) or tender lower abdomen with a dull backache.
- *Bright red bleeding per vaginum:* The bleed is usually bright red and contains foetal and placental parts which the patient may describe as thick dark red blood clots.
- *Her cervical os is fully open:* This is the only feature that differentiates between threatened (os remains closed) and inevitable abortion.

CONFUSA

Incomplete abortion is a difficult entity to differentiate from inevitable abortion. The diagnosis of incomplete abortion is only possible after a detailed clinical examination (small for date uterus, retained products, patulous os), so it is safe to term as such cases as inevitable abortion before the clinical examination.

Investigation of Choice

Complete clinical examination.

Immediate Management

Morphine IM + Methergin

Note: Methergin not to be give in second trimester inevitable abortion.

Treatment of Choice

- *First trimester:* Dilatation and evacuation followed by curettage under GA.
- *Second trimester:* Oxytocin drip.

27. A 16-year-old girl with right iliac fossa pain has a vaginal ultrasound which demonstrates an echogenic cystic mass just superior to the right fornix.

Diagnosis: Torted ovarian cyst.

Clinchers

- *16-year-old girl:* Although there is no particular age incidence, usually it is seen in teenage girls.
- *Right iliac fossa pain:* Torted right ovarian cyst can mimic appendicits and ectopic pregnancy. Twisting occludes the venous return but arterial supply continues to engorge the cyst and cause great pain.
- *Echogenic cystic mass just superior to the right fornix:* This is the typical position of an ovarian cyst. Also it appears as a cystic mass on USG (24% of all ovarian tumours are functional cysts).

CONFUSA

The main differential diagnosis in this question is ectopic pregnancy which can be safely ruled out as there is no given history of any amenorrhoea. Note that neither USG nor bimanual examination can confirm the difference between ectopic pregnancy/appendicitis or torted cysts.

Investigation of Choice

Only laparoscopy can distinguish a cyst from an ectopic pregnancy or appendicitis (contraindicated in malignancy).

Immediate Management

FNAC to rule out malignancy.

Treatment of Choice

Urgent laparotomy.

Your notes:

29. A 22-year-old girl with a history of two terminations complains of right iliac fossa pain, a watery brownish vaginal discharge and fever. She is found to have an elevated white cell count. She uses tampons.

Diagnosis: Pelvic inflammatory disease (PID).

Clinchers

- *22-year-old girl:* Sexually active women under 25 years of age have the highest prevalence of PID (especially Chlamydia).
- *History of two terminations:* PID can cause repeated abortions ectopic pregnancy and tubal infertility.
- *Right iliac fossa pain:* An adnexal mass and iliac fossa pain (either side) may be present in 20% of woman, usually those who are most systemically unwell (as is this case).
- *Watery brownish vaginal discharge:* A watery brown vaginal discharge always signifies endometrial inflammation (endometritis). So it is more in favour of PID rather than an ectopic.
- *Fever:* In more severe cases of PID, pyrexia, a raised neutrophil count and a raised ESR can be present.
- *Elevated white cell count:* Due to severe infection as explained above. This episode is most probably an "acute on chronic PID."

CONFUSA

Ectopic pregnancy can be the main confusing diagnosis in this question but is ruled out as its patient usually present with a hyperacute history, amenorrhoea and shock. Moreover, it is not there in the list of options.

Investigation of Choice

Gold standard: Laparoscopy.

Immediate Management

Urine pregnancy test to rule out ectopic.

Treatment of Choice

Antibiotics (after proper culture)

- Endocervical swabs
  - *Chlamydia*
  - *Neisseria*
- High vaginal swabs
  - *Trichomonas*
  - Bacterial vaginosis

Your notes:

69. A woman had a caesarean section done in the morning presented with a blood pressure of 80/65 mmHg and pulse rate of 120 beats/min.

Diagnosis: Hypovolaemic shock.

Clinchers

- *Caesarean section:* It is a major operation and may lead to hypovolaemia if the patient has bleed extensively during the surgery or postoperative intrauterine bleeding due to uterine atonia (common after a caesarean section).
- *BP of 80/65 mmHg:* Reduction in circulating blood volume results in a reduction fo stroke volume and cardiac output. BP is initially maintained (as in cardiogenic shock), with increased sympathetic activity raising the peripheral vascular resistance leading to the clinical picture of a cold, clammy patient with a tachycardia (and hence a pulse rate of 120 bpm). As volume losses increase, the blood pressure falls. So most probably the patient is still bleeding (most probably intrauterine).
  (Note: There is no tachycardia in a spinal shock).

CONFUSA

In young and fit, the systolic BP may remain normal, although the pulse pressure will narrow, with upto 30% of blood volume depletion.

Investigation of Choice

BP/CVP/urine output.

Immediate Management

If bleed already—Colloid.
If bleeding—Blood.

Treatment of Choice

Treatment of underlying cause.

Your notes:

121. A woman in the eight-week of her pregnancy develops bright red bleeding of four hours duration. On examination her cervical os is completely closed.

Diagnosis: Threatened abortion.

Clinchers

- *Eight-week of her pregnancy:* This can well be a case of first trimester abortion. Abortion is the loss of pregnancy before 24 week gestation.
- *Develops bright red bleeding;* In threatened abortion the bleeding is usually slight and bright red in colour.
- *Cervical oS is completely closed:* This is the most important point in this question. If the symptoms are mild and cervical os is closed, it is a threatened abortion.

In this case we go for ultrasonography. On USG a well-formed gestational ring and positive cardiac activity state 98% chance of continuation of pregnancy.

USG gestational ring + cardiac activity → 98% chances of survival

Investigation of Choice

Ultrasonography (USG)

Immediate Management

Rest (until bleeding stops)

Treatment of Choice

Advice rest, 75% will settle. In others sedation and relief of pain may be ensured by phenobarbitone 30 mg or diazepam 5 mg twice daily.

Your notes:

122. A woman in the twelfth week of her pregnancy develops bright red bleeding of four hours duration with large clots. On examination the cervical os is wide open.

Diagnosis: Inevitable abortion.

Clinchers

- *Twelfth week of pregnancy:* Abortion is loss of pregnancy before 24 weeks gestation.
- *Bright red bleeding with clots:* Increased vaginal bleeding with clots and increased pain that is colicky in nature is a sign of inevitable abortion.
- *Cervical os is wide open:* This is again the most important point in this question, because internal examination revealing dilated internal os of the cervix through which the products of conception can be felt is diagnostic of inevitable abortion.

Diagnosis can be confirmed an ultrasonography. On USG if it is found that most of the products of conception have already been passed, it is incomplete abortion.

Investigation of Choice

USG (ultrasonography).

Immediate Management

If bleeding is profuse consider ergometrine 0.5 mg IM.

Treatment of Choice

Take appropriate measures to look after general condition (e.g. bleeding, shock, etc). Accelerate the process of expulsion.

Your notes:

123. A woman in the tenth week of her pregnancy develops bright red bleeding of one day duration. Her Gp organises an ultrasound examination which reveals heart contractions.

Diagnosis: Probable threatened abortion.

Clinchers

➢ *Tenth week:* After 24 weeks (and effectively after 20 weeks for the purpose of management in A and E department), vaginal bleeding is classed as an antepartum haemorrhage. Before this time it may be:
- A threatened abortion
- An incomplete abortion
- A complete abortion
- Other local causes

➢ *USG reveals heart contractions:* Formal scanning may detect a heart beat at 7 weeks gestation. A presence of contracting fetal heart rules out fetal loss. Other indications for fetal loss can be:
- Significant pain and tenderness
- Heavy of continuing bleeding
- Passage of placental material in addition to blood clots.

CONFUSA

Vaginal bleeding occurs in upto one-fifth of all pregnant women but in over 50% of cases the pregnancy will continue successfully. A fresh bleed can due to local trauma to vaginal walls or cervix. So always rule it out by colposcopic examination.

Investigation of Choice

Colposcopy to rule out local bleeding.

Immediate Management

Early USG (aldready done in this case).

Treatment of Choice

Patients with threatened abortion without symptoms or signs of fetal loss may be referred back to the GP for bed-rest at home.

Your notes:

156. A pregnant woman has a vaginal discharge. The pH is 2 and mycelia are seen.

Diagnosis: Candidiasis.

Clinchers

➢ *Pregnant woman has vaginal discharge:* Pregnancy favours candidial infection becomes of increased vaginal acidity and high glycogen content. Other risk factors for candidial infections are:
- Hormonal contraceptive pills
- Diabetes
- Immunodeficiencies
- Antibiotics
- Steroids

➢ *pH is 2:* Gram-positive fungus *'Candida albicans'* flourishes in an acid medium with an abundant supply or carbohydrates.

➢ *Mycelia are seen:* In candidial infection, microscopy reveals strings of mycelium or typical oval spores. Culture or Sabouraud's medium.

CONFUSA

If still any confusion, the diagnosis of thrush (*Candia albicans*) can be established by following features
- Candidial discharge is classically white curds
- Vulva and vagina may be red, fissured and rose.

Investigation of Choice

Microscopy + culture

Treatment of Choice

A single imidazole pessary, e.g. clotrimazole 500 mg. For further treatment you may refer page 48 (OHCS), 5th edn.

Your notes:

157. A woman has a vaginal discharge. The pH is 8 and clue cells are seen.

Diagnosis: Bacterial vaginosis.

Clinchers

- *Vaginal discharge:* The character of discharge is not specified, so let us have an idea of type, of vaginal discharges:
  - White curdy discharge—Thrush (*Candida albicans*)
  - Thin, bubbly, fishy smelling discharge—*Trichomonas vaginalis*
  - Offensive discharge with fishy odour—bacterial vaginosis.
- *pH is 8:* Vaginal pH > 5.5 is seen in bacterial vaginosis, candidiasis occurs in acidic vaginal pH.
- *Clue cells:* Stippled vaginal epithelia 'clue cells' seen on met microscopy supports the diagnosis of bacterial vaginosis.

CONFUSA

Though the diagnosis is settled for bacterial vaginosis, the nature of vaginal discharge should have been mentioned. In bacterial vaginosis offensive discharge with fishy odour occurs.

Investigation of Choice

Wet microscopy and culture.

Treatment of Choice

Metronidazole 2 g PO once or clindamycin 2% vaginal cream. If recurrent treat the partner also. And in pregnant females use metronidazole alone 200 mg/8 hr PO for 7 days.

Your notes:

158. A woman has severe right sided abdominal pain and fever. She has a foul smelling vaginal discharge. She has a palpable right sided firmness.

Diagnosis: Pelvic inflammatory disease (PID).

Clinchers

- *Right sided abdominal pain and fever:* PID presents with pain which is usually bilateral but may be localized to one side, with fever. Most of the cases are because of *Chlamydia* but rarely gonococcus and *Streptococcus* may be the culprits.
- *Foul smelling vaginal discharge:* Along with pain and fever PID presents with cervicals with profuse purulent or blood vaginal discharge.
- *Palpable right sided firmness:* In chronic cases inflammation leads to fibrosis, so adhesions may develop between pelvic organs. The tubes may get distended with pus (pyosalpinx) or fluids (hydrosalpinx).

CONFUSA

In endometeriosis, pelvic pain is the most common symptom (classically cyclical during periods), but foul smelling vaginal discharge is not seen. Here secondary dysmenorrhoea and deep dyspareuria are common.

Investigation of Choice

Endocervical and urethral swabs if practicable. Check for *Chlamydia*. Later we can go for blood culture if fever is present.

Immediate Management

Admit for blood culture and IV antibiotics if very unwell.

Treatment of Choice

Refer page 50 (OHCS) 5th end.

Your notes:

159. A woman on the contraceptive pill for several years has a slight whitish vaginal discharge. On inspection she is found to have a pinkish colouration of the outer cervix.

Diagnosis: Cervical erosion (cervical ectropion).

Clinchers

- *On contraceptive pills:* Ectropions extend temporarily under the influence of hormones in following conditions:
  - During puberty
  - With the combined pill and during pregnancy
- In this case endocervical epithelium extends its territory over paler epithelium of ectocervix. Endocervical canal is lined by mucus columnar epithelium and vaginal cervix with squamous epithelium, therefore columnar epithelium in ectocervix giving if pinkish colouration.

Columnar epithelium is soft and glandular therefore ectropion is prone to bleeding and there is excess mucus production, and hence they are also prone to infection.

CONFUSA

History of women being an contraceptive pills with vaginal discharge may point towards thrush (*Candida albicans*), but the discharge of thrush is white curdy. In candidiasis microscopy will reveal stringe of mycelium.

Treatment of Choice

Generally no treatment is required. But in case it creates nuisance, cautery can be done.

Your notes:

160. A middle-aged woman with a vaginal disharge is found to have several ulcers at the vaginal introitus.

Diagnosis: Herpes simplex.

Clinchers

- *Vaginal discharge:* Vaginal discharge occurs in herpes due to exudation from the lesion in the cervix and vagina.
- *Several ulcers at vaginal introitus:* In herpes simplex the vulva is ulcerated and exquisitely painful. Herpes type II is sexually acquired, this classically causes genital infections. This may be caused by type I transferred from cold sores. Several ulcers at vaginal introitus are characteristically seen in herpes.

Immediate Management

If painful give strong analgesia.

Treatment of Choice

Analgesia, lidocaine gel 2%, salt baths (and micturating in the bath) help. Acyclovir topically and 200 mg 5 times daily PO for 5 days shortens symptoms and infectivity.

Reassure the patient that subsequent attacks are shorter and less painful.

Your notes:

171. A couple aged 25 years have been trying for a baby for six months.

Diagnosis: Normal

Clinchers

- *Trying for a baby for six months:* Infertility cannot be a diagnosis before one year of unprotected intercourse in healthy couples of child-bearing age. Usually 80% couples achieve a pregnancy after 12 months and 90% after two years (in young couples it is 90% within one year).
- *25 years age:* Infertility decreases with age, but this is a young couple and this age factor is ruled out. They must be given more time to try for a baby.

CONFUSA

Infertility is a symptom and not a diagnosis. High fertility in one partner can compensate low fertility in the other. Investigations of infertility can be a tremendous strain on patients. So, sympathetic management is crucial.

Investigation of Choice

Infertility investigations are not initiated before one year.

Immediate Management

Reassurance.

Treatment of Choice

None.

Your notes:

172. Useful in determining ovulation.

Diagnosis: Day 21 progesterone.

Clinchers

Tests for ovulation are often asked in the themes on investigation of infertility. So lets discuss them.

- *Indication:* Infertility with regular menstrual cycles.

  Eamples:
  - *USG:* Visualization of follicle development or change to secretory endometrium
  - *Midcycle mucus test:* Ovulatory mucus is like raw egg white.
  - *Clear plan kit:* detects LH surge
  - *21 day progesterone test:* detect a luteal rise in progesterone to >30 nmol/L 7 days before the onset of menstruation at 21st day.
  - *BBT:* Detecting a rise in basal body temperature at midcycle.

CONFUSA

The only proof of ovulation is pregnancy. It is possible for a follicle to luteinize without rupturing, so tests may be positive in the absence of an ovum. Negative results imply failure to ovulate.

Investigation of Choice

Day 21 progesterone test is the best test.

Your notes:

173. An essential investigation for all heterosexual infertile couples.

Diagnosis: Semen analysis.

Clinchers

Semen analysis is an essential investigation and can be perforemd in a primary care setting.

Requirements:
- 3 days abstinence
- Two samples at one month interval

Normal values in semen analysis:
- Volume—mean 2.75 ml
- Count > 20 million sperm/mL
- Mortility > 40% motile
- Form > 60% normal morphology

Impaired sperm production can be a side effect of:
- Psychotropic drugs
- Antiepileptics
- Antihypertensive
- Chemotherapy

CONFUSA

A satisfactory postcoital test can obviate the need for a semen analysis, so it should be done first.

Interesting fact: Mean sperm count is 66 million/mL and this is falling at a rate of 100 sperms/mL/hour worldwide.

Immediate Management

Reduced counts require specialist referral.

Your notes:

174. This investigation is of little value in infertility.

Diagnosis: Bacteriological examination of urine.

Clinchers

It is a non-specific question, so let us see the role of pelvic inflammatory diseases and venereal diseases in causing infertility.

Tubal dysfunction: If affects the normal transport of oocyte and embryo. PID is a major cause of tubal infertility. Sexually transmitted diseases with chlamydia-trachomatis, gonococci and other microorganisms may lead to tubal damage (*Chlamydia* is most common). Tuberculosis is a leading cause of tubal damage in developing countries.

CONFUSA

Either acute or chronic urinary tract infections rarely produce infertility. Bacteriological examination of urine can tell about any UTI but signify almost nothing about a possible cause of infertility.

Your notes:

175. It is an essential investigation of the female partner.

Diagnosis: Tubal patency test.

Clinchers

It is an essential investigation as it is important to exclude tubal causes which account to 14% cases of infertility. It interfers with meeting of sperm and ova and assisted reproductive technique may required to help in conception. Main tests of tubal patency are:

1. Laparoscopy with dye
2. Hysterosalpingogram (constant X-ray)
3. High contrast ultrasonography (HyCoSy)

Note:

- HyCoSy is a modern, ultrasound based investigation using a negative (normal saline) and positive (Echovist) contrast media to outline the uterine cavity and fallopian tubes, tubal patency and avoid exposure to X-rays.
- Hysterosalpingogram is done within first ten days of menstruation in order to avoid inadvertent exposure of the early embryo to X-rays.

CONFUSA

Tubal patency tests are same of the few investigations in context of infertility that yield a definitive result and are potentially remediable. That makes them essential to either exclude or treat.

Investigation of Choice

HyCoSy.

Immediate Management

Reassurance.

Treatment of Choice

Tubal problems may be remedied by surgery but the results are poor. So in vitro fertilization (IVF) is a better option.

Note: Gamete intrafallopian transfer (GIFT) can be used only when tubes are potent.

Your notes:

182. A 37-year-old woman presents with a sudden onset of severe left iliac fossa pain. On vaginal USG, 2 cm echogenic masses are seen in the broad ligament. She says this pain seems to come every month.

Diagnosis: Endometriosis

Clinchers

- *37-year-old woman:* Endometriosis is typically seen in those with postmenstrual exposure, common in fourth decade of life.
- *Severe left iliac fossa pain (comes every month):* Pelvic pain classically cyclical at the time if periods is the most common symptoms. Periods are usually heavy and frequent.
- *On USG, 2 cm echogenic masses seen in broad ligament:* Foci if endometrial tissue may be found on an ovary, rectovaginal pouch, uterosacral ligaments, surface if pelvic peritoneum, broad ligament and sometimes in distant organs like lungs.
- *On vaginal examination*
  - Fixed retroverted uterus
  - Nodules in uterosacral ligament
  - General tenderness.

Investigation of Choice

Laparoscopy shows

- Types cysts
- Peritoneal deposits

Treatment of Choice

- Danazol 400-800 mg OD
- Gestrinone 2.5-5 mg PO twice weekly
- Buserelin/goserelin (LHRH analyses)

Surgical local exicision or diathermy of endometriotic tissue or hysterectomy may depend upon site of lesion and women's with for future fertility.

Your notes:

183. A 23-year-old woman just had an intrauterine device fitted. She complains of a watery brown vaginal discharge and abdominal pain.

Diagnosis: Pelvic inflammatory disease (PID).

Clinchers

- *Intrauterine device fitted:* 10% of cases of PID follow childbirth or instrumentation (insertion of IUCD, TOP) though 90% are sexually acquired (mostly due to *Chlamydia*).
- *Watery brown vaginal discharge:* PID present with abdominal pain and vaginal discharge. Discharge is come times profuse and purulent, or it may be bloody. These is spasm of lower abdominal muscles.

In chronic cases abdominal mass may also be palpated because the inflammation leads to fibrosis, so adhesions develop between pelvic organs.

Investigation of Choice

Endocervical and urethral swabs if practicable. Always check for chlamydia. Go for blood culture if febrile.

Immediate Management

Admit for blood culture and IV antibiotics if very unwell.

Treatment of Choice

Page 50 (OHCS), 5th edn.

Your notes:

184. An 18 weeks pregnant female presents with lower abdominal pain and tenderness, with offensive vaginal discharge. She has high grade fever since last two days.

Diagnosis: Septic abortion

Clinchers

- *Lower abdominal pain:* In this question this pain may be due to pelvic infection.
- *Offensive vaginal discharge with high grade fever:* This point towards the infection (probably uterus). To support the diagnosis of septic abortion, fever more than 38°C for more than 24 hours (with or withour chills and rigors) should be present. Offensive and purulent vaginal discharge support the diagnosis of infection.

Majority of infection occurs following illegal induced abortion (rare in UK) in developing countries.

Any abortion associated with clinical evidence of infection of the uterus and it content is called septic abortion.

Investigation of Choice

Cervical or high vaginal swab for culture. Ultrasonography.

Treatment of Choice

Hospitalization. Aim at

- To control sepsis
- Remove source of infection
- Supportive therapy

Go for analgesia, sedatives and antibiotics.

Your notes:

185. A 32-year-old who conscientiously uses the oral contraceptive pill, has experienced monthly vaginal bleeding. On abdominal examination she is comfortable. Her temperature is 37°C. She is otherwise healthy.

Diagnosis: Break through bleeding.

Clinchers

- *Conscientiously uses—OCP:* It means she is a regular in taking the pills.
- *Monthly vaginal bleeding:* Menstruation is initiated by the withdrawal of oestrogen and progesterone. Such as effect is produced in women receiving oestrogens and progestogens in the form of the combined contraceptive pill or hormone replcement therapy—withdrawal bleeding on completion of a pack.
- *On abdominal examination she is comfortable:* This rules out any pelvic inflammatory disease. Otherwise also OCP use decreases the risk of PID. The only infection whose incidence is increased by using OCP is monoilial vaginitis (candidiasis).

CONFUSA

Intermenstrual spotting is common in the first three months of the start of the pills, but it gradaully disappears. Heavy spotting can be stopped by increasing the dose for a few months.

Investigation of Choice
None required.

Immediate Management
Reassurance.

Treatment of Choice
None required.

Your notes:

186. A patient in her third pregnancy presents to her GP at 12 weeks gestation. She was mildly hypertensive in both of her previous pregnancies. Her BP is 150/100 mmHg. Two weeks later at the hospital antenatal clinic her BP is 150/95 mmHg.

Diagnosis: Essential hypertension (EH)

Clinchers

- *Third pregnancy:* EH is common in older multiparas, and present before pregnancy or in first trimester (in this case 12 weeks).
- *Mildly hypertensive in both of her previous pregnancies:* Those with EH are five times more likely to develop pre-eclampsia. Also increased BP is a positive risk factor for PIH.
- *BP is 150/100 mmHg, two weeks later 150/95 mmHg:* Isolated BP measurements are never reliable in pregnancy. So BP has to be recorded on at least two occasions (at least >4 hr apart) to make a diagnosis. In this case the BP is more of less the same on two occasions (two weeks apart). Also the diastolic BP is > 90 mmHg on both occasions.

CONFUSA

If the symptoms are episodic, think of phaeochromocytoma. PIH by definition does not present before 20 weeks for the first-time.

Investigation of Choice
24 hours urinary proteins (to screen for pre-eclampsia).

Immediate Management
BP monitoring (biweekly).

Treatment of Choice
Oral antihypertensive (as BP should be kept < 140/90 mmHg).

Your notes:

187. A 22-year-old Nigerian woman has an uneventful first pregnancy to 30 weeks. She is then admitted as an emergency with epigastric pain. During the first two hours her BP rises from 150/105 to 170/120 mmHg. On dipstick test she is found to have 3+ proteinuria. The fetal cardiotocogram (CTG) is normal.

Diagnosis: Fulminating PIH.

Clinchers

- *First pregnancy:* 70% cases of pre-eclampsia occur in primigravidas. A recurrence rate of 20% is present for multigravidas (with same partner). With a new partner the incidence of recurrence increases.
- *30 weeks:* By definition PIH present for the first-time after 20 weeks.
- *Epigastric pain:* It is due to stretching of liver capsule.
- *BP rises from 150/105 to 170/120 mmHg in two hours:* A rapid rise in BP is a characteristic feature of fulminant PIH and require immediate IV antihypertensives.
- *3+ proteinuria:* It signifies significant proteinuria and hence qualifies for the diagnosis of fulminant PIH.
- *CTG is normal:* Abnormal CTG signifies foetal distress and warrants an immediate caesarean section. In this case it is not required as CTG is normal. Still regular CTG monitoring (1 to 2 per day of one hour each) must be done.

CONFUSA

In severe (fulminating) PIH, delivery is the only definitive treatment (Note: PIH regress by delivery of placenta and not only fetus). The delivery is often vaginal, except in conditions given below where a caesarean section is preferred (A B C D E)

A—Abruption
B—BP unctrollable; breech
C—Cervix unfavourable
D—Distress of foetus
E—Error in induction of delivery (failed induction)

Note: Delivery criteria in PIH
Mild PIH—can continue till 40 weeks
Moderate PIH—can continue till 37 weeks
Severe PIH—as soon as possible
and eclampsia

Investigation of Choice
CTG (already done in this case).

Immediate Management
IV hydralazine/Labetalol.

Treatment of Choice
Intravenous antihypertensive (hydralazine/labetalol) immediately + Regular monitoring

188. At an antenatal clinic visit at 38 weeks gestation, a 36-year-old multiparous woman has a BP of 140/90 mmHg. She has no proteinuria and is otherwise well.

Diagnosis: Normal.

Clinchers

- *38 weeks gestation:* PIH usually present in the second trimester and not this late.
- *36-year-old:* Age > 35 years (or < 20 years) is a positive risk factor for PIH/eclampsia).
- *Multiparous:* Usually multiparous females are not affected by PIH if there is no history of it in the previous pregnancies.
- *BP 140/90 mmHg:* By definition the diastolic BP has to cross 90 to qualify for a diagnosis of PIH. The classification criteria of PIH are given in next question (Q 189). This BP does not classify as a criteria for diagnosis.
- *No proteinuria:* Excludes pre-eclampsia/severe PIH.
- *Otherwise well:* Excludes other medical disorders.

CONFUSA

In cases of PIH (pregnancy induced hypertension), admit if

- BP rises by >30/20 mmHg over booking BP
- BP reaches
  - 160/100 without proteinuria
  - 140/90 with proteinuria

PIH can be diagnosed only with BP elevation above in criteria on at least 2 occasions (> 4 hours apart).

Investigation of Choice
Biweekly BP monitoring.

Immediate Management
Take second BP measurement after four hours.

Treatment of Choice
A period of observation for blood pressure.

Your notes:

189. At 32 weeks, a 22-year-old primigravida is found to have a BP of 145/100 mmHg. She has no proteinuria but is found to have edema of her knees.

Diagnosis: Pregnancy induced hypertension (PIH).

Clinchers

- *32 weeks:* By definition PIH called so only if it appears for first-time after 20 weeks. Hypertension occurring before is usually due to an existing and non-pregnancy induced condition.
- *Primigravida:* PIH is an almost exclusive disease of primigravidas.
- *BP of 145/100 mmHg with no proteinuria:* PIH is classified according to BP and proteinuria.
  Mild PIH—BP upto 140/100 mmHg without proteinuria
  Moderate PIH—BP upto 160/110 mmHg without proteinuria
  Severe PIH—BP more than 160/110 mmHg with proteinuria
  (Proteinuria is > 300 mg excretion of proteins in urine in 24 hours).
- *Oedema of her knees:* Peripheral oedema in pregnancy has little significance if it occurs as an isolated finding. But it signifies severe PIH if it occurs along with hypertension and proteinuria.

CONFUSA

PIH is almost exclusively seen in primigravidas. But in multiparous women its risk is increased if the existing pregnancy is with a new partner. Other risk factors for PIH in multigravidas are: history of first pregnancy, H. mole, multiple pregnancy, gestational diabetes mellitus.

Investigation of Choice
Foetal USG.

Immediate Management
Admit in first instance for assessment and monitoring.

Treatment of Choice
Since the disease in question is a moderate PIH, its management is:

- Care in day assessment until/hospital
- Oral antihypertensives if—BP > 160/100 mmHg (sustained)
  Note: It is > 170/110 mmHg according to OHCS.
- Can continue upto 37 weeks with regular monitoring of:
  Daily—urinary proteins
  Bi-weekly—LFT
  Weekly—Plasma U and E, plasma urate, total urinary proteins.

Indications of delivery in moderate disease

- Progression to pre-eclampsia
- Declining maternal renal function
- Foetal distress
  - Abnormal CTG (cardiotocogram)
  - Absence of end diastolic flow in doppler of umbilical circulation
- Placental abruption.

Your notes:

190. At 34 weeks, an 86 kg woman complains of persistent headaches and 'flashing lights'. There is no hyperreflexia and her BP is 150/100 mmHg. Urinalysis is negative but she has finger edema.

Diagnosis: Pre-eclampsia

Clinchers

Preclampsia is a syndrome of sings and when the symptoms occurs, it is usually too late.

- *34 weeks:* It develops after 20 weeks and usually resolves within 10 days of delivery.
- *86 kg woman:* Predisposing factors of pre-eclampsia are

Maternal	*Fetal*
• Primiparity • History of severe pre-eclampsia • Positive family history • Height <155 cm • Overweight • Age < 20 or > 35 yrs • Pre-existing migraine • BP - or renal disease	• H mole • Multiple pregnancy • Placental hydrops (e.g. Rh disease)

- *Persisting headaches:* Frontal>occipital, reason is cerebral oedema. It is of dragging/throbbing type
  - Worsen on
    - Supine position
    - Morning
  - Resolves on—mobility
- *Flashing lights:* Visual symptoms are common in pre-eclampsia. They are due to oedema of neural layer in retina.

  The most common visual symptoms are
  - Black holes
  - Double vision
  - Flashing lights
- *No hyperreflexia:* Hyperreflexia is said to be present when a reflex can be obtained away from the tendon that usually causes it, e.g. knee reflex by tapping anterior surface of tibia (rather than the tendon). It is an important sign of impending eclampsia.
- *BP is 150/100 mmHg:* A diastolic BP exceeding 90 mmHg on at least two occasions in the second half of pregnancy, where the blood pressure was previously normal, accompanied by significant proteinuria (> 300 mg/24 h) qualifies for a diagnosis of pre-eclampsia.
- *Urinalysis negative:* It means no proteinuria. Proteinuria is the last feature of pre-eclampsia to appear. It may be trace or at times coupious. There may be few hyaline casts, epithelial cells or even few red cells. It is considered significant only when >300 mg/24 h. Proteinuria may also be missed in an isolated urinary examination, so do a 24 hours total urinary protein excretion measurement to rule it out.
- *Finger oedema:* Traditionally the presence of peripheral oedema has been included in the definition, however, this is a common finding in otherwise normal pregnancy and its absence does not preclude the diagnosis (nor does its presence makes the diagnosis). However, tightness of the ring on the finger (finger oedema) is an early manifestation of pre-eclampsia oedema. Gradually the swelling may extend to face, abdominal wall, vulva and even the whole body.

CONFUSA

In the UK, high quality antenatal care has reduced the problems of pre-eclamptic toxaemia to such an extent that 75% of cases of eclampsia now occur in the post-partum period and a similar proportion occur without pre-existing hypertension.

Investigation of Choice

24 hours urinary protein.

Immediate Management

BP control by IB hydralazine/Labetalol if there is an acute or progressive increase in BP.

Treatment of Choice

Oral antihypertensive are given in case of sustained rise of BP till > 160/100 mmHg or at lower levels if cerebral edema is present (i.e. in this case). Antihypertensives that can be uses are;

- Methyldopa—contraindicated in liver disease
- Labetalol—contraindicated in asthma
- Magnesium sulfate—(preferred drug in USA)

Your notes:

PAPER 4

51. A 14-year-old girl has just started having sexual relationship with her boyfriend of 2 months.

Best option: OCPs + condom

Clinchers

- *14-year-old girl:* OCP's are not preferral over 35 years of age, as it increases the risk of thromboembolism (more common if they smoke). Smokers: stop pill at 30 years.
- *With her boyfriend:* In steady relationships only OCPs would be the fine, but here to reduced risk of transmission of most STDs, condom together with OCP would help.

When prescribing OCPs tell her about the risks. Look for any contraindications.

Contraindications to OPCs

Absolute contraindications

A. Circulatory diseases (past/present)
- Arterial or venous thrombosis
- Severe hypertension
- Angina/valvular heart disease/ischaemic heart diseases
- Migraine
- Hyperlipidaemia

B. Diseases of liver
- Active liver disease
- Liver adenoma, carcinoma
- History of cholestatic, jaundice in pregnancy

C. Others
- Pregnancy
- Breast cancer (estrogen dependent neoplasms)
- Undiagnosed genital tract bleeding

Relations contraindications
- Obesity
- Epilepsy
- Age over 35 years
- Varicosities
- Bronchial asthma
- Smoking

CONFUSA

Condoms would not only prevent pregnancy, but will also give protection against STDs.

Your notes:

52. 35-year-old female after her third child wants reliable contraception. She is a smoker and does not want to gain weight.

Best option: IUCD.

Clinchers

- Death due to the pill in 35-year-old is 8 times more common if they smoke. At 30 years either stop smoking or stop the pills.
- *35-year-old female:* A relative contraindications for OCPs. For other contraceptives refer previous question.
- *She is a smoker:* Smoking is contraindication for OCPs. Increases the risk of thromboembolism.
- *Does not want to gain weight:* Weight gain is an adverse effect of OCPs. The progestin have got an anabolic effect due its chemical relation to testosterone which results in a positive nitrogen balance and fat deposition.

CONFUSA

Sterilization would have been a better option, since she already has three children. If this female is quite sure that she does not want further children, then sterilization is the most effective form of contraception for this female.

IUCD is the best form of contraception after sterilization for older women.

Side effects of OCPs
- Nausea, vomiting, headache
- Mastalgia
- Weight gain
- Chloasma and acne
- Menstrual abnormalities
- Libido may be diminished

Major complications are:
- Depression
- Hypertension
- Thromboembolism/coronary thrombosis
- Cholestatic jaundice.

Your notes:

53. An 18-year-old girl has been on OCPs since 2 years ,has to have rifampicin prophylaxis since her room-mate has meningitis.

Best option: OCPs + condom.

Clinchers

- *Rifampicin prophylaxis:* Liver enzyme inducers, e.g. rifampicin, anticonvulsants and griseofulvin reduce the efficacy of oral contraceptives by decreasing circulating, oestrogen. For rifampicin take precaution besides OCPs whilst use and four weeks after. Best alternatives would be to change the contraceptives method if on long-term rifampicin.

Barrier method along with OCPs can be used here. With long-term use of these drugs consider using 50 Hg estrogen pills with higher doses of progesterone, e.g. Norinyl-I.

Your notes:

54. Girl with learning disorder begins to find males attractive. Her parents and teachers are worried.

Best option: Depovera.

Clinchers

Depovera 150 mg given deep IM is given 12 weekly, started during the first 5 days of a cycle. It is medroxyprogesterone acetate, simple, safe and very effective.

Since it is given once in 12 weeks it has following advantages.

- Secret
- No compliance problems
- No oestrogen content
- Reduced for menstrual syndrome
- Suppresses ovulation.

Therefore in a girl with learning disorder depovera is the best option.

Your notes:

55. Female after her first-child wants reliable contraception but wants no chemicals in her body, complains of heavy periods and dysmenorrhoea, husband does not want to use condoms.

Best option: Mirena coil.

Clinchers

- Mirena coil (carries levonorgesterol) is an IUCD carrying hormone. It has been shown to be *helpful in dysmenorrhoea.* Local effects make implantation less likely, and *periods lighter.* It lasts 3 years. There may be less risk of ectopic pregnancy.
- *Heavy periods and dysmenorrhoea:* Mirena coil is beneficial in both of these conditions.

CONFUSA

Diaphragm (intravaginal device made of rubber), could have been the answer, but it is not a popular method. Complaints of dysmenorrhoea favours mirena coil.

Your notes:

142. Young girl has put on weight, hirsutism, oligomenorrhoea.

Diagnosis: Polycystic ovary syndrome (PCOS).

Clinchers

- *Young girl:* 5-10% of the premenopausal women are affected by this common syndrome.
- *Put on weight:* PCOS is related to insulin resistance, so hyperinsulinemia is a feature. As a result the patient can become obese.
- *Hirsutism:* In PCOS, hormonal cycling is disrupted because of ovarian, hypothalamic-pituitary and adrenal dysfunction. As a result virilisation with hirsutism and acne usually occurs.
- *Oligomenorrhoea:* It is also a component of virilization. Often there is amenorrhoea (secondary) (Stein-Leventhal syndrome). The patient may present with infertility.

CONFUSA

Hirsutism is common (10% of women) and is usually benign. It implies hair growth in women in male pattern. Differential diagnosis of hirsutism depends on menses:

- Menstruation abnormal—cause is - testosterone
- Menstruation normal—cause is other than of - testosterone

Investigation of Choice

- *Screening:* LH -, testosterone -
- *Definitive:* USG/laparoscopy (characteristic ovaries)

Immediate Management

Advice weight loss

Treatment of Choice

Symptomatic

- Infertility—clomiphene
- Bleeding—combined pill
- Hirsutism—cyproterone
- Insulin resistance—metformin

Your notes:

143. Female on OCPs complains of postcoital bleeding.

Diagnosis: Cervical ectropion

Clinchers

- *OCP:* Ectocervix contain a transformation zone, where the stratified squamous epithelium of the vagina meets the columnar epithelium of the cervical canal. The anatomical site of this squamocolumnar junction fluctuates under hormonal influence, and the high turnover of this tissue is important in the pathogenesis of cervical carcinoma. The columnar epithelium is normally visible with the speculum during
  - Ovulatory phase of menstrual cycle
  - Pregnancy
  - OCP use
- *Postcoital bleeding:* It may give rise to postcoital bleeding, as fine blood vessels, within the columnar epithelium are easily traumatised.

CONFUSA

Cervical ectropion is sometimes termed as cervical erosion. Usually the main complaint of cervical ectropion is excessive nonpurulent discharge, as the surface area of the columnar epithelium containing mucus glands is increased. It may give rise to spotting during pregnancy in which case it is usually left untreated till after the pregnancy.

Investigation of Choice

Per speculum exam (red ring around OS because the endocervical epithelium has extended its territory over the paler epithelium of the ectocervix).

Immediate Management

Reassurance about cause and treatment.

Treatment of Choice

Usually none required.
If symptoms are distressing

- Thermal cautery (sometimes confusingly called cold coagulation).

Your notes:

145. A woman on the contraceptive pill for several years has a slight whitish vaginal discharge. On inspection she is found to have a pinkish coloration of the outer cervix.

Diagnosis: Cervical ectropion

Clinchers

Note: See Q 143 of this theme also.

- *Contraceptive pill:* It increases the incidence of cervical ectropion as the hormonal inthence imparted by it causes to squamocolumnar junction to shift due to outgrowth of columnar epithelium.
- *Discharge:* Discharge in cervical ectropion is due to excessive mucus secretion as the surface area of the columnar epithelium containing mucus glands is increased. If the discharge becomes troublesome to the patient, discontinuing the contraceptive pill, or alternatively ablative treatment under local anaesthesia using a thermal probe can reduce it.
- *Pinkish colouration of outer cervix:* This is the typical appearance of the columnar epithelium on ectocervix. Other than ectropion, columnar epithelium is visible during pregnancy and ovulatory phase of menstrual cycle.

CONFUSA

The appearance of the cervix in ectropion is sometimes inappropriately termed as cervical erosion. It should be avoided as it conveys quite the wrong impression of what is really a normal phenomenon.

Investigation of Choice

Per speculum examination (already done in this patient)

Immediate Management

Reassurance (that it is a completely normal phenomenon)

Treatment of Choice

Indicated only if the discharge is troublesome

- Thermal ablation under LA (heat the tissue to 100°C, destroying epithelium to a depth of 3-4 mm)

Note: It is also known as cold agglutination.

Your notes:

169. An 80-year-old sexually active woman with dyspareunia and recurrent dysuria.

Diagnosis: Atrophic vaginitis

Clinchers

- *80-year-old:* This condition is always seen post-menopausally because of lack of oestrogens.
- *Sexually active women:* Because of vaginal wall dryness and thinning, there can be discomfort during intercourse. If the woman would not have been sexually active, atrophic vaginitis, if mild, would have been asymptomatic.
- *Dyspareunia:* There is *superficial* dyspareunia in this condition.
- *Recurrent dysuria:* Low grade infection can coexist with atrophic vaginitis.

CONFUSA

Hormone replacement therapy postmenopausally produces withdrawal bleeds. Topical oestorgens are enough to thicken the epithelium and reduce the pH, but insufficient to produce excessive endometrial stimulation or other causes of bleeding.

Investigation of Choice

Urine culture and sensitivity

Immediate Management

Advice topical lubrication during coitus.

Treatment of Choice

- If there is secondary infection, antibiotics to which the organism is sensitive may be given
- Topical oestrogen creams or pessaries (e.g. dienoestrol or premarin (once or twice a week)

Your notes:

170. A middle-aged woman with a vaginal discharge is found to have several ulcers at the vaginal introitus.

Diagnosis: Herpes labialis

Clinchers

- *Middle-aged woman:* Herpes labialis is most common in sexually active females, so its incidence is characteristically minimal in children and elderly.
- *Vaginal discharge:* Pain, itching, dysuria, vaginal and urethral discharge, and tender inguinal lymphadenopathy are the predominant local symptoms.
- *Several ulcers of the vaginal introitus:* Widely spaced bilateral lesions of the external genitalia are characteristic. In it painful vesicles develop initially which then coalesce into multiple ulcers.

CONFUSA

First episodes of genital herpes in patients who have had prior HSV-1 infection are associated with less frequent systemic symptoms and faster healing than primary genital herpes. In primary herpes, if the case is seen very early it may only affect a small part of the vulva appearing to be a recurrent episode. It is sensible therefore to routinely prescribe a course of antiviral medication for five days for all patients presenting with first attack, even if the clinical suspicion is of a secondary episode.

Investigation of Choice

Culture/electron microscopy.

Immediate Management

Rule out any past history of genital herpes.

Treatment of Choice

Acyclovir 200 mg, 5 times a day for five days
\+ Analgesics
\+ bathing in salt water
\+ lignocaine gel.

Your notes:

PAPER 5

82. A 39-year gravida 3 para 2 + 0, presents at 39-weeks. Her cervix is 8 cm dilated but she complains of severe pain. Her baby is in occipitoposterior position.

Diagnosis: Occipitoposterior presentation

Preferred analgesia: Epidural anaesthesia

Clinchers

- *Gravida 3 para 2+0:* Currently pregnant, with two live births and no miscarriages.
- 73% occipitoposterior delivery will be spontaneous vaginal delivery, 22% will require forceps and 5% a caesarean section.

  In occipitoposterior deliveries, labour tends to be prolonged, because of the degree of rotation needed, so adequate hydration and analgesia (consider epidural) are important.

  During labour (occipitoposterior presentation):

- 65% rotate 130° to become occipitoanterior
- 20% rotate to transverse and then arrest (deep transverse arrest)
- 15% rotate so that occiput lies posterior, here birth is be flexion of head

CONFUSA

Pudendal block is used for instrumental delivery, but analgesia is insufficient for rotational forceps.

Epidurals may be helpful in:

- Occipitoposterior position
- Breech/multiple pregnancies
- Preterm delivery
- Pre-eclampsia
- Forceps delivery, and
- Incoordinate uterine contractions

Problems with epidural anaesthesia

- Postural hypotension
- Urinary retention (catheterize irregularly)
- Paralysis
- After delivery
  - urinary retention
  - headache.

Your notes:

85. A 31-year-old woman has a retained placenta, following a spontaneous vaginal delivery.

Diagnosis: Retained placenta

Preferred anaesthesia: General anaesthesia

Clinchers

Placenta not delivered in 30 minutes after delivery will probably not be expelled. Physiological third stage takes 30 minutes.

Danger with retained placenta is haemorrhage, therefore active intervention is required.

For manual removal, call on anaesthetist. Manual removal can be done under epidural if *in situ,* halothane assists by relaxing the uterus.

CONFUSA

Retained placenta is an emergency. Delay may precipitate postpartum haemorrhage.

Immediate Management

Set up IVI and cross match blood (24)

Treatment of Choice

Remove placenta manually. This can be done under epidural anaesthesia, if *in situ,* halothane assists by relaxing the uterus. Rarely placenta does not separate manually (placenta accreta) and hysterectomy may be necessary.

Ref page 223, Holland and Brews

Placanta Retained

- Placenta separated but retained
  - Manual removal under GA
- Morbid adhesion
  - Manual removal if separation possible
  - Hysterectomy

Your notes:

142. A 22-year-old Nigerian woman has an uneventful first pregnancy to 30 weeks. She is then admitted with epigastric pain. During the first two hours her BP rises from 150/105 to 170/120 mmHg. On dipstick test she is found to have 3+ proteinuria. The foetal cardiotocogram (CTG) is normal.

Diagnosis: Fulminating PIH.

Clinchers

- *First pregnancy:* 70% cases of pre-eclampsia occur in primigravidas. A recurrence rate of 20% is present for multigravidas (with same partner). With a new partner the incidence of recurrence increases.
- *30 weeks:* By definition PIH present for the first-time after 20 weeks.
- *Epigastric pain:* It is due to stretching of liver capsule.
- *BP rises from 150/105 to 170/120 mmHg in two hours:* A rapid rise in BP is a characteristic feature of fulminant PIH and require immediate IV antihypertensives.
- *3 + proteinuria:* It signifies significant proteinuria and hence qualifies for the diagnosis of fulminant PIH.

CTG is normal: Abnormal CTG signifies foetal distress and warrants an immediate caesarean section. In this case it is not required as CTG is normal. Still regular CTG monitoring (1 to 2 per day of one hour each) must be done.

CONFUSA

In severe (fulminating) PIH, delivery is the only definitive treatment (Note: PIH regress by delivery of placenta and not only fetus). The delivery is often vaginal, except in conditions given below where a caesarian section is preferred (A B C D E)

A—Abruption
B—BP unctrollable; breech
C—Cervix unfavourable
D—Distress of fetus
E—Error in induction of delivery (failed induction)

Note: Delivery criteria in PIH
Mild PIH—can continue till 40 weeks
Moderate PIH—can continue till 37 weeks
Severe PIH—as soon as possible
and eclampsia

Investigation of Choice
CTG (already done in this case).

Immediate Management
IV hydralazine/Labetalol.

Treatment of Choice
Intravenous antihypertensive (hydralazine/labetalol) immediately + Regular monitoring.

143. At an antenatal clinic visit at 38 weeks gestation, a 36-year-old multiparous woman has a BP of 140/90 mmHg. She has no proteinuria and is otherwise well.

Diagnosis: Normal.

Clinchers

- *38 weeks gestation:* PIH usually present in the second trimester and not this late.
- *36-year-old:* Age > 35 years (or < 20 years) is a positive risk factor for PIH/eclampsia).
- *Multiparous:* Usually multiparous females are not affected by PIH if there is no history of it in the previous pregnancies.
- *BP 140/90 mmHg:* By definition the diastolic BP has to cross 90 to qualify for a diagnosis of PIH. The classification criteria of PIH are given in next question (Q 189). This BP does not classify as a criteria for diagnosis.
- *No proteinuria:* Excludes pre-eclampsia/severe PIH.
- *Otherwise well:* Excludes other medical disorders.

CONFUSA

In cases of PIH (pregnancy induced hypertension), admit if

- BP rises by >30/20 mmHg over booking BP
- BP reaches
  - 160/100 without proteinuria
  - 140/90 with proteinuria

PIH can be diagnosed only with BP elevation above in criteria on at least 2 occasions (> 4 hours apart).

Investigation of Choice
Biweekly BP monitoring.

Immediate Management
Take second BP measurement after four hours.

Treatment of Choice
A period of observation for blood pressure.

Your notes:

144. At 32 weeks, a 22-year-old primigravida is found to have a BP of 145/100 mmHg. She has no proteinuria but is found to have oedema of her knees.

Diagnosis: Pregnancy induced hypertension (PIH).

Clinchers

- *32 weeks:* By definition PIH called so only if it appears for first-time after 20 weeks. Hypertension occurring before is usually due to an existing and non-pregnancy induced condition.
- *Primigravida:* PIH is an almost exclusive disease of primigravidas.
- *BP of 145/100 mmHg with no proteinuria:* PIH is classified according to BP and proteinuria.
  Mild PIH—BP upto 140/100 mmHg without proteinuria
  Moderate PIH—BP upto 160/110 mmHg without proteinuria
  Severe PIH—BP more than 160/110 mmHg with proteinuria
  (Proteinuria is > 300 mg excretion of proteins in urine in 24 hours).
- *Oedema of her knees:* Peripheral oedema in pregnancy has little significance if it occurs as an isolated finding. But it signifies severe PIH if it occurs along with hypertension and proteinuria.

CONFUSA

PIH is almost exclusively seen in primigravidas. But in multiparous women its risk is increased if the existing pregnancy is with a new partner. Other risk factors for PIH in multigravidas are: history of first pregnancy, H. mole, multiple pregnancy, gestational diabetes mellitus.

Investigation of Choice
Foetal USG.

Immediate Management
Admit in first instance for assessment and monitoring.

Treatment of Choice
Since the disease in question is a moderate PIH, its management is:

- Care in day assessment until/hospital
- Oral antihypertensives if—BP > 160/100 mmHg (sustained)
  Note: It is > 170/110 mmHg according to OHCS.
- Can continue upto 37 weeks with regular monitoring of:
  Daily—urinary proteins
  Bi-weekly—LFT
  Weekly—Plasma U and E, plasma urate, total urinary proteins.

Indications of delivery in moderate disease

- Progression to pre-eclampsia
- Declining maternal renal function
- Foetal distress
  - Abnormal CTG (cardiotocogram)
  - Absence of end diastolic flow in doppler of umbilical circulation
- Placental abruption.

Your notes:

145. At 34 weeks, an 86 kg woman complains of persistent headaches and 'flashing lights'. There is no hyper-reflexia and her BP is 150/100 mmHg. Urinalysis is negative but she has finger oedema.

Diagnosis: Pre-eclampsia

Clinchers

Preclampsia is a syndrome of sings and when the symptoms occurs, it is usually too late.

- *34 weeks:* It develops after 20 weeks and usually resolves within 10 days of delivery.
- *86 kg woman:* Predisposing factors of pre-eclampsia are

Maternal	*Fetal*
• Primiparity • History of severe pre-eclampsia • Positive family history • Height <155 cm • Overweight • Age < 20 or > 35 years • Pre-existing migraine • BP - or renal disease	• H mole • Multiple pregnancy • Placental hydrops (e.g. Rh disease)

- *Persisting headaches:* Frontal>occipital, reason is cerebral oedema. It is of dragging/throbbing type
  - Worsen on
    - Supine position
    - Morning
  - Resolves on—mobility
- *Flashing lights:* Visual symptoms are common in pre-eclampsia. They are due to oedema of neural layer in retina.

  The most common visual symptoms are
  - Black holes
  - Double vision
  - Flashing lights
- *No hyperreflexia:* Hyperreflexia is said to be present when a reflex can be obtained away from the tendon that usually causes it, e.g. knee reflex by tapping anterior surface of tibia (rather than the tendon). It is an important sign of impending eclampsia.
- *BP is 150/100 mmHg:* A diastolic BP exceeding 90 mmHg on at least two occasions in the second half of pregnancy, where the blood pressure was previously normal, accompanied by significant proteinuria (> 300 mg/24 h) qualifies for a diagnosis of pre-eclampsia.
- *Urinalysis negative:* It means no proteinuria. Proteinuria is the last feature of pre-eclampsia to appear. It may be trace or at times coupious. There may be few hyaline casts, epithelial cells or even few red cells. It is considered significant only when >300 mg/24 h. Proteinuria may also be missed in an isolated urinary examination, so do a 24 hours total urinary protein excretion measurement to rule it out.
- *Finger oedema:* Traditionally the presence of peripheral oedema has been included in the definition, however, this is a common finding in otherwise normal pregnancy and its absence does not preclude the diagnosis (nor does its presence makes the diagnosis). However, tightness of the ring on the finger (finger oedema) is an early manifestation of pre-eclampsia oedema. Gradually the swelling may extend to face, abdominal wall, vulva and even the whole body.

CONFUSA

In the UK, high quality antenatal care has reduced the problems of pre-eclamptic toxaemia to such an extent that 75% of cases of eclampsia now occur in the post-partum period and a similar proportion occur without pre-existing hypertension.

Investigation of Choice

24 hours urinary protein.

Immediate Management

BP control by IB hydralazine/Labetalol if there is an acute or progressive increase in BP.

Treatment of Choice

Oral antihypertensive are given in case of sustained rise of BP till > 160/100 mmHg or at lower levels if cerebral oedema is present (i.e. in this case). Antihypertensives that can be uses are;

- Methyldopa—contraindicated in liver disease
- Labetalol—contraindicated in asthma
- Magnesium sulfate—(preferred drug in USA)

Your notes:

162. A 30-year-old woman presents with a three month history of amenorrhoea.

Diagnosis: Pregnancy

Clinchers

- 30-year-old woman: Since pregnancy is the first thing to be excluded as a cause of amenorrhoea in women of the fertile age group.

CONFUSA

Pregnancy produces a physiological hypercoagulable state inspite of the haemodilution effect it produces. In the late pregnancy limited mobility and prolonged bed-rest can precipitate deep vein thrombosis.

Investigation of Choice

Urine pregnancy test

Immediate Management

Refer to a physiotherapist to teach her the required exercises

Treatment of Choice

Regular exercises.

Your notes:

PAPER 6

57. A 37-year-old woman presents with a sudden onset of severe left iliac fossa pain. On vaginal USG, 2 cm echogenic masses are seen in the broad ligament. She says this pain seems to come every month.

Diagnosis: Endometriosis

Clinchers

- *37-year-old woman:* Endometriosis is typically seen in those with postmenstrual exposure, common in fourth decade of life.
- *Severe left iliac fossa pain (comes every month):* Pelvic pain classically cyclical at the time if periods is the most common symptoms. Periods are usually heavy and frequent.
- *On USG, 2 cm echogenic masses seen in broad ligament:* Foci if endometrial tissue may be found on an ovary, rectovaginal pouch, uterosacral ligaments, surface if pelvic peritoneum, broad ligament and sometimes in distant organs like lungs.
- *On vaginal examination*
  - Fixed retroverted uterus
  - Nodules in uterosacral ligament
  - General tenderness.

Investigation of Choice

Laparoscopy shows
- Types cysts
- Peritoneal deposits

Treatment of Choice
- Danazol 400-800 mg OD
- Gestrinone 2.5-5 mg PO twice weekly
- Buserelin/goserelin (LHRH analyses)

Surgical local exicision or diathermy of endometriotic tissue or hysterectomy may depend upon site of lesion and women's with for future fertility.

Your notes:

58. A 23-year-old woman just had an intrauterine device fitted. She complains of a watery brown vaginal discharge and abdominal pain.

Diagnosis: Pelvic inflammatory disease (PID).

Clinchers

- *Intrauterine device fitted:* 10% of cases of PID follow childbirth or instrumentation (insertion of IUCD, TOP) though 90% are sexually acquired (mostly due to *Chlamydia*).
- *Watery brown vaginal discharge:* PID present with abdominal pain and vaginal discharge. Discharge is some times profuse and purulent, or it may be bloody. These is spasm of lower abdominal muscles.

In chronic cases abdominal mass may also be palpated because the inflammation leads to fibrosis, so adhesions develop between pelvic organs.

Investigation of Choice

Endocervical and urethral swabs if practicable. Always check for chlamydia. Go for blood culture if febrile.

Immediate Management

Admit for blood culture and IV antibiotics if very unwell.

Treatment of Choice

Page 50 (OHCS), 5th edn.

Your notes:

59. An 18 weeks pregnant female presents with lower abdominal pain and tenderness, with offensive vaginal discharge. She has high grade fever since last two days.

Diagnosis: Septic abortion

Clinchers

- *Lower abdominal pain:* In this question this pain may be due to pelvic infection.
- *Offensive vaginal discharge with high grade fever:* This point towards the infection (probably uterus). To support the diagnosis of septic abortion, fever more than 38°C for more than 24 hours (with or without chills and rigors) should be present. Offensive and purulent vaginal discharge support the diagnosis of infection.

Majority of infection occurs following illegal induced abortion (rare in UK) in developing Countries.

Any abortion associated with clinical evidence of infection of the uterus and it content is called septic abortion.

Investigation of Choice

Cervical or high vaginal swab for culture. Ultrasonography.

Treatment of Choice

Hospitalization. Aim at

- To control sepsis
- Remove source of infection
- Supportive therapy

Go for analgesia, sedatives and antibiotics.

Your notes:

60. A 32-year-old who conscientiously uses the oral contraceptive pill, has experienced monthly vaginal bleeding. On abdominal examination she is comfortable. Her temperature is 37°C. She is otherwise healthy.

Diagnosis: Break through bleeding.

Clinchers

- *Conscientiously uses—OCP:* It means she is a regular in taking the pills.
- *Monthly vaginal bleeding:* Menstruation is initiated by the withdrawal of oestrogen and progesterone. Such as effect is produced in women receiving oestrogens and progestogens in the form of the combined contraceptive pill or hormone replcement therapy—withdrawal bleeding on completion of a pack.
- *On abdominal examination she is comfortable:* This rules out any pelvic inflammatory disease. Otherwise also OCP use decreases the risk of PID. The only infection whose incidence is increased by using OCP is monoilial vaginitis (candidiasis).

CONFUSA

Intermenstrual spotting is common in the first three months of the start of the pills, but it gradually disappears. Heavy spotting can be stopped by increasing the dose for a few months.

Investigation of Choice
None required.

Immediate Management
Reassurance.

Treatment of Choice
None required.

Your notes:

161. An 85-year-old with 14 children,severe heart failure, complains of dysuria, feeling of pressure in lower abdomen.

Diagnosis: Genital prolapse

Clinchers

- *85-year-old:* Prolapse is more evident in older age (i.e. late after menopause) when there is general weakening and shrinking of the supports of the pelvic organs.
- *With 14 children:* Each labour increases the risk of prolapse. It is due to overstretching of the uterine supports during labour.
- *Severe heart failure:* This patient is unfit for operation on medical grounds. So pessary treatment is indicated here.
- *Dysuria:* Urinary symptoms in genital prolapse are:
  - *Frequency of* micturition is common and is often only at day time. Nocturnal frequency may be present if there is added cystitis
  - *Urgency* of micturition due to weakness of the bladder sphincter mechanism and urge incontinence may occur in some cases
  - *Difficulty in emptying:* The bladder completely
  - *Retention of urine* following urethral overstretch
  - *Stress incontinence.*
- *Feeling of pressure in lower abdomen:* A dragging sensation or bearing down in the back or lower abdomen is a common complaint in prolapse. Other associated complaints can be:
  - A feeling of fullness of vagina
  - A lump coming down

CONFUSA

Symptoms similar to those of prolapse may be caused by:

- Varicose veins of the vulva
- Haemorrhoids
- Rectal prolapse
- Cystitis
- Vaginitis with congestion of vulva
- Pressure form a large abdominal tumor

There are a few cases where a ring pessary fails to control prolapse and operation cannot be performed. In these cases use: *Cup and stem pessary.*

Investigation of Choice

- Colposcopy
- Urine microscopy and culture if UTI is also suspected

Immediate Management
Reassurance that the condition is treatable

Treatment of Choice Plastic ring pessary.

164. An 80-year-old sexually active woman with dyspareunia and recurrent dysuria.

Diagnosis: Atrophic vaginitis

Clinchers

- *80-year-old:* This condition is always seen postmenopausally because of lack of oestrogens.
- *Sexually active women:* Because of vaginal wall dryness and thinning, there can be discomfort during intercourse. If the woman would not have been sexually active, atrophic vaginitis, if mild, would have been asymptomatic.
- *Dyspareunia:* There is *superficial* dyspareunia in this condition.
- *Recurrent dysuria:* Low grade infection can coexist with atrophic vaginitis.

CONFUSA

Hormone replacement therapy postmenopausally produces withdrawal bleeds. Topical oestorgens are enough to thicken the epithelium and reduce the pH, but insufficient to produce excessive endometrial stimulation or other causes of bleeding.

Investigation of Choice
Urine culture and sensitivity

Immediate Management
Advice topical lubrication during coitus.

Treatment of Choice

- If there is secondary infection, antibiotics to which the organism is sensitive may be given
- Topical oestrogen creams or pessaries (e.g. dienoestrol or premarin (once or twice a week)

Your notes:

165. A middle-aged woman with a vaginal discharge is found to have several ulcers at the vaginal introitus.

Diagnosis: Herpes labialis

Clinchers

- *Middle-aged woman:* Herpes labialis is most common in sexually active females, so its incidence is characteristically minimal in children and elderly.
- *Vaginal discharge:* Pain, itching, dysuria, vaginal and urethral discharge, and tender inguinal lymphadenopathy are the predominant local symptoms.
- *Several ulcers of the vaginal introitus:* Widely spaced bilateral lesions of the external genitalia are characteristic. In it painful vesicles develop initially which then coalesce into multiple ulcers.

CONFUSA

First episodes of genital herpes in patients who have had prior HSV-1 infection are associated with less frequent systemic symptoms and faster healing than primary genital herpes. In primary herpes, if the case is seen very early it may only affect a small part of the vulva appearing to be a recurrent episode. It is sensible therefore to routinely prescribe a course of antiviral medication for five days for all patients presenting with first attack, even if the clinical suspicion is of a secondary episode.

Investigation of Choice
Culture/electron microscopy.

Immediate Management
Rule out any past history of genital herpes.

Treatment of Choice
Acyclovir 200 mg, 5 times a day for five days
+ Analgesics
+ bathing in salt water
+ lignocaine gel.

Your notes:

166. A 20-year-old woman who has been on oral contraceptive develops bright red postcoital bleeding (PCB).

Diagnosis: Cervical ectropion

Clinchers

- *OCP:* Ectocervix contain a transformation zone, where the stratified squamous epithelium of the vagina meets the columnar epithelium of the cervical canal. The anatomical site of this squamocolumnar junction fluctuates under hormonal influence, and the high turnover of this tissue is important in the pathogenesis of cervical carcinoma. The columnar epithelium is normally visible with the speculum during
  - Ovulatory phase of menstrual cycle
  - Pregnancy
  - OCP use
- *Postcoital bleeding:* It may give rise to postcoital bleeding, as fine blood vessels, within the columnar epithelium are easily traumatised.

CONFUSA

Cervical ectropion is sometimes termed as cervical erosion. Usually the main complaint of cervical ectropion is excessive nonpurulent discharge, as the surface area of the columnar epithelium containing mucus glands is increased. It may give rise to spotting during pregnancy in which case it is usually left untreated till after the pregnancy.

Investigation of Choice

Per speculum exam (red ring around OS because the endocervical epithelium has extended its territory over the paler epithelium of the ectocervix).

Immediate Management

Reassurance about cause and treatment.

Treatment of Choice

Usually none required.
If symptoms are distressing
- Thermal cautery (sometimes confusingly called cold coagulation).

Your notes:

167. A 55-year-old female develops a single episode of postmenopausal bleeding. She stopped menstruation 7 years ago. Ultrasound shows endometrial thickness.

Diagnosis: Endometrial carcinoma

Clinchers

- *55 years old:* It usually presents after the menopause.
- *Single episode of postmenopausal bleeding:* Any post-menopausal vaginal bleeding must be investigated as the cause may be endometrial carcinomas.
- *Stopped menstruation 7 years ago:* Occasional bleeding is common upto 1 year after menopause but not upto 7 years.
- *USG shows endometrial thickness:* This clearly suggest endometrial growth and hence indicate a need to obtain the tissue diagnosis.

CONFUSA

Postmenopausal bleeding is an early sign and generally leads a woman to see her doctor, but examination is usually normal. Endometrial carcinoma is less common than carcinoma of cervix. Most endometrial tumours are adenocarcinomas and are related to excessive exposure to oestrogens unopposed by progesterone.

Investigation of Choice

Uterine sampling or curettage

Immediate Management

Take detailed history

Treatment of Choice

- Stage I and II—total hysterectomy with bilateral salpingo-oophorectomy
- Inoperable cases—radiotherapy

168. A 49-year-old woman with complaint of hot flushes, vaginal dryness and her menstruation become irregular 5 months ago.

Diagnosis: Menopause

Clinchers

- *49-year-old:* The manopause or cessation of periods, naturally occurs about the age of 45-55 years.
- *Hot flushes, vaginal dryness:* Features of oestrogen deficiency are hot flushes (which occurs in most women and can be disabling), vaginal dryness and atrophy of the breasts. There may also be vague symptoms of loss of libido, loss of self-esteem, nonspecific, aches and pains, irritability, depression, loss of concentration and weight gain.
- *Menstruation become irregular 5 months ago:* Most women notice irregular scanty periods carrying on over a variable period, though in some sudden amenorrhoea or menorrhagia occur.

CONFUSA

Menopause may also occur surgically with radiotherapy to the ovaries and with ovarian disease (e.g. premature menopause).

Investigation of Choice

Urinary FSH concentration (-)-Just to reassure her that these are not symptoms of some pathology.

Immediate Management

Reassurance and counselling.

Treatment of Choice

Option of hormone replacement therapy

169. A 14-year-old women with painless vaginal bleeding.

Diagnosis: Menarche

Clinchers

- *14-year-old:* Menarche usually occurs at age of 11-15 years.
- *Painless vaginal bleeding:* In this age group it most commonly represents menarche though any traumatic bleed must also be excluded.

CONFUSA

In girls events of puberty start age of 9-13 years with breast bud enlargement and continues to 12-18 years. Pubic hair commences at ages 9-14 years and is completed at 12-16 years. Menarche occurs relatively late (11-15 years) but peak height velocity is reached much earlier than in boys (10-13 years). Growth is completed earlier than in boys.

Investigation of Choice

None required usually

Immediate Management

Exclude traumatic bleed

Treatment of Choice

None

PAPER 7

42. Woman history of 8/52 amenorrhoea presents with abdominal pain rigidity and is pale. Pain radiating to tip of shoulder.

Diagnosis: Ruptured ectopic pregnancy

Clinchers

- *8 weeks amenorrhoea:* Ectopic pregnancy generally presents at around 8 weeks amenorrhoea, but it may present before a period is missed.
- *Abdominal pain, rigidity, pale:* Always think of ectopic in a sexually active women with abdominal pain and bleeding. Ectopic can rupture, and cause severe pain, may radiate to tip of shoulder (diaphragmatic irritation) abdominal rigidity (peritonitis) and shock, (excessive bleeding-hence pale).

Ectopic pregnancy is one outside the uterine cavity, the most common site being the fallopian tube.

The tubal pregnancy can terminate in following ways:

- *Absorption:* Embryo dies in the tube, with a small amount of bleeding and is partly absorbed.
- *Tubal abortion:* Part or all of the products of conception are expelled from the tube, into the peritoneal cavity.
- *Tubal rupture:* Most dramatic and best known termination of tubal pregnancy (there is acute intraperitoneal haemorrhage from erosion of an artery.
- *Secondary abdominal pregnancy:* Rare outcome. Here embryo gets attached in the peritoneal cavity. (In West Indies, many cases of children delivered from the peritoneal cavity by laparotomy has been reported).

CONFUSA

Other causes of abdominal pain to be kept in mind are: perforation of peptic ulcer, sigmoid diverticulum, or the appendix, acute pancreatitis, leaking aortic aneurysm; intra-abdominal sepsis with septic shock; acute salpingitis.

Investigation of Choice

Ultrasonography

Immediate Management

Patient must be taken immediately to the operation theatre. Do not waste time in attempting resuscitation which can prove useless and only increase bleeding step up IV drip and transfuse blood immediately and the affected tube should be removed.

156. Female on OCPs complains of postcoital bleeding.

Diagnosis: Cervical ectropion

Clinchers

- *OCP:* Ectocervix contain a transformation zone, where the stratified squamous epithelium of the vagina meets the columnar epithelium of the cervical canal. The anatomical site of this squamocolumnar junction fluctuates under hormonal influence, and the high turnover of this tissue is important in the pathogenesis of cervical carcinoma. The columnar epithelium is normally visible with the speculum during
  - Ovulatory phase of menstrual cycle
  - Pregnancy
  - OCP use
- *Postcoital bleeding:* It may give rise to postcoital bleed–ing, as fine blood vessels, within the columnar epithelium are easily traumatised.

CONFUSA

Cervical ectropion is sometimes termed as cervical erosion. Usually the main complaint of cervical ectropion is excessive nonpurulent discharge, as the surface area of the columnar epithelium containing mucus glands is increased. It may give rise to spotting during pregnancy in which case it is usually left untreated till after the pregnancy.

Investigation of Choice

Per speculum exam (red ring around OS because the endocervical epithelium has extended its territory over the paler epithelium of the ectocervix).

Immediate Management

Reassurance about cause and treatment.

Treatment of Choice

Usually none required.

If symptoms are distressing

- Thermal cautery (sometimes confusingly called cold coagulation).

Your notes:

158. A 49-year-old woman with complaint of hot flushes, vaginal dryness and her menstruation become irregular 5 months ago.

Diagnosis: Menopause

Clinchers

- *49-year-old:* The menopause or cessation of periods, naturally occurs about the age of 45-55 years.
- *Hot flushes, vaginal dryness:* Features of oestrogen deficiency are hot flushes (which occur in most women and can be disabling), vaginal dryness and atrophy of the breasts. There may also be vague symptoms of loss of libido, loss of self-esteem, nonspecific, aches and pains, irritability, depression, loss of concentration and weight gain.
- *Menstruation become irregular 5 months ago:* Most women notice irregular scanty periods carrying on over a variable period, though in some sudden amenorrhoea or menorrhagia occur.

CONFUSA

Menopause may also occur surgically with radiotherapy to the ovaries and with ovarian disease (e.g. premature menopause).

Investigation of Choice

Urinary FSH concentration (-)—Just to reassure here that these are not symptoms of some pathology

Immediate Management

Reassurance and counselling

Treatment of Choice

Option of hormone replacement therapy

Your notes:

159. A 14-year-old women with painless vaginal bleeding.

Diagnosis: Menarche

Clinchers

- *14-year-old:* Menarche usually occurs at age of 11-15 years.
- *Painless vaginal bleeding:* In this age group it most commonly represent menarche though any traumatic bleed must also be excluded.

CONFUSA

In girls events of puberty start age of 9-13 years with breast bud enlargement and continues to 12-18 years. Pubic hair commences at ages 9-14 years and is completed at 12-16 years. Menarche occurs relatively late (11-15 years) but peak height velocity is reached much earlier than in boys (10-13 years). Growth is completed earlier than in boys.

Investigation of Choice

None required usually

Immediate Management

Exclude traumatic bleed

Treatment of Choice

None

Your notes:

160. A 55-year-old lady with history of intermittent postmenopausal bleeding. Vaginal and speculum examinations are normal.

Diagnosis: Endometrial carcinoma

Clinchers

- *A 55-year-old:* Mean age of presentation is 56 years. It is rare under the age of 40.
- *Intermittent postmenopausal bleeding:* This symptom should always be assumed to be caused by carcinoma of endometrium until proven otherwise.
- *Vaginal and speculum examination are normal:* This has ruled out any local cause of bleeding (e.g. vaginal trauma) so this warrants examination of the endometrium now.

CONFUSA

Endometrial carcinoma is associated with hyperestrogenic states, i.e.
- Obesity
- Diabetes
- Late menopause
- Prolonged use of unopposed oestrogens
- Oestrogen secreting tumours

Investigation of Choice

- *Screening:* Ultrasound (to assess dimensions of any tumour and to show endometrial thickness)
- *Definitive:* Uterine sampling or curettage

Immediate Management

Perform staging to decide the line of treatment.

Treatment of Choice

Usually surgical

Uterus	*Tumour*	*Surgery*
Small	Well differentiated	*Total abdominal hysterectomy* + bilateral salpingo-oophorectomy + internal iliac node frozen section biopsy
Enlarged	Confined to upper part of corpus	*Extended hysterectomy* + bilateral salpingo-oophorectomy + removal of a cuff of vagina + lymph node sampling
Cervix invaded		*Wertheim's* (Removal of upper lost half of the vagina and pelvic lymph node)

- *Radiotherapy*
  - If node is involved
  - If there is deep invasion of myometrium
- *Hormone therapy:* Progestogens inhibit the rate of growth and spread of endometrial carcinoma.

15 Oncology

PAPER 1

Serial No. 8

Subject: Medicine

Topic: Oncology

Question: A young male with recent onset seizures. Brain Biopsy performed gives a diagnosis of Glioblastoma multiforme.

Diagnosis: Glioblastoma multiforme (GBM)

Clinchers

- *Young Male:* GBM may manifest at any age, but it affects adults preferentially, with a peak incidence at 45-70 years.
- *Recent Onset seizures:* The most common mode of presentation of most intracranial space occupying lesion are headache and recent onset seizures. Nausea and vomiting and cognitive impairment due to raised intracranial tension and neurological deficits can also occur.
- *Glioblastoma Multiforme:* The histopathology of glioblastoma multiforme is extremely variable. These are composed of poorly differentiated, often pleomorphic astrocytic cells with marked nuclear atypia and brisk mitotic activity. Necrosis is an essential diagnostic feature, and prominent microvascular proliferation is common. Macroscopically, glioblastomas are poorly delineated, with peripheral grayish tumour cells, central yellowish necrosis from myelin breakdown, and multiple areas of old and recent haemorrhages. Most glioblastomas of the cerebral hemispheres are clearly intraparenchymal with an epicenter in the white matter.

CONFUSA

- On CT scans, glioblastomas usually appear as irregularly shaped hypodense (NOT hyperdense; its because of central necrosis) lesions with a peripheral ringlike zone of contrast enhancement surrounded by an area of cerebral oedema.
- Despite the short duration of symptoms, these tumours often are surprisingly large at the time of presentation, occupying much of a cerebral lobe.
- Glial fibrillary acidic protein (GFAP) is the most valuable marker for neoplastic astrocytes.

Investigation of Choice

MRI with and without contrast is the study of choice. These lesions typically have an enhancing ring and a broad surrounding zone of oedema.

The central hypodense core represents necrosis, the contrast-enhancing ring is composed of highly dense neoplastic cells with abnormal vessels permeable to contrast agents, and the peripheral zone of nonenhancing low attenuation is vasogenic oedema containing varying numbers of invasive tumour cells.

Immediate Management

For seizures, the patient usually is started on phenytoin or carbamazepine .

Vasogenic cerebral oedema typically is managed with dexamethasone, usually in combination with some form of antiulcer agent .

Treatment of Choice

The treatment of patients with malignant gliomas is mainly palliative and encompasses surgery, radiotherapy, and chemotherapy.

Radiation therapy in addition to surgery has been shown to prolong survival in patients with glioblastoma multiforme compared to surgery alone.

Carmustine and cisplatin have been the primary chemotherapeutic agents used against malignant gliomas.

Because these tumours cannot be cured with surgery, the surgical goals are to establish a pathological diagnosis, relieve mass effect, and, if possible, achieve a gross total resection to facilitate adjuvant therapy.

Stereotactic biopsy followed by radiation therapy may be considered in certain circumstances.

According to recent NICE guidelines, treatment with temozolamide should be considered in patients with recurrent malignant glioma who have failed first-line chemotherapy treatment with other agents (either because of lack of efficacy or because of side effects).

Your notes:

Serial No. 94

Subject: Surgery

Topic: Bladder

Question: A 67-year-old man with painless haematuria.

Diagnosis: Carcinoma bladder

Clinchers

- *67-year-old man:* Carcinoma bladder is more common in males with male-to-female ratio of 3: 1. However, women generally have a worse prognosis than men. The median age at diagnosis is 68 years, and the incidence increases directly with age.
- *Painless haematuria:* Bladder cancer classically presents as total, gross, painless haematuria. Consider all patients with gross haematuria to have bladder cancer, until proven otherwise.

CONFUSA

- Both microscopic and macroscopic haematuria, when caused by a urothelial cancer are intermittent. Therefore repeat urine testing can be negative for haematuria in the presence of a tumour.
- 90% of bladder cancers are transitional cell carcinomas; Squamous cell carcinomas are typically associated with *Schistosoma haematobium infestation.*
- Epidemiologic data present a strong link between bladder cancer and environmental exposures (smoking, aromatic dyes, drugs, schistosomiasis and more), suggesting that bladder cancer is a potentially preventable disease.

Investigation of Choice

Diagnostic cystoscopy with biopsy is the most important procedure.

Further staging investigations may be necessary: CT, chest X-ray, and possibly MRI and/or bone scan

Immediate Management

Stage the disease (TNM Staging):

Tumor:

- Tis: carcinoma *in situ*
- T1: no palpable tumour:
  - pTa: tumour confined to epithelium
  - pT1: invasion of subepithelial connective tissue
- T2: no mass or thickening palpable:
  - pT2: invasion of superficial bladder muscle
- T3: palpable hard, mobile mass:
  - pT3a: invasion of deep muscle (outer half)
  - pT3b: invasion beyond bladder wall:
    - pT3bI: microscopically
    - pT3bII: macroscopically
- T4: palpable hard, fixed mass:
  - pT4a: invasion of prostate, uterus, vagina
  - pT4b: invasion of pelvic wall, abdominal wall

Nodes:

- No - no nodal involvement
- N1 - single ipsilateral regional node
- N2 - contralateral or multiple regional nodes
- N3 - fixed regional nodes
- N4 - extra-regional nodes
- Nx - nodal status not known

Metastases:

- M0 - no metastases evident
- M1 - metastases present
- Mx - metastatic status not known

Treatment of Choice

pTa and pT1

Treated mainly by transurethral resection.

Intravesical cytotoxic chemotherapy using agents such as thiotepa, mitomycin, doxorubicin, and epirubicin, may be given as adjuvant therapy, as they reduce the multiplicity and frequency of recurrence.

Intravesical BCG immunotherapy may be required for carcinoma in situ and pT1G3 cancer.

In all cases, regular endoscopic follow up is essential.

T2

External radiotherapy or less commonly in the UK, by cystectomy.

Life-long endoscopic follow-up is indicated. If tumour is present in the bladder 6 months after radiotherapy, or recurs, treatment by total cystectomy with urinary diversion is indicated.

T3

External radiotherapy is the Treatment of Choice for T3 bladder cancer as complete resection carries the risk of bladder perforation.

T4

Palliative radiotherapy only can be offered to control pain and haematuria with T4 staged bladder cancer.

Your notes:

Serial No. 117

Subject: Surgery

Topic: Infectious Diseases

Question: A-40-year old lady from Asia with lumps in her neck, FNAC of which revealed centre of casseous material with graulomas, surrounded by fibrosis.

Diagnosis: Tuberculous lymphadenopathy

Clinchers

- *40-year-old lady:* Tuberculosis more commonly flares up in elderly, however, it can affect almost any age. Female: Male ratio is 2: 1 It is commoner amongst the homeless, drug addicts and alcoholics.
- *From Asia:* Countries of Asia such as India, China, Indonesia, Pakistan and Bangladesh have the largest number of cases. Recently there have been striking increases in the number of cases in the former Soviet Union and in sub-Saharan Africa also. Migration from these highly endemic area predisposes an individual for infection.
- *With lumps in her neck:* Cervical tuberculous lymphadenitis or scrofula classically presents as painless enlarging persistent mass in the neck. Associated systemic symptoms like low grade fever, weight loss and malaise can also be present.
- *FNAC of which revealed centre of casseous material with graunolmas. surrounded by fibrosis:* This is the classical description of infection by tuberculosis.Caseating granulomas are almost diagnostic, however, demostration of acid fast bacilli (AFB) is required for a definitive diagnosis.

CONFUSA

- As TB is an AIDS-defining illness, current guidelines state that it may be appropriate to offer HIV testing to patients if they are from an area or background with increased risk of HIV co-infection.
- Note that lymphoma can also present as cervical lymphadenopathy, low grade fever and weight loss. Histological diagnosis would be definitive.
- In the developed world, the disease is more common in some sections of society eg alcoholics, undernourished, ethnic communities, the elderly, and HIV+ve individuals.
- The disease is also more common in patients after gastrectomy for peptic ulcer

Investigation of Choice

Excision biopsy

Immediate Management

- All patients should be referred for specialist advice and management usually involving a team approach including Consultant and specialist nurses.
- Disease Notification is compulsory under the Public Health Act 1984. This will trigger contact tracing and provide surveillance data. Usually this is initiated by the Specialist or doctor initiating treatment.

Treatment of Choice

Antituberculous therapy

Your notes:

Serial No. 118

Subject: Surgery

Topic: GIT

Question: A 60-year-old man with a lump in supra-clavicular region and decreased appetite. He has lost 5 kg weight recently.

Diagnosis: Carcinoma Stomach

Clinchers

- *A 60-year-old man:* The incidence of carcinoma stomach in England and Wales for men is 20 per 100,000, and for women 7 per 100 000. 99% of cases of upper gastrointestinal cancer (oesophagus, stomach, pancreas) occur over in patients over 40 years old and over 90% of gastric cancers occur in patients over 55 years old. The risk of carcinoma stomach in those below 55 years is extremely low.
- *Lump in supra-clavicular region:* The enlarged left supraclavicular node in cases of carcinoma stomach is known as Virchow's node and the sign is called Troisier's sign. This is the sign of advanced disease and inoperability.
- *Decreased appetite, lost 5 kg weight recently:* This is the most common presenting symptoms, with more than 95% patients presenting with anorexia and weight loss. Dyspepsia and anaemia are among other common symptoms.

CONFUSA

- For any patient above 55 years, with dyspeptic symptoms, endoscopy is essential before starting on anti secretory drugs. Proton pump inhibitors may appear to heal malignant ulcers thus delaying the diagnosis or result in a misdiagnosis on first endoscopy.
- Again, all gastric ulcers should be biopsied as most mimic benign ulcers with even positive response to anti secretory treatment.
- Sister Joseph Nodule is a metastatic tumour deposit in the umbilicus, the anatomical region where the peritoneum is closest to the skin. It is rare, but its presence signifies inoperability.

Investigation of Choice

Endoscopy and biopsy

CT/ MRI required for staging

Immediate Management

Stage the disease.

TNM staging (carcinoma stomach)

T0	No evidence of primary tumour
Tis	Carcinoma *in situ* (intraepithelial)
T1	Invades lamina propira or submucosa
T2	Invades muscularis propria or suberosa (not visceral peritoneum)
T3	Penetrates visceral peritoneum but not adjacent structures
T4	Invades adjacent structures (spleen, colon etc)
N0	No LN metastasis
N1	1-6 lymph nodes
N2	7-15 lymph nodes
N3	more than 15 lymph nodes
M0	No distant metastasis
M1	Distant metastasis, in portal LN, mesenteric, retroperitoneal distant

TX, NX or MX indicates "not assessed"

STAGE OF DISEASE

Stage I—	T1N0M0	T1N1M0	T2N0M0
Stage II—	T1N2M0	T2N1M0	T3N0M0
Stage III—	T2N2M0	T3N1M0	T4N0M0
Stage IV—	T3N2M0	T4N1M0	

Treatment of Choice

Surgery is the treatment of choice for gastric cancer. Distal (antral) tumours should be treated by subtotal gastrectomy and proximal tumours by total gastrectomy.

Your notes:

Serial No. 119

Subject: Surgery

Topic: Thyroid

Question: A man comes with a lump in front of his neck which moves up on swallowing. Scan shows a mass replacing the left lobe of thyroid and spreading to sternomastoid and adjacent muscles.

Diagnosis: Thyroid Carcinoma

Clinchers

- *A man:* Thyroid carcinoma is more common in women than men especially in the women of reproductive age group. However, in solitary thyroid nodules, cancer risk is more in males.The risk of malignancy rises with age.
- *Lump in front of his neck which moves up on swallowing:* Lump in front of neck which rises on swallowing is the characteristic description of a mass attached to the thyroid. Most closest differential being thyroglossal cyst.
- *A mass replacing the left lobe of thyroid:* This signify that the mass is arising from the left lobe of thyroid.
- *Spreading to sternomastoid and adjacent muscles:* This signifies the malignant nature of the mass as it has infiltrated the adjacent muscles.

CONFUSA

- A slow growing thyroid tumour with lymphatic metastasis is usually Papillary carcinoma (Most common, best prognosis).
- For patients with features of phaeochromocytoma, a thyroid mass usually signify medullary carcinoma (MEN 2A or MEN 2B syndrome).
- Thyroid tumours with pulsating bony metastasis is usually follicular carcinoma.
- Rapidly expanding thyroid mass with local pressure effects can be either lymphoma or anaplastic carcinoma.

Investigation of Choice

FNAC most useful

Immediate Management

refer for expert opinion

Treatment of Choice

Most thyroid tumours are treated surgically with follow up radioiodine ablation if the tumour will concentrate I-131.

Serial No. 121

Subject: Medicine

Topic: Chest

Question: A shipyard worker develops shortness of breath and a lump in his supraclavicular fossa.There is a small pleural effusion noted on the same side of the lump.

Diagnosis: Mesothelioma

Clinchers

- *A shipyard worker:* Asbestosis and the associated mesothelioma is an industrial disease, Most commonly seen in those who have worked in construction and ship repair but also seen in other trades brining regular exposure to asbestos such as laggers and plumbers.
- *Shortness of breath:* Asbestos exposure most commonly causes pleural mesothelioma (rarely, peritoneal mesothelioma). The effection of pleura causes thickening and the patient most commonly presents with shortness of breath which is usually progressive.
- *A lump in his supraclavicular fossa:* This signify the metastasis and secondary enlargement of supracalvicular lymph nodes.
- *Small pleural effusion noted on the same side of the lump:* Unilateral pleural effusion is almost always a constant finding.

CONFUSA

- The fullness in the neck can be mistaken for Pancoast's Tumour and students may get wrongly illusioned towards carcinoma lung as the most probable diagnosis for such a presentation, as above.
- However, do not forget that Pancoast's tumour is usally associated with pain in the inner surface of the arm and the fourth and fifth fingers (ulnar distribution) and paralysis and wasting of the muscles of the hand and forearm.
- Morever, for it to be lung carcinoma, question should have given hints on the smoking history than occupational exposure to asbestos.

Investigation of Choice

Pleural biopsy required for a definitive diagnosis.
Chest radiography/CT shows a pleural thickening and an associated pleural effusion.

Immediate Management

Stage the disease

Staging of Mesothelioma

Stage I: Disease confined inside the capsule of the parietal pleura: ipsilateral pleura, lung, pericardium, and diaphragm.

Stage II: As described for stage I with intrathoracic (N1 or N2) lymph nodes.

Stage III: This signifies local extension of disease into the following: chest wall or mediastinum; heart or through the diaphram, peritoneum; with or without extra-thoracic or contralateral (N3) lymph node involvement.

Stage IV: Distant metastases.

Treatment of Choice

- Usually only symptomatic treatment is possible.
- Curative surgical treatment may be possible with stage 1 disease.
- Extrapleural pneumonectomy may be used to lengthen time of recurrence.
- Pleurectomy and decortication is used for palliative pain relief and recurrent pleural effusions.
- No evidence that radiotherapy or chemotherapy improves survival.
- Radiotherapy may help with pain management.

Your notes:

Serial No. 131

Subject: Medicine

Topic: Arrhythmias

Question: A woman experiences 'thumping' in her chest associated with breathlessness, while asleep. She sits up to get symptoms resolve in few minutes time.

Diagnosis: Atrial myxoma

Clinchers

- *A woman:* Atrial myxomas predominantly occur in females, with more than 75% sporadic cases seen females. The usual age of presentation is anywhere between 3 and 86 years, however, highest incidence is observed around 40-60 years.
- *'Thumping', with breathlessness, while asleep:* The most common symptom patients present with is dyspnoea, whether exertional, nocturnal or posture specific.
- *She sits up to get symptoms resolve in few minutes time:* This appears to be most typical of atrial myxoma, as the tumour obstructing the outflow tract of heart (usually left sided) can cause increase severity of symptoms. As soon as the patient gets up to assume an erect posture, the obstruction is relieved and the symptoms resolve out.

CONFUSA

The symptoms of atrial myxoma can vary from totally symptom free to sudden death. Patient may present with unusual palpitations or features of right/left heart failure, which usually resolve by the changing postures (until and unless the tumour is too large). It can also present with features of thromboembolism, dizziness or syncope. Constitutional symptoms like fever, weight loss, arthralgias, and Raynaud phenomenon are observed in 50% of patients.

Investigation of Choice

ECHO – Transthoracic or Transesophageal

Immediate Management

Consult expert advice

Treatment of Choice

Surgical Resection

Your notes:

Serial No. 146

Subject: Medicine

Topic: Gastro

Question: A 55-year-old man with epigastric pain and haematemesis. Endoscopy confirms adenocarcinoma stomach.

Diagnosis: Carcinoma stomach

Clinchers

- *55-year-old man:* The incidence of carcinoma stomach in England and Wales for men is 20 per 100,000, and for women 7 per 100 000. 99% of cases of upper gastrointestinal cancer (oesophagus, stomach, pancreas) occur over in patients over 40 years old and over 90% of gastric cancers occur in patients over 55 years old. The risk of carcinoma stomach in those below 55 years is extremely low.
- *Epigastric pain and haematemesis* The is most common presenting symptoms, with more than 95% patients, are anorexia and weight loss. Dyspepsia and anaemia are among other common symptoms. Hematemesis and an upper abdominal mass is observed in advanced cases.
- *Endoscopy confirms adenocarcinoma stomach:* 95% of gastric carcinomas are adenocarcinomas, with around 64% of carcinomas located in the prepyloric region.

CONFUSA

- For any patient above 55 years, with dyspeptic symptoms, endoscopy is essential before starting on anti secretory drugs. Proton pump inhibitors may appear to heal malignant ulcers thus delaying the diagnosis or result in a misdiagnosis on first endoscopy.
- Again, all gastric ulcers should be biopsied as most mimic benign ulcers with even positive response to anti secretory treatment.
- Sister Joseph Nodule is a metastatic tumour deposit in the umbilicus, the anatomical region where the peritoneum is closest to the skin. It is rare, but its presence signifies inoperability.

Investigation of Choice

Endoscopy and biopsy
CT/ MRI required for staging

Immediate Management

Stage the disease.

TNM staging (carcinoma stomach)

T0	No evidence of primary tumour
Tis	Carcinoma in situ (intraepithelial)
T1	Invades lamina propira or submucosa
T2	Invades muscularis propria or suberosa (not visceral peritoneum)
T3	Penetrates visceral peritoneum but not adjacent structures
T4	Invades adjacent structures (spleen, colon etc)
N0	No LN metastasis
N1	1-6 lymph nodes
N2	7-15 lymph nodes
N3	more than 15 lymph nodes
M0	No distant metastasis
M1	Distant metastasis, in portal LN, mesenteric, retroperitoneal distant

TX, NX or MX indicates "not assessed"

STAGE OF DISEASE

Stage I—	T1N0M0	T1N1M0	T2N0M0
Stage II—	T1N2M0	T2N1M0	T3N0M0
Stage III—	T2N2M0	T3N1M0	T4N0M0
Stage IV—	T3N2M0	T4N1M0	

Treatment of Choice

Surgery is the Treatment of Choice for gastric cancer. Distal (antral) tumours should be treated by subtotal gastrectomy and proximal tumours by total gastrectomy.

Your notes:

Serial No. 147

Subject: Gynaecology

Topic: Gynaecological malignancy

Question: A 46-year-old lady with family history of ovarian carcinoma. Pelvic USG fails to reveal any abnormality.

Diagnosis: Carcinoma Ovary (suspected)

Clinchers

- *46-year-old lady:* Ovarian carcinoma most commonly present between 3rd and 8th decades with peak incidence at 58 years.
- *Family history of ovarian carcinoma:* Family history is one most important factor which puts the patient in the high risk group and the need for screening in such cases with the aim of early diagnosis.
- *Pelvic USG fails to reveal any abnormality:* Pelvic ultrasound is useful only when the suspected carcinoma has produced has a mass large enough to be caught by the USG.

CONFUSA

Family risk of ovarian cancer:
- woman with a mother with ovarian cancer - relative risk = 6
- woman with a sister with ovarian cancer - relative risk = 3.8
- woman with a daughter with ovarian cancer - relative risk = 1.1
- if a woman has two close relatives with ovarian cancer then her risk of developing ovarian cancer is approximately 40%

Investigation of Choice

Serum CA-125 antigen >35IU/ml is suggestive of early ovarian carcinoma in high-risk cases.

Ultrasound is of use only when the carcinoma has advanced to such a stage, which produces an evident mass in the pelvis.

Look for BRCA1 or BRCA2, if such genes were identified in the effected relatives.

Immediate Management

Refer to oncology unit or gynaecological cancer unit if tests found positive.

Treatment of Choice

If positive -Total abdominal hysterectomy with bilateral salpingoophorectomy.
If negative- Reassurance

Serial No. 148

Subject: Gynaecology

Topic: Gynaecology malignancy

Question: A lady had undergone total abdominal hysterectomy with bilateral salpingo-oophorectomy and omentectomy for carcinoma ovary, now comes for follow up. Her CA 125 had come to normal levels after surgery.

Diagnosis: Ca ovary (follow up)

Clinchers

- *Total abdominal hysterectomy with bilateral salpingo-oophorectomy:* This is the standard procedure of surgical management of ovarian carcinoma, leaving apart those grossly advanced stages where only debulking surgery can be possible.
- *Omentectomy:* The total abdominal hysterectomy with bilateral salpingo-ophorectomy is usually combined with infracolic omentectomy, with thorough examination of all serosal surfaces and biopsing any doubtful lesions. This is necessary for staging of the disease, and positive biopsy may require a further debulking surgery.
- *For follow-up:* Continuous follow-up is essential for all ovarian cancer patients. This includes patients whose disease is in remission after treatment. Although most women who develop a recurrence do so within the first 2 years after treatment, ovarian cancer can reappear up to 20 years later.
- *CA 125 had come to normal levels after surgery:* This denotes that complete resection of the tumor was obtained.

CONFUSA

- CA-125 determine the activity of the cancer.
- If the CA125 level is increased during the follow up visits, a CT scan, biopsy, and peritoneal lavage may be required to locate the new cancer site.
- Recurrent cancer may require additional chemotherapy and, possibly, secondary debulking surgery

Investigation of Choice

CA-125 levels

Immediate Management

If levels doubled or more than 35IU/L, further investigations are required. (see confusa above).

Treatment of Choice

Recurrent cancer may require additional chemotherapy and, possibly, secondary debulking surgery.

Serial No. 150

Subject: Gynaecology

Topic: Gynaecological malignancy

Question: A lady with history of treated ovarian carcinoma, attends clinic to rule out recurrence.

Diagnosis: Carcinoma ovary (follow up)

Clinchers

- *History of treated ovarian carcinoma:* Total abdominal hysterectomy with bilateral salpingoophorectomy is the standard procedure of surgical management of ovarian carcinoma. This is usually combined with infracolic omentectomy, with thorough examination of all serosal surfaces and biopsing any doubtful lesions. This is necessary for staging of the disease, and positive biopsy may require a further debulking surgery.
- *Attends clinic to rule out recurrence:* Continuous follow-up is essential for all ovarian cancer patients. This includes patients whose disease is in remission after treatment. Although most women who develop a recurrence do so within the first 2 years after treatment, ovarian cancer can reappear up to 20 years later.

CONFUSA

- Post surgical status of CA 125 should to be obtained, to make it an efficient tool in monitoring recurrence. A single measurement of CA 125 is not useful as it can be elevated due to various other causes than just recurrence. Doubling of CA 125 levels after surgery or persistent high values suggest recurrence or incomplete removal. Hence, stressing the value of serial measurment of CA 125.

Investigation of Choice

CA-125 levels

CT scan is indicated if previous CA 125 levels are not known.

Immediate Management

If levels doubled or more than 35 IU/L, further investigations are required.

Treatment of Choice

Recurrent cancer may require additional chemotherapy and, possibly, secondary debulking surgery.

Your notes:

Serial No. 155

Subject: Medicine

Topic: Gastro

Question: A 46-year-old man with recent change of bowel habits, weight loss and occult blood in stools positive.

Diagnosis: Carcinoma Caecum

Clinchers

- *46-year-old man:* Right sided colon carcinoma involving caecum, more commonly effects women and those above 40 years of age.
- *Recent change of bowel habits:* Change in bowel habit can occur in the form of diarrhoea or constipation, but this is more classically observed in the growth involving the left colon.
- *Weight loss:* The right sided growth usually present late, most commonly detected during investigation for unusual weight loss or severe anaemia.
- *Occult blood in stools positive:* Occult bleeding is more common for the right sided growth than the left sided growth which generally presents as frank rectal bleeding.

CONFUSA

Often it is difficult to differentiate between rectal carcinoma and carcinoma ceacum. While both can present with weight loss and iron deficiency anaemia, rectal carcinoma will have typical 'rectal' symptoms associated like, tenesmus, colicky pain, frank rectal bleeding and an early change in bowel habit.

Carcinoma caecum is usually silent for long and present with vague symptoms of fatigue, weight loss associated with positive occult blood in stools. Bowel habits change quite late.

Investigation of Choice

Barium enema for screening

Colonoscopy is the gold standard for diagnosis

Immediate Management

Refer immediately, anyone of over 50 years of age with any of the following symptoms over a period of six weeks:

- Rectal bleeding with a change in bowel habit to looseness or increased frequency.
- Rectal bleeding without anal symptoms.
- Palpable abdominal or rectal mass.
- Intestinal obstruction.

All patients with iron-deficiency anaemia without other obvious cause should be thoroughly investigated for colorectal cancer.

Treatment of Choice

Right hemicolectomy

NICE has recommended that open rather than laparoscopic surgery should be used for the treatment of colorectal cancer and laparoscopic surgery should be restricted to randomised controlled clinical trials.

Your notes:

Serial No. 157

Subject: Medicine

Topic: Gastro

Question: A 42-year-old man with recent change in bowel habits, tenesmus and bloody stools. Sigmoidoscopy shows ulcerative mass in rectum.

Diagnosis: Carcinoma rectum

Clinchers

- *42-year-old man:* Most patients with rectal carcinoma are above 40 years with men slightly more commonly affected than women. (Compare with right sided growths, which is more common in women).
- *Recent change in bowel habits:* Change in bowel habit can occur in the form of diarrhoea or constipation, is more classically observed in the growth involving the left colon than right colon. The change in bowel habits occur due to obstruction. Initially there is constipation, due to the obstructed passage at the tumour site, which then liquefies and accompany with large amount of mucous, which the patient describes as early morning spurious diarrhoea, which is difficult to hold.
- *Tenesmus and bloody stools:* These are typical 'rectal' symptoms occur due to the mass irritating the rectal mucosa.
- *Sigmoidoscopy shows ulcerative mass in rectum:* This is the typical macroscopic appearance of the growth, most being ulcerated because of repeated impaction with the fecal matter.

CONFUSA

Solitary rectal ulcer is one diagnosis, which can grossly confuse the picture of carcinoma rectum. It also presents with constipation, blood and mucus from rectum, change in bowel habits. However, pain and long history of constipation is the most characteristic feature. Sigmoidoscopy shows well-demarcated irregular ulcer, more commonly on the anterior wall. Again the solitary ulcer of rectum presents early (20-30 years of age) and more common in women.

The absence of history of long standing constipation and older age of the patient in the question, suggests more towards the diagnosis of carcinoma rectum than solitary ulcer of rectum.

Investigation of Choice

Sigmoidoscopy and biopsy

Immediate Management

Patients presenting with acute obstruction need require immediate surgery with relief of obstruction and a colostomy.

Treatment of Choice

- Local resection is indiacted if the patient is too old or frail to withstand a major operation.
- Anterior resection of rectum is indicated for growths more than 10 cm from the anal verge but below the recto-sigmoid junction.
- Abdomino-perineal resection of rectum is indicated for growths less than 10 cm from the anal verge.
- Hartmann's procedure is required if the tumour is unresectable.

Your notes:

Serial No. 169

Subject: Medicine

Topic: Chest

Question: A 40-year-old chronic smoker presents with chest pain, hemoptysis and headache.

Diagnosis: Carcinoma lung (with cerebral metastasis)

Clinchers

- *40-year-old:* Lung cancer is the most common cause of cancer death for men, who account for 60% of lung cancer cases. In women, lung cancer is the second most common cause of cancer death after breast cancer. Peak incidence is in sixth decade in males and seventh decade in females.
- *Chronic smoker:* Smoking is the most important factor associated with the occurrence of lung cancer present in about 90% cases. The second most important factor associated is occupational exposire to asbestos.
- *Chest pain, hemoptysis:* Cough and hemoptysis are the most common presenting complaints and usually denote a luminal mass. Involvement of pleura causes chest pain, while involvement of mediastinum is usually associated with dyspnoea.
- *Headache:* This is suggesting intracranial metastasis, brain being included among the common sites of extra-thoacic metastasis. Other common sites for metastasis are hilar lymph nodes, liver, bones and adrenals.

CONFUSA

Cough and hemoptysis are also common presenting symptoms of tuberculosis, which is again associated with weight loss and fatigue. However, cough in tuberculosis is usually productive compared to that seen in carcinoma, which is dry and irritating. Again, travel history (to or from an endemic area) is an important point to distinguish as tuberculosis is not a common disease in UK.

Investigation of Choice

Screening: Chest X ray

Definitive Diagnosis: Bronchoscopy with biopsy

Staging: CT scan

Immediate Management

Immediate referral for expert advise

Treatment of Choice

NICE has recommended following treatment protocol for lung carcinoma:

- *Surgical treatment*
  Lobectomy is the procedure of choice for for Stages I and II; limited resection or radical radiotherapy should be considered for those who cannot tolerate lobectomy because of pulmonary compromise.
  Complete resection of the tumour is recommended for Stages II and III.
- *Radical Radiotherapy*
  Indicated for patients with stage I, II or III NSCLC with have good performance status
- *Chemotherapy*
  Indicated for patients with NSCLC (stages III and IV). A single third-generation drug (docetaxel, gemcitabine, paclitaxel or vinorelbine), is usually combined with a platinum drug – carboplatin or cisplatin. Single-agent chemotherapy with a third-generation drug can be offered to patients who cannot tolerate a platinum combination.

Note: Small cell lung carcinomas (SCLC) metastasise early so surgical treatment is not indicated. In this case radiotherapy and combination chemotherapy is tried.

Your notes:

PAPER 2

Serial No. 7

Subject: Medicine

Topic: Renal

Question: A 62-year-old man with recurrent painless hematuria and loss of weight.

Diagnosis: Carcinoma bladder

Clinchers

- *62-year-old man:* Carcinoma bladder is more common in males with male-to-female ratio of 3: 1. However, women generally have a worse prognosis than men. The median age at diagnosis is 68 years, and the incidence increases directly with age.
- *Recurrent painless haematuria:* Bladder cancer classically presents as total, gross, painless haematuria. Consider all patients with gross haematuria to have bladder cancer, until proven otherwise.
- *Loss of weight:* Loss of weight occurs as the most common paraneoplastic syndrome associated with most malignancies, and is again going in favour of diagnosis of carcinoma bladder in this setting.

CONFUSA

Both microscopic and macroscopic haematuria, when caused by a urothelial cancer are intermittent. Therefore repeat urine testing can be negative for haematuria in the presence of a tumour. 90% of bladder cancers are transitional cell carcinomas; Squamous cell carcinomas are typically associated with Schistosoma haematobium infestation. Epidemiologic data present a strong link between bladder cancer and environmental exposures (smoking, aromatic dyes, drugs, schistosomiasis and more), suggesting that bladder cancer is a potentially preventable disease.

Investigation of Choice

Diagnostic cystoscopy with biopsy is the most important procedure.

Further staging investigations may be necessary: CT, chest X-ray, and possibly MRI and/or bone scan

Immediate Management

Stage the disease (TNM Staging):

Tumour:

Tis : carcinoma *in situ*

T1 : no palpable tumour
pTa : tumour confined to epithelium

pT1 : invasion of subepithelial connective tissue
T2 : no mass or thickening palpable :
pT2 : invasion of superficial bladder muscle

T3 : palpable hard, mobile mass :
pT3a : invasion of deep muscle (outer half)
pT3b : invasion beyond bladder wall :
pT3bI : microscopically
pT3bII : macroscopically

T4 : palpable hard, fixed mass :
pT4a : invasion of prostate, uterus, vagina
pT4b : invasion of pelvic wall, abdominal wall

Nodes:

No - no nodal involvement
N1 - single ipsilateral regional node
N2 - contralateral or multiple regional nodes
N3 - fixed regional nodes
N4 - extra-regional nodes
Nx - nodal status not known

Metastases:

M0 - no metastases evident
M1 - metastases present
Mx - metastatic status not known

Treatment of Choice

pTa and pT1

Treated mainly by transurethral resection.

Intravesical cytotoxic chemotherapy using agents such as thiotepa, mitomycin, doxorubicin, and epirubicin, may be given as adjuvant therapy, as they reduce the multiplicity and frequency of recurrence.

Intravesical BCG immunotherapy may be required for carcinoma *in situ* and pT1G3 cancer.

In all cases, regular endoscopic follow-up is essential.

T2

External radiotherapy or less commonly in the UK, by cystectomy.

Life-long endoscopic follow-up is indicated. If tumour is present in the bladder 6 months after radiotherapy, or recurs, treatment by total cystectomy with urinary diversion is indicated.

T3

External radiotherapy is the Treatment of Choice for T3 bladder cancer as complete resection carries the risk of bladder perforation.

T4

Palliative radiotherapy only can be offered to control pain and haematuria with T4 staged bladder cancer.

Your notes:

Serial No. 9

Subject: Medicine

Topic: Renal

Question: A 42-year-old man presents with flank pain and gross haematuria. His left flank appears full.

Diagnosis: Renal cell carcinoma

Clinchers

- *42-year-old:* Renal cell carcinoma is more common in incidence after 40 years of age with a peak around the sixth decade. It is twice as common in men than women. It accounts for 2% of all cancers in the UK
- Flank pain, gross haemturia, left flank full: This is the classical triad of renal cell carcinoma-haematuria, flank pain and palpable flank mass. The complete triad of features is present in 10-15% cases.

CONFUSA

A number of paraneoplastic syndromes are associated with renal cell carcinoma:
- Polycythaemia - due to secretion of erythropoietin
- Hypercalcaemia - due to secretion of PTH related peptide
- Hypertension - due to secretion of renin
- Neuromyopathy
- Feminising/masculinising syndromes

Investigation of Choice

Screening - Intravenous urography
Staging- CT scan

Immediate Management

Urgent referral

Stage the disease:

TNM Staging:

T1 - Tumour confined to the capsule
T2 - Tumour with calyceal deformity
T3a -Tumour extension to perirenal fat or ipsilateral adrenal gland
T3b- Tumour extension to renal vein
T3c- Tumour extension to inferior vena
T4a- Tumour extension to neighbouring organs
T4b- Tumour extension to inferior vena cava (above diaphragm)
N1-N4- Lymphatic involvement
M1-Distant metastases

Treatment of Choice

Nephrectomy is the Treatment of Choice for renal adenocarcinoma in the absence of distant metastases. Can be combined with Post-operative radiotherapy, chemotherapy or hormonal therapy (with medroxy-progesterone acetate).

Your notes:

Serial No. 97

Subject: Urogenital

Topic: Prostate

Question: A 60-year-old man with complaints of frequency and dysuria. PSA is 120 ng/ml. He also has back pain.

Diagnosis: Carcinoma prostate

Clinchers

- *60-year-old man:* Prostatic carcinoma is the second most common cancer in men in the UK, with the peak of presentation between 65 and 85 years of age.
- *Frequency and dysuria:* Most cases of carcinoma prostate present with symptoms signifying bladder outlet obstruction like hesitancy, or acute retention, urgency, frequency or dribbling.
- *PSA is 120 ng/ml:* Prostate-specific antigen (PSA) is a serine protease which is usually specifically expressed in the prostate, and thus is an useful tumour marker. A PSA of more than 4 ng/ml in a 60-year-old should initiate investigation for carcinoma prostate. A PSA of more than 100 signifies metastatic spread of the disease.
- *Back pain:* This is again pointing towards the metastatic spread of the cancer to the bones.

CONFUSA

Levels of Prostate Specific Antigen (PSA) change with age. The following cut-off levels indicates further investigation:

AGE (YEARS)	PSA CUT OFF (ng/ml)
50-59	>=3.0
60-69	>=4.0
70 and over	>5.0

Investigation of Choice

Screening: PSA

Definitive: Transrectal ultrasound of prostate (TRUSP) with needle biopsy of nodular or hard areas for histological confirmation.

Immediate Management

Specialist referral

Treatment of Choice

Locally Advanced Disease

- Watch and wait: In very old patients or if there is a poor life-expectancy

- Bilateral surgical orchidectomy: not preferred
- Chemical orchidectomy with an LHRH agonist or with non steriodal anti androgen(flutamide).
- Radiotherapy with adjuvant LHRH agonist is the most widely used treatment.

Metastatic Disease
- Bilateral orchidectomy
- LHRH agonist
- Maximal androgen blockade by performing bilateral orchidectomy plus anti-androgen

Note that in men with asymptomatic localised well-differentiated disease, radical treatments (prostatectomy, radiotherapy, brachytherapy or a combination of these) have not been shown to reduce overall mortality compared with conservative management, and may introduce more morbidity than the disease itself might cause.

Your notes:

Serial No. 117

Subject: Surgery

Topic: GIT

Question: A 65-year-old male with weight loss, right-sided abdominal pain and tenesmus. On examination-a granular mass is seen in the rectum.

Diagnosis: Carcinoma rectum

Clinchers
- *65-year-old, weight loss:* An elderly with unexpalanble weight loss always suggests first towards carcinoma, the site of which is usually suggested by the associated symptoms and later confirmed by an appropriate investigation.
- *Right sided abdominal pain and tenesmus:* The presence of tenesmus and also right sided abdominal pain suggest involvement of rectum. A per rectal examination or microscopic examination of the stools would have shown the presence of blod as well.
- *A granular mass in the rectum:* This adds further to our diagnosis.

CONFUSA

Although an inflammatory bowel disease (especially, ulcerative colitis) can present with a similar picture of weight loss, abdominal pain and tenesmus, the presence of mass per rectum leaves no suspicion for carcinoma rectum as diagnosis. However, for questions like, *'A 68-year-old man with weight loss, abdominal pain, tenesmus'*, its always safe to go with carcinoma as diagnosis keeping in view of the age of the patient. Always look for other hints in the question which may suggest a different diagnosis.

Investigation of Choice
Definitive diagnosis: Biopsy of suspicious masses
Spread: CT Scan

Immediate Management
Urgent referral

Treatment of Choice
High Rectal tumours: Anterior resection
Low rectal tumours (<8 cm from anal verge): Abdomino perineal resection

Your notes:

Serial No. 147

Subject: Surgery

Topic: GIT

Question: A 60-year-old man with a lump in supra-clavicular region and decreased appetite. He has lost 5 kg weight recently.

Diagnosis: Carcinoma stomach

Clinchers

- *A 60-year-old man:* The incidence of carcinoma stomach in England and Wales for men is 20 per 100,000, and for women 7 per 100 000. 99% of cases of upper gastrointestinal cancer (oesophagus, stomach, pancreas) occur over in patients over 40 years old and over 90% of gastric cancers occur in patients over 55 years old. The risk of carcinoma stomach in those below 55 years is extremely low.
- *Lump in supra-clavicular region:* The enlarged left supraclavicular node in cases of carcinoma stomach is known as Virchow's node and the sign is called Troisier's sign. This is the sign of advanced disease and inoperability.
- *Decreased appetite, lost 5 kg weight recently:* This is the most common presenting symptoms, with more than 95% patients presenting with anorexia and weight loss. Dyspepsia and anaemia are among other common symptoms.

CONFUSA

- For any patient above 55 years, with dyspeptic symptoms, endoscopy is essential before starting on anti secretory drugs. Proton pump inhibitors may appear to heal malignant ulcers thus delaying the diagnosis or result in a misdiagnosis on first endoscopy.
- Again, all gastric ulcers should be biopsied as most mimic benign ulcers with even positive response to anti secretory treatment.
- Sister Joseph Nodule is a metastatic tumour deposit in the umbilicus, the anatomical region where the peritoneum is closest to the skin. It is rare, but its presence signifies inoperability.

Investigation of Choice

Endoscopy and biopsy

CT/ MRI required for staging

Immediate Management

TNM staging (carcinoma stomach)

T0	No evidence of primary tumour
Tis	Carcinoma in situ (intraepithelial)
T1	Invades lamina propira or submucosa
T2	Invades muscularis propria or suberosa (not visceral peritoneum)
T3	Penetrates visceral peritoneum but not adjacent structures
T4	Invades adjacent structures (spleen, colon etc)
N0	No LN metastasis
N1	1-6 lymph nodes
N2	7-15 lymph nodes
N3	more than 15 lymph nodes
M0	No distant metastasis
M1	Distant metastasis, in portal LN, mesenteric, retroperitoneal distant

TX, NX or MX indicates "not assessed"

STAGE OF DISEASE

Stage I—	T1N0M0	T1N1M0	T2N0M0
Stage II—	T1N2M0	T2N1M0	T3N0M0
Stage III—	T2N2M0	T3N1M0	T4N0M0
Stage IV—	T3N2M0	T4N1M0	

Stage the disease.

Treatment of Choice

Surgery is the Treatment of Choice for gastric cancer. Distal (antral) tumours should be treated by subtotal gastrectomy and proximal tumours by total gastrectomy.

Your notes:

Serial No. 148

Subject: Surgery

Topic: Thyroid

Question: A man comes with a lump in front of his neck which moves up on swallowing. Scan shows a mass replacing the left lobe of thyroid and spreading to sternomastoid and adjacent muscles.

Diagnosis: Thyroid Carcinoma

Clinchers

- *A man:* Thyroid carcinoma is more common in women than men especially in the women of reproductive age group. However, in solitary thyroid nodules, cancer risk is more in males.The risk of malignancy rises with age.
- *Lump in front of his neck which moves up on swallowing:* Lump in front of neck which rises on swallowing is the characteristic description of a mass attached to the thyroid. Most closest differential being thyroglossal cyst.
- *A mass replacing the left lobe of thyroid:* This signify that the mass is arising from the left lobe of thyroid.
- *Spreading to sternomastoid and adjacent muscles:* This signifies the malignant nature of the mass as it has infiltrated the adjacent muscles.

CONFUSA

- A slow growing thyroid tumour with lymphatic metastasis is usually Papillary carcinoma (Most common, best prognosis).
- For patients with features of phaeochromocytoma, a thyroid mass usually signify medullary carcinoma (MEN 2A or MEN 2B syndrome).
- Thyroid tumours with pulsating bony metastasis is usually follicular carcinoma.
- Rapidly expanding thyroid mass with local pressure effects can be either lymphoma or anaplastic carcinoma.

Investigation of Choice

FNAC most useful

Immediate Management

refer for expert opinion

Treatment of Choice

Most thyroid tumours are treated surgically with follow up radioiodine ablation if the tumour will concentrate I-131.

Serial No. 150

Subject: Medicine

Topic: Chest

Question: A shipyard worker develops shortness of breath and a lump in his supraclavicular fossa.There is a small pleural effusion noted on the same side of the lump.

Diagnosis: Mesothelioma

Clinchers

- *A shipyard worker:* Asbestosis and the associated mesothelioma is an industrial disease, Most commonly seen in those who have worked in construction and ship repair but also seen in other trades brining regular exposure to asbestos such as laggers and plumbers.
- *Shortness of breath:* Asbestos exposure most commonly causes pleural mesothelioma (rarely, peritoneal mesothelioma). The effection of pleura causes thickening and the patient most commonly present with shortness of breath which is usually progressive.
- *A lump in his supraclavicular fossa:* This signify the metastasis and secondary enlargement of supracalvicular lymph nodes.
- *Small pleural effusion noted on the same side of the lump:* Unilateral pleural effusion is almost always a constant finding.

CONFUSA

- The fullness in the neck can be mistaken for Pancoast's tumour and students may get wrongly illusioned towards carcinoma lung as the most probable diagnosis for such a presentation, as above.
- However, do not forget that Pancoast's tumour is usally associated with pain in the inner surface of the arm and the fourth and fifth fingers (ulnar distribution) and paralysis and wasting of the muscles of the hand and forearm.
- Morever, for it to be lung carcinoma, question should have given hints on the smoking history than occupational exposure to asbestos.

Investigation of Choice

Pleural biopsy required for a definitive diagnosis. Chest radiography/CT shows a pleural thickening and an associated pleural effusion.

Immediate Management

Stage the disease

Staging of Mesothelioma

Stage I: Disease confined inside the capsule of the parietal pleura: ipsilateral pleura, lung, pericardium, and diaphragm.

Stage II: As described for stage I with intrathoracic (N1 or N2) lymph nodes.

Stage III: This signifies local extension of disease into the following: chest wall or mediastinum; heart or through the diaphram, peritoneum; with or without extra-thoracic or contralateral (N3) lymph node involvement.

Stage IV: Distant metastases.

Treatment of Choice

- Usually only symptomatic treatment is possible.
- Curative surgical treatment may be possible with stage 1 disease.
- Extrapleural pneumonectomy may be used to lengthen time of recurrence.
- Pleurectomy and decortication is used for palliative pain relief and recurrent pleural effusions.
- No evidence that radiotherapy or chemotherapy improves survival.
- Radiotherapy may help with pain management

Your notes:

PAPER 3

42. A 58-year-old man with fever and an area of consolidation on his chest X-ray is treated with antibiotics. His fever resolves but four weeks later but he still has a large area of consolidation.

Diagnosis: Bronchial carcinoma.

Clinchers

- *58-year-old man:* Elderly males with lung symptoms should be investigated to rule out lung cancer especially if they have history of smoking.
- *Fever:* This is because of the secondary pneumonia. Carcinoma causing partial obstruction of a bronchus interrupts the mucociliary escalator, and bacteria are retained within affected lobe.
- *An area of consolidation on his chest X-ray:* Secondary pneumonia due to above described mechanism appears as a lobar consolidation on CXR.
- *Is treated with antibiotics:* Treatment with antibiotics usually clears the pneumonia and resolves the fever within few days.
- *His fever resolves but four weeks later:* Any opacity secondary to inflammation should have been resolved in four weeks.
- *He still has a large area of consolidation:* Any opacity persisting beyound this time should make one strongly suspicious of a neoplastic lesion in this age group.

CONFUSA

The only confusion in this question can exist if one overlook the age of the patient and remain focussed only on the complications of pneumonia.

Investigation of Choice

- *Screening:* CXR (already done in this case)
- *Definitive:* Bronchoscopy with biopsy.

Immediate Management

Assess operability.

Treatment of Choice

- Non-small cell tumours: Surgery (avoided in > 65 years with metastatic disease as rate of mortality is more than expected five-year survival)
- Radiotherapy: For bronchial obstruction (as in this case).

Your notes:

61. Carcinoma of the right main bronchus.

Diagnosis: Already stated as the question.

Clinchers

Hemoptysis is the second most common symptom of presentation of a bronchial carcinoma, occurring in 70% of cases. (The most common symptom is cough, occurring in 80%).

Bronchial carcinoma is a frequent carcinoma asked in PLAB exams. So let us seen some most frequently occurring clinchers in such questions

- Elderly
- Smoker
- Male
- Cough
- Hemoptysis
- Dyspnoea
- Chest pain
- Recurrent/slowly resolving pneumonia
- Anorexia
- Weight loss
- Clubbing
- Hypertrophic pulmonary osteoarthritis (wrist pain)
- Supraclavicular or axillary lymphadenopathy.

CONFUSA

Most of the neurological signs caused by a bronchial carcinoma are due to brain metastases. Nonmetastatic neurological signs do occur and can be confusing, there are: confusion, fits, cerebellar syndrome, proximal myopathy, peripheral neuropathy, polymyositis, Eatan-Lambert syndrome.

Investigation of Choice

- *Screening:* CXR (often normal).
- *Definitive:* Fibreoptic bronchoscopy (as it gives a histological diagnosis also and can assess operatibility)

Treatment of Choice

Depends on stage: Surgical excision in operable cases, otherwise palliative radiotherapy.

Your notes:

63. Bronchial carcinoid.

Diagnosis: Already stated as the question.

Clinchers

Questions about bronchial carcinoids are a rarity in PLAB exam. Still let us review some salient features of them.

- Usually follow a benign course
- May secrete other hormones, effects of whom constitute the common presenting complaints of this condition. They can secrete
  - ACTH
  - Arginine vasopressin
- Carcinoid syndrome is only produce when any carcinoid has liver metastases. It is characterised by:
  - Cutaneous flush
  - Bronchoconstrition
  - Diarrhoea.

CONFUSA

Bronchial carcinoids and small cell carcinoma both develops from the same cells (kulchitsky cell in bronchial epithelium). But carcinoid can be differentiated by presence of carcinoid syndrome (only in presence of liver metastases) and cardiac valvular lesions—both of these are absent in small cell carcinoma of lung. Paraneoplastic syndromes are not a criteria for differentiation as both can cause them (especially ACTH).

Investigation of Choice

- *Screening:* 24 hours urine 5HIAA increase.
- *Definitive:* CXR/CT—usually done only if liver metastases are absent as only then a curative resection is possible.

Immediate Management

High dose octreotide for crises + careful fluid balance.

Treatment of Choice

- Crises—Octreotide
- Flushing—Ketanserin
- Diarrhoea—Loperamide/cyproheptadine
- Hepatic metastases—embolisation
- Bronchial obstruction—surgical debulking

Your notes:

107. A middle-aged man develops constipation with overflow diarrhoea and bright red bleeding per rectum. A barium enema reveals an ulcerated stricture in the sigmoid colon.

Diagnosis: Sigmoid carcinoma.

Clinchers

- *Middle-aged man:* Carcinoma of colon usually occurs in patients over 50 years of age but it is not rare earlier in adult life.
- *Constipation with overflow diarrhoea:* In the carcinoma of left side of colon (sigmoid), alteration of basal habit is seen. The episodes of constipation are followed by attacks of diarrhoea.
- *Bright red bleeding per rectum:* Low tumours may result in tenesmus accompanied by the passage of mucus and blood, especially in the early morning.
- *An ulcerated stricture in the sigmoid colon:* Ulcerated stricture is a sign of malignancy, but it may well be Crohn's involvement of the colon. Sigmoidoscopic examination becomes important here. Biopsy should be taken to ascertain the diagnosis.

CONFUSA

This question may be confused with Crohn's involvement of the colon. Sigmoidoscopy and biopsy should be performed.

Investigation of Choice

- Sigmoidoscopy
- *Barium enema*: It shows 'apple core' appearance, i.e. a short, irregular stenosis with sharp shoulders at each end (look at Figure 57.43, page 1051, Bailey and Love, 23rd edn).

Treatment of Choice

Preoperative treatment: Bowel is cleared by enemas and oral stimulant laxatives (e.g. picolax). Principle of operative treatment is wild resection of the growth together with a regional lymphatics.

In obstructed cases, where bowel preparation is contraindicated the primary goal is to relieve obstruction.

Your notes:

110. An elderly woman is found anaemic. As part of her examination, she has a barium enema, which reveals a mass lesion in the ascending colon.

Diagnosis: Caecal carcinoma.

Clinchers

- *Elderly woman:* Caecal carcinoma presents in older age group with a long history.
- *Anaemia:* Carcinoma of caecum presents with anaemia diarrhoea weight loss, and sometimes as right iliac fossa mass. Anaemia occurs due to occult blood loss.
- *Mass in the ascending colon:* Barium enema showing mass in ascending colon confirms our diagnosis of caecal carcinoma.
- *Ascending colon:* Right sided colonic carcinoma typically presents with constipation with or without diarrhoea, whereas left sided colonic carcinoma presents with anorexia, weight loss and constipation.

CONFUSA

Young parents with diarrhoea and right iliac fossa a mass focus on Crohn's disease and there should be no confusion with an appendicular mass.

Investigation of Choice

Barium enema and occult blood test.

Immediate Management

Estimate haemoglobin.

Your notes:

PAPER 4

115. A 58-year-old man with fever and an area of consolidation on his chest X-ray is treated with antibiotics. His fever resolves but four weeks later but he still has a large area of consolidation.

Diagnosis: Bronchial carcinoma.

Clinchers

- *58-year-old man:* Elderly males with lung symptoms should be investigated to rule out lung cancer especially if they have history of smoking.
- *Fever:* This is because of the secondary pneumonia. Carcinoma causing partial obstruction of a bronchus interrupts the mucociliary escalator, and bacteria are retained within affected lobe.
- *An area of consolidation on his chest X-ray:* Secondary pneumonia due to above described mechanism appears as a lobar consolidation on CXR.
- *Is treated with antibiotics:* Treatment with antibiotics usually clears the pneumonia and resolves the fever within few days.
- *His fever resolves but four weeks later:* Any opacity secondary to inflammation should have been resolved in four weeks.
- *He still has a large area of consolidation:* Any opacity persisting beyound this time should make one strongly suspicious of a neoplastic lesion in this age group.

CONFUSA

The only confusion in this question can exist if one overlook the age of the patient and remain focussed only on the complications of pneumonia.

Investigation of Choice

- *Screening:* CXR (already done in this case)
- *Definitive:* Bronchoscopy with biopsy.

Immediate Management

Assess operability.

Treatment of Choice

- Non-small cell tumours: Surgery (avoided in > 65 yrs with metastatic disease as rate of mortality is more than expected five-year survival)
- Radiotherapy: For bronchial obstruction (as in this case).

Your notes:

126. An 80-year-old with prostatic carcinoma comes with 4 month history of low backache.

Diagnosis: Metastatic disease.

Clinchers

- *Carcinoma prostate:* Carcinoma of prostate is more usually discovered at a stage when it has already spread beyond its capsule and may have invaded pelvic cellular tissues, bladder base and bone.
- *Low backache for 4 months:* Once the diagnosis of prostate carcinoma has been established, it would be normal to perform a bone scan as part of the staging procedure if the PSA is >20 nmol/mL. If the PSA is < 29 nmol/mL than a bone scan would only be performed on clinical indications (like low backache). So a bone scan is must in this case.

CONFUSA

The bone scan is performed by the injection of technetium-99m, which is then monitored using a gamma camera. It is more sensitive in the diagnosis of metastases than a skeletal survey, but false positives occur in areas of arthritis, osteomyelitis or a healing fracture.

Investigation of Choice

^{99}Tc bone scan.

Immediate Management

TNM staging of tumour.

Treatment of Choice

The main stay of treatment of metastatic prostatic carcinoma is androgen suppression or the use of specific androgen antagonists, which produce symptomatic relief in 75% cases.

Your notes:

128. Man on GnRH's for prostate cancer comes after 2 months for a follow-up.

Diagnosis: Follow-up case of hormone therapy for prostate carcinoma.

Clinchers

- *GnRH for prostate cancer:* GnRH agonists, e.g. buserilin and goserilin, which inhibit the release of luteinizing hormone (LH) from the anterior pituitary, with consequent reduction of testicular production of testosterone. The exact mechanism is

  GnRH agonists
  ↓
  Initially stimulate hypothalamic GnRH receptors
  ↓
  Later down regulation of hypothalamic GnRH receptors
  ↓
  Cessation of pituitary LH production
  ↓
  Decrease in testosterone production to levels akin to castration levels

- *Comes after 2 months for a follow-up:* GnRH agonists are usually given in 2-3 month depot injection so the patient has to come every 2 months for follow-up. PSA (prostate specific antigen) is the best way to follow the response after hormone therapy.

CONFUSA

Though transrectal USG can also be used for follow-up and to measures response to treatment, PSA is the accurate and best way. Transrectal USG will also be used, but as an additional investigation to measure the size and regression.

Investigation of Choice
PSA

Immediate Management
Check for gynaecomastia or other such side effects of GnRH therapy.

Treatment of Choice
Give second depot injection of GnRH agonist.

Your notes:

129. Man with prostate Ca which has extended outside the capsule presenting with features of renal failure.

Diagnosis: Bladder outflow obstruction (BOO).

Clinchers

- *Prostate carcinoma which has extended outside capsule:* It means that it is a locally advanced disease. Bladder base is a frequent site of prostatic metastases. Otherwise also, prostatic enlargement due to carcinomatous growth can produce BOO.
- *Features of renal failure:* The obstruction to outflow of the bladder may result in renal failure with drowsiness, headache and impairment of intellect due to uraemia.

CONFUSA

Pain is not a symptom of BOO and its presence should prompt the exclusion of acute retention, urinary infection stones carcinoma of the prostate and carcinoma *in situ* of the bladder (1242, Bailey and Love, 23rd edn).

Investigation of Choice
Pressure-flow urodynamic studies

Immediate Management
Suprapubic catheterisation

Treatment of Choice
Prostatectomy.

Your notes:

130. A man having adenocarcinoma prostate which has already spread to pelvic side walls has to be given chemotherapy.

Diagnosis: Metastatic prostate carcinoma

Clinchers

- *Adenocarcinoma:* This is the most common variety of carcinoma prostate and is usually well-differentiated. Occasionally anaplastic variety is seen.
- *Spread to pelvic side walls:* Carcinoma prostate is more usually discovered at a stage when it has already spread beyond its capsule and may well have involved other organs, particularly the pelvic cellular tissues, bladder base and bone. The mainstay of this disease is androgen suppression or the use of specific androgen antagonists, which will produce symptomatic relief in disseminated prostatic cancer is about 75% of patients.

CONFUSA

This chemotherapy in this case is most probably stilbesterol, an oestrogen analogue, which is used as primary therapy is majority of cases. It may have feminising side effects such as gynaecomastia, nipple and scrotal pigmentation and testicular atrophy. More importantly, it may result in fluid retention and precipitate congestive cardiac failure, so that in elderly patients with cardiovascular disease bilateral orchidectomy should be performed.

Investigation of Choice

Transrectal USG (can assess extracapsular spread)

Immediate Management

Rule out heart disease

Treatment of Choice

Stilbesterol.

Your notes:

135. A 55-year-old man, history of altered bowel habit from 2 months, anaemia, loss of weight.

Diagnosis: Colon carcinoma.

Clinchers

- *55-year-old man:* Colon carcinoma are the second most common cause of death from malignancy in UK. Tumours may occur at any age. Females are affected more than males (Note: The incidence of rectal cancer is roughly equal in two sexes). The peak in incidence occurs after 50 years.
- *Altered bowel habit for two months:* The most common symptom is a change in bowel habits, either constipation, diarrhoea or two alternating with each other.
- *Anaemia and loss of weight:* More common in caecal carcinoma (see confusa below).

CONFUSA

Tumours of the left side of the colon, where the contained stool is solid, are typically constricting growths, so obstructive symptoms predominate along with constipation. In contrast, tumours of the right side tend to be proliferative and here the stools are semi-liquid, therefore obstructive symptoms are relatively uncommon and the patient with a carcinoma of the caecum or ascending colon often presents with anaemia and loss of weight.

Investigation of Choice

- *Screening:* Barium enema
- *Definitive:* Colonoscopy with biopsy.

Immediate Management

Correct anaemia with haematinics or blood transfusion.

Treatment of Choice

Surgical excision.

Your notes:

141. A 55-year-old lady with history of intermittent postmenopausal bleeding. Vaginal and speculum examinations are normal.

Diagnosis: Endometrial carcinoma

Clinchers

- *A 55-year-old:* Mean age of presentation is 56 years. It is rare under the age of 40.
- *Intermittent postmenopausal bleeding:* This symptom should always be assumed to be caused by carcinoma of endometrium until proven otherwise.
- *Vaginal and speculum examination are normal:* This has ruled out any local cause of bleeding (e.g. vaginal trauma) so this warrants examination of the endometrium now.

CONFUSA

Endometrial carcinoma is associated with hyperestrogenic states, i.e.
- Obesity
- Diabetes
- Late menopause
- Prolonged use of unopposed oestrogens
- Oestrogen secreting tumours

Investigation of Choice

- *Screening:* Ultrasound (to assess dimensions of any tumour and to show endometrial thickness)
- *Definitive:* Uterine sampling or curettage

Immediate Management

Perform staging to decide the line of treatment.

Treatment of Choice

Usually surgical

Small	Well differentiated	*Total abdominal hysterectomy* + bilateral salpingo-oophorectomy + internal iliac node frozen section biopsy
Enlarged	Confined to upper part of corpus	*Extended hysterectomy* + bilateral salpingo-ophorectomy + removal of a cuff of vagina + lymph node sampling
Cervix invaded		*Wertheim's* (Removal of upper half of the vagina and pelvic lymph node)

- *Radiotherapy*
  - If node is involved
  - If there is deep invasion of myometrium
- *Hormone therapy:* Progestogens inhibit the rate of growth and spread of endometrial carcinoma.

158. Patient after radiotherapy for bowel adenocarcinoma comes with bright red rectal bleeding.

Diagnosis: Radiation proctitis

Clinchers

- *Radiotherapy for bowel adenocarcinoma:* It means that pelvic irradiation was given in this patient. Radiation proctitis, which may present as a localized area of colitis, is usually found in the setting of radiation prcotitis.
- *Bright red rectal bleeding:* Whenever rectal bleeding is the presenting complaint, a colonic source should be considered. Radiation damage to rectum (proctitis) produces diarrhoea, with or without blood and tenesmus.

CONFUSA

The onset of radiation proctitis may be months to years after irradiation. Characteristic features on sigmoidoscopy include:
- Mucosal atrophy
- Telangiectasia
- Friability
- Small ulceration

GI desquamation after radiation can be differential diagnosis but its main presenting feature is a profuse non-bloody diarrhoea.

Investigation of Choice

Sigmoidoscopy (proctoscopy is seldom sufficient in proctitis due to any cause).

Immediate Management

Blood transfusion if anaemic and massive blood loss.

Treatment of Choice

- Symptomatic
- Local steroids sometimes help (per rectal prednisolone)

Your notes:

159. Patient with superior vena cava obstruction after radiotherapy.

Diagnosis: Superior vena cava (SVC) obstruction

Clinchers

➢ *SVC obstruction after radiotherapy:* It is commonly due to:
- Lung carcinoma
- Lymphoma

Since for lymphoma and small cell lung carcinoma chemotherapy is generally is used, the condition must be a radiosensitive lung carcinoma, i.e. non-small cell lung cancer.

Signs and symptoms of SVC obstruction are:
- Dyspnoea
- Orthopnoea
- Facial and upper limb swelling
- Cough
- Plethora
- Cyanosis
- Headache
- Venous enlargement.

CONFUSA

Bronchoscopy should be avoided in all cases of SVC obstruction as it can be hazardous and can lead to vena caval perforation.

Investigation of Choice
Venography (SVC stenting)

Immediate Management
Dexamethasone 4 mg/6h PO

Treatment of Choice
SVC stenting + debulking of tumour later on

Your notes:

160. Female with fungating breast carcinoma with a bad odour.

Diagnosis: Fungating breast carcinoma

Clinchers

➢ *Fungating breast carcinoma:* This must be an inoperable tumour and may require palliative surgery and radiotherapy.

➢ *Bad odour:* Metronidazole 400 mg/8h PO mitigates unpleasant odours from tumours. Charcol dressings such as actisorb also absorb the bad odour. The aetiology of bad odour in a fungating carcinoma invariably is infection by anaerobic organisms. The odour can be very distressing to the patient, attendants and health care workers.

CONFUSA

Occasionally toilet mastectomy or radiotherapy is required to control a fungating tumour, but often incision through microscopically permeated tissues makes the outcome worse than original.

Investigation of Choice
None required

Immediate Management
Charcoal dressing

Treatment of Choice
Metronidazole (400 mg/8h PO or gel)

Your notes:

191. Female, 41-year-old, presents with hard, irregular fixed swelling, stridor, dysphagia since 3 months.

Diagnosis: Anaplastic carcinoma thyroid

Clinchers

- *Female:* E: G » 3: 1
- *41-year-old:* Its risk and incidence increases with age and mainly occurs in elderly women.
- *Hard, irregular fixed swelling:* It is a typical presentation from anaplastic carcinoma. It needs to be differentiated from sarcoma or lymphoma. Multinodular goitre can also present like this.

  Note: Anaplastic carcinoma tissues do not concentrate iodine.
- *Stridor:* Due to tracheal compression by the rapid internal growth of the tumour. It may also invade the trachea.
- *Dysphagia:* Due to oesophageal compression due to mass effect of the tumour.
- *Since 3 months:* Anaplastic carcinomas are very fast growing and highly malignant.

CONFUSA

Usually the more malignant tumors of thyroid occur in younger age and tumors occurring in elderly patients are usually benign. But anaplastic carcinoma is an exception to this state of affairs as it occurs more in the elderly and is highly malignant (both locally and hematogeneously). Always make it a point to rule out thyroid lymphoma and sarcoma because their presentation is very similar.

Investigation of Choice

Biopsy.

Immediate Management

Tracheostomy for stridor (if it worsens).

Treatment of Choice

- Radical thyroidectomy
- Inoperable tumours palliative radiotherapy.

Your notes:

195. A 35-year-old woman who was diagnosed as having coeliac disease at the age of 12 years has had good control of her abdominal symptoms for a number of years. She presents with a recent history of weight loss, tiredness, diarrhoea and abdominal pain.

Diagnosis: Small bowel lymphoma (probable).

Clinchers

- *35-year-old:* Incidence of lymphomas peak after 30 years
- *Coeliac disease:* The risk of small bowel lymphoma is increased in patients with a prior history of:
  - Malabsorption conditions (e.g. celiac sprue)
  - Regional enteritis
  - Depressed immune function
    - Congenital immunodeficiencies
    - Prior organ transplantation
    - Autoimmune disorders
    - AIDS
- *Good control of abdominal symptoms for a number of years:* Coeliac disease symptoms are very amenable to diet control and since the symptoms are in control in this patient for many years, there is no reason that they should relapse. Considering her age and high risk, lymphoma should be ruled out.
- *Weight loss, tiredness, diarrhoea and abdominal pain:* Characteristic of any malabsorption syndrome (in this case induced by lymphoma).

CONFUSA

Primary intestinal lymphoma accounts for 20% of malignancies of small bowel. Essentially all these neoplasms are non-Hodgkin's lymphoma. Its incidence is: Ileum > jejunum > duodenum (mirrors the relative amount of normal lymphoid cells in these anatomic areas).

Investigation of Choice

- *Screening:* Contrast radiographs (infiltration and thickening of mucosal folds, mucosal nodules, ulcerations)
- *Definitive:* Surgical exploration and resection for tissue diagnosis.

Immediate Management

Rule out ethnic relation (Jews and Arabs) which produce a nonresectable immunoproliferative small intestinal disease and any non-compliance on gluten free diet.

Treatment of Choice

Surgical exploration +
Postresection radio/chemotherapy.

196. Female with breast carcinoma 3 years back, was treated with mastectomy and lymph node clearance on the left side, presents with a swollen limb and decreased hand movements.

Diagnosis: Acquired lymphoedema of arm.

Clinchers

- *Breast carcinoma:* The late oedema of the arm is a troublesome complication of breast cancer treatment. It is seen more commonly when radical axillary lymph node dissection and radiotherapy are combined.
- *3 years back:* It usually presents late but can occur any-time from months to years after treatment.
- *Mastectomy and lymph node clearance on left side:* It involves massive removal of lymphatics which hampers the lymphatic drainage of arm. Radical axillary dissection is now rarely combined with radiotherapy (radiotherapy produced postradiation fibrosis which when compounded by impaired lymphatic drainage due to block dissection, increases the risk of lymphoedema by several times) because of this complication, but still it does occur with either modality of treatment alone.
- *Swollen arm:* Due to impaired lymphatic drainage.
- *Decreased hand movements:* It is due to compression of the nerves supplying the hand in compartments of arm and forearm.

CONFUSA

There is usually no precipitating cause but recurrent tumour must be excluded as neoplastic infiltration on the axilla can cause arm swelling due to both lymphatic and venous blockage. The differentiating features is that the neoplastic infiltrations are often painful due to nerve involvement. The diagnosis of lymphoedema also depends on exclusion of other causes of oedema, e.g. venous oedema. Lymphoedema cannot be differentiating from venous oedema by "pitting sign" in acute stage (as both will pit on pressure). However, when lymphoedema becomes chronic the subcutaneous tissue become indurated from fibrous tissue replacement, the pitting will not then occur.

Investigation of Choice

Lymphangiography using radiopaque contrast or radioactive isotope will confirm lymphatic obstruction, and contrast lymphangiography may demonstrate megalymphatics.

Immediate Management

Rule out recurrence of carcinoma.

Treatment of Choice

Treatment of late oedema is difficult but limb-elevation, elastic arm stockings and pneumatic compression devices can be useful.

Your notes:

197. Presents with thirst, confusion, constipation.

Diagnosis: Hypercalcaemia of malignancy.

Clinchers

- *Thirst, confusion, constipation:* signs and symptoms of hypercalcaemia of malignancy are:
  - Lethargy
  - Anorexia
  - Nausea
  - Polydipsia
  - Polyuria
  - Constipation
  - Dehydration
  - Confusion
  - Weakness

These signs and symptoms are most obvious with serum calcium > 3 mmol/L.

Hypercalcaemia of malignancy is the most common paraneoplastic endocrine syndrome and is responsible for about 40% of all hypercalcaemia.

CONFUSA

Hypercalcaemia of malignancy can occur by one of the two mechanisms:

1. Humoral hypercalcaemia—caused by circulating hormones (e.g. PTH)
2. Local osteolytic hypercalcaemia—caused by local paracrine factors secreted by cancers within bone. This type occurs in relation with breast carcinoma which produces lytic bone metastases. Other cancers involved are kidney, ovary and skin.

Investigation of Choice

Serum calcium.

Immediate Management

Rehydrate with 3-4 litres of 0.9% saline IV (over 24 hours).

Note: Avoid diuretics

Treatment of Choice

Bisphosphonate pamidronate (60-90 mg IV) decreases osteoclastic bone resorption.

Alteration of mental status (as in this case) is indicated of severe hypercalcaemia and require treatment with calcitonin in addition to all of the above measures.

Your notes:

PAPER 5

51. For the past two weeks a middle aged railway engineer has complained of acute constipation. His stools are dark, but not apparently blood stained. Abdominal palpation detects a mass with moderate tenderness.

Diagnosis: Colonic cancer (left side)

Clinchers

- *Middle aged railway engineer:* Colon cancer may occur at any age, but it more common after 40.
- *Acute constipation for past two weeks:* In it, typically an adult with presiously regular bowel habit suddenly develops irregularity. There may be increasing difficulty in getting the bowels to move, requiring laxatives. The episodes of constipation may be followed by attacks of diarrhoea.
- *Stools are dark, but not apparently blood stained:* This is malaena, signifying blood loss high in the colon. Otherwise bleed may be bright, malaena or occult.
- *Mass with moderate tenderness:* This confirms our suspicious as there is usually a mass palpable either per abdomen or per rectum.

CONFUSA

Tumours of the left side of the colon, where the contained stool is solid, are typically constricting growths, so obstructive features predominate. In contrast, tumours of the right side tend to be proliferative and here the stools are semi-liquid therefore obstructive symptoms are relatively uncommon and the patient with a carcinoma of the caecum or ascending colon often presents with anaemia and loss of weight. In carcinoma of left side of colon, the lump that is felt on abdominal, rectal or bimanual palpation is sometimes not the tumour itself, but impacted faeces above it. When the tumour is situated in a pendulous pelvic colon, a hard movable swelling may be felt in the rectovesical pouch on rectal examination.

Investigation of Choice

Colonoscopy

Immediate Management

Laxatives for constipation

Treatment of Choice

Surgery

52. **A 43-year-old man says he cannot finish his stool and that what he does pass is streaked with blood. He says he has always been regular. He wants to know if a laxative will help.**

Diagnosis: Rectal carcinoma

Clinchers

- *43-year-old man:* The sexes are equally affected and it occurs in any age group from the twenties onwards, but is particularly common in age range 50-70 years.
- *He cannot finish his stool:* The patients bowels open but there is a sensation that there are more faeces to be passed. This sense of incomplete defecation is typical of rectal carcinoma.
- *What he does pass is streaked with blood:* The patient may endeavour to empty the rectum several times a day (spurious diarrhoea), often with the passage of flatus and a little blood stained mucus (blood slime).
- *He says he has always been regular:* This signify that the alteration in bowel habits is of recent onset and excludes any pre-existing pathology.
- *Wants to know if a laxative will help:* The patient may find it necessary to start taking an aperient, or to supplement the usual dose and as a result the tendency towards diarrhoea ensues.

CONFUSA

Sence of incomplete defaecation results in tenesmus which is a painful straining to empty the bowels without resultant evacuation. This "sense" is a very important early symptom and is almost invariably present in tumours of the lower half of the rectum. Pain is a late symptom. Weight loss is suggestive of hepatic metastases. In approximately 90% of cases the neoplasm can be felt digitally.

Investigation of Choice

- *Screening:* Proctosigmoidoscopy
- *Definitive:* Biopsy

Immediate Management

Laxatives

Treatment of Choice

Surgery —upper 1/3—Anterior resection
—middle 1/3—± Anterior resection
—lower 1/3—Abdominoperineal resection

69. **A young woman complains of weakness, fatigue, and anorexia. Her cervical lymph nodes are enlarged, painless, and rubbery. Her skin itches and she sometimes has night sweats. On physical examination you find her spleen and liver to be enlarged.**

Diagnosis: Hodgkin's disease (HD)

Clinchers

- *Young woman:* In Hodgkin's disease the age-specific incidence curve is characteristically bimodal, with an initial peak in young adults (15 to 35 years) and a second peak after age 50. There is increased male prevalence which is most prominent in young adults.
- *Weakness, fatigue and anorexia:* 25 to 30 per cent of patients have some constitutional symptoms at presentation. The most common is low grade fever, which can be associated with recurrent night sweats. Another important presenting symptom is unexplained weight loss of greater than 10 percent over 6 months or less. Fatigue, malaise and weakness are other frequent symptoms.
- *Cervical lymph nodes are enlarged, painless and rubbery:* HD commonly presents with a newly-detected mass or group of lymph nodes that are firm, freely movable and usually nontender. Approximately half of the patients presents with adenopathy in the neck or supraclavicular area, and over 70% of patients present with superficial lymph node enlargement. Because these are frequently non-painful, detection by the patient may be delayed until the lymph nodes are quite large
- *Skin itches:* Pruritus occurs in approximately to 10 per cent of patients of initial diagnosis; it is usually generalised may be associated with a skin rash, and rarely may be the only disease manifestation.
- *Night sweats:* Most common constitutional symptom at presentation is a low grade fever, which can be associated with recurrent night sweats, for same patients night sweats may be the sole complaint. These symptoms ar more commonly seen in older patients and in those with more advanced stage disease.
- *Spleen and liver enlarged:* In HD, primary abdominal disease with hepatomegaly, splenomegaly and massive adenopathy is uncommon, and other neoplastic diseases, especially non-Hodgkin's lymphoma must be excluded under these circumstances.

CONFUSA

Nodes involved by HD tend to be contiguous and or axila in contrast to non-Hodgkin's lymphomas, which have a tendency to be noncontinuous and centrifungal and involve epitrochlear, Waldeyer's and abdominal nodes.

Investigation of Choice
Lymph node biopsy.

Immediate Management
Immediate symptomatic management.

Treatment of Choice
Radiotherapy for stages IA and IIA
Chemotherapy for IIA to IVB (ABVD regimen)

Your notes:

70. A 44-year-old man presents with ill health. He complains of wasting, fever and sweats. He does not have a skin rash, but he does have skin nodules. On physical examination you find disparate groups of lymph nodes to be enlarged.

Diagnosis: Non-Hodgkin's lymphoma (NHL)

Clinchers

- *44-year-old man:* Can occur at any age and with variable expressions in sexes as it constitutes a heterogeneous group of lymphomas.
- *Presents with ill health + wasting, fever and sweats:* Unlike patients with Hodgkin's disease who present with weight loss, fever or night sweats, fewer than 20 percent of patients with NHL present with mediastinal adenopathy.
- *Does not have a skin rash, but the does have skin nodules:* Absence of skin rash excludes HD. Skin nodules represent cutaneous lesions found in aggressive NHLs.
- *Disparate groups of lymph nodes to be enlarged:* Unlike HD, which have centripetal (axial) and contiguous lymphadenopathy. NHL is characterised by centripetal (non-axial) and non-contiguous (disparate) lymphadenopathy.

CONFUSA

In teenages and young adults, infections mononucleosis and HD should be placed high in the differential diagnosis. Regarding any lymphadenopathy, it is generally agreed that a firm lymph node larger than 1 cm that is not associated with a documentable infection and that persists longer than 4 weeks should be considered for biopsy.

Investigation of Choice
Histology (lymph node biopsy).

Immediate Management
Staging of the disease.

Treatment of Choice
Since this tumour is appearing to be of a high grade—CHOP regimen chemotherapy.

Your notes:

149. A 60-year-old man with a history of weight loss, presents with bleeding per rectum. He also reports a history of diarrhoea which seems to alternate with constipation. His haemoglobin is 10 g/dl.

Diagnosis: Carcinoma of the colon

Clinchers

- *60-year-old man:* Females are affected more than males (carcinoma colon). More common in elderly females.
- *History of weight loss:* Sign of malignancy.
- *Bleeding per rectum:* Diarrhoea in colonic carcinoma is accompanied by mucus (produced by the excessive secretion of mucus from the tumour), or bleeding which may be bright, melaena, or occult.
- *Diarrhoea alternative with constipation:* This is the most common local effect, produced by carcinoma of colon (local effect).

CONFUSA

The most important differential diagnosis is from diverticulosis of colon. It is impossible to be certain of this differentiation clinically or even on special investigations unless a positive biopsy is obtained by flexible sigmoidoscopy or colonoscopy. Ulcerative colitis should also be kept in mind.

Investigation of Choice

- Sigmoidoscopy/colonoscopy
- U and E, barium enema (look for filling defect apple core appearance).

Immediate Management

Monitor U and E

Treatment of Choice

Principle of operative treatment is wide resection of the growth together with it regional lymphatics.

Your notes:

164. A 70-year-old man presents with back pain and jaundice.

Diagnosis: Malignancy

Clinchers

- *70-year-old man:* Incidence of malignancy cotinually increases with age. If any old person present with some suggestive symptoms, a malignancy has to be ruled out first.
- *Back pain and jaundice:* Most probably it is carcinoma prostate as it usually presents with metastases to liver (thus producing jaundice) and spine (back pain).

CONFUSA

It should always be kept in mind that only an extensive involvement of liver by metastases can produce jaundice. Usually the presence of liver metastases causing jaundice suggest inoperatibility and a grave prognosis.

The combination of back pain and jaundice may also suggest a haematological malignancy – back pain due to the extra medullary hematopoiesis and jaundice due to rapid turnover of red blood cells. In most cases, the hint goes towards multiple myeloma, however, also look for other hints in the question (viz, anaemia, electrophoresis – M Band, Bence Jones Proteinuria).

Investigation of Choice

Pelvic USG

Immediate Management

Take micturition history

Treatment of Choice

Palliative.

Your notes:

171. A fit 55-year-old gentleman, complains of recurrent episodes of 'seeing visible veins on his body', which are tender. He has started to lose weight and attributes this to his diarrhoea. The consultant dermatologist thinks he has thrombophlebitis migrans.

Diagnosis: Carcinoma of tail of pancreas.

Clinchers

- *Fit 55-year-old gentleman:* Incidence of neoplasia increases with age.
- *Recurrent episodes of 'seeing visible veins on his body':* Local findings of thrombophlebitis migrans consist of induration of redness and tenderness along the course of a vein. Long saphenous vein is most commonly involved. This is Trousseau's syndrome.
- *Started to lose weight:* It is for any unobvious reason, then in this age it is mostly due to malignancy.
- *Diarrhoea:* This suggest carcinoma pancreas which is characteristically associated with thrombophlebitis migrans.
- *Thrombophlebitis migrans:* It strongly indicates our suspicion.

CONFUSA

Thrombophlebitis migrans is successive crops of tender nodular affecting blood vessels throughout the body, associated with carcinoma of the pancreas (especially body and tail tumours).

Investigation of Choice
CT scan

Immediate Management
Exclude DVT as it frequently accompanies.

Treatment of Choice
Symptomatic.

Your notes:

176. The time span over which a percentage of women with cervical intraepithelial neoplasia (CIN) untreated will develop cancer.

Diagnosis (Answer): 3-10 years

Clinchers
The proportion of severe dysplasia and carcinoma *in situ* that progresses to invasive cancer is uncertain , and such an assessment becomes difficult as recognized cases are treated promptly. It is probable that about 10-30% of cases ultimately progress to cancer in 3-10 years time.

CONFUSA

Initially it was believed that CIN III tended to develop from CIN I and II and only CIN III lesions would progress to invasive cancer. Most authors now believe that CIN III lesions probably arise as such. Apparent progression from CIN I to CIN III is explained on the basis of a smaller area of CIN III only becoming apparent with time as the lesions enlarge. The risk of invasion of CIN I and II abnormalities has not been clearly defined.

Investigation of Choice

- *Screening:* Pap smear
- *Definitive:* Colposcopic directed biopsy

Immediate Management
Seek specialist advise

Treatment of Choice
Completely removing abnormal epithelium of CIN and yearly follow-up smears for five years.

Your notes:

177. The age at which the peak incidence of cervical carcinoma occurs.

Diagnosis (Answer): 30 years

Clinchers

Cervical carcinoma was once a disease of the over-50s it is now seen in under 40s (OHCS, page 34, 5th edn). Cervical cancer occurs almost exclusively among women who are, or have been, sexually active. There is increasing evidence that infection by certain strains of human papilloma virus (HPV) is a factor. Studies have shown that between 10 and 30 percent of sexually active women have acquired HPV infection of the genital tract by the age of 30 years. The proportion of women infected is higher if the woman or her partner have had several sexual partners.

CONFUSA

There is a bit of confusion about age of peak incidence according to various books, e.g.

Lecture notes (Gyn and Obs)	45-55 years
OHCS	under 40s
Ten teachers (Gyn)	younger women

But since the latest evidence points towards younger women in their 30s, we can safely mark this option.

178. The interval for cervical smears to be taken in a woman treated one year previously for cervical intraepithelial neoplasia.

Diagnosis (Answer): 12 months

Clinchers

The follow-up of patients treated for CIN is controversial. In some areas one or two follow-up colposcopies are offered but in others follow-up is entirely by cytology. Women who have undergone treatment for CIN III have approximately a three-fold incidence of invasive carcinoma compared with the background population. Whether this justifies more intensive screening programmes in the long-term has not been clearly defined. Certainly for the first five years women should be offered smears every year and possibly for longer than this.

CONFUSA

Cervical cytological screening is designed to detect over 90 per cent of cytological abnormalities. In theory cervical screening fulfils many of the criteria of a successful screening procedure. The cervical smear test will diagnose the vast majority of cytological abnormalities and the treatment of precancer is simple, safe, non-destructive and usually curative. As a result of women having regular cervical screening the incidence of cervical carcinoma has fallen.

Investigation of Choice

Yearly pap smears.

Immediate Management

Counselling.

Your notes:

179. The age at which screening stops for women with a normal smear history.

Diagnosis (Answer): 65 years

Clinchers

- The cervical screening programme includes:
  - Start with 2 smears in the first year of sexual activity
    - Then 3 yearly smears
    - Stop at 65 years age if smear history is normal.

CONFUSA

A successful cervical screening programme can reduce the incidence of invasive carcinoma by 90%. The trouble is those most at risk are the hardest to trace and persuade to have screening, e.g.

- Older woman
- Smoking
- Inner cities

Papanicolaou test (Pap smear) is used for cervical screenings. Positive test require further investigations like:

- Colposcopy
- Cervical biopsy
- Fractional curettage

A pap test can detect about 98% of the cancer cervix, and about 80% of endometrial cancer.

Your notes:

180. The time scale within which the 50% of patients with recurrent disease will present, following treatment for stage 1B cervical cancer.

Diagnosis (Answer): 12 months.

Clinchers

- In stages IB and IIA there is little difference between the results of surgery and radiotherapy. When the disease recurs it does so:
  - Within one year in 50 percent of patients
  - Within two years in 75 percent
  - Within five years in 90 percent

  (Source: Ten teachers (Gyn), 18th edn)

CONFUSA

The prognosis of invasive cervical carcinoma varies depending on the method of treatment chosen, the experience of the radiotherapist or surgeon, and on the country. Expectation of five years survival is:

- Stage I > 85%
- Stage II 50%
- Stage III 25%
- Stage IV 5%

Your notes:

PAPER 6

26. For the past two weeks a middle aged railway engineer has complained of acute constipation. His stools are dark, but not apparently blood stained. Abdominal palpation detects a mass with moderate tenderness.

Diagnosis: Colonic cancer (left side)

Clinchers

- *Middle aged railway engineer:* Colon cancer may occur at any age, but it more common after 40.
- *Acute constipation for past two weeks:* In it, typically an adult with presiously regular bowel habit suddenly develops irregularity. There may be increasing difficulty in getting the bowels to move, requiring laxatives. The episodes of constipation may be followed by attacks of diarrhoea.
- *Stools are dark, but not apparently blood stained:* This is malaena, signifying blood loss high in the colon. Otherwise bleed may be bright, malaena or occult.
- *Mass with moderate tenderness:* This confirms our suspicious as there is usually a mass palpable either per abdomen or per rectum.

CONFUSA

Tumours of the left side of the colon, where the contained stool is solid, are typically constricting growths, so obstructive features predominate. In contrast, tumours of the right side tend to be proliferative and here the stools are semi-liquid therefore obstructive symptoms are relatively uncommon and the patient with a carcinoma of the caecum or ascending colon often presents with anaemia and loss of weight. In carcinoma of left side of colon, the lump that is felt on abdominal, rectal or bimanual palpation is sometimes not the tumour itself, but impacted faeces above it. When the tumour is situated in a pendulous pelvic colon, a hard movable swelling may be felt in the rectovesical pouch on rectal examination.

Investigation of Choice
Colonoscopy

Immediate Management
Laxatives for constipation

Treatment of Choice
Surgery

27. A 43-year-old man says he cannot finish his stool and that what he does pass is streaked with blood. He says he has always been regular. He wants to know if a laxative will help.

Diagnosis: Rectal carcinoma

Clinchers

- *43-year-old man:* The sexes are equally affected and it occurs in any age group from the twenties onwards, but is particularly common in age range 50-70 years.
- *He cannot finish his stool:* The patients bowels open but there is a sensation that there are more faeces to be passed. This sense of incomplete defecation is typical of rectal carcinoma.
- *What he does pass is streaked with blood:* The patient may endeavour to empty the rectum several times a day (spurious diarrhoea), often with the passage of flatus and a little blood stained mucus (blood slime).
- *He says he has always been regular:* This signify that the alteration in bowel habits is of recent onset and excludes any pre-existing pathology.
- *Wants to know if a laxative will help:* The patient may find it necessary to start taking an aperient, or to supplement the usual dose and as a result the tendency towards diarrhoea ensues.

CONFUSA

Sence of incomplete defecation results in tenesmus which is a painful straining to empty the bowels without resultant evacuation. This "sense" is a very important early symptom and is almost invariably present in tumours of the lower half of the rectum. Pain is a late symptom. Weight loss is suggestive of hepatic metastases. In approximately 90% of cases the neoplasm can be felt digitally.

Investigation of Choice

- *Screening:* Proctosigmoidoscopy
- *Definitive:* Biopsy

Immediate Management
Laxatives

Treatment of Choice
Surgery —upper 1/3—Anterior resection
—middle 1/3—± Anterior resection
—lower 1/3—Abdominoperineal resection

35. A patient with difficulty in swallowing, filling defect, he has a long standing history of Barret's oesophagus.

Diagnosis: Oesophageal carcinoma.

Clinchers (Note: See Q 33 of this theme also)

- *Difficulty in swallowing:* Dysphagia is a hallmark of oesophageal carcinoma but it is often an indication of inoperable lesion.
- *Filling defect:* A filling defect evident on radiograph after barium swallow can be produced by carcinoma oesophagus, pharyngeal pouch and achalasia (in the given list of options).
- *Long-standing history of Barret's oesophagus:* It is a recognized risk factor for development of adenocarcinoma in lower 1/3 of the oesophagus. Other definitive risk factors are: spices, alcohol, tobacco, achalasia, tylosis and Plummer-Vinson syndrome.

CONFUSA

Plummer-Vinson syndrome is seen mostly in postmenopausal females. Most common site of occurrence of oesophageal carcinoma is middle 1/3 of oesophagus for squamous cell carcinoma and lower 1/3 of oesophagus for adenocarcinoma.

Investigation of Choice

Barium swallow, CXR

Oesophagoscopy with biopsy/brushings.

Immediate Management

Treat the complications.

Treatment of Choice

Radiotherapy and surgery complete for dismal statistics (6% vs 4% 5 year survival).

Your notes:

51. Female, 41-year-old, presents with hard, irregular fixed swelling, stridor, dysphagia since 3 months.

Diagnosis: Anaplastic carcinoma thyroid

Clinchers

- *Female:* E: G » 3: 1
- *41-year-old:* Its risk and incidence increases with age and mainly occurs in elderly women.
- *Hard, irregular fixed swelling:* It is a typical presentation from anaplastic carcinoma. It needs to be differentiated from sarcoma or lymphoma. Multinodular goitre can also present like this.

  Note: Anaplastic carcinoma tissues do not concentrate iodine.
- *Stridor:* Due to tracheal compression by the rapid internal growth of the tumour. It may also invade the trachea.
- *Dysphagia:* Due to oesophageal compression due to mass effect of the tumour.
- *Since 3 months:* Anaplastic carcinomas are very fast growing and highly malignant.

CONFUSA

Usually the more malignant tumours of thyroid occur in younger age and tumours occurring in elderly patients are usually benign. But anaplastic carcinoma is an exception to this state of affairs as it occurs more in the elderly and is highly malignant (both locally and hematogeneously). Always make it a point to rule out thyroid lymphoma and sarcoma because their presentation is very similar.

Investigation of Choice

Biopsy.

Immediate Management

Tracheostomy for stridor (if it worsens).

Treatment of Choice

- Radical thyroidectomy
- Inoperable tumours

  palliative radiotherapy.

Your notes:

75. A 58-year-old man with fever and an area of consolidation on his chest X-ray is treated with antibiotics. His fever resolves but four weeks later but he still has a large area of consolidation.

Diagnosis: Bronchial carcinoma.

Clinchers

- *58-year-old man:* Elderly males with lung symptoms should be investigated to rule out lung cancer especially if they have history of smoking.
- *Fever:* This is because of the secondary pneumonia. Carcinoma causing partial obstruction of a bronchus interrupts the mucociliary escalator, and bacteria are retained within affected lobe.
- *An area of consolidation on his chest X-ray:* Secondary pneumonia due to above described mechanism appears as a lobar consolidation on CXR.
- *Is treated with antibiotics:* Treatment with antibiotics usually clears the pneumonia and resolves the fever within few days.
- *His fever resolves but four weeks later:* Any opacity secondary to inflammation should have been resolved in four weeks.
- *He still has a large area of consolidation:* Any opacity persisting beyound this time should make one strongly suspicious of a neoplastic lesion in this age group.

CONFUSA

The only confusion in this question can exist if one overlook the age of the patient and remain focussed only on the complications of pneumonia.

Investigation of Choice

- *Screening:* CXR (already done in this case)
- *Definitive:* Bronchoscopy with biopsy.

Immediate Management

Assess operability.

Treatment of Choice

- Non-small cell tumours: Surgery (avoided in > 65 years with metastatic disease as rate of mortality is more than expected five-year survival)
- Radiotherapy: For bronchial obstruction (as in this case).

Your notes:

86. Female with breast carcinoma 3 years back, was treated with mastectomy and lymph node clearance on the left side, presents with a swollen limb and decreased hand movements.

Diagnosis: Acquired lymphoedema of arm.

Clinchers

- *Breast carcinoma:* The late oedema of the arm is a troublesome complication of breast cancer treatment. It is seen more commonly when radical axillary lymph node dissection and radiotherapy are combined.
- *3 years back:* It usually present late but can occur anytime from months to years after treatment.
- *Mastectomy and lymph node clearance on left side:* It involves massive removal of lymphatics which hampers the lymphatic drainage of arm. Radical axillary dissection is now rarely combined with radiotherapy (radiotherapy produced postradiation fibrosis which when compounded by impaired lymphatic drainage due to block dissection, increases the risk of lymphoedema by several times) because of this complication, but still it does occur with either modality of treatment alone.
- *Swollen arm:* Due to impaired lymphatic drainage.
- *Decreased hand movements:* It is due to compression of the nerves supplying the hand in compartments of arm and forearm.

CONFUSA

There is usually no precipitating cause but recurrent tumour must be excluded as neoplastic infiltration on the axilla can cause arm swelling due to both lymphatic and venous blockage. The differentiating features is that the neoplastic infiltrations are often painful due to nerve involvement. The diagnosis of lymphoedema also depends on exclusion of other causes of oedema, e.g. venous oedema. Lymphoedema cannot be differentiating from venous oedema by "pitting sign" in acute stage (as both will pit on pressure). However, when lymphoedema becomes chronic the subcutaneous tissue become indurated from fibrous tissue replacement, the pitting will not then occur.

Investigation of Choice

Lymphangiography using radiopaque contrast or radioactive isotope will confirm lymphatic obstruction, and contrast lymphangiography may demonstrate megalymphatics.

Immediate Management

Rule out recurrence of carcinoma.

Treatment of Choice

Treatment of late oedema is difficult but limb-elevation, elastic arm stockings and pneumatic compression devices can be useful.

87. Presents with thirst, confusion, constipation.

Diagnosis: Hypercalcaemia of malignancy.

Clinchers

➢ *Thirst, confusion, constipation:* signs and symptoms of hypercalcaemia of malignancy are:

- Lethargy
- Anorexia
- Nausea
- Polydipsia
- Polyuria
- Constipation
- Dehydration
- Confusion
- Weakness

These signs and symptoms are most obvious with serum calcium > 3 mmol/L.

Hypercalcaemia of malignancy is the most common paraneoplastic endocrine syndrome and is responsible for about 40% of all hypercalcaemia.

CONFUSA

Hypercalcaemia of malignancy can occur by one of the two mechanisms:

1. Humoral hypercalcaemia—caused by circulating hormones (e.g. PTH)
2. Local osteolytic hypercalcaemia—caused by local paracrine factors secreted by cancers within bone. This type occurs in relation with breast carcinoma which produces lytic bone metastases. Other cancers involved are kidney, ovary and skin.

Investigation of Choice

Serum calcium.

Immediate Management

Rehydrate with 3-4 litres of 0.9% saline IV (over 24 hours).

Note: Avoid diuretics

Treatment of Choice

Bisphosphonate pamidronate (60-90 mg IV) decreases osteoclastic bone resorption.

Alteration of mental status (as in this case) is indicated of severe hypercalcaemia and require treatment with calcitonin in addition to all of the above measures.

Your notes:

88. Presents with weakness of both legs, difficulty walking, urine retention.

Diagnosis: Vertebral compression fracture due to metastases.

Clinchers

➢ *Breast carcinoma:* Bone is a common site for the disposition of secondary tumours usually of epithelial origin. Breast metastases are common in
- Ribs
- Thoracic vertebrae
- Clavicles

➢ *Weakness of both legs:* Vertebral fractures involving the cord may entrap cord to produce paraplegia below the level of the fracture. Usually legs are involved in fracture of thoracic vertebrae. Upper limbs are also involved if there is cervical vertebral fracture.

➢ *Difficulty walking:* Due to paraplegia.

➢ *Urinary retention:* Bladder tone is lost immediately after cord injury. Distension leads to ureteric reflux and renal damage. Later on the bladder may become automatic or neurogenic bladder. Bowel dysfunction will also be present.

CONFUSA

Causes of spinal cord compression can be either extension of tumor from vertebral body (osteoblastic metastases) or crush fracture (osteoclastic metastases). Breast carcinoma commonly produces osteoclastic metastases though it can produce osteoblastic metastases too. Prostatic carcinoma produces osteoblastic metastases.

Investigation of Choice
- *Screening:* Urgent plain X-ray spine
- *Definitive:* MRI/myelogram

Immediate Management

Get neurosurgery and clinical oncology opinions.

Treatment of Choice

Dexamethasone 8-16 mg IV then 4 mg/6h PO

Surgical decompression is the definitive treatment.

Your notes:

96. Patient with a pulsatile hard mass fixed under the upper 1/3 of the sternomastoid muscle.

Diagnosis: Chemodectoma

Clinchers

➢ *Hard mass:* Chemodectomas arise from carotid body and usually firm. Occasionally they are soft and pulsatile. It does not usually cause bruits.

➢ *Fixed:* These tumours more from side to side but not up and down. Most behave in a benign fashion, in a few patients the tumour becomes locally invasive and may metastasise.

➢ *Under the upper 1/3 of the sternomastoid muscle:* This tumour must be suspected in masses just anterior or under the upper third of sternomastoid.

CONFUSA

The tumour presents as a slowly growing enlarging mass in a patient over the age of 30 years. Occasionally, pressure on the carotid sinus from the tumour produces attacks of faintness. Extension of the tumour may lead to cranial nerve palsies (VII, IX, X, XI and XII), resulting in dysphagia and hoarseness.

Investigation of Choice

Digital substraction angiography

Immediate Management

Check the opposite side as the tumour is often bilateral.

Treatment of Choice

Extirpation by vascular surgeon.

151. 80-year-old with prostatic carcinoma comes with 4 month history of low backache.

Diagnosis: Metastatic disease.

Clinchers

- *Carcinoma prostate:* Carcinoma of prostate is more usually discovered at a stage when it has already spread beyond its capsule and may have invaded pelvic cellular tissues, bladder base and bone.
- *Low backache for 4 months:* Once the diagnosis of prostate carcinoma has been established, it would be normal to perform a bone scan as part of the staging procedure if the PSA is >20 nmol/mL. If the PSA is < 29 nmol/mL than a bone scan would only be performed on clinical indications (like low backache). So a bone scan is must in this case.

CONFUSA

The bone scan is performed by the injection of technetium-99m, which is then monitored using a gamma camera. It is more sensitive in the diagnosis of metastases than a skeletal survey, but false positives occur in areas of arthritis, osteomyelitis or a healing fracture.

Investigation of Choice
Tc^{99} bone scan.

Immediate Management
TNM staging of tumour.

Treatment of Choice
The main stay of treatment of metastatic prostatic carcinoma is androgen suppression or the use of specific androgen antagonists, which produce symptomatic relief in 75% cases.

Your notes:

152. Patient with prostatic cancer has been treated, now complains of confusion, thirst, body aches, constipation.

Diagnosis: Hypercalcaemia

Clinchers

- *Prostate carcinoma:* It produces osteoblastic metastases to the bone.
- *Has been treated:* The patient might have been operated upon to remove the local disease. The metastases to bone would either have been missed then or have now presented as a recurrence.
- *Confusion, thirst, body aches, constipation:* These all are symptoms of hypercalcaemia. Other symptoms and signs can be:
  - Lethargy
  - Anorexia
  - Nausea
  - Polydipsia
  - polyuria
  - Dehydration
  - Weakness.

CONFUSA

Hypercalcaemia is produced by following cancers:
- Myeloma (40% cases of hypercalcaemia in malignancy)
- Breast
- Prostate
- Bronchus
- Kidney
- Thyroid

Investigation of Choice
Serum calcium.

Immediate Management
Rehydrate (3-4 litres of 0.9% saline IV over 24 hours)

Treatment of Choice
Bisphosphonate IV
- Best treatment is control of underlying malignancy
- Resistant hypercalcaemia—calcitonin

Your notes:

153. Man on GnRH's for prostate cancer comes after 2 months for a follow-up.

Diagnosis: Follow-up case of hormone therapy for prostate carcinoma.

Clinchers

- *GnRH for prostate cancer:* GnRH agonists, e.g. buserilin and goserilin, which inhibit the release of luteinizing hormone (LH) from the anterior pituitary, with consequent reduction of testicular production of testosterone. The exact mechanism is

  GnRH agonists

  ↓

  Initially stimulate hypothalamic GnRH receptors

  ↓

  Later down regulation of hypothalamic GnRH receptors

  ↓

  Cessation of pituitary LH production

  ↓

  Decrease in testosterone production to levels akin to castration levels

- *Comes after 2 months for a follow up:* GnRH agonists are usually given in 2-3 month depot injection so the patient has to come every 2 months for follow up. PSA (prostate specific antigen) is the best way to follow the response after hormone therapy.

CONFUSA

Though transrectal USG can also be used for follow up and to measures response to treatment, PSA is the accurate and best way. Transrectal USG will also be used, but as an additional investigation to measure the size and regression.

Investigation of Choice
PSA

Immediate Management
Check for gynaecomastia or other such side effects of GnRH therapy.

Treatment of Choice
Give second depot injection of GnRH agonist.

Your notes:

155. A man having adenocarcinoma prostate which has already spread to pelvic side walls has to be given chemotherapy.

Diagnosis: Metastatic prostate carcinoma

Clinchers

- *Adenocarcinoma:* This is the most common variety of carcinoma prostate and is usually well-differentiated. Occasionally anaplastic variety is seen.
- *Spread to pelvic side walls:* Carcinoma prostate is more usually discovered at a stage when it has already spread beyond its capsule and may well have involved other organs, particularly the pelvic cellular tissues, bladder base and bone. The mainstay of this disease is androgen suppression or the use of specific androgen antagonists, which will produce symptomatic relief in disseminated prostatic cancer is about 75% of patients.

CONFUSA

This chemotherapy in this case is most probably stilbesterol, an oestrogen analogue, which is used as primary therapy is majority of cases. It may have feminising side effects such as gynaecomastia, nipple and scrotal pigmentation and testicular atrophy. More importantly, it may result in fluid retention and precipitate congestive cardiac failure, so that in elderly patients with cardiovascular disease bilateral orchidectomy should be performed.

Investigation of Choice
Transrectal USG (can assess extracapsular spread)

Immediate Management
Rule out heart disease

Treatment of Choice
Stilbesterol.

Your notes:

157. A 70-year-old man inoperable gastric cancer causing obstruction, and multiple liver metastases, is taking a large dose of oral analgesia. Despite this, his pain is currently unrelieved.

Diagnosis: Inoperable gastric carcinoma.

Clinchers

- *70-year-old man:* Gastric carcinoma can affect any age but particularly common in 50-70 years age groups (Incidence of most solid organ malignancies increases with age). In general men are more affected.
- *Inoperative gastric cancer:* Unequivocal evidence of incurability are
  - Hematogenous metastases
  - Involvement of distant peritoneum
  - N4 nodal disease
  - Disease beyond N4 nodes
  - Fixation to structures that cannot be removed (It is important to note that the involvement of another organ *per se* does not imply incurability provided it can be removed).
- *Causing obstruction:* The active medial management of malignant bowel obstruction includes:
  - The relief of intestinal colic using an antispasmodic such as hyoscine butylbromide 60-80 mg daily.
  - Treating continuous pain with adequate analgesia such as diamorphine.
  - Treating vomiting if nausea is a problem with a centrally acting antiemetic such as cyclizine 150 mg daily or haloperidol 5-10 mg daily.
- *Multiple liver metastases:* Liver metastases occur hematogenously and hematogenous spread implies inoperability.
- *Taking large dose of oral analgesia but ineffective pain relief:* It can be due to—non-absorption of oral dry due to obstruction

This necessitates the change of mode of administration. For cancer patients, who need long-term analgesia, continuous subcutaneous infusion is the preferred route.

CONFUSA

Diamorphine is preferred for subcutaneous infusion because of its greater solubility). By subcutaneous or intramuscular injection, diamorphine is approximately twice as potent as morphine orally.

Investigation of Choice

USG (for obstruction).

Immediate Management

Subcutaneous opiate infusion (diamorphine).

Treatment of Choice

In patients suffering from significant symptoms of either obstruction or bleeding, palliative resection is appropriate.

170. A 55-year-old lady with history of intermittent postmenopausal bleeding. Vaginal and speculum examinations are normal.

Diagnosis: Endometrial carcinoma

Clinchers

- *A 55-year-old:* Mean age of presentation is 56 years. It is rare under the age of 40.
- *Intermittent postmenopausal bleeding:* This symptom should always be assumed to be caused by carcinoma of endometrium until proven otherwise.
- *Vaginal and speculum examination are normal:* This has ruled out any local cause of bleeding (e.g. vaginal trauma) so this warrants examination of the endometrium now.

CONFUSA

Endometrial carcinoma is associated with hyperestrogenic states, i.e.

- Obesity
- Diabetes
- Late menopause
- Prolonged use of unopposed oestrogens
- Oestrogen secreting tumours

Investigation of Choice

- *Screening:* Ultrasound (to assess dimensions of any tumour and to show endometrial thickness)
- *Definitive:* Uterine sampling or curettage.

Immediate Management

Perform staging to decide the line of treatment.

Treatment of Choice

Usually surgical

Small	Well differentiated	*Total abdominal hysterectomy* + bilateral salpingo-ophorectomy + internal iliac node frozen section biopsy
Enlarged	Confined to upper part of corpus	*Extended hysterectomy* + bilateral salpingo-ophorectomy + removal of a cuff of vagina + lymph node sampling
Cervix invaded		*Wertheim's* (Removal of upper half of the vagina and pelvic lymph node)

- *Radiotherapy*
  - If node is involved
  - If there is deep invasion of myometrium
- *Hormone therapy:* Progestogens inhibit the rate of growth and spread of endometrial carcinoma.

PAPER 7

27. A 65-year-old male with weight loss, right-sided pain, tenesmus. On examination-mass in the rectum

Diagnosis: Carcinoma rectum.

Clinchers

- *65-year-old male:* It occurs in any age group from the twenties onwards, but is particularly common in the age range 50-70 years. The sexes are equally affected.
- *Weight loss, right side pain and tenesmus:* Bowel disturbance (constipation and/or diarrhoea in 80%) and bleeding, which is almost 60% of patients. There may also be mucus discharge rectal pain and tenesemus.
- *Mass in rectum:* Rectal examination reveals the tumour in 90% of cases.

CONFUSA

Abdominal palpation is negative in early cases but careful attention must be paid to the detection of hepatomegaly, ascites or abdominal distension. Other general featurs that may be detected in lead cases are enlarged supraclavicular nodes, nodes in the groin or jaundice.

Investigation of Choice

Sigmoidoscopy.

Immediate Management

Rule out faecal impaction and plevic abscess.

Treatment of Choice

Surgery

- Upper 1/3 tumours: Anterior resection
- Middle 1/3 tumours: Anterior resection if
  - female
  - satisfactory distal clearing
- Lower 1/3—Abdominal perineal resection.

Your notes:

32. A 60-year-old man with complaint of frequency, dysuria. PSA is 120 ng/ml, also has back pain.

Diagnosis: Carcinoma prostate.

Clinchers

- *60-year-old man:* Incidence of prostatic carcinoma increases with age. It is the most common malignant tumour in men over the age of 65 years. In England and Wales in 1998, 11000 men were registered and 8000 died from it.
- *Frequency, dysuria:* These are the symptoms of BOO, along with nocturia, hesitancy, poor stream and terminal dribbling. These symptoms can be seen in BPH, bladder neck stenosis, *prostate carcinoma,* urethral strictures, bladder neck hypertrophy and functional obstruction due to neuropathic conditions.
- *PSA is 120 ng/ml:* Prostate-specific antigen is good at following the course of advanced disease. Finding of a PSA > 10 ng/ml diagnostic of advanced prostate cancer.
  Decrease of PSA to the normal range following hormonal ablation is a good prognostic sign.
- *Back pain:* Bone pain, malaise, arthritis, anaemia are other clinical features of prostatic carcinoma. Weight loss and bone pain indicate metastatic disease, spread by the bloodstream.
- *Digital rectal examination:* May reveal hard, irregular prostate gland.

CONFUSA

These complaints may be present in BPH, but PSA value of 120 ng/ml is diagnostic of advanced carcinoma.

Investigation of Choice

- Prostate-specific antigen (PSA)
- Transrectal ultrasound
- Bone X-ray/bone scan.

Treatment of Choice

- *Local disease:* Nerve sparing radical prostatectomy (maintains erectile function) is widely used in USA, but there is a considerable defate over relative merits of prostatectomy, radiotherapy or watchful waiting with monitoring of PSA.
- *Metastatic disease:* Hormonal drugs (gonadotropin-releasing analogues) may give benefit for 1-2 years.

Case history

A 72-year-old man presents with 2 month history of haematuria and low back pain. Osteosclerotic lesions seen on pelvic X-ray.

- **Metastatic prostatic neoplasia:** This is suggested by haematuria, metastasis, hypercalcaemia and raised ESR.

157. A 55-year-old female develops a single episode of postmenopausal bleeding. She stopped menstruation 7 years ago. Ultrasound shows endometrial thickness.

Diagnosis: Endometrial carcinoma

Clinchers

- *55-year-old:* It usually presents after the menopause.
- *Single episode of postmenopausal bleeding:* Any post-menopausal vaginal bleeding must be investigated as the cause may be endometrial carcinomas.
- *Stopped menstruation 7 years ago:* Occasional bleeding is common upto 1 year after menopause but not upto 7 years.
- *USG shows endometrial thickness:* This clearly suggest endometrial growth and hence indicate a need to obtain the tissue diagnosis.

CONFUSA

Postmenopausal bleeding is an early sign and generally leads a woman to see her doctor, but examination is usually normal. Endometrial carcinoma is less common than carcinoma of cervix. Most endometrial tumours are adenocarcinomas and are related to excessive exposure to oestrogens unopposed by progesterone.

Investigation of Choice

Uterine sampling or curettage

Immediate Management

Take detailed history

Treatment of Choice

- Stage I and II—total hysterectomy with bilateral salpingo-oophorectomy
- Inoperable cases—radiotherapy

Your notes:

16 Ophthalmology

PAPER 1

Serial No. 19

Subject: Ophthalmology

Topic: Red Eye

Question: Acute Bacterial Conjunctivitis

Diagnosis: Acute Bacterial Conjunctivitis

Clinchers

- Conjunctivitis typically is a self-limited process; however, depending on the immune status of the patient and the etiology, conjunctivitis can progress to increasingly severe and sight-threatening infections.
- Purulent bacterial conjunctivitis in the neonate usually is caused by *Neisseria gonorrhoeae.* This type of conjunctivitis can be invasive and can lead to rapid corneal perforation.
- Ocular surface disease (e.g., keratitis sicca, trichiasis, chronic blepharitis) predisposes the patient to bacterial conjunctivitis.
- Staphylococcal and streptococcal species are the most common pathogens.
- The conjunctiva is usually hyperemic, however, cornea should be clear. Presence of corneal clouding suggests an alternative diagnosis such as glaucoma.

CONFUSA

DDs of Red Eye:

- Grittiness (not pain) with conjunctival hyperemia and mucopurulent discharge suggests conjunctivitis.
- Dull pain with photophobia, corneal deposits and fixed small pupils suggest Iritis.
- Acute severe pain, hazy cornea and fixed dilated pupils suggest Acute Glaucoma.
- Periauricular Lymphadenopathy is more common with viral conjunctivitis than bacterial conjunctivitis.

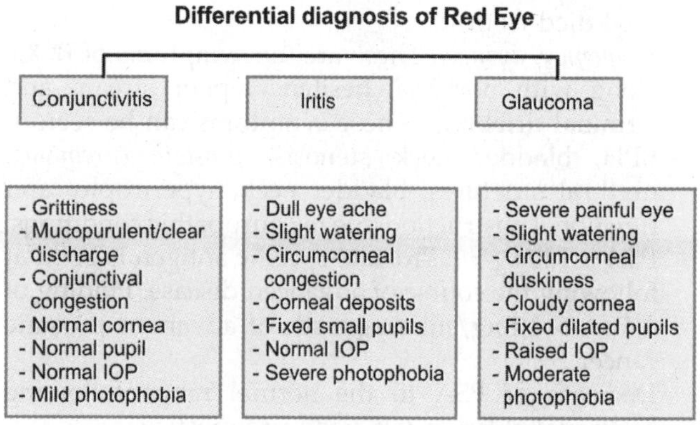

Investigation of Choice

- Gram stain is considered the criterion standard for determining the bacterial cause of conjunctivitis. Simple conjunctivitis does not require a Gram stain. Eosinophils seen on Gram stain are indicative of allergic conjunctivitis (also seen in parasitic causes).
- Conjunctival exudate culture is required in all newborns, neonates, persons who are immunosuppressed, or when *N. gonorrhoeae* is suspected as the offending organism.
  (exudate is collected from lower conjunctival fornix).

Immediate Management

Attention to personal hygiene to prevent spread of disease;

Irrigation of the conjunctival sac with saline to remove secretions

Treatment of Choice

Broad spectrum antibiotic drop or ointment, e.g. chloramphenicol ointment applied twice daily for five days. If culture or Gram stain has been undertaken, treatment is as for the organism identified.

Your notes:

Serial No. 20

Subject: Ophthalmology

Topic: Red Eye

Question: Acute allergic conjunctivitis

Diagnosis: Acute Allergic conjunctivitis

Clinchers

- *Seasonal Allergic Conjunctivitis:* Occurs due to Common airborne antigens including pollen, grass, and weeds. The symptoms are typically present in a defined period of time (i.e., in spring when the predominant airborne allergen is tree pollen; in summer when the predominant allergen is grass pollen; or in fall when the predominant allergen is weed pollen. Typically, patients are symptom-free during the winter months in cooler climates because of the decreased airborne transmission of these allergens.
- *Perennial Allergic Conjunctivitis:* Similar to seasonal allergic conjunctivitis, just that they have symptoms throughout the year because the implicated allergens are usually household allergens such as dust mite, cockroaches or pets.
- *Vernal Keratoconjunctivitis:* This is usually associated with a personal or family history of atopy. More than 90% of patients exhibit one or more atopic conditions such as asthma, eczema, or seasonal allergic rhinitis.
- *Atopic Keratoconjunctivitis:* Strongly associated with atopic dermatitis.
- *Giant Papillary Conjunctivitis:* Immune-mediated inflammatory disorder of superior tarsal conjunctiva. Occurs due to immunologic reaction to a variety of foreign bodies, especially contact lenses. Other associated 'foreign bodies' include ocular prostheses, extruded scleral buckles, and exposed sutures following previous surgical intervention.

CONFUSA

- Atopic and Vernal Keratoconjunctivitis, though may look very similar, look specifically for ATOPIC DERMATITIS to come to a diagnosis of atopic keratoconjunctivitis.
- Trachoma is also associated with formation of papillae in superior tarsal conjunctiva, but there the etiology is infective *(Chlamydia trachomatis)* not allergic.

Investigation of Choice

- Superficial conjunctival scrapings may reveal eosinophils.
- Skin testing may provide definitive diagnosis and pinpoint the offending allergen.
- In vernal keratoconjunctivitis, conjunctival scrapings of the superior tarsal conjunctiva and of Horner-Trantas dots show an abundance of eosinophils.

Immediate Management

- Antihistamine drops and tablets, with cold compresses relieve the itching.
- Local vasoconstrictors such as adrenaline may relieve the chemosis in the acute phase.

Treatment of Choice

- Avoid offending allergen
- Remove offending agent (viz, contact lenses)
- **Mast Cell Stabilizers**

Your notes:

Serial No. 21

Subject: Ophthalmology

Topic: Red Eye

Question: Acute angle closure glaucoma

Diagnosis: Acute angle closure glaucoma

Clinchers

- Acute angle closure glaucoma usually presents as painful red eye.
- The attacks are precipitated by factors which cause pupillary dilatation viz, night or drugs causing pupillary dilatation.
- Old age also increases the frequency of attacks because gradual thickening of lens causes papillary block.

CONFUSA

- Although pilocarpine was once the 1st line of treatment in acute attacks of glaucoma, currently the 1st line of management is aimed at instant lowering of intraocular pressure (carbonic anhydrase inhibitors, like acetazolamide).
- Because most of the attacks are also associated with nausea and vomiting, intravenous route for acetazolamide is more preferred than the oral route.
- Beta Blockers are the 2nd line treatment options.

Investigation of Choice

- Intraocular Pressure Measurement

Immediate Management

- Reduction of intra-ocular pressure by reducing aqueous secretion—acetazolamide, usually IV (see Confusa)
- Pupillary constriction—topical pilocarpine or thymoxamine, an alpha receptor antagonist.

Treatment of Choice

Surgical or laser iridectomy is indiacted once the attack has been controlled.

Your notes:

Serial No. 22

Subject: Ophthalmology

Topic: Cornea

Question: Keratitis (non-infective)

Diagnosis: Keratitis (non-infective)

Clinchers

- Keratitis is inflammation of cornea brought about various factors, infective and non-infective.
- Common infectious agents are: *Staphylococcus*, *Streptococcus*, herpes (both simplex and zoster), adenovirus, rubeola, rubella, mumps, trachoma, infectious mononucleosis, and pneumococcus;
- Also Vitamin A deficiency or broad spectrum antibiotic drug reactions may lead to keratitis.
- It may also follow trauma, may be associated with other eye infections (e.g., conjunctivitis),
- It may be related to other corneal disorders (e.g., degenerative conditions, or ptosis, which may cause a "dry eye" like Neuroparalytic keratitis, Sjögren's syndrome, Bell's Palsy.
- It may be associated with a variety of systemic disorders, especially those of autoimmune origin.
- It commonly presents as a painful red eye with reduced visual acuity due to cellular infiltration and later, corneal oedema.

CONFUSA

- Marginal Keratitis: This is ocular hypersensitivity reaction to conjunctival infection with bacteria, especially *Staphylococcus aureus*.
- Disciform Keratitis: Due to Herpes Simplex infection; corneal grafting is the only treatment.
- Interstitial Keratitis: Late feature of congenital syphilis.
- Rosacea Keratitis: Associated feature of acne rosacea.

Investigation of Choice

Fluorescein staining will show corneal ulceration. Culture and scrapings may be needed for suspected bacterial keratitis.

Immediate Management

- Protect eyes with pad and bandage or dark goggles
- Cycloplegics (1% atropine ointment/drops) to reduce pain from ciliary spasm and prevent the formation of posterior synechiae.

- Systemic analgesics and anti-inflammatory drugs like paracetamol.

Treatment of Choice

Depending on the cause of the keratitis.

- Infective (bacterial/fungal/viral) Keratitis: Antibiotic/ antifungal/viral drops.
- Keratitis Associated with autoimmune diseases: Steroids.
- Neuroparalytic Keratitis and Sjögren's Syndrome: Artificial Tears and Keratoplasty.

Your notes:

Serial No. 23

Subject: Ophthalmology

Topic: Cornea

Question: Corneal Abrasion

Diagnosis: Corneal Abrasion

Clinchers

- Extremely painful condition.
- It's a superficial injury, involving only the epithelium of cornea.
- Symptoms include pain, photophobia, lacrimation, blepharospasm.
- Always examine the under surface of the upper lid to rule out any foreign body.

CONFUSA

Recurrent corneal erosion is a syndrome affecting young mothers who are prone to injure their cornea with finger nails of their baby. The injured corneal heals by itself, however, the new epithelium is weak and gets abraded by itself, due to friction with the upper eyelids.

Typically the picture is of a young mother with previous history of corneal injury, wakes up in the morning with watering, pain, photophobia and blurred vision.

Investigation of Choice

Fluorescein staining

Immediate Management

Firm padding for 24-48 hrs to allow healing of epithelium

Instill cycloplegic to relieve ciliary spasm

Systemic analgesics

Treatment of Choice

Prophylactic antibiotics;

Evert the upper conjunctiva and examine carefully to rule out the possibility of foreign body.

Your notes:

Serial No. 24

Subject: Ophthalmology

Topic: Uveal Tract

Question: Uveitis

Diagnosis: Uveitis

Clinchers

- Uveitis is inflammation of the uveal tract.
- Anterior uveitis includes iritis and iridocyclitis; posterior uveitis refers to choroiditis, and since the retina is almost always secondarily affected, chorio-retinitis. Iritis describes an acute non-granulomatous anterior uveitis.
- Anterior Uveitis is known for its association with Juvenile Rheumatoid arthritis (pauciarticular form) and ankylosing spondylitis.
- Intermediate uveitis is defined as intraocular inflammation that predominantly involves the peripheral retina, pars plana, and vitreous. It is associated with 'snowballs' or 'cotton wool balls' - small, fluffy, vitreous inflammatory foci at the extreme periphery, often overlying the pars plana.
- Posterior uveitis is associated with Behcet's syndrome, CMV, Toxoplasmosis, Tuberculosis, Sarcoidosis.

CONFUSA

Heterochromic uveitis is an idiopathic form of anterior uveitis associated with depigmentation of iris of the affected eye. The typical picture is usually of a young male presenting with slight clouding of vision with floating spots, not associated with any pain or redness. On careful examination irises would be found to be of different colours (hence, heterochromic uveitis).

Investigation of Choice

Depending upon the cause of the disease.

Immediate Management

Cycloplegics
Corticosteroids

Treatment of Choice

Depending on the cause of the disease.

Your notes:

Serial No. 103

Subject: Ophthalmology

Topic: Loss of Vision

Question: A diabetic and hypertensive with sudden painless loss of vision. On examination, fundus appears pale.

Diagnosis: Central Retinal Artery Occlusion

Clinchers

- *Diabetic and hypertensive:* Atherosclerosis being one most important risk factor for thrombotic occlusion of retinal artery, diabetics and hypertensive are both at high risk as, both these conditions are known to accelerate the process of atherosclerosis. Men are affected more than women and is usually seen in elderly, above 60 years of age.
- *Sudden painless loss of vision:* It characteristically presents as painless, almost instantaneous loss of vision in one eye. In 90% of cases visual acuity is reduced only to counting fingers or light perception. The patient might give histories of earlier transient visual loss (amaurosis fugax).
- *Fundus appears pale:* Retina is usually pale and opaque because of oedema, only the choroid or retinal pigment epithelium are seen through very thin overlying foveola as the typically described, "cherry red spot". However, these fundal changes take hours to develop. Afferent pupillary defect appears immediately after the occlusion.

CONFUSA

- Embolic occlusion can also occur in atherosclerosis, however, diseased heart valves and atrial fibrillation are remain the more common causes.
- Embolic occlusion is typically preceded by episodes of amaurosis fugax as minute emboli interrupt blood flow before disintegrating and passing to the periphery.
- Occlusion due to vasospastic disease is transient, and vision usually returns within a few hours.
- Occlusion due to giant cell arteritis typically has history of headaches, jaw claudication, scalp tenderness, proximal muscle and joint aches, anorexia, weight loss, or fever.

Investigation of Choice

Fluorescein angiography.

Immediate Management

This is an ophthalmological emergency.
Immediate referral to the eye emergency department.

Treatment of Choice

Treatment aims at rapid reduction of intraocular pressure. This must be done within the first 2 hours, the principle being to dislodge the emboli into a more peripheral branch.

Firm ocular massage may dislodge embolus.

Anterior chamber paracentesis, isovolaemic haemodilution, reduction of arterial hypertension and acetazolamide 500 mg IV are all used to decrease intraocular tension.

Your notes:

PAPER 2

Serial No.86

Subject: Ophthalmology

Topic: Conjunctiva

Question: Allergic conjunctivitis

Diagnosis: Allergic conjunctivitis

Clinchers

- *Seasonal Allergic Conjunctivitis:* Occurs due to Common airborne antigens including pollen, grass, and weeds. The symptoms are typically present in a defined period of time i.e., in spring when the predominant airborne allergen is tree pollen; in summer when the predominant allergen is grass pollen; or in fall when the predominant allergen is weed pollen. Typically, patients are symptom-free during the winter months in cooler climates because of the decreased airborne transmission of these allergens.
- *Perennial Allergic Conjunctivitis:* Similar to seasonal allergic conjunctivitis, just that they have symptoms throughout the year because the implicated allergens are usually household allergens such as dust mite, cockroaches or pets.
- *Vernal Keratoconjunctivitis:* This is usually associated with a personal or family history of atopy. More than 90% of patients exhibit one or more atopic conditions such as asthma, eczema, or seasonal allergic rhinitis.
- *Atopic Keratoconjunctivitis:* Strongly associated with atopic dermatitis.
- *Giant Papillary Conjunctivitis:* Immune-mediated inflammatory disorder of superior tarsal conjunctiva. Occurs due to immunologic reaction to a variety of foreign bodies, especially contact lenses. Other associated 'foreign bodies' include ocular prostheses, extruded scleral buckles, and exposed sutures following previous surgical intervention.

CONFUSA

- Atopic and Vernal Keratoconjunctivitis, though may look very similar, look specifically for ATOPIC DERMATITIS to come to a diagnosis of atopic keratoconjunctivitis.
- Trachoma is also associated with formation of papillae in superior tarsal conjunctiva, but there the etiology is infective *(Chlamydia trachomatis)* not allergic.

Investigation of Choice

Superficial conjunctival scrapings may reveal eosinophils.

Skin testing may provide definitive diagnosis and pinpoint the offending allergen.

In vernal keratoconjunctivitis, conjunctival scrapings of the superior tarsal conjunctiva and of Horner-Trantas dots show an abundance of eosinophils.

Immediate Management

Antihistamine drops and tablets, with cold compresses relieve the itching.

Local vasoconstrictors such as adrenaline may relieve the chemosis in the acute phase.

Treatment of Choice

Avoid offending allergen
Remove offending agent (viz, contact lenses)
Mast Cell Stabilizers

Your notes:

Serial No. 87

Subject: Ophthalmology

Topic: Conjunctiva

Question: Ophthalmia neonatorum

Diagnosis: Ophthalmia neonatorum

Clinchers

- The infection of a neonate's eye occurring within one month of birth is known as ophthalmia neonatorum. Though most cases of ophthalmia neonatorum is in the form of bacterial conjunctivitis, it can also be due to viral conjunctivitis or rarely penetrating keratitis.
- Most cases of ophthalmia neonatorum are due to gonococcal infection and present within 48 hours of birth as severe conjunctivitis.
- The conjunctival infection can also be associated with fulminating disseminated gonococcal infection.

CONFUSA

Though we commonly relate the term ophthalmia neonatorum with gonococcal infection, it can occur due to variety of other causes like chlamydia or Group B beta hemolytic Streptococci. The chlamydial infection usually presents later than the gonococcal infection (3-13 days after birth) and is associated with the formation of pseudomembrane. However, the follicle formation which so characteristically seen with chlamydial infection in adults (recall trachoma), is not seen in infants because of the lack of adenoid tissue in the infant conjunctiva.

Investigation of Choice

If baby well: Eye swab for Gram stain smear and culture.
If baby is unwell: Full sepsis screen.

Immediate Management

Its an ocular emergency—Refer Immediately

Treatment of Choice

Topical chloramphenicol 0.5% eye drops and intramuscular benzylpenicillin or cefotaxime.

Fusidic acid is an alternative antibacterial to chloramphenicol.

Your notes:

Serial No. 88

Subject: Ophthalmology

Topic: Conjunctiva

Question: Trachoma

Diagnosis: Trachoma

Clinchers

- Trachoma is one of the commonest causes of blindness worldwide affecting more than one hundred million people affected.
- The condition is due to chlamydial infection—types A-C—leading to a chronic suppurative eye disease with follicular keratoconjunctivitis, eutropion and trichiasis.
- The disease is endemic in North Africa and the Middle East. Poverty, dry and sandy conditions, chronic childhood exposure to C. Trachomatis (A-C), and lack of access to medical care act as contributory factors.

CONFUSA

Because the main predisposing factors are close contacts, poverty and lack of personal hygiene, the World Health Organisation has implemented a policy of prevention of trachoma by 4 main steps—SAFE Strategy:

- Surgery for trichiasis
- Antibiotics, especially azithromycin to eradicate infection
- Facial cleansing and attention to hygiene.
- Environmental improvement

Investigation of Choice

Clinical diagnosis—Papillary hypertrophy and large follicles under upper eyelids are typical.

Immediate Management

Trace all family members who may have been in contact with the patient since they may harbour the disease.

Treatment of Choice

Oral azithromycin is the antibiotic of choice. Other drugs used are tetracycline, doxycycline or erythromycin.

If a child is infected the entire family should be treated.

Your notes:

Serial No. 89

Subject: Ophthalmology

Topic: Conjunctiva

Question: Reiter's Disease

Diagnosis: Reiter's Disease

Clinchers

- A triad of urethritis, conjunctivitis and a seronegative arthritis is known as Reiter's Disease.
- It usually follows an initial genital infection (urethritis) or enteric infection by Salmonella or Yersinia.
- Most affected patients are HLA B27 positive.

CONFUSA

For any question with features of arthritis involving the large joints (typically affecting the knees, ankles, feet & hands) always look carefully for a hints on a previous urethral infection, unprotected sexual intercourse or an episode of gastroenteritis. Seronegative arthritis and HLA B27 positivity are other strong hints in favor of Reiter's Syndrome.

Investigation of Choice

Urethral swab for culture (if urethritis present)
Stool culture (if enetral infection present)

Immediate Management

None

Treatment of Choice

Urethritis-Tetracycline;
Conjunctivitis-Chloramphenicol.
Arthritis-Rest, immobilisation of the joint, aspiration of the effusion, NSAIDs, and possibly steroids.
Physiotherapy should be given.
Keratodermia blenorrhagica—1% hydrocortisone.

Your notes:

Serial No. 90

Subject: Ophthalmology

Topic: Red Eye

Question: Acute Bacterial Conjunctivitis

Diagnosis: Acute Bacterial Conjunctivitis

Clinchers

- Conjunctivitis typically is a self-limited process; however, depending on the immune status of the patient and the etiology, conjunctivitis can progress to increasingly severe and sight-threatening infections.
- Purulent bacterial conjunctivitis in the neonate usually is caused by *Neisseria gonorrhoeae*. This type of conjunctivitis can be invasive and can lead to rapid corneal perforation.
- Ocular surface disease (e.g., keratitis sicca, trichiasis, chronic blepharitis) predisposes the patient to bacterial conjunctivitis.
- Staphylococcal and streptococcal species are the most common pathogens.
- The conjunctiva is usually hyperemic, however, cornea should be clear. Presence of corneal clouding suggests an alternative diagnosis such as glaucoma.

CONFUSA

DDs of Red Eye:

- Grittiness (not pain) with conjunctival hyperemia and mucopurulent discharge suggests conjunctivitis.
- Dull pain with photophobia, corneal deposits and fixed small pupils suggest Iritis.
- Acute severe pain, hazy cornea and fixed dilated pupils suggest Acute Glaucoma.
- Periauricular Lymphadenopathy is more common with viral conjunctivitis than bacterial conjunctivitis.

Investigation of Choice

- Gram stain is considered the criterion standard for determining the bacterial cause of conjunctivitis. Simple conjunctivitis does not require a Gram stain. Eosinophils seen on Gram stain are indicative of allergic conjunctivitis (also seen in parasitic causes).
- Conjunctival exudate culture is required in all newborns, neonates, persons who are immunosuppressed, or when *N. gonorrhoeae* is suspected as the offending organism.
  (exudate is collected from lower conjunctival fornix).

Differential diagnosis of Red Eye

Conjunctivitis	Iritis	Glaucoma
- Grittiness - Mucopurulent/clear discharge - Conjunctival congestion - Normal cornea - Normal pupil - Normal IOP - Mild photophobia	- Dull eye ache - Slight watering - Circumcorneal congestion - Corneal deposits - Fixed small pupils - Normal IOP - Severe photophobia	- Severe painful eye - Slight watering - Circumcorneal duskiness - Cloudy cornea - Fixed dilated pupils - Raised IOP - Moderate photophobia

Immediate Management

Attention to personal hygiene to prevent spread of disease;

Irrigation of the conjunctival sac with saline to remove secretions.

Treatment of Choice

Broad spectrum antibiotic drop or ointment, e.g. chloramphenicol ointment applied twice daily for five days. If culture or Gram stain has been undertaken, treatment is as for the organism identified.

Your notes:

PAPER 3

7. A 75-year-old has difficulty watching television complaining of a peripheral constriction of vision. On examination there is cupping of both optical discs.

Diagnosis: Chronic simple glaucoma (CSG).

Clinchers

- *75-year-old:* CSG risk increases with increasing age.
- *Difficulty watching television:* CSG can produce intermittent blurring of vision or peripheral constriction of visual field, both of which can interfere in sight.
- *Complaining of a peripheral constriction of vision:* Characteristic of CSG. Nasal and superior fields are lost first with the last vision remaining in the temporal field. Since the central field is intact, good acuity is maintained.
- *On examination there is cupping of both optical discs:* Intraocular pressure >21 mmHg causes optic disc cupping ± capillary closure, hence nerve damage, with sausage-shaped field defects (scotomata) near the blind spot, which may then coalesce to form major defects. Normal optic cups are similar in both eyes in shape and occupy < 50% of optic disc. In glaucoma these enlarge (widens and deepens) and optic disc pales (atrophy).

CONFUSA

Simple glaucoma is asympatomatic until visual fields are severely and irreversibly impaired. Some people may get glaucoma with normal intraocular pressure (IOP).

Investigation of Choice

IOP measurement + perimetry.

Immediate Management

Dorzolamide (if IOP -)

Treatment of Choice

- Medical reduction of IOP (i.e. timolol)
- Surgery if medical intervention fails (flap valve trabeculectomy)

Note: In older patient (like this case) Argon laser trabeculoplasty is preferred over surgery.

Your notes:

8. A 50-year-old with a history of SLE complains of loss of vision. On examination he is found to have multiple opacities in the lens of his eyes.

Diagnosis: Cataract.

Clinchers

- *History of SLE:* SLE is nonorgan specific due to immune disease in which antinuclear antibodies (ANA) occurs. There is no direct relationship between SLE and opacities in the lens. Though retinal exudates are sometimes seen in SLE patients.
- *In this question, since it is a diagnosed case of SLE:* We presume that patient is on treatment. Steroids are the most commonly prescribed drugs in SLE. This question could be explained on this basis (corticosteroid induced cataract).
- *Multiple opacities in the lens of his eyes:* These are associated with the use of topical as well as systemic steroids. Prolonged use of steroids may result in cataract formation.

CONFUSA

Since the patient is 50-year-old, it can well be a senile cataract also.

Immediate Management

- Decrease the dose of steroids.
- Low dose steroids have value in chronic disease.

Treatment of Choice

For cataract: ECCE with PCIOL.

Your notes:

9. A diabetic on oral hypoglycaemics complains of sudden deterioration in vision of his right eye. On examination he is found to have bilateral proliferative retinopathy with retinal haemorrhage on the right side.

Diagnosis: Vitreous haemorrhage.

Clinchers

- *Diabetic:* The most common and characteristic form of involvement of eye in diabetes is retinopathy. Diabetes is the leading cause of blindness in UK in those aged 20-65.
- *On oral hypoglycemics:* Oral hypoglycaemics does not have any specific visual side effects.
- *Complains of sudden deterioration in vision of his right eye:* The cause of it must be vitreous haemorrhage.
- *Bilateral proliferative retinopathy with retinal haemorrhage on the right side:* High retinal blood flow induces a microangiopathy in capillaries, precapillary arterioles and venules, causing occlusion and leakage. Occlusion causes ischaemia which leads to new vessel formation in the retina, the optic disc and on the iris, i.e. proliferative retinopathy. New vessels can bleed, causing vitreous haemorrhage. Rupture of micro-aneurysms causes retinal haemorrhages, flame haemorrhages when at nerve root level, blot haemorrhage when deep in retina.

CONFUSA

Although retinal detachment (which is also common in diabetic retinopathy) can present with same picture, it will be evident on fundoscopy which has been done in this case.

Investigation of Choice

Fundus fluorescein angiography to elucidate areas of neovascularisation, leakage and capillary nonperfusion.

Immediate Management

Control of hypertension (usually associated and can deteriorate a case of vitreous haemorrhage) + refer urgently to ophthalmologist.

Treatment of Choice

If vitreous haemorrhage is massive and does not clear, surgical vitrectomy may be needed. Otherwise do photocoagulation.

Your notes:

10. An 80-year-old has markedly decreased visual acuity. On fundoscopy she is found to have bilateral macular pigmentation.

Diagnosis: Senile macular degeneration (SMD).

Clinchers

- *80-year-old:* As the name suggests it occurs in elderly people. It is the most common cause of registrable blindness in UK. Usually it occurs above 65 years age.
- *Markedly decreased visual acuity:* Loss of central vision (hence visual acuity) is the main presenting complaint in SMD. Visual fields are unaffected.
- *Bilateral macular pigmentation:* SMD is a bilateral disease. The disc appears normal but there is pigment, fine exudate and haemorrhage at the macula. It is of two types—exudative and nonexudative. Drusen of Bruch's membrane is one of the earliest findings in the macula, varying in size, shape and colour. Drusen need not result in visual loss, and visual impairment may occur associated with a generalised pigmentary granularity and/or with atrophy of retinal pigment epithelium, photoreceptors and choriocapillaries.

CONFUSA

Though it is a bilateral disease, the fellow eye may appear quite different in its fundus appearance. Macula holes are an uncommon type of macula degeneration, which may present with distorted vision as well as visual loss.

Investigation of Choice

Fundoscopy by an expert.

Immediate Management

None except counselling.

Treatment of Choice

For most there is no effective treatment (especially for nonexudative SMD).

Laser photocoagulation is indicated in patients with exudative SMD having foveal choroidal neovascularisation to prevent further loss of vision.

Your notes:

191. A 35-year-old man presents with pain in the right eye, vomiting and loss of vision.

Diagnosis: Acute glaucoma

Clinchers

- *Painful loss of vision:* In this question the presentation seems to be acute. Let us see the causes of sudden painful loss of vision.
  - Acute congenital glaucoma
  - Acute iridocyclitis
  - Chemical/mechanical injuries to the eyeball.
- *Vomiting:* Severe pain in eye with loss of vision associated is the typical attack of acute congestive glaucoma.

CONFUSA

In iridocyclitis there is painful deterioration of vision, along with circumcorneal congestion. The onset is usually gradual. Moreover history of coloured haloes is present in glaucoma and not in iridocyclitis.

Immediate Management

Injectable analgesics (pethidine) to relieve pain. Systemic hyperosmotics (mannitol IV) given initially to lower IOP.

Treatment of Choice

It is essential surgical. However, medical therapy is instituted as an emergency and temporary measure before the eye is ready for operation.

Surgical treatment may consists of either

- peripheral iridectomy
- filtration surgery.

Your notes:

192. A 55-year-old known diabetic and hypertensive wakes up in the morning with diminished vision.

Diagnosis: Retinal detachment (RD).

Clinchers

- *55-year-old:* RD is most common in 40-60 years of age.
- *Diabetic:* Diabetes induces a high retinal blood flow—microangiopathy in capillary, precapillary arterioles and venules—occlusion and leakage—ischaemia—new vessel formation in retina (proliferative retinopathy)—new vessels carry along them fibrous tissue—increased traction—separation of neurosensory retina proper from pigment epithelium (as there are loosely attached)—retinal detachment.
- *Hypertensive:* It predisposes to accumulation of fluid beneath retina and a hypertensive retinopathy, both of which can potentially produce RD.
- *Wakes up in morning with diminished vision:* RD usually present as a sudden painless loss of vision.

CONFUSA

Only 50% of patients developing detachment have premonitary symptoms—flashing lights or the sensation of spots before the eyes as the retina has been abnormally stimulated prior to detachment. Detachment of lower half of the retina tends not to pull of the macula, whereas upper half detachments do (if the macula becomes detached, central vision is lost and does not recover completely even if the retina is successfully replaced). RD is sometimes described as a curtain falling over the vision.

Investigation of Choice

Retinoscopy (grey opalescent retina, ballooning forward).

Immediate Management

Urgent ophthalmology referral.

Treatment of Choice

Scleral silicone implants, cryotherapy, pneumatic retinopathy or argon or laser coagulation.

Your notes:

193. A 25-year-old man present to the accident and emergency department with pain in the right eye associated with backache.

Diagnosis: Uveitits.

Clinchers

- *25-year-old man:* Ankylosing spondylitis is more common in men, in second and third decades of life.
- *Pain in right eye with backache:* In ankylosing spondylitis patient (young man) typically presents with morning stiffness, backache, sacroiliac pain, progressive loss of spinal movement. Other features are uveitis, carditis, thoracic excursion, chest pain, plantar fascitis, lung fibrosis, etc.

Diagnosis is clinically supported by radiological findings. Though the clinical findings in this question are hard to find, but then this is what PLAB is all about.

Investigation of Choice

Radiology.

Treatment of Choice

Exercise not rest, for backache. NSAIDs may relieve pain and stiffness. Rarely spinal osteotomy is useful.

Your notes:

194. An elderly woman presents with a history of visual loss and scalp soreness.

Diagnosis: Cranial arteritis.

Clinchers

- *Elderly woman:* Cranial arteritis is rare under 55 years,
- *History of visual loss and scalp soreness:* Typical symptom of giant cell (cranial/temporal) arteritis are:
  - Headache
  - Scalp tenderness (e.g. on combing hair)
  - Jaw claudication
  - Sudden blindness in one eye

Tests: ESR-, CRP-, platelets, alkaline phosphatase - and Hb is decreased.

Investigation of Choice

Erythrocyte sedimentation rate.

Immediate Management

Start prednisolone 40-60 mg/24 hr PO immediately.

Treatment of Choice

Reduce prednisolone after 5-7 days in light of symptoms and ESR.

Your notes:

195. An elderly man who is an inpatient (for hypertension) wakes in the morning note that he cannot see his breakfast. He has no other complaints. He has a carotid bruit.

Diagnosis: Central retinal artery occlusion.

Clinchers

- *In patient (for hypertension):* Long-term complications of hypertension are:
  - Cardiac: MI, CHF
  - Cerebrovascular: TIA, stroke
  - Renal proteinuria: Microscopic haematuria,—BUN/creatinine
  - Retinopathy: Haemorrhage, exudates, arteriolar narrowing, papilloedema
- *Carotid bruit:* May signify stenosis (>30%) often near the internal carotid origin. Usual cause: athroma.
- *Cannot see his breakfast:* In central retinal artery occlusion, there is dramatic vision loss within seconds. The occlusion is usually due to thromboembolism (listen to carotid bruit).

Investigation of Choice

Carotid Doppler.

Treatment of Choice

If stenosis (carotid) is > 80%, go for surgery.

Your notes:

PAPER 4

125. Patient gets diplopia when he works very hard.

Diagnosis: Myasthenia gravis (MG)

Clinchers

- *Gets diplopia when he works very hard:* Fatiguability is the single most important feature of MG. Muscles are not commonly affected in the early stages:
  - Proximal limb muscles
  - Extraocular muscles
  - Muscles of mastication, speech and facial expression.

Complex extraocular palsies, ptosis and a typical fluctuating proximal weakness are found.

CONFUSA

The reflexes are initially preserved in MG but may be fatiguable. Muscle wasting is sometimes seen late in the disease. The clinical picture of fluctuating weakness may be diagnostic. Early symptoms of weakness and fatigue are frequently dismissed by attending doctors.

Investigation of Choice

Tensilon test (only do if resuscitation facilities available)

Immediate Management

Rule out

- Thymic tumour
- Hyperthyroidism
- Rheumatoid arthritis
- SLE

Treatment of Choice

Pyridostigmine + prednisolone.

Your notes:

PAPER 5

17. A 50-year-old woman complains of sudden loss of vision in one eye. She describes the incident, like a curtain coming down.

Diagnosis: Retinal detachment

Clinchers

- *50-year-old woman:* Retinal detachment is most common between 40 and 60 years, though it may occur at any age. F : M (3 : 2) ratio.
- *Sudden painless loss of vision:* Causes of sudden painless loss of vision are:
  - Retinal detachment
  - Central retinal artery/vein occlusion
  - Vitreous haemorrhage
  - Central serous retinopathy
  - Optic neuritis
  - Methyl alcohol amblyopia
- *Curtain coming down (in one eye):* Appearance of dark cloud, or veil like curtain in front of eye suddenly is the sign of retinal detachment (large and central).

CONFUSA

Retinal detachment should be differentiated from the other causes of sudden painless loss of vision (given above). In early cases of retinal detachment patient notices a localised relative loss in the field of vision (of detached retina) which progresses as detachment proceeds towards the macular area.

Investigation of Choice

- *Ophthalmoscopy:* Detached retina gives grey reflex instead of normal pink reflex
- *Visual field charting*
- *USG* confirms the diagnosis.

Treatment of Choice

- Sealing of retinal breaks
- Bring the sclerochoroid and detached retina near to each other.

High risk factors for retinal detachment: Myopia, aphakia, retinal detachment in fellow eye, history of retinal detachment in family.

Your notes:

19. A 68-year-old smoker suddenly notices markedly reduced vision in one eye. He cannot read any letter on visual acuity chart but can count fingers. The fundus is pale.

Diagnosis: Central retinal artery occlusion (CRAO).

Clinchers

- *68-year-old smoker:* These are the risk factors for CRAO. More commonly seen in patients suffering from hypertension and other cardiovascular diseases. It is usually unilateral, but rarely be bilateral (1-2% cases).
- *Notices reduced vision in one eye:* CRAO is usually unilateral. Sudden painless loss of vision is suggestive of central retinal artery occlusion.
- *Fundus is pale:* Retina becomes milky white due to oedema. Retinal arteries are markedly narrowed. Fundus is pale.

CONFUSA

Sudden painless loss of vision occur in central retinal artery occlusion, vitreous haemorrhage, retinal detachment, central retinal vein occlusion, central serous retinopathy, optic neuritis and methyl alcohol amblyopia.

Investigation of Choice

Investigate for the cause.

Immediate Management

- Immediate lowering of IOP (IV mannitol)
- Vasodilators and inhalation of a mixture of 5% CO_2 and 95% O_2 (may help in relieving angiospasm)
- Anticoagulants
- Intravenous steroids.

Treatment of Choice

Treatment is unsatisfactory as retinal tissue cannot survive ischaemia for more than a few hours. Emergency treatment (as above) should be followed.

Your notes:

20. A 30-year-old man has recurrent episodes of an acutely painful red eye with reduced vision.

Diagnosis: Uveitis

Clinchers

- *Acutely painful red eye reduced vision:* These symptoms are suggestive of anterior uveitis (iridocyclitis).
- *Pain:* It is a dominating symptom of anterior uveitis, typically worsen at right.
- *Redness:* It is due to circumcorneal congestion, which is a result of active hyperaemia of anterior ciliary, vessels.
- *Reduces vision:* Defective vision in patient with iridocyclitis may vary from slight blur in early phase to marked deterioration in late phase.
- Look for corneal oedema and keratic precipitates (KP) at back of cornea.

CONFUSA

Acute congestive glaucoma and acute conjunctivitis should be kept in mind here, and should be differentiated from iridocyclitis. Other conditions that may cause sudden painful visual loss are chemical or mechanical injuries to the eyeball.

Investigation of Choice

Includes battery of tests due to its varied etiology.

Immediate Management

1 per cent atropine sulphate eye ointment or drops 2-3 times day. In case of atropine allergy other cycloplegics should be used.

Treatment of Choice

Local treatment with mydriatic-cycloplegic drugs and corticosteroids (reduce inflammation).

Systemic therapy with corticosteroids (especially in non-granulomatous iridocyclitis). NSAIDs where steroids contraindicated. Adrenocorticotrophic hormone where steroids fail to act.

Finally treat the cause.

Your notes:

61. A 69-year-old patient presented to his GP with sudden onset of redness in the right eye. There was no pain and vision was unaffected.

Diagnosis: Subconjunctival haemorrhage.

Most appropriate management: No treatment.

Clinchers

Red eye may be due to variety of conditions, but here since there is no pain and the vision is unaffected, no active intervention is required. Though in this case we must check the blood pressure of the patient. No need to go for coagulation studies, as one of the options in this questions suggests.

Subconjunctival haemorrhage may be due to rupture of conjunctival capillaries, due to raised pressure, e.g. in whooping cough, strangulation, epileptic fits, etc. May also be seen in vascular diseases such as arterio-sclerosis, hypertension and diabetes mellitus.

CONFUSA

Checking the blood pressure and observation are the main line of treatment in this patient. If any underlying cause is established or suspected, it should be investigated and managed.

Investigation of Choice

Not required.

Immediate Management

No treatment.

Treatment of Choice

Treat the cause when discovered. Assurance to the patient is must. No other active intervention required. Cold compresses can be given in the beginning if bleeding.

Your notes:

62. A 60-year-old patient complains of severe pain in his left eye with severe deterioration of vision. He had noticed haloes around street lights at night for a few days before the onset of the pain.

Diagnosis: Angle closure glaucoma (ACG).

Most appropriate management: 3% pilocarpine drops and acetazolamide.

Clinchers

- *69-year-old patient:* Angle closure glaucoma is comparatively most common in 5th to 6th decades of life.
- *Severe pain and deterioration of vision:* Causes of painful (sudden) loss of vision are:
  - Acute congestive glaucoma
  - Acute iridocyclitis
  - Chemical injury to eyeball
  - Mechanical injury to eyeball
- *Coloured haloes:* These are seen around the light due to corneal oedema.

CONFUSA

Though the management in this case is essentially surgical, medical therapy of 3% pilocarpine drops and acetazolamide is instituted as an emergency.

Investigation of Choice

Gonioscopy

Immediate Management

3% pilocarpine and acetazolamide

Treatment of Choice

Peripheral iridectomy or filtration surgery. In the interval between confirmation of the diagnosis and surgery use give 3% pilocarpine drops and acetazolamide.

Your notes:

63. A mother brings her 2-year-old child with a squint. On examination a leucokoric right pupil is seen with an absent red reflex.

Diagnosis: Retinoblastoma

Most appropriate management: Enucleation

Clinchers

- *2-year-old child:* Retinoblastoma is the most common intraocular tumour of childhood. Though congenital, it is not recognised at birth, and is usually seen between 1-2 years of age, with no sex predisposition.
- *Squint:* Usually convergent may develop in retinoblastoma.
- *Leucokoric right pupil:* Conditions other than retinoblastoma that present as leucocoria are: congenital cataract, inflammatory deposits in vitreous following a plastic cyclitis or choroiditis, coloboma of the choroid, retrolental fibroplasia, toxocara endophthalmitis and exudative retinopathy of coats.

CONFUSA

Retinoblastoma should be differentiated from other conditions that present as leucocoria.

Investigation of Choice

Fundus examination and ophthalmoscopy
Plain X-ray orbit shows calcification
USG and CT are very useful.

Treatment of Choice

Enucleation (excision of the eyeball)
Absolute indications of enucleation are:

- retinoblastoma, and
- malignant melanoma

Indications of evisceration (removal of the contents of the eyeball leaving behind the sclera) are—

- panophthalmitis
- expulsive choroidal haemorrhage, and
- bleeding anterior staphyloma.

Your notes:

64. A 12-year-old Libyan boy gave a two-week history of discomfort, redness and mucopurulent discharge affecting both eyes. His two siblings have a similar problem.

Diagnosis: Acute mucopurulent conjunctivitis

Most appropriate management: Immediate antibiotic therapy.

Clinchers

- *12-year-old Libyan boy:* Infective conjunctivitis is still common in developing countries.
- *Discomfort, redness, mucopurulent discharge:* There are the symptoms of acute mucopurulent conjunctivitis. Discomfort and foreign body sensation due to engorgement of vessels.
- *Time siblings have similar problem:* Mucopurulent conjunctivitis may be caused by *Staphylococcus aureus* Koch-Weeks bacillus, Pneumococcus or Streptococcus. It is infective in nature.

CONFUSA

Conjunctival congestion is more marked in palpebral conjunctiva, fornices and peripheral part of bulbar conjunctiva. Circumcorneal congestion is seen in iridocyclitis.

Investigation of Choice

Conjunctival cytology and bacterial examination of secretions and scrapings.

Immediate Management

Topical broad spectrum antibiotics to control the infection.

Treatment of Choice

Topical antibiotics

- Irrigation of conjunctival sac with sterile warm saline once or twice a day
- Dark goggles
- No bandage
- No steroids (infection may flare up).

Your notes:

PAPER 6

1. A 69-year-old patient presented to his GP with sudden onset of redness in the right eye. There was no pain and vision was unaffected.

Diagnosis: Subconjunctival haemorrhage.

Most appropriate management: No treatment.

Clinchers

Red eye may be due to variety of conditions, but here since there is no pain and the vision is unaffected, no active intervention is required. Though in this case we must check the blood pressure of the patient. No need to go for coagulation studies, as one of the options in this questions suggests.

Subconjunctival haemorrhage may be due to rupture of conjunctival capillaries, due to raised pressure, e.g. in whooping cough, strangulation, epileptic fits, etc. May also be seen in vascular diseases such as arteriosclerosis, hypertension and diabetes mellitus.

CONFUSA

Checking the blood pressure and observation are the main line of treatment in this patient. If any underlying cause is established or suspected, it should be investigated and managed.

Investigation of Choice

Not required.

Immediate Management

No treatment.

Treatment of Choice

Treat the cause when discovered. Assurance to the patient is must. No other active intervention required. Cold compresses can be given in the beginning if bleeding.

Your notes:

2. A patient presents with metal pieces to his eyes.

Diagnosis: Intraocular foreign bodies (IOFB).

Clinchers

➢ *Metal pieces to his eyes:* A careful history about of mode of injury may give a clue about the type of IOFB. A thorough ocular examination with slit-lamp including gonioscopy should be carried out. The signs which may give some indication about IOFB are:
- Subconjunctival haemorrhage
- Corneal scar
- Holes in the iris
- Opaque track through the lens

With clear media, sometimes IOFB may be seen on ophthalmoscopy in the vitreous or on the retina. IFOB lodged in the angle of anterior chamber may be visualized by gonioscopy.

CONFUSA

Anteroposterior and lateral X-rays of the orbit are indispensable for the location of IOFB, as metallic foreign body are radiopaque. Its exact localization is mandatory to plan proper removal.

Investigation of Choice

Plain X-rays of orbit

Immediate Management

Ophthalmology referral

Treatment of Choice

Magnetic foreign body is removed with a hand held magnet.

Nonmagnetic foreign body is picked up with a toothless forceps.

Your notes:

3. A mother brings her 2-year-old child with a squint. On examination a leucokoric right pupil is seen with an absent red reflex.

Diagnosis: Retinoblastoma

Most appropriate management: Enucleation

Clinchers

➢ *2-year-old child:* Retinoblastoma is the most common intraocular tumour of childhood. Though congenital, it is not recognised at birth, and is usually seen between 1-2 years of age, with no sex predisposition.

➢ *Squint:* Usually convergent may develop in retinoblastoma.

➢ *Leucokoric right pupil:* Conditions other than retinoblastoma that present as leucocoria are: congenital cataract, inflammatory deposits in vitreous following a plastic cyclitis or choroiditis, coloboma of the choroid, retrolental fibroplasia, toxocara endophthalmitis and exudative retinopathy of coats.

CONFUSA

Retinoblastoma should be differentiated from other conditions that present as leukocoria.

Investigation of Choice

Fundus examination and ophthalmoscopy

Plain X-ray orbit shows calcification

USG and CT are very useful.

Treatment of Choice

Enucleation (excision of the eyeball)

Absolute indications of enucleation are:
- retinoblastoma, and
- malignant melanoma

Indications of evisceration (removal of the contents of the eyeball leaving behind the sclera) are
- panophthalmitis
- expulsive choroidal haemorrhage, and
- bleeding anterior staphyloma.

Your notes:

4. A 12-year-old Libyan boy gave a two-week history of discomfort, redness and mucopurulent discharge affecting both eyes. His two siblings have a similar problem.

Diagnosis: Acute mucopurulent conjunctivitis

Most appropriate management: Immediate antibiotic therapy.

Clinchers

➢ *12-year-old Libyan boy:* Infective conjunctivitis is still common in developing countries.

➢ *Discomfort, redness, mucopurulent discharge:* There are the symptoms of acute mucopurulent conjunctivitis. Discomfort and foreign body sensation due to engorgement of vessels.

➢ *Time siblings have similar problem:* Mucopurulent conjunctivitis may be caused by *Staphylococcus aureus* Koch-Weeks bacillus, Pneumococcus or streptococcus. It is infective in nature.

CONFUSA

Conjunctival congestion is more marked in palpebral conjunctiva, fornices and peripheral part of bulbar conjunctiva. Circumcorneal congestion is seen in iridocyclitis.

Investigation of Choice

Conjunctival cytology and bacterial examination of secretions and scrapings.

Immediate Management

Topical broad spectrum antibiotics to control the infection.

Treatment of Choice

Topical antibiotics

- Irrigation of conjunctival sac with sterile warm saline once or twice a day
- Dark goggles
- No bandage
- No steroids (infection may flare up).

Your notes:

5. A 23-year-old woman has a history of recurrent attacks of blurring of vision associated with redness, pain and photophobia. Both eyes have been affected in the past. She is currently being investigated for bowel disease and a severe backache.

Diagnosis: Multiple sclerosis

Most appropriate management: 0.5% prednisolone drops 2 hourly and cyclopentolate drops.

Clinchers

➢ *23-year-old man:* Multiple sclerosis has female preponderance. Mean age of onset is 30 years.

➢ *Recurrent attacks of blurring of vision:* Early picture of multiple sclerosis is usually one of relapses followed by remissions become incomplete. In multiple sclerosis, plaques of demyelination are seen at the sites through at the CNS.

➢ *Bowel disease of severe backache:* Bowel (constipation), fatigue, motor weakness, optic neuritis, incontinence, numbness, tingling in limbs, cerebellar symptoms may be seen in multiple sclerosis.

CONFUSA

Isolated neurological deficits are never diagnostic, but may become so, if a careful history reveals previous episodes.

Investigation of Choice

MRI is sensitive

Immediate Management

Treat the complication

Treatment of Choice

No cure but following may help

- Methylprednisolone (shortens relapses), use sparingly. It does no alter overall prognosis.
- β-*interferon:* Relapse rate by 1/3.

Your notes:

7. A 50-year-old woman complains of sudden loss of vision in one eye. She describes the incident, like a curtain coming down.

Diagnosis: Retinal detachment

Clinchers

- *50-year-old woman:* Retinal detachment is most common between 40 and 60 years, though it may occur at any age. F : M (3 : 2) ratio.
- *Sudden painless loss of vision:* Causes of sudden painless loss of vision are:
  - Retinal detachment
  - Central retinal artery/vein occlusion
  - Vitreous haemorrhage
  - Central serous retinopathy
  - Optic neuritis
  - Methyl alcohol amblyopia
- *Curtain coming down (in one eye):* Appearance of dark cloud, or veil like curtain in front of eye suddenly is the sign of retinal detachment (large and central).

CONFUSA

Retinal detachment should be differentiated from the other causes of sudden painless loss of vision (given above). In early cases of retinal detachment patient notices a localised relative loss in the field of vision (of detached retina) which progresses as detachment proceeds towards the macular area.

Investigation of Choice

- *Ophthalmoscopy:* Detached retina gives grey reflex instead of normal pink reflex
- *Visual field charting*
- *USG* confirms the diagnosis.

Treatment of Choice

- Sealing of retinal breaks
- Bring the sclerochoroid and detached retina near to each other.

High risk factors for retinal detachment: Myopia, aphakia, retinal detachment in fellow eye, history of retinal detachment in family.

Your notes:

8. An 84-year-old woman notices sudden increased visual impairment. She is found to have homonymous hemianopia.

Diagnosis: Cerebral haemorrhage

Clinchers

- *84-year-old woman:* Incidence of rupture of cerebral vessel aneurysms increases with age. These aneurysms are common in females.
- *Sudden increased visual impairment:* Since the defect is of sudden onset, it rules out tumours or other chronic disease processes as a causation. There is no given history of trauma cerebral embolism can be ruled out as it usually do not produce permanent changes.
- *Homonymous hemianopia:* Most commonly it results from lesions in optic tract (tumours pressing it), geniculate body and optic radiations (cerebral haemorrhage). Since we have ruled out tumours to be cause, cerebral haemorrhage is a safe answer.

CONFUSA

Hemianopia denotes loss of half of the field of vision. The most common clinical form is homonymous hemianopia, in which the right of left half of the binocular field of vision is lost, owing to loss of the temporal half of one field and the nasal half of the other, a condition due to a lesion situated in any part of the visual paths from the chiasma to the occipital lobe. Right hemianopia is more quickly discovered than left owing to the fact that reading is impossible; left hemianopia is often discovered when the patient does not see food on the left side of the plate.

Investigation of Choice

MRI/CT

Immediate Management

Admit and specialist evaluation

Treatment of Choice

Symptomatic + as per radiological findings.

Your notes:

9. A 68-year-old smoker suddenly notices markedly reduced vision in one eye. He cannot read any letter on visual acuity chart but can count fingers. The fundus is pale.

Diagnosis: Central retinal artery occlusion (CRAO).

Clinchers

- *68-year-old smoker:* These are the risk factors for CRAO. More commonly seen in patients suffering from hypertension and other cardiovascular diseases. It is usually unilateral, but rarely be bilateral (1-2% cases).
- *Notices reduced vision in one eye:* CRAO is usually unilateral. Sudden painless loss of vision is suggestive of central retinal artery occlusion.
- *Fundus is pale:* Retina becomes milky white due to oedema. Retinal arteries are markedly narrowed. Fundus is pale.

CONFUSA

Sudden painless loss of vision occur in central retinal artery occlusion, vitreous haemorrhage, retinal detachment, central retinal vein occlusion, central serous retinopathy, optic neuritis and methyl alcohol amblyopia.

Investigation of Choice

Investigate for the cause.

Immediate Management

- Immediate lowering of IOP (IV mannitol)
- Vasodilators and inhalation of a mixture of 5% CO_2 and 95% O_2 (may help in relieving angiospasm)
- Anticoagulants
- Intravenous steroids

Treatment of Choice

Treatment is unsatisfactory as retinal tissue cannot survive ischaemia for more than a few hours. Emergency treatment (as above) should be followed.

Your notes:

10. A 30-year-old man has recurrent episodes of an acutely painful red eye with reduced vision.

Diagnosis: Uveitis

Clinchers

- *Acutely painful red eye reduced vision:* These symptoms are suggestive of anterior uveitis (iridocyclitis).
- *Pain:* It is a dominating symptom of anterior uveitis, typically worsen at right.
- *Redness:* It is due to circumcorneal congestion, which is a result of active hyperaemia of anterior ciliary, vessels.
- *Reduces vision:* Defective vision in patient with iridocyclitis may vary from slight blur in early phase to marked deterioration in late phase.
- Look for corneal oedema and keratic precipitates (KP) at back of cornea.

CONFUSA

Acute congestive glaucoma and acute conjunctivitis should be kept in mind here, and should be differentiated from iridocyclitis. Other conditions that may cause sudden painful visual loss are chemical or mechanical injuries to the eyeball.

Investigation of Choice

Includes battery of tests due to its varied etiology.

Immediate Management

1 per cent atropine sulphate eye ointment or drops 2-3 times day. In case of atropine allergy other cycloplegics should be used.

Treatment of Choice

Local treatment with mydriatic-cycloplegic drugs and corticosteroids (reduce inflammation).

Systemic therapy with corticosteroids (especially in non-granulomatous iridocyclitis). NSAIDs where steroids contraindicated. Adrenocorticotrophic hormone where steroids fail to act.

Finally treat the cause.

Your notes:

113. Patient has repeated attacks of multiple sclerosis, and now has pale temporal disc.

Diagnosis (of anatomical site): Optic nerve

Clinchers

- *Pale temporal disc:* Disc pallor following an attack of multiple sclerosis is a sign of optic atrophy. It is first seen in temporal region.

  The optic disc appearance depends upon the site of the plaque of multiple sclerosis, within the optic nerve. If the lesion is in the nerve head, there is disc swelling (optic neuritis). If the lesion is several millimeters behind the disc, there is generally no ophthalmoscopic feature. Here the doctor sees nothing and the patient sees nothing.

  After the attack subsides, usually there is no residual symptom, but small scotoma or defects in colour vision can be demonstrated. Disc pallor is a late sequelae of multiple sclerosis and a sign of optic atrophy.

CONFUSA

Disc swelling from optic neuritis causes early and measurably visual acuity loss, thus distinguishing it from disc swelling from raised intracranial pressure.

Investigation of Choice

MRI (magnetic resonance imaging)

Immediate Management

Refer to neurology

Treatment of Choice

When diagnosed, inform the patient of the diagnosis. There is no cure.

- *Polyunsatured fats*—may help.
- *Methylprednisolone*—shortens relapses
- β-interferon 1b
  - Relapse rate by 1/3
  - Lesion accumulation on MRI
  - Slow accumulation of disability.

114. Patient with complaint of blurring of vision, papilloedema and pain in eye.

Diagnosis (of anatomical site): Optic nerve

Clinchers

- *Blurring of vision:* Optic neuritis produces variable loss. It usually begins as blurring of the central visual field, which may remain mild or progress to severe visual loss, or rarely, to complete loss of light perception. In mild cases, the patient may complain only of a subjective loss of brightness in the affected eye. Symptoms are generally monocular, but attacks may be bilateral.
- *Papilloedema:* This is due to optic neuritis fundoscopic examination in it may be normal or with swelling of optic disc.
- *Pain in eye:* Pain, localized to the orbit or supraorbital area is frequently present and may precede visual loss. The pain typically worsens with eye movement.

CONFUSA

Visual blurring in MS may result from optic neuritis or diplopia. They are distinguished by asking the patient to cover each eye sequentially and observing whether the visual difficulty clears. Diplopia in MS is often due to an internuclear ophthalmoplegia (INO) or to a sixth nerve palsy; ocular muscle palsies due to involvement of the third or fourth cranial nerve are rare.

Investigation of Choice

MRI

Immediate Management

Refer to neurology

Treatment of Choice

When diagnosed, inform the patient of the diagnosis. There is no cure.

- *Polyunsatured fats*—may help
- *Methylprednisolone*—shortens relapses
- β-interferon 1b
  - Relapse rate by 1/3
  - Lesion accumulation on MRI
  - Slow accumulation of disability.

172. A 75-year-old has difficulty watching television complaining of a peripheral constriction of vision. On examination there is cupping of both optical discs

Diagnosis: Chronic simple glaucoma (CSG).

Clinchers

- *75-year-old:* CSG risk increases with increasing age.
- *Difficulty watching television:* CSG can produce intermittent blurring of vision or peripheral constriction of visual field, both of which can interfere in sight.
- *Complaining of a peripheral constriction of vision:* Characteristic of CSG. Nasal and superior fields are lost first with the last vision remaining in the temporal field. Since the central field is intact, good acuity is maintained.
- *On examination there is cupping of both optical discs:* Intraocular pressure >21 mmHg causes optic disc cupping ± capillary closure, hence nerve damage, with sausage-shaped field defects (scotomata) near the blind spot, which may then coalesce to form major defects. Normal optic cups are similar in both eyes in shape and occupy < 50% of optic disc. In glaucoma these enlarge (widens and deepens) and optic disc pales (atrophy).

CONFUSA

Simple glaucoma is asymptomatic until visual fields are severely and irreversibly impaired. Some people may get glaucoma with normal intraocular pressure (IOP).

Investigation of Choice

IOP measurement + perimetry.

Immediate Management

Dorzolamide (if IOP -)

Treatment of Choice

- Medical reduction of IOP (i.e. timolol)
- Surgery if medical intervention fails (flap valve trabeculectomy)

Note: In older patient (like this case) Argon laser trabeculoplasty is preferred over surgery.

Your notes:

173. A 50-year-old with a history of SLE complains of loss of vision. On examination he is found to have multiple opacities in the lens of his eyes.

Diagnosis: Cataract.

Clinchers

- *History of SLE:* SLE is nonorgan specific due to immune disease in which antinuclear antibodies (ANA) occurs. There is no direct relationship between SLE and opacities in the lens. Though retinal exudates are sometimes seen in SLE patients.
- *In this question, since it is a diagnosed case of SLE:* We presume that patient is on treatment. Steroids are the most commonly prescribed drugs in SLE. This question could be explained on this basis (corticosteroid induced cataract).
- *Multiple opacities in the lens of his eyes:* These are associated with the use of topical as well as systemic steroids. Prolonged use of steroids may result in cataract formation.

CONFUSA

Since the patient is 50-year-old, it can well be a senile cataract also.

Immediate Management

- Decrease the dose of steroids.
- Low dose steroids have value in chronic disease.

Treatment of Choice

For cataract: ECCE with PCIOL.

Your notes:

174. A diabetic on oral hypoglycaemics complains of sudden deterioration in vision of his right eye. On examination he is found to have bilateral proliferative retinopathy with retinal haemorrhage on the right side.

Diagnosis: Vitreous haemorrhage.

Clinchers

- *Diabetic:* The most common and characteristic form of involvement of eye in diabetes is retinopathy. Diabetes is the leading cause of blindness in UK in those aged 20-65.
- *On oral hypoglycaemics:* Oral hypoglycaemics does not have any specific visual side effects.
- *Complains of sudden deterioration in vision of his right eye:* The cause of it must be vitreous hemorrhage.
- *Bilateral proliferative retinopathy with retinal haemorrhage on the right side:* High retinal blood flow induces a microangiopathy in capillaries, precapillary arterioles and venules, causing occlusion and leakage. Occlusion causes ischaemia which leads to new vessel formation in the retina, the optic disc and on the iris, i.e. proliferative retinopathy. New vessels can bleed, causing vitreous haemorrhage. Rupture of micro-aneurysms causes retinal haemorrhages, flame haemorrhages when at nerve root level, blot hemorrhage when deep in retina.

CONFUSA

Although retinal detachment (which is also common in diabetic retinopathy) can present with same picture, it will be evident on fundoscopy which has been done in this case.

Investigation of Choice

Fundus fluorescein angiography to elucidate areas of neovascularisation, leakage and capillary non-perfusion.

Immediate Management

Control of hypertension (usually associated and can deteriorate a case of vitreous haemorrhage) + refer urgently to ophthalmologist.

Treatment of Choice

If vitreous haemorrhage is massive and does not clear, surgical vitrectomy may be needed. Otherwise do photocoagulation.

Your notes:

175. An 80-year-old has markedly decreased visual acuity. On fundoscopy she is found to have bilateral macular pigmentation.

Diagnosis: Senile macular degeneration (SMD).

Clinchers

- *80-year-old:* As the name suggests it occurs in elderly people. It is the most common cause of registrable blindness in UK. Usually it occurs above 65 years age.
- *Markedly decreased visual acuity:* Loss of central vision (hence visual acuity) is the main presenting complaint in SMD. Visual fields are unaffected.
- *Bilateral macular pigmentation:* SMD is a bilateral disease. The disc appears normal but there is pigment, fine exudate and haemorrhage at the macula. It is of two types—exudative and nonexudative. Drusen of Bruch's membrane is one of the earliest findings in the macula, varying in size, shape and colour. Drusen need not result in visual loss, and visual impairment may occur associated with a generalised pigmentary granularity and/or with atrophy of retinal pigment epithelium, photoreceptors and choriocapillaries.

CONFUSA

Though it is a bilateral disease, the fellow eye may appear quite different in its fundus appearance. Macula holes are an uncommon type of macula degeneration, which may present with distorted vision as well as visual loss.

Investigation of Choice

Fundoscopy by an expert.

Immediate Management

None except counselling.

Treatment of Choice

For most there is no effective treatment (especially for nonexudative SMD).

Laser photocoagulation is indicated in patients with exudative SMD having foveal choroidal neovascularisation to prevent further loss of vision.

Your notes:

PAPER 7

137. 60-year-old develops tunnel vision. There is enlargement of the optic cup.

Diagnosis: Chronic simple glaucoma (CSG).

Clinchers

- *60-year-old:* The risk of CSG increases with increasing age.
- *Tunnel vision:* Isopter contraction is the earliest visual field defect occurring in glaucoma. It refers to mild generalized constriction of the central as well as peripheral field. However, it is of limited diagnostic value, as it may also occur in many other conditions.
- *Enlargement of optic cup:* Normal optic cups are similar (left and right) in shape and occupy less than 50% of the optic disc. In glaucoma these enlarge, especially along the vertical axis.

CONFUSA

Ocular hypertension is the term used when a patient has an IOT constantly more than 21 mm Hg but no optic disc or visual field changes. These patients should be carefully monitored by an ophthalmologist.

Investigation of Choice
Visual field mapping

Immediate Management
Refer to ophthalmologist

Treatment of Choice
There is medical treatment to reduce IOT to less than 21 mmHg. Surgery is used if medical treatment fails.

Your notes:

140. A woman who is a Visual Display Operator develops headache when she works for several hours.

Diagnosis: Hypermetropia

Clinchers

- *Woman:* There is no as such sexual discrimination in the incidence.
- *Visual display unit operator develops headache when she works severel hours:* This is most probably an exacerbation of the asthenopic symptoms in a fully corrected hypermetropia due to sustained accomodative efforts. The vision is otherwise normal as the hypermetropia is fully corrected at all other times.

CONFUSA

Astheopic symptoms are
- Tiredness of eyes
- Frontal or fronto-temporal headache
- Watering
- Mild photophobia

These asthenopic symptoms are especially associated with near work and increase towards evening.

Investigation of Choice
Test visual acuity

Immediate Management
Refer to an opticians

Treatment of Choice
Convex spectacle lenses.

Your notes:

17 Orthopaedics

PAPER 1

Subject: Orthopaedics

Topic: Fractures

Question: An 8-month-baby brought to Accident and Emergency with bronchiolitis. He has 6 posterior rib healing fractures.

Diagnosis: Osteogenesis Imperfecta

Clinchers

- *8-month-baby:* Osteogenesis imperfecta can present with easy bruising and multiple fractures most commonly in infancy.
- *Brought to Accident & Emergency with bronchiolitis:* Bronchiolits was just the illness due to which the child was brought to hospital and attention drawn towards the latest discovered fractures.
- *6 posterior ribs healing fractures:* The description is very consistent with the presentation of osteogenesis imperfecta where the fractures occur at points of stress (though minimal). For a 8 month old baby the maximum point of stress is his back on which he laid. Once the child starts walking, the points of stress change to the lower limb bones.

CONFUSA

- Non-accidental Injury is an important differential diagnosis here and should be ruled out with caution.
- When both of these conditions can present with multiple fractures and skin bruising, the osteogenesis imperfecta is associated with decreased bone mineral density and here lies the importance of doing a skeletal survey.

Investigation of Choice
Skeletal Survey

Immediate Management
Fractures usually heal easily—however in severe cases the long bones may become increasingly bent and the child may become unable to walk.

Treatment of Choice
Bisphosphonate treatement, under specialist centre supervision, is emerging as a useful treatment for bone pain and recurrent fracture, particularly in type III osteogenesis imperfecta.

Your notes:

Serial No. 5

Subject: Orthopaedics

Topic: Fractures

Question: An 8-year-old boy sustained a wrist fracture following a fall in rugby match. He has a history of 6 fractures in previous 3 years. Father is deaf.

Diagnosis: Osteogenesis Imperfecta

Clinchers

- *8-year-old boy:* Osteogenesis Imperfecta usually presents in infancy. This boy seems to have milder form of the disease and hence presenting late. Osteogenesis Imperfecta Type I and III are relatively mild forms of disease, compatible with survival and near normal stature.
- *History of 6 fractures in previous 3 years:* Multiple fractures are hallmarks of the disease process. Most consistent with diagnosis.
- *Father is deaf:* This further substantiates the diagnosis of Osteogenesis Imperfecta which is usually runs in families with autosomal dominant inheritance. Associated features of the disease include deafness, dental deformities, skeletal deformities, joint laxity, easy bruising and blue sclerae.

CONFUSA

- Osteogenesis imperfecta is basically a clinical diagnosis. With all the features in this patient so consistent with the disease, presence of blue sclera would make the picture complete.
- Although, Non-accidental injury is the most common differential here (as explained in the previous question), in this boy, there is always a history of trauma before fractures which makes Non-Accidental Injury unlikely.
- Hence, looking for Blue sclera is most apt next step to follow in this patient, rather than going for skeletal survey.

Investigation of Choice

Look for Blue Sclera

Immediate Management

Fractures usually heal easily—however in severe cases the long bones may become increasingly bent and the child may become unable to walk.

Treatment of Choice

Bisphosphonate treatement, under specialist centre supervision, is emerging as a useful treatment for bone pain and recurrent fracture, particularly in type III osteogenesis imperfecta.

Your notes:

Serial No. 79

Subject: Orthopaedics

Topic: Rheumatology

Question: More common in females; with incidence of 20% in elderly Caucasian females and associated with change in body shape.

Diagnosis: Osteoporosis

Clinchers

- *More common in females:* Osteoporosis more commonly affects females, especially postmenopausal age group because oestrogen (or testosterone) deficiency, regardless of age of occurrence, results in accelerated bone loss.
- *20 % incidence in elderly Caucasian females:* Severe osteoporosis is present in 20% of women between 75 and 85 years of age. The incidence of vertebral fractures in women increases markedly from the age of 50 years; by the age of 70 years, about one third of white Caucasian women will have at least one vertebral fracture.
- *Associated with change in body shape:* Osteoporosis is basically 'thinning' of bones which pre-disposes affected individuals for 'easy' fractures. The affected female gradually suffers from loss of height, and a stooping posture. This is due to fractured vertebrae which become 'squashed' with the weight of the body.

CONFUSA

The incidence of femoral neck fractures increases after the age of 65 years, more markedly in women than in men

- The incidence is more in Caucasians females than Blacks. It is suggested to be due to a reduction in the rate of skeletal remodeling which provide a means for maintaining and preserving bone mass in blacks. Also, the lower femoral neck BMD and longer femoral neck axis length in whites predispose them to more fractures.
- The lifetime risk of fracture for a 50-year-old Caucasian woman is about 3 times that for a man of the same age.

Investigation of Choice

Dual energy X-ray absorptiometry (DEXA scan).

The World Health Organisation has defined osteoporosis to be present when the bone density as measured by dual energy X-ray absorptiometry is more than 2.5 standard deviations below the young adult mean (i.e. T score < -2.5).

Immediate Management

Any fracture requires immediate orthopaedic attention.

Treatment of Choice

- Prevent falls
- Advise not to smoke or drink excessive alcohol
- Adequate dietary calcium and vitamin D and regular exercise.
- HRT is frequently used to prevent osteoporosis
- In patients who are unwilling to take HRT, bisphosphonates or combined calcium and vitamin D should be used
- In cases of established osteoporosis Bisphosphonates are the drugs of choice.

Your notes:

Serial No. 80

Subject: Orthopaedics

Topic: Rheumatology

Question: More common in females, affecting 1% of population, associated with loss of activity within 10 years of onset of disease in 10% of the affected.

Diagnosis: Rheumatoid arthritis

Clinchers

- *More common in females:* Women are affected three times more often than men with rheumatoid arthritis. The peak incidence is between the ages of 25 and 55 years.
- *Affecting 1 % of population:* RA affects from 1-3% of the population.
- *Loss of activity within 10 years of onset in 10% of the affected:* Rheumatoid arthritis follows a very unpredictable course. Most patients have relapses and remissions. After a 10 year period about 25% of patients will have complete remission. About 40% of patients will have moderate impairment. The remainder of patients will have either severe impairment (25%) or will be crippled by their disease (10%).

CONFUSA

- Rheumatoid arthritis affects about 1% of the population
- The female:male ratio is 2.5 : 1
- The onset of the disease is usually between the ages of 40 and 70 years of age
- Rheumatoid arthritis is a worldwide disease but:
  - It is rare in rural Africa
  - It is common in Pima and Chippewa native Americans.

Investigation of Choice

- Raised ESR and CRP during active disease
- Rheumatoid factor is present in 80% of cases
- X-rays of affected joints may show typical erosions

Immediate Management

Analgesics, NSAIDs and steroids are used for symptomatic relief of pain and stiffness.

Treatment of Choice

- The mainstay of medical management consists of early introduction of a disease-modifying anti-rheumatic drug (DMARD). The most commonly prescribed first-line DMARD is low-dose weekly methotrexate.
- Disease-modifying anti-rheumatic drugs (DMARDs) are used as monotherapy in early rheumatoid arthritis and in combination in patients with potential for progressive disease.

Your notes:

Note: GMC is changing the pattern of questions by including more of epidemiology and such hints which are typical, but ought to be ignored when we read texts. Read everything in OHCM/ OHCS you can, with the new stresses on prognosis of the disease, incidence and age-sex /racial preponderance.

Serial No. 81

Subject: Orthopaedics

Topic: Rheumatology

Question: More common in males, associated with stiff back and joints and positive HLA B27.

Diagnosis: Ankylosing spondylitis (AS), also known as Marie-Strümpell arthritis, Bechterew disease.

Clinchers

- *More common in males:* Male Caucasians are affected more severely and more often (3 : 1) than females. The mean age of onset is between 26 years of age. About 1 in 1000 people in the UK have AS.
- *Stiff back and joints:* Back pain is the main symptom. The pain usually starts in the lower back and more pronounced upon awakening and improves with activity. The most common joints affected are: vertebrae, hips, knees, ankles, and shoulders. Affected joints can become painful, stiff, and swollen.
- *Positive HLA B27:* This is the most striking feature of ankylosing spondylitis. Most patients with ankylosing spondylitis are HLA-B27 positive—the risk of transmitting the antigen to his/ her children is 50%. If a child is HLA-B27 positive then the chance of developing ankylosing spondylitis is 1 in 3.

CONFUSA

- Ankylosing spondylitis tends to run in families with close relatives suffering from either ankylosing spondylitis itself or one of the other seronegative spondarthritides such as Reiter's disease, psoriatic arthritis or enteropathic arthritis. The presence of HLA B 27 predisposes an individual for manifesting the disease.
- Usually a genitourinary or bowel infection may trigger the development of the disease in these individuals. Klebsiella bacteria carry antigens which mimic B27.

Investigation of Choice

- The diagnosis is usually made by the typical symptoms, negative rheumatoid factor and positive HLA B 27.
- Clinical assessment be based mainly on validated questionnaires usually completed by patients such as the Bath Ankylosing Spondylitis Disease Activity Index (BASDAI), which measures pain, tenderness, stiffness and fatigue, and the Bath Ankylosing Spondylitis Functional Index (BASFI), which measures activities of daily living.

Immediate Management

- NSAIDs and analgesics control pain.
- Sulphasalazine is useful in peripheral arthritis.
- Tumour necrosis factor antagonists like etanercept and infliximab, may be offered to patients with moderate or severe ankylosing spondylitis who have had an inadequate response to NSAIDs.

Treatment of Choice

The most important item of self-management is that the patient must exercise and keep moving.
Postural training can help prevent serious deformity.
Vertebral osteotomy (to correct severe flexion deformity).
Total hip replacement to treat affected hip joints.

Your notes:

Serial No. 82

Subject: Orthopaedics

Topic: Back Pain

Question: Associated with heavy work; pulling and pushing and psychosocial factors.

Diagnosis: Intervertebral Disc Prolapse (IVDP).

Clinchers

- *Associated with heavy work, pulling and pushing:* Most cases of prolapsed discs occur when excess pressure is suddenly put on the disc. This can occur due to weight lifting, especially when lifting in an awkward position. Factors that may increase the risk of developing a slipped disc include: a job involving lots of lifting, a job involving lots of sitting (especially driving), weight bearing sports (weightlifting, etc), smoking, obesity, and increasing age (a disc is more likely to prolapse if it has become weaker which occurs with increasing age).
- *Psychosocial factors:* Psychosocial factor may be defined as a measurement that potentially relates psychological phenomena to the social environment and to pathophysiological changes. It has been hypothesised that exposure to suboptimal psychosocial factors may lead to altered spinal loading due to increased muscle tension. This then possibly affects the nutrition of intervertebral discs, nerve roots, and other spinal tissues. Hence, such individuals are more prone for disc prolapse and low backache.

CONFUSA

In the past, advice had been to rest until the pain eases. This approach is now discarded taking the fact that the patients are more likely to develop chronic back pain if they rest a lot rather than keep active. As a rule, patients are advised to keep up with normal activities.

Investigation of Choice

Radiograph—may show disc space narrowing and osteophytes in cases of chronic recurrence; can show herniation of nucleus pulposus into the vertebral bodies (Schmorl's nodes).

Most useful is MRI scan in locating the exact site and size of the prolapse.

Immediate Management

Cauda equina syndrome or progressive neurological deficits may require immediate decompression surgeries.

Treatment of Choice

Get back into normal activities as soon as possible.

Pain killers.

Physiotherapy may be beneficial in certain cases.

Your notes:

Serial No. 83

Subject: Orthopaedics

Topic: Backache

Question: Associated with incidence of more than 70% and more than 90% show complete recovery.

Diagnosis: Benign backache

Clinchers

- *Incidence of more than 70%:* Back pain is the largest single cause of lost working hours amongst both manual and sedentary workers; and an important cause of disability. About 3 in 4 people have one or more bouts of back pain.
- *90% show complete recovery:* 90% of acute episodes of low back pain will resolve within 6 weeks.

CONFUSA

- About 19 in 20 cases of acute back pain are classed as 'simple or benign back pain'. There is no underlying disease process. The cause of most cases is thought to be a sprain or small tear to a ligament or muscle. This may be caused by heavy lifting, an awkward twisting movement, or bad posture.
- Peak prevalence is in those aged 45-59 years.
- Men and women are equally affected; however, work related back pain is more common among males.
- 90% of acute episodes of low back pain will resolve within 6 weeks.

Investigation of Choice

Careful history to rule out other serious causes is important.

Routine lumbar spine X-rays or blood tests are not indicated.

Immediate Management

Reassurance
Analgesics
Avoid Bed Rest

Treatment of Choice

Posture management: Patients are advised to avoid standing or walking in a bent-forward position. Wherever possible, walk or stand with shoulders and head slightly back. When sitting at a desk, maintain right chair height for the desk. Sleeping on a bed with a firm mattress is thought to be best.

Your notes:

PAPER 2

Serial No. 5

Subject: Surgery

Topic: Breast

Question: A 60-year-old woman is admitted to the accident and emergency department having fallen in the street. She is complaining of pain in the right hip and the right lower limb is lying in external rotation. She had breast conserving surgery, radiotherapy and chemotherapy eight years ago for breast cancer.

Diagnosis: Bony metastases

Clinchers

- *60-year-old woman.....external rotation:* These all signify a fracture neck of the femur. It can be due to osetoporosis (since she is 60-year-old) or bony metastasis (as in this case).
- *breast conserving surgery, radiotherapy and chemotherapy:* Since there is a positive history of breast cancer (which is known for osteolytic bony metastasis), the patient should be investigated for a recurrence and bony metastasis.

CONFUSA

Skeletal metastases in breast carcinoma occur via bloodstream. In order of frequency they are found in:
- Lumbar vertebrae
- Femur (as in this case)
- Thoracic vertebrae
- Rib
- Skull

Investigation of Choice

Bone Scan (whole body)

Immediate Management

Splinting

Treatment of Choice

Open reduction and internal fixation
Palliative treatment of breast carcinoma

Your notes:

PAPER 3

32. A young man involved in a motorcycle accident has a secure airway and a normal Glasgow Coma Scale. He is noted to have a swollen right thigh.

Diagnosis: Right femoral shaft fracture.

Clinchers

- *Young man involved in a motorcycle accident:* Most of the motorcycle accident victims are young males who are out to take an adventurous ride.
- *Has a secure airway:* That means that immediate management of ABC (airway, breathing and circulation) has been done.
- *Normal Glasgow Coma Scale:* This rules out any head injury (except subdural haematoma).
- *Swollen right thigh:* This could be soft tissue injury or a fracture femur. However, fracture femur is more common in a motorcycle accident.

CONFUSA

This is a simple question which is testing your knowledge of basic rules of management of trauma. These are divided into primary survey and secondary survey. Primary survey is based on ABC approach and AVPU scoring is done. Glasgow scoring is done only in secondary survey. Since it has been done in this patient it means secondary survey has been done and hence it is time for splinting.

Investigation of Choice

Femoral shaft fracture should be clinically evident without immediate resort to radiographs. X-rays are mainly used to excluded other injuries and to check the position of bone after application of a splint.

Immediate Management

Effective analgesia. Initially nitrous oxide mixture and then IV opiates—if not contraindicated—or femoral nerve block.

Treatment of Choice

Thomas or other traction splint.

Your notes:

33. A young man involved in a motorcycle accident has a secure airway, is ventilated, immobilised and anaesthesized after admission with a Glasgow Coma Scale of 9. He is noted to have a swollen right thigh.

Diagnosis: Right femoral shaft fracture with moderate head injury.

Clinchers

- *Young man involved in a motorcycle accident:* Young men are more often victims of two wheeler accidents.
- *Has a secure airway:* It means that primary survey is over.
- *Ventilated, immobilised and anaesthesized:* It means that secondary survey is also over.
- *Glasgow Coma Scale of 9:* It denotes moderate head injury (GCS range 9-12).
- *Swollen right thigh:* It is most probably femoural shaft fracture as it is very common in such accidents.

CONFUSA

Now the question boils down to what next to do? Like in the preveious question, we shall have to follow a sequential management. Anaesthesia is usually not given in a case of head injury except when femoral fracture needs to splinted (Entonox) or cranial haematoma is to be evacuated. Since there are no given symptoms/signs of a cranial haematoma, it has to be the reduction of femoural fracture.

Investigation of Choice

Femoural shaft fracture should be clinically evident without immediate resort to radiographs. X-rays are mainly used to excluded other injuries and to check the position of bone after application of a splint.

Immediate Management

Effective analgesia. Initially nitrous oxide mixture and then IV opiates—if not contraindicated—or femoral nerve block.

Treatment of Choice

Thomas or other traction splint.

Your notes:

115. A 67-year-old woman complains of right hip pain. On examination the right hip is aducted, externally rotated and flexed.

Diagnosis: Fracture neck of femur.

Clinchers

- *67-year-old woman:* Osteoporosis is the main cause of spontaneous fractures of neck of femur in elderlies (as it is a weight bearing joint). Usually females are more prone to fracture neck of femur in old age.
- *Right hip pain:* There is pain in the hip, thigh or knee but may be little to see on local examination.
- *Right hip is adducted, externally rotated and flexed:* The affected leg may be shortened and externally rotated but this classical appearance is dependent on the grade of the fracture. A more valuable sign is pain on gental passive rotation of the extended leg. If the fracture has impacted, other movements may be good with minimal pain including even straight leg raising. Tenderness is most marked posteriorly.

CONFUSA

There are three circumstances in which fracture neck of femur occurs:

1. At any age: Associated with major violence and multiple injuries
2. In the elderly: After a simple fall.
3. Spontaneously: As a result of osteoporosis or bony secondary deposits.

Investigation of Choice

X-ray

- AP view of hips and pelvis
- Lateral view of affected hip.

Immediate Management

A box splint to control leg movements + Analgesia.

Treatment of Choice

Internal fixation or hemiarthroplasty is usually performed within 24 hours.

Your notes:

161. Man involved in road traffic accident is found to have communited fractures of the tibia and fibula. He develops rapid swelling of the lower limb below the knee. Arterial pulses are absent below the knee.

Diagnosis: Compartment syndrome.

Clinchers

- *Communited fractures of tibia and fibula:* A communited fracture will cause much more swelling and local inflammation than a simple fracture. Also polytrauma usually causes obstructed venous outflow from a compartment.
- *Rapid swelling of the lower limb below the knee:* Swelling of the leg in any compartment of the leg produces the pressure to rise gradually within the compartment. The situation is compounded by an obstructed venous outflow from the compartment due to trauma. When the pressure reaches a critical level any nerves passing through the compartment cease to function, causing paraesthesiae intially, followed by loss of sensation in the area supplied by nerve. As the pressure continues to rise, tissue perfusion may cease, particularly in the muscles, and rarely a point can be reached when the pressure rises above arterial level and all structures within the compartment rises above arterial level and all structures within the compartment becomes ischaemic.

CONFUSA

Since the fractures involve both tibial compartment and fibular compartment, there will be no arterial pulses on either side. Otherwise the findings are limited to the affected compartment only.

Investigation of Choice

Measure intracompartmental pressures using a simple manometer (pressure higher than 30 mm Hg are an indication for urgent decompression).

Immediate Management

Orthopaedics referral.

Treatment of Choice

Immediate decompression by fasciotomy to prevent impending muscle necrosis and to save the leg (since even arterial pulses are blocked, the intracompartmental pressure must be much higher than 30 mmHg).

Your notes:

170. A 55-year-old roofer complains of lower back pain radiating into the right leg having fallen from a scaffold. He has no loss of power or sensation when examined.

Diagnosis: Lumbar fracture

Clinchers

- *55-year-old:* Elderlies can have osteoporotic bones which can fracture on slightest trauma or spontaneously. Spine, especially lumbar region, is most prone to sustain an osteoporotic fracture.
- *Lower back pain radiating into right leg:* Trapped nerve roots of lumbar plexus can lead to pain in right leg. Lower back pain is directly attributable to the presence of fracture in that region.
- *Having fallen from a scaffold:* This is the reason for his lumbar fracture. He is entitled to compensation under UK laws as this injury qualifies as a professional hazard.
- *No loss of power or sensation:* Lumbar fractures are not usually associated with paraplegia, but they are variably unstable, so neurological deficits can be a complication any time.

CONFUSA

In the absence of any neurological deficit a plain X-ray should be the first investigation. Subsequently a CT scan or MRI can be done to assess the stability of the injured vertebra and integrity of the spinal canal.

Investigation of Choice

X-ray lumbar spine.

Immediate Management

Orthopaedics (spinal injury unit) referral.

Treatment of Choice

If there is no paraplegia, external support with a moulded polythene or plaster jacket until union occurs is adequate.

Your notes:

177. A tall young man developed sharp chest pain on his right, following a road traffic accident. On palpation, this area is tender. A chest X-ray shows his lungs are not injured.

Diagnosis: Fracture rib.

Clinchers

- *Tall young man:* Nothing of much significance in this question.
- *RTA:* Fracture ribs result from direct blows or falls an are a common component of polytrauma in RTAs.
- *Tender on palpation:* It is present in the area of fracture and is inevitable. Moreover there is pain on inspiration and coughing along with considerable difficulty with trunk movements.
- *Lungs are not injured (on CXR):* The chest should be examined thoroughly to exclude underlying pneumo/haemothorax and contusion in any case of rib fracture. A clear CXR rules out these.

CONFUSA

A chest X-ray (CXR) is mandatory in the presence of dyspnoea or past history of respiratory problems. There are usually more tibs fractured than you can easily see on the X-ray. Multiple rib fractures on an adults CXR usually indicate past episodes of alcohol abuse; in case of a child—nonaccidental injury should be considered.

Investigation of Choice

Chest X-ray.

Immediate Management

Analgesia.

Treatment of Choice

> 3 ribs fractured:

- High concentration O_2 by mask
- Monitor SaO_2, BP, ECG, respiratory rate and blood gases
- Request anaesthetic opinion for intensive care.

< 3 ribs fractured: Exclude underlying problems and respiratory difficulties and discharge with adequate analgesia.

Your notes:

196. A six-year-old boy complains of intermittent hip pain for several months. Haematological investigations are normal. X-rays show flattening of the femoural head.

Diagnosis: Perthes' disease (Legg-Calve-Perthes disease).

Clinchers

- *Six-year-old boy:* Perthes' disease is commonly present in the 3-11 years age group though the usual presentation is at age 4-7 years.

  It is more common in boys and about 15% cases are bilateral. There is a definite familiar tendency and the condition has been described in identical twins.
- *Intermittent hip pain for several months:* In the initial stages, the symptoms tend to be relatively minor. Pain and a limp are usual presenting features. Pain is often slight and may have been present over several weeks or months.
- *Haematological investigations are normal:* Since the disease is secondary to epiphyseal ischaemia and infarction and not due to inflammation, the haematological investigations are usually normal.
- *X-rays show flattening of the femoral head:* This specific feature is caused by localized osteonecrosis. The X-ray changes are characteristic and it is often obvious that the condition has been present for time prior to presentation.

Radiological progression of Perthes' disease:

Earliest signs—increased density of epiphyses
—widening of medial joint space
↓
Fragmented epiphyses + flattened femoral head
↓
Healing + new bone formation
↓
Flat femoral head + wider neck
↓
Remodelling
↓
Osteoarthritis (in adults life)

CONFUSA

The prognosis is better in
- Younger child
- Partial involvement of head of femur
- Boys.

Investigation of Choice

Early X-rays (lateral view)

Immediate Management

Admission for observation and rest.

Treatment of Choice

Depends upon femoral head involvement:
- *<½ of femoral head affected + joint space depth well preserved*—bed rest until pain subsides, followed by X-ray surveillance.
- *>½ of femoral head affected + narrowing of total joint space*—surgery may be considered.

Your notes:

197. A two-year-old girl with one day history of increasing hip pain has become unable to weight bear. Her WCC is 21/fl, with an ESR of 89 mm/hr and a CRP of 300 mg/l. A radiograph of the hip shows a widened joint space.

Diagnosis: Septic arthritis.

Clinchers

- *Two-year-old girl:* It occurs most commonly below the age of four years. When it occurs in neonates it is known as Smith's arthritis.
- *One day history of increasing hip pain:* In older child it usually presents as an acute fever with extensive pain and spasm in the joint. It is rapid in onset (difference from Perthes' disease).
- *Unable to weight bear:* Child is unable to walk in septic arthritis because of pain (difference from Perthes' disease in which child can walk but with a limb).
- *WCC 21/fl, ESR 89 mm/hr, CRP 300 IU/l:* Normal WCC is 4-11/fl, ESR < 20 mm/hr and CRP < 10 IU/L. Any increase in these inflammatory markers denotes a sepsis somewhere in the body.
- *Radiograph of the hip shows a widened joint space:* Fluid in joint makes the joint space look wide on radiographs. An aspiration will confirm the presence of fluid.

CONFUSA

Differential diagnosis of septic arthritis is from 'irritable hip' and acute onset of Perthes' disease. Rheumatic fever and Still's disease occasionally present initially as a monoarthritis.

Investigation of Choice

Diagnostic aspiration and culture of joint.

Immediate Management

Joint aspiration, as it relieves pain also + Analgesia.

Treatment of Choice

Open surgical drainage and appropriate antibiotics.

Your notes:

198. A 12-year-old boy with left groin pain for 6 weeks is noticed to stand with the left leg externally rotated. Examination reveals negligible internal rotation of the hip.

Diagnosis: Slipped upper femoral epiphyses (SUFE).

Clinchers

- *12-year-old boy:* SUFE is found in older children. The child is frequently overweight and may have delayed sexual development.
- *Boys > girls:* It is a bilateral in 24% of patients.
- *Left groin pain for 6 weeks:* Classically symptoms are insiduous in onset, as the displacement is gradual. It is often associated with a limp (like Perthes' disease).
- *Stand with the left leg externally rotated:* External rotation of the limb at rest is pathognomic. Also the limb may be slightly short.
- *Negligible internal rotation of the hip:* Passive internal rotation is characteristically diminished in SUFE.

CONFUSA

The condition may not be apparent in early stages on an AP X-ray, but is detectable on a lateral film. A line drawn through the centre of the femoral neck in any X-ray projection should pass through the centre of the head. If it does not then some displacement has occurred.

Investigation of Choice

Special lateral X-ray view

(Findings: Posterior displacement of the upper femoral epiphysis)

Immediate Management

Orthopaedics referral.

Treatment of Choice

- *Acute symptoms*
  - Traction in internal rotation
  - Alternatively manipulation under GA
- *Chronic symptoms*
  - Pinning
  - If not possible—osteotomy.

Your notes:

199. A four-year-old boy complains of right hip pain a few days following an upper respiratory tract infection. Blood tests are as follows: WCC 12/fl, ESR 10 mm/hr and CRP 2 mg/L.

Diagnosis: Irritable hip syndrome (transient synovitis).

Clinchers

- *Four-year-old boy:* It is essentially a disease of childhood.
- *Right hip pain:* It is because of a sterile effusion in the hip (as it is a type of reactive arthritis).
- *A few days following an upper respiratory tract infection:* It often follows an upper respiratory tract infection.
- *WCC 12/fl, ESR 10 mm/hr and CRP 2 mg/L:* Blood tests are usually normal in irritable hip syndrome. Moreover the children are not systemically ill. Also there are no X-ray changes.

CONFUSA

When there has been unilateral limitation of all hip movements but a spontaneous recovery after bed-rest in the presence of normal X-rays, a retrospective diagnosis of transient synovitis is made. If other joints are involved, consider the diagnosis of juvenile rheumatoid arthritis. Rarely in irritable hip, an X-ray taken several weeks later may show the early changes of Perthes' disease.

Investigation of Choice

Microscopy of hip joint aspirate.
(Typical findings: fluid containing WBC but no organisms).

Immediate Management

Aspiration of the hip joint (as it reduces pain).

Treatment of Choice

Bed-rest + observation.

Your notes:

200. A five-year-old girl complains of progressively increasing severe pain in her left hip and upper leg for 6 days. She is able to walk but limps visibly. Blood tests are as follows: WCC 19/fl, ESR 72 mm/hr and CRP 94 mg/L. X-rays and ultrasound scans of the hip are normal.

Diagnosis: Osteomyelitis (acute).

Clinchers

- *Five-year-old girl:* Acute osteomyelitis occur mainly in children. Poor lining conditions predispose to it, and there may be an obvious primary focus of infection such as a boil, sore throat, etc.
- *Progressively increasing severe pain in her left hip and upper leg for 6 days:* Pain is usually localized to the metaphyseal region of the bone.
- *Able to walk but limps visibly:* There is an unwillingness to move because of pain. There may be a visible limp if area of hip and femur and involved.
- *WCC 19/fl, ESR 72 mm/hr and CRP 94 mg/l:* All the inflammatory markers rise as it is as infective condition.
- *X-rays and ultrasound scans of the hip are normal:* X-ray changes are not apparent for few days but then shows haziness and loss of density of affected bone—subperiosteal reaction—sequestrum and involucrum.

CONFUSA

Osteomyelitis can be difficult to differentiate clinically from septic arthritis. But a typical difference between the two is in walking. In osteomyelitis the child may still be able to walk which is not the case with septic arthritis. Also the pain in osteomyelitis is more chronic in onset and less severe than septic arthritis.

Investigation of Choice

MRI.

Immediate Management

Send blood culture (positive in 60%).

Treatment of Choice

Flucloxacillin 250-500 mg/6 hr IVI or IM till sequesterum culture reports are known.

Open surgery to drain abscess and remove sequestera.

Your notes:

PAPER 4

81. A 16-year-old boy falls from a tree. Complains of pain in left anatomical fossa. X-rays are normal.

Diagnosis: Fracture scaphoid (left hand).

Clinchers

- *16-year-old:* The relative compressibility of the bone in children makes scaphoid fracture uncommon under the age of 14 years. It is most common in men between the ages of 20 and 50 years.
- *Falls from a tree:* It is often sustained in falls when the impact is beared by hand.
- *Pain in left anatomical fossa:* Tenderness is typically found in the anatomical snuff box between the long and short extensors of the thumb and also on the dorsal and volar aspects of the scaphoid bone.
- *X-rays are normal:* Structures it is merely a crack fracture of scaphoid and not visible on initial X-rays until bone resorption at 10-14 days have widened the fracture line. Ultrasound and bone scan have been associated in such cases.

CONFUSA

A missed scaphoid fracture may cause more long-term morbidity than many major trunk injuries. In fracture scaphoid, swelling is usually minimal. Movements may be good, but forced thumb adduction and extension are usually painful. Unfortunately, many injuries to the soft-tissues may present a similar picture. Avascular necrosis may fellow a scaphoid fracture.

Investigation of Choice
Isotope scan

Immediate Management
Plaster cast is applied extending from the thumb interphalangeal joint to the elbow in all cases of suspected fracture scaphoid.

Treatment of Choice
Plaster cast for 3 months in confirmed scaphoid fracture.

Your notes:

82. Man falls on hand. X-ray shows perilunate dislocation.

Diagnosis: Perilunate dislocation.

Clinchers

- *Falls on hand:* This is a common mode of injury in lunate or perilunate dislocations.
- *Perilunate dislocations:* In this dislocation, the lunate remains in position and the rest of the carpal bones dislocate dorsally.

CONFUSA

Perilunate and lunate dislocations are rare injuries of the wrist. In lunate dislocation the lunate dislocates anteriorly but the rest of the carpals remain in position. In both types severe loss of wrist movements is inevitable. Avascular necrosis of the lunate is a common complication.

Investigation of Choice
Wrist X-ray.

Immediate Management
Urgent orthopaedics referral.

Treatment of Choice
Open reduction.

Your notes:

83. A 43-year-old man after a fall, pain in anatomical snuff-box and X-ray shows impacted distal radius fracture.

Diagnosis: Colle's fracture.

Clinchers

- *43-year-old man:* It is the most common fracture in people above 40 years of age and is particularly common in women because of postmenopausal osteoporosis. It is much less common in young adults.
- *Fall:* A Colle's fracture is almost always produced by a fall on an outstretched hand.
- *Pain in anatomical snuff box:* The patient usually presents with pain, swelling and deformity of the wrist. On examination, tenderness and irregularity of the lower end of the radius is found which can be felt in anatomical snuff box.
- *X-ray shows impacted distal radius fracture:* Colle's fracture mean a fracture within 2-3 cm of the lower end of the radius with backward tilt, backward displacement and, often impaction of the distal fragment producing shortening of the radius and radial deviation of the wrist. The fracture may be comminuted. The styloid process of the ulnar is often avulsed by the triangular articular disc. So that the inferior radio-ulnar joint is disrupted.

CONFUSA

If Colle's fracture is only minimally displaced reduction is not necessary. A useful way of assessing the need for reduction is to draw a line between the two lips of the articular surface of the radius on the lateral film.

Reduction	drawn line relative to line of radial shaft
• not necessary	at right angle slight forward tilt
• necessary	any backward tilt

Investigation of Choice

Lateral and anteroposterior X-ray wrist.

Immediate Management

Urgent ortho referral.

Treatment of Choice

- *Undisplaced fracture:* below elbow plaster cast for 6 weeks.
- *Displaced fracture:* manipulative reduction followed by immobilization in Colle's cast.

84. Man falls on hand, pain in anatomical fossa.

Diagnosis: Fracture scaphoid (probably).

Clinchers (Note: See question 81 in his theme also)

- *Fall on hand:* A common mode of injury for scaphoid fracture.
- *Pain in anatomical fossa:* Pain in this area with no obvious deformity or swelling following a fall on the outstretched hand, in an adult, should make one suspect strongly about the possibility of a scaphoid fracture.

Note: A force transmitted along the axis of second metacarpal may produce pain the region of the scaphoid bone.

CONFUSA

A scaphoid fracture is more common in young adults. It is rare in children and elderly. Commonly fracture occurs through the waist of the scaphoid. Rarely, it occurs through the tuberosity. It may be either a crack fracture or a displaced fracture.

Investigation of Choice

X-ray wrist including oblique view of scaphoid.

Immediate Management

A scaphoid cast for at least 2 weeks in all suspected cases (irrespective of whether they are visible or not on X-ray—if invisible do a repeat X-ray after 2 weeks).

Treatment of Choice

Scaphoid cast for 3 months in a confirmed scaphoid fracture.

Your notes:

85. Young girl tripped while holding mother's hand. Now cannot use arm at all.

Diagnosis: Pulled elbow.

Clinchers

- *Young girl:* This condition occurs in children between 1-4 years of age.
- *Tripped while holding mother's hand:* It occurs when pulled up by the arms, while being lifted in play. The head of the radius is pulled partly out of the annular ligament when a child is lifted by the wrist.
- *Now cannot use arm at all:* The child starts crying and is unable to move the affected limb. The forearm lies in an attitude of pronation. There may be mild swelling at the elbow.

CONFUSA

It is not possible to see the subluxated head on an X-ray because it is still cartilaginous. X-rays are taken only to rule out any other bony injury. Do not attempt to reduce a pulled elbow if there is any doubt about the diagnosis.

Investigation of Choice

Entirely clinical diagnosis.

Immediate Management

Refer to orthopaedics.

Treatment of Choice

Elbow rotation (forced supination with a thumb over the radial head). A click will be heard on reduction. Final reassurance for the doctor, and doubling parents, is obtained by letting the child play and watching normal movements return. This may take sometime.

Your notes:

151. An elderly busy man with indigestion, acute pain lateral side of hip.

Diagnosis: Probable osteoarthritis (OA).

Clinchers

- *Elderly:* The peak incidence of OA is in 6th decade. The disease is frequently bilateral, usually with more advanced pathology or more severe symptoms on one side. It is symptomatic three times more in women.
- *Busy man:* This require immediate pain relief so that the disease does not affect his day to activities.
- *Indigestion:* This is a contraindication for NSAID use which are often used for pain relief in OA.
- *Acute pain lateral side of hip:* Pain is the predominant symptom in OA and although the disease is bilateral in manifest earlier on one side. The most common joints to involves in OA are the weight bearing joints, i.e. hip and knee joints. Pain is felt over greater trochanter (as in this case) or groin.

CONFUSA

OA management also involves use of walking aids. It is held in:
- Contralateral hand—for hip arthritis
- Ipsilateral hand—for knee arthritis

for nocturnal pain in OA, low dose tricyclics can be used.

Investigation of Choice

Radiology (loss of joint space; subchondral sclerosis and cysts marginal osteophytes).

Immediate Management

Local steroid injection (although it may complicate things if used for long-time).

Treatment of Choice

Exercises and physiotherapy
Arthrodesis/osteotomy/arthroplasty in severe disease.

Your notes:

152. Patient with symmetrical polyarthritis, pain does not decrease with simple analgesia.

Diagnosis: Rheumatoid arthritis.

Clinchers

- *Symmetrical:* Since RA is a systemic autoimmune disease, it ought to be symmetrical.
- *Polyarthritis:* Small bones of the hand bilaterally are involved initially in RA bringing a picture of polyarthritis.
- *Pain does not decrease with simple analgesia:* This mean that an additional drug is required to bring pain relief. NSAIDs are the first line drug in RA and control pain and stiffness (but do not reducing the underlying inflammatory relapse or the acute flare reactants in the serum).

CONFUSA

"Simple analgesic" in UK paracetamol (or a combination of dextropropoxyphene and paracetamol). Drugs used in RA does not qualify as simple analgesia. While starting with NSAIDs in RA, always start with a familiar drug. Methotrexate is drug of choice is USA and not much used in UK.

Investigation of Choice

ESR and Hb.

Immediate Management

Refer to physiotherapy unit for occupational therapy and regular exercise (counselling).

Treatment of Choice

Ibuprofen 400-800 mg/8h after food.

Your notes:

200. Presents with features of fracture femur.

Diagnosis: Metastatic tumour producing pathological fracture.

Clinchers

- *Fracture femur:* Breast carcinoma (and most other epithelial tumours) commonly metastasizes to bone. Usually it is the local bones which are involved but arterial spread may result in deposition anywhere in the skeleton, particularly the flat bones, vertebrae and proximal ends of femur and humerus. Usually the breast carcinoma produces osteolytic (clastic) metastases which increases the risk of fractures especially in weight bearing bones like femur and vertebrae.

CONFUSA

Presence of bony metastases usually means a poor prognosis for life. So the priority in treating any pathological fracture is not restoration of bone congruity but the improvement of life's quality.

Investigation of Choice

- *Screening:* X-ray femur (radiolucency)
- *Definitive:* Whole body bone scan

Immediate Management

Splinting and take opinion of an orthopaedician and a clinical oncologist.

Treatment of Choice

Pathological fractures are normally best treated by internal fixation to enable the patient to mobilize early. Still the best treatment is to treat the primary. Breast carcinoma may respond to hormone therapy, e.g. oophorectomy, androgen or steroid treatment. Tamoxifen is a common antioestrogen drug used for this purpose.

Your notes:

PAPER 5

32. A 22-year-old motorist arrives in the Accident and Emergency Department after an accident. His airway is patent. He is noted to have a splinted right leg.

Diagnosis: Normal saline infusion.

Clinchers

- *22-year-old motorist:* Young motorists constitute a high risk group for RTA.
- *Airway patent:* This suggest that management of primary survey is over.
- *Splinted right leg:* This suggests that there may be a femoral fracture and also the fact that secondary survey is also over. Femoral fractures are associated with profuse blood loss and no time should be wasted in restoring the blood volume.

CONFUSA

Restoration of blood volume is best done by blood transfusion but arranging blood and cross-matching have taken time. So the first priority in such patients should be to start with a plasma expander immediately (i.e. haemacell) and transfuse blood later on. But since it is not given as an option, infusion of normal saline is the safest answer here.

Investigation of Choice
X-ray (right thigh).

Immediate Management
Haemacell/Normal saline
+
Admit.

Treatment of Choice
Surgical/conservative management of fracture femur.

Your notes:

35. An 18-year-old girl is being resuscitated after an accident. Her airway is secure. She complains of neck pain. Her pulse rate is 100 beats/min and blood pressure is 110/70 mmHg. Glasgow Coma Scale is 13. She has a deformed left thigh.

Diagnosis: Polytrauma

Clinchers

- *18-year-old girl:* Young patients can be resuscitated successfully most of the time after RTA. All she needs is urgent and coordinated medical care.
- *Airway secure:* This means that primary survey is over and we now need to focus on secondary survey.
- *Neck pain:* This could be due to spinal, vertebral or soft tissue injuries of neck which are very common after RTA, e.g Whiplash injuries. Since primary survey has been over the neck must have been stabilised. This complaint thus does not require any urgent intervention
- *Pulse 100 bpm:* This is tachycardia and an indication to rule out hypovolemia or continuing blood loss.
- *BP 110/70:* This is normal but can be deceptive as BP does not fall till about 25% of circulating blood volume is lost.
- *GCS 13:* This may indicate a concussion injury or a severe head injury. Definitive care will require urgent evaluation of neurological condition and head injuries by a neurosurgeon after stabilising ABC (Airway, breathing and circulation).
- *Deformed left thigh:* This could be the source of continuing blood loss so its splintage now has a priority over almost everything (as it constitutes management of C in ABC).

CONFUSA

Gross swelling of thigh after RTA should always arouse suspicion of a rupture of the femoral artery. Otherwise shock is rare with an isolated fracture, but blood replacement may be necessary. Sciatic nerve injury occasionally occurs.

Investigation of Choice.
X-ray cervical spine and femur.

Immediate Management
Splint the limb +
Neurosurgical referral +
Haemacell.

Treatment of Choice
Fixation of fracture + treatment of other injuries.

56. A 7-year-old boy presents with a history of acute onset of pain in the knee. On examination, the left lower limb is flexed, abducted, internally rotated.

Diagnosis: Perthes' disease.

Clinchers

- *7-year-old:* The condition usually presents at age 7-8, although it may occur at any age from 3 years (or occasionally younger) upto 11 to 12.
- *Boy:* Boys are affected more commonly than girls. 15% of cases are bilateral.
- *History of acute of pain in the knee:* Pain and limb are the usual presenting features. Pain is often slight and may have been present over several weeks.
- *Left lower limb is flexed, abducted and internally rotated:* The clinical signs are usually minor, perhaps slight restriction of movements of the hip, especially internal rotation associated with some spasm.

CONFUSA

The prognosis of perthes' disease which is sometimes known as Legg-Calve-Perthes disease, is better in younger child and when only part of the head is involved. Girls fare worse than boys for any given age. Many of the difficulties centre around treating a condition which quickly becomes symptom-free and is then only manifest as a sense of changes on X-rays.

Investigation of Choice
Radiology.

Immediate Management
Bed rest + refer to specialist.

Treatment of Choice
Traction (in bed or an abduction frame).

Your notes:

57. A 67-year-old woman complains of right hip pain. On examination the right hip is adducted, externally rotated and flexed.

Diagnosis: Fracture neck of femur.

Clinchers

- *67-year-old:* In elderly people, the fracture occurs with a seemingly trivial fall. Osteoporosis is considered an important contributory factor at this age.
- *Woman:* Incidence of osteoporosis is more in post-menopausal females.
- *Right hip pain:* The elderly patient with fracture neck of femur is usually brought to the casualty department with complaints of pain in the groin and inability to move his limb or bear weight on the limb following a 'trivial' injury like slipping on the floor, missing a step, etc.
- *Right hip is adducted, externally rotated are flexed:* The affected leg may be shortened and externally rotated but this classical appearance is dependent on the grade of the fracture.

CONFUSA

A more valuable sign in fracture neck of femur is pain on gentle passive rotation of the extended leg. If the fracture has impacted, other movements may be good with minimal pain including even straight leg raising. Tenderness is most marked posteriorly.

Investigation of Choice
AP and lateral views of hips.

Immediate Management
Admit + box splint + analgesia.

Treatment of Choice
Internal fixation/hemiarthroplasty.

Your notes:

58. A 10-year-old girl is febrile. On examination it is difficult to abduct the thighs.

Diagnosis: Septic arthritis.

Clinchers

- *10-year-girl:* In children the most common cause of septic arthritis is osteomyelitis. Minor trauma, soft tissue infection or a non-specific joint inflammation can also lead to it.
- *Difficult to abduct the thighs:* The most common joints to become infected are the interphalangeal joints and the knee. The joint is held in flexion and all movements are restricted by intense pain.
- *Febrile:* This denotes the systemic reaction to sepsis.

CONFUSA

If there is doubt then the patient should be assumed to have a septic arthritis until provided otherwise. Diagnostic joint aspiration is not recommended in the ED. Admission must be arranged under the care of either the orthopaedic or the rheumatology departments, as seems most appropriate from the likely underlying pathology.

Investigation of Choice

Radiograph + joint aspiration under specialist care.

Immediate Management

Admit.

Treatment of Choice

Antibiotics.

Your notes:

59. A child presents with right hip pain. On examination the hip is flexed, abducted and externally rotated.

Diagnosis: Slipped femoral epiphyses

Clinchers

- *Child:* It occurs more commonly in very fat and sexually underdeveloped or tall, thin sexually normal children. It occurs at puberty, between 12-14 years.
- *Right hip pain:* Pain in the groin, often radiating to the thigh and the knee is the common presenting complaint.
- *Hip is flexed, abducted and externally rotated:* On examination, the leg is found to be externally rotated and 1-2 cm short. A limitation of the hip movements is characteristic—there is limited abduction and internal rotation. When the hip is flexed, the knee goes towards the ipsilateral axilla. Muscle bulk may be reduced. Trendelenburg's sign may be positive.

CONFUSA

Often in the initial stages, the symptoms are considered due to a 'sprain', and disregarded. They soon disappear only to recur. Limp occurs early and is more constant. It is more common in boys and in patients with endocrine abnormalities.

Investigation of Choice

Radiology.

Immediate Management

Prophylactic pinning of the unaffected side.

Treatment of Choice

Closed reduction + pinning.

Your notes:

60. A five-year-old girl complains of progressively increasing severe pain in her left hip and upper leg for 6 days. She is able to walk but limps visibly. Blood tests are as follows: WCC 19/fl, ESR 72 mm/hr and CRP 94 mg/l. X-rays and ultrasound scans of the hip are normal.

Diagnosis: Osteomyelitis (acute).

Clinchers

- *Five year old girl:* Acute osteomyelitis occur mainly in children. Poor lining conditions predipose to it, and there may be an obvious primary focus of infection such as a boil, sore throat etc.
- *Progressively increasing severe pain in her left hip and upper leg for 6 days:* Pain is usually localized to the metaphyseal region of the bone.
- *Able to walk but limps visibly:* There is an unwillingness to move because of pain. There may be a visible limp if area of hip and femur and involved.
- *WCC 19/fl, ESR 72 mm/hr and CRP 94 mg/l:* All the inflammatory markers rise as it is as infective condition.
- *X-rays and ultrasound scans of the hip are normal:* X-ray changes are not apparent for few days but then shows haziness and loss of density of affected bone—subperiosteal reaction—sequesterum and involucrum.

CONFUSA

Osteomyelitis can be difficult to differentiate clinically from septic arthritis. But a typical difference between the two is in walking. In osteomyelitis the child may still be able to walk which is not the case with septic arthritis. Also the pain in osteomyelitis is more chronic in onset and less severe than septic arthritis.

Investigation of Choice

MRI.

Immediate Management

Send blood culture (positive in 60%).

Treatment of Choice

Flucloxacillin 250-500 mg/6 hr IVI or IM till sequesterum culture reports are known.

Open surgery to drain abscess and remove sequestera.

121. A 16-year-old mother brings her baby for immunization. The nurse notices the baby has multiple bruises along both arms and legs. The baby is crying excessively. The house officer notices multiple fractures and that the baby has blue sclerae.

Diagnosis: Osteogenesis imperfecta.

Clinchers

- *16-year-old mother:* Not of much significance except the fact that battered baby condition is more prevalent among teenage mothers.
- *Multiple bruises along both arms and legs:* Because of connective tissue involvement, the skin scars extensively.
- *Crying excessively:* Because of pain induced by fractures and generalised illness.
- *Multiple fractures:* It is the hallmark of severe osteogenesis imperfecta. But these are also found in battered baby syndrome (non-accidental injury).
- *Blue sclerae:* It is the differentiating feature from non-accidental injury as blue sclerae are almost pathognomic of osteogenesis imperfecta with this clinical profile.

CONFUSA

Non-accidental injury is the main differential diagnosis in this case. Other thing to be noted is that osteogenesis imperfecta is known by many different names and they can appear in the options as such, i.e. fragilitas ossium, brittle bone syndrome, Adair-Dighton syndrome.

Investigation of Choice

Screening: X-ray (decrease in bone density)
Definitive: Absorptiometry (X-ray/photon)

Immediate Management

Symptomatic treatment (i.e. fractures—traction followed by light cast).

Treatment of Choice

Judicious exercise programme to prevent loss of bone mass secondary to physical inactivity.

Your notes:

PAPER 6

90. Presents with features of fracture femur.

Diagnosis: Metastatic tumour producing pathological fracture.

Clinchers

➢ *Fracture femur:* Breast carcinoma (and most other epithelial tumours) commonly metastasizes to bone. Usually it is the local bones which are involved but arterial spread may result in deposition anywhere in the skeleton, particularly the flat bones, vertebrae and proximal ends of femur and humerus. Usually the breast carcinoma produces osteolytic (clastic) metastases which increases the risk of fractures especially in weight bearing bones like femur and vertebrae.

CONFUSA

Presence of bony metastases usually means a poor prognosis for life. So the priority in treating any pathological fracture is not restoration of bone congruity but the improvement of life's quality.

Investigation of Choice

- *Screening:* X-ray femur (radiolucency)
- *Definitive:* Whole body bone scan

Immediate Management

Splinting and take opinion of an orthopaedician and a clinical oncologist.

Treatment of Choice

Pathological fractures are normally best treated by internal fixation to enable the patient to mobilize early. Still the best treatment is to treat the primary. Breast carcinoma may respond to hormone therapy, e.g. oophorectomy, androgen or steroid treatment. Tamoxifen is a common anti-oestrogen drug used for this purpose.

Your notes:

91. A 16-year-old mother brings her baby for immunization. The nurse notices the baby has multiple bruises along both arms and legs. The baby is crying excessively. The house officer notices multiple fractures and that the baby has blue sclerae.

Diagnosis: Osteogenesis imperfecta.

Clinchers

➢ *16-year-old mother:* Not of much significance except the fact that battered baby condition is more prevalent among teenage mothers.

➢ *Multiple bruises along both arms and legs:* Because of connective tissue involvement, the skin scars extensively.

➢ *Crying excessively:* Because of pain induced by fractures and generalised illness.

➢ *Multiple fractures:* It is the hallmark of severe osteogenesis imperfecta. But these are also found in battered baby syndrome (non-accidental injury).

➢ *Blue sclerae:* It is the differentiating feature from non-accidental injury as blue sclerae are almost pathognomic of osteogenesis imperfecta with this clinical profile.

CONFUSA

Non-accidental injury is the main differential diagnosis in this case. Other thing to be noted is that osteogenesis imperfecta is known by many different names and they can appear in the options as such, i.e. fragilitas ossium, brittle bone syndrome, Adair-Dighton syndrome.

Investigation of Choice

Screening: X-ray (decrease in bone density)
Definitive: Absorptiometry (X-ray/photon)

Immediate Management

Symptomatic treatment (i.e. fractures—traction followed by light cast).

Treatment of Choice

Judicious exercise programme to prevent loss of bone mass secondary to physical inactivity.

Your notes:

126. A six-year-old boy complains of intermittent hip pain for several months. Haematological investigations are normal. X-rays show flattening of the femoral head.

Diagnosis: Perthes' disease (Legg-Calve-Perthes disease).

Clinchers

- *Six-year-old boy:* Perthes' disease is commonly present in the 3-11 years age group though the usual presentation is at age 4-7 years.

  It is more common in boys and about 15% cases are bilateral. There is a definite familiar tendency and the condition has been described in identical twins.
- *Intermittent hip pain for several months:* In the initial stages, the symptoms tend to be relatively minor. Pain and a limp are usual presenting features. Pain is often slight and may have been present over several weeks or months.
- *Haematological investigations are normal:* Since the disease is secondary to epiphyseal ischaemia and infarction and not due to inflammation, the haematological investigations are usually normal.
- *X-rays show flattening of the femoral head:* This specific feature is caused by localized osteonecrosis. The X-ray changes are characteristic and it is often obvious that the condition has been present for time prior to presentation.

Radiological progression of perthes disease:

Earliest signs—Increased density of epiphyses
—Widening of medial joint space
↓
Fragmented epiphyses + flattened femoral head
↓
Healing + new bone formation
↓
Flat femoral head + wider neck
↓
Remodelling
↓
Osteoarthritis (in adults life)

CONFUSA

The prognosis is better in
- Younger child
- Partial involvement of head of femur
- Boys.

Investigation of Choice

Early X-rays (lateral view)

Immediate Management

Admission for observation and rest

Treatment of Choice

Depends upon femoral head involvement:
- *<½ of femoral head affected + joint space depth well preserved*—bed rest until pain subsides, followed by X-ray surveillance.
- *>½ of femoral head affected + narrowing of total joint space*—surgery may be considered.

Your notes:

127. A two-year-old girl with one day history of increasing hip pain has become unable to weight bear. Her WCC is 21/fl, with an ESR of 89 mm/hr and a CRP of 300 mg/l. A radiograph of the hip shows a widened joint space.

Diagnosis: Septic arthritis.

Clinchers

- *Two-year-old girl:* It occurs most commonly below the age of four years. When it occurs in neonates it is known as Smith's arthritis.
- *One day history of increasing hip pain:* In older child it usually presents as an acute fever with extensive pain and spasm in the joint. It is rapid in onset (difference from Perthes' disease).
- *Unable to weight bear:* Child is unable to walk in septic arthritis because of pain (difference from Perthes' disease in which child can walk but with a limb).
- *WCC 21/fl, ESR 89 mm/hr, CRP 300 IU/l:* Normal WCC is 4-11/fl, ESR < 20 mm/hr and CRP < 10 IU/L. Any increase in these inflammatory markers denotes a sepsis somewhere in the body.
- *Radiograph of the hip shows a widened joint space:* Fluid in joint makes the joint space look wide on radiographs. An aspiration will confirm the presence of fluid.

CONFUSA

Differential diagnosis of septic arthritis is from 'irritable hip' and acute onset of Perthes' disease. Rheumatic fever and Still's disease occasionally present initially as a monoarthritis.

Investigation of Choice

Diagnostic aspiration and culture of joint.

Immediate Management

Joint aspiration, as it relieves pain also + Analgesia.

Treatment of Choice

Open surgical drainage and appropriate antibiotics.

Your notes:

128. A 12-year-old boy with left groin pain for 6 weeks is noticed to stand with the left leg externally rotated. Examination reveals negligible internal rotation of the hip.

Diagnosis: Slipped upper femoral epiphyses (SUFE).

Clinchers

- *12-year-old boy:* SUFE is found in older children. The child is frequently overweight and may have delayed sexual development
- *Boys > girls:* It is a bilateral in 24% of patients.
- *Left groin pain for 6 weeks:* Classically symptoms are insiduous in onset, as the displacement is gradual. It is often associated with a limp (like Perthes' disease).
- *Stand with the left leg externally rotated:* External rotation of the limb at rest is pathognomic. Also the limb may be slightly short.
- *Negligible internal rotation of the hip:* Passive internal rotation is characteristically diminished in SUFE.

CONFUSA

The condition may not be apparent in early stages on an AP X-ray, but is detectable on a lateral film. A line drawn through the centre of the femoral neck in any X-ray projection should pass through the centre of the head. If it does not then some displacement has occurred.

Investigation of Choice

Special lateral X-ray view

(Findings: Posterior displacement of the upper femoral epiphysis).

Immediate Management

Orthopaedics referral.

Treatment of Choice

- *Acute symptoms*
  - Traction in internal rotation
  - Alternatively manipulation under GA
- *Chronic symptoms*
  - Pinning
  - If not possible—osteotomy.

Your notes:

129. A four-year-old boy complains of right hip pain a few days following an upper respiratory tract infection. Blood tests are as follows: WCC 12/fl, ESR 10 mm/hr and CRP 2 mg/L.

Diagnosis: Irritable hip syndrome (transient synovitis).

Clinchers

- *Four-year-old boy:* It is essentially a disease of childhood.
- *Right hip pain:* It is because of a sterile effusion in the hip (as it is a type of reactive arthritis).
- *A few days following an upper respiratory tract infection:* It often follows an upper respiratory tract infection.
- *WCC 12/fl, ESR 10 mm/hr and CRP 2 mg/l:* Blood tests are usually normal in irritable hip syndrome. Moreover the children are not systemically ill. Also there are no X-ray changes.

CONFUSA

When there has been unilateral limitation of all hip movements but a spontaneous recovery after bed-rest in the presence of normal X-rays, a retrospective diagnosis of transient synovitis is made. If other joints are involved, consider the diagnosis of juvenile rheumatoid arthritis. Rarely in irritable hip, an X-ray taken several weeks later may show the early changees of Perthes' disease.

Investigation of Choice

Microscopy of hip joint aspirate.
(Typical findings: fluid containing WBC but no organisms).

Immediate Management

Aspiration of the hip joint (as it reduces pain).

Treatment of Choice

Bed-rest + observation.

Your notes:

130. A five-year-old girl complains of progressively increasing severe pain in her left hip and upper leg for 6 days. She is able to walk but limps visibly. Blood tests are as follows: WCC 19/fl, ESR 72 mm/hr and CRP 94 mg/L. X rays and ultrasound scans of the hip are normal.

Diagnosis: Osteomyelitis (acute).

Clinchers

- *Five-year-old girl:* Acute osteomyelitis occur mainly in children. Poor lining conditions predipose to it, and there may be an obvious primary focus of infection such as a boil, sore throat, etc.
- *Progressively increasing severe pain in her left hip and upper leg for 6 days:* Pain is usually localized to the metaphyseal region of the bone.
- *Able to walk but limps visibly:* There is an unwillingness to move because of pain. There may be a visible limp if area of hip and femur and involved.
- *WCC 19/fl, ESR 72 mm/hr and CRP 94 mg/l:* All the inflammatory markers rise as it is as infective condition.
- *X-rays and ultrasound scans of the hip are normal:* X-ray changes are not apparent for few days but then shows haziness and loss of density of affected bone—subperiosteal reaction—sequestrum and involucrum.

CONFUSA

Osteomyelitis can be difficult to differentiate clinically from septic arthritis. But a typical difference between the two is in walking. In osteomyelitis the child may still be able to walk which is not the case with septic arthritis. Also the pain in osteomyelitis is more chronic in onset and less severe than septic arthritis.

Investigation of Choice

MRI.

Immediate Management

Send blood culture (positive in 60%).

Treatment of Choice

Flucloxacillin 250-500 mg/6 hr IVI or IM till sequesterum culture reports are known.

Open surgery to drain abscess and remove sequestera.

Your notes:

180. A 67-year-old woman complains of right hip pain. On examination the right hip is adducted, externally rotated and flexed.

Diagnosis: Fracture neck of femur.

Clinchers

- *67-year-old woman:* Osteoporosis is the main cause of spontaneous fractures of neck of femur in elderlies (as it is a weight bearing joint). Usually females are more prone to fracture neck of femur in old age.
- *Right hip pain:* There is pain in the hip, thigh or knee but may be little to see on local examination.
- *Right hip is adducted, externally rotated and flexed:* The affected leg may be shortened and externally rotated but this classical appearance is dependent on the grade of the fracture. A more valuable sign is pain on gental passive rotation of the extended leg. If the fracture has impacted, other movements may be good with minimal pain including even straight leg raising. Tenderness is most marked posteriorly.

CONFUSA

There are three circumstances in which fracture neck of femur occurs:

1. At any age: Associated with major violence and multiple injuries
2. In the elderly: After a simple fall.
3. Spontaneously: As a result of osteoporosis or bony secondary deposits.

Investigation of Choice

X-ray

- AP view of hips and pelvis
- Lateral view of affected hip.

Immediate Management

A box splint to control leg movements + Analgesia.

Treatment of Choice

Internal fixation or hemiarthroplasty is usually performed within 24 hours.

Your notes:

PAPER 7

22. Girl in road traffic accident (RTA). Neck is immobilised and IV line established. Has deformed, swollen thigh, pale.

Diagnosis: Fracture shaft of femur and severe blood loss.

Clinchers

- *RTA:* Fracture of long bones is very common in victims of RTA.
- *Neck is immobilised and IV line established:* These suggest that primary survey is over.
- *Deformed, swollen thigh:* This is most probably a fracture of femoral shaft. Such fractures are often associated with massive blood loss (especially if there is concomitant pelvic fractures).
- *Pale:* This confirms the presence of blood loss and indicate urgent blood transfusion.

CONFUSA

In the primary survey the state of the circulation is quickly assessed by observation of:

- Skin colour and temperature
- Pulse rate and volume
- Capillary refill time at a finger pulp or nail bed
- JVP
- BP

Investigation of Choice

X-ray thigh.

Immediate Management

Blood transfusion and orthopaedic referral.

Treatment of Choice

Splinting of the thigh and then evaluation by orthopaedicians. But these has to be done after blood transfusion.

Your Notes

56. A 7-day-old baby cries whenever lifted. Labour was difficult.

Diagnosis: Fracture shaft femur.

Clinchers

- *7-day-old:* Since the baby is only of 7 days, he will not have any obvious features of fracture shaft femur (i.e. impaired mobility, etc.). It also suggest the fracture to be consequence of difficult labour.
- *Cries whenever lifted:* This may be the only feature of skeletal injuries in a newborn.
- *Labour was difficult:* Prolonged labour can produce foetal hypoxia and some powerful uterine contract ons or bearing down efforts can cause fracture of clavicle or femur.

CONFUSA

Neonatal mortality rises with prolonged labour as does material mortality (especially with infection).

Investigation of Choice
X-ray femur.

Immediate Management
Splinting.

Your notes:

57. Young girl tripped while holding mother's hand. Now cannot use arm at all.

Diagnosis: Pulled elbow.

Clinchers

- *Young girl:* This condition occurs in children between 1-4 years of age.
- *Tripped while holding mother's hand:* It occurs when pulled up by the arms, while being lifted in play. The head of the radius is pulled partly out of the annular ligament when a child is lifted by the wrist.
- *Now cannot use arm at all:* The child starts crying and is unable to move the affected limb. The forearm lies in an attitude of pronation. There may be mild swelling at the elbow.

CONFUSA

It is not possible to see the subluxated head on an X-ray because it is still cartilagineous. X-rays are taken only to rule out any other bony injury. Do not attempt to reduce a pulled elbow if there is any doubt about the diagnosis.

Investigation of Choice
Entirely clinical diagnosis.

Immediate Management
Refer to orthopaedics.

Treatment of Choice
Elbow rotation (forced supination with a thumb over the radial head). A click will be heard on reduction. Final reassurance for the doctor, and doubling parents, is obtained by letting the child play and watching normal movements return. This may take sometime.

Your notes:

58. Young boy fell off horse onto his hand. Now with complaint of mild tenderness over the clavicle but able to use forearm.

Diagnosis: Green stick injury.

Clinchers

- *Young boy:* Young soft bones may partially break after bending. This is called green stick fracture.
- *Fell off horse onto his hand:* Greenstick fractures of clavicle are common after childhood falls.
- *Mild tenderness over the clavicle but able to use forearm:* There may be minimal symptoms, i.e. little deformity and tenderness. There is also remarkably good movements of arm and shoulder girdle.

CONFUSA

In green stick fracture of clavicle, sometimes the child may refuse to use the whole arm on the affected side and thus mimic a pulled elbow.

Investigation of Choice
Anteroposterior radiograph.

Immediate Management
Appropriate analgesia.

Treatment of Choice
Broad arm sling.

Your notes:

59. Young child fell on outstretched hand and now has absent radial pulse.

Diagnosis: Supracondylar fracture.

Clinchers

- *Young child:* This injury occurs in older children (peak incidence at age 8 years). It is one of the most serious fractures in childhood as it is often associated with complications.
- *Fell on outstretched hand:* This is typical of supracondylar fracture. As the hand strikes the ground the elbow is forced into hyperextension resulting in fracture of the humerus above the condyles.
- *Absent radial pulse:* This implies vascular damage which is common in this injury. It suggests that the fracture is complicated with gross displacement (usually of the distal fragment posteriorly).

CONFUSA

Reduction under GA by the orthopaedic team and subsequent monitoring of distal neurovascular function is essential. Failure to do this may result in Volkmann's ischaemic contracture of the forearm muscles with permanent disability in the hand. Some undisplaced fractures may be treated on an outpatient basis, but this decision should be left to the orthopaedic staff.

Investigation of Choice
Radiography (AP + lateral view) with radiograph of opposite elbow for comparison.

Immediate Management
Orthopaedics referral

Treatment of Choice
Reduction under GA
Internal fixation if articular surface is implicated.

Your notes:

60. A 12-year-old boy with left groin pain for 6 weeks is noticed to stand with the left leg externally rotated. Examination reveals negligible internal rotation of the hip.

Diagnosis: Slipped upper femoral epiphyses (SUFE).

Clinchers

- *12-year-old boy:* SUFE is found in older children. The child is frequently overweight and may have delayed sexual development.
- *Boys > girls:* It is a bilateral in 24% of patients.
- *Left groin pain for 6 weeks:* Classically symptoms are insiduous in onset, as the displacement is gradual. It is often associated with a limp (like Perthes' disease).
- *Stand with the left leg externally rotated:* External rotation of the limb at rest is pathognomic. Also the limb may be slightly short.
- *Negligible internal rotation of the hip:* Passive internal rotation is characteristically diminished in SUFE.

CONFUSA

The condition may not be apparent in early stages on an AP X-ray, but is detectable on a lateral film. A line drawn through the centre of the femoral neck in any X-ray projection should pass through the centre of the head. If it does not then some displacement has occurred.

Investigation of Choice

Special lateral X-ray view

(Findings: Posterior displacement of the upper femoral epiphysis)

Immediate Management

Orthopaedics referral.

Treatment of Choice

- *Acute symptoms*
  - Traction in internal rotation
  - Alternatively manipulation under GA
- *Chronic symptoms*
  - Pinning
  - If not possible—osteotomy.

Your notes:

18 Paediatrics

PAPER 1

Serial No. 134

Subject: Obstetrics

Topic: Prenatal Screening

Question: A lady at 16 weeks gestation, scan shows nuchal folds and double bubble sign; the most reliable way to diagnose Down's syndrome.

Diagnosis: Down's syndrome

Clinchers

- *At 16 weeks gestation:* Definitive diagnosis of requires karyotyping. Cells can be obtained by either amniocentesis or chorionic villous sampling. However, at 14-16 weeks of gestation amniocentesis is more sensitive and safe for the prenatal diagnosis.
- *Scan shows nuchal folds:* This is actually nuchal oedema, reflecting fetal heart failure which can be due to serious anomaly of heart and great vessels. Although this is strongly suggestive of Down's syndrome. It is apparent that it can occur in several other conditions associated with fetal heart failure.
- *Double bubble sign:* This is suggesting duodenal atresia, again a very common anomaly associated with Down's syndrome.
- *The most reliable way to diagnose Down's syndrome:* Amniocentesis (at 14-16 weeks) is 99.5% accurate (However, it can miss rare cases of mosaicism and will provide inaccurate results if there is maternal cell contamination. Chorionic villous sampling can be performed earlier (10-13 weeks) but accuracy is less (96-98%) because greater risk of maternal cell contamination and missing mosaicism.

CONFUSA

- Triple test: It is particularly offered to at risk mothers, in the antenatal period. The test measures alpha-fetoprotein, human chorionic gonadotrophin and unconjugated oestriol.
- Low maternal serum alpha-fetoprotein (MSAFP), elevated human chorionic gonadotropin (hCG) and low unconjugated oestriol are markers for Down's syndrome.
- Quadruple test: A fourth component–Inhibin-A, when added to the above test, improves the detection rate from 78% (standard triple test) to 82% and reduces the false positive rate from 7.8 to 6.9%.

Investigation of Choice

Amniocentesis with karyotyping.

Immediate Management

Necessary counselling and information to the parents.

Treatment of Choice

Genetic counselling; discuss the risk with subsequent pregnancies.

Your notes:

Serial No. 137

Subject: Obstetrics

Topic: Prenatal screening

Question: A lady 24 weeks pregnant with a previous child dead from congenital heart disease.

Diagnosis: Congenital Heart Disease.

Clinchers

- *Twenty-four weeks pregnant:* Two-dimensional echo examination of the fetus can be readily performed as early as 16-17 weeks of gestation. This can detect nearly all forms of structural congenital heart disease *in utero*.
- *Previous child dead from congenital heart disease:* By far this is the most common indication for performing a fetal echocardiography. Although the increased risk of congenital cardiac disease in fetuses with first-order relatives who have congenital heart disease is low (2-5%), there is a significant increase in risk over the general population. More importantly, parents' anxiety about whether they will have a second child with heart disease may be very high. For this reason, fetal echocardiography is usually offered to parents with previous child having congenital heart disease.

CONFUSA

Fetal heart studies is restricted to situations which pose the fetus with a risk of having a congenital heart disease:

- Extracardiac anomalies like omphalocele which are know to co-exist with ventricular septal defect or tetralogy of Fallot.
- Abnormal fetal growth and fetal distress: To rule out congestive heart failure and fetal arrythmias.
- Chromosomal anomalies: Most chromosomal anomalies are associated with cardiac structural abnormalities, like endocardial cushion defect with trisomy 21.
- Irregular rhytm of fetal heart
- Maternal diseases, like diabetes or exposure to anti-epileptics or other 'cardiac' teratogens
- History of previous children with heart disease.

Investigation of Choice

Fetal Echo

Immediate Management

Treat any life-threatening arrythmias or CHF

Treatment of Choice

According to the condition identified.

Serial No. 138

Subject: Paediatrics

Topic: Neonatal Screening.

Question: A pregnant lady wants to know if her baby will be suffering from hypothyroidism.

Diagnosis: Congenital Hypothyroidism (suspected).

Clinchers

- Infants are usually normal at birth due to maternal hormone. Hypothyroid infants present in first month of life with feeding difficulties, respiratory difficulties with little crying, sleeps a lot, has poor appetite and is generally sluggish.
- Screening for congenital hypothyroidism involves looking for high concentrations of neonatal blood TSH - this test is found to be better than measuring blood thyroxine levels.
- The 'Blood Spot Test' is done in infants to screen for both congenital hypothyroidism and phenylketonuria.

CONFUSA

- Screening for congenital hypothyroidism is part of the screening programme for all newborn babies. The UK Newborn Screening Programme Centre has beeen set up to monitor this and screening for other inborn errors of metabolism (PKU).
- Both the test above are included in the Blood Spot Programme accoding to the National Screening Committee Policy.

Investigation of Choice

Fetal blood at birth.

Immediate Management

None

Treatment of Choice

Hormone replacement with L-thyroxine.

Your notes:

PAPER 2

Serial No. 12

Subject: Pediatrics

Topic: Rash

Question: A 12-year-old girl develops a fine macular rash after taking ampicillin prescribed to her for sore throat and fever. She has enlarged cervical lymph nodes.

Diagnosis: Infectious Mononucleosis(IMN)

Clinchers

- *12-year-old girl:* While in developed countries, IMN is more common between ages 15-25 yrs, in developing countries it is more common in children under 3 years of age.
- *Sore throat, fever, enlarged cervical lymph nodes:* IMN initially presents with non specific features like anorexia, fatigue, malaise, fever, sore throat, and enlarged cervical lymph nodes. There is often mild hepatosplenomegaly.
- *A fine macular rash after taking ampicillin:* The appearance of macular rash after taking ampicillin is almost characteristic of the condition.

CONFUSA

Prognosis of IMN–Although in most cases symptoms resolve in 2-4 weeks, in few fatigue, malaise, and anorexia may last for weeks or even months. There is evidence that, in patients with infectious mononucleosis, the chronic symptom of fatigue is reported in up to one half of patients. Poor physical functioning consistently predicts delayed recovery.

Investigation of Choice

Screening: FBC, Bood film(atypical T lymphocytes)
Paul Bunnell Test
Specific tests: Serology

Immediate Management

None

Treatment of Choice

There is no specific treatment available for glandular fever.

Ampicillin and amoxycillin should not be used if there is any possibility of EBV infection as they cause a rash. Penicillin is apparently safer.

Your notes:

Serial No. 13

Subject: Pediatrics

Topic: Rash

Question: A 7-month-old infant is brought with a rose-pink macular rash over the trunk. The baby was febrile before the onset of rash.

Diagnosis: Roseola Infantum

Clinchers

- *Seven month old infant:* Roseola is a benign condition is most probably due to infection with human herpes virus type 6. It is most common in infants between 6 and 18 months.
- *Rose-pink macular rash over the trunk:* The roseola presents with pyrexia, mild pharyngitis and lymphadenopathy. The incubation period varies from 10-15 days.
- *Was febrile before the onset of rash:* Rash typically appears after disappearance of fever; starts first involving the trunk and later may spread to the face and extremities. Its most prominent over the thighs and buttocks. It disappears within two days without desquamation or pigmentation.

CONFUSA

The closest differential diagnosis for roseola are rubella and measles. While measles have a predominant prodromal phase characterised by the catarrhal stage where there may be cough, coryza, conjunctivitis and the presence of Koplik spots. Rubella is chatacterised by post auricular lymphadenopathy and a not so prominent, pink macular rash.

Investigation of Choice

None

Immediate Management

Control fever with anti-pyretics.

Treatment of Choice

None; its a self limiting disease associated with full recovery.

Your notes:

Serial No. 14

Subject: Paediatrics

Topic: Rash

Question: A 6-year-old child develops fever, arthralgias and a confluent rash on the face with a "slapped cheek" appearance.

Diagnosis: Erythema Infectiosum (Fifth Disease)

Clinchers

- *Six-year-old child:* Erythema Infectiosum occurs due to infection with human erythrovirus B19, in school-aged children.
- *Fever, arthralgias:* The prodrome consists of mild fever with a sore throat and gastrointestinal disturbance. Occasionally, cervical lymphadenopathy and arthralgia may also be present.
- *"Slapped cheek" appearance:* This is perhaps the most characteristic of the condition. The rash is bright, erythematous and macular starts on the face giving the appearance of a slapped cheek. Later this spreads down to involve proximal arms and extensor surfaces of the legs. Palms and soles are rarely involved.

CONFUSA

While this disease rarely have any consequences in the healthy, in those with sickle cell anaemia, spherocytosis, or leukaemia, the disease may precipitate an aplastic crisis. The complications of this condition are based on the fact that it tends mostly to affect cells with a rapid turnover.

Investigation of Choice
Serology: IgM antibody to parvovirus B19

Immediate Management
None

Treatment of Choice
None; Its a benign self-limited disease.

For patients with arthralgias or pruritus, symptomatic relief can be obtained using oral analgesics and antihistamines or topical antipruritic lotions.

Your notes:

Serial No. 15

Subject: Paediatrics

Topic: Rash

Question: A 4-year-old child presents with a generalised blanching and an erythematous rash. He also has fever, conjunctivitis, photophobia and coryza. Red lesions with white centers are present on the buccal mucosa.

Diagnosis: Measles

Clinchers

- *4-year-old:* Measles is an infectious illness, predominantly affecting the school going children and is caused by an RNA paramyxovirus.
- *fever, conjunctivitis, photophobia and coryza:* Measles have a predominat prodromal phase characterised by the catarrhal stage where there may be cough, coryza, conjunctivitis and fever. Photophobia can be due to the aseptic meningitis commonly seen with the condition.
- *generalised blanching and an erythematous rash:* The exanthematous stage begins by rash, appearing 3 to 5 days later which is maculopapular, firstly behind the ears, then down the body, becoming confluent, fading by the third day.
- *Red lesions with white centres are present on the buccal mucosa:* This is the characteristic description of Koplik's Spots, seen in infectious pre-eruptive and catarrhal stage of measles infection, usually seen on the mucous membrane opposite the second molar tooth.

CONFUSA

The picture can be easily confused with menigococcal meningitis, which can also present as fever with rash along with photophobia and neck stiffness. However, a child with meningococcemia tends to be more toxic and the rash is non-blanching, purpuric.

Investigation of Choice
None: it is a clinical diagnosis.

Immediate Management
Isolate the child.
Measles is a notifiable disease in the UK.

Treatment of Choice
Symptomatic:

- Analgesics for headache and backache

- Treatment of bacterial superinfection
- Monitor and correct nutritional and hydrational changes; measles may produce dramatic weight reduction
- Non-vaccinated contacts should be given live measles vaccine, best within 3 days of the exposure, but up to 6 days in particular patients such as immunocompromised; alternatively, immunodeficient contacts or those under the age of nine months may be given intravenous immunoglobulin.

Your notes:

Serial No. 61

Subject: Obstetrics

Topic: Prenatal diagnosis

Question: A pregnant lady with previous male child affected with this disorder want to know whether this child is also affected.

Diagnosis: Duchenne's Muscular Dystrophy (DMD)

Clinchers

Previous male child affected with this disorder: The only hint provided in question is that the disease is congenital and is prevalent in males.

The most likely disease with this pattern (among the listed options) is the one which follows X-linked pattern, is Duchenne's Muscular Dystrophy(DMD).

DMD is inherited an X-linked manner, severely affecting males while female carriers only show mild myopathy features.

The gene for Duchenne's muscular dystrophy is the dystrophin locus at Xp21.

The disease typically manifests by 5 years of age and the affected child presents with features of gradually worsening muscle power, psuedohypertrophy of calf muscles, cardiomyopathy and scoliosis.

CONFUSA

Genetic counselling is an important aspect of dealing with families with a child diagnosed with DMD. Here, the female relatives are tested to see if they are carriers. However, note that 10-20% cases of DMD occur due to spontaneous mutation and is not inherited. So, even if the mother (with already one child diagnosed with DMD) is not a carrier of dystrophin mutation, there is still a high possibility of the second child to be affected because of other eggs carrying the same mutation.

Investigation of Choice

Screening: Serum creatinine kinase
Definitive: Muscle biopsy
Prenatal diagnosis: Chorionic villous sampling and looking for dystrophin mutation.

Immediate Management

None

Treatment of Choice

Genetic counselling

Your notes:

Serial No. 63

Subject: Obstetrics

Topic: Prenatal diagnosis

Question: A pregnant lady with high hCG and low AFP.

Diagnosis: Down's syndrome

Clinchers

- *High hCG, low AFP:* This forms the basis of the triple test, particularly offered to at risk mothers, in the antenatal period. The test measures alpha-fetoprotein, human chorionic gonadotrophin and unconjugated estriol. Low maternal serum alpha-fetoprotein (MSAFP), elevated human chorionic gonadotropin (hCG) and low unconjugated oestriol are markers for Down's syndrome.
- *Definitive diagnosis of requires karyotyping.* Cells can be obtained by either amniocentesis or chorionic villous sampling. However, at 14-16 weeks of gestation amniocentesis is more sensitive and safe for the prenatal diagnosis.

CONFUSA

Although it is widely known that the incidence of Down's syndrome, increases with maternal age, always remember that mothers of any age can have infants with Down's syndrome and, because fewer women over the age of 40 years have babies, the majority of Down's syndrome babies are born to younger mothers.

Also note that, for definitive diagnosis, karyotyping is a must; rest all tests are only suggestive of Down's syndrome.

Investigation of Choice

Amniocentesis with karyotyping

Immediate Management

Necessary counselling and information to the parents.

Treatment of Choice

Genetic counselling: Discuss the risk with subsequent pregnancies.

Your notes:

Serial No. 109

Subject: Paediatrics.

Topic: Respiratory.

Question: A 2-year-old child presents with acute fever, drowsiness, stridor and drooling. He looks shocked and unwell.

Diagnosis: Acute Epiglottitis

Clinchers

- *Two-years-old child:* Patient is usually 2-6 years of age. In comparison, croup generally occurs in children less than 2 years of age.
- *Acute fever, drowsiness, stridor and drooling:* Stridor is the most important feature, and could be expiratory or inspiratory. The child looks sick and usually sits up-forwards to maintain the airway.
- *He looks shocked and unwell:* The condition is caused by *Haemophilus* influneza virus and is known for its aggressiveness and association with septic shock. However, the most urgent emergency to avoid in this condition is respiratory obstruction.

CONFUSA

Acute laryngotracheobronchitis or croup can be quite confusing with the above mentioned picture. However, note that croup occurs in children younger than 2 years of age, the clinical course is not as rapid as seen in epiglottitis and barking cough is characteristic. Hoarseness can e present, but there is no dysphagia. The child prefers to lie down than to sit up and drool. The stridor associated with croup is typically inspiratory.

Investigation of Choice

Diagnosis is mainly clinical. Any investigation can delay the immediate resuscitation measures.

If the epiglottis neeeds to be visualized, it is done with a laryngoscope or bronchoscope in an operating room with complete cardiorespiratory support. Visualization of the epiglottis in other settings by depressing the tongue is contraindicated because of the possibility of inducing airway obstruction.

Immediate Management

Immediate referal for expert advise.

Treatment of Choice

Intubate—If respiratory obstruction becomes unavoidable
Give nebulised adrenaline.
Get IV access–symptomatic support
Antibiotic of choice–chloramphenicol or cefotaxime.

PAPER 3

1. A 16-year-old mother brings her baby for immunization. The nurse notices the baby has multiple bruises along both arms and legs. The baby is crying excessively. The house officer notices multiple fractures and that the baby has blue sclerae.

Diagnosis: Osteogenesis imperfecta.

Clinchers

- *16-year-old mother:* Not of much significance except the fact that battered baby condition is more prevalent among teenage mothers.
- *Multiple bruises along both arms and legs:* Because of connective tissue involvement, the skin scars extensively.
- *Crying excessively:* Because of pain induced by fractures and generalised illness.
- *Multiple fractures:* It is the hallmark of severe osteogenesis imperfecta. But these are also found in battered baby syndrome (non-accidental injury).
- *Blue sclerae:* It is the differentiating feature from non-accidental injury as blue sclerae are almost pathognomic of osteogenesis imperfecta with this clinical profile.

CONFUSA

Non-accidental injury is the main differential diagnosis in this case. Other thing to be noted is that osteogenesis imperfecta is known by many different names and they can appear in the options as such, i.e. fragilitas ossium, brittle bone syndrome, Adair-Dighton syndrome.

Investigation of Choice

Screening: X-ray (decrease in bone density)
Definitive: Absorptiometry (X-ray/photon)

Immediate Management

Symptomatic treatment (i.e. fractures—traction followed by light cast).

Treatment of Choice

Judicious exercise programme to prevent loss of bone mass secondary to physical inactivity.

Your notes:

46. A four-year-old boy walks with a prominent lordosis. He has goood speech, can build objects using blocks and has good social awareness.

Diagnosis: Duchenne muscular dystrophy (DMD).

Clinchers

- *Four-year-old boy:* DMD is present at birth, but the disorder usually becomes apparent between ages 3 and 5. It occurs exclusively in boys as it is a X-linked recessive disease.
- *Walks with a prominent lordosis:* Contractures of the heel cords and iliotibial bands forces the child to walk on toes, thereby producing a lordotic posture (This happens before the progressive loss of muscle strength makes him wheelchair bound).
- *He has good speech, can build objects using blocks, has good social awareness:* Intellectual development in DMD is common, the average IQ is approximately one standard deviation below the mean. Impairment of intellectual function appears to be nonprogressive and performance is least affected.

CONFUSA

Bilateral congenital dysplasia/dislocation of hip (CDH) can be a confusing option in this case but it can be safely excluded by the fact that CDH is 6 times more common in girls and usually diagnosed well before 4 years. Although the findings in bilateral CHD can be similar, i.e. lordosis and wide perineum. Becker muscular dystrophy can be a clinical differential, especially because of less incidence of mental retardation in it, but it usually presents after 5 years of age.

Investigation of Choice

- *Screening:* Serum creatine phosphokinase (CK)
- *Definitive:* EMG and biopsy (abnormal fibres surrounded by fat and fibrous tissues).

Immediate Management

Screen for any chest infection (usually present in DMD) and treat if present.

Treatment of Choice

- Prednisolone 0.75 mg/kg
- Aim to keep boy walking by using knee-ankle-foot orthoses
- Spinal fixation (Luque operation) or bracing reduces scoliosis.

47. A nine-month-baby born at term has a weight in the 97th percentile. His development is delayed.

Diagnosis: Hypothyroidism.

Clinchers

- *Nine-month-baby:* Hypothyroidism can be easily diagnosed at this age as before this age it manifest as very nonspecific features, i.e. excessive sleeping, inactivity, slow feeding and little crying.
- *Born at term:* There may be no signs at birth, the first sign is often prolonged neonatal jaundice. A term delivery in this case also exclude prematurity as a cause of developmental delay.
- *Has a weight in the 97th percentile:* Hypothyroidism produces a decrease in BMR, thereby resulting in weight gain.
- *His development is delayed:* Delayed growth and mental development, hypotonia and slowly relaxing reflexes are characteristic in hypothyroidism. Other features are coarse dry hair, flat nasal bridge, protruding tongue, umbilical hernia and slow pulse. Other late signs: IQ decrease, delayed puberty (occasionally precocious), short stature and delayed dentition).

CONFUSA

Differential diagnosis of large tongue are

- Hypothyroidism
- Amyloidosis
- Storage disorders

Investigation of Choice

- *Screening:* Heel prick test (filter paper blood spots at 5-7 days of age)
- *Definitive:* TSH/wrist X-ray (bone age is less than chronological age).

Treatment of Choice

Thyroxine 10 μg/kg/day (≤ 50 μg/day)—infants
100 μg/day—5 years age

- Start adult doses at 12 years
- Adjust according to growth rate and clinical response.

Your notes:

48. A nine-month-baby born at term has a weight in the 3rd percentile. His development is delayed. His head and body size are both small.

Diagnosis: Constitutional Delay.

Clinchers

- *Nine-month-baby:* Earliest possible age to make a diagnosis of constitutional delay.
- *Born at term*: Rules out any growth delay due to prematurity.
- *Has a weight in the 3rd percentile:* Third percentile is the lowest cut off of weight in normal range (highest is 97th percentile). This signifies a delay in weight gain although he is considered normal.
- *His development is delayed:* There could be many causes for delayed development which could not be ascertained here because of lack of detailed history and information in the question.
- *His head and body size are both small:* Since both head and body are small, there is a uniform all round delay—by definition this is constitutional delay. He might have been a small for gestation age baby.

CONFUSA

Microcephaly is a feature of many congenital disorders resulting in developmental delay (e.g. fetal alcohol syndrome, intrauterine infections, chromosomal disorders, etc.). But in it body size is usually normaly.

Investigation of Choice

Detailed work up to find a cause.

Immediate Management

Ensure proper nutrition.

Treatment of Choice

Depends upon cause, otherwise no treatment required as he is in normal range.

Your notes:

PAPER 4

41. Child who is HIV positive is due for MMR.

Diagnosis: Balanced risk.

Clinchers

- *MMR vaccines:* Those age 18 months to 5 years who have not had the vaccine (even if they have had single measles vaccine) may have MMR with the pre-school of DPT. There is no upper age limit.
- As per the UK schedule, first dose of MMR (0.5 ml SC) is given between 12-18 months.
- *HIV positive:* Immunodeficiencies are a contraindication for MMR vaccination but these include only primary immunodeficiencies and not HIV or AIDS (208, OHCS, 5th edn).

CONFUSA

Contraindications for MMR vaccination

Condition	Delay for
Fever	till fever resolves
Pregnancy	till one month postpartum
Previous line vaccine	till 3 weeks
Previous Ig	till 3 months
Primary immunodeficiencies (except HIV and AIDS)	not given
Steroid therapy	till 3 months after discontinuation
Leukaemia	not given
Lymphoma	not given
Recent radiotherapy	till 6 months to one year
Anaphylaxis history by • egg • neomycin • kanamycin	not given

- Steroid therapy implies prednisolone ≥ 2 mg/kg/day from > 1 week (or equivalent doses)
- Neomycin or kanamycin are the vaccine preservatives
- The vaccine is chick embryo based, so a history of anaphylaxis by egg protein (and not egg allergy) is a contraindication

Investigation of Choice
None required.

Immediate Management
None required.

Treatment of Choice
Continue as per schedule.

Your notes:

42. Child due for Hib, DPT, etc. suffering from acute febrile illness.

Diagnosis: Risk of febrile convulsions.

Clinchers

Note: An acute febrile illness is a contraindication for any vaccine.

- *HiB vaccine:* It is a bacterial polysaccharide protein conjugate vaccine for *Haemophilus influenza* type V strain. It has a few insignificant local effects and no serious reactions.
- *DPT vaccination:* It is a combination vaccine against diphtheria, pertussis and tetanus. In them diphtheria and tetanus are toxoids and pertussis is an a cellular vaccine. According to UK schedule the first dose is given at 2 months of age (in preterm babies—2 month postnatally).
- *Acute febrile illness:* It is a contraindication for DPT vaccination (not so for Hib) as the pertussis component in it produces a post vaccination fever of >39.5°C within 48 hours. Since the child is already febrile, it can compound the problem and can lead to febrile convulsions. Its better to delay the vaccine till the fever resolves or at least 2 weeks.

CONFUSA

The only other contraindication for pertussis vaccination is a past severe reaction to pertussis vaccine—i.e. indurated redness most of the way around the arm, or over most of the anterolateral thigh (depending on the site of injection) or a generalised reaction.

Note: According to BNF (British National Formulary) website, evolving neurological problems are also a contraindication untill the condition is stable.

Investigation of Choice
Fever workup.

Immediate Management
Paracetamol ± tepid sponging.

Treatment of Choice
Delay by 2 weeks.

Your notes:

43. Child cried for 2 hours after Hib, DPT, etc.

Diagnosis: No risk from further vaccination.

Clinchers

- *Cried for 2 hours after Hib, DPT:* Persistent, inconsolable crying lasting ≥ 3 hours within 48 hours after DPT vaccination is a valid *precaution* for further vaccination. Since this child does not meet this criteria, the rest of the immunization schedule can be safely continued.

CONFUSA

Since the above criterion is only a precaution and not a contraindication, it warrants further vaccination after careful review. The benefits and risk of administering a specific vaccine to an individual under the circumstances are considered. It benefits outweigh the risk, e.g. during on outbreak or foreign travel, the vaccine should be administered.

Investigation of Choice

A complete work up to find the cause of inconsolable crying.

Immediate Management

A complete work up to find the cause of inconsolable crying.

Treatment of Choice

Continue as per schedule.

Your notes:

44. Family history of egg allergy. Child due for MMR.

Diagnosis: Insignificant risk of anaphylaxis.

Clinchers

- *Family history of egg allergy:* The only contraindication for MMR (a chick embryo based vaccine) is previous history of anaphylaxis by egg intake. History of other egg allergies in the subject to be vaccinated or in his family is a contraindication.

Note: Other vaccine which can produce complications in previous history of egg allergy is Hib vaccine.

CONFUSA

Persons with a history of anaphylactic reactions (and not just history of egg allergy in himself or in family) following egg ingestion be vaccinated only with caution. Protocols have been developed for vaccinating such persons and should be consulted.

Investigation of Choice

None.

Immediate Management

Cautions–vaccination and monitoring thereafter.

Treatment of Choice

Continue as per schedule.

Your notes:

45. History of convulsions. Child due for HiB, DPT, etc.

Diagnosis: Insignificant risk of febrile convulsions.

Clinchers

- *History of convulsions:* The parents of children with a tendency to have convulsions should be counselled on the management of any fever developing after immunization. Febrile convulsions may occur 5-10 days after measles vaccination (or MMR) whereas they may take place in the first 72 hours after pertussis immunization. Suggestion may include paracetamol, sponge with tepid water, give extra fluids, dress in thin clothing and place in a cool room. In high-risk children, an antipyretic drug may be suggested routinely for the first 72 hours after immunization. Where the tendency is severe, the parents may be instructed on rectal diazepam administration (source: BNF website).
- *Hib, DPT*–Only the pertussis component is known to produce a febrile syndrome postvaccination (Hence increase the risk of febrile convulsions).

CONFUSA

Presence of history of convulsions (personal/family) is a special consideration (i.e. require individual care review) and not a contraindication for vaccination. Most children with idiopathic epilepsy, or a family history of epilepsy (sibling or parent) should be vaccinated. If in doubt, seek expert advice rather than withholding the vaccine. Those with special CNS conditions (e.g. cerebral palsy, spina bifida) are *especially recommended* for vaccination.

Investigation of Choice

None required.

Immediate Management

Counsel and teach the parents about the prevention and management of febrile convulsions.

Treatment of Choice

Continue as per schedule.

Your notes:

86. A 12-month-old child of unemployed parents, did not gain weight from 6 months.

Diagnosis: Failure to thrive

Clinchers

- *Twelve-month-old:* Failure to thrive means poor weight gain in infancy. In 95% cases this is due to not enough food being offered, or not enough food being taken.
- *Unemployed parents:* This titles the suspicion more towards not enough food being offered.
- *Did not gain weight from 6 months:* This is a serious finding as infants usually gain 2-3 kg during this period.

CONFUSA

Failure to thrive is mainly because of poverty in developing countries. In UK it is:

- Difficulty at home
- Emotional deprivation
- Unskilled feeding techniques

While investigating, focus on there points:

- Signs of abuse
- Family finances
- Chart family heights
- Feeding patterns
- Dysmorphic face
- Parenteral illness
- Activity level; behaviour
- General health and happiness

Investigation of Choice

Nutrition assessment

Immediate Management

Rule out any malabsorption disease.

Treatment of Choice

Correct nutritional deficiencies in diet.

Your notes:

136. A 4-year-old boy has fever since 2 days, presents with convulsions since 5 min, still convulsing in the ambulance, IV line has been established.

Diagnosis: Febrile convulsions.

Clinchers

- *Boy:* Febrile convulsions occur in about 3% of children between the ages of 5 months and 5 years.
- *Fever:* They are thought to be caused by viraemia and often recurrent.
- *Convulsions × 5 min:* The child may present with prolonged fitting or there may have been a short period of clonic or tonic activity.
- *Still convulsing in the ambulance IV line has been established:* The first preference is to protect the convulsing child from harm If the child is still convulsing, give diazepam (or larazepam) emulsion 0.3 mg per kg slow IV. This can be repeated after a few minutes if fitting continues.

CONFUSA

Give 0.5 mg diazepam per rectally if IV access is delayed. The usual progression of treatment (if fitting does not stop) should be

Diazepam—IV/per rectal

↓

Paraldehyde—per rectum (diluted 50: 50 with arachis oil)

↓

Phenytoin—18 mg/kg IV over 15 minutes (with EEG monitoring

↓

IV thiopentone—for intractable fitting

Investigation of Choice

Blood glucose (all cases)

Immediate Management

IV lorazepam

Treatment of Choice

- Criteria for hospital admission
  - Prolonged
  - Recurrent — Febrile convulsion
  - First
- Paracetamol or Ibuprofen after fitting has stopped.

Your notes:

137. A 2-year-old boy with past and family history of febrile convulsions. He is OK now.

Diagnosis: Recurrent febrile convulsions.

Clinchers

- *History of febrile convulsions:* A febrile convulsion is diagnosed if the following occur together:
  - A tonic/clonic, symmetrical generalised with no focal feature
  - Occurring as the temperature rises rapidly in a febrile illness
  - In a normally developing child between 5 months and 5 years of age
  - With no signs of CNS infection or previous history of epilepsy
  - When there are less than 3 seizures, each lasting < 5 min.
- *He is OK now:* This means that he require no active treatment now.
- *Family history positive:* The chances of recurrence of a febrile convulsion are about 50% if first degree relative is also affected.

CONFUSA

Apart from being taught the use of rectal diazepam, the patient should be explained to bring down any future fever promptly with oral paracetamol and tepid sponging. Since the child is only 2-year-old, he will undergo MMR and pertussis vaccination at 4 years age, both of which can cause fever. Explain them to be ready for immediate intervention then.

Immediate Management

Rectal diazepam use explained to parents especially the mother, e.g. with one 5 mg tube (stesolid).

Treatment of Choice

Control of convulsions have been explained in previous question.

Your notes:

PAPER 5

36. A nine-year-old boy has a mild cough and wheeze after playing football in the cold weather.

Diagnosis: Exercise induced asthma

Clinchers

- *Nine-year-old boy:* Exercise induced asthma is most commonly present in childhood.
- *Mild cough and wheeze:* These are the diagnostic symptoms of asthma.
- *After playing football in cold weather:* Cold weather and exercise are both precipitants of asthma. Exercise is one of the most common precipitants of acute episodes of asthma. Exercise probably provokes bronchospasm to some extent in every asthmatic patients, and in some it is the only trigger that produces symptoms. There is a significant interaction between the ventilation produced by exercise, the temperature, and the water content of the inspired air and the magnitude of the postexertional obstruction.

CONFUSA

Cromoglycate is used prophylaxis is mild and exercised asthma (always inhaled), especially in children. Note that it may precipitate asthma. Exercise induction differs from other naturally occurring provocations of asthma, such as antigens or viral infections, in that it does not evoke any long-term sequelae nor does it change airway reactivity.

Investigation of Choice

PEFR

Immediate Management

Nebulisation.

Treatment of Choice

Prophylactic inhaled sodium cromoglycate.

If PEFR is > 75% of the predicted, patient is mild and can be discharged with usual inhaled bronchodilator. If PEFR is between 50 and 75% of predicted, give neubulized salbutamol with oxygen.

Your notes:

37. A six-year-old girl with asthma uses her bronchodilator twice a day to relieve her mild wheeze. Her parents refuse to give her any treatment containing corticosteroids

Diagnosis: Asthma

Clinchers

- *Six-year-old girl:* Sodium cromoglycate is preferred treatment for mild cases of asthma in children.
- *Uses her bronchodilator twice a day to relieve her mild wheeze:* If occasional short acting bronchodilators are required for symptom relief for more than once daily or night time symptoms, go to step 2 of British Thoracic Society guidelines (BTS guidelines).
- *Refuse to give her any treatment containing corticosteroids:* Since step 2 and step 3 of BTS guidelines are based on steroids, we will proceed to step 4 which recommends sodium cromoglycate for children.

CONFUSA

Usually all the questions pertaining to treatment of asthma in PLAB exam are based upon BTS guidelines. Refer to them on page 172, OHCM, 5th edn or www.bnf.org.

Investigation of Choice

PEFR monitoring.

Immediate Management

Evaluate for antigens precipitants.

Treatment of Choice

Inhaled sodium cromoglycate

(addition of it to the existing bronchodilator treatment).

Your notes:

38. **A nine-year-old girl with chronic asthma presents to the A and E department with rapidly worsening wheeze not relieved with inhaled bronchodilators.**

Diagnosis: Acute episode of severe asthma.

Clinchers

- *Nine-year-old girl:* In childhood there is a 2:1 male/female preponderance, but the sex ratio equalizes by age 30.
- *Chronic asthma:* This increases the risk of status asthmatics.
- *Rapidly worsening wheeze:* This suggest urgent intervention as the condition is worsening.
- *Not relieved with inhaled bronchodilators:* Acute attacks need to be treated with steroids if bronchodilators are not effective.

CONFUSA

Glucocorticoids are not bronchodilators, and their major use in asthma is in reducing airway inflammation. Systemic or oral steroids are most beneficial in acute illness when severe airway obstruction is not resolving or is worsening despite intense optimal bronchodilator theory, and in chronic disease when there has been failure of a previously optimal regimen with frequent recurrences of symptoms of increasing severity.

Investigation of Choice
None required.

Immediate Management
Nebulised bronchodilators.

Treatment of Choice
Oral steroids.

Your notes:

39. **A four-year-old boy with eczema and recurrent wheeze whenever he gets a viral infection has now developed night cough, there as been no improvement in spite of using inhaled bronchodilator twice each night.**

Diagnosis: Asthma.

Clinchers

- *Four-year-old boy:* In young children, the most important infections agents are respiratory syncytial virus and parainfluenza virus.
- *Eczema and recurrent wheeze:* Well-controlled studies have demonstrated that respiratory viruses and not bacteria or allergy are the major etiologic factors. Although asthma is most commonly associated with atropy (e.g. eczema).
- *Viral infection:* Respiratory viral infections, are the most common of the stimuli that evoke acute exacerbations of asthma.
- *Night cough despite bronchodilators twice each night:* This suggest that the bronchodilators should be changed to long acting ones or additional drugs are required.

CONFUSA

Cromolyn and nedocromil, like the inhaled steroids, improve lung function and reduce symptoms and lower airway reactivity in asthmatics. They are most effective in atopic patients who have either seasonal disease or perennial airway stimulation.

Investigation of Choice
PEFR before sleep.

Immediate Management
Rule out any heart disease.

Treatment of Choice
Inhaled sodium cromoglycate (Additional).

Your notes:

40. A 14-year-old boy, with well controlled asthma, using inhaled steroids and a bronchodilator comes to the A and E. Department with breathlessness and swollen lips after eating a peanut, butter-sandwich.

Diagnosis: Anaphylaxis.

Clinchers

- *Well controlled asthma, using inhaled steroids and a bronchodilator:* This is step 2 treatment in BTS guidelines. Since it is well controlled a severe acute attack of asthma is unlikely is this patient.
- *Breathlessness and swollen lips after eating a peanut butter-sandwich:* This is an anaphylactic reaction to peanut which is common among caucasians. It requires management on its guidelines. But since he is an asthmatic, oral bronchodilator can be added on as required basis.

CONFUSA

It is a type I IgE mediated hypersensitivity reaction to peanut. Release of histamine and other agents.
Causes: Capillary leak, wheeze, cyanosis, oedema of larynx, lids, tongue and lips, urticaria. These more common in atopic individuals. Other foods which are commonly involved are eggs, fish and strawberries.

Investigation of Choice
ECG monitoring

Immediate Management
Admit + IM adrenaline (Not IV unless the patient is severely ill or has no pulse).

Treatment of Choice
As required oral bronchodilator.

Your notes:

118. A baby has a number of fits, each occurring in the morning on four consecutive days. On physical examination you find the liver to be enlarged. His fasting blood sugar is low and his uric acid is high.

Diagnosis: G6PD deficiency.

Clinchers

- *Baby:* G6PD deficiency presents at a young age. Among the congenital shunt defects, it is the most common.
- *Number of fits each occurring in the morning on four consecutive days:* These suggest severe haemolytic crises. Since they are occurring at same time every day, the cause should be searched for which could be a breakfast of fava beans or simply circardias stress.
- *Liver to be enlarged:* It is a common finding in G6PD deficiency.
- *Fasting blood sugar low:* It could also be the stress as in newborns (age is not given in this questions), hypoglycemia can precipitate attacks.
- *Uric acid high:* Due to haemolysis.

CONFUSA

Although we are also not 100% convinced by this answer, among the given list of options it is the closest guess. May be some points in either the question or the options is missing. But if the question repeats in this form only, then you can safely mark it as an answer.

Investigation of Choice
Characteristic cells in peripheral smear during an attack (Screening: Dye reduction tests).

Immediate Management
Consider blood transfusion.

Treatment of Choice
As per the cause + symptomatic.

Your notes:

135. An anxious mother called you to say that her son's best friend in school has caught meningitis.

Diagnosis: Immediate 'contact' of meningitis.

Clinchers

Meningitis prophylaxis

Talk to your consultant in community disease control. Offer prophylaxis is:

- Household/nurser contacts (i.e. within droplet range)
- Those who have kissed the patient's mouth.

CONFUSA

If the student suffering from meningitis is just a classmate and the best friend of her son, then there is no need of any chemoprophylaxis.

Investigation of Choice

None required except screening the skin for any nonblanching petechiae.

Immediate Management

Reassure mother.

Treatment of Choice

Rifampicin prophylaxis

- 600 mg/12 h PO for 2 days
- Children > 1 yr 10 mg/kg/12 h
  < 1 yr 10 mg/kg/12 h

  or

  Ciprofloxacin
- 500 mg PO, 1 dose, adult only.

Your notes:

181. A 15-year-old boy has very poor grades at school despite being very attentive and hard working. His mother reckons its because he is teased at school because his breasts look like a girl's. On further examination he is found to have small firm testes. He is mildly asthmatic.

Diagnosis: Klinefelter's syndrome.

Clinchers

- *15-year-old:* Patient usually present in adolescence with poor sexual development
- *Poor grades despite being very attentive and hard working:* Patients are occasionally mentally retarded.
- *Breasts look like a girls and small firm testes:* Gynaecomastia and small peanut size but firm testes are signs of androgen deficiency found in Klinefelter's.
- *Mildly asthmatic:* Obesity and varicose veins occur in one-third to one-half and abnormalities of thyroid function, diabetes mellitus, and pulmonary disease may be present in Klinefelter's.

CONFUSA

Gynaecomastia ordinarily develops during adolescence, is generally bilateral and painless, and may become disfiguring. The risk of breast cancer is 20 times that of normal men, but only about a fifth that in women. Most have male psychosexual orientation and function sexually as normal men.

Investigation of Choice

Karyotyping.

Immediate Management

Genetic counselling.

Treatment of Choice

Androgen replacement therapy (if patient is mentally subnormal, use it carefully).

Your notes:

PAPER 6

95. An 8-year-old girl is noted to have fresh bloody staining of her pants. She also suffers from eneuresis. She has recently started horse-riding lessons.

Diagnosis: Accidental injury.

Clinchers

- *Fresh bloody staining of her pant:* Most probably from trauma as the history given in question does not potray any illness.
- *She also suffers from eneuresis:* Bedwetting occurs on most nights in 15% of 5-year-old, and is still a problem in upto 3% of 15-year-old (usually from delayed maturation of bladder control). So, it is probably normal.
- *She has recently started horse-riding lessons:* It can be reason for trauma, most probably rupture of hymen, which is common in horse riding training for adolescent girls.

CONFUSA

GMC has tried to mislead us by putting the history of eneuresis in this question. But eneuresis has nothing to do with bleeding anywhere. So the question is still straight enough.

Investigation of Choice

For bleeding: Local examination.
For eneuresis: Test for UTI, GU abnormality and DM.

Immediate Management

Reassurance.

Treatment of Choice

Desmopressin nasal spray.

Your notes:

106. Copies circle, can say 4 words.

Answer: Three years

Clinchers

Apart from these a 3 year child can do:

- Jumps
- Can stand on one foot
- Can build an 8-cube tower
- Knows his first and last name
- Dress with help
- Imitate bridges with cubes
- Imitates vertical line within 30°
- Recognizes 3 colours
- Plays interactive games like TAG.

CONFUSA	
Copies circle	3 years
Copies cross	4 years
Copies square	5 years

Your notes:

107. Smiles responsively, Head lags.

Answer: 6 weeks

Clinchers

At 6 weeks, an infant can:

- Vocalizes, not crying
- Smiles responsively
- Move eyes 90° to midline
- Regards face

CONFUSA	
Smiles responsively	6 weeks
Smiles spontaneously	4 months

Your notes:

108. Can walk 4 steps upstairs.

Answer: 2 years

Clinchers

Other milestones seen in a 2 years old child

- Dons shoes not tied
- Washes and dries hands
- Jumps in place
- Kicks a ball
- Over arm bowling
- Gets undressed

CONFUSA	
Walks holding on to furniture	9 months
Walks well	12 months
Walks backwards	14 months
Walks up steps	17 months
Heel to toe walk	3½ years

Your notes:

109. Holds head up at 45° when prone, vocalise.

Answer: Two months

Clinchers

Things that a 2 months old child can do

- Holds head at 45° when prone
- Vocalizes
- Smiles responsively
- Move eyes 90° to midline and past midline
- Laughs
- Hands together.

CONFUSA	
Lifts head when prone	1 month
Holds head at 45° when prone	2 months
Holds head at 90° when prone	2½ months
Sits with head steady	4 months

Your notes:

110. Pincer grip; can say "Mummy" ± "Daddy"

Answer: One year.

Clinchers

Other things that a 1 year old child can do is:

- Just stands
- Walks using a table's support
- Clashes cubes
- Plays 'pat a cake'
- Indicates wants (not cry)
- Drinks from cup.

CONFUSA	
Dada or mama (nonspecific)	7 months
Dada or mama (Specific)	9 months
2 words other than mama, dada	13 months
Combines 2 different words	19 months
Defines 6 words	4 ½ years

Your notes:

186. 24-month-old child, brought with a history of having been accidentally locked up in a car for about 3 hours. On examination in the A and E child is crying but his vitals are stable. What is the next step.

Diagnosis: Insignificant fluid loss.

Clinchers

- *Twenty-four months of child:* Dehydration in a child, if not corrected, can end up fatally.
- *Accidentally locked up in a car for about 3 hours:* The existence of dehydration in this case depends upon the weather conditions. If it is sunny outside, the child can loose a significant amount of fluid in perspiration. But nothing of that sort has been mentioned in the question.
- *Crying but vitals are stable:* In mild dehydration, the only feature usually is the irritable child. Stable vitals exclude severe dehydration though they can often be deceptive in case of children.

CONFUSA

The body loses about 125 ml of fluids in urine, stools, exhaled air and perspiration and gains 15 ml of fluid endogenously as a metabolic by product for every 100 calories metabolized. In case of accidental locking of a child in car for prolonged periods on a sunny day, sunburns should also be excluded.

Investigation of Choice

None required.

Immediate Management

Check skin turgor and urine output.

Treatment of Choice

Give water to sip.

Your notes:

188. Mother comes to the A and E with her child of 3 years, history of D and V. On examination the child appears mildly dehydrated.

Diagnosis: Mild dehydration.

Clinchers

- *Three years old child:* The key to effective fluid management in childhood diarrhoea is early replacement of fluid losses, starting with the first sign of liquid stool.
- *Diarrhoea and vomiting:* Diarrhoea and vomiting (D and V) are common but potentially serious illnesses in early childhood. In most cases of acute diarrhoea, electrolytes such as chloride and sodium besides water are actively secreted from the gut mucosa and are thus lost in stools.
- *Mild dehydration:* In cases of mild to moderate dehydration, fluid, electrolyte and acid-base homeostasis should be preserved and maintained. Usually if renal function is maintained, such imbalances can not occur.

CONFUSA

A child may lose almost as much water and electrolytes from the body during an episode of diarrhoea as an adult, since the length and surface area of intestinal mucosa of a child, from where the diarrhoeal fluids are secreted, are fairly large. Loss of one litre of fluid from the body of a child weighing 7 kg is much more hazardous compared with a similar depletion from an adult of 70 kg weight.

Investigation of Choice

Stool culture and microscopy.

Immediate Management

Give anti-emetics.

Treatment of Choice

ORS 90 meE (This is WHO ORS and provides 90 mEq/L of Na^+, 20 mEq/L of K^+, 80 mEq/L of Cl^- and 30 mEq/L of HCO_3 or citrate).

Your notes:

196. Child who is HIV positive is due for MMR.

Diagnosis: Balanced risk.

Clinchers

- *MMR vaccines:* Those age 18 months to 5 years who have not had the vaccine (even if they have had single measles vaccine) may have MMR with the preschool of DPT. There is no upper age limit.
- As per the UK schedule, first dose of MMR (0.5 ml SC) is given between 12-18 months.
- *HIV positive:* Immunodeficiencies are a contraindication for MMR vaccination but these include only primary immunodeficiencies and not HIV or AIDS (208, OHCS, 5th edn).

CONFUSA

Contraindications for MMR vaccination

Condition	Delay for
Fever	till fever resolves
Pregnancy	till one month postpartum
Previous line vaccine	till 3 weeks
Previous Ig	till 3 months
Primary immunodeficiencies (except HIV and AIDS)	not given
Steroid therapy	till 3 months after discontinuation
Leukaemia	not given
Lymphoma	not given
Recent radiotherapy	till 6 months to one year
Anaphylaxis history by • Egg • Neomycin • Kanamycin	not given

- Steroid therapy implies prednisolone $\geq$ 2 mg/kg/day from > 1 week (or equivalent doses)
- Neomycin or kanamycin are the vaccine preservatives
- The vaccine is chick embryo based, so a history of anaphylaxis by egg protein (and not egg allergy) is a contraindication

Investigation of Choice
None required.

Immediate Management
None required.

Treatment of Choice
Continue as per schedule.

Your notes:

197. Child due for HiB, DPT, etc. suffering from acute febrile illness.

Diagnosis: Risk of febrile convulsions.

Clinchers

Note: An acute febrile illness is a contraindication for any vaccine.

- *HiB vaccine:* It is a bacterial polysaccharide protein conjugate vaccine for Haemophilus influenza type V strain. It has a few insignificant local effects and no serious reactions.
- *DPT vaccination:* It is a combination vaccine against diphtheria, pertussis and tetanus. In them diphtheria and tetanus are toxoids and pertussis is an a cellular vaccine. According to UK schedule the first dose is given at 2 months of age (in preterm babies—2 month postnatally).
- *Acute febrile illness:* It is a contraindication for DPT vaccination (not so for Hib) as the pertussis component in it produces a post vaccination fever of >39.5°C within 48 hours. Since the child is already febrile, it can compound the problem and can lead to febrile convulsions. Its better to delay the vaccine till the fever resolves or at least 2 weeks.

CONFUSA

The only other contraindication for pertussis vaccination is a past severe reaction to pertussis vaccine—i.e. indurated redness most of the way around the arm, or over most of the anterolateral thigh (depending on the site of injection) or a generalised reaction.

Note: According to BNF (British National Formulary) website, evolving neurological problems are also a contraindication untill the condition is stable.

Investigation of Choice
Fever workup.

Immediate Management
Paracetamol ± tepid sponging.

Treatment of Choice
Delay by 2 weeks.

Your notes:

198. Child cried for 2 hours after Hib, DPT, etc.

Diagnosis: No risk from further vaccination.

Clinchers

- *Cried for 2 hours after Hib, DPT:* Persistent, inconsolable crying lasting ≥ 3 hours within 48 hours after DPT vaccination is a valid *precaution* for further vaccination. Since this child does not meet this criteria, the rest of the immunisation schedule can be safely continued.

CONFUSA

Since the above criterion is only a precaution and not a contraindication, it warrants further vaccination after careful review. The benefits and risk of administering a specific vaccine to an individual under the circumstances are considered. It benefits outweigh the risk, e.g. during on outbreak or foreign travel, the vaccine should be administered.

Investigation of Choice

A complete work up to find the cause of inconsolable crying.

Immediate Management

A complete work up to find the cause of inconsolable crying.

Treatment of Choice

Continue as per schedule.

Your notes:

199. Family history of egg allergy. Child due for MMR.

Diagnosis: Insignificant risk of anaphylaxis.

Clinchers

- *Family history of egg allergy:* The only contraindication for MMR (a chick embryo based vaccine) is previous history of anaphylaxis by egg intake. History of other egg allergies in the subject to be vaccinated or in his family is a contraindication.

Note: Other vaccine which can produce complications in previous history of egg allergy is Hib vaccine.

CONFUSA

Persons with a history of anaphylactic reactions (and not just history of egg allergy in himself or in family) following egg ingestion be vaccinated only with caution. Protocols have been developed for vaccinating such persons and should be consulted.

Investigation of Choice

None.

Immediate Management

Cautions vaccination and monitoring thereafter.

Treatment of Choice

Continue as per schedule.

Your notes:

200. History of convulsions. Child due for Hib, DPT, etc.

Diagnosis: Insignificant risk of febrile convulsions.

Clinchers

- *History of convulsions:* The parents of children with a tendency to have convulsions should be counselled on the management of any fever developing after immunization. Febrile convulsions may occur 5-10 days after measles vaccination (or MMR) whereas they may take place in the first 72 hours after pertussis immunization. Suggestion may include paracetamol, sponge with tepid water, give extra-fluids, dress in thin clothing and place in a cool room. In high-risk children, an antipyretic drug may be suggested routinely for the first 72 hours after immunization. Where the tendency is severe, the parents may be instructed on rectal diazepam administration (source: BNF website).
- *Hib, DPT*—Only the pertussis component is known to produce a febrile syndrome postvaccination (Hence increase the risk of febrile convulsions)

CONFUSA

Presence of history of convulsions (personal/family) is a special consideration (i.e. require individual care review) and not a contraindication for vaccination. Most children with idiopathic epilepsy, or a family history of epilepsy (sibling or parent) should be vaccinated. If in doubt, seek expert advice rather than withholding the vaccine. Those with special CNS conditions (e.g. cerebral palsy, spina bifida) are *especially recommended* for vaccination.

Investigation of Choice
None required.

Immediate Management
Counsel and teach the parents about the prevention and management of febrile convulsions.

Treatment of Choice
Continue as per schedule.

Your notes:

PAPER 7

10. A one and half year old girl, was brought with complaint of dysuria. Culture of urine reveals mixed bacteria.

Diagnosis: UTI

Clinchers

- *One and half year old girl:* Incidence of UTI in girls is more after then neonatal age.
- *Dysuria:* At such age, dysuria suggests only a UTI. It could be secondary to some GU tract abnormality.
- *Culture of urine reveals mixed bacteria:* This suggests contamination of the urine sample. A repeat clean midstream catch should be sent again for culture. Genitals should be washed with water and tap repeatedly (in cycles of 1 min) before the "catch."

CONFUSA

In infants, suprapubic aspiration is definitive and any organisms found in it are significant.

Investigation of Choice
MSU culture.

Immediate Management
Counsel parents about keeping local hygiene of the child.

Treatment of Choice
Trimethoprim.

Your Notes

11. A 3-week-old week presents with projectile vomiting, appearing hungry after each emesis. On examination, dehydration is present and there is a mass in abdomen.

Diagnosis: Pyloric stenosis

Clinchers

- *Three-week-old:* Pyloric stenosis is not present at birth, but develops during the first month of life.
- *Projectile vomiting:* Vomiting typically occurs after feeds, and becomes projectile, e.g. vomiting over far end of cot.
- *Appearing hungry after each emesis:* Even though the patient is ill, he is rarely obtunded; he is alert, anxious, and hungry—and possibly malnourished, dehydrated and always hungry.
- *Dehydration:* It is almost invariably present because of the inability to take oral fluids (i.e. milk).
- *Mass in abdomen:* An olive-sized pyloric mass is present in this condition.

CONFUSA

Congenital pyloric stenosis is distinguished from other causes of vomiting (e.g. gastric reflux) by 3 important points:

1. The vomit does not contain bile, as the obstruction, is so high.
2. No diarrhoea: Constipation is likely (occasionally starvation stools).
3. Even though patient is ill, he does not look so.

Investigation of Choice
USG

Immediate Management
Wide bore nasogastric tube

Treatment of Choice
Ramstedt's pyloromyotomy

Your Notes:

13. A 3-month-old child is brought with recurrent vomiting, but is otherwise thriving well and healthy. The symptom seems to subside when the child is strapped in baby's seat.

Diagnosis: Physiological gastro-oesophageal reflux (GFR).

Clinchers

- *3-month-old:* GFR usually presents in the first year of age. GE reflux persisting after that is always pathological.
- *Recurrent vomiting:* Recurrent regurgitation and vomiting is a common symptoms initially.
- *Otherwise thriving well and healthy:* Since it is a physiological condition, the child will have minimal or no effect on its health.
- *Symptom seems to subside when the child is strapped in baby's seat:* The cause of physiologic GER is inadequate development of lower oesophageal pressure regurgitation (dysmotility). This results in spontaneous effortness regurgitation of gastric contents into the oesophagus. Obviously these symptoms can subside if there is a firm strap over the lower chest (baby's seat).

CONFUSA

GER persisting after one year is always pathological. Most such cases are associated with inappropriate transient relaxation of lower oesophageal sphincter. These transient relaxation episodes may occur along with swallowing and pharyngeal contractions. There is also delayed clearance of acid from the distal oesophagus. Such a patient may have complications like:

- Recurrent lower respiratory infections (aspiration)
- GI blood loss (hematemesis)
- Anaemia
- Failure to thrive

Investigation of Choice
Esophageal pH monitoring but usually none required till one year of age.

Immediate Management
Counselling of mother to nurse child in semi-upright position.

Treatment of Choice
Observation till one year of age.

Your Notes:

14. A 6-year-old girl presents with fever, frequency, dysuria and abdominal pain.

Diagnosis: Urinary tract infection (UTI)

Clinchers

- *Six-year-old girl:* Prevalence of covert bacteriuria in school going girls in UK is 3%. Recurrence is 35% if more than 2-year-old. Overall the annual incidence of UTI in girls is more in UK (Girls: 0.31-1%, Boys: 0.17-0.23%).
- *Fever, frequency, dysuria and abdominal pain:* Suprapubic tenderness. Occurs in symptomatic bacteriuria unequivocally suggests UTI especially distal GU tract (i.e. cystitis).

CONFUSA

In the newborn period the incidence of UTI is about the same in boys and girls, since:

- The route of infection may be hematogenous.
- Boys have a higher incidence of urinary tract anomalies.

Beyond infancy the incidence of UTI is higher in girls. Asymptomatic bacteriuria is also more frequent in girls.

Investigation of Choice

Urinalysis and culture.

Immediate Management

Exclude reflux (with MCU).

Treatment of Choice

Trimethoprim.

Your Notes:

40. An anxious mother called you to say that her son's best friend in school has caught meningitis.

Diagnosis: Immediate 'contact' of meningitis.

Clinchers

Meningitis prophylaxis

Talk to your consultant in community disease control.
Offer prophylaxis is:

- Household/nurser contacts (i.e. within droplet range)
- Those who have kissed the patient's mouth.

CONFUSA

If the student suffering from meningitis is just a classmate and the best friend of her son, then there is no need of any chemoprophylaxis.

Investigation of Choice

None required except screening the skin for any non-blanching petechiae.

Immediate Management

Reassure mother.

Treatment of Choice

Rifampicin prophylaxis

- 600 mg/12 h PO for 2 days
- Children > 1 yr 10 mg/kg/12 h
  < 1 yr 10 mg/kg/12 h

  or

  Ciprofloxacin
- 500 mg PO, 1 dose, adult only

Your notes:

103. An 18-month-old patient is still says a few words, mother is worried.

Diagnosis: Speech delay (probable).

Clinchers

➢ *Eighteen-month-old:* The normal pattern of speech development is:
- At 1 year—few meaningful words
- At 18 months—2 words utterances
- At 2 years—subject-verb-object sentences
- At 3½ years—mastered thought, language, abstraction and elements of reason, with a 1000 word vocabulary.

➢ *Mother is worried:* If this is not her first child, she might be having knowledge of normal pattern of speech development as there will be a sound basis of her worries which require assessment.

CONFUSA

If a child reaches 3-year-old with a vocabulary of less than 50 words one should suspect a pathology. In children presenting before that an assessment of developmental milestones is done. If that is satisfactory there is no need for detailed investigations usually.

Investigation of Choice

Milestone assessment.

Immediate Management

Reassurance to mother.

Treatment of Choice

Usually none required except observation till 3 years of age.

Your notes:

19 Pharmacology

PAPER 3

51. A middle-aged woman remains unconcious 12 hours following a cholecystectomy. On examination both pupils are seen to be pinpoint.

Diagnosis: Opiate overdosage.

Clinchers

- *Middle-aged woman:* Maximum incidence of gallstones is in middle-aged women. In the UK they are found in approximately 10% of women in their forties increasing to 30% after the age of 60 years. They are about half as common in men (aphorism: fair, fat, fertile, females of forty).
- *Remains unconcious 12 hours following a cholecystectomy:* Opiate overdosage (prescribed postoperatively for analgesia) can produce coma, respiratory depression and acidosis.
- *Both pupils are seen to be pinpoint:* Pinpoint pupils are seen in opiate overdose and hence our suspicion is confirmed.

CONFUSA

The other common etiology of pinpoint is pontine hemorrhage. But that is very unlikely in postoperative middle-aged patient. Moreover no indication of any hypertensive disease is given in this question (Hypertension is associated with pontine haemorrhage).

Investigation of Choice
Respiratory rate.

Immediate Management
Respiratory support (oxygen/IPPV)

Treatment of Choice
Immediate reversal by naloxone.

CASE HISTORY: HYPOGLYCAEMIA

- A 36-year-old male returns from holiday in Laos. He becomes febrile, drowsy, confused and complains of headache. Blood glucose is low.
  - Hypoglycaemia
  - Do thick blood film
- This patent has developed hypoglycaemia, secondary to plasmodium falciparum malaria.

55. A 25-year-old found deeply unconscious is brought to the accident and emergency (A and E) department. He has an abrasion over his left temple and puncture marks on his left forearm.

Diagnosis: Narcotic overdose.

Clinchers

- *Twenty-five-year-old:* Maximum incidence of drug addiction in UK is in teens and twenties.
- *Deeply unconscious:* Opiates the most common drugs of abuse which produces unconsciousness. Other drugs are:
  - Barbiturates
  - Solvents
  - Benzodiazepines.
- *Abrasion over his left temple:* It might be sustained secondarily due to a fall on being knocked out of consciousness by the "kick" of the drug of abuse.
- *Puncture marks on his left forearm:* It suggests IV drug abuse. There will be several puncture marks varying ages along the line of veins. Since most people are right handed, it is usual to find out such marks on left forearm. Next most common site is feet.

CONFUSA

Abrasion over his left temple could suggest an intracranial injury also. But first priority will always be to give Naloxone IV (flumazenile if BZD abuse suspected) and then to evaluated for head injury.

Investigation of Choice
Pupil size (pinpoint pupil in opiate overdose).

Immediate Management
Naloxone IV.

Treatment of Choice
According to local guidelines for drug abusers, i.e.

- If willing to leave the habit—refer to local deaddiction centre
- If not willing—enrol in needle exchange programme.

Your notes:

96. A 70-year-old woman has taken 20 mg of temazepam at night for the last 30 years. She has begun to suffer with falls and has agreed that the temazepam might be contributing to the falls.

Diagnosis: Benzodiazepine addiction.

Clinchers

- *Seventy-year-old:* A large number of older patients take benzodiazepines regularly, particularly temazepam and nitrazepam.
- *Falls:* There is good evidence in published trials that sedative medications increase the risk of falls and that sedative withdrawal reduces this risk.

CONFUSA

Benzodiazepine withdrawal symptoms are very common if the drug has been taken regularly for longer than six months (30 years in this case). But in this case the symptoms are due to sedative action and not due to withdrawal. Withdrawal is easier from long acting benzodiazepines, such as diazepam or chlordiazepoxide.

Investigation of Choice

Neurological examination to rule out it as a cause for falls.

Immediate Management

Counselling.

Treatment of Choice

Patient converted to an equivalent dose of diazepam, which is then reduced by 3 mg every one or two weeks.

Your notes:

136. Cimetidine.

Diagnosis: Impotence

Clinchers

As it is a direct question, lets discuss cimetidine in particular,

- It is a H_2 blocker
- Cimetidine crosses placenta and reaches milk, but penetration in brain is poor.
- Well-tolerated by most patients: adverse effects occur in 5% people. Main side effects is evident in males because of:
  - *Antiandrogenic action*
    It displaces dihydrotestosterone from its cystoplasmic receptor.
  - *Increases plasma prolactin*
  - *Inhibits degradation of estradiol by liver*

So, high doses of cimetidine for long periods have produce.

- Gynaecomastia
- Loss of libido
- Impotence
- Temporary decrease in sperm count.

CONFUSA

This antiandrogenic profile of side effects of cimetidien is not shared by any other H_2 blocker.

Investigation of Choice

Serum estradiol.

Immediate Management

Reassure.

Treatment of Choice

Discontinue cimetidine.

Your notes:

137. Cyclophosphamide.

Diagnosis: Haemorrhagic cystitis.

Clinchers

Haemorrhagic cystitis can develop in patients receiving cyclophosphamide or ifosphamide. Both these drugs are metabolized to acrolein (a strong chemical irritant) excreted in urine. Prolonged contact or high concentrations may lead to bladder irritation and haemorrhage.

Other side effects of cyclophosphamide:
- Bone marrow suppression
- Bladder carcinoma
- Gonadal suppression
- GI intolerance
- Hypogammaglobulinaemia
- Pulmonary fibrosis
- Myelodysplasia
- Oncogenesis

Immediate Management

In haemorrhagic cystitis, the maintenance of a high urine flow may be sufficient supportive care.

Treatment of Choice

Conservative management. If it fails irrigation of the bladder with 0.37 to 0.74 per cent formalin solution for 10 min stops bleeding in most cases.

In extreme cases, cystectomy may be necessary.

Your notes:

138. Diamorphine.

Diagnosis: Constipation.

Clinchers

Opioid analgesia is a leading cause of constipation in herpitalized patients. It is aggravated by low fluid fibres intake. Diamorphine is a semisynthetic opiate. It is 3 times more potent than morphine. It is considered to be more euphorient and highly addicting. This drug is favoured in illcit drug trafficking. This drug has been banned in most countries except UK.

Constipation is a prominent side effec of diamorphine.

CONFUSA

Drugs that lead to constipation are:
- Opiate analgesics (e.g. morphine, diamorphine, codiene)
- Anticholinergics (tricyclics, phenothiazines)
- Iron

Immediate Management

Laxative.

Treatment of Choice

Treat the cause. Advice high fibre diet with adequate fluid intake (unless cause is GI obstruction, megacolon or colonic hypotonia). Encourage exercise.

Drugs used rarely
- Bulking agents (ispaghula husk)
- Stool softners (arachis oil enema)
- Osmotic laxative
- Stimulated laxatives.

Your notes:

139. Amoxycillin.

Diagnosis: Stevens-Johnson syndrome.

Clinchers

Drugs like amoxycillin (penicillins), sulfonamides and sedatives, may induce a systemic illness with fever, arthralgia, myalgia ± pneumonitis and conjunctivitis. The skin develops typical target lesions of erythema multiforme often on plams.

Other causes of Stevens-Johnson syndrome include viruses or other infection (e.g. of herpes simplex) and neoplasm.

Treatment of Choice

Calamine lotion for the skin, steroids (systemic and eye-drops) were once used, but ask a dermatologist and ophthalmologist.

Your notes:

140. Oral contraceptive pill.

Diagnosis: Deep vein thrombosis.

Clinchers

The older preparations of oral contraceptives increased the incidence of venous thromboembolism, but this is found to be only marginal with the newer reduced steroid content pills. However, even these phase significant risk in woman > 35 years age diabetics, hypertensives and those who smoke.

The most common symptoms of DVT are of pain in the calf, with varying degree of redness and swelling.

Investigation of Choice

Venography, or Doppler ultrasound. Venography is invasive technique. Colour Doppler ultrasound is now preferred first line method of investigating suspected DVT.

Immediate Management

In any women with suspicion of DVT, heparin or low molecular weight heparin should be given in treatmet doses, until the diagnosis is confirmed or refuted.

Your notes:

PAPER 4

1. Man treated with gentamicin for peritonitis for 10 days presents with deafness.

Diagnosis: Ototoxicity.

Clinchers

Various drugs and chemicals can damage the inner ear and cause sensorineural deafness and tinnitus.

Symptoms of ototoxicity are—hearing loss, tinnitus, and/or giddiness, may manifest during treatment or after completion of treatment.

Ototoxic drugs: *Aminoglycoside antibiotics*: Gentamicin is the most important of all. Other includes—streptomycin, tobramycin, neomycin, etc.

- *Diuretics*: Furosemide, ethacrinic, etc.
- *Antimalarials*: Quinine, chloroquine.
- *Cytotoxic drugs*: Nitrogen, mustard, cisplatin
- *Analgesics*: Salicylates, indomethacin, ibuprofen.
- *Chemicals*: Alcohol, tobacco, marijuana, carbon monoxide poisoning.

Investigation of Choice

Rinne test (positive), i.e. air conduction < bone conduction.

Immediate Management

Weber lateralised to better ear.

Treatment of Choice

Stop gentamicin at once.

Your notes:

11. β_2 agonist.

Diagnosis: Salbutamol.

Clinchers

Salbutamol is a sedative β_2 adrenergic receptor agonist (other example: terbutaline).

β_2 receptors are present in brochi, blood vessels, uterus, GIT, urinary tract, eye.

β_2 stimulation causes—bronchodilatation, vasodilatation and uterine relaxation, without producing significant cardiac stimulation.

Salbutamol is primarily and in bronchial asthma.

Other uses are:

- Uterine relaxant: to delay premature labour
- In hyperkalaemic familial periodic, paralysis—cause increased uptake of K^+ by muscles.

Side effects

Most important side effects is muscle tremor. Tachycardia and arrhythmias are less likely.

Your notes:

12. Antimuscarinic

Diagnosis: Ipratropium bromide.

Clinchers

Ipratropium bromide is a semisynthetic anticholinergic drug. It blocks the action of acetylcholine on autonomic effectors and in the CNS exerted through muscarinic receptor.

Ipratropium bromide 40-80 µg by inhalation, acts selectively on bronchial muscles without altering volume on consistency of respiratory secretions.

It is suitable for regular prophylactic use rather than rapid symptomatic relief during an attack, because of gradual onset and late peak (at 60-90 min) of bronchodilator effect in comparision to inhaled sympathomimetics.

Ipratropium bromide is more effective in COPD (chronic obstructive pulmonary disease), since parasympathetic tone is the major reversible factor here.

CONFUSA

Atropine is highly selective for musurinic receptors, the synthetic derivatives do passes significant nicotinic blocking property in addition.

Your notes:

13. Interferes with cell wall synthesis.

Diagnosis: Beta-lactum antibiotics.

Clinchers

- Amoxicillin is a semisynthetic penicillin, with extended spectrum of activity, containing a beta-lactum ring.
  All the beta-lactum antibiotics interfere with the synthesis of bacterial cell wall.
  Beta-lactum antibiotics inhibit the transpeptidase so that cross linking (which maintains the does knit structure of the cell wall) does not take place.
- *Mechanism of action:* When bacteria divide in the pressure of a beta-lactum antibiotic, cell wall deficient (CWD) forms are produced. Because the interior of the bacterium is hyperosmotic, CWD forms smell and burst—bacteriolysis.

CONFUSA

Drugs that inhibit cell wall synthesis are: penicillin, cephalosporins, cycloserine, vancomycin, bacitracin.

Your notes:

14. Increases the activity of respiratory muscles.

Diagnosis: Analeptics.

Clinchers

- *Doxapram:* At low doses it is more selective for the respiratory centre than other analeptics. It stimulates respiration through carotid and arotic body chemoreceptors as well.

  Its role in therapeutics is very narrow, with narrow safety margin. Mechanical support to respiration and other measures to improve circulation are more effective.
- *Mechanism of action:* Doxapram acts by promoting excitation of central neurons, thus stimulating respiration.
- *Other analeptics:* Ethyl and propyl butamide, Nikethamide.

Your notes:

15. Urinary antiseptic.

Answer: Trimethoprim

Clinchers

Trimethoprim is a diaminopyrimidine, a structural analogue of pteridine moiety of folic acid. It is a competitive inhibitor of dihyrofolate reductase, the enzyme responsible for reduction of dihydrofolic acid to tetrahydrofolic acid, the essential final component in the folic acid synthesis pathway that is necessary for all one-carbon transfer reactions like the sulfonamides, timethoprim is bactericidal in the absence of thymine but is only bacteriostatic when this pyrimidine is present in high concentration. The selective antibacterial activitiy of trimethoprim is based on the extreme sensitivity of bacterial dihydrofolate reductase to inhibition by this drug in comparison with the mammalian enzyme. The bacterial enzyme is approximately 50,000 times more sensitive to such inhibition.

CONFUSA

Trimethoprim is used for treatment of UTI, i.e. for acute cases, suppressive treatment of chronic and recurrent cases—specially in females.

Your notes:

17. Not given in a chronic asthmatic after a myocardial infarction.

Diagnosis: Myocardial infarction in chronic asthmatic.

Clinchers

β-adrenergic blockers reduce myocardial O_2 consumption, limit infarct size, and reduce mortality. But is contraindicated in asthmatic patient.

β_2-receptors induces peripheral vasoconstriction and bronchoconstriction.

Important contraindications of β-blockers are:

- Asthma/COPD
- Peripheral vascular disease
- Heart failure/heart block.

Immediate Management

Aspirin 300 mg PO. Analgesia, e.g. morphine 5-10 mg IV + metoclopromide 10 mg IV

Treatment of Choice

Stop smoking and avoid precipitants. Follow British Thoracic Society guidelines refer page 172 (OHCM), 5th edn for chronic asthma. For management of MI refer to page 781 (OHCM), 5th edn.

Your notes:

18. Used to control acute severe asthma in a 15-year-old with severe breathlessness in A and E.

Diagnosis: Acute severe asthma.

Clinchers

- *Control acute severe asthma:* Acute severe asthma is a medical emergency, presented with acute breathlessness and wheeze. The first step in management is to sit patient up and give high-dose O_2.

  Nabulised β_2 agonist (salbutamol or terbutaline) nebulised with O_2 is the fastest acting bronchodilator, therefore used to control acute severe asthma.
- *15-year-old:* 15-year-old can receive a full dose of β_2 agonists (i.e. salbutamol 5 mg or terbutalin 10 mg). Half dose is given in very young children.

  In very young children add ipratrapium 0.25 mg to nabulized beta-agonist.

CONFUSA

Hydrocortisone 200 mg IV or prednisolone 30 mg PO are both added if the patient is very ill, but they are no substitute to nabulised beta-agonists.

In life-threatening conditions nabulised ipratropium and IV aminophylline can be added.

Investigation of Choice

In acute asthma PEFR, sputum culture, U and E, blood culture and ABG. In chronic cases look for obstructive defects (↓ FEV_1/FVC, ↑ residual volume).

Your notes:

19. Used to control intermittent night wheeze in a person using inhaled high dose steroids presently.

Diagnosis: Asthma.

Clinchers

- *Control intermittent night wheeze:* Salmeterol is a long acting inhaled β_2-agonist that can help nocturnal symptoms and reduce morning dips.
- *Inhaled high dose steroids presently:* Long acting inhaled β_2-agonists (salmetrol) is an alternative to ↓ steroid dose when symptoms are uncontrolled (rinse mouth after inhaled steroid to prevent and candidiasis).

Therefore, intermittent night wheeze in a person using inhaled high dose steroids presently can be controlled by long acting (inhaled) β_2-agonists like salmetrol.

Do refer to the British Thoracic Society guidelines for control of asthma in page 172 (OHCM), 5th edn.

CONFUSA

Aminophylline may be tried as prophylaxis, at night PO, to prevent morning dipping, but not in this question.

Immediate Management

Long acting inhaled β_2-agonists (salmetrol).

Your notes:

61. A schizophrenic on long-term treatment complains of impotence, has high prolactin levels,extrapyramidal side effects (EPS).

Diagnosis: Side effects (Chlorpromazine)

Clinchers

- *Schizophrenic on long-term treatment:* After a single episode of schizophrenia, medication is continued for 12-24 months. If the person remains week it should be tailed off because there is little evidence that further medication is beneficial and because of the risk of tardive dyskinesia. Patients who have had multiple episodes or persistent symptoms usually remain on medication for many years, though the need for it should remain under regular review.
- *Impotence:* Inhibition of ejaculation is more common with low potency phenothiazines and is due to α-adrenergic blockade.
- *High prolactic levels:* It occurs infrequently after prolonged use and is associated with low levels of gonadotrophins which may also be responsible for impotence. It is due to blockade of hypothalamic dopamine receptors.
- *Extrapyramidal side effects:* These are the major dose limiting side effects—more prominent with high potency drugs.

CONFUSA

Akathisia is an EPS which can be mistaken for exacerbation of psychosis—differentiation may be helped by an IM injection of benzotropin (2 mg): akathesia will respond but not exacerbation of psychosis. Parkinsonism is another EPS that can be mistaken for depression or for negative symptoms in schizophrenia.

Investigation of Choice

Serum prolactin (already done in this case).

Immediate Management

Reduce dose of antipsychotics.

Treatment of Choice

Symptomatic:

- Acute dystonia—IM/IV anticholinergics
- Parkinsonism—reduce dose or add anticholinergic
- Alkathesia—reduce dose + propranolol
- Tardine dyskinesia—reduce! stop drug
- Impotence—α agonist

Your notes:

62. Drug with anticholinergic side effects, dry mouth, blurred vision, tremor.

Diagnosis: Side effects of tricyclics.

Clinchers

- Anticholinergic side effects: These can be
  - Dry mouth
  - Bad taste
  - Constipation
  - Epigastric distress
  - Urinary retention/heritancy (especially in males with enlarged prostate)
  - Blurred vision
  - Palpitation.

CONFUSA

Though anticholinergic side effects can also occurs with antipsychotics, they are more characteristic and common with tricyclics. Amitriptyline especially produce sedation, mental confusion and weakness in addition.

Investigation of Choice

None required.

Immediate Management

Reduce dose.

Treatment of Choice

Stop or change dry if troublesome.

Your notes:

63. Patient on treatment for bipolar disorder, now present with weight gain and loss of appetite.

Diagnosis: Lithium side effects.

Clinchers

- *Bipolar disorder treatment:* Its first line prophylactic treatment is lithium. Majority of patients stabilizes on lithium and usually do not need alternative or second line drugs.
- *Weight gain and loss of appetite:* This suggests hypothyroidism which is infact a prominent yet rare side effects of lithium. It is due to interference with iodination of tyrosine—decreased thyroxine synthesis.

CONFUSA

Lithium induced hypothyroidism is seen in 20% women. In men it is rare. Other main side effect of lithium on long-term usage is renal diabetes insipidus. Lithium induces granulocytosis and infact sometimes used to treat agranulocytosis (e.g. chemotherapy induced leukopenia and agranulocytosis).

Investigation of Choice

TSH.

Immediate Management

Rule out primary thyroid disease.

Treatment of Choice

Thyroxine administration.

Your notes:

64. Schizophrenic patient under treatment presents with sore throat, decreased WBC, agranulocytosis.

Diagnosis: Clozapine side effects.

Clinchers

- *Schizophrenic patient:* Clozapine is an atypical antipsychotic and is pharmacologically distinct from other in that it has only weak D_2 blocking action and produces few extrapyramidal symptoms; tardive dyskinesia is also rare with it. It suppresses both positive and negative symptoms of schizophrenia and many patients refractory to typical neuroleptics respond.
- *Sore throat:* It is due to infections secondary to agranulocytosis.
- *Decreased WBC and agranulocytosis:* The major limitation of clozapine is higher incidence of agranulocytosis and other blood dyscrasias.

CONFUSA

Clozapine is used only as a reserve drug in resistant schizophrenia (who have not responded to, or are intolerant of, two other antipsychotics). In UK it is given on a named patient basis and weekly white cell counts are mandatory. It is very expensive (~£ 3000 per year in UK)—though cost benefit analyses are favourable as in-patient care is reduced.

Investigation of Choice

Weekly white cell counts.

Immediate Management

Stop drug.

Treatment of Choice

Change clozapine with new antipsychotics, i.e. risperidone, olanzapine and questiapine which do not have EPS like clozapine but do not need blood tests.

Your notes:

65. Schizophrenic patient under treatment presents with fever, increased WCC, increased muscle creatinine kinase levels.

Diagnosis: Neuroleptic malignant syndrome (NMS).

Clinchers

- *Schizophrenic patient under treatment:* Most probably he is taking some high potency antipsychotics with whom this syndrome is common.
- *Fever:* Pyrexia is pathognomonic of this condition.
- *Increased WCC:* Investigations invariably show increased WCC.
- *Increased muscle creatinine kinase levels:* Increased creatinine phosphokinase and myoglobin may be present in blood. It lasts 5-10 days after drug withdrawal and may be fatal.

CONFUSA

NMS occurs in 0.2% of patients on antipsychotics (particularly with high potency drugs i.e. Haloperidol). Its symptoms appear a few days to a few weeks after initiation of therapy. Its main presenting symptoms are:

- Hyperthermia
- Muscle rigidity
- Autonomic instability (tachycardia, labila BP, pallor)
- Fluctuating level of consciousness.

Investigation of Choice

CPK (↑); WCC (↑); LFT (deranged)

Immediate Management

Stop drug immediately and give symptomatic treatment (e.g. temperature reduction)

Treatment of Choice

Bromocriptine (to enhance dopaminergic activity)

+

Dantrolene (to reduce muscle tone).

Your notes:

93. Unconscious boy with pin point pupils, respiratory rate—4/min.

Diagnosis: Opiate overdose.

Clinchers

- *Unconscious:* Delayed reflexes, thready pulse and coma may occur in case of a large overdose.
- *Pinpoint pupil:* It is characteristic of opioid overdose. Other conditions in which pin point pupils can be seen are:
  - Positive haemorrhage
  - Heat stroke
- *Respiratory rate is 4/min:* Respiratory depression is the main fatal complication of opioid overdose as it suppresses the respiratory centres [tip: k (*k*appa) receptors are involved in "kick" effects and μ (*m*u) receptors are involved in medical effects like respiratory depression].

CONFUSA

In severe intoxication, mydriasis (instead of miosis) may occur due to hypoxia. Tolerance to all opioids rapidly develops (except to constipation and miotic effects). Because of this (and because of batch-to-batch variation in purity), overdose is common and frequently fatal due to respiratory depression. On the other hand, opioid withdrawal is rarely life-threatening although the symptoms are severe.

Investigation of Choice

Urinary opioids test (but treatment is the first priority, testing follow it).

Immediate Management

Ventilatory support.

Treatment of Choice

Naloxane 0.8-2 mg IV

Repeat every 2 min until breathing adequate.

Your notes:

138. Young girl on Na valproate, parents come with complaints of increased seizure frequency and frequent absences from school. On examination, she is mildly obese.

Diagnosis: Side effects of valproate.

Clinchers

- *Young girl:* Valproate is often not the first line drug in children. Carbamazepine is a recommended effective first line drug for partial and generalized tonic-clonic seizures. It has the advantage of very few side effects.
- *Increased seizure frequency:* This signifies the refractiveness of valproate in this patient. If any drug fail to relieve seizures with monotherapy, addition of a second drug is necessary. If there is presence of side effects to first drug, then it should be discontinued after tapering the dose gradually.
- *Frequent absences from school:* Do not confuse this with absence seizures. This only signify increased frequency of the illness.
- *Mildly obese:* Sodium valproate causes weight gain as its adverse effect. So, this case requires a replacement of sodium valproate with another drug.

CONFUSA

If seizures continue despite gradual increases to the maximum tolerated dose and documented compliance, then it becomes necessary to switch over to another antiepileptic drug. This is usually done by maintaining the patient on the first drug while a second drug is added. The dose of the second drug should be adjusted to decrease seizures frequency without causing toxicity. Once this is achieved, the first drug can be gradually withdrawn (usually over weeks unless there is significant toxicity). The dose of the second drug is then further optimized based on seizures response and side effects.

Investigation of Choice

Drug levels.

Immediate Management

Evaluation by an expert.

Treatment of Choice

Replace valproate with an appropriate drug.

Your notes:

157. Patient cannot cough up bronchial secretions. Noise is distressing to attendants.

Diagnosis: Bronchial rattles.

Clinchers

- *Bronchial secretions:* In palliative exaggerated bronchial secretions are there in case of bronchial malignancies. It is due to increase in surface area and number of glands in bronchial epithelium. Such patients are usually debilitated and cannot cough up the secretions. Such profuse secretions require regular endotracheal suction to keep the passages clear and provide symptomatic relief to the patient. Often it produces noisy bronchial rattles which can be quite distressing to the patient and the attendant. To prevent these problems and to give symptomatic relief to the patient, anticholinergics can be given to dry up the respiratory secretions.

CONFUSA

Partial bronchial obstruction can also produce noisy breathing. But that needs palliative surgery to treat the condition, although prednisolone can provide symptomatic relief.

Investigation of Choice

Chest X-ray.

Immediate Management

Endotracheal suction.

Treatment of Choice

Hyoscine hydrobromide 0.4-0.8 mg/8 h Sc

or

0.3 mg sublingual.

Your notes:

PAPER 5

26. A 60-year-old woman hypertensive was started on antihypertensive 2 weeks ago. Now has a creatinine level of 500 micromol/L.

Diagnosis: Acute renal failure.

Clinchers

- *On antihypertensive 2 week ago:* Angiotensin converting enzyme activity inhibition (ACE inhibitors) and renal prostaglaind biosynthesis (cyclooxygenase inhibitor) inhibitors are the major culprits, leading to renal hypoperfusion, leading to prerenal azotemia.

  Captopril is an ACE inhibitor that lowers the BP.

  Captopril induces hypotension as a result of decrease in total peripheral resistance. Both systolic and diastolic BP falls.
- *Creatinine level of 500 Hmol/L:* Normal value of creatinine in plasma ranges between 70-$\leq$ 150 mmol/L. Recent increase in the plasma urea and creatinine concentration are the biochemical indictors of acute renal failure.

CONFUSA

On captopril, renal blood flow is not compromised even when BP falls substantially, but for in patients with bilateral renal artery stenosis due to dilatation of efferent arterioles and fall in glomerular filtration pressure, therefore contraindicated in such patients.

Investigation of Choice

- Blood tests: U and E, FBC, creatinine, blood culture.
- Urine: Microscopy and biochemical tests.
- ECG (hyperkalaemia).

Immediate Management

- Change in antihypertensive therapy.
- Adjust doses of renally excreted drugs.

Manage complications, (hyperkalaemia, pulmonary edema, bleeding). Seek specialist help sooner rather than later.

Drug producing this condition

Captopril.

Your notes:

27. A child with recurrent nephrotic syndrome is brought for treatment. Three weeks after start of treatment, he now has massive haematuria.

Diagnosis: Haemorrhagic cystitis.

Clinchers

- *Child with recurrent nephrotic syndrome:* Minimal change disease accounts for 80% of nephrotic syndrome in children. MCD is highly steroid responsive, but relapses occur in 50% of cases following withdrawal of glucocorticoids. In such patients upto fail to achieve lasting remission, alkylating agents are usual. *Cyclophosphamide* (2 to 3 mg/kg per day) or chlorambucil (0.1 to 0.2 mg/kg per day) is started after steroid induced remission and continued for 8 to 12 weeks.
- *Now develops massive haematuria:* Microscopic haematuria may be present in MCD (in 20-30 percent cases). But massive haematuria here is a sign of cystitis, which may occur with the use of cyclophosphamide.

CONFUSA

The benefits of cyclophosphamide must be balanced against risk of infertility, cystitis, alopecia, infection and secondary malignancies.

Investigation of Choice

Cystoscopy

Immediate Management

Stop cyclophospamide

Treatment of Choice

Long term renal and patient survival is excellent in MCD. Titrate the risk of cyclophosphide, otherwise MCD is highly steroid.

Drug producing this condition

Cyclophosphamide

Your notes:

29. Patient with complaint of ataxia and tinnitus with mild hearing loss. He has moderate renal failure.

Diagnosis: Ototoxicity (Answer: Gentamycin).

Clinchers

Aminoglycoside antibiotics (gentamycin) have a narrow therapeutic index. Most important side effects being nephrotoxocity and ototoxicity. Rarely respiratory depression may be observed.

Nephrotoxicity is manifested clinically by a gradual rise in serum creatinine levels after a few days of therapy.

Ototoxicity from aminoglycosides therapy presents as either auditory or vestibular damage.

CONFUSA

Fear to toxicity should not prevent the use of aminoglycosides for a legitimate indication, since toxicity is usually mild and reversible.

Investigation of Choice

- Serum concentration of gentamycin
- Blood urea or Serum creatinine.

Immediate Management

Stop gentamycin. When serum concentration are monitored and duration of therapy kept minimum, then adverse effect are unlikely.

Treatment of Choice

Substitute gentamicin with a safe drug.

Your notes:

72. This drug competes with vitamin K.

Most appropriate answer: Warfarin.

Clinchers

Warfarin is the most commonly used coumarin. It is used twice daily (oral) as long-term anticoagulation. It has a narrow therapeutic range, which varies with the condition being treated. It is measured as a ratio compared with standard prothrombin time (international normalized ratio, INR).

Warfarin produces a state analogous to vitamin K deficiency, by inhibiting the reductase enzyme responsible for regenerating the active form of vitamin K. In UK warfarin tablets are 1 mg (brown), 3 mg (blue), 5 mg (pink).

Contraindications for warfarin

- Peptic ulcer
- Bleeding disorders
- Severe hypertension
- Liver failure
- Endocarditis
- Cerebral aneurysms.

Main indications for anticoagulation

- DVT; pulmonary emboli
- Stroke prevention: AF, or prosthetic heart valves (treat indefinitely).
- Prevention of thromboembolism postoperatively in high risk patient.

Your notes:

74. A patient who has overdosed on an unknown medication presents with palpitations. What is the most likely cause?

Diagnosis: Tricyclic antidepressants overdose.

Clinchers

Acute poisoning due to overdose of tricyclic antidepressant is not infrequent and it may endanger life. It is usually self-attempted by the depressed patients.

Manifestations include ECG changes, ventricular arrhythmia, tachycardia.

Excitement, delirium and other anticholinergic symptom as seen in atropine poisoning along with respiratory depression with low BP may be present.

CONFUSA

Atropine poisoning should be kept in mind, as it also presents with anticholinergic symptoms.

Investigation of Choice

Blood tests
ECG.

Immediate Management

Physostigmine (0.5-2 mg IV), reversed central and peripheral anticholinergic effects.

Treatment of Choice

Treatment is primary supportive

- Correct acidosis by bicarbonate infusion
- Physostigmine
- Propranolol/lidocaine (for arrhythmias)
- Diazepam IV (for convulsions and delirium).

Your notes:

81. A 20-year-old primigravida at 40 weeks, is 6 cm is dilated and she requests pain relief. She dislikes injections.

Management of pain: Nitrous oxide.

Clinchers

Relaxation is the best nondrug analgesia that is safe for mother and fetus, but this is not always sufficient. Epidural anaesthesia can be set up once labour is established (cervix > 3 cm).

Nitrous oxide (inhaled) can be used throughout the labour. Nitrous oxide 50% in oxygen is self-administered using demand value. It is contraindicated in pneumothorax.

CONFUSA

This female dislikes injections, therefore injectable forms of anaesthesia can be ruled out. Nitrous oxide (an inhalational agent) should be the best option here. Contraindication of nitrous oxide: **Pneumothorax.**

Treatment of Choice

In this question, the best option seem to be nitrous oxide. (Entonox).

Your notes:

83. A 28-year-old woman wants to be able to move around during labour, pain free.

Preferred analgesia: Pudendal nerve block.

Clinchers

Block pudendal nerve with xylocaine 0.5 or 1% as its two or three branches circumnavigate the ischial spine. It numbs the area on right only. Here women can more around freely, without pain.

Pudendal block is used with perineal infiltration, for instumental delivery, but analgesia is insufficient for rotational forceps. It is basically used for outlet manipulation in second stage of labour.

CONFUSA

Nitrous oxide due to its effect on consciousness (impaired) and sedative affect can be ruled out in this question.

OHCS (page 115) 6th edn says that combined spinal epidural (CSE) anaesthesia gives quicker pain relief with little or no motor blockade in most mothers allowing standing, walking, sitting and voiding urine.

Your notes:

84. **A Gravida 4 para 2 + 1, has been in labour for 4 hours. She is 3 cm dilated and has already received 2 injections of pethidine. She stills complains of pain.**

Preferred analgesia: Epidural anaesthesia.

Clinchers

Pethidine 50-150 mg IM can be tried in labour pain, but not when birth is expected in < 2-3 hours as neonatal respiratory depression may occur (reversible with naloxone).

Since cervix is 3 cm dilated epidural anaesthesia can be considered. In anaesthetizes the fibers carried by T_{11}-S_5. Constant monitoring is required once epidural is set up. She has been in labour for four hours, so epidural will be of great help. For other indications of epidural refer to Q 82, Nov. 2001 paper.

CONFUSA

Narcotic injections (pethidine) are tried in the first stage, with onset of analgesia within 20 minutes and lasts 3 hours. They are contraindicated in mothers on MAOIs (page 340, OHCS).

Problems with epidural

Refer question no 82, (PLAB November 2001).

Your notes:

104. A middle-aged woman remains unconcious 12 hours following a cholecystectomy. On examination both pupils are seen to be pinpoint.

Diagnosis: Opiate overdosage.

Clinchers

- *Middle-aged woman:* Maximum incidence of gallstones is in middle-aged women. In the UK they are found in approximately 10% of women in their forties increasing to 30% after the age of 60 years. They are about half as common in men (aphorism: fair, fat, fertile, females of forty).
- *Remains unconcious 12 hours following a cholecystectomy:* Opiate overdosage (prescribed postoperatively for analgesia) can produce coma, respiratory depression and acidosis.
- *Both pupils are seen to be pinpoint:* Pinpoint pupils are seen in opiate overdose and hence our suspicion is confirmed.

CONFUSA

The other common a etiology of pinpoint pupils is pontine hemorrhage. But that is very unlikely in post-operative middle-aged patient. Moreover no indication of any hypertensive disease is given in this question (Hypertension is associated with pontine hemorrhage).

Investigation of Choice

Respiratory rate.

Immediate Management

Respiratory support (oxygen/IPPV)

Treatment of Choice

Immediate reversal by naloxone.

Your notes:

196. Three gm sachet of amoxicillin one hour before the procedure.

Answer: Dental treatment of cardiac patients.

Clinchers

Endocarditis prophylaxis before dental procedures:
Local or no anaesthetic.

- Amoxicillin 3 g PO, 1 hour before the procedure
- Clindamycin 600 mg PO if: allergic to penicillin, > 1 dose of penicillin in previous month

General anaesthetic, no special risk

- Amoxicillin 1g IV at induction, followed by 500 mg PO 6 hours later.
- OR amoxicillin 3 g PO 4 hours before induction, followed by 3 g PO as soon as possible after procedure.

General anaesthetic, special risk patients

(NOTE: Special risk signify = prosthetic valves
= previous endocarditis)

- Amoxicillin 1g IV + gentamicin 120 mg IV at induction followed by Amoxicillin 500 mg PO 6 hours later.
- Consider alternatives if,
  = History of penicillin allergy
  = > 1 dose of penicillin in previous month
- Alternatives are
  - Vancomycin 1g IV over 100 min
    +
    Gentamicin 120 mg IV at induction
  - Teicoplanin 400 mg IV
    +
    Gentamicin 120 mg IV at induction
  - Clindamycin 300 mg IV over 10 min at induction followed by clindamycin 150 mg IV 6 hours later.

CONFUSA

The principal of prophylaxis is to treat before contamination occurs, and this is particularly important with antibiotics, where as adequate antibiotic concentration needs to be present in the blood at the time of exposure of infection. Anyone with congenital heart disease, acquired valve disease or prosthetic valve is at risk of infective endocarditis and should take prophylactic antibiotics before procedures which may result in bacteraemia. The dental procedures considered fit for prophylaxis include extractions, scaling, polishing or gingival surgery.

Investigation of Choice

Echocardiography to rule out congenital and often heart diseases if suspected.

Immediate Management: Prophylactic antibiotics.

Treatment of Choice: Stated as the question itself.

197. Three days of intravenous broad spectrum antibiotics beginning with induction of anaesthesia.

Diagnosis (Answer): Heart valve replacement

Clinchers

- The required prophylactic regimen is—
  Amoxicillin 1g IV + gentamicin 120 mg IV
- First dose is given at induction of anaesthesia and is continued upto 3 days.

CONFUSA

Infection of valve postoperatively is a situation akin to infective endocarditis of a native valve. For more detailed notes on chemoprophylaxis in various disease states refer to British national formularly or www.bnf.org.

Investigation of Choice

As per the requirements of the operation.

Immediate Management

Antimicrobial chemoprophylaxis.

Treatment of Choice

Stated as the question itself.

198. Clear fluids by mouth and two sachets of sodium picosulphate on the day before the operation plus broad spectrum intravenous antibiotics at induction.

Diagnosis (Answer): Sigmoid colectomy.

Clinchers

- *Sodium picosulfate*: Before any colorectal surgery, give 1 sachet of picolax (sodium picosulfate 10 mg + magnesium citrate) each, at:
  - On the morning before surgery.
  - During the afternoon before surgery
- *Broad spectrum IV antibiotics at induction*: Cefuroxime 1.5 g 18 h, 3 doses IV/IM + Metronidazole 500 mg/8 h, 3 doses IV.

CONFUSA

Sodium picosulfate should be used with care if there is any risk of bowel perforation. Otherwise bowel preparation is of utmost importance before colorectal surgery. Antibiotics used should kill anaerobes and coliforms especially.

Investigation of Choice

As per the requirements for the operation.

Immediate Management

Meticulous bowel preparation.

Treatment of Choice

States as the question itself.

Your notes:

199. Long-term oral penicillin and immunization against pneumococcal infection.

Diagnosis (Answer): Splenectomy

Clinchers

- Removal of the spleen predisposes the patient, especially the child, to infection with organisms such as the pneumococcus. The clinical course is of a fulminant bacterial infection, with shock and circulatory collapse, termed overwhelming post splenectomy sepsis (OPSS).
- Prophylactic immunization with:
  = Pneumococcal
  = Meningococcal
  = *Haemophilus influenzae* type of vaccine should be administered, preoperatively where possible. In addition, children should have prophylactive daily low dose oral penicillin until they reach adulthood.

CONFUSA

The major aim of antibiotic prophylaxis in splenectomy is to present serious pneumococcal sepsis. Regarding oral penicillin, the duration of treatment is,

- Children—till adult hood
- Adult—for first year after splenectomy
- Immunosuppressed—life-long.

Investigation of Choice

Usually none.

Immediate Management

Vaccination (if possible preoperatively).

Treatment of Choice

Stated as the question itself. Preoperatively also phenoxymethyl penicillin is given (500 mg/12 hourly).

Your notes:

200. One dose of metronidazole at induction of anaesthesia.

Diagnosis (Answer): Emergency appendicectomy.

Clinchers

- The prophylactive antibiotic regimen for as emergency appendicectomy is:
  Metronidazole 1g 18 h + Cefuroxime 1.5 g/8 h
- These are given in 3 doses IV, the first dose is given 1 hour preoperatively or at the induction of anaesthesia.

CONFUSA

If it is an elective appendicectomy, then give+ 3 dose regimen of metronidazole suppositories 1g/8 h + Cefuroxime 1.5/8 h IV or Gentamicin IV

Investigation of Choice
None required usually.

Immediate Management
Shift patient to OT.

Treatment of Choice
Stated as the question itself.

Your notes:

PAPER 6

21. Schizophrenic patient under treatment presents with fever, increased WCC, increased muscle creatinine kinase levels.

Diagnosis: Neuroleptic malignant syndrome (NMS).

Clinchers

- *Schizophrenic patient under treatment:* Most probably he is taking some high potency antipsychotics with whom this syndrome is common.
- *Fever:* Pyrexia is pathognomonic of this condition.
- *Increased WCC:* Investigations invariably show increased WCC.
- *Increased muscle creatinine kinase levels:* Increased creatinine phosphokinase and myoglobin may be present in blood. It lasts 5-10 days after drug withdrawal and may be fatal.

CONFUSA

NMS occurs in 0.2% of patients on antipsychotics (particularly with high potency drugs i.e. Haloperidol). Its symptoms appear a few days to a few weeks after initiation of therapy. Its main presenting symptoms are:

- Hyperthermia
- Muscle rigidity
- Autonomic instability (tachycardia, labila BP, pallor)
- Fluctuating level of consciousness.

Investigation of Choice
CPK (↑); WCC (↑); LFT (deranged)

Immediate Management
Stop drug immediately and give symptomatic treatment (e.g. temperature reduction).

Treatment of Choice
Bromocriptine (to enhance dopaminergic activity)
+
Dantrolene (to reduce muscle tone).

Your notes:

23. Schizophrenic patient under treatment presents with sore throat, decreased WBC, agranulocytosis.

Diagnosis: Clozapine side effects.

Clinchers

- *Schizophrenic patient:* Clozapine is an atypical antipsychotic and is pharmacologically distinct from other in that it has only weak D_2 blocking action and produces few extrapyramidal symptoms; tardive dyskinesia is also rare with it. It suppresses both positive and negative symptoms of schizophrenia and many patients refractory to typical neuroleptics respond.
- *Sore throat:* It is due to infections secondary to agranulocytosis.
- *Decreased WBC and agranulocytosis:* The major limitation of clozapine is higher incidence of agranulocytosis and other blood dyscrasias.

CONFUSA

Clozapine is used only as a reserve drug in resistant schizophrenia (who have not responded to, or are intolerant of, two other antipsychotics). In UK it is given on a named patient basis and weekly white cell counts are mandatory. It is very expensive (~£ 3000 per year in UK)—though cost benefit analyses are favourable as in-patient care is reduced.

Investigation of Choice

Weekly white cell counts.

Immediate Management

Stop drug.

Treatment of Choice

Change clozapine with new antipsychotics, i.e. risperidone, olanzapine and questiapine which do not have EPS like clozapine but do not need blood tests.

Your notes:

25. A patient who has overdosed on an unknown medication presents with palpitations. What is the most likely cause?

Diagnosis: Tricyclic antidepressants overdose.

Clinchers

Acute poisoning due to overdose of tricyclic antidepressant is not infrequent and it may endanger life. It is usually self-attempted by the depressed patients.

Manifestations include ECG changes, ventricular arrhythmia, tachycardia.

Excitement, delirium and other anticholinergic symptom as seen in atropine poisoning along with respiratory depression with low BP may be present.

CONFUSA

Atropine poisoning should be kept in mind, as it also presents with anticholinergic symptoms.

Investigation of Choice

Blood tests
ECG

Immediate Management

Physostigmine (0.5-2 mg IV), reversed central and peripheral anticholinergic effects.

Treatment of Choice

Treatment is primary supportive

- Correct acidosis by bicarbonate infusion
- Physostigmine
- Propranolol/lidocaine (for arrhythmias)
- Diazepam IV (for convulsions and delirium).

Your notes:

138. Man with prosthetic heart valve presents with epistaxis.

Diagnosis: Anticoagulant overdose.

Clinchers

- *Prosthetic heart valve:* Patients with prosthetic heart valves are treated with anticoagulants, indefinitely.
- *Epistaxis:* Littles area is very prone to bleeding. Here there is convergence of the anterior ethmoidal artery, the septal branches of the sphenopalatine and the superior labial arteries and greater palatine.

Anticoagulant overdose is an important cause of bleeding tendency (e.g. Warfarin anticoagulation)

Other causes of epistaxis are degenerative arterial disease and hypertension in older people, and local causes are atrophic rhinitis, hereditary telangiectasia and tumours of the nose of sinuses.

Investigation of Choice

INR.

Immediate Management

Treat shock and replace blood if necessary.

Treatment of Choice

Titrate the dose of anticoagulant for prosthetic heart valve. For epistaxis:

- Apply firm uninterrupted pressure of nostrils f/w finger and thumb for 10 minutes, possibly with ice pack over bridge of nose.
- If still bleeding spray—2.5-10% cocaine solution over mucosa. This will anaesthetize the mucosa and reduce bleeding by constricting vessels. Cauterize any bleeding points.
- Pack the nose.
- If bleeding recurs, further packs.
- Rarely arterial ligation.
- In severe, resistant bleeds, consider embolization of the feeding vessel.

Your notes:

145. A 38-year-old woman presents with cervical lymphadenopathy. Mature lymphoblasts are seen on the blood film. Examination reveals a mild splenomegaly. She is on phenytoin for epilepsy.

Diagnosis: Phenytoin side effects.

Clinchers

- *Cervical lymphadenopathy:* It can occur as a syndrome of hypersensitivity to phenytoin. It includes rashes, DLE and neutropenia. It is rare but requires discontinuation of therapy.
- *Mature lymphoblasts.* It is also a component of the above mentioned hypersensitivity syndrome. It manifest as leukocytosis often with atypical lymphocytes and eosinophils.
- *Mild splenomegaly:* Can occur in phenytoin treatment as a response to various blood dyscrasias phenytoin causes as side effects.

CONFUSA

Acute myeloid leukemia can be excluded as the presenting cells are not myeloblasts. Plus it need bone marrow biopsy for definitive diagnosis. Nevertheless, gum hyperplasia can occur in this condition also in addition to phenytoin therapy. (So even if you are confused, you would not be wrong). Acute lymphoblastic leukemia is characterised by immature lymphoblasts and not mature lymphoblasts (as in this case).

Note: Ciclosporin also causes gum hypertrophy.

Investigation of Choice

Phenytoin blood levels (Normal: 40-80 μmol/L).

Immediate Management

Systemic steroids to reduce symptoms.

Treatment of Choice

Discontinue phenytoin.

Your notes:

191. 3 gm sachet of amoxicillin one hour before the procedure.

Answer: Dental treatment of cardiac patients.

Clinchers

Endocarditis prophylaxis before dental procedures:

Local or no anaesthetic.

- Amoxicillin 3 g PO, 1 hour before the procedure
- Clindamycin 600 mg PO if: allergic to penicillin, > 1 dose of penicillin in previous month.

General anaesthetic, no special risk

- Amoxicillin 1g IV at induction, followed by 500 mg PO 6 hours later or
- Amoxicillin 3g PO 4 hours before induction, followed by 3 g PO as soon as possible after procedure.

General anaesthetic, special risk patients:

(NOTE: Special risk signify = prosthetic valves
= previous endocarditis)

- Amoxicillin 1g IV + gentamicin 120 mg IV at induction followed by amoxicillin 500 mg PO 6 hours later.
- Consider alternatives if,
  = history of penicillin allergy
  = > 1 dose of penicillin in previous month
- Alternatives are
  - Vancomycin 1g IV over 100 min
    +
    Gentamicin 120 mg IV at induction.
  - Teicoplanin 400 mg IV
    +
    Gentamicin 120 mg IV at induction.
  - Clindamycin 300 mg IV over 10 min at induction followed by clindamycin 150 mg IV 6 hour later.

CONFUSA

The principal of prophylaxis is to treat before contamination occurs, and this is particularly important with antibiotics, where as adequate antibiotic concentration needs to be present in the blood at the time of exposure of infection. Anyone with congenital heart disease, acquired valve disease or prosthetic valve is at risk of infective endocarditis and should take prophylactic antibiotics before procedures which may result in bacteraemia. The dental procedures considered fit for prophylaxis include extractions, scaling, polishing or gingival surgery.

Investigation of Choice

Echocardiography to rule out congenital and often heart diseases if suspected.

Immediate Management: Prophylactic antibiotics.

Treatment of Choice: Stated as the question itself.

192. Three days of intravenous broad spectrum antibiotics beginning with induction of anaesthesia.

Diagnosis (Answer): Heart valve replacement.

Clinchers

- ➢ The required prophylactic regimen is Amoxicillin 1g IV + gentamicin 120 mg IV
- ➢ First dose is given at induction of anaesthesia and is continued upto 3 days.

CONFUSA

Infection of valve postoperatively is a situation akin to infective endocarditis of a native valve. For more detailed notes on chemoprophylaxis in various disease states refer to British National Formularly or www.bnf.org.

Investigation of Choice

As per the requirements of the operation.

Immediate Management

Antimicrobial chemoprophylaxis.

Treatment of Choice

Stated as the question itself.

193. Clear fluids by mouth and two sachets of sodium picosulphate on the day before the operation plus broad spectrum intravenous antibiotics at induction.

Diagnosis(Answer): Sigmoid colectomy.

Clinchers

➢ *Sodium picosulfate*: Before any colorectal surgery, give 1 sachet of picolax (sodium picosulfate 10 mg + magnesium citrate) each, at:
- On the morning before surgery
- During the afternoon before surgery.

➢ *Broad spectrum IV antibiotics at induction*: Cefuroxime 1.5 g 18 h, 3 doses IV/IM + metronidazole 500 mg/ 8 h, 3 doses IV.

CONFUSA

Sodium picosulfate should be used with care if there is any risk of bowel perforation. Otherwise bowel preparation is of utmost importance before colorectal surgery. Antibiotics used should kill anaerobes and coliforms especially.

Investigation of Choice

As per the requirements for the operation.

Immediate Management

Meticulous bowel preparation.

Treatment of Choice

States as the question itself.

Your notes:

194. Long-term oral penicillin and immunization against pneumococcal infection.

Diagnosis (Answer): Splenectomy

Clinchers

➢ Removal of the spleen predisposes the patient, especially the child, to infection with organisms such as the pneumococcus. The clinical course is of a fulminant bacterial infection, with shock and circulatory collapse, termed overwhelming post splenectomy sepsis (OPSS).

➢ Prophylactic immunization with:
= pneumococcal
= meningococcal
= *Haemophilus influenzae* type of vaccine should be administered, preoperatively where possible. In addition, children should have prophylactive daily low dose oral penicillin until they reach adulthood.

CONFUSA

The major aim of antibiotic prophylaxis in splenectomy is to present serious pneumococcal sepsis. Regarding oral penicillin, the duration of treatment is:
- Children—till adult hood
- Adult—for first year after splenectomy
- Immunosuppressed—life-long.

Investigation of Choice

Usually none.

Immediate Management

Vaccination (if possible preoperatively).

Treatment of Choice

Stated as the question itself. Preoperatively also phenoxymethyl penicillin is given (500 mg/12 hourly).

Your notes:

195. One dose of metronidazole at induction of anaesthesia.

Diagnosis (Answer): Emergency appendicectomy.

Clinchers

- The prophylactive antibiotic regimen for as emergency appendicectomy is:
  Metronidazole 1g 18 h + cefuroxime 1.5 g/8 h
- These are given in 3 doses IV, the first dose is given 1 hour preoperatively or at the induction of anaesthesia.

CONFUSA

If it is an elective appendicectomy, then give 3 dose regimen of metronidazole suppositories 1g/8 h + Cefuroxime 1.5/8 h IV or Gentamicin IV

Investigation of Choice
None required usually.

Immediate Management
Shift patient to OT.

Treatment of Choice
Stated as the question itself.

Your notes:

PAPER 7

44. Patient admitted with suspected tetanus and is given tetanus immunoglobulin and an antibiotic to which he is not allergic. Ten hours later the patient is breathless with tachycardia.

Diagnosis: Anaphylaxis.

Clinchers

- *Given tetanus Ig:* Tetanus Ig can produce anaphylaxis.
- *An antibiotic to which he is not allergic:* Anaphylaxis occurs via a different mechanism—it is due to induction of an IgE antibody response that causes a generalized release of mediators from mast cells.
- *Ten minutes later the patient is breathless:* Anaphylaxis is a life-threatening hypersensitivity reaction to contact with an allergen; it may appear within minutes to exposure to the offending substance. Manifestations include respiratory distress, pruritus, urticaria; mucous membrane swelling; GI disturbances including nausea, vomiting, pain and diarrhoea; and vascular collapse.
- *Tachycardia:* Its presence exclude a vasovagal syncope.

CONFUSA

Virtually any allergen may incite an anaphylactic reaction, but among the more common agents are proteins such as antisera, hormones, pollen extracts, hymenoptera venom, foods (peanuts), drugs (especially antibiotics), and diagnostic agents. Atopy does not seem to predispose to anaphylaxis from penicillin or venom exposures.

Investigation of Choice
Purely clinical diagnosis.

Immediate Management
Summon skilled anaesthetic help.

Treatment of Choice
Parenteral adrenaline + IV hydrocortisone + IV chlorpheniramine.

Your notes:

88. Interfere with the function of vitamin K.

Diagnosis (Answer): Warfarin

Clinchers

The coumarin anticoagulants, which include warfarin and dicoumarol, present the reduction of vitamin K epoxides in liver microsomes and induce a state of analogous to vitamin K deficiency.

CONFUSA

Warfarin slows thrombin generation and clot formation by impairing the biologic activity of the prothrombin complex proteins and are used to prevent the recurrence of venous thrombosis and pulmonary embolism.

Investigation of Choice

PT (prolonged).

Immediate Management

Evaluate for any spontaneous bleed.

Treatment of Choice

Vitamin K supplements if toxicity is clinically confirmed.

Your notes:

95. Not given in a chronic asthmatic after a myocardial infarction.

Diagnosis: β blockers

Clinchers

- *Chronic asthmatic:* β-blockers worsens chronic obstructive lung disease and can precipitate life threatening attack of bronchial asthma due to their bronchocontricting action. They are absolutely contraindicated in asthmatics.
- *Myocardial infarction:* They decreases heart rate, force of contraction (at relatively higher doses) and cardiac output. They prolong systole by retarding conduction so that synergy of contraction of ventricular fibres is disturbed. The effects on a normal resting subject are not appreciable, but becomes prominent under sympathetic overactivity e.g. exercise or emotion. Cardiac work and oxygen consumption are reduced as the product of heart rate and aortic pressure decreases. Total coronary blood flow is reduced because of blockade of dilator β-receptors, but this is largely restricted to the subepicardial region, while the subendocardial area (which is the site of ischaemia) is not affected. Overall effect in angina patients is improvement of O_2 supply) demand status and exercise tolerance is increased.

CONFUSA

The broncho-constriction effect is hardly discenible in normal individuals because sympathetic broncho-dilator tone is minimal and β-blockers increase bronchial resistance by blocking $β_2$-receptors. In asthmatics, however, the condition is consistently worsened and a severe attack may be precipitated.

Your notes:

123. Anticholinergic effects, arrhythmias.

Diagnosis: Tricyclic antidepressant (TCA) poisoning.

Clinchers

- *Anticholinergic effects:* The effects of TCA are largely related to their anticholinergic activity and so include:

  Peripheral effects
  - Blurred vision
  - Dry mouth
  - Dilated pupils
  - Urinary retention
  - Diverse GI symptoms
  - Tachycardia
  - Dysrhythmia

  Central effects:
  - Agitation
  - Anxiety
  - Hyperactivity
  - Disorientation
  - Confusion
  - Drowsiness
  - Lethargy
  - Hallucinations
  - Nystagmus
  - Dysarthria
  - Ataxia
  - Movement disorders
  - Hyper-reflexia
  - Extensor plantar response
  - Hyperthermia.
- *Arrhythmias:* Cardiac dysrhythmias are the most common cause of death. Tachycardia (rate > 120 bpm) is worrying, especially with ECG change. Prolongation of the QRS complex >100 ms suggests cardiotoxicity. A QRS duration of more than 160 ms is associated with a very high risk of life threatening dysrhythmia.

CONFUSA

Poisoning with TCAs is implicated in over one-fifth of all fatal ingestions. Dothiepin is the most common drug involved. Ingested amounts are usually significant as the patient who need TCAs will often have a mental state compatible with suicide. An ingestion of 35 mg/kg is the median lethal dose for an adult. TCAs are the most common cause of VF in children in UK. Anti-dysrhythmic drugs are best avoided in TCA poisoning as conduction deficits may make the ECG difficult to interpret. Moreover, some of these drugs will produce a synergistic cardiotoxicity. Mild hypotension usually responds to IV fluids; for more severe hypotension alkali therapy is required.

Investigation of Choice

12 lead ECG.

Immediate Management

ICU admission

\+

Gastric emptying (upto 8 hours)

\+

Activated charcoal (may be repeated)

\+

IV benzodiazepine (for agitation or convulsions).

Treatment of Choice

IV sodium bicarbonate.

Your notes:

124. Patient on treatment for atrial fibrillation, now has palpitations.

Diagnosis: Digoxin poisoning.

Clinchers

- *On treatment for atrial fibrillation:* The patient is most probably on digoxin which is indicated in acute AF (i.e. ≤ 72 h) to control the ventricular rate.
- *Palpitations:* They represent to the patient the sensation of feeling his heart beat. Generally, they can be classified etiologically into four types (according to patient's description).
  - *Irregular fast palpitations:* due to:
    - Paroxysmal AF (as in this case)
    - Flutter with variable block.
  - *Dropped or missed beats*—related to rest, recumbency or eating, due to—
    - Atrial/ventricular ectopics.
  - *Regular pounding:* Due to anxiety
  - *Slow palpitations:* Due to
    - drugs, i.e. β blockers
    - Bigeminus

CONFUSA

The elderly and patients with hyperthyroidism are more prone to digoxin toxicity. But in patients with fluctuating renal function, digoxin, which is metabolized by the liver, may be preferable. The most common features of digoxin toxicity are:

- Anorexia, nausea, altered vision
- Arrhythmia (e.g. ventricular premature beats especially
  - Bigeminy
  - VT
  - AV block)
- Digoxin levels >2.5 nmol/L

Investigation of Choice

Serum digoxin level and potassium

Immediate Management

Discontinue digoxin + management of arrhythmias

Treatment of Choice

Digoxin antibodies (Fab fragments)
Dose: 60 × total digoxin load
[load (mg) = plasma digoxin concentration (ng/ml) × body weight (kg) × 0.0056].

Your notes:

20 Psychiatry

PAPER 1

Serial No.31

Subject: Psychiatry

Topic: Antipsychotics

Question: A chronic schizophrenic on treatment develops sore throat and agranulocytosis.

Diagnosis: Clozapine side effect

Clinchers

- *A chronic schizophrenic on treatment:* A chronic patient would need continued long-term prophylaxis with antipsychotics to prevent acute exaggeration of the condition. Long-term use of antipsychotics are generally associated with varied side effects out of which, extrapyramidal side effects are most common and distressing. In such cases, the prophylaxis is usually switched over to atypical antipsychotics.
- *Develops sore throat and agranulocytosis:* Clozapine is one atypical antipsychotic which is classically associated with neutropenia and agranulocytosis.

CONFUSA

- Olanzapine, also a thienbenzodiazepine, closely related to clozapine but does not cause agranulocytosis.
- In its latest guidelines, NICE has recommended that the oral atypical antipsychotic drugs amisulpride, olanzapine, quetiapine, risperidone and zotepine should be considered in the choice of first-line treatments for individuals with newly diagnosed schizophrenia.
- NICE also recommends that in individuals with evidence of treatment-resistant schizophrenia (TRS), clozapine should be introduced at the earliest opportunity. (TRS is suggested by a lack of satisfactory clinical improvement despite the sequential use of the recommended doses for 6 to 8 weeks of at least two antipsychotics, at least one of which should be an atypical).

Investigation of Choice

Leucocyte and differential blood counts

Immediate Management

If leucocyte count below 3000/mm^3 or

If absolute neutrophil count below 1500/mm^3, discontinue drug permanently and refer to haematologist.

Treatment of Choice

Start prophylactic antibiotic at slightest evidence of infection (viz fever or sore throat).

Refer to haematologist.

Change drug.

Your notes:

Serial No. 32

Subject: Psychiatry

Topic: Antipsychotics

Question: A schizophrenic on treatment develops galactorrhea and loss of libido.

Diagnosis: Hyperprolactinaemia (secondary to chlorpromazine therapy)

Clinchers

- *Schizophrenic on treatment:* Chlorpromazine remains the widely used drug for the treatment of schizophrenia. Only the patients developing intolerable side effects or resistance to this are switched over to other drugs like clozapine.
- *Galactorrhaea and loss of libido:* Chlorpromazine blocks the D2 dopamine receptor, releasing the inhibition on prolactin production and cause hyperprolactinaemia.

CONFUSA

- In a male on antipsychotics, developing impotence, loss of libido, decreased seminal fluid volume or gyneacomastia/galactorrhea, suspect hyperprolactinemia.
- In a female on antipsychotics, developing hirsuitism, infertility, breast engorgement, oilgomennorhea or inappropriate galactorrhea (non-puerperal), suspect hyperprolactinaemia.

Investigation of Choice

- Check serum prolactin levels. Drug-induced increases in serum prolactin do not generally lead to levels above 2500 mU/L
- In cases of suspected drug-induced hyperoprolactinaemia where very high levels of prolactin are seen (over 2500 mU/L) then detailed physical examination (including visual fields), pituitary imaging and measurement of pituitary hormone levels are indicated.

Immediate Management

Withdraw the suspected drug and remeasure prolactin level 4-6 weeks later;

If there is no symptomatic improvement or prolactin levels remain high then nondrug causes of hyperprolactinaemia should be considered

Treatment of Choice

In cases of confirmed drug induced hyperprolactinaemia, substitute the offending drug with the closest substitute.

Serial No. 33

Subject: Psychiatry

Topic: Antipsychotics

Question: A schizophrenic on treatment develops fever, stiffness of limbs and raised creatinine levels.

Diagnosis: Neuroleptic Malignant Syndrome (NMS)

Clinchers

- *Schizophrenic on treatment:* Chlorpromazine remains the widely used drug for the treatment of schizophrenia. Only the patients developing intolerable side effects or resistance to this are switched over to other drugs like clozapine.
- *Develops fever:* In a patient on antipsychotics developing raised temperature, neuroleptic malignant syndrome should be suspected in the absence of any other obvious cause.
- *Stiffness of limbs:* Muscular rigidity developing in the form of stiffness of limbs or jaws remain the most important feature.
- *Raised creatinine levels:* This further confirms muscle toxicity. Antipsychotics lead to increased calcium release from the sarcoplasmic reticulum, resulting in increased contractility, which can contribute to hyperthermia, rigidity, and muscle cell breakdown.

CONFUSA

- Limb stiffness can also occur as a part of extrapyramidal side effects associated with antipsychotics, viz. acute dystonia, Parkinosonism.
- Causes of fever (viz, infections) should always be ruled out especially when the patient is on atypical antipsychotics like clozapine.
- Raised creatinine levels can also occur following electroconvulsive therapy.
- Lethal catatonia is a similar condition that might be confused with NMS. It occurs in people with schizophrenia or during manic episodes. Neuroleptics usually improve the symptoms of lethal catatonia. A detailed history usually reveals episodes of catatonia while a patient is not taking neuroleptics. The condition also also tends to have a prodrome of excitement and agitation prior to the onset of rigidity, while NMS tends to begin with rigidity.

Investigation of Choice

NMS is basically a clinical diagnosis. The key to diagnosis is that symptoms occur only after exposure to

antipsychotics. In addition to hyperthermia and rigidity, at least 2 other clinical features of NMS, including leukocytosis and laboratory evidence of muscle injury, should be present.

Immediate Management

- Discontinue all antipsychotics.
- Supportive measures:
  - Circulatory and ventilatory support.
  - Cooling blankets and antipyretics to control temperature.
  - Aggressive fluid resuscitation and alkalization of urine to prevent acute renal failure

Treatment of Choice

- Rechallenge with neuroleptics is probably safe if a gap of 2 weeks has been left between resolution of the neuroleptic syndrome and the reintroduction of the drug
- Use of dantrolene and bromocriptine is unproven

Your notes:

Serial No. 34

Subject: Medicine

Topic: Psychiatry

Question: A patient on long-term treatment for bipolar disorder complains of lethargy, weight gain and hypothermia.

Diagnosis: Lithium induced Hypothyroidism

Clinchers

➢ *Long-term treatment for bipolar disorder:* lithium salts are used in the prophylaxis and treatment of mania, in the prophylaxis of bipolar disorder and in the prophylaxis of recurrent depression.This patient most probably was on lithium for his bipolar disorder.

➢ *Lethargy, weigth gain and hypothermia:* These are the features typical for hypothyroidism. Lthium inhibits the secretion of T4 and T3 and is associated with thyroiditis, goitre, hypothyroidism and possibly hyperthyroidism also.

CONFUSA

- Documenting the duration of lithium therapy is important.
- Symptoms of hypothyroidism or thyrotoxicosis can be easily confused as a part of spectrum of symptoms seens with bipolar disorder or mania.
- Thyroid function should be checked every 6–12 months on stabilised regimens.

Investigation of Choice

Thyroid function tests.

However, all the tests should be read in the light of prolonged lithium therapy.

Immediate Management

- If the diagnosis of hypothyroidism is established, early initiation of levothyroxine therapy is indicated, especially when discontinuation of lithium is inadvisable because of the patient's psychiatric status.
- For patients who develop goitre over time, even in the absence of hypothyroidism (clinical or subclinical), also consider levothyroxine therapy aimed at restoring normal serum thyrotropin levels.

Treatment of Choice

Levothyroxine remains the treatment of choice for lithium incuded hypothyroidism.

Serial No. 35

Subject: Medicine

Topic: Psychiatry

Question: A 40-year-old lady on treatment for depression develops dry skin and mouth.

Diagnosis: Antimuscarinic side effect

Clinchers

- *A 40-year-old:* Incidence of depression usually increases with advancing age.
- *lady:* women are twice more commonly affected than men with depression.
- *On treatment for depression:* Tricyclic antidepressants are most effective for treating moderate to severe endogenous depression associated with psychomotor and physiological changes such as loss of appetite and sleep disturbances.
- *Develops dry skin and mouth:* These are characteristic antimuscarinic side effects associated with tricyclic antidepressants. Associated features also include disturbance of accommodation, difficulty in micturition, constipation, paralytic ileus, postural hypotension, tachycardia, increased sweating, orgasmic impotence, precipitation of glaucoma

CONFUSA

- For routine care, a selective serotonin reuptake inhibitor (SSRI) is the first choice drug - because SSRIs are as effective as tricyclic antidepressants and are less likely to be discontinued because of side effects.
- Also, when there is a risk of the patient taking an overdose it is usually preferable to choose an SSRI, because tricyclic antidepressants are more dangerous in overdose than other equally effective drugs recommended for routine use in primary care.

Investigation of Choice

Confirm the medication and if it is liable to cause to such side effects.

Rule out other possibility of xerostomia like Sjögren's Syndrome(not always essential).

Immediate Management

The patient should be encouraged to persist with treatment as some tolerance to these side-effects usually develop.

Treatment of Choice

The dose can be initially and then gradually increased, but this must be balanced against the need to obtain a full therapeutic effect as soon as possible.

Serial No. 46

Subject: Medicine

Topic: Psychiatry

Question: A 68-year-old man refuses to talk and avoids eye contact. Says that there is no point talking to him as he is a complete failure and that his memory has given up.

Diagnosis: Pseudodementia

Clinchers

- *A 68-year-old man:* Pseudodementia more common in elderly with increased incidence in females.
- *Refuses to talk, avoids eye contact:* Patient gets socially withdrawn avoiding any sort of interaction.
- *Says there is no point talking to him:* He is describing his deficits; suggesting pseudodementia.
- *As he is a complete failure:* Highlighting his negative points; again suggesting a component of depression in his symptoms.
- *His memory has given up:* He is aware of the problem and accepts that there are lapses in the memory.

CONFUSA

Pseudodementia is the term applied to apparent cognitive impairment associated with psychiatric disorders, most often depression (50-100%). This is often reversible and responds to antidepressants. See figure to differentiate between dementia and pseudodementia.

Investigation of Choice

Rule out organic brain diseases, epilepsy and schizophrenia which can present with similar picture.
Diagnosis is mainly on clinical features.

Pseudodentia Vs Dementia

Clinical Features	Pseudodementia	Dementia
1. Patient's complaint	Describe deficit in detail	Complains little try conceal deficit
2. Attitude	Emphasize disability highlight failures	Shows delight in accomplishments
3. Effort	Make little effort perform even simple tasks	Struggle to perform tasks. Rely on notes. Calendars to keep up
4. Concern about	Very concerned	Appear unconcerned
5. Social Skills	Loss prominent and early on	Social skills retained
6. Nocturnal accentuation of dysfunction	Uncommon	Common
7. Attention & concentration	Often well preserved	Faulty
8. Response to questions	"Don't know" answers typical	Frequently provide near miss answers
9. Memory loss	Memory gaps for periods	Loss of recent more severe than remote events
10. Performance on tasks of similar difficulty	Marked variability	Consistently poor performance
11. History of psychiatric dysfunction	Common	Unusual

Immediate Management
Carefully rule out other causes of dementia

Treatment of Choice
Antidepressants

Your notes:

Serial No. 47

Subject: Medicine

Topic: Psychiatry

Question: A 66-year-old man admitted in hospital develops features of disorientation and visual hallucinations on third day of admission.

Diagnosis: Acute delirium (also known as acute confusional state, acute cognitive dysfunction, toxic metabolic encephalopathy)

Clinchers

- *66-year-old man admitted in hospital:* Acute delirium presents in about 10% of all admissions aged above 65 yrs of age. This is usually associated with psychosocial stress and sleep deprivation associated with in-patients.
- *Disorientation:* Characteristic of delirium; impaired awareness of self and also the surroundings may be present.
- *Visual hallucinations:* Patients may have visual hallucinations or persecutory delusions as well as grandiose delusions.

CONFUSA

- Delirium tremens is a similar state of acute confusion, occurring as a part of severe withdrawl reaction in a chronic heavy alcoholic.
- It usually develops within one week following the cessation of heavy ingestion of alcohol or a reduction in the amount of alcohol ingested. Hence, most commonly gets precipitated when a heavy drinker is admitted in hospital for other usual minor ailments.
- Always look for a history of alcoholism in such questions to come to a diagnosis of delirium tremens.

Investigation of Choice
History and examination, including mental status questionnaire, are vital parts of the investigation of an acutely confused patient. Extensive investigations to rule out any primary abnormality which could have precipitated the episode.

Immediate Management
Sedate the patient with drugs such as haloperidol or chlorpromazine.

Treatment of Choice
Treat the primary cause.

Serial No. 48

Subject: Medicine

Topic: Psychiatry

Question: A man brought to OPD with features of disorientation and visual hallucinations. Wife says he was alright till few days before when he caught cold.

Diagnosis: Acute Delirium

Clinchers

- *Features of disorientation:* Characteristic of delirium; impaired awareness of self and also the surroundings may be present.
- *Visual hallucinations:* Patients may have visual hallucinations or persecutory delusions as well as grandiose delusions.
- *He was alright till few days before when he caught cold:* Several factors can cause delirium. Most common factors can be remembered by the popular mnemonic - HIDE MAP [Hypoxia, Infection, Drugs, Endocrine (Diabetes), Metabolic, Alcohol, Psychosis).

CONFUSA

- Delirium tremens is a similar state of acute confusion, occurring as a part of severe withdrawl reaction in a chronic heavy alcoholic.
- It usually develops within one week following the cessation of heavy ingestion of alcohol or a reduction in the amount of alcohol ingested. Hence, most commonly gets precipitated when a heavy drinker is admitted in hospital for other usual minor ailments.
- Always look for a history of alcoholism in such questions to come to a diagnosis of delirium tremens.

Investigation of Choice

History and examination, including mental status questionnaire, are vital parts of the investigation of an acutely confused patient. Extensive investigations to rule out any primary abnormality which could have precipitated the episode.

Immediate Management

Sedate the patient with drugs such as haloperidol or chlorpromazine.

Treatment of Choice

Treat the primary cause.

Your notes:

Serial No. 74

Subject: Psychiatry

Topic: Depression

Question: More common in females; associated with low mood and recurring depression which lasts for not more than 2 weeks.

Diagnosis: Recurrent brief depression

Clinchers

- *More common in females:* Recurrent brief depression shows only slight preponderance in females with the sex ratio of 1: 1.3, compared to major depression which is 16 times more common in female population.
- *Low mood:* Low mood can be associated with any depressive disorder.
- *Recurring depression which lasts for not more than 2 weeks:* The most characteristic feature of RBD which differentiates it from other similar conditions. Recurrent brief depression is characterised by frequently occurring brief depressive episodes, lasting less than two weeks

CONFUSA

- Recurrent brief depression is characterised by frequently occurring brief depressive episodes, lasting less than two weeks,
- It is now recognised as a common and disabling illness with a chronic relapsing course and a significant suicide risk.
- The episodes have a mean duration of 3 days, but otherwise fulfill the symptomatic criteria for DSM III-R major depression.
- They recur erratically with a mean period of 18 days between the start of one episode and the next.
- Because of the frequency of the episodes patients may report longer continuous periods of depression than was the case and may be mistakenly perceived as dysthymia as major depression.

Investigation of Choice

Rule out other similar conditions as dysthymia or major depression.

Immediate Management

Identify suicide risks; RBD is associated with considerable suicidality and treatment-seeking and is comorbid with anxiety disorders

Treatment of Choice

Optimal treatment regime for RBD is, at present, unclear. It has been suggested that:

- A prescription with modern antidepressants seems to be appropriate first-line treatment. [Note that longer response rates (weeks to a few months) are characteristic for RBD since symptoms are occurring less frequently in comparison to major depressive episodes.]

Your notes:

Serial No.75

Subject: Psychiatry

Topic: Depression

Question: More common in females; characterized by low mood, insomnia, palpitations and sweating.

Diagnosis: Mixed anxiety and depressive disorder (MADD, also known as, cothymia)

Clinchers

- *More common in females:* As goes with depression and anxiety, the syndrome of mixed anxiety and depressive disorder is more common in females.
- *Low mood, insomnia:* These signify the depressive symptoms;
- *Palpitations, sweating:* These symptoms signify anxiety;

The most specific symptoms signifying mixed anxiety and depressive disorder include:

- difficulty in concentrating,
- feeling mentally tense,
- feeling of hopelessness or despair,
- shortening of breath,
- lowered mood,
- feeling dizzy, unsteady, faint, or light headed;
- early waking up,
- nightmares,
- dry mouth,
- hot flushes or cold chills,
- frequent tearfulness.

CONFUSA

Generalized anxiety disorder is the closest differential diagnosis here and refers to a residual category of psychiatric disorders, where patients have anxiety symptoms without panic attacks, agoraphobia or other marked phobic symptoms. Although, it can be associated with features of insomnia and early morning awakening, other typical features of depression are usually absent.

Investigation of Choice

Careful history; rule out psychoactive substance abuse, physical diseases affecting mental state, and mental disorders other than anxiety or mood disorders.

Immediate Management

Suicidal tendencies demand immediate attention.

Treatment of Choice

Treatment tends is mainly aimed at easing depression. The anxiety symptoms often resolve with that.

It is interesting to note that some investigators have found that up to one third of patients with anxiety neuroses have mitral valve pathology. This may be due to the excess demands placed on the heart by anxiety.

Serial No. 76

Subject: Psychiatry

Topic: Depression

Question: More common in females; charactersied by annual recurrence of depressive symptoms.

Diagnosis: Seasonal Affective disorder (SAD)

Clinchers

- *More common in females:* SAD usually first begins between the ages of 20 to 30, but it can develop at any age. It affects four times as many women as men.
- *Annual recurrence of depressive symptoms:* The diagnosis of SAD is based on having episodes of depression which have occurred on at least two consecutive in a specific season of the year. The symptoms usually clear in other seasons. Winter depression is the most common type. In the UK and other countries north of the equator the symptoms usually develop sometime between September and November and continue until March or April. Symptoms tend to be worse in December, January and February. Summer depression is extremely rare.

CONFUSA

- People with SAD tend to have 'atypical' symptoms of depression. They tend to put on weight rather than lose weight. This is because many people with SAD develop craving for sweet things and have an increased appetite. Rather than difficulty sleeping, they tend to be more sleepy and sleep more. Some people with SAD report a feeling of heaviness in the arms and legs.
- Without treatment, the symptoms tend to improve and go fairly abruptly in the spring, over a week or so. Some people develop great bursts of energy and creativity in the spring. In a small number of cases, as spring arrives the mood changes from depression into an abnormal 'high' and elated mood (mania or hypomania).
- Some people who work in buildings without windows may have SAD symptoms throughout the year.

Investigation of Choice

The diagnosis of SAD is based on having episodes of depression which have occurred on at least two consecutive years in the winter months, with symptoms clearing in the spring. Also, associated 'atypical' features of depression (see confusa above).

Immediate Management

Suicidal tendencies demand immediate attention.

Treatment of Choice

- Light Therapy: Light therapy (sitting in front of a special bright light for scheduled a time each day) is an effective treatment in many cases. This is often the first treatment tried.
- Antidepressants
- Cognitive Behaviour Therapy

Your notes:

Serial No. 77

Subject: Psychiatry

Topic: Mood Disorder

Question: More common in females, characterized by profound depression that alternate with periods of excessively elevated and / or irritable mood.

Diagnosis: Bipolar affective disorder (also known as Manic depression, Bipolar illness)

Clinchers

- *More common in females:* Bipolar Disorder I occurs equally in both sexes; however, rapid-cycling bipolar disorder (4 or more episodes a year) is more common in women than in men. Incidence of Bipolar Disorder II is higher in females than in males.
- *Profound depression that alternate with periods of excessively elevated mood:* These are typical feature of bipolar disorder. Bipolar affective disorder is a lifelong condition. There is no usual pattern. However, without treatment, the average length for an episode of mania is 4 months and the average length for an episode of depression is 6-9 months. Some people may have 'mixed states' where symptoms of both mania and depression occur at the same time. For example, a low mood, but with racing thoughts.

CONFUSA

- Maniac depressive illness constitutes one pole of a spectrum of mood disorders including bipolar I (BPI), bipolar II (BPII), cyclothymia (oscillating high and low moods), and major depression.
- BPI also is referred to as classic manic-depression, characterized by distinct episodes of major depression contrasting vividly with episodes of mania, which lead to severe impairment of function.
- In comparison, BPII is a milder disorder consisting of depression alternating with periods of hypomania. Hypomania may be thought of as a less severe form of mania that does not include psychotic symptoms or lead to major impairment of social or occupational function.

Investigation of Choice

Rule out substance abuse or dug induced mania (antidepressants can propel a patient into mania; other medications may include captopril, cimetidine, corticosteroids, cyclosporine, disulfiram, hydralazine,

isoniazid, levodopa). Rule out cerebrovascular disease or encephalitis.

Immediate Management

Inpatient hospital treatment is indicated when there is a possibility of:

- *Danger to self:* A patient, especially one in a depressive episode, may present with a significant risk for suicide. Alternately, a person in extreme mania, who foregoes rest, sleep, or food, may be in a state of serious exhaustion.
- *Danger to others:* Patients with bipolar disorder can become a threat to others.
- *Total inability to function:* Occasionally, depression is so profound that the person cannot function at all. Leaving such a person alone would be dangerous and not therapeutic.
- *Totally out of control:* This is true especially during a manic episode.
- *Medical conditions that warrant medication monitoring:* For example, patients with certain cardiac conditions should be in a medical environment where the effects of the psychotropic medications can be monitored and observed

Treatment of Choice

Lithium remains the drug of first choice.

Your notes:

Serial No.78

Subject: Psychiatry

Topic: Mood disorders

Question: More commonly seen in males; characterized by elevated mood inflated self-esteem, overspending grandiosity and increased libido.

Diagnosis: Mania

Clinchers

- *More commonly seen in males:* Mania slightly more common in males than females.
- *Elevated mood, inflated self esteem, overspending, grandiosity, increased libido:* An episode of mania may begin abruptly, over the space of a few hours or days, or gradually, over some weeks. The subjective experience of mania in its minor forms usually includes heightened feelings of well-being with increased alertness and drive, inflated self-esteem, and expansive sociability. In addition to a general elevation of mood, instability or lability is typical. Irritability may easily be evoked, and other mood states such as anxiety or sadness, fleetingly but intensely expressed, may become apparent.

CONFUSA

- Increased sexual drive and socially embarrassing behaviour may be mistaken for frontal lobe syndrome.
- It is sometimes difficult to distinguish between mania and schizophrenia, especially if psychotic symptoms are prominent, incongruent with the underlying mood, or persist after the overactivity subsides. Such diagnostic difficulties are commonly found in cases presenting in adolescence. When affective and schizophrenic symptoms are evenly balanced and prominent enough such that a diagnosis of each can be made independently, then the term schizoaffective disorder is used.

Investigation of Choice

It's a clinical diagnosis.

Rule out substance abuse, alcohol and drugs causing acute mania.

Drugs commonly noted to induce mania include corticosteroids and androgenic steroids, L-dopa and antidepressants.

Immediate Management

Admit; Consider benzodiazepines for sedation
Lithium

Treatment of Choice

Lithium

Serial No. 158

Subject: Medicine

Topic: Substance Abuse

Question: Male with needle marks, is brought in coma state with pinpoint pupils.

Diagnosis: Heroine abuse

Clinchers

- *Male:* While it is being considered that substance abuse is more common in males, addiction among females appears to be grossly underreported.
- *Needle marks:* The locally manufactured heroine contain variety of impurities which limit their absorption through mucous membranes. Hence, rather than sniffing or snorting, the most popular way it is used among the dependent persons is by intravenous injections ('mainlining').
- *Coma state, pinpoint puplis:* Like any other opiate, heroine exerts its action by acting on mu, kappa and delta receptors. The most common clinical presentation for heroin overdose is the accidental injection of a highly concentrated crude product. Patients usually present with coma, respiratory depression, and miosis, which occur as fast as, 10 minutes of an intravenous injection.

CONFUSA

While the combination of needle marks with coma state, respiratory depression goes well with heroine toxicity in a suspected case of substance abuse, always consider a possibility to rule out head injury as falls and assaults are very common in the group and pontine haemorrhage also would present as coma, respiratory depression and pin point pupils. Look out for key words in the question, which can signify a head injury in such patients.

Investigation of Choice

Urine screen for drugs of abuse (remember the possibility of multiple drug ingestion).

Immediate Management

Give naloxone intravenously (0.4 to 2 mg for an adult and 0.01 mg/kg body weight for children) if coma or respiratory depression is present. Give IM if no vein is available. Repeat the dose if there is no response within two minutes.

Treatment of Choice

Counseling for de addiction

Register with regional drug misuse database/ notification of addicts

PAPER 2

Serial No. 46

Subject: Psychiatry

Topic: Psychosis

Question: A 26-year-old woman with established schizophrenia since age 15 lives with her very supportive parents, but has never fully recovered. She has been on a range of appropriate medication in adequate dosage since diagnosis.

Diagnosis: Chronic Schizophrenia

Clinchers

- *A 26-year-old woman with established schizophrenia since age 15:* Onset of schizophrenia before 20 years of age is a poor prognostic factor. She is being suffering from the disease for longer than 10 years now. Course of disease more than 2 years is also a poor prognostic factor.
- *never recovered fully:* In the presence of adverse prognostic factors, full recovery is usually not possible.
- *Family very supportive:* So this patient can be treated at home after educating the family regarding the nature of illness, its course and treatment. It is being shown that a supportive family can reduce this relapse rate to below 10 percent.

CONFUSA

Family therapy can significantly decrease relapse rates for the schizophrenic family member.This therapy encourages the family to convene a family meeting whenever an issue arises, in order to discuss and specify the exact nature of the problem, to list and consider alternative solutions, and to select and implement the consensual best solution.

Investigation of Choice

None required

Immediate Management

Rule out tardive dyskinesia (side effect of antipsychotics)

Treatment of Choice

Supportive Family Therapy

Your notes:

Serial No. 47

Subject: Psychiatry

Topic: Psychoses

Question: A 28-year-old man has been detained in hospital and is being treated for paranoid schizophrenia with depot anti-psychotic medication. He had stabbed his mother in the hand with a screwdriver. He is now symptom free and ready to be discharged home to live with his mother, who is worried.

Diagnosis: Chronic Schizophrenia

Clinchers

- *Schizophrenic:* means a previously diagnosed case.
- *Stabbed his mother's hand, treated with depot injection:* This particular patient is presenting with acute psychosis with paranoid hallucinations. It was adequately controlled with the antipsychotics then and the ideal management would have been to continue these antipsychotics orally to prevent further such further events. However, the fact that he was violent during this particular event puts his family (and others as well) at risk of future injuries.

CONFUSA

In the UK, the National Health Service has suggested that best practice should include a documented risk assessment before any patient is discharged to the community (which becomes more important for this patient who comes with a positive history of violent behaviour). Risk management items address feasibility of plans, exposure to destabilizers, social supports, treatment compliance, and stress. The risk management process is dynamic and iterative; it changes over time,depending on such factors as response to treatment, treatment compliance, and manipulation of environmental factors.

Investigation of Choice
None required

Immediate Management
Rule out tardive dyskinesia (side effect of antipsychotics)

Treatment of Choice
Risk Management Strategy

Your notes:

Serial No. 48

Subject: Psychiatry

Topic: Psychoses

Question: A 64-year-old man with eight admissions to hospital in the last five years is again brought to hospital by his son. It is known that he always stops taking his antipsychotic tablets at home. His wife died 6 months ago and he has been depressed and threatening to kill himself and refused any treatment.

Diagnosis: Chronic Relapsing Schizophrenia

Clinchers

- *Eight admissions to hospital in the last five years:* Hospitalization in schizophrenia is indicated if there is:
  - -Neglect of food and water intake
  - -Danger to self or others
  - -Poor drug compliance
  - -Significant neglect of self care
  - -Lack of social support
- *he always stops taking his antipsychotic tablets at home:* This apparently explains his cause for relapses. Non-compliance with the antipsychotics is mainly treated with cognitive therapy and using depot preparations of antipsychotics.
- *His wife died 6 months ago and he has been depressed and threatening to kill himself and refused any treatment:* He is showing features of major depression and refusal to take treatment leaves only electroconvulsive therapy as the major intervention required here, keeping in view of his suicidal threats.

CONFUSA

Upto two-thirds of schizophrenics would relapse if antipsychotic medication is discontinued within the first 5 years of treatment. So the best plan is to offer prophylaxis to everyone in the lowest effective dose and by depot injections if concordance/compliance is a problem.

Investigation of Choice
None

Immediate Management
Electroconvulsive Therapy (ECT)

Treatment of Choice
Continue with antipsychotics
Cognitive therapy to maintain compliance.

Serial No. 49

Subject: Psychiatry

Topic: Psychoses

Question: An 80-year-old man has a paranoid psychosis and mild cognitive decline. He is hard of hearing and says his neighbours are killing his cattle, but the authority has already announced that there is an outburst of some disease due to which cows are dying. He is continuously observing the neighbours by binoculars.

Diagnosis: Paranoid Schizophrenia

Clinchers

- *An 80-year-old man:* The onset of paranoid schizophrenia is usually insidious and occurs later in life (i.e. late 3rd and early 4th decade) as compared to other types of schizophrenia.
- *He is hard of: by binoculars:* Paranoid delusions are the typical features of the condition. These are delusions which concern the relationship between self and others.

CONFUSA

Examples of other paranoid delusions seen are:
- Delusion of reference:Patient is extremely self-conscious and thinks that everybody is talking about him. They may even see references to themselves in newspapers and on TV which are not there.
- Delusions of persecution: commonest type; patient thinks that someone or some organisation is out to harm them in some way.
- Delusions of grandeur: primarily associated with mania; here patient thinks too high of himself.

Investigation of Choice

Clinical Diagnosis

Immediate Management

Admit (always in paranoid schizophrenia as the patient is in a danger to self and others).

Treatment of Choice

Antipsychotics + Benzodiazepines for paranoid episodes.

Your notes:

Serial No. 50

Subject: Psychiatry

Topic: Psychoses

Question: An 89-year -old woman presents with a three-week history of not eating and not sleeping. She is convinced that she is about to be investigated by the government for spying, which is not the case. She refuses to eat or drink and her physical state is deteriorating. She is agreeable to treatment.

Diagnosis: Paranoid Schizophrenia

Clinchers

- three -week history of not eating and not sleeping: her paranoid delusions are making her anxious enough to hamper with her daily routines, eating and sleeping.
- She is convinced that she is about to be investigated by the government for spying, which is not the case: This is typical delusion of persecution seen most commonly with long standing cases of schizophrenia.
- She is agreeable to treatment: This is showing that she is still having the insight that something is wrong with her that she needs treatment.

CONFUSA

With her presenting symptoms of not eating and sleeping for 3 weeks might as well be confused with depression and you could have chosen ECT as an answer. However, the diagnosis of depression should be made in the light of other features like low mood, ideas of guilt, worthlessness, recurrent thoughts of death and suicide, etc.

Investigation of Choice

None

Immediate Management

Admit

Treatment of Choice

Antipsychotics + Benzodiazepines for paranoid episodes

Your notes:

Serial No. 60

Subject: Psychiatry

Topic: Dementia

Question: A 42-year-old man brought to OPD with features of disorientation and visual hallucinations. Wife says he was alright till few days before when he caught cold.

Diagnosis: Acute Delirium

Clinchers

- *Features of disorientation:* Characteristic of delirium; impaired awareness of self and also the surroundings may be present.
- *Visual hallucinations:* Patients may have visual hallucinations or persecutory delusions as well as grandiose delusions.
- *He was alright till few days before when he caught cold:* Several factors can cause delirium. Most common factors can be remembered by the popular mnemonic - HIDE MAP [Hypoxia, Infection, Drugs, Endocrine (Diabetes), Metabolic, Alcohol, Psychosis).

CONFUSA

Delirium tremens is a similar state of acute confusion, occurring as a part of severe withdrawl reaction in a chronic heavy alcoholic.

It usually develops within one week following the cessation of heavy ingestion of alcohol or a reduction in the amount of alcohol ingested. Hence, most commonly gets precipitated when a heavy drinker is admitted in hospital for other usual minor ailments.

Always look for a history of alcoholism in such questions to come to a diagnosis of delirium tremens.

Investigation of Choice

History and examination, including mental status questionnaire, are vital parts of the investigation of an acutely confused patient. Extensive investigations to rule out any primary abnormality which could have precipitated the episode.

Immediate Management

Sedate the patient with drugs such as haloperidol or chlorpromazine.

Treatment of Choice

Treat the primary cause.

Your notes:

Serial No. 167

Subject: Medicine

Topic: Neurology

Question: A 48-year-old man has normal memory on examination; wife complaints of him becoming aggressive lately and talking about their sexual life publicly.

Diagnosis: Frontal lobe dementia

Clinchers

- *48-year-old man:* can present in any age or gender. However, it closely follows cerebrovascular risk of age and sex preference, being more common in males and increasing with age.
- *Normal memory on examination:* cognitive function and behaviour may seem entirely normal.
- *Becoming aggressive lately:* Frontal lobe syndrome usually presents with alteration in personality and social conduct. Patients usually lose sensitivity to the effects of their behaviours on others.
- *Talking about their sexual life publicly:* This is disinhibition, the most charactersitic of frontal lobe pathology. Other frontal lobe behavioural abnormalities include hyperorality, utilization behaviour (i.e., picking up and manipulating any object in the environment, appropriate or not), and inappropriate sexuality.

CONFUSA

- Patients with frontal lobe dementia usually have preserved memory and visuospatial functions, while those with Alzheimer's have nearly universal involvement of these functions.
- Frontal lobe patients perform worse than Alzheimer's Disease patients on syntactic and speech fluency tasks and have more severe impairment of attention (e.g., digit span).
- These differences between frontal lobe dementia and Alzheimer's reflect the pathologic involvement of the frontal and temporal lobes, particularly in the left hemisphere, as compared to the early involvement in Alzheimer's of the hippocampus and parietal lobes.

Investigation of Choice

CT scan shows cerebral atrophy, usually of the frontal lobe and helps to rule out causes like stroke or any space occupying lesions.

Neuropsychological testing and evaluation by a speech/language pathologist with standardized

language batteries is diagnostic.

Immediate Management
Identify any treatable causes of dementia.

Treatment of Choice
Symptomatic drug treatment.
Behaviour Therapy
Treat any associated depression

Your notes:

Serial No. 168

Subject: Medicine

Topic: Neurology

Question: A 65-year-old lady with no medical complaints is found entering a shop at odd hours of early morning.

Diagnosis: Alzheimer's Disease (AD)

Clinchers

- *A 65-year-old lady*: The risk of AD is significantly higher in women than in men. AD is most prevalent in individuals older than 60 years
- *with no medical complaints:* This rules out any possibility of vascular dementia which can closely resembles AD.
- *found entering a shop at odd hours of early morning:* She is showing visualspatial disorientation, characteristic of AD; there may also be an impairment of topographical memory and patients may become disoriented and get lost easily.

CONFUSA

Lewy Body dementia may appear same as AD, but differs in following aspects:

- Memory loss: memory may be relatively normal in the early stages of Lewy body dementia, however its usually the presenting feature in AD.
- There is marked fluctuations of memory in patients with Lewy Body dementia and patient may appear severely demented and totally normal in different times of the same day. In AD, course is usually progressive; no fluctuations observed.
- Parkinsonism is an early feature of Lewy Body dementia; observed late in AD.
- Hallucinations is a major feature in Lewy body, not seen in AD.

Investigation of Choice
Apart from histology there are no specific tests for the diagnosis of Alzheimer's disease. Therefore, the principle is to rule out the differential diagnoses, and to diagnose Alzheimer's by exclusion.

Immediate Management
Avoid alcohol and drugs and treat any other disease which may exacerbate confusion.
Social and community support

Treatment of Choice

- Cholinesterase inhibitors: Donepezil, rivastigmine, galantamine and tacrine .These drugs are available for the treatment of mild to moderate AD. There may be a slowing or even arrest of cognitive decline for about 8-9 months ; however the underlying disease process is not halted
- Memantine is the first N-methyl-D-aspartate receptor antagonist to be licensed for the treatment of patients with moderately severe to severe Alzheimer's disease

Your notes:

Serial No. 169

Subject: Medicine

Topic: Psychiatry

Question: A 68-year-old man refuses to talk and avoids eye contact. Says that there is no point talking to him as he is a complete failure and that his memory has given up.

Diagnosis: Pseudodementia

Clinchers

- *68-year-old man:* Pseudodementia more common in elderly with increased incidence in females.
- *Refuses to talk, avoids eye contact:* Patient gets socially withdrawn avoiding any sort of interaction.
- *Says there is no point talking to him:* He is describing his deficits; suggesting pseudodementia.
- *As he is a complete failure:* Highlighting his negative points; again suggesting a component of depression in his symptoms.
- *His memory has given up:* He is aware of the problem and accepts that there are lapses in the memory.

CONFUSA

Pseudodementia is the term applied to apparent cognitive impairment associated with psychiatric disorders, most often depression (50-100%). This is often reversible and responds to antidepressants. See figure to differentiate between dementia and psuedo-dementia.

Investigation of Choice

Rule out organic brain diseases, epilepsy and schizophrenia which can present with similar picture. Diagnosis is mainly based on clinical picture.

Immediate Management

Carefully rule out other causes of dementia

Treatment of Choice

Antidepressants

Pseudodentia Vs Dementia

Clinical Features	Pseudodementia	Dementia
1. Patient's complaint	Describe deficit in detail	Complains little try conceal deficit
2. Attitude	Emphasize disability highlight failures	Shows delight in accomplishments
3. Effort	Make little effort perform even simple tasks	Struggle to perform tasks. Rely on notes. Calendars to keep up
4. Concern about	Very concerned	Appear unconcerned
5. Social Skills	Loss prominent and early on	Social skills retained
6. Nocturnal accentuation of dysfunction	Uncommon	Common
7. Attention & concentration	Often well preserved	Faulty
8. Response to questions	"Don't know" answers typical	Frequently provide near miss answers
9. Memory loss	Memory gaps for periods	Loss of recent more severe than remote events
10. Performance on tasks of similar difficulty	Marked variability	Consistently poor performance
11. History of psychiatric dysfunction	Common	Unusual

Serial No. 170

Subject: Medicine

Topic: Psychiatry

Question: A 66-year-old man admitted in hospital develops features of disorientation and visual hallucinations on third day of admission.

Diagnosis: Acute delirium (also known as acute confusional state, acute cognitive dysfunction, toxic metabolic encephalopathy)

Clinchers

- *66-year-old man admitted in hospital:* Acute delirium presents in about 10% of all admissions aged above 65 yrs of age. This is usually associated with psychosocial stress and sleep deprivation associated with in-patients.
- *disorientation:* Characteristic of delirium; impaired awareness of self and also the surroundings may be present.
- *visual hallucinantions:* Patients may have visual hallucinations or persecutory delusions as well as grandiose delusions.

CONFUSA

- Delirium tremens is a similar state of acute confusion, occurring as a part of severe withdrawl reaction in a chronic heavy alcoholic.
- It usually develops within one week following the cessation of heavy ingestion of alcohol or a reduction in the amount of alcohol ingested. Hence, most commonly gets precipitated when a heavy drinker is admitted in hospital for other usual minor ailments.
- Always look for a history of alcoholism in such questions to come to a diagnosis of delirium tremens.

Investigation of Choice

History and examination, including mental status questionnaire, are vital parts of the investigation of an acutely confused patient. Extensive investigations to rule out any primary abnormality which could have precipitated the episode.

Immediate Management

Sedate the patient with drugs such as haloperidol or chlorpromazine.

Treatment of Choice

Treat the primary cause.

PAPER 3

56. A middle-aged woman has had several admissions for severe depression. She now turns up with a very severe depression despite all treatment.

Diagnosis: Refractory depression.

Clinchers

- *Middle-aged woman:* Middle-aged females are most prone to depression.
- *Has had several admissions for severe depression:* This proves that the depression is persistent and many different treatment approaches have been tried.
- *She now turns up with a very severe depression despite all treatment:* This means that the depression is severe and refractory to drug treatment. The condition can lead to a serious risk of health and may be the patient can go into a depressive stupor if left untreated.

CONFUSA

ECT is the Treatment of Choice in depression where,
- The patient is dangerously suicidal
- Delay in treatment represents a serious health risk
- The patient is refusing food and drink
- Patient is in depressive stupor

Investigation of Choice

Preanaesthetic checkup (as patient will be given ECT under GA, usually thiopental).

Treatment of Choice

Electroconvulsive therapy (ECT).

Your notes:

57. A woman has bouts of depression alternating with bouts of mania. She has had first line antidepressants but they have not worked.

Diagnosis: Manic depressive illness (MDI)
(Bipolar affective disorder)

Clinchers

- *Woman:* Depression is more common in females especially those in middle-age group.
- *Bouts of depression alternating with bouts of mania:* This fulfils the criteria to be diagnosed as MDI. Usually there is also a history of MDI in a close relative.
- *She has had first line antidepressants but they have not worked:* In MDI antidepressants work only in the depressive phases. For prophylaxis lithium is required.

CONFUSA

Cyclothymic disorders is less severe manic depressive illness (i.e. instead of manic episodes, there will be euphoric or hypomanic episodes. Note: Mania has delusions as a sign, hypomania does not). Cyclothymia is basically cyclical mood swings without the more florid features.

Investigation of Choice

Plasma creatinine and TSH (to exclude kidney or thyroid disease, necessary before starting lithium therapy).

Immediate Management

Sedation if manic (chlorpromazine or benzodiazepine).

Treatment of Choice

Lithium prophylaxis.

Your notes:

58. A young dentist, successful at work lacks confidence in himself. He finds that he is unable to socialise properly and has early morning waking. He is on no treatment.

Diagnosis: Mild depression

Clinchers

- *Young dentist:* Mild episodes of depression are very common among young professionals. The usual precipitants in them are over realisation of thier shortcomings in their professional field.
- *Successful at work:* It proves that the depression is not major as it is not interfering with his work and efficiency.
- *Lacks confidence in himself:* This signifies a personality problem and can be a reason for his depression.
- *He finds that he is unable to socialise properly:* It is a feature of a personality disorder and could be the precipitating cause of depression.
- *Early morning waking:* It is a pathognomic feature of depression.
- *He is on no treatment:* It means that first line antidepressant therapy can be used in this case.

CONFUSA

The main confusion in this question lies in choosing the answer. Since he has a personality disorder, it needs to be corrected for complete cure of his depression. But a definitive indication for antidepressant therapy is present (early morning awakening), so it has to be initiated first. Psychoanalysis and counselling will follow it.

Investigation of Choice

Detailed history.

Immediate Management

Trycyclic antidepressants (presence of biological features or stressful life events suggets a good response to antidepressants). Give imipramine as it is more effective for early moring awakening as it less sedating—less interference with work).

Treatment of Choice

Tricyclic antidepressants + psychoanalysis.

Your notes:

59. A 44-year-old has repeated episodes of depressed mood in response to feeling rejected, and a craving for sweets and chocolate. These reactive mood changes are accompanied by lethargy and increased appetite, particularly with a preference for carbohydrates.

Diagnosis: Depression.

Clinchers

- *A 44-year-old:* Depression is most common among middle-aged people (especially females).
- *Repeated episodes of depressed mood in response to feeling rejected:* It proves that the depression is recurrent and has a basis, i.e. it is not endogenous depression.
- *Craving for sweets and chocolate:* Usually depression causes poor appetite and weight loss, but in some rare cases it may produce increased appetite.

CONFUSA

Bulimia nervosa is characterised by binge eating and vomiting afterwards. Depression is a feature in it also but it typically follows the episodes of vomiting and is absolutely never precipitate by feeling of rejection. MAO inhibitors are the antipsychotics which stimulate appetite and help in gaining weight (by increasing a craving for carbohydrates, fluoxetine is an antidepressant which helps in losing weight and hence is preferred in obese patients with depression.

Investigation of Choice

Detailed history.

Immediate Management

Cognitive therapy (for feeling of rejections).

Treatment of Choice

Fluoxetine.

Your notes:

60. A 20-year-old previously healthy girl is waiting for her college exam result. The result is arriving that day by post and she is suffering from acute anxiety due to the importance of the results for her future career. Her mother consults their general practitioners.

Diagnosis: Acute anxiety neurosis.

Clinchers

- *Previously healthy:* Rules out any past history of any psychiatric or organic disorder.
- *College exam result due:* Causes of acute anxiety are usually stress and life events (e.g. gaining a spouse, losing a job, moving a house, results, etc).
- *Mother consults their general practitioner:* Acute anxiety before such an important event is normal. It remains physiological until it does not affect one's performance or social life. If her mother has consulted a GP for the anxiety, it must be significant and affecting her life/personality in some way. Since anxiety neurosis is characterised by a response out of proportion to the stress that precipitates them (an exaggeration of personality), this case seems more as a neurosis rather than a normal response.

CONFUSA

- Before diagnosing a neurosis, always rule out any underlying depression
- Panic attacks (hyperventilation syndromes) are also common in young females but are not precipitated usually by any obvious cause and have a totally different symptomatic profile.

Investigation of Choice

Detailed psychiatric history.

Immediate Management

Symptom control (best way is through simple listening and reassurance).

Treatment of Choice

Behaviour therapy + diazepam/lorazepam.

Your notes:

98. A 40-year-old man has become increasingly dependent on alcohol since his wife died last year. He admits that he has a problem and wishes to stop drinking. He does not with to take antidepressants.

Diagnosis: Alcohol dependence.

Clinchers

- *Since his wife died:* Alcohol dependence is often precipitated by breavment, in the false belief that it alleviates the symptoms of depression. But infact, alcohol does the opposite, as it a depressant and will exacerbate the problem.
- *Admits problem drinking and wishes to stop drinking:* Treatment of any dependency is only beneficial if the patient recognises the problem and wants to give up drinking. But even so, the relapse rates are very high. Supportive counselling and group psychotherapy (e.g. alcoholics anonymous) is of most benefit.
- *Does not wish to take antidepressants:* Since the patient is aware of the problem and has insight in it, antidepressants may not be needed (group psychotherapy alone can help). If he still experience difficulty abstaining, disulfiram may be used. It produces an unpleasant reaction (flushing and nausea) when taken with alcohol and will discourage a patient from drinking.

CONFUSA

Drugs which help in abstinence:

- Disulfiram—makes drinking unpleasant
- Naltrexone—takes pleasure out of drinking (halve the relapse rates)
- Acamprosate—mitigates anxiety, insomnia and craving.

Investigation of Choice

Gamma GT (increased); LFTs to rule out liver damage.

Immediate Management

Admit.

Treatment of Choice

Group psychotherapy.

Your notes:

99. A 63-year-old retired surgeon is admitted with a short history of bizarre behaviour. He claims that GMC are investigating him for murder and have hired a private detective to follow him. He has evidence of a coarse tremour, horizontal nystagmus and an ataxic gait. His wife says that the story about GMC is untrue but is worried about the amount of gin that her husband has drunk since retirement.

Diagnosis: Wernicke's encephalopathy + Korsakoff's psychosis.

Clinchers

- *Bizzare behaviour:* Due to dementia in Korsakoff's psychosis.
- *"GMC are investigating him for murder and have hired a private detective to follow him":* It is a delusion (a false, unshakeable belief). Delusions and paranoia are commonly features of Korsakoff's psychosis. Other features can be impairement of new learning and confabulations.
- *Coarse tremour, horizontal nystagmus and ataxic gait:* These are features of Wernicke's encephalopathy. It usually presents as a traid of nystagmus, ophthalmoplegia (commonly external recti) and ataxia. Other eye signs such as ptosis, abnormal pupillary reactions and altered consciousness may also occur. It may present with headache, anorexia, vomiting, and confusion.
- *Wife is worried about alcohol (gin) intake:* it substantiates our diagnostic suspicious of alcohol abuse.

CONFUSA

Wernicke's encephalopathy appears before Korsakoff's psychosis in patients of alcohol abuse. Wernicke's encephalopathy is a potentially reversible stage with thiamine treatment. Korsakoff's psychosis is irreversible.

Investigation of Choice

Red cell transketolase (decrease).

Immediate Management

IV thiamine amine urgently.

Treatment of Choice

Thiamine 200-300 mg/24 h PO.

Note: Give Pabrinex (2-3 pairs of high potency ampoules every 8 hr IV over 10 min for ≤ 2 days) if—oral route is impossible.

100. A 37-year-old retired professional footballer admits of using cocaine and heroin for the last three years. He has recently signed a contract to present a sports show on television and wishes to 'clean his life up' first. His wife and family are very supportive of this.

Diagnosis: Narcotic drug abuse.

Clinchers

- *Cocaine and heroin addiction:* They are common drugs of abuse.
- *Wishes to clean his life up first:* i.e. he is willing to leave drug addiction. Any patient who is clearly willing to leave drug addiction should be provided proper medical deaddiction. Even those patient's who are not willing to leave should be counselled for enrolement in deaddiction programmes.
- *His wife and family are very supportive:* Since this patient had adequate social support, there is not reason for his receiving in patient treatment only. Drug dependency teams can arrange supported outpatient withdrawal programmes.

CONFUSA

Abuse of drugs is a criminal offence in UK, but still patient confidentiality does not allow you to inform the police. Although it is the duty of the doctor to make sure that the patient is registered as a drug addict in the confidential registers of the regional health authorities.

Investigation of Choice

A complete health check up to ensure risk-free out patient treatment.

Immediate Management

Outpatient referral to drug dependency team.

Treatment of Choice

Drug withdrawal programme (outpatient).

Your notes:

151. A female lawyer is becoming anxious when she has to speak in front of people. This is affecting her work as she needs to speak out in court

Diagnosis: Anxiety.

Clinchers

- *Becoming anxious when she has to speak in front of people:* It is a type of performance anxiety and has a recognised anxiety provoking stimulus.
- *Affecting her work:* Anxiety is acceptable and require no treatment until and unless it becomes symptomatic, i.e.
  - Affect work/social life
  - Somatization symptoms

CONFUSA

If not treated, she may become less efficient because of her constant performance anxiety. This might lead to more interference with her work more and hence may be predisposed to develop anxiety neurosis.

Investigation of Choice

A detailed psychiatric history.

Immediate Management

Reassurance.

Treatment of Choice

Desensitization, i.e. a graded exposure to the anxiety provoking stimulus (behaviour therapy). Anxiolytics may be needed to enable effective work to be done with the patient.

Your notes:

152. A student approaching her secondary level exams is becoming increasingly anxious a few days ahead of her exam.

Diagnosis: Anxiety.

Clinchers

- *Approaching her secondary level exams:* This is an anxiety provoking stimulus in this patient. Usually sterss and life events precipitate anxiety which can be exaggerated in some individuals, thus producing symptoms.
- *Becoming increasingly anxious:* Since the condition is progressive, she need treatment. This will also ensure that the anxiety will not hamper her preparation and performance in the exams.

CONFUSA

Desensitization cannot work in this patient as the anxiety provoking stimulus is an isolated event in future and not something she has to cope up with every day.

Investigation of Choice

Detailed psychiatric history.

Immediate Management

Anxiolytics indicated if the condition is hampering her studies.

Treatment of Choice

Progressive relaxation training (the patient is taught to tense and relax groups of muscles in an orderly way—e.g., starting with the toes and working up the body. By concentrating on this, anxiety and muscle tone are reduced).

Your notes:

153. A 20-year-old woman attends A and E complaining of sudden breathlessness and anxiety. She describes palpitations and paraesthesiae of her hands, feet and lips. ECG shows sinus tachycardia and O_2 saturation is normal.

Diagnosis: Panic attacks.

Clinchers

- *A 20-year-old female:* young females are most prone to have panic attacks.
- *Sudden breathlessness and anxiety:* Classically the symptoms begin unexpectedly or 'out-of-the-blue'. Usually there is no apparent precipitating factor. The patient becomes increasingly frightened by an apparent inability to breath adequately. Attempts to breadth rapidly results in dizziness and further anxiety.
- *Palpitations:* It is due to sympathetic overactivity. Other symptoms attributed to sympathetic stimulation are—tachycardia, sweating, flushes, dyspnoea, hyperventilation, dry mouth, frequency and hesitancy of micturition, dizziness, diarrhoea, mydriasis.
- *Paraesthesiae of her hands, feet and lips:* Tachypnoea blows off CO_2 and the resultant respiratory alkalosis causes a fall in ionised calcium. This hypocalcaemia manifest as paraesthesiae in the fingers and perioral area.
- *Sinus tachycardia:* Due to sympathetic stimulation.
- *O_2 saturation is increased:* Due to hyperventilation.

CONFUSA

The most important differential diagnosis in a female is from MVPS (mitral valve prolapse syndrome). This syndrome, more commonly seen in young females (like panic disorder), presents with classical symptoms of panic disorder occurring in episodes. It is caused by prolapse, usually congenital, of the mitral valve into the atrium during ventricular systole. On auscultation, a mid systolic click and a systolic murmur can be heard sometimes. The clininical differentiation between MVPS and panic disorder is difficult. The diagnosis is usually established on echocardiography.

Investigation of Choice

To rule out organic respiratory problems (ECG, CXR, ABG).

Immediate Management

Confirmation of normality with warm reassurance to the patient.

Treatment of Choice

Re-breathing into a closed bag and mask system without oxygen.

154. This treatment is very effective in endogenous anxiety and phobias.

Diagnosis: Panick attacks associated with phobias.

Clinchers

The drug of choice of panic attacks associated with phobias is MAO inhibitor.

MAO inhibitors act on mono amine oxidase which is responsible for the degradation of catecholamines after reuptake. Their final effects is the same as tricyclic antidepressants, i.e. functional increase in the NE and/or 5HT levels at the receptor site. The increase in brain amine levels is probably responsible for their action.

CONFUSA

It takes 5-10 days before a MAO inhibitor has any evident action. Therefore it is useless to give it on a SOS basis. They must be administered regularly in sufficient doses to achieve desired effect.

Investigation of Choice

A detailed psychiatric history.

Immediate Management

Lorazepam if immediate agitation is present.

Treatment of Choice

MAO inhibitors (phenelzine).

Your notes:

155. A 25-year-old woman finds it difficult to leave her house. She becomes very agitated in supermarkes and describes palpitations and difficult breathing when in crowds.

Diagnosis: Agoraphobia.

Clinchers

- *A 25-year-old woman:* All phobic disorders are more common in females.
- *Difficult to leave her house:* This is fear of open places, public places, crowded places, any other place from where there is not easy escape to a safe place (safe place is usually home according to the patients).
- *Becomes very agitated in super and describes palpitations and difficult breathing when in crowds:* If patient of agoraphobia finds herself/himself in a crowded place like supermarkets, he/she will suddenly develop incapaciating symptoms of palpitations or a full blown panic attack, which can lead to agitation. Difficulty breathing leading to hyperventilation is a typical symptoms of panic attacks.

CONFUSA

As the agoraphobia increases in severity, there is a gradual restriction in normal day to day activities. The activity may become so severely restricted that the person becomes self-imprisoned at home. One or two persons (usually close relations) may be relied upon, with whom the patient can leave home. Claustrophobia is just the opposite—fear of closed spaces from where there is no easy escape to a safe place.

Investigation of Choice

Detailed psychiatric history.

Immediate Management

Rebreathing into a bag if panic attack is present.

Treatment of Choice

Behaviour therapy

Your notes:

PAPER 4

35. A 21-year-old female found unconscious next to her 22-year-old husband, who was found dead. Her ECG shows evidence of acute MI.

Diagnosis: Cocaine abuse

Clinchers

- *A 21-year-old female and a 22-year-old husband:* The experimentation with recreational drugs of abuse is highest amongst young persons. Also it is very rare to have a MI at this young age.
- *Husband dead:* It is most probably due to drug overdose. This couple might be the first times on drugs and most probably did not know how much is enough for them.
- *Female—ECG shows acute MI + is unconscious:* MI per se do not produce unconsciousness. She might be unconscious due to the effect of drug. As cocaine is a potent vasoconstrictor, it can cause MI by inducing coronary artery spasm.

CONFUSA

Cocaine is rarely used for homicide or suicide. Accidental cases occur from addiction, hypodermic injection and from urethral, vesical and rectal injection. It is believed to be an aphrodisiac and to increase the duration of sexual act by paralysing sensory nerves of glans penis. Sudden death by cocaine is due to cardiac arrhythmias due to direct action on myocardium and cardiopulmonary arrest.

Investigation of Choice

Toxicology screen

Immediate Management

Airway and circulatory stabilization.

Treatment of Choice

Amyl nitrate is an antidote and is given by inhalation.

Your notes:

56. Most common form of dementia in the UK.

Diagnosis: Alzheimer's disease (AD)

Clinchers

About 25% of the elderly population suffer from a psychiatric disability, mainly anxiety and depression. However, dementia affects about 10% of those aged over 65 years and 20% of those over 80 years of age a total of 650 thousand people in England and Wales. Seventy percent are due to Alzheimer's disease.

CONFUSA

Neurotransmitter changes with disease

- Depression—decreased NE and 5-HT
- Alzheimer's—decreased Ach
- Huntingtons's disease—decreased GABA and ACh
- Schizophrenia—increased dopamine
- Parkinsonism—decreased dopamine

Investigation of Choice

AD is a diagnosis of exclusion

- MRI or CT—exclude
  - Multiinfarct dementia
  - Subdural haemorrhage
  - Abscess
  - Tumour

Immediate Management

Usually none required, otherwise symptomatic.

Treatment of Choice

Donepezil

Your notes:

57. Characterised by neurofibrillary tangles and senile plaques.

Diagnosis: Alzheimer's disease (AD)

Clinchers

- ➢ *Neurofibrillary tangles and senile plaques:* Neuropathological changes include neuronal reduction, neurofibrillary tangles, senile neuritic plaques and a variable amyloid angiopathy. These changes are particularly seen in the hippocampus, substantia innominate, locus cenuleus and the tempoparietal and frontal cortices.
- ➢ *TIP:* 6 A's of dementia
  - Aphasia
  - Apraxia
  - Agnosia
  - Amnesia
  - Abstract thought
  - Agitation

CONFUSA

Usually pathophysiology questions are not asked in PLAB exam, but there may be a couple of questions or whole theme on these features. So do not skip these topics during your first reading.

Investigation of Choice

See previous question.

Immediate Management

See previous question.

Treatment of Choice

See previous question.

Your notes:

58. May respond to antidepressants.

Diagnosis: Pseudodementia.

Clinchers

Depression can produce cognitive impairment, called pseudodementia contributed to by lack of motivation, concentration and self-confidence.

CONFUSA

Pseudodementia must be differentiated from dementia, as the foramen can respond to antidepressants. Two questions can help in distinguishing them:

- Did low mood or poor memory come first?
- Is the failure to answer questions due to lack of ability or lack of motivation?

Note that dementia and depression can also occur together.

Investigation of Choice

Clinical diagnosis.

Immediate Management

Rule out delirium by checking level of consciousness.

Treatment of Choice

Antidepressants.

Your notes:

59. Increased disinhibition,preservation of intellect

Diagnosis: Frontal dementia.

Clinchers

- *Increased disinhibition:* Frontal lobe lesions produces personality changes and disinhibition increases, i.e. the patient becomes
  - Indecent
  - Indolent
  - Indiscreet
- *Preservation of intellect:* There is no intellectual impairment in frontal lobe dementia. Psychosis is never present in frontal lobe dementia.

CONFUSA

Intellectual deterioration is a hallmark of corpus callosum lesions. Also do not confuse increased disinhibition with hypersexuality which is a feature of temporal lobe lesions.

Investigation of Choice

CT/MRI.

Immediate Management

None required.

Treatment of Choice

- Conservative and symptomatic
- Surgery if SOL present.

Your notes:

66. Man living in a hostel,brought to hospital after he collapsed. On the 3rd day, he points out things other people cannot see, disorientation in time and place.

Diagnosis: Delirium tremens (DT).

Clinchers

- *Living in a hostel:* Alcoholism or binges drinking is more prevalent in hostels and young people. Often they do not drink in moderation resulting in withdrawal symptoms.
- *Brought to hospital after he collapsed:* He must have collapsed because of a heavy prolonged drinking session (alcohol intoxication)
- *On 3rd day:* Onset of DT is typically 24-72 hours after prolonged drinking.
- *Points out things other people cannot see:* Visual hallucinations are characteristic (e.g. pink elephants) in DT.
- *Disorientation in time and place:* Clouding of consciousness and disorientation is a feature of DT.

CONFUSA

In alcoholic hallucinosis, heavy drinker experiences recurrent auditory hallucinations, usually of threatening or derogatory nature. In contract to delirium tremens, the hallucinations typically occur in clear consciousness.

Investigation of Choice

The diagnosis is purely clinical.

Immediate Management

Adequate sedation + intensive monitoring.

Treatment of Choice

Supportive therapy.

Your notes:

67. An 80-year-old female is on no medication. Cause of concern is that she was trying to get into a shop at 6: 00am. Neighbours say she is ok except her memory is not as good as it used to be since 2 years. She is otherwise well.

Diagnosis: Alzheimer's dementia (AD).

Clinchers

- *An 80-year-old:* The onset of AD can be in middle adult life or even earlier (of presenile onset) but the incidence is higher in later life. It is the most common cause of dementia in elderly. The frequency of AD increases with each decade of adult life to reach 20 to 40% of population over the age of 85.
- *Female:* Female gender may also be a risk factor independent of the greater longevity of women. Unconfirmed studies have suggested that postmenopausal oestrogen use is associated with a decreased frequency of AD.
- *She was trying to get into a shop at 6: 00 AM:* AD produced cognitive problems which interfere with daily activities, such as keeping track of finances, following instructions on the job, driving, shopping and house keeping. In this case the patient seem to have completely lost sense of judgement and forgot the opening time of the shop.
- *Memory is not as good as it used to be:* Failing memory is the most common presenting feature of AD.
- *Otherwise well:* This rules out any acute cause for confusional state.

CONFUSA

Rarely AD patients may have a form of cortical blindness in which they deny their inability to see. In AD, social graces, routine behaviour and superficial conversation may be surprisingly retained. Patients at risk of developing AD are with:

- Family history
- Down's syndrome
- ALL
- Head injury.

Investigation of Choice

Neuroimaging (rule out frontal lobe dementia, Lewy body dementia and Pick's disease).

Immediate Management

Usually none required, otherwise symptomatic.

Treatment of Choice

Donepezil.

70. A 70-year-old man says his life is not worth living, his existence is a waste, he performs all his work very slowly, he has lost weight.

Diagnosis: Depression.

Clinchers

- *A 70-year-old man:* The incidence of depression increases with age; the disorder is approximately twice as prevalent in women as in men, regardless of age.
- *Say his life is not worthlining, his existence is a waste:* In depression thoughts are negative and pessimistic, centring upon unpleasant memories, past failings and a bleak future. Hopelessness, helplessness and worthlessness readily supervene, not only reinforcing the depressed mood but leading to suicidal thoughts. Mood is infact a criterion to differentiate minor (transiently low mood) and major (persistently low mood) depression.
- *Performs all his work very slowly:* This is *psychomotor retardation* a typical feature of depression.
- *Lost weight:* Loss of appetite in depression leads to loss of weight. Rarely some patients have increased appetite leading to weight gain.

CONFUSA

Many depressed patients do not complain of or admit to, low mood, but present because of the associated cognitive, behaviourly or somatic symptoms. Somatic presentations of depression are particularly common in Asian cultures. In depression, pcyhomotor retardation can increase to the point where the person sits motionless and mute—depressive stupor. This used to end in death from dehyhdration; it now calls for emergency ECT.

Investigation of Choice

A detailed psychiatric history.

Immediate Management

Exclude suicidal ideation.

Treatment of Choice

Fluoxetine.

Your notes:

91. 40-year-old lady stops talking suddenly, says someone took away her thoughts.

Diagnosis: Schizophrenia

Clinchers

- *A 40-year-old lady:* As compared to males, the onset of schizophrenia is usually late in females and often runs a more benign course.
- *Stops talking suddenly:* Thought blocking is a characteristic feature of schizophrenia. There is a sudden interruption of stream of speech before the thought is completed. After a pause, the subject cannot recall what she had meant to say.
- *Say someone took away her thoughts:* Thoughts blocking is characteristically associated with thoughts withdrawn in schizophrenia. This is perception of removal of thoughts by an external force. This is a diagnostic first rank symptom of schizophrenia.

CONFUSA

Thought blocking can also be seen in complex partial seizures (temporal lobe epilepsy; absence seizures). But they are more commonly seen in children and extremely unusual to present at this age. In temporal lobe epilepsy, the subject continues to speak after a pause, from where he/she have left but not in schizophrenia.

Investigation of Choice

Schizophrenia is a clinical diagnosis. Physical investigations are mainly used to rule out the organic disorders. Brain imaging is considered if there are neurological symptoms or signs.

Immediate Management

Admission: The mental health act may be needed, since patients are at risk from neglect or dangerous acts.

Treatment of choice

After a single episode of schizophrenia continue treatment for 12-24 months with antipsychotic drugs (lozapine/risperidone).

Your notes:

92. A 17-year-old girl comes anxious and tearful to A and E. She is unkempt and dishevelled, says she lost her medication, says she aches all over and demand immediate pain relief.

Diagnosis: Opioid withdrawal.

Clinchers

- *A 17-year-old girl:* Substance misuse is more prevalent in teens and twenties.
- *Anxious and tearful:* Opioid withdrawal leads to an extremely unpleasant withdrawal syndrome (cold turkey) involving:
  - Craving (presents in this case)
  - Myalgia
  - Restlessness and insomnia
  - Sweating
  - Abdominal pain, vomiting, diarrhoea
  - Dilated pupils, running nose and eyes
  - Tachycardia
  - Yawning and
  - Goose bumps
- *Unkempt and dishevelled:* A typical condition of a drug addict.
- *Says she lost her medication:* The unbearable withdrawal syndrome forces the patient to steal, lie or do almost anything in order to get the drug. However, if you question her about the medication or the disease she is suffering from, she will have no answer and may respond with agitation.
- *Demand immediate pain relief:* This confirms that the substance being misused is opioid. It is so as its withdrawal produces pain to myalgia or the patients having knowledge of opioids being used in hospital for pain relief.

Investigation of Choice

Toxicology screen—because she might have consumed large doses of analgesics in order to get pain relief.

Immediate Management

Admission

Treatment of Choice

Counselling to get enrolled in systematic withdrawal programme. If not agreeing, enrol in harm reduction and maintenance therapy. Report all patients for registration in confidential register of NHS.

Your notes:

95. A 20-year-old woman attends A and E complaining of sudden breathlessness and anxiety. She describes palpitations and paresthesiae of her hands, feet and lips. ECG shows sinus tachycardia and O_2 saturation is normal.

Diagnosis: Panic attacks.

Clinchers

- *A 20-year-old female:* young females are most prone to have panic attacks.
- *Sudden breathlessness and anxiety:* Classically the symptoms begin unexpectedly or 'out-of-the-blue'. Usually there is no apparent precipitating factor. The patient becomes increasingly frightened by an apparent inability to breath adequately. Attempts to breadth rapidly results in dizziness and further anxiety.
- *Palpitations:* It is due to sympathetic overactivity. Other symptoms attributed to sympathetic stimulation are—tachycardia, sweating, flushes, dyspnoea, hyperventilation, dry mouth, frequency and hesitancy of micturition, dizziness, diarrhoea, mydriasis.
- *Paraesthesiae of her hands, feet and lips:* Tachypnoea blows off CO_2 and the resultant respiratory alkalosis causes a fall in ionised calcium. This hypocalcaemia manifest as paraesthesiae in the fingers and perioral area.
- *Sinus tachcycardia:* Due to sympathetic stimulation.
- *O_2 saturation is increased:* due to hyperventilation.

CONFUSA

The most important differential diagnosis in a female is from MVPS (mitral valve prolapse syndrome). This syndrome, more commonly seen in young females (like panic disorder), presents with classical symptoms of panic disorder occurring in episodes. It is caused by prolapse, usually congenital, of the mitral valve into the atrium during ventricular systole. On auscultation, a mid systolic click and a systolic murmur can be heard sometimes. The clininical differentiation between MVPS and panic disorder is difficult. The diagnosis is usually established on echocardiography.

Investigation of Choice

To rule out organic respiratory problems (ECG, CXR, ABG).

Immediate Management

Confirmation of normality with warm reassurance to the patient.

Treatment of choice

Re-breathing into a closed bag and mask system without oxygen.

144. An 18 -year-old university student with history of 3 months of amenorrhoea and starvation.

Diagnosis: Anorexia nervosa

Clinchers

- *A 18-year-old:* Anorexia mainly affects females (sex ratio 10: 1). The average age of onset is 15-16 years. The prevalence in the UK is about 1% in females aged 12-18.
- *University students:* It precipitates because of well-marked stressors, such as new school or colleges, first sexual encounters and examinations.
- *3 months of amenorrhoea:* Anorexia nervosa may lead to pituitary damage and thus to permanent amenorrhoea and sterility. The endocrinal disturbances include elevated cortisol and growth hormone levels.
- *Starvation:* There is deliberately weight loss, induced primarily by restriction of food intake. Weight is > 15% below normal and BMI is < 17.5.

CONFUSA

In anorexia nervosa, periods cease before weight loss becomes apparent (lecture notes, gynae-obs, pg 29, 1st Edn). If the onset is before puberty, there is delay in secondary sexual development. In menstruating females, always rule out amenorrhoea due to OCP usage. In early stages the weight loss must be distinguished from other causes of weight loss.

The psychiatric differential diagnosis include:

- Depressive disorder
- Substance misuse
- Obsessive-compulsive disorder

The medical disorders in differential diagnosis as:

- Inflammatory bowel disease
- Malabsorption syndromes
- Hypopituitarism
- Cancer.

Investigation of Choice

BMI

Immediate Management

If extreme weakness, fainting, K^{+} $^{-}$ or glucose $^{-}$, then prompt admission to hospital.

Treatment of choice

Cognitive-behavioural therapy.

Your notes:

PAPER 5

1. A 20-year-old man keeps cleaning his hands every time he shakes his partners' hands. He was a high achiever in high school.

Diagnosis: Obsessive compulsive personality disorder (OCD).

Clinchers

- *A 20-year-old:* The onset of OSD is usually in early 20's. It is slightly more common in unmarried people.
- *Man:* OCD is equally common in men and women.
- *Keeps cleaning his hands every time he shakes his partners' hands:* Washers are the most common type. Here the obsession is of contamination with dirt, germs, body excretions and the like. The compulsion is washing of hands or the whole hand, repeatedly many times a day. It usually spreads on to washing of clothes, washing of bathroom, door knobs and personal articles, gradually. The person tries to avoid contamination but is unable to, so washing becomes a ritual.
- *High achiever in school:* This disorder is more common in persons from upper social strata and with high intelligence.

CONFUSA

The differential diagnosis is from depressive disorder (in which obsessional symptoms are common), psychotic disorder (since obsessions can be hard to distinguish from delusions) and anankastic personality disorder.

Investigation of Choice

Clinical diagnosis.

Immediate Management

Specialist evaluation.

Treatment of choice

Behavioural therapy

+

Drug treatment

(TCA/SSRI/clomipramine).

Your notes:

2. A 56-year-old farmer believes his 34-year-old neighbour is killing his farm animals despite the local veterinary's advice that the death is due to an outbreak of anthrax. He spends hours watching his neighbour through pair of binocular lens, hoping to catch in the act.

Diagnosis: Paranoid personality disorder.

Clinchers

- *A 56-year-old farmer:* It occurs at early age in adult life with a stable course over the years.
- *Believes his 34-year-old neighbour is killing his farm animals despite the local veterinary's advice that the death is due to an outbreak of anthrax:* In it, the person may have excessive sensitiveness to setbacks and rebuffs. There is tendency to bear grudges persistently, e.g. refusal to forgive insults and injuries or slights. There may be recurrent suspicious, with out justification and contrary to evidence (as in this case).
- *Spends hours watching his neighbour:* There is preoccupation with unsubstantiated conspirational explanation of events and the patient may go to any length to prove them.

CONFUSA

Paranoid personality disorder is more common in men. It is more common in minority groups and immigrants. Psychodynamically the underlying defense mechanism is projection. For the diagnosis of this disorder, clear evidence is usually required of the presence of at least three of the traits or behaviours given in clinical description by ICD-10 (CDDG). This disorder is found premorbidly in some patients of paranoid schizophrenia.

Investigation of Choice

Clinical diagnosis.

Immediate Management

Exclude delusional (paranoid) disorder.

Treatment of choice

Individual and supportive psychotherapy.

Your notes:

3. A 16-year-old girl is described as 'queer' by her mates. She is unfriendly and has no close friends despite numerous attempts by boys in her college. She lacks empathy and is largely introspective.

Diagnosis: Schizoid personality disorder.

Clinchers

- *A 16-year-old girl:* Like all personality disorder, schizoid personality disorder has an onset in early childhood with stable course over the years. It is more common in men.
- *Described as 'queer' by her mates:* There is almost invariable preference for solitary activities in this disorder. The patient lacks close friends or confiding relationships (or having only one) and of desire of such relationships. There is also marked insensitivity to prevailing social norms and conventions.
- *Unfriendly and has no close friends:* See above.
- *Despite numerous attempts by boys in her college:* There is little interest on the part of the patient in having sexual experiences with another person (taking into account her age).
- *Lacks empathy:* There is emotional coldness, detached or flattened affectivity and limited capacity to express either warm, tender feelings or anger towards others.
- *Largely introspective:* There is excessive preoccupation with fantasy and introspection.

CONFUSA

The features of this disorder may overlap with paranoid and schizotypal personality disorders, but can be differentiated clinically as psychotic features are absent. Psychodynamically it is supposed to result from 'cold and aloof' parenting in a child with introverted temperament. However, this hypothesis is far from proven in the research conducted so far.

Investigation of Choice

Clinical diagnosis.

Immediate Management

Specialist evaluation.

Treatment of choice

Individual psychotherapy.

+

Psychoanalysis

+

Gradual involvement in group psychotherapy

4. A 16-year-old girl in high school always comes late to class wearing strong perfume in a vain attempt to attract attention. She laughs loudly at jokes, many of her mates do not find particularly hilarious.

Diagnosis: Histrionic personality disorder

Clinchers

- *A 16-year-old:* Like all personality disorders, it has an onset in early childhood with stable course over the years.
- *Girls:* More common in females.
- *Always comes late + strong perfume + laughs loudly:* These are exhibitionistic traits which signify an attention seeking attitude, a characteristic feature. There is also continual seeking for excitement and appreciation by others. Dramatic emotionally, i.e. self dramatization, theatricality and exaggerated expression of emotions is usually present. There is an attempt to look charming, beautiful and seductive. Suicidal gestures may be made.

CONFUSA

Associated features may include egocentricity, self-indulgence, continuous longing for appreciation, feelings that are easily hurt and persistent manipulative behaviour to achieve own needs. Interpersonal relationships of such persons are often stormy and ungratifying. Psychodynamically, there are intense dependency needs. The defence mechanisms used most are acting out and dissociation.

Investigation of Choice

Clinical diagnosis.

Immediate Management

Specialist evaluation.

Treatment of choice

Psychoanalysis

+

Psychoanalytic psychotherapy.

Your notes:

5. A 32-year-old man always gives in to his wife over any decision even when he knows this is not right. He insists on having his wife prepare his every meal, wash him and put him to sleep. He cries whenever his wife is away.

Diagnosis: Dependent personality disorder

Clinchers

- *A 32-year-old man:* Like all personality disorders, it has an onset in early childhood with sable course over the years.
- *Always gives in to his wife over any decision even when he knows this is not right:* In this disorder the patient encourage or allow others to make most of one's important life decisions. There is limited capacity on the patient's part to make everyday decisions without an excessive amount of advice and reassurance from others.
- *Insists on having his wife prepare his every meal, wash him and put him to sleep:* These suggest dependence on her wife as the patient usually think himself as incompetent.
- *Cries whenever his wife is away:* There is feeling of being uncomfortable or helplessness when alone or abandoned by person with who he has a close relationship. It is because of exaggerated fears of inability to care for onself.

CONFUSA

Dependent personality disorders may overlap with avoidant and passive aggressive personality disorders. Some patients exhibit masochistic character. They repetitively establish close interpersonal relationships which result in punishment.

Investigation of Choice

Clinical diagnosis

Immediate Management

Specialist evaluation

Treatment of choice

Individual psychotherapy

+

Group psychotherapy

+

Behaviour therapy in the form of assertiveness training is useful

21. A 56-year-old man with no previous history is brought to the Accident and Emergency Department by his wife who says that he has become progressively more forgetful, tends to lose his temper and is emotionally labile. There is no history of infectious diseases or trauma.

Diagnosis: Alzheimer's dementia (AD)

Clinchers

- *A 56-year-old":* The onset can be in middle adult life or even earlier (of presenile onset) but the incidence is higher in later life.
- *No previous history:* It is insidious in onset and usually have no precipitating or prodromal symptoms.
- *Brought by wife:* The patients are not insightful enough to present themselves.
- *Progressively more forgetful:* There is impaired ability to learn new information or to recall previously learned information.
- *Tends to lose his temper and is emotionally labile:* Behavioural changes are common and include wandering, agitation and aggression. Paranoia with persecutory delusions occurs in upto 50% of patients.
- *No history of infectious diseases or trauma:* Though AD can develop long after head trauma, majority have no risk factors.

CONFUSA

Apraxia (as impaired ability to carry out motor activities despite intact motor function) and agnosia (the failure to recognize or identify objects despite intact sensory functions) are characteristic of AD.

Investigation of Choice

Histology (rarely used)

Immediate Management

Rule out other dementia (with neuroimaging, B_{12}, TSH).

Treatment of choice

MRC menu (see page 536, OHCM, 5th edn).

Your notes:

71. A homeless patient presents to A and E with drowsiness. On examination, abrasions and puncture marks were found on his arm. He has pin-point pupil.

Diagnosis: Opioid poisoning

Antidote: Naloxone

Clinchers

- *Homeless patient:* Risk factor for drug addiction.
- *Drowsiness:* Stupor, coma, fall in BP, shallow and occasional breathing are all signs of acute opioid poisoning.
- *Abrasions and puncture marks:* Further support the diagnosis of drug injection.
- *Pin-point pupil:* This confirms the diagnosis of opioid poisoning.

CONFUSA

Drowsiness, coma can be caused by benzodiazepines, alcohol, opiates, tricyclic or barbiturates.

Constricted pupils are seen opiates or insecticides (organophosphates). On the other hand dilated pupils are seen in amphetamines, cocaine, quinine or tricyclic.

Investigation of Choice

Take blood. Always check for paracetamol and salicylate levels. Diagnosis is mainly from history.

Immediate Management

Naloxone, e.g. 0.8-2 mg IV repeat every 2 minutes, until breathing adequate.

Treatment of choice

Advocate supportive measures

Start the antidote

Referral to psychiatrist.

Your notes:

148. A 16-year-old frail girl coplains of constipation. Her Body Mass Index (BMI) is found to be 17. She is extremely afraid of eating and admits to sticking a finger down her throat to induce vomiting after meals. She is unusually sensitive to cold.

Diagnosis: Anorexia noervosa

Clinchers

- *A 16-year-old girl:* Anorexia mainly affects females (sex ratio 10: 1). The average age of onset is 15-16 years. The prevalence in the UK is about 1% in females aged 12-18.
- *Frail:* It signifies the weight loss.
- *Constipation:* It is due to reduced food intake and not due to any other pathology.
- *BMI 17:* BMI < 17.5 is diagnostic of anorexia in this typical clinical profile.
- *Extremely afraid of eating:* This is found as there is a profound fear of getting fat.
- *Admits to sticking a finger down her throat to induce vomiting after meals:* It social circumstances or binge eating causes more intake than usual, vomiting induced as soon as possible, often in a public rest room.
- *Unusually sensitive to cold:* Cold intolerance is presumable due to a defect in regulatory thermogenesis secondary to hypothalamic dysfunction.

CONFUSA

Patients with anorexia nervosa are vulnerable to sudden death from ventricular tachyarrhythmias. ECG shows prolonged QT intervals. The risk of death becomes high when weight declines 35% below ideal, probably because of protein deficiency.

Investigation of Choice

Clinical diagnosis

Immediate Management

Admit

Treatment of choice

Cognitive-behaviour therapy.

Your notes:

151. A 23-year-old woman has been using heroin (IV) for 4-years. She is not willing to stop using the heroin.

Diagnosis: Risk for HIV and hepatitis B

Clinchers

- *A 23-year-old woman:* Highest incidence and prevalence of drug abuse is in teens and twenties.
- *IV heroin for 4 years:* She is at high risk of acquiring serious communicable disease like HIV and hepatitis B.
- *Not willing to stop using the heroin:* Although it is the duty of the doctor to counsel the patient for deaddiction, but he can not force it. For patients unwilling to stop drug abuse, the doctor should arrange for enrolment in the local needle exchange programme. The heatlh office maintain a confidential register for that purpose.

CONFUSA

The practice of sharing needles and syringes for IV drug use continues to be a major route for transmission of HIV in both developed countries and parts of South-east Asia and latin America. In some areas successful education and needle exchange schemes have reduced the rate of transmission by this route. Needle exchange is successful as the drug abusers often do not have enough money to spend on needles and thus extremely share and reuse them.

Investigation of Choice

HIV screening after consent

Immediate Management

Needle exchange

Treatment of choice

De-addiction counselling and enrolment.

Your notes:

PAPER 6

78. A 20-year-old woman attends A and E complaining of sudden breathlessness and anxiety. She describes palpitations and paresthesiae of her hands, feet and lips. ECG shows sinus tachycardia and O2 saturation is normal.

Diagnosis: Panic attacks.

Clinchers

- *A 20-year-old female:* young females are most prone to have panic attacks.
- *Sudden breathlessness and anxiety:* Classically the symptoms begin unexpectedly or 'out-of-the-blue'. Usually there is no apparent precipitating factor. The patient becomes increasingly frightened by an apparent inability to breath adequately. Attempts to breadth rapidly results in dizziness and further anxiety.
- *Palpitations:* It is due to sympathetic overactivity. Other symptoms attributed to sympathetic stimulation are—tachycardia, sweating, flushes, dyspnoea, hyperventilation, dry mouth, frequency and hesitancy of micturition, dizziness, diarrhoea, mydriasis.
- *Paraesthesiae of her hands, feet and lips:* Tachypnoea blows off CO_2 and the resultant respiratory alkalosis causes a fall in ionised calcium. This hypocalcaemia manifest as paraesthesiae in the fingers and perioral area.
- *Sinus tachcycardia:* Due to sympathetic stimulation.
- *O_2 saturation is increased:* due to hyperventilation.

CONFUSA

The most important differential diagnosis in a female is from MVPS (mitral valve prolapse syndrome). This syndrome, more commonly seen in young females (like panic disorder), presents with classical symptoms of panic disorder occurring in episodes. It is caused by prolapse, usually congenital, of the mitral valve into the atrium during ventricular systole. On auscultation, a mid systolic click and a systolic murmur can be heard sometimes. The clininical differentiation between MVPS and panic disorder is difficult. The diagnosis is usually established on echocardiography.

Investigation of Choice

To rule out organic respiratory problems (ECG, CXR, ABG).

Immediate Management

Confirmation of normality with warm reassurance to the patient.

Treatment of choice

Re-breathing into a closed bag and mask system without oxygen.

PAPER 7

78. A 20-year-old woman attends A and E complaining of sudden breathlessness and anxiety. She describes palpitations and paresthesiae of her hands, feet and lips. ECG shows sinus tachycardia and O2 saturation is normal.

Diagnosis: Panic attacks.

Clinchers

- *A 20-year-old female:* Young females are most prone to have panic attacks.
- *Sudden breathlessness and anxiety:* Classically the symptoms begin unexpectedly or 'out-of-the-blue'. Usually there is no apparent precipitating factor. The patient becomes increasingly frightened by an apparent inability to breath adequately. Attempts to breadth rapidly results in dizziness and further anxiety.
- *Palpitations:* It is due to sympathetic overactivity. Other symptoms attributed to sympathetic stimulation are—tachycardia, sweating, flushes, dyspnoea, hyperventilation, dry mouth, frequency and hesitancy of micturition, dizziness, diarrhoea, mydriasis.
- *Paraesthesiae of her hands, feet and lips:* Tachypnoea blows off CO_2 and the resultant respiratory alkalosis causes a fall in ionised calcium. This hypocalcaemia manifest as paraesthesiae in the fingers and perioral area.
- *Sinus tachcycardia:* Due to sympathetic stimulation.
- *O_2 saturation is increased:* due to hyperventilation.

CONFUSA

The most important differential diagnosis in a female is from MVPS (mitral valve prolapse syndrome). This syndrome, more commonly seen in young females (like panic disorder), presents with classical symptoms of panic disorder occurring in episodes. It is caused by prolapse, usually congenital, of the mitral valve into the atrium during ventricular systole. On auscultation, a mid systolic click and a systolic murmur can be heard sometimes. The clininical differentiation between MVPS and panic disorder is difficult. The diagnosis is usually established on echocardiography.

Investigation of Choice

To rule out organic respiratory problems (ECG, CXR, ABG).

Immediate Management

Confirmation of normality with warm reassurance to the patient.

Treatment of choice

Re-breathing into a closed bag and mask system without oxygen.

25. A 15-year-old girl has cut her wrist and bled profusely. She is pale, tachycardiac and does not want to live.

Diagnosis: Suicide attempt with hypovolaemic shock.

Clinchers

- *Has cut her wrist:* Lacerations in this area frequently involve deep structures and accurate diagnosis is essential. History is usually unhelpful in suicide attempts.
- *Bled profusely:* This suggest a massive blood loss and so a search for features of hypotensive shock should be started.
- *Pale, tachycardiac:* This confirms the hypovolaemic shock. Tachycardia is usually manifest after at least 15-30% loss of circulating blood.
- *Does not want to live:* She needs continuous monitoring and appropriate sedation as she may repeat the attempt to suicide.

CONFUSA

In wrist lacerations, a full assessment of the distal neurovascular function is essential. Test all tendons and nerves individually. Any positive finding of deep structure involvement must be discussed with a senior colleague at once. Further exploration must be carried out:

- In an operating theatre
- Under adequate anaesthesia (GA usually)
- With a bloodless field
- By an experienced surgeon

Note:

- A divided nerve may continue to conduct some sensation for several hours if the nerve ends are touching.
- Abductor pollices brevis is paralysed in T_1 root lesions but not in ulnar nerve lesions. To test this muscle the thumb is moved vertically upwards against resistance with the hand in supine position.

Investigation of Choice

Urine output.

Immediate Management

External compression to prevent further blood loss then start treating the shock

Treatment of choice

Microvascular surgery

+

Psychiatric referral later.

111. A schizophrenic who stabbed his mother's hand with a screw driver was recently admitted and treated with depot injection antipsychotic. He is now symptom -free and ready for discharge.

Diagnosis: Chronic schizophrenia

Clinchers

- *Schizophrenic:* It means that it is a previously diagnosed case.
- *Stabbed his mother's hand:* It must be an acute exacerbation of schizophrenic episode.
- *Recently admitted and treated with depot injection:* Patients who have had multiple episodes or persistent symptoms usually remain on medication for many years, though the need for it (and the effect of cautions reductions in dose) should remain under regular review. Medication is often given in depot form.

CONFUSA

The main specific psychological intervention is a form of family therapy. This arose from the finding that patients living with families who have high expressed emotion (EE) had a much higher chance of relapse than those exposed to low EE. EE is the intensity and amount of emotional involvement by the family with the patient. It was then found that high EE families could be taught to lower EE, and relapse rates fell.

Investigation of Choice

None except observation.

Immediate Management

Rule out tardive dyskinesia.

Treatment of choice

Family therapy.

Your notes:

112. Patient (schizophrenia) has had about 8 admissions in the last 5 years. He is uncompliant with drugs.

Diagnosis: Chronic relapsing schizophrenia.

Clinchers

- *8 admissions in last 5 years:* Hospitalization in schizophrenia is indicated if there is:
  1. Neglect of food and water intake
  2. Danger to self or others
  3. Poor drug compliance
  4. Significant neglect of self care
  5. Lack of social support.
- *He is uncompliant with drugs:* To ensure drug compliance depot preparation with long duration of action can be used. Cognitive therapy is used to reduce symptoms and to increase treatment adherence (118, Lecture notes, psychiatry, 8th edn).

CONFUSA

Upto two-thirds will relapse if antipsychotic medication is discontinued within the first 5 years of treatment. So the best plan is to offer prophylaxis to everyone in the lowest effective dose and by depot infections if concordance/compliance is a problem.

Investigation of Choice
None

Immediate Management
Depot antipsychotic injections.
Treatment of choice
Cognitive therapy.

Your notes:

113. Young patient now 25 years was diagnosed with schizophrenia at 15, but despite different medications has not recovered fully. The family is very supportive.

Diagnosis: Chronic schizophrenia

Clinchers

- *Young patient: Diagnosed with schizophrenia at 15.* Onset of schizophrenia before 20 years of age is a poor prognostic factor.
- *Total duration: 10 years:* Course of disease more than 2 years is also a poor prognosis factor.
- *Not recovered fully:* In the presence of prognostic factors, the recovery is usually not fully possible.
- *Family is very supportive:* So this patient can be treated at home after educating the family regarding the nature of illness, its course and treatment.

CONFUSA

Apart from education, family is also given social skills training to enhance communication and decrease family tensions. Family is taught to decrease expectations and to give emotional over-involvement, critical comments and hostility.

Investigation of Choice
None-required.

Immediate Management
Rule out tardive dyskinesia (a side effect of antipsychotics).
Treatment of choice
Education of the patient and family.

Your notes:

114. A 25-year-old patient is admitted. He is depressed and has not been eating/drinking for many days. Has lost weight.

Diagnosis: Severe depression (depressive stupor).

Clinchers

- *A 35-year-old:* In younger patient (<40 years old), psychomotor retardation is more common which is characterised by slowed thinking and activity, decreased energy and monotonous voice.
- *Has not been eating/drinking for many days:* Psychomotor retardation can increase to the point where the person sits motionless and mute—depressive stupor. The person does not eat or drink anything for many days and usually ends in death from dehydration. It calls for an emergency ECT.
- *Lost weight:* This corroborates the diagnosis.

CONFUSA

In older patients agitation is common with marked anxiety, restlessness (inability to sit still, hand-wriggling, picking at body parts or other objects) and subjective feeling of unease.

Investigation of Choice

A routine screening for medical disorders before ECT.

Immediate Management

Parenteral nutrition.
Treatment of choice
Emergency ECT.

Your notes:

115. A 40-year-old patient with features of paranoid schizophrenia.

Diagnosis: Paranoid schizophrenia

Clinchers

- *A 40-year-old:* The onset of paranoid schizophrenia is usually insidious and occurs later in life (i.e. later 3rd and early 4th decade) as compared to other types of schizophrenia.
- *Paranoid schizophrenia:* The course is usually progressive and complete recovery usually does not occur. There may be frequent remissions and relapses. At times, the functional capability may be only slightly impaired.

CONFUSA

Differential diagnosis is from delusional (paranoid) disorders and paranoid personality disorders.

Investigation of Choice

Purely clinical diagnosis however neuroimaging may be done especially in late onset of schizophrenia to rule out a brain lesion.

Immediate Management

Admit (always in paranoid schizophrenia as the patient is a danger to self and others).
Treatment of choice
Antipsychotics
+
Benzodiazepine for paranoid episodes.

Your notes:

116. Arachnophobia.

Diagnosis: Already stated as the question itself.

Clinchers

- Arachnophobia is irrational fear of spiders. Anticipatory anxiety leads to persistant avoidant behaviour, while confrontation with the avoided object or situation leads to panic attack. Gradually, the phobia may spread to other objects or situations. The disorder is diagnosed only if there is marked distress and/or disturbance in daily functioning in addition to fear and avoidance of the specified object or situation.

CONFUSA

Arachnophobia is a specific or simple phobia. Examples of simple a pbobia are:

- Acrophobia—fear of high places
- Zoophobia—fear of animals
- Xenophobia—fear of strangers
- Algopobia—fear of pain
- Claustrophobia—fear of closed placed.

In contrast to agoraphobia and social phobia where the stimuli are generalized, in specific phobia the stimulus is usually circumscribed.

These phobias are more common in women with an onset in late second decade or early third decade. Typically, the onset is sudden without any apparent cause. The cause is usually chronic with gradually increasing restriction of daily activities.

Investigation of Choice

None

Immediate Management

Rebreathing into paper bag if panic attack occurs.

Treatment of choice

Not well established; CBT or MAOI are used.

Your notes:

117. Post-traumatic Stress Disorder (PTSD)

Diagnosis: Already stated as the question

Clinchers

PTSD is a delayed response to an exceptionally severe event (e.g., serious road accident, major disasters like earthquakes). The major symptoms are (according to components).

- Emotion—anxiety, irritability.
- Cognition—flashbacks, nightmares.
- Behaviour—avoidance (of situations associated with trauma).
- Bodily symptoms—exaggerated startle response.
- Associations—substance misuse, depression.

Onset of PTSD is usually after 6 months of the event.

CONFUSA

PTSD became topical in UK and USA because of its prevalence in Vietnam war veterrans. It can be a legal basis for personal injury compensation claims. While diagnosing PTSD in PLAB EMQ never forget to ascertain whether the patient was personally involved in the event himself or not (If not, then it can never be PTSD).

Investigation of Choice

A detailed psychiatric history

Immediate Management

Exclude associated depression or substance misuse.

Treatment of choice

Cognitive behaviour therapy (CBT).

Your notes:

118. Bereavement.

Diagnosis: Grief reaction

Clinchers

Bereavement induces a grief reaction as a normal response and a depressive illness as abnormal response. Three stages of grief have been described.

I. Shock and disbelief
II. Preoccupation and depression
III. Acceptance and resolution.

Note: Recurrence of grief is common around anniversaries.

CONFUSA

Before diagnosis grief reaction always exclude depression which may also follow bereavement.

	Depression	*Grief*
Onset	Delayed	Immediate
Duration	Weeks to years	Weeks to months
Pattern	Denies loss	Gradually accepts loss
Adjustment	Absent	Ultimately ensues
Expression of grief	Difficult	Open
Guilt	Masked	Mild
Psychomotor retardation	+	Absent
Symptom course	Pervasive	Fluctuating
Suicidal thoughts	Common	Transient
Psychotic features	In severe cases	No

Investigation of Choice

A detailed psychiatric history

Immediate Management

Exclude associated depression and anorexia

Treatment of choice

No active intervention requires as it is a normal process, though counselling and support may be required. Antidepressants require only if there is associated depression.

Your notes:

119. A female lawyer is becoming anxious when she has to speak in front of people. This is affecting her work as she needs to speak out in court.

Diagnosis: Anxiety.

Clinchers

- *Becoming anxious when she has to speak in front of people:* It is a type of performance anxiety and has a recognised anxiety provoking stimulus.
- *Affecting her work:* Anxiety is acceptable and require no treatment until and unless it becomes symptomatic, i.e.
  - Affect work/social life
  - Somatization symptoms

CONFUSA

If not treated, she may become less efficient because of her constant performance anxiety. This might lead to more interference with her work more and hence may be predisposed to develop anxiety neurosis.

Investigation of Choice

A detailed psychiatric history.

Immediate Management

Reassurance.

Treatment of choice

Desensitization, i.e. a graded exposure to the anxiety provoking stimulus (behaviour therapy). Anxiolytics may be needed to enable effective work to be done with the patient.

Your notes:

120. This treatment is very affective in endogenous anxiety and phobias.

Diagnosis: Panick attacks associated with phobias.

Clinchers

The drug of choice of panic attacks associated with phobias is MAO inhibitor.

MAO inhibitors act on mono amine oxidase which is responsible for the degradation of catecholamines after reuptake. Their final effects is the same as tricyclic antidepressants, i.e. functional increase in the NE and/or 5HT levels at the receptor site. The increase in brain amine levels is probably responsible for their action.

CONFUSA

It takes 5-10 days before a MAO inhibitor has any evident action. Therefore it is useless to give it on a SOS basis. They must be administered regularly in sufficient doses to achieve desired effect.

Investigation of Choice

A detailed psychiatric history.

Immediate Management

Lorazepam if immediate agitation is present.

Treatment of choice

MAO inhibitors (phenelzine).

Your notes:

155. An elderly man found wandering aimlessly, brought to the A and E by neighbours, who inform that his GP had called on his yesterday.

Diagnosis: Acute psychiatric disturbances

Clinchers

- *Elderly man:* Episodes of acute psychiatric disturbance are much more common in the elderly patients who may have associated dementia or concurrent chronic medical problems or treatments which may precipitate it.
- *Wandering aimlessly:* This signifies disorientation and confusional state.
- *Brought to the A and E by neighbours:* This signifies lack of insight on the part o the patient and thus qualifies as a psychoses. Also it indicates lack of family support at home.
- *His GP had called on him yesterday:* This suggest that he is under some medical treatment. One should contact the GP immediately to enquire about it.

CONFUSA

Behaviour is influenced by the interplay between the environment and psyche and is modified by drugs. A disturbed patient may be suffering from a psychiatric condition, an organic brain lesion, a personality disorder or an emotional upset. The task of the emergency department is to:

- Identify those patients who need immediate therapy
- Support the coping strategies of the patient
- Liaise with the appropriate agency for further care

Investigation of Choice

Blood glucose + EEG

Immediate Management

Contact the GP

Treatment of choice

As per the diagnosis but mainly symptomatic

Your notes:

21 Renal Medicine

PAPER 1

Serial No. 88

Subject: Medicine

Topic: Renal
Question:
Normocytic normochromic anaemia (Hb- 8g/dl)
Reticulocytosis
Fragmented Red Cells
Thrombocytopenia
Urea 7.9mmol/L creatinine 180 micromol/L

Diagnosis: Haemolytic Uremic Syndrome

Clinchers

- *Normocytic normochromic anaemia:* This refers to anaemia with MCV in the range of 76-96 femtolitres. The most common cause for normocytic normochromic anaemia is anaemia of chronic disease, however, the results are interpreted in the light of other lab findings.
- *Hb- 8g/dl:* In HUS, anaemia is severe with haemoglobin in the range of 7-9 g/dl.
- *Reticulocytosis:* Recticulocytosis signify haemolysis as the cause for decreased haemoglobin and subsequent anaemia.
- *Fragmented red cells:* Now, this is signifying the cause of haemolysis being some microangiopathy which is causing intravascular haemolysis and thus, mechanical obstruction causing narrowing of the microvasculature. Fragmented red cells or schistiocytes are typical. In HUS it occurs due to endothelial injury.
- *Thromobocytopenia:* The thrombocytopenia is thought to be a consequence of platelet consumption at sites of endothelial injury.
- *Urea 7.9 mmol/L, creatinine 180 micromol/L:* This is signifying acute renal failure. The triad of acute renal failure with microangiopathic haemolytic anaemia and thrombocytopenia suggests haemolytic uraemic syndrome.

CONFUSA

- Thrombotic Thromobocytopenic purpura also produces a similar picture of thrombocytopenia, microangiopathic haemolytic anaemia with renal and neurological abnormalities. This is usually accompanied by fever.
- While in TTP, the micrangiopathy is usually due aggregation of platelets, obstructing the capillaries, the cause in HUS is due to extensive thrombosis, subsequent to endothelial injury.
- A female(pregnant or on OCPs) presenting with fever, purpura with altered level of consciousness or other neurological abnormality, think of TTP.
- A child presenting with features of renal failure after acute diarrhoeal illness, think of HUS. Purpura not as common feature in HUS than TTP.

Investigation of Choice
Stool culture and detection of 0157: H7 antigen

Immediate Management
Supportive:
Renal failure- maintain adequate fluid; dialysis may be required in severe cases.
Anaemia- small repeated blood transfusions
Hypertension- ACE inhibitors

Treatment of Choice
Volume plasmapheresis with fresh frozen replacement is the treatment of choice

Your notes:

Serial No. 89

Subject: Medicine

Topic: Renal

Question:

Normochromic Normocytic Anaemia

Oliguria

Hypertension

Low erythropoietin

Diagnosis: Chronic renal failure

Clinchers

- *Normochromic normocytic anaemia:* This refers to anaemia with MCV in the range of 76-96 femtolitres. The most common cause for normocytic normochromic anaemia is anaemia of chronic disease, however, the results are interpreted in the light of other lab findings.
- *Oliguria:* This is suggesting impaired renal function, may be the probable cause of the above mentioned findings; normochromic normocytic anaemia being a close accompaniment of chronic renal failure due to decreased renal erythropoietin and accumulating nitrogenous toxins suppressing the bone marrow functions.
- *Hypertension:* Hypertension is very closely related to chronic renal failure. While uncontrolled hypertension can lead to renal failure in the long process, renal insufficiency itself can lead to hypertension usually due to hypervolaemia and occasionally to activation of the renin-angiotensin-aldosterone system.
- *Low erythropoietin:* This is most suggestive of renal parenchymal damage which decreases the renal production of erythropoietin.

CONFUSA

- The most common cause of end-stage renal disease is diabetic nephropathy, followed by hypertensive nephroangiosclerosis and various primary and secondary glomerulopathies.
- Anaemia due to chronic renal failure is different from other causes of anaemia due to chronic disease when it comes to erythropoietin levels. While in CRF erythropoietin levels are low, in other causes of anaemia due to chronic disease, erythropoietin levels are in the higher range.

Investigation of Choice

Serial urea and serum creatinine shows a steady decline in renal function over months or years. FBC, U and Es, urinalysis.

Ultrasound – typically shows small echogenic bilateral kidneys.

Renal biopsy - this investigation may be undertaken, e.g. in patients with chronic renal failure and normal sized kidneys

Immediate Management

Protein restricted diet

Control blood pressure: ACE inhibitors (Target BP <130/80 mm Hg)

Treat anaemia: Human recombinant erythropoietin

Treat Renal osteodystrophy: Phosphate restricted diet, phosphate binders, Vitamin D analogues and calcium supplementation to reduce the risk of tissue calcification

Treat Hyperlipidemia: Statins

Any electrolyte abnormality requires immediate attention.

Treatment of Choice

Long-term renal dialysis

Renal transplantation

Your notes:

Serial No.91

Subject: Medicine

Topic: Renal

Question:

Protaeinuria

Hypercholesterolemia

Generalised oedema

Diagnosis: Nephrotic Syndrome

Clinchers

- *Proteinuria:* The nephrotic syndrome is a renal disorder characterised by heavy urinary protein losses. Proteinuria is usually greater than 3.0 g per 24 hours in adults and 0.05 g/kg/24 hours in children. Hypoalbuminaemia seen in the condition, results mainly from increased catabolism and is not caused only by urinary loss of albumin;
- *Hypercholesterolaemia:* Hypercholesterolaemia is a consistent feature of nephrotic syndrome. It is thought that it results from hypoalbuminaemia due to inhibition of the reaction catalysed by lecithin cholesterol acyltransferase converting cholesterol of high density lipoproteins to cholesterol esters and to an inhibition of high density lipoprotein particle formation from very low density lipoproteins due to reduced activity of lipoprotein lipase.
- *Generalised oedema:* It is mainly due to hypoalbuminaemia and salt-water retention by the kidneys.

CONFUSA

- In severe cases of nephrotic syndrome the proteinuria may be less than 3 g/24 hr (because of low plasma proteins).
- The most common cause of nephrotic syndrome in children is Minimal Change Disease.
- The most common cause of nephrotic syndrome in adults is Memebranous Nephropathy.

Investigation of Choice

Renal function tests to confirm nephrotic syndrome and the severity of conditions.

Battery of tests required to find out the aetiology behind nephrotic syndrome.

Renal biopsy will usually give a definite diagnosis.

Immediate Management

- Treat edema: Diuretics (frusemide 80-250 mg/day PO), Intravenous albumin
- Treat hypertension: ACE inhibitors
- Penicillin prophylaxis.
- Subcutaneous heparin, for the prevention of venous thromboses in the bedbound; warfarin is indicated for symptomatic thrombosis
- Hyperlipidaemia - may resolve with treatment of nephrotic syndrome but may require specific lipid lowering medication.
- Salt restricted diet.

Treatment of Choice

- In children, The standard treatment is with daily with prednisolone 60 mg per square metre for four weeks followed by 40 mg per square metre on 3 of 7 days for a further four weeks.
- In adults, treatment is aimed at treating the underlying condition.

Renal transplantation may be considered in end stage cases.

Your notes:

Serial No. 92

Subject: Medicine

Topic: Renal

Question:

Haematuria, proteinuria

Raised Urea and Creatinine

Hypertension

Diagnosis: Acute Glomerulonephritis

Clinchers

- *Haematuria, proteinuria:* The cardinal feature of all glomerulonephritides is haematuria (microscopic or macroscopic) with red cell casts in the urine. It is usually associated with proteinuria, however, the degree of protein loss is less than what is seen in nephrotic syndrome.
- *Raised urea and creatinine:* This is suggesting acute onset azotemia bcause of decreased glomerulofiltration rate secondary to glomerular damage, usually secondary to immunological causes.
- *Hypertension:* The decreased GFR and avid distal nephron salt and water retention result in expansion of intravascular volume, oedema, and, systemic hypertension.

CONFUSA

- In nephritic syndrome, oedema is usually facial and not as severe as seen in nephritic syndrome.
- Fall in glomerulofiltration rate (GFR) is more characteristic of nephritic syndrome than nephrotic.
- In cases with features of acute glomerulonephritis with haemoptysis, search for autoantibodies directed against the alpha 3 chain of type IV collagen - to rule out Goodpasture's Syndrome.

Investigation of Choice

Extensive investigations required to confirm glomerulonephritis as well as to find out the cause for it.

- Blood tests - FBC; ESR; U+Es; LFTs; CRP; immunoglobulins; serum electrophoresis; complement (C3,C4); autoantibodies - antinuclear antibody (ANA), antineutrophil cytoplasmic antibody (ANCA), anti-double stranded DNA (anti-dsDNA), antiglomerular basement membrane (anti-GBM); HBsAg; antiHCV; antistreptolysin O titre (ASOT); blood culture
- Urine analysis, microscopy (red cell casts - may also be dysmorphic red cells) and culture
- Urine collection — 24 hours collection for creatinine clearance and protein excretion
- Radiological investigation - renal ultrasound, chest X-ray
- Renal biopsy

Immediate Management

Supportive to relieve oedema and hypertension.

Steroids have no role

Treatment of Choice

Aimed at treating/ controling the underlying condition.

Treat the underlying infections when acute glomerulonephritis is associated with chronic infections.

Your notes:

Serial No. 93

Subject: Medicine

Topic: Renal

Question: A 12-year-old boy suffered a blow to his flank during a rugby match. He later complained of one episode of frank haematuria. He is normal otherwise.

Diagnosis: Blunt Injury Kidney

Clinchers

- *12-year-old boy:* Renal trauma in children is more common than in adults, possibly because children tend to have less developed musculoskeletal protection and proportionally larger kidneys than adults.
- *Blow to his flank:* A direct blow to the flank or back is the most common mechanism of injury, and 80% of all renal injuries occur as a result of blunt trauma.
- *Rugby match:* Contact and collision sports are more likely to produce a renal injury, but any sport in which trauma can affect the abdomen or back is risky. Activities most often implicated include skiing, bicycle and motorcycle activities, equestrian sports, football, rugby and mountain climbing.
- *One episode of frank haematuria:* Haematuria is the most common sign following renal injury.It may also be accompanied by flank pain and ecchymosis.
- *Normal otherwise:* This rules out any serious consequences of blunt trauma to the kidney, viz, renal laceration or renal vascular injury. However, initial stable condition may be deceptive and requires high index of suspcion and continuous monitoring.

CONFUSA

- Haematuria in athletes following vigorous activity is not uncommon (don't forget rhabdomyolysis and transient haematuria which is also commonly associated with athletes).
- The first time an athlete is evaluated for this condition, whether it be gross or microscopic in nature, a serial urinalysis at 24 and 48 hours is important. If the urine clears, no further evaluation is necessary.
- Those with progressive symptoms such as flank pain, haematuria lasting more than 48 hours, gross haematuria, prolonged oliguria, or urinary casts need further evaluation with urine culture, imaging studies, and serum renal studies.

Investigation of Choice

CT is the most informative radiologic study and the method of choice in cases of severe renal trauma.

Immediate Management

Rule out any other associated injury to abdominal organs.

Treatment of Choice

Most urologists generally advocate conservative management of renal injury for haemodynamically stable patients who do not have concomitant organ involvement.

Conservative management consists of monitoring the patient's vital signs in a controlled hospital environment.

If coexisting intraperitoneal trauma is present, surgical intervention may be recommended.

Injury to the renal pedicle requires immediate surgical intervention.

Your notes:

Page Kidney:

Page kidney is an accumulation of blood in the perinephric or subcapsular space that results in compression of the involved kidney, renal ischaemia and hypertension.

The name comes from a 1955 report by Engel and Page of a football player who suffered a subcapsular haematoma and subsequently developed hypertension.

Page kidney tends to be found in previously well individuals who develop hypertension and who often have a history of blunt renal trauma.

The pathophysiology of Page kidney is caused by effects on the renin (aldosterone) system.

Surgery is rarely necessary, but fluid should be drained.

PAPER 2

Serial No. 6

Subject: Medicine

Topic: Renal

Question: A 40-year-old man was investigated with cystoscopy which was normal, for recurrent haematuria 15 years ago. He now presents with haematuria and his BP is found to be 180/110.

Diagnosis: Polycystic Kidney Disease (Adult)

Clinchers

- *40-year-old man:* Polycystic Kidney disease is a common inherited(autosomal dominant) disease with a prevalence of about 1 in 1000. It usually presents in adult life in 4th-5th decade.
- *Cystoscopy normal:* This rules out any bladder or urethral pathology which can also present as recurrent hematuria.
- *Recurrent haematuria:* The disease usually presents as gross haematuria due to haemorrhage into a cyst with or without loin pain or discomfort, hypertension and features of uraemia. It is usually self-limited (lasting <1 wk) but recurrent.
- *BP is found to be 180/110:* More than 60-70% of adults are hypertensive before the onset of renal failure.

CONFUSA

The presentation can be easily confused with chronic glomerulonephritis. However, note that, chronic glomerulonephritis presents with gradually worsening renal function characterised by gradually reducing glomerular filtration rate and appearance of features of uraemia. Haematuria which can be present in acute glomerulonephritis is rarely seen in the chronic stage (esp. GROSS haematuria); The triad of recurrent haematuria with loin pain/mass and hypertension is typical for polycystic kideny disease.

Investigation of Choice

Ultrasound

Immediate Management

Control Blood Pressure- ACE inhibitors
Treat UTIs- Antibiotics
Large Cysts - Unroofing of cyst wall helps in decreasing loin pain

Treatment of Choice

Renal Transplant

Serial No. 8

Subject: Medicine

Topic: Renal

Question: A 4-year-old deaf child presents with recurrent haematuria.

Diagnosis: Alport's syndrome (Familial hereditary nephritis)

Clinchers

- *4-year-old:* Alport's syndrome is a familial nephritis characterised by haematuria, progressive renal failure, neurosensory hearing loss, and a group of ocular abnormalities.
- *Deaf child:* Sensorineural deafness begins initially in the high frequency range but progresses to involve the speech range and eventually causes complete deafness.
- *Recurrent haematuria:* Haematuria is the most common presenting symptom.Persistent microscopic haematuria is usually present from early childhood. Episodic gross haematuria, at times precipitated by upper respiratory infections, is common during the first 2 decades of life.

CONFUSA

10% of patients with Alport's syndrome have eye abnormalities including:
-Cataracts
-Anterior lenticonus
-Macular lesions

Investigation of Choice

Urinalysis and microscopy- haematuria and proteinuria
Renal biopsy - light microscopy shows mesangial cell proliferation and capillary wall thickening, progressing to glomerular sclerosis and tubulointerstitial changes. Electron microscopy shows glomerular basement membrane changes (splitting of lamina densa, lamellation)

Immediate Management

None

Treatment of Choice

No treatment is curative.
Control blood pressure
Renal dialysis and transplantation
Arrange genetic counselling

Prognosis: Males usually require renal replacement therapy by age 20-30 years. Females have a normal life span and subclinical hearing loss, but may develop haematuria during the stress of illness or pregnancy.

Serial No. 10

Subject: Medicine

Topic: Renal

Question: A six-year-old has a number of episodes of painless microscopic haematuria with no evidence of a UTI and a normal IVU.

Diagnosis: Benign recurrent haematuria (also known as Essential Haematuria, Thin-Basement-Membrane Nephropathy)

Clinchers

- *Six-year-old:* Thin-Basement-Membrane Nephropathy is a nonprogressive genetic kidney disease that usually begins during childhood.
- *Painless microscopic haematuria:* The disorder is characterized by the presence of haematuria. The blood in the urine may be present in microscopic amounts (microscopic haematuria) and not visible to the eye, present in small amounts that give the urine a "cloudy" or "smoky" appearance, or easily visible (macroscopic).
- *No evidence of a UTI, a normal IVU:* This is a benign condition and usually there is no infection, no proteinuria, renal function is normal and no structural abnormality is present on ultrasound.

CONFUSA

Many individuals with the disorder have abnormalities of the renal glomeruli. In such cases, the basement membrane supporting the loops of capillaries that make up the renal glomeruli may be abnormally thin, thus allowing easy passage of the red blood cells.

Investigation of Choice

Rule out infection or other structural abnormality or glomerulonephritis as a cause for the presenting haematuria.

Immediate Management

Reassurance

Treatment of Choice

None

Your notes:

Serial No. 27

Subject: Medicine

Topic: Anaemia

Question: A 7-year-old child had recurrent urinary tract infection in childhood. He looks pale with a yellowish complexion and his height is at present at the third centile.

Diagnosis: Chronic Renal Failure

Clinchers

- A 7-year-old child: Urinary tract infections are not uncommon in childhood. About 8% or more of girls and about 2% of boys will have a urinary tract infection at some time during childhood. The majority of urinary tract infections occur in the first year of life.
- Recurrent urinary tract infection in childhood: Recurrent urinary tract infection and reflux causes scarring of renal tissue ultimately leading to chronic renal failure.
- Looks pale: Chronic renal failure causes normocytic anaemia with normal reticulocyte count due to lack of erythropoietin
- Yellowish complexion: Yellow brown itchy skin is a characteristic feature of chronic renal failure and occurs due to cutaneous deposition of retained nitrogenous wastes.
- Height is at present at the third centile: Growth failure among patients with chronic renal failure is multifactorial, relating to the age at which chronic renal insufficiency develops, the degree of acidosis, insufficient caloric intake, renal osteodystrophy, and abnormalities of the growth hormone/insulin-like growth factor axis in renal failure.

CONFUSA

Urinary tract infection is an important diagnosis in a child not to be missed because infection may damage the developing kidney.Each year in the UK, 10-20 children enter endstage renal failure programmes because of complications from reflux and chronic pyelonephritis.

Investigation of Choice

USG

Immediate Management

Specialist referral

Treatment of Choice

Symptomatic Treatment:
- Protein restricted diet
- Control of blood pressure- ACE inhibitors are the agents of choice.
- Anaemia - Human recombinant erythropoietin
- Renal osteodystrophy - phosphate binders (e.g. Calcichew (R)) and reduce dietary intake of phosphate (less cheese, eggs, milk);
- Hyperlipidaemia - Statins

Peritoneal dialysis or haemodialysis - required when the patient is in end-stage renal failure
The ultimate treatment is renal transplantation.

Your notes:

Serial No. 98

Subject: Urogenital

Topic: Urolithiasis

Question: A 27-year-old female patient comes to A and E with complaints of severe flank pain. She is restless. The pain radiates to the groin.

Diagnosis: Ureteric Colic

Clinchers
- *27-year-old female:* Urinary calculi prevalence in UK is just 3% and more common in males affecting mainly young in their mid 20s. A later peak is seen at 50 years of age especially in the females.
- *Severe flank pain, radiates to the groin:* Ureteric colic arises due to passage of a solid (commonly, calculi or blood clot) substance from the kidney through the ureters. The pain typically originates in the flanks (loin) and radiates to the groin and testicle in men, and the labia majora in women ('Loin to groin' pain).
- *Restless:* The patient is typically restless and writhing in an attempt to find the most comfortable position, in contrast to acute peritonitis, when the patient lies as still as possible as even slightest movement exaggerates the pain.

CONFUSA

The flank pain in such a setting can also be due to acute pyelonephritis. It also begins similarly, with an acute onset of pain in the loin which radiates to the iliac fossa and suprapubic area. Look carefully for the hints in the question, like fever, chills and rigor, vomiting or renal angle tenderness, which suggest the diagnosis of acute pyelonephritis than just ureteric colic.

Investigation of Choice

X-ray KUB - Screening
Abdominal Ultrasound - to rule out complications like pyelonephritis/ hydronephrosis

Immediate Management

Pain relief - Diclofenac 150 mg orally or per rectal (if vomiting present).
Adequate fluid replacement

Treatment of Choice

Adequate fluid may help most stones pass off the tract by itself.
Larger stones may require surgical interventions like lithotripsy, endoscopy and percutaneous techniques.

Serial No. 104

Subject: Urogenital

Topic: Urolithiasis

Question: A 47-year-old female with bilateral pelvic masses and terminal haematuria.

Diagnosis: Bladder Calculi

Clinchers

- *47-year-old female:* Bladder stones are common in developing countries and rare in UK. It usually affects males more than females with peak at 20 years. A later peak at around 50 years is observed in females and is attributed to infective stones.
- *Bilateral pelvic masses:* The site of impaction if being at the neck of bladder, it can cause back pressure and reflux leading first to bilateral hydronephrosis and later when infection ensues, bilateral pyelonephritis.
- *Terminal haematuria:* This is the most important sign of bladder stone. The haematuria is usually at the end of the micturation, when the stone tries to follow the urethral tract with the flow of the urine and injuring the mucosa on its way. The haematuria in bladder cancer occurs throughout the flow (not terminal).

CONFUSA

The presence of upper urinary tract calculi is not necessarily a predisposition to the formation of bladder stones. Stones in the bladder are often formed *in situ*, rather than originating from the upper tracts. Stones that DO reach the bladder from the upper tracts are likely to pass easily down the urethra.

Investigation of Choice

X-ray KUB - Screening

Abdominal Ultrasound - to rule out complications like pyelonephritis/ hydronephrosis

Immediate Management

Urinary analysis to know the nature of stones - oxalate, uric acid or pigment stones.

Analgesics to control associated pain.

Adequate fluid to maintain hydration.

Treatment of Choice

The only potentially effective medical treatment for bladder calculi is urinary alkalinization for the dissolution of uric acid stones. Stone dissolution may be possible if the urinary pH is greater than or equal to 6.5. Potassium citrate at 60 mEq/d is commonly used. Endoscopy is the surgical intervention of choice. Small stones may simply be washed out of the bladder via a cystoscope. Larger stones must first be fragmented. Traditionally, this is done by litholapaxy or ESWL (requires full bladder).

Your notes:

PAPER 3

12. A febrile 39-year-old woman with hypertension, has a history of recurrent urinary tract infections. Abdominal ultrasound showed a dilated calyx.

Diagnosis: Pyonephrosis.

Clinchers

- *Febrile:* It signifies a purulent infection.
- *39-year-old:* Pyonephrosis is most commonly secondary to an obstructing ureteral stone. It produces hydronephrosis which in turn gets infected (especially by Proteus) due to stagnation of urine. The peak age of incidence is 20-50 years.
- *Woman:* The incidence of renal calculi in females is four times less than males. In this case there is history of recurrent UTI which can produce a benign ureteral stricture/functional obstruction to produce an infected hydronephrosis (pyonephrosis).
- *Dilated calyx:* It is due to back pressure due to obstruction and is a characteristic finding in hydronephrosis.

CONFUSA

The contentious feature in this case can be the presence of hypertension. It could be totally unrelated to this condition or due to scarring by previous episodes of nephritis secondary to UTI.

Investigation of Choice

IVU

- Little or no function
- Enlarged renal shadow

DMSA scintigraphy—will quantify residual function in the kidney after treatment.

Immediate Management

Antipyretics.

Treatment of Choice

- Urgent drainage by percutaneous nephrostomy.
- If no residual renal function—nephrectomy.

Your notes:

34. A man involved in a mining accident presents with oliguria and passing dark brown urine.

Diagnosis: Acute tubular necrosis secondary to rhabdomyolysis.

Clinchers

- *Mining accident:* Mining accident can produce urinary symptoms commonly in two ways:
  1. Direct urethral injury (due to pelvic fracture)
  2. Rhabdomyolysis secondary to crush injury.
- *Oliguria:* Oliguria in this case can be due to either:
  1. Urethral trauma and hence rentention
  2. ATN
- *Dark brown urine:* It is due to appearance of myoglobin (a muscle protein) in urine. It is released on muscle injury (crush injury) or necrosis or reperfusion of an ischaemic limb.

CONFUSA

Dark urine which is positive for blood on dipstick but without RBCs on microscopy can be confusing, but it is a characteristic finding in rhabdomyolysis. Urethral trauma can be safely excluded as there will be retention and fresh red blood on meatus.

Investigation of Choice

Dipstick test and microscopy for urine.

Immediate Management

Large volumes of IV fluids

+

IV mannitol/IV bicarbonate

Treatment of choice

Haemodialysis/filtration if required.

Your notes:

37. A 40-year-old man with a blood pressure of 180/115 is found to have a loud bruit in his right upper abdomen.

Diagnosis: Right renal artery stenosis.

Clinchers

- *A 40-year-old:* The most common causes of renal artery stenosis is atherosclerosis. It is common in age > 50 years though cases may be seen in younger ages (as in this case). Fibromuscular dysplasia is another cause seen in younger females (20-30 yrs).
- *Blood pressure of 180/115:* Unilateral renal ischaemia results in reduction in the pressure in afferent glomerular arterioles. This leads to an increase in the production and release of renin from the juxta-glomerular apparatus with a consequent increase in angiotensin II. This leads to systemic hypertension.
- *Loud bruit in his right upper abdomen:* It is due to stenosis in the involved renal artery. Coexistent carotid or femoral bruits are present if the cause is atherosclerosis. Leg pulses may be absent due to coexistent peripheral vascular disease.

CONFUSA

The presence of a loud bruit in right upper abdomen clinches the diagnosis here. But if there is no mention of it in a question with suggestion towards renal hypertension, then the only other differential (for unilateral disease) is reflux nephropathy.

Investigation of Choice

- *Screening:* Spiral CT/MRI
- *Definitive:* Renal angiography (Gold standard)

Immediate Management

Hypotensive therapy (ACE inhibitors contraindicated).

Treatment of Choice

Percutaneous transluminal renal angioplasty or surgery.

Your notes:

141. Middle-aged man with haematuria and colicky left loin pain.

Diagnosis: Renal colic.

Clinchers

- *Middle-aged man:* Fifty percent of patients of renal colic present between the ages of 30 until and 50 years. The male: female ratio is 4: 3.
- *Haematuria:* Haematuria is sometimes a leading symptom of stone disease and occasionally the only one. As a rule the amount of feeding is small. Other causes of haematuria are:
  - Kidney
    - Glomerular diseases
    - Polycystic kidney
    - Carcinoma
    - Stone
    - Trauma (including renal biopsy)
    - Vacuolar malformation
    - Embolism
    - Renal vein thrombosis
  - Ureter
    - Stone
    - Neoplasm
  - Bladder
    - Carcinoma
    - Stone
    - Trauma
    - Inflammatory, e.g. TB, cystitis, schistosomiasis
  - Prostate
    - Benign prostatic hypertrophy
    - Carcinoma
  - Urethra
    - Trauma
    - Stone
    - Urethritis
    - Neoplasm
  - General
    - Anticoagulant therapy
    - Thrombocytopenia
    - Haemophilia
    - Sickle cell disease
    - Malaria
    - Exercise (heavy)
  - Red urine
    - Haemoglobinuria
    - Myoglobinuria
    - Acute intermittent prophyria
    - Beet root
    - Senna

- Phenolphthalein
- Rifampicin

➢ *Colicky left loin pain:* Ureteric colic is an agonising pain passing from loin to groin. It starts suddenly and may be associated with strangury (painful passage of few drops of urine). Colic pain is the result of smooth muscle contraction against a resistance. Common causes of colicky pain are

- Biliary tract
  - Stone in Hartmann's pouch
  - Stone in cystic duct
  - Stone in ampula of Vater
- Renal tract
  - Ureteric colic due to stone, blood clot or tumour
- Intestinal tract
  - Mechanical obstruction
  - Appendicular colic as appendix lumen occludes
- Uterus
  - Parturition
  - Menstruation
  - Ectopic pregnancy in fallopian tube

Investigation of Choice

Radiography (plain films of kidneys, ureter and bladder) [KUB film]. Following radiography, excretion urography may be done to confirm calculus and its location. USG scanning can be performed in locating stones.

Your notes:

PAPER 4

22. Man who is not able to pass urine, tired, complains of hiccups.

Diagnosis: Renal failure.

Clinchers

➢ *Not able to pass urine:* Oliguria (urine output < 400 ml/d) is a frequent but not invariable feature of acute renal failure.

➢ *Complains of hiccups:* Hiccups occur when there is increased retention of nitrogenous waste products. In renal failure, there is increase in plasma urea and creatine concentration.

Features suggestive of chronic renal failure include anaemia, neuropathy, radiological evidence of renal osteodystrophy or small scared kidney.

CONFUSA

Renal failure may cause high anion gap acidosis, poor filtration and reabsorption of organic onions contribute to the pathogenesis. In this question the answer could have been metabolic acidosis, if renal failure was not amongst the options.

Investigation of Choice

- Blood urea and S creatinine
- Arterial blood gas (ABG) analysis
- Selectrolyte

Immediate Management

In case of acidosis, replace alkali ($NaHCO_3$), to maintain (CHO_3^-) between 20 and 24 mmol/L.

Treatment of choice

- Identify the cause of ARF
- Eliminate triggering insult (e.g., nephrotoxin) and/or institute disease specific therapy.
- Prevent and manage uraemic complications
- Metabolic acidosis is not treated unless, serum bicarbonate concentration falls below 15 mmol/L or arterial pH falls below 7.2.

Your notes:

107. Autosomal dominant.

Diagnosis: Polycystic kidney disease (PKD)

Clinchers

Adult polycystic kidney disease is an autosomal dominant disease characterised by multiple expanding cysts of both kidneys that ultimately destroy the renal parenchyma and cause renal failure. It is a common condition affecting roughly 1 out of every 400 to 1000 live births an accounting for about 10% of cases of chronic renal failure requiring transplantation or dialysis. The pattern of inheritance is autosomal dominant with high penetrance. The disease is universally bilateral, reported unilateral cases probably represent multicystic dysplasia.

➢ *Clinical features*
- Episodic flank pain
- Haematuria (often gross)
- Hypertension
- Urinary infection in third or fourth decade

➢ *Associations*
- Hepatic cysts
- Intracranial berry aneurysms

➢ *Genes of chromosome*
- 16 (PKD 1)
- 4 (PKD 2)

CONFUSA

The cysts intially involve only portions of the nephrons, so that the renal function is retained until about the fourth or fifth decade of life. The likelihood of developing renal failure is less than 2% in affected individuals younger than 40 years but rises to 25% by age 50 years, 40% by 60 years, and 75% by age 70 to 75 years.

Investigation of Choice

USG

Immediate Management

Monitor BP and U and E

Treatment of Choice
- Treat infections
- Dialysis/transplantation for end stage renal failure

Your notes:

109. Deposition of immune complexes on basement membrane.

Diagnosis: Glomerulonephritis

Clinchers

Renal disease is the most common secondary cause of hypertension. 3/4 cases are from intrinsic renal disease of which glomerulonephritis is the most common. In glomerulonephritis, IgA; nephropathy is the most common one worldwide and is characterised by deposition of immune complexes on the basement membranes.

CONFUSA

The cardinal feature of glomerulonephritis is haematuria (which may be microscopic), with red cells casts in urine.

Investigation of Choice
- *Screening:* Urine analysis and microscopy (red cell casts ± dysmorphic red cells)
- *Definitive:* Biopsy and immunofluorescence

Immediate Management

Refer to a nephrologist for management

Keep BP $\leq$ 130/80.

Treatment of Choice

Depends upon underlying condition.

Your notes:

PAPER 5

48. An elderly man underwent an emergency repair of an abdominal aortic aneurysm. He had been severely hypotensive before and during surgery. After surgery, his blood pressure was satisfactory, but urine output only 5 ml/hr in the first 2 hours.

Diagnosis: Acute tubular necrosis (Ischaemic).

Clinchers

- *Emergency repair of an abdominal aortic aneurysm:* This means that the repair was undertaken after an aneurysmal rupture or acute aortic expansion. Either of these produce a severe hypotension. Moreover, during the surgery the renal arterial ostia are often compressed when the aorta is clamped and are thus rendered ischaemic for the duration of cross clamping. The left renal vein may be ligated and divided as part of the operative procedure. Hypotension pre-or postoperatively may exacerbate the renal injury.
- *Severely hypotensive before and during surgery:* Circulatory compromise produces renal hypoperfusion and thence ischaemic necrosis of the tubules.
- *After surgery, his BP was satisfactory:* This rules out any continuing ischaemia and a need for urgent intervention. Also it suggests a definitive injury to the kidney.
- *Urine output only 5 ml/hr in first 2 hours:* Urine output should be >30 mL/hr postoperatively. A value significantly lower than this suggests renal dysfunction (due to hypoperfusion or ATN).

CONFUSA

Low urine output (if there is no ATN) postoperatively is almost always due to inadequate infusion of fluid. One should check JVP, and review for sings of cardiac failure. Treat by increasing IVI rate unless patient is in heart or renal failure, or profusely bleeding (in that case, blood should be transfused). If in doubt a fluid challenge may be indicated: ½-1 L over 30-60 minutes, with monitoring of urine output. Then the IVI rate may be increased to 1 litre/h for 2-3 h. Only if output does not increase should a diuretic be considered; a CVP line may be needed if estimation of fluid balance is difficult. A normal value is 0-5 cm of water relative to the sternal angle.
Note: If not catheterised exclude retention.

Investigation of Choice

Urinary sodium concentration (It differentiates whether the oliguria is prerenal and amenable to fluid therapy or a result of acute tubular necrosis—urinary Na >40 mmol/L.

Immediate Management

Perform an aseptic catheterisation
+
early specialist (nephrologist and interminist) referral

Treatment of choice

Supportive until spontaneous recovery of renal function occurs.

Your notes:

116. A 45-year-old man is diagnosed as having a kidney condition and treated. He soon develops postural hypotension with ankle oedema. His serum sodium is high, his potassium normal, his urea normal, and he has heavy proteinuria.

Diagnosis: Nephrotic syndrome (NS)

Clinchers

- *A 45-year-old man:* Although proliferative glomerulonephritis is more common than membranous disease, the later is the most common form of glomerulonephritis to cause nephrotic syndrome in UK. Diabetic glomerular disease can also cause it in a middle aged person.
- *Having a kidney condition and treated:* It must be a glomerular nephritis which was treated.
- *Postural hypotension:* It can occur due to autonomic dysfunction and hypovolaemia.
- *Ankle oedema:* It is characteristically seen and is due to hypoalbuminaemia.
- *Serum Na^+ high, potassium normal, urea normal:* Activation of renin-angiotensin-aldosterone system produces hyperaldosteronism which promotes sodium and water reabsorption in the distal nephron.
- *Heavy proteinuria:* It occurs partly because structural damage to the glomerular basement membrane leads to an increase in size and number of pores, allowing passage of more and larger molecules. Reduction of fixed negative charge occurs in glomerular disease and is an important factor in genesis of heavy proteinuria.

CONFUSA

Neither elevation of JVP nor pulmonary oedema are features of nephrotic syndrome, through they either or both may be present if renal and/or cardiac failure are present in the nephrotic patient.

Investigation of Choice

- *Screening:* 24-hour urinary protein (>3-4 g/day)
- *Definitive:* Transcutaneous renal biopsy

Immediate Management

Diuresis (but is contraindicated here because of postural hypotension).

Treatment of Choice

Dietary sodium restriction + albumin infusion

159. An 83-year-old man with small cell lung cancer presents with ankle oedema and is found to have 8 g/day, urine proteinuria. He is started on frusemide. 10 days later his blood pressure is 115/75 mmHg lying and 85/65 mmHg standing. Serum biochemistry was; Sodium 121 mmol/L, bicarbonate 24 mmol/L, potassium 3.6 mmol/L, Creatinine 113 mmol/L, chloride 95 mmol/L, Urea 11.5 mmol/L, Glucose 5.7 mmol/L, albumin 27 g, osmolality 263 mOs m/L, urine osmolality 417 mOs m/L.

Diagnosis: Dilutional hyponatremia with nephrotic syndrome

Clinchers

- *A 83-year-old woman:* Incidence of most of the malignancies increases with increasing age.
- *Small cell lung cancer:* SIADH is mostly associated with four malignancies, i.e.
  - Small cell lung carcinoma
  - Pancreas
  - Prostate
  - Lymphoma
- *Ankle oedema + 8g/day urine proteinuria:* Daily urinary protein excretion is < 150 mg in normal persons. This massive proteinuria along with ankle oedema is characteristic of nephrotic syndrome.
- *Frusemide:* Excess diuretics administration can produce a dilutional hyponatremia with electrolyte profile similar to SIADH.
- *10 days later:* Dilutional hyponatraemia develops after repeated administration of the offending diuretic over days.
- *Sodium 121 mmol/L:* Low, as it is dilutional hyponatraemia.
- *BP 115/75 mmHg lying and 85/65 mmHg standing:* Orthostatic hypotension is present in nephrotic syndrome usually.
- *Bicarbonate 24 mmol/L:* Normal.
- *Potassium 3.6 mmol/L:* Normal.
- *Creatinine 113 µmol/L:* Normal.
- *Chloride 95 mmol/L:* Normal.
- *Urea 11.5 mmol/L:* Increased owing to nephrotic syndrome.
- *Glucose 5.7 mmol/L:* Normal.
- *Albumin 27 g:* Low, owing to nephrotic syndrome.
- *Serum osmolality 263 mOsm/L:* Low (normal 278-305) but do not quality for SIADH which is < 260 osmol/L. It is low because of dilutional hyponatraemia.
- *Urine osmolality 417 mOsm/L:* It suggest concentrated urine but not > 500 mOsm/L to suggest SIADH.

CONFUSA

SIADH is an important, but overdiagnosed, caused of hyponatraemia. The diagnosis of SIADH requires, the absence of hypovolaemia oedema, or diuretics. SIADH must always be distinguished from dilutional hyponatremia.

Investigation of Choice
Serum electrolytes.

Immediate Management
Stop diuretics or reset their dose.

Treatment of Choice
Treat the cause + fluid restriction.

Your notes:

PAPER 6

67. Man who is not able to pass urine, tired, complains of hiccups.

Diagnosis: Renal failure.

Clinchers

- *Not able to pass urine:* Oliguria (urine output < 400 mL/d) is a frequent but not invariable feature of acute renal failure.
- *Complains of hiccups:* Hiccups occur when there is increased retention of nitrogenous waste products. In renal failure, there is increase in plasma urea and creatine concentration.

Features suggestive of chronic renal failure include anaemia, neuropathy, radiological evidence of renal osteodystrophy or small scared kidney.

CONFUSA

Renal failure may cause high anion gap acidosis, poor filtration and reabsorption of organic onions contribute to the pathogenesis. In this question the answer could have been metabolic acidosis, if renal failure was not amongst the options.

Investigation of Choice

- Blood urea and S creatinine
- Arterial blood gas (ABG) analysis
- S electrolyte

Immediate Management
In case of acidosis, replace alkali ($NaHCO_3$), to maintain (CHO_3^-) between 20 and 24 mmol/L.
Treatment of choice

- Identify the cause of ARF
- Eliminate triggering insult (e.g. nephrotoxin) and/or institute disease specific therapy.
- Prevent and manage uraemic complications
- Metabolic acidosis is not treated unless, serum bicarbonate concentration falls below 15 mmol/L or arterial pH falls below 7.2.

Your notes:

154. Man with prostate Ca which has extended outside the capsule presenting with features of renal failure.

Diagnosis: Bladder outflow obstruction (BOO).

Clinchers

- *Prostate carcinoma which has extended outside capsule:* It means that it is a locally advanced disease. Bladder base is a frequent site of prostatic metastases. Otherwise also, prostatic enlargement due to carcinomatous growth can produce BOO.
- *Features of renal failure:* The obstruction to outflow of the bladder may result in renal failure with drowsiness, headache and impairment of intellect due to uraemia.

CONFUSA

Pain is not a symptom of BOO and its presence should prompt the exclusion of acute retention, urinary infection stones 3carcinoma of the prostate and carcinoma *in situ* of the bladder (1242, Bailey and Love, 23rd Edn).

Investigation of Choice

Pressure-flow urodynamic studies

Immediate Management

Suprapubic catheterisation

Treatment of choice

Prostatectomy.

Your notes:

PAPER 7

1. A 60-year-old woman hypertensive was started on antihypertensive 2 weeks ago. Now has a creatinine level of 500 micromol/L.

Diagnosis: Acute renal failure

Clinchers

- *On antihypertensive 2 week ago:* Angiotensin converting enzyme activity inhibition (ACE inhibitors) and renal prostaglandin biosynthesis (cyclooxygenase inhibitor) inhibitors are the major culprits, leading to renal hypoperfusion, leading to prerenal azotemia.

  Captopril is an ACE inhibitor that lowers the BP.

  Captopril induces hypotension as a result of decrease in total peripheral resistance. Both systolic and diastolic BP falls.
- *Creatinine level of 500 Hmol/L:* Normal value of creatinine in plasma ranges between 70-≤ 150 mmol/L. Recent increase in the plasma urea and creatinine concentration are the biochemical indictors of acute renal failure.

CONFUSA

On captopril, renal blood flow is not compromised even when BP falls substantially, but for him patients with bilateral renal artery stenosis due to dilatation of efferent arterioles and fall in glomerular filtration pressure; contraindicated in such patients.

Investigation of Choice

- Blood tests: U and E, FBC, creatinine, blood culture.
- Urine: Microscopy and biochemical tests.
- ECG (hyperkalemia).

Immediate Management

- Change in antihypertensive therapy.
- Adjust doses of renally excreted drugs.

  Manage complications, (hyperkalemia, pulmonary oedema, bleeding). Seek specialist help sooner rather than later.

Drug producing this condition

Captopril.

Your Notes

2. A child with recurrent nephrotic syndrome is brought for treatment. 3 weeks after start of treatment, he now has massive haematuria.

Diagnosis: Haemorrhagic cystitis

Clinchers

- *Child with recurrent nephrotic syndrome:* Minimal change disease accounts for 80% of nephrotic syndrome in children. MCD is highly steroid responsive, but relapses occur in 50% of cases following withdrawal of glucocorticoids. In such patients upto fail to achieve lasting remission, alkylating agents are usual. *Cyclophosphamide* (2 to 3 mg/kg per day) or chlorambucil (0.1 to 0.2 mg/kg per day) is started after steroid induced remission and continued for 8 to 12 weeks.
- *Now develops massive haematuria:* Microscopic haematuria may be present in MCD (in 20-30 percent cases). But massive haematuria here is a sign of cystitis, which may occur with the use of cyclophosphamide.

CONFUSA

The benefits of cyclophosphamide must be balanced against risk of infertility, cystitis, alopecia, infection and secondary malignancies.

Investigation of Choice

Cystoscopy.

Immediate Management

Stop cyclophospamide.

Treatment of Choice

Long-term renal and patient survival is excellent in MCD. Titrate the risk of cyclophosphamide, otherwise MCD is highly steroid.

Drug producing this condition

Cyclophosphamide.

Your Notes

3. A patient in severe renal failure has potassium level of 2.5 mmol/L.

Diagnosis: Hypokalemia (Answer: frusemide)

Clinchers

- *Severe renal failure:* May be due to glomerulonephritis, pyelonephritis, interstitial nephritis, DM, hypertension, cystic diseases, etc. In CRF there is usually, irreversible and long-standing loss of renal function. In CRF treatment is aimed at treating reversible causes (relieve obstruction, stop nephrotoxic drugs, treat hypercalcaemia). High does of loop diuretics (furosemide) are used to treat oedema.
- *Potassium level of 2.5:* Normal range of potassium is 3.5-5 mmol/L. Hypokalaemia is the most significant problem with high ceiling diuretics (frusemide) and thiazides. Usual manifestations of hypokalaemia are weakness, fatigue, muscle cramps and cardiac arrhythmias.

CONFUSA

Hypokalaemia is less common with standard doses of high ceiling diuretics (frusemide), than with thiazides, possibly because of shorter duration of action of the former which permits intermittent operation of compensatory reflection mechanism.

Investigation of Choice

- Blood: FBC, ESR, U and E, Creatinine, S calcium
- Urine: Microscopy, creatinine clearance
- Renal ultrasound

Immediate Management

Change frusemide with potassium sparing Diuretics

Treatment of Choice

For hypokalaemia: Attempt to maintain serum K^+ at or above 3.5 mEq/L, by:

- High dietary K^+ intake
- Supplements of KCl (24-72 mEq/day) or
- Concurrent use of K^+ sparing diuretics

Your Notes

4. Patient with complaint of ataxia and tinnitus with mild hearing loss. He has moderate renal failure.

Diagnosis: Ototoxicity (Answer: Gentamicin)

Clinchers

Aminoglycoside antibiotics (gentamicin) have a narrow therapeutic index. Most important side effects being nephrotoxicity and ototoxicity. Rarely respiratory depression may be observed.

Nephrotoxicity is manifested clinically by a gradual rise in serum creatinine levels after a few days of therapy.

Ototoxicity from aminoglycosides therapy presents as either auditory or vestibular damage.

CONFUSA

Fear to toxicity should not prevent the use of aminoglycosides for a legitimate indication, since toxicity is usually mild and reversible.

Investigation of Choice

- Serum concentration of gentamicin
- Blood urea and serum creatinine

Immediate Management

Stop gentamicin. When serum concentrations are monitored and duration of therapy kept minimum, then adverse effect are unlikely.

Treatment of choice

Stop gentamicin. No other intervention required, since the toxicity is usually mild and reversible.

Your Notes

5. A fit 50-year-old man is prescribed oral acetazolamide by an ophthalmologist for suspected glaucoma. He presents with lethargy and shortness of breath on exertion. Sodium 140 mmol/L, potassium 3.2 mmol/L, bicarbonate 18 mmol/L, chloride 115 mmol/L, urea 6.7 mmol/L, creatinine 114 mmol/L.

Diagnosis: Type II renal tubular acidosis (Proximal RTA).

Clinchers

- *Fit 50-year-old man:* Excludes any pre-existing pathology to be the cause of this condition.
- *Oral acetazolamide:* Acetazolamide causes increased renal bicarbonate losses. Hence it is the most probable cause in this case.
- *Lethargy and shortness of breath on exertion:* These are due to hypokalemia and acidosis respectively.
- *Sodium 140 mmol/L:* Normal.
- *Potassium 3.5 mmol/L:* Low, as hypokalaemia is a feature.
- *Bicarbonate 18 mmol/L:* Low as acetazolamide - renal losses.
- *Urea 6.7 mmol/L:* Normal, but still on higher side (range 2.5-6.7 mmol/L).
- *Creatinine 114 mmol/L:* Normal.

CONFUSA

Renal tubular acidosis generally may be secondary to immunological drug-induced or structural damage to the tubular cells, an inherited abnormality, or an isolated (primary) abnormality. As with most disorders which are not well-understood, the nomenclature is confusing.

Investigation of Choice

Urinary pH and serum electrolytes.

Immediate Management

Discontinue acetazolamide if still taking.

Treatment of choice

Sodium bicarbonate (massive doses may be required to overcome the renal 'leak').

Your Notes

33. Female patient with complaint of sever flank pain, is restless and the pain radiates to the groin.

Diagnosis: Uraeteric colic.

Clinchers

- *Female:* Renal calculi is four times more common in males, than females (E: G » 4: 1). And therefore female, cannot be excluded here. With peak age between 20-50 years.
- *Flank pain, restless, radiating to groin:* Stone in kidney cause loin pain. Stones in ureter cause ureteric colic. Here pain classically radiates from loin to the groin and is associated with nausea and vomiting.

Some important risk factors for renal calculi are: dehydration, UTI, hypercalcaemia, hypercalciuria, -dietary oxalate.

CONFUSA

The diagnosis should be confirmed by abdominal KUB film and ultrasound. In KUB film 80% of stones are visible (97% on CT).

Investigation of Choice

- Abdominal KUB film
- Ultrasound
- Blood: U and E, Ca^{2+}, PO_4^{3-}
- 24 h urine: Creatinine, Ca^{2+}, oxalate, urate.

Immediate Management

- IV fluids (if not accepting orally)
- Analgesia
- If evidence of obstruction, seek urological help urgently

Treatment of Choice

Increase fluid intake. If no obstruction f/w attacks, manage conservatively.

- *Ureteric stones:* Usually pass spontaneously or remove endoscopically
- *Pelvicalyceal stones*
  - < 5 mm—no treatment, unless obstruction/ infection
  - < 2 cm—lithotripsy
  - 2-4 cm—with normal collecting ducts—go for lithotripsy (take measure to prevent obstruction)
- *Renal colic:* IV fluids (oral if tolerating) + analgesia
- *Evidence of obstruction*: Seek urological help (retrograde stent insertion, nephrostomy and antegrade pyelography).

Your notes:

22 Respiratory Medicine

PAPER 1

Serial No. 64

Subject: Medicine

Topic: Chest Medicine

Question: Man with right lower lobe pneumonia, is allergic to penicillin.

Diagnosis: Right lower lobe pneumonia

Clinchers

- *Right lower lobe pneumonia:* Community acquired pneumonia is a common disease with a reducing incidence. It usually occurs in children or the elderly, or in people with an underlying pathology. Most common cause of community acquired pneumonia is pneumococcal pneumonia.
- *Allergic to penicillin:* For uncomplicated community-acquired pneumonia, amoxicillin remains the first choice in the UK. In patients allergic to penicillin, a suitable alternative is erythromycin 500 mg qds PO or clarithromycin 500 mg bd.

CONFUSA

- Erythromycin is also preferred when atypical pneumonia is suspected.
- When staphylococcal pneumonia suspected (i.e. post influenza or post measles pneumonia), add flucloxacillin.
- Substitute erythromycin with clarithromycin in cases of gastrointestinal intolerance to oral erythromycin.

Investigation of Choice

Chest X-ray

Immediate Management

Start blind therapy before culture/Gram stain reports:

- For community acquired:
  Mild cases: treated with oral amoxycillin 500 mg tds and erythromycin 500 mg qds.
  Severe cases: treated with I.V. ampicillin 1 g and erythromycin 500 mg qds, if no previous influenza epidemic; otherwise, with I.V. cefuroxime 1.5 g qds and erythromycin 500 mg qds.
- For hospital acquired:
  Cefuroxime is the drug of first choice. Include metronidazole if the clinical state does not improve because of the likelihood of anaerobes. Immunosuppressed patients may require high dose broad spectrum antibiotics, antifungal and antiviral agents.

Treatment of Choice

According to culture report.

Your notes:

Serial No. 65

Subject: Medicine

Topic: Chest Medicine

Question: A HIV positive drug abuser with shortness of breath and bilateral expanding shadows on CXR.

Diagnosis: Pneumocystis carinii Pneumonia (PCP)

Clinchers

- *Drug abuser:* drug abuser (intravenous) are more at the risk of contracting HIV and develop complications resulting from that. However, intravenous drug abuse can also predispose individuals to pneumonia (or other infections) from the skin commensals like Staphylococcous, fungi, etc.
- *HIV positive:* This confirms our suspect that the patient is in an immunocompromised state. PCP is more common in HIV positive individuals with CD 4 count less than 200 and not on PCP prophylaxis.
- *Shortness of breath:* It classically presents with dyspnoea on exertion and dry cough.
- *Bilateral expanding shadows on CXR:* The classic finding is diffuse perihilar alveolar or interstitial infiltrates. However, it can present from almost no findings on CXR to extensive bilateral consolidation.

CONFUSA

- PCP is an AIDS defining illness.
- PCP prophylaxis is indicated if CD 4 counts fall below 200/microlitre or less than 20% of total lymphocyte count or after an episode of PCP.
- Most effective agent for both treatment and prophylaxis is Cotrimoxazole. Pentamidine is used only if cotrimoxazole is not tolerated.

Investigation of Choice

Bronchioalveolar lavage with silver staining to demonstrate organisms.

Gallium scan help in diagnosisng relapse.

Immediate Management

Patients with hypoxaemia with a PO_2 less than 60 mmHg should be hospitalised.

Administer oxygen.

Treatment of Choice

- First-line treatment: IV co-trimoxazole
- Second line treatment: pentamidine I
  However, note that pentamidine has serious adverse effects including cardiac arrhythmias, hypotension, pancreatitis, thrombocytopaenia, neutropaenia, hypoglycaemia, hypocalcaemia and acute renal failure and should be monitored carefully.
- In cases of moderate or severe PCP (i.e. patient is hypoxic) then patients should also receive prednisolone 40 mg bd for 5 days - then withdrawn over 2 weeks. This has been shown to reduce the mortality and morbidity.

Your notes:

Serial No. 66

Subject: Medicine

Topic: Chest Medicine

Question: An alcoholic comes with haemoptysis and chronic cough; CXR shows right upper lobe consolidation.

Diagnosis: Tuberculosis

Clinchers

- *Alcoholic:* The risk of tuberculosis increases in states of poor health and poor immune system. Malnutrition and alcoholism usually go together.
- *Haemoptysis, chronic cough:* Pulmonary tuberculosis is hallmarked by chronic productive cough, haemoptysis, breathlessness and systemic features of fever, malaise and night sweats.
- *Right upper lobe consolidation:* The mycobacteriae classically like the 'airy' areas of the lung; Upper lobe cavitation/consolodation is almost pathognomoic of tuberculosis.

CONFUSA

- Tuberculosis is a notifiable disease in UK. In all suspected cases it is necessary to obtain relevant clinical samples (sputum, pleural fluid) to establish the diagnosis.
- Tuberculosis usually does not occur in immunocompetent individuals; rule out causes of immunosuppression among the affected. Advise HIV testing.
- TB is an AIDS definig illness.

Investigation of Choice

CXR - typical radiological features diagnostic of tuberculosis

Sputum AFB to confirm diagnosis.

Heaf and Tine tests and Mantoux test is only for screening.

Immediate Management

Rule out immunosuppression.

Contact tracing of household members and close contacts.

Treatment of Choice

Antituberculous therapy

Your notes:

Serial No. 67

Subject: Medicine

Topic: Chest

Question: A 53-year-old business executive develops acute onset breathlessness, myalgia and dry cough. Chest X-ray shows bibasal consolidation.

Diagnosis: Legionella Pneumonia

Clinchers

- *53-year-old:* Men are more commonly affected than females; mean age of affection being around 52 years, incidence and mortality associated with the disease increases with age.
- *Business executive:* This puts him at high risk for developing the disease as Legionella is an airborne infection with the bacterium living in air-conditioning systems, whirlpool spas and domestic hot water systems in large buildings. The typical presentation is of a previously fit adult male falling sick after attending some meeting/ seminar.
- *Acute onset breathlessness, myalgia:* The disease begins classically after an icubation period of 2-10 days with features similar to that of flu. Some patients may also complain of gastrointestinal symptoms of nausea, vomiting and diarrhoea; altered mental status and cranial/ peripheral neuropathy are not uncommon. Occasionally haematuria and renal failure may be associated.
- *Dry cough:* Cough is initially dry and non-productive, later becoming productive and patient may even develop haemoptysis.
- *CXR shows bibasal consolidation:* classical presentation; but radiological features are usually mild or even absent compared to physical findings.

CONFUSA

- Pontiac fever is a milder illness caused by this same legionella bacteria.
- It causes a flu-like illness which lasts just a few days. Symptoms include: fever, shivers, headache, muscle aches, tiredness and a dry cough.
- The infection does not affect the lung.
- No treatment is needed other than paracetamol or ibuprofen to ease a fever and muscle aches.

Investigation of Choice

- Urinary antigen detection
- Four fold increase in antibody titre, at 2 to 5 weeks

- Immunoflourescent staining of the organism in the pleural fluid, sputum or bronchial washings

Immediate Management

- Oxygen therapy is the mainstay of prehospital therapy.
- Intravenous (IV) access and fluid therapy may be indicated for dehydration.
- Restraints may be required for patients with altered mental status.

Treatment of Choice

- Erythromycin (or clarithromycin) is the Treatment of Choice
- Severe infections may require the addition of rifampicin
- Support must be given in the event of any system failure - ventilation in respiratory failure, dialysis in renal failure

Your notes:

Serial No. 68

Subject: Medicine

Topic: Pneumonia

Question: An elderly man with COPD having attacks of pneumonia every winter for the past 2 years. He wants your advice for this winter.

Diagnosis: Influenza

Clinchers

- *Elderly:* Risk of complications due to influenza, hospitalisation and death are higher among those age >65 years, very young children and those at risk factors (see confusa). Residents of nursing homes are particularly at risk of serious complications because of their age, high rate of chronic disease and living in a closed community.
- *With COPD:* Any sort of chronic respiratory tract disease puts the patient in high risk category.
- *Attacks of pneumonia every winter:* This seasonal variation typically suggests influenza; epidemics of influenza occur mainly in the winter months.
- *Wants your advise:* The patient is in question is an ideal candidate for flu vaccine;
  National policy in the UK is that vaccinations should be offered to:
  - All patients aged >65 years
  - All patients aged over 6 months with the risk factors
  - All those living in long-stay facilities including residential or nursing homes.

CONFUSA

At-risk patients include those with:

- Chronic respiratory disease, including asthma
- Chronic heart disease (excluding uncomplicated, controlled hypertension)
- Chronic renal disease
- Diabetes mellitus
- Immunosuppression – including asplenia or splenic dysfunction or have received systemic steroids equivalent to 20 mg prednisolone daily for more than 2 weeks.

Investigation of Choice

Diagnosis is on clinical grounds and accuracy may be determined by prevalence of influenza.

The criterion standard for diagnosing influenza A and B is a viral culture of nasal-pharyngeal and/or throat samples.

Direct immunofluorescent tests may offer rapid diagnosis but is not readily available.

Immediate Management

- Self-management is recommended including rest, increased fluid intake, analgesics and antipyretics
- Patients should be advised to stay at home and keep away from 'at-risk' individuals.

Treatment of Choice

Three antiviral drugs are licensed for the treatment of influenza:

- Zanamivir – licenced for influenza A and B in patients age >12 years when given within 48 hours of onset of symptoms and influenza is circulating.
- Oseltamivir – licenced for influenza A and B in patients aged >1 year with same conditions as zanivir. Also licensed for prophylaxis in patients age >13 years.
- Amantadine – licensed for treatment of and prophylaxis against influenza A in patients at risk of complications. Should also be started within 48 hours of symptoms.
- All three above have been shown to reduce duration of symptoms by approximately 1 day.
- NICE recommends the use of zanamivir for the treatment of at-risk adults.

Your notes:

Serial No. 69

Subject: Medicine

Topic: Pneumonia

Question: An 18-year-old girl comes with fever, myalgia and shortness of breath. Half of her hostel is similarly ill.

Diagnosis: Influenza/ flu like illness

Clinchers

- *18-year-old girl:* Though any age can contract the disease, elderly are more at risk for developing complications.
- *Fever, myalgia, shortness of breath:* Typical presentation of influenza or flu like illness. Children may also develop pleuritic chest pain, dry cough or diarrhoea.
- *Half her hostel is similarly ill:* Influenza typically occurs in epidemics and those in residential stay or in crowded places are typically at risk.

CONFUSA

- Although *Staphylococcus aureus* is typically known to be associated with post- influenza pneumonia, the most common pathogen to cause in pneumonia in such patients is pneumococcous.
- Zanamivir or Oseltamivir may be prescribed when:
  - in a residential care home outbreak of flu, or
  - in those at increased risk of complications and have close contact with a person with flu.

Investigation of Choice

Diagnosis is on clinical grounds and accuracy may be determined by prevalence of influenza.

The criterion standard for diagnosing influenza A and B is a viral culture of nasal-pharyngeal and/or throat samples.

Direct immunofluorescent tests may offer rapid diagnosis but is not readily available.

Immediate Management

- Self-management is recommended including rest, increased fluid intake, analgesics and antipyretics
- Patients should be advised to stay at home and keep away from 'at-risk' individuals.

Treatment of Choice

Three antiviral drugs are licensed for the treatment of influenza:

- Zanamivir – licenced for influenza A and B in patients age >12 years when given within 48 hours of onset of symptoms and influenza is circulating.

- Oseltamivir – licenced for influenza A and B in patients aged >1 year with same conditions as zanivir. Also licensed for prophylaxis in patients age >13 years.
- Amantadine – licensed for treatment of and prophylaxis against influenza A in patients at risk of complications. Should also be started within 48 hours of symptoms.
- All three above have been shown to reduce duration of symptoms by approximately 1 day.
- NICE recommends the use of zanamivir for the treatment of at-risk adults.

Your notes:

Serial No. 111

Subject: Medicine

Topic: Chest

Question:
Temp 37 °C
JVP raised
CXR normal
ECG- T inversion in L3
BP 100/60; PR 130 bpm

Diagnosis: Pulmonary Embolism (PE)

Clinchers

- *Temp 37 °C:* Normal temperature rules any infective cause of this presentation. However, atypically pulmonary embolism can also present as fever.
- *JVP raised:* PE reduces the cross-sectional area of the pulmonary vascular bed, resulting in an increment in pulmonary vascular resistance, which, in turn, increases the right ventricular afterload leading to right heart failure and thus an increased JVP.
- *CXR normal*: The chest X-ray is usually normal in early stages. However, later, Westermark sign (dilatation of pulmonary vessels and a sharp cutoff), atelectasis, a small pleural effusion, and an elevated diaphragm may become evident.
- *ECG- T inversion in L3:* The ECG findings in pulmonary embolism are variable and include non-specific ST-T changes. The classical S1-Q3-T3 pattern with right axis deviation and right bundle branch block is seen only in 20% cases.
- *BP 100/60; PR 130 bpm:* With massive pulmonary embolism, patients are usually in shock with systemic hypotension, tachycardia, tachypnoea and poor perfusion of the extremities.

CONFUSA

- In case of patient developing swollen painful legs (especially unilateral) and breathing difficulties, after air travel, always rule out pulmonary embolism.
- The UK Department of Health (DH) recommends that patients with a personal or family history of venous thromboembolism or clotting abnormalities, a history or current treatment of cancer, those who have suffered a stroke or have had recent major surgery, should obtain medical advice before travelling.
- It is also adviced that patients who have had a hip or knee replacement should avoid long haul flights for three months.

- Patients who are in a high-risk group (including women taking the pill or HRT) should be considered for the use of elastic stockings during air travels.

Investigation of Choice

- Ventilation-perfusion scan - demonstrate areas of ventilation-perfusion mismatch.
- Spiral computed tomography with contrast is the investigation of choice in patients with lung disease; enables direct visualisation of PE in pulmonary vessels as filling defects. Excellent for central or lobar PE's.
- Digital subtraction pulmonary angiography is the "gold standard". Sensitivity is ~98%, specificity 95-98%.
- Blood gases show impaired gas exchange with arterial hypoxaemia and hypocapnia.
- Rapid plasma D-dimer ELISA assay: This is a highly sensitive but not specific test for diagnosing pulmonary embolism. When levels of D-dimer are less than 500 µg/l, it reliably excludes PE (sensitivity >99%). However, a level of _500 µg/L is of no use diagnostically.

Immediate Management

See Flow chart 22.1

Treatment of Choice

Fibrinolysis: A standard regimen is -
Loading dose: streptokinase 250,000 u IVI over 30 min
Maintenance dose: streptokinase 100,000 u/h IVI for 24-48 hours, followed by heparin. TPA - bolus 0.6 mg/kg over 5 minutes or 100 mg over 2 hours followed by heparin.

Your notes:

Flow chart 22.1: Emergency management of pulmonary embolism

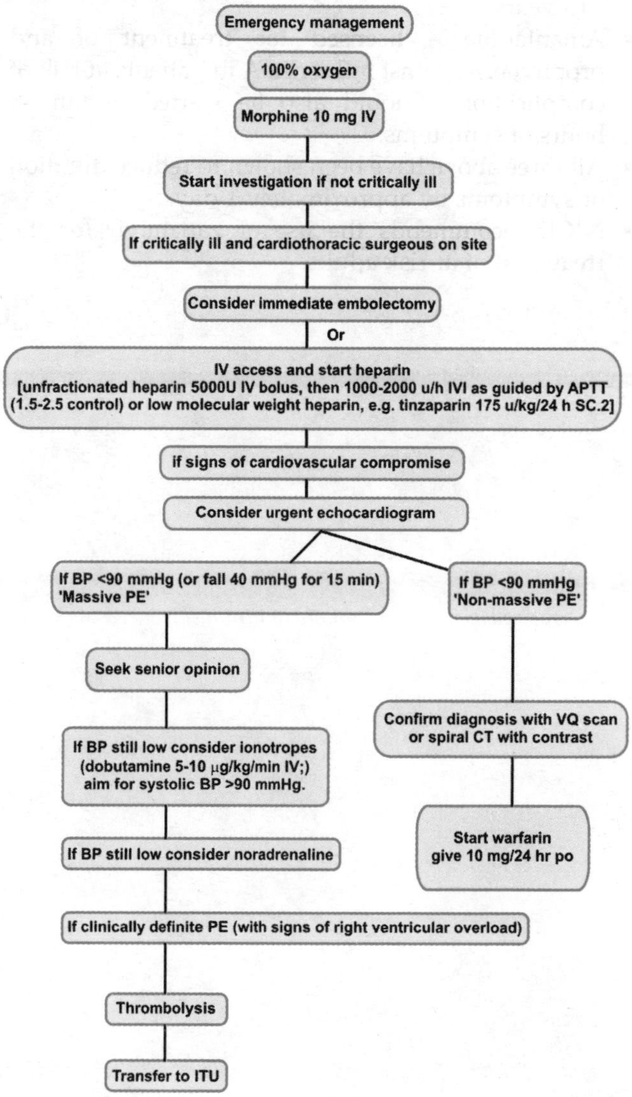

Serial No. 113

Subject: Medicine

Topic: Chest

Question:
Temp 39 °C
JVP normal
CXR shows consolidation of right middle lobe
BP 120/90 PR 100 bpm/irregular

Diagnosis: Pneumonia (right middle lobe)

Clinchers

- *Temp 39 °C:* Pneumonia presentation is usually sudden with a dramatic onset of fever and rigor as first symptoms especially in the young. However, in older patients, there might be no fever at all.
- *JVP normal:* JVP is usually normal in pneumonia until and unless the picture is complicated by acute septicaemia and high output cardiac failure or even decompensated heart due to associated atrial fibrillation.
- *CXR shows consolidation of right middle lobe:* This is the typical description of lobar pneumonia most commonly caused by *Streptococous pneumoniae.*
- *BP 120/90 PR 100 bpm/irregular:* This is suggesting normotension. Tachycardia is usually due to febrile state and infectious aetiology of the condition. Irregular pulse rate is suggesting associated atrial fibrillation.

CONFUSA

CXR findings can give a clue to the causative microorganisms in pneumonia:

- Focal opacity (segment or lobar pneumonia)- *Streptoccous pneumoniae*
- Interstitial pattern- *Mycoplasma pneumoniae, Pneumocystis carinii, Chlamydia psittaci*
- Interstitial pattern with hilar and/or mediastinal lymphadenopathy - Epstein-Barr virus, *Francisella tularensis, Chlamydia psittaci, Mycoplasma pneumoniae,* fungi
- Cavitation or necrotizing pneumonia - Mixed aerobic-anaerobic infection (lung abscess), *Staph aureus,* aerobic gram-negative bacilli, *Mycobacterium tuberculosis*
- Bulging oblique or horizontal fissure - *Klebsiella pneumoniae*
- Multifocal bilateral segment or lobar opacities - *Staph aureus, Coxiella burnetii, Legionella pneumophila,*
- Miliary (diffuse micronodular) pattern - *Mycobacterium tuberculosis, Histoplasma capsulatum*
- Pneumatoceles (thin-walled cavities) - *Staph aureus*
- "Round" pneumonia (often presents as solitary pulmonary nodule) - *Coxiella burnetii, Streptococcous pneumoniae, Legionella pneumophila, Staph aureus*

Investigation of Choice

CXR
Microbiological specimens may be necessary in patients who fail to respond to conventional treatment.

Immediate Management

- Admit, if patient fulfils criteria for admission.
- The decision to admit is based on a variety of factors including severity of illness, age, underlying health problems and social circumstances. The British Thoracic Society guidelines for community acquired pneumonia in adults recommend use of the CURB-65 score.
- CURB-65 score is a 6-point score system, one point for each of:
  - Confusion,
  - Urea >7 mmol/L,
  - Respiratory rate 30/min or more,
  - Systolic Blood pressure below 90 mmHg (or diastolic below 60 mmHg),
  - Age 65 years or older.
- Patients who have a CURB-65 score of 0 are at low risk of death and do not normally require hospitalisation for clinical reasons.
- Patients who have a CURB-65 score of 1 or 2 are at increased risk of death and hospital referral and assessment should be considered, particularly with a score of 2.
- Patients who have a CURB-65 score of 3 or more are at high risk of death and require urgent hospital admission.

Treatment of Choice

Start blind therapy immediately and adjust as the underlying organism becomes more certain. The choice of antibiotic regime will be governed by updated local guidelines. Following are the current recommendations in the BNF.

- *Uncomplicated community-acquired pneumonia*
  - Amoxicillin (or benzylpenicillin if previously healthy chest or erythromycin if penicillin-allergic)
- *Severe community-acquired pneumonia of unknown aetiology*
  - Cefuroxime (or cefotaxime) plus erythromycin

- *Pneumonia possibly caused by atypical pathogens*
  - Erythromycin
  - Severe Legionella infections may require addition of rifampicin;
  - Tetracycline is an alternative for chlamydial and mycoplasma infections
- *Hospital-acquired pneumonia*
  - Cefuroxime is the drug of first choice. Include metronidazole if the clinical state does not improve because of the likelihood of anaerobes. Immunosuppressed patients may require high dose broad spectrum antibiotics, antifungal and antiviral agents.

Note: In all the cases above add flucloxacillin if staphylococci suspected, e.g. in influenza or measles; Add erythromycin if atypical pathogens suspected

Your notes:

Serial No. 114

Subject: Medicine

Topic: Chest

Question:
Temp 37 °C
JVP normal
CXR reduced markings on right side
BP 130/80 PR 90 bpm/regular

Diagnosis: Simple Pneumothorax (right sided)

Clinchers

- *Temp 37 °C:* Pneumothorax (simple) usually occurs due to spontaneous rupture of subpleural blebs. Patient is usually non-febrile with underlying healthy lungs.
- *JVP normal:* Raised JVP mediastinal shift and haemodynamic instability denote tension pneumothorax.
- *CXR reduced markings on right side:* The presence of air in the pleural space causes the collapse of lung which classically appears as reduced markings on the affected lungs. No markings denote complete collapse or 100% pneumothorax.
- *BP 130/80 PR 90 bpm/regular:* Haemodynamic instability denotes tension pneumothorax. Simple pneumothorax rarely produce haemodynamic changes except for slight tachycardia, which is evident in this patient.

CONFUSA

- Pneumomediastinum is a similar condition where patient presents with retrosternal chest pain, usually radiating to the neck, back, or shoulders, exacerbated by deep inspiration, coughing, or when supine.
- Often it is associated with surgical emphysema and Hamman's sign (clicking noise synchronous with heartbeat; also seen in left sided pneumothorax).
- No treatment is necessary as the air is gradually reabsorbed.

Investigation of Choice
Chest X-ray.

- Don't wait for CXR if you suspect a tension pneumothorax - Aspirate first.
- CT scanning is recommended to differentiate pneumothorax from complex bullous lung disease; if surgical emphysema obscures the CXR, or assessing tube placement is difficult.

- Arterial blood gases are only required if the patient is clinically in respiratory failure.

Immediate Management

- Ascertain if active management is required; Small, closed, mildly symptomatic spontaneous pneumothoraces can be observed (don't require admission). Advise the patients to return for reassessment if their symptoms worsen, and arrange repeat CXR in a few days to check resolution or improvement.
- Active management is required for all primary pneumothoraces if patient is breathless and/or there is a rim of air >2 cm on CXR (i.e. "large" pneumothorax).

Treatment of Choice

See Flow chart 22.2 active management of simple pneumothorax

Flow chart 22.2: Active management of simple pneumothorax

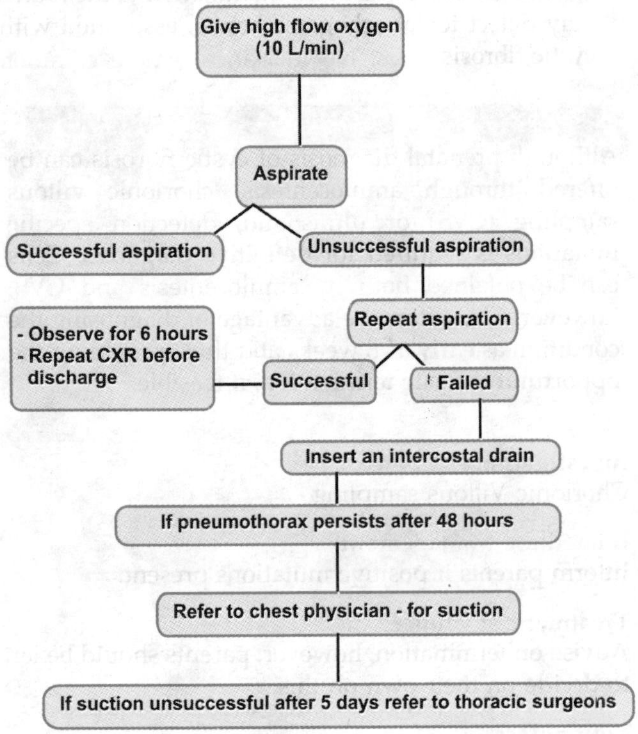

Your notes:

Serial No. 116

Subject: Medicine

Topic: Chest

Question:
Temp 37 ºC
JVP raised
PR 90 bpm/regular
BP 100/90
CXR bilateral shadows
Basal creptitions

Diagnosis: Pulmonary oedema

Clinchers

- *Temp 37 ºC:* Normal temperature rules out infectious causes for the pulmonary edema viz, saepticaemia, infective endocarditis.
- *JVP raised:* Raised JVP along with signs like tachycardia and peripheral oedema are highly suggestive of congestive cardiac failure as the cause of pulmonary oedema.
- *PR 90 bpm/regular, BP 100/90:* Tachycardia and hypotension are again pointing towards a cardiac cause for pulmonary oedema.
- *CXR bilateral shadows:* Pulmonary oedema is classically represented on CXR as perihilar infiltrates in the typical butterfly pattern reflecting a PCWP greater than 25 mm Hg.
- *Basal creptitions:* Fine crackles heard on chest auscultation located mainly on the basal areas of the lung fields bilaterally are characteristic of pulmonary oedema.

CONFUSA

- Drug abuser presenting with pulmonary oedema-always rule out heroine (opioids) as the most important cause.
- Scorpion sting can cause massive pulmonary oedema especially in children.
- High altitude is another cause of unexplained pulmonary oedema.
- Acute breathlessness in an elderly with pink sputum is most likely due to pulmonary oedema precipitated by left ventricular failure.
- Pulmonary oedema secondary to altered capillary permeability–includes acute respiratory deficiency syndrome (ARDS), infectious causes, inhaled toxins, circulating exogenous toxins, vasoactive substances, disseminated intravascular coagulopathy (DIC), immunologic processes reactions, uremia, near drowning, and other aspirations.

Investigation of Choice

- Confirm pulmonary oedema: CXR (signs of pulmonary oedema);
- Find out a cause for pulmonary oedema: ECG (look for signs of myocardial infarct); blood gases; U&E; glucose, 'cardiac' enzymes.

Immediate Management

- Propped up position.
- 100% O_2, if no pre-existing lung disease.
- Insert an IV cannula.

Drugs:

- Furosemide = Frusemide 40–80 mg IV (slowly) - produces transient venodilatation and subsequent diuresis. It also increases the production of vasodilator prostaglandins in the kidneys (avoid NSAIDs as they antagonise this action).
- Parenteral opiates or opioids, e.g. Diamorphine 2.5 - 5 mg IV slowly, (care in liver failure or chronic obstructive airways disease). This relieves anxiety, pain and distress as well as both producing transient venodilatation and reducing myocardial oxygen demand.
- Nitrates (buccally, SL or IV) eg. GTN spray 2 puffs SL or 2 x 0.3mg tablets SL. They reduce venous filling pressure (preload), output impedence and improve coronary filling. They are particularly appropriate if the patient has episodes of angina. Consider Isosorbide dinitrate 2–7mg/h IVI provided systolic BP >110 mmHg.
- If there is fast AF, give digoxin 0.75–1.25 mg PO (or 0.5 mg IV, slowly, if very urgent). Treat other arrhythmias.

Treatment of Choice

Treat the cause

Prognosis of pulmonary oedema

Killip classification

Class	*Clinical features*	*Hospital mortality*
I	No signs of left ventricular dysfunction	6%
II	S3 gallop with mild/moderate pulmonary congestion	30%
III	Severe pulmonary oedema	40%
IV	Cardiogenic shock	80-90%

Serial No. 135

Subject: Obstetrics

Topic: Prenatal Screening

Question: Pregnant lady with previous baby affected with cystic fibrosis, wants to confirm if her present baby is alright.

Diagnosis: Cystic Fibrosis

Clinchers

- *With previous baby affected with cystic fibrosis:* parents with an affected child need to be informed that there is a 25% risk of having another child with cystic fibrosis.
- *Wants to confirm if her present baby is alright:* The diagnosis of cystic fibrosis can be made during pregnancy as long as the CF mutations are known (usually obtained from the affected sibling). Samples are obtained by chorionic villous sampling (CVS) or amniocentesis. Ultrasound examination of the foetus may detect foetal echogenic bowel, associated with cystic fibrosis.

CONFUSA

Although prenatal diagnosis of cystic fibrosis can be offered through amniocentesis, chorionic villous sampling (CVS) or ultrasound, detection specific mutations is required for definitive diagnosis. Cells can be obtained both by amniocentesis and CVS, however, CVS offers the advantage of diagnosing the condition as early as 8 weeks and thus, providing the opportunity of safe termination, if feasible.

Investigation of Choice

Chorionic Villous sampling

Immediate Management

Inform parents if positive mutations present.

Treatment of Choice

Advise on termination, however, parents should be left to decide on their own on this.

Your notes:

PAPER 2

Serial No. 65

Subject: Obstetrics

Topic: Prenatal diagnosis

Question: A pregnant lady with previous child affected with recurrent chest infections and diarrhoea wants to know whether this child is affected too.

Diagnosis: Cystic fibrosis

Clinchers

- *Previous child affected with recurrent chest infections, diarrhoea:* Cystic fibrosis is an autosomal recessive, inherited disease. Presents in neonates with complications like meconium ileus, in early infancy as wheezing, coughing, and/or recurrent respiratory infections and pneumonia or gastrointestinal manifestations. Patients presenting late usually have predominant pulmonary symptoms.
- Gastrointestinal tract presentation in early infancy may be in the form of steatorrhoea, failure to thrive, or both. This is due to pancreatic insufficiency.
- Whether this child is affected too: parents with an affected child need to be informed that there is a 25% risk of having another child with cystic fibrosis. The diagnosis of cystic fibrosis can be made during pregnancy as long as the CF mutations are known (usually obtained from the affected sibling). Samples are obtained by chorionic villous sampling (CVS) or amniocentesis. Ultrasound examination of the foetus may detect foetal echogenic bowel, associated with cystic fibrosis.

CONFUSA

Although prenatal diagnosis of cystic fibrosis can be offered through amniocentesis, chorionic villous sampling (CVS) or ultrasound, detection specific mutations is required for definitive diagnosis. Cells can be obtained both by amniocentesis and CVS, however, CVS offers the advantage of diagnosing the condition as early as 8 weeks and thus, providing the opportunity of safe termination, if feasible.

Investigation of Choice
Chorionic Villous Sampling

Immediate Management
Inform parents if positive mutations present.

Treatment of Choice
Advise on termination, however, parents should be left to decide on their own on this.

Your notes:

Serial No. 107

Subject: Medicine

Topic: Infection

Question: A 40-year-old man has cough, fever and mild dyspnoea. He has reduced air entry and is dull to percussion at the left lung base. He is neither systemically unwell nor hypoxic. He has a documented penicillin murmur.

Diagnosis: Pulmonary Infarction

Clinchers

- *40-year-old man:* The risk of pulmonary embolism and infarction increases with age as the incidence of cardiac and pulmonary diseases as well as the risk of venous thromboembolism increases exponentially with age.
- *Cough, fever and mild dyspnoea:* Pleuritic chest pain is the most common symptom associated with pulmonary infarction. Other symptoms are fever, cough, dyspnoea, tachypnoea and haemoptysis.
- *Reduced air entry and is dull to percussion at the left lung base:* This is denoting the infarcted zone of the lung. The infarcted area is usually filled with an infiltrate (similar as 'consolidation' in lobar pneumonia).
- *He is neither systemically unwell nor hypoxic:* The pulmonary embolism is nearly always submassive when present as pulmonary infarction. The patient shows no systemic features of illness. Arterial blood gases are not diagnostic. PCO_2 is usually decreased (owing to dyspnoea/ hyperventilation). PO_2 is often normal or near normal because usually only a small percentage of the pulmonary circulation is obstructed.
- *He has a documented penicillin murmur:* This relates to the source of the emboli which has apparently caused this infarct. His underlying rheumatic heart disease is the most significant clincher in the diagnosis.

CONFUSA

It is easy to confuse this picture with 'Atypical Pneumonia' as the theme is regarding treatment of infection. However, note that in atypical pneumonia, there is never a lobar consolidation (as signified hereby, 'dull to percussion at the left lung base'). In atypical pneumonia, typically, consolidation is absent and chest radiograms are patchy and densely shadowed out of proportion to the severity of clinical features.

Investigation of Choice

CXR is the most useful investigation here. It will show infiltrate/consolidation of the involved lobe, elevated hemidiaphragm and/or a small pleural effusion.

Immediate Management

Anticoagulation: Heparin infusion should be started immediately, with the introduction of warfarin

Symptomatic support to the heart or lungs in the form of ionotropics or oxygen, if required.

Treatment of Choice

Anticoagulation to prevent further episodes.

Infarcted area can either resolve by itself in few weeks or evolve into a scar.

Your notes:

Serial No. 110

Subject: Medicine

Topic: Infections

Question: A 60-year-old male smoker presents with severe dyspnoea, dry cough and fever. He is unwell, tachycardiac and cyanosed.

Diagnosis: Atypical pneumonia

Clinchers

- *A 60-year-old male:* Atypical pneumonia is more common in males and rare in children younger than 4 years of age.
- *Smoker:* Elderly individuals, smokers, and people with chronic illnesses and weakened immune systems are at higher risk for atypical of pneumonia.
- *Severe dyspnoea, dry cough and fever:* The condition starts with an initial influenza like picture. The cough is dry initially and later becomes productive with a mucoid and purulent sputum.
- *He is unwell, tachycardiac and cyanosed:* Cyanosis is seen in advanced cases and requires immediate intervention in the form of oxygen therapy.

CONFUSA

The above picture can be very well confused with a normal community acquired pneumonia. However, the hints of old age and chronic smoker goes more in favour of community acquired atypical pneumonia. Moreover, an otherwise 'typical' pneumonia would present with a productive cough.

Investigation of Choice

Chest X-Ray — Typically, consolidation is lacking and chest radiograms are patchily and densely shadowed out of proportion to the severity of clinical features.

Immediate Management

Symptomatic

Treatment of Choice

Erythromycin (or clarithromycin/azithromycin)

Your notes:

Serial No. 161

Subject: Medicine

Topic: Chest Medicine

Question: A 47-year-old man was brought to the emergency room after having experienced chest discomfort and shortness of breath, followed by a syncopal episode. He was short of breath (breathing at 40 and requiring 100% oxygen to maintain an adequate saturation) and had a depressed level of consciousness. He was pale, diaphoretic, and in shock with a pulse of 120 bpm and a blood pressure of 70 mmHg systolic.

Diagnosis: Pulmonary embolism

Clinchers

- *A 47-year-old man:* the risk of pulmonary embolism increases with age and although its more commonly seen related to pregnancy, sex does not appear to be an independent risk factor for pulmonary embolism.
- *Chest discomfort, Shortness of breath:* The presenting symptoms are vague and usually misleading to a different diagnosis. Patient may complain of chest pain, dyspnoea, haemoptysis or most cases remain asymptomatic.
- *Syncopal episode:* This could be one of the presenting features of the PE, the cause could a compromised left ventricular output due to a massive embolism.
- *Breathing at 40, requiring 100% oxygen:* This especially signifies that there is some degree of ventilation-Perfusion mismatch that the patients is so tachypnoeic yet the oxygen saturation is so difficult to maintain.
- *Depressed level of consciousness:* Hypoxia, resulting from the depressed cardiac output and the V-P mismatch causes impaired consciousness, especially in those with a massive embolism.
- *Pale, diaphoretic, and in shock:* This is suggesting increased sympathetic activity. However, the features can be easily misinterpreted as an Acute Myocardial Infarction.
- *Pulse of 120 bp, a blood pressure of 70 mmHg systolic:* Tachycardia, tachypnoea, hypotension, raised JVP, cyanosis, impaired oxygen saturation are all seen with pulmonary embolism.

CONFUSA

The above picture typically is of a cardiogenic shock which can occur either due to a massive pulmonary embolism or a massive myocardial infarct. The clinical pictures when correlated with the provided ECG, clearly shows a Right Bundle Branch Block (RBBB) and absence of any significant ST elevation or hyperacute T waves.

Flow chart 22.3: Emergency management of pulmonary embolism

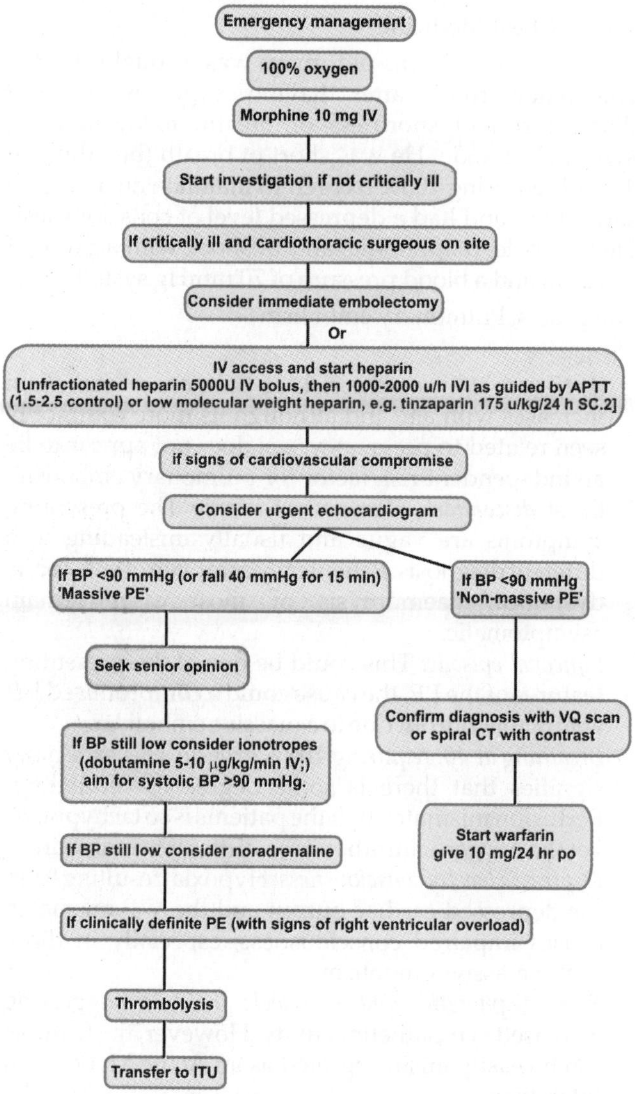

Investigation of Choice

- Ventilation-perfusion scan - demonstrate areas of ventilation-perfusion mismatch.
- Spiral computed tomography with contrast is the investigation of choice in patients with lung disease; enables direct visualisation of PE in pulmonary vessels as filling defects. Excellent for central or lobar PE's.
- Digital subtraction pulmonary angiography is the "gold standard". **Sensitivity is ~98%, specificity 95-98%.**
- Blood gases show impaired gas exchange with arterial hypoxaemia and hypocapnia.
- Rapid plasma D-dimer ELISA assay: This is a highly sensitive but not specific test for diagnosing pulmonary embolism.When levels of D-dimer are less than 500 μg/L, it reliably excludes PE (sensitivity >99%). However, a level of 500 μg/L is of no use diagnostically.

Immediate Management

See Flow Chart: 22.3.

Treatment of Choice

Fibrinolysis: A standard regimen is -
Loading dose: streptokinase 250,000 u IVI over 30 min
Maintenance dose: streptokinase 100,000u/h IVI for 24-48 hours, followed by heparin.TPA - bolus 0.6 mg/kg over 5 minutes or 100 mg over 2 hours followed by heparin

Your notes:

Serial No. 163

Subject: Medicine

Topic: Chest

Question: A 40-year-old male presents with an irregular pulse rate (100 bpm). His BP is 120/90 mm Hg , JVP is not elevated and Temperature is 39 ºC. The chest X-ray taken in the A & E shows positive findings.

Diagnosis: Pneumonia (right middle lobe)

Clinchers

- *Temp 39ºC:* Pneumonia presentation is usually sudden with a dramatic onste of fever and rigor as first symptoms especially in the young. However, in older patients, there might be no fever at all.
- *JVP normal:* JVP is usually normal in pneumonia until and unless the picture is complicated by acute septicaemia and high output cardiac failure or even decompensated heart due to associated atrial fibrillation.
- *CXR shows consolidation of right middle lobe:* This is the typical description of lobar pneumonia most commonly caused by *Streptococous pneumoniae*.
- *BP 120/90 PR 100 bpm/irregular:* This is suggesting normotension. Tachycardia is usually due to febrile state and infectious aetiology of the condition. Irregular pulse rate is suggesting associated atrial fibrillation.

CONFUSA

CXR findings can give a clue to the causative microorganisms in Pneumonia:

- Focal opacity (segment or lobar pneumonia) - *Streptococcus pneumoniae*
- Interstitial pattern- *Mycoplasma pneumoniae, Pneumocystis carinii, Chlamydia psittaci*
- Interstitial pattern with hilar and/or mediastinal lymphadenopathy - Epstein-Barr virus, Franciscella tularensis, *Chlamydia psittaci, Mycoplasma pneumoniae*, fungi
- Cavitation or necrotizing pneumonia - Mixed aerobic-anaerobic infection (lung abscess), *Staph aureus*, aerobic gram-negative bacilli, *Mycobacterium tuberculosis*
- Bulging oblique or horizontal fissure - *Klebsiella pneumoniae*
- Multifocal bilateral segment or lobar opacities - *Staph aureus, Coxiella burnetii, Legionella pneumophila,*
- Miliary (diffuse micronodular) pattern - *Mycobacterium tuberculosis, Histoplasma capsulatum*
- Pneumatoceles (thin-walled cavities) - *Staph aureus*
- "Round" pneumonia (often presents as solitary pulmonary nodule) - *Coxiella burnetii, Streptococcous pneumoniae, Legionella pneumophila, Staph aureus.*

Investigation of Choice

CXR

Microbiological specimens may be necessary in patients who fail to respond to conventional treatment.

Immediate Management

- Admit, if patient fulfils criteria for admission.
- The decision to admit is based on a variety of factors including severity of illness, age, underlying health problems and social circumstances. The British Thoracic Society guidelines for community acquired pneumonia in adults recommend use of the CURB-65 score.
- CURB-65 score is a 6-point score system, one point for each of:
  - Confusion,
  - Urea >7 mmol/L,
  - Respiratory rate 30/min or more,
  - Systolic blood pressure below 90 mmHg (or diastolic below 60 mmHg),
  - Age 65 years or older.
- Patients who have a CURB-65 score of 0 are at low risk of death and do not normally require hospitalisation for clinical reasons.
- Patients who have a CURB-65 score of 1 or 2 are at increased risk of death and hospital referral and assessment should be considered, particularly with a score of 2.
- Patients who have a CURB-65 score of 3 or more are at high risk of death and require urgent hospital admission.

Treatment of Choice

Start blind therapy immediately and adjust as the underlying organism becomes more certain. The choice of antibiotic regime will be governed by updated local guidelines. Following are the current recommendations in the BNF.

- *Uncomplicated community-acquired pneumonia*
  - Amoxicillin (or benzylpenicillin if previously healthy chest or erythromycin if penicillin-allergic)
- *Severe community-acquired pneumonia of unknown aetiology*
  - Cefuroxime (or cefotaxime) plus erythromycin
- *Pneumonia possibly caused by atypical pathogens*
  - Erythromycin

- Severe Legionella infections may require addition of rifampicin;
- Tetracycline is an alternative for chlamydial and mycoplasma infections

• *Hospital-acquired pneumonia*
  - Cefuroxime is the drug of first choice. Include metronidazole if the clinical state does not improve because of the likelihood of anaerobes. Immunosuppressed patients may require high dose broad spectrum antibiotics, antifungal and antiviral agents.

Note: In all the cases above add flucloxacillin if staphylococci suspected, e.g. in influenza or measles; Add erythromycin if atypical pathogens suspected

Your notes:

Serial No. 164

Subject: Medicine

Topic: Chest

Question: A 22-year-old tall male presents with acute onset breathlessness. His temperature is 37ºC and his JVP appears to be normal. His BP is 130/80 PR 90 bpm/regular and the CXR taken shows reduced markings on right side.

Diagnosis: Simple Pneumothorax (right sided) (Flow chart 22.4)

Clinchers

➢ *Temp 37ºC:* Pneumothorax (simple) usually occurs due to spontaneous rupture of subpleural blebs. Patient is usually non-febrile with underlying healthy lungs.

➢ *JVP normal:* Raised JVP mediastinal shift and haemodynamic instability denote tension pneumothorax.

➢ *CXR reduced markings on right side:* The presence of air in the pleural space causes the collapse of lung which classically appears as reduced markings on the effected lungs. No markings denote complete collapse or 100% pneumothorax.

➢ *BP 130/80 PR 90 bpm/regular:* Haemodynamic instability denotes tension pneumothorax. Simple pneumomothorax rarely produce haemodynamic changes except for slight tachycardia, which is evident in this patient.

CONFUSA

• Pneumomediastinum is a similar condition where patient presents with retrosternal chest pain, usually radiating to the neck, back, or shoulders, exacerbated by deep inspiration, coughing, or when supine.
• Often it is associated with surgical emphysema and Hamman's sign (clicking noise synchronous with heartbeat; also seen in left sided pneumothorax).
• No treatment is necessary as the air is gradually reabsorbed.

Investigation of Choice

Chest X-ray.

• Don't wait for CXR if you suspect a tension pneumothorax - Aspirate first.
• CT scanning is recommended to differentiate pneumothorax from complex bullous lung disease; if surgical emphysema obscures the CXR, or assessing tube placement is difficult.

- Arterial blood gases are only required if the patient is clinically in respiratory failure

Immediate Management

- Ascertain if active management is required; Small, closed, mildly symptomatic spontaneous pneumothoraces can be observed (don't require admission). Advise the patients to return for reassessment if their symptoms worsen, and arrange repeat CXR in a few days to check resolution or improvement.
- Active management is required for all primary pneumothoraces if patient is breathless and/or there is a rim of air >2 cm on CXR (i.e. "large" pneumothorax).

Treatment of Choice

Flow chart 22.4: Active management of simple pneumothorax

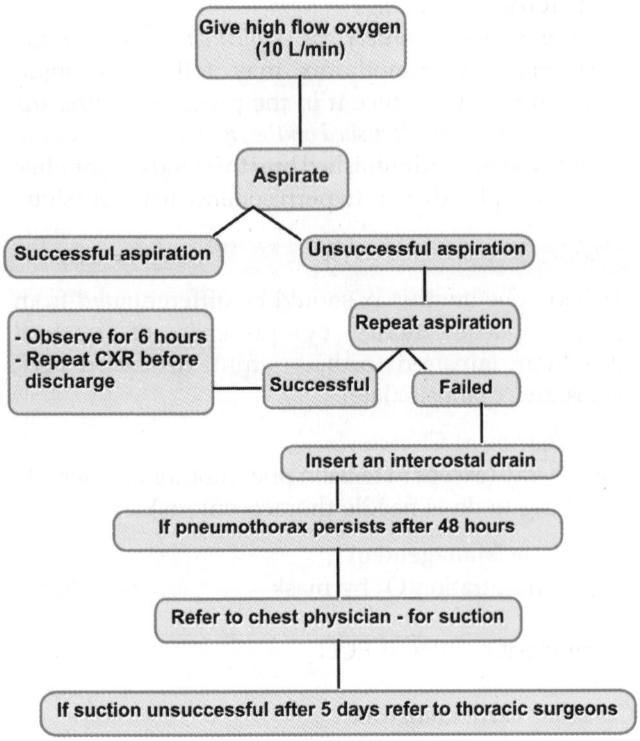

Your notes:

Serial No. 165

Subject: Medicine

Topic: Chest

Question: An 85-year-old female presents with breathlessness. On examination her temperature is 37 °C and JVP is raised. Her PR is 90 bpm/regular and BP 100/90. CXR shows bilateral shadows.

Diagnosis: Pulmonary oedema

Clinchers

- *Temp 37 °C:* Normal temperature rules out infectious causes for the pulmonary oedema viz, septicaemia, infective endocarditis.
- *JVP raised:* Raised JVP along with signs like tachycardia and peripheral oedema are highly suggestive of congestive cardiac failure as the cause of pulmonary oedema.
- *PR 90 bpm/regular, BP 100/90:* Tachycardia and hypotension are again pointing towards a cardiac cause for pulmonary oedema.
- *CXR bilateral shadows:* Pulmonary oedema is classically represented on CXR as perihilar infiltrates in the typical butterfly pattern reflecting a PCWP greater than 25 mm Hg.
- *Basal creptitions:* Fine crackles heard on chest auscultation located mainly on the basal areas of the lung fields bilaterally are characteristic of pulmonary oedema.

CONFUSA

- Drug abuser presenting with pulmonary oedema-always rule out heroine (opioids) as the most important cause.
- Scorpion sting can cause massive pulmonary oedema especially in children.
- High altitude is another cause of unexplained pulmonary oedema.
- Acute breathlessness in an elderly with pink sputum is most likely due to pulmonary oedema precipitated by left ventricular failure.
- Pulmonary oedema secondary to altered capillary permeability–includes acute respiratory deficiency syndrome (ARDS), infectious causes, inhaled toxins, circulating exogenous toxins, vasoactive substances, disseminated intravascular coagulopathy (DIC), immunologic processes reactions, uremia, near drowning, and other aspirations.

Investigation of Choice

- Confirm pulmonary oedema: CXR (signs of pulmonary oedema);
- Find out a cause for pulmonary oedema: ECG (look for signs of myocardial infarct); blood gases; U&E; glucose, 'cardiac' enzymes.

Immediate Management

- Propped up position.
- 100% O_2, if no pre-existing lung disease.
- Insert an IV cannula.

Drugs:

- Furosemide = Frusemide 40–80 mg IV (slowly) - produces transient venodilatation and subsequent diuresis. It also increases the production of vasodilator prostaglandins in the kidneys (avoid NSAIDs as they antagonise this action).
- Parenteral opiates or opioids, e.g. Diamorphine 2.5 - 5mg IV slowly, (care in liver failure or chronic obstructive airways disease). This relieves anxiety, pain and distress as well as both producing transient venodilatation and reducing myocardial oxygen demand.
- Nitrates (buccally, SL or IV) e.g. GTN spray 2 puffs SL or 2 x 0.3 mg tablets SL. They reduce venous filling pressure (preload), output impedence and improve coronary filling. They are particularly appropriate if the patient has episodes of angina. Consider Isosorbide dinitrate 2–7 mg/h IVI provided systolic BP >110 mmHg.
- If there is fast AF, give digoxin 0.75–1.25 mg PO (or 0.5 mg IV, slowly, if very urgent). Treat other arrhythmias.

Treatment of Choice

Treat the cause

Your notes:

Prognosis of pulmonary oedema

Killip classification

Class	*Clinical features*	*Hospital mortality*
I	No signs of left ventricular dysfunction	6%
II	S3 gallop with mild/moderate pulmonary congestion	30%
III	Severe pulmonary oedema	40%
IV	Cardiogenic shock	80-90%

PAPER 3

31. A young man involved in a motorcycle accident is stable in the casualty department. His neck is cleared but when he sits up he develops sudden shortness of breath. His breath sounds are dimished on the right side.

Diagnosis: Simple right sided pneumothorax.

Clinchers

- *Young man:* Young man usually has uncomplicated pneumothoraces as they have no add on lung pathologies.
- *Involved in a motorcycle accident:* Motorcycle accident injuries are mostly sustained on head, chest (rib fractures) and legs.
- *Is stable in the casualty department:* Rules out any life-threatening injury.
- *His neck is cleared:* It gives him a reason to sit straight. The overworked SHO might have missed the rib fractures.
- *When he sits up he develops sudden shortness of breath:* Traumatic pneumothorax may follow rib injury which might produce it in the proces of sitting up.
- *Breath sounds are dimished on the right side:* In pneumothorax there are diminished breath sounds on the affected side (plus there is hyperresonance to percussion).

CONFUSA

Tension pneumothorax should be differentiated from simple pneumothorax by presence of tracheal deviation, impaired cardiac output, distended neck veins and cyanosis (late).

Investigation of Choice

Chest X-ray (except in tension pneumothorax where the first thing to do is needle thoracocentesis).

Immediate Management

High concentration O_2 by mask

\+

Monitor SaO_2, BP and ECG

\+

Consider early analgesia

Treatment of Choice

Needle aspiration

↓ if fails

Chest drain

- Other indications for chest drain
  - Recurrence within 24 hours
  - Haemopneumothorax
  - IPPV

41. A patient is suspected of having bronchiectasis.

Diagnosis: Bronchiectasis (as given in the question).

Clinchers

- *Suspected of having bronchiectasis:* Bronchiectasis does not cause hoarseness per se. It can be secondary to:
  1. *Persistent and recurrent cough:* Which may produce laryngeal trauma to produce hoarseness.
  2. *Steroid inhaler use:* Which have a direct effect on laryngeal musculature to produce hoarseness. Or it can predisposes to laryngeal candidiasis on prolonged use which may produce hoarseness. Steroid inhalers (or oral steroids) can decrease the rate of progression of bronchiectasis by acting as anti-inflammatory agents.

CONFUSA

The only confusion in this question is whether to first confirm the diagnosis of bronchiectasis or to seen for laryngeal pathology secondary to bronchiectasis (as described above). It will be safe to go for the confirmation of the diagnosis first as the second option is dependent on it.

Investigation of Choice

High resolution CT scan.

Immediate Management

- Bronchodilators if demonstrable airflow limitation.
- Antibiotics if infection is present.

Treatment of Choice

- *Conservative* i.e. postural drainage + antibiotics + bronchodilators + steroids
- *Surgery*
  - In localised disease (left lower lobe and lingual are most common sites for localised disease)
  - To control severe haemoptysis.

Case History

A 37-year-old woman has long standing pleural effusions (recurrent), lymphoedema, dystrophic nails and severe productive cough.

Diagnosis: Yellow nail syndrome

Yellow nail syndrome: Associated with lymphatic hypoplasia, bronchiectasis, pleural effusions, COPD and carcinoma. The nails are grossly thickened and yellowish brown.

44. A 55-year-old smoker complains of shortness of breath and a cough. Laryngoscopy is normal.

Diagnosis: Suspected bronchial carcinoma.

Clinchers

- *A 55-year-old smoker:* A 55-year-old smoker would have been smoking for about 30-35 years and that makes him a high-risk case for bronchial carcinoma.
- *Shortness of breath:* It can be a presenting complaint of a bronchial carcinoma but is only for less than 5% cases. Other symptoms that can occur as a presenting complaint in < 5% cases are chest infection, malaise, weight loss, hoarseness and distant spread.
- *Cough:* It is the most common presenting symptom of bronchial carcinoma. Other common presenting complaints are haemoptysis and chest pain.
- *Laryngoscopy is normal:* This rules out any laryngeal pathology resulting in this presentation, i.e. carcinoma of larynx which is also common in male smokers (carcinoma larynx presents as dysphagia and hoarseness).

CONFUSA

Because of their common aetiology COPD is also frequently present in elderly smokers. So it always need to be ruled out preoperatively by lung function tests and gas transfer tests.

Investigation of Choice

- *Screening:* CXR is the most valuable test.
- *Definitive:* CT chest.

Immediate Management

Symptomatic.

Treatment of Choice

Surgery (see Q 42).

Your notes:

62. Pulmonary embolism.

Diagnosis: Already stated as the question.

Clinchers

Since the question, has not given any clinical profile, let us see the most common 'clinchers', that GMC uses in their exams for this condition.

- *Precipitants:* Air travel, recent operation, pregnancy, OCP, hormone replacement therapy, disseminated malignancy, DVT.
- *Symptoms:* Acute breathlessness, pleuritic chest pain, haemoptysis.
- *Signs:* Tachypnoea, tachycardia, hypotension, raised JVP, pleural rub.
- *CXR:* Usually normal (in GMC questions).
- *ECG:* Usually normal (in GMC questions), $S_IQ_{III}T_{III}$ pattern, sinus tachycardia, right bundle branch block.

CONFUSA

Pulmonary embolism produces central cyanosis due to decreased oxygen saturation which is produced by only three other common conditions, i.e.
- Pulmonary oedema
- Severe respiratory disease
- Congenital cyanotic heart disease.

Investigation of Choice

Investigation of pulmonary embolism is a point of major confusion in PLAB examination. Consider following points while choosing the investigation for PE:
- *Screening*
  - V/Q scan—only if the patient is stable and not severely breathless
  - Spiral CT with contrast—if facilities are available patient's general state do not allow a V/Q scan to be done
- *Definitive:* Pulmonary angiogram—but not usually done because of risk of complications and it being an invasive test.

Note: Always look in the "instructions" to the theme about the type of investigation being asked for, i.e. is it "definitive" or "screening". It is important as the answer is usually different for both and you will end up losing marks for something you know.

Immediate Management

Anticoagulation with LMW heparin (Dalteparin 200 U/kg/24 hr SC; max dose 18,000 IU/24h)
- Stop when INR > 2

Treatment of Choice

Oral warfarin 10 mg for minimum 3 months.

64. Bronchiectasis.

Diagnosis: Already stated as the question.

Clinchers

Bronchiectasis is a frequent question in PLAB exam. The most frequent 'clinchers' used by GMC to describe this condition are:

- *Secondary to:* Cystic fibrosis, kartageneger's syndrome, pertussis in the childhood, allergic bronchopulmonary aspergillosis.
  "Non-GMC" conditions—Young's syndrome (primary ciliary dyskinesia), measles, bronchiolitis, pneumonia, TB, HIV, bronchial obstruction (tumour, foreign body), hypogammaglobulinaemia, rheumatoid arthritis, ulcerative colitis, idiopathic.
- *Symptoms:* Persistent cough, copious purulent sputum, intermittent haemoptysis.
- *Signs:* Finger clubbing, coarse inspiratory, crackles, wheeze.
- *Complications:* Pneumonia, pleural effusion, pneumothorax, haemoptysis, cerebral abscess, amyloidosis.

CONFUSA

Spirometry is bronchiectasis shows an obstructive pattern. Reversability should be assessed to differentiate from asthma.

Investigation of Choice
- *Screening:* CXR—Tramline and ring shadows.
- *Definitive:* High resolution CT chest—to assess extent and distribution.

Immediate Management

Antibiotics if infection (usually pseudomonas) is present.

Treatment of Choice

Postural drainage + bronchodilators (if asthma, COPD, cystic fibrosis, ABPA present) + steroids (if ABPA present).

Indications for surgery are:
- Localized bronchiectasis
- To control severe haemoptysis.

Your notes:

101. A middle-aged woman develops a purulent cough with some haemoptysis. A chest X-ray reveals right upper lobe consolidation.

Diagnosis: *Streptococcus pneumoniae.*

Clinchers

- *Middle-aged woman:* Streptococcal pneumonia affects all ages, but is more common in middle-aged and elderly.
- *Purulent cough:* Mycoplasma, *Legionella, Chlamydia* and *Pneumocystis carinii* characteristically presents with dry cough. Streptococcal and staphylococcal generally presents with purulent cough.
- *Some haemoptysis:* Acute bronchitis, pneumonia, neoplasm (primary) haemoptysis in the United Kingdom. TB is common in third world countries.
- *Right upper lobe consolidation:* Lobar consolidation is sign of streptococcal pneumonia, more commonly on right side.

CONFUSA

When there is history of hemoptysis, always think of TB and malignancy first.

Investigation of Choice
Chest X-ray.

Treatment of Choice
Ampicillin or cefuroxime.

Your notes:

102. A young woman with no relevant medical history develops a severe purulent cough. A chest X-ray reveals multiple cavitating bilateral lung lesions.

Diagnosis: Staphylococcal pneumonia.

Clinchers

- *Young woman:* Staphylococcal pneumonia occurs in young and elderly patients.
- *No relevant medical history:* Helps rule out any chronic condition like tuberculosis, though not that significant.
- *Severe purulent cough:* History of severe purulent cough is common is staphylococcal pneunomia.
- *Multiple cavitating bilateral lung lesions:* Bilateral cavitating bronchopneunomia is characteristic of *Staphylococcal pneumonia.*

Investigation of Choice
Chest X-ray.

Treatment of Choice
Flucloxacillin.

Your notes:

CXR: Pneumonia

CONSOLIDATION				CAVITATION	
LOBAR	BIBASAL	PATHCY		BILATERAL	UPPER LOBE
Pneumococcal	Legionella	Bilateral	As Such	Staphylococcus	Klebsiella
		Mycoplasma	Chlamydia Psittaci		

* Bilateral Perihilar *interstitial* shadowing—Pneuomocystis Carinii Pneumonia

103. A young male prostitute develops a dry cough. A chest X-ray reveals bilateral interstitial infiltrates.

Diagnosis: *Pneumocystis carinii* pneumonia (PCP).

Clinchers

- *Young male prostitute: Pneumocystis carinii* causes pneumonia in the immunosuppressed (e.g. HIV).
- *Dry cough: Pneumocystis carinii* presents with fever, dry cough, exertional dyspnoea, and bilateral crepitation.
- *Bilateral interstitial infiltrates:* In PCP chest X-ray may be normal or bilateral interstitial (perihilar) infiltration can be seen.

Investigation of Choice
Chest X-ray.

Treatment of Choice
High dose co-trimoxazole IV or pentamidine by slow IV for 2-3 weeks. In case of severe hypoxaemia, steroids can be added.

Your notes:

104. A young man has recently suffers from a bout of influenza. He now develops a purulent cough.

Diagnosis: Staphylococcal pneumonia.

Clinchers

- *Young man:* Staphylococcal pneumonia occurs in young and elderly patients.
- *Recently suffers from a bout of influenza:* Staphylococcal pneumonia, very commonly present as a complication of influenza infection. More commonly seen in intravenous drug users or patients with underlying disease (e.g. leukemia, lymphoma, cystic fibrosis).
- *He now develops a purulent cough:* History of purulent cough supports the diagnosis of staphylococcal pneumonia.

CONFUSA

Though there should be no confusion in this question, but the diagnosis should be supported with chest X-ray findings. In staphylococcal pneumonia typical bilateral cavitating bronchopneumonia is seen.

Investigation of Choice
Chest X-ray.

Treatment of Choice
Flucloxacillin.

Your notes:

105. Man comes back from a holiday in Malaysia and he develops malaise, fever and dry cough. Chest X-ray reveals bilateral consolidation.

Diagnosis: Legionella pneumophila.

Clinchers

- *Back from holiday to Malaysia:* Legionella pneumophila colonizes water tanks kept at < 60°C (e.g. hotel airconditioning and hot water system). Therefore, this is a very good clincher in this question.
- *Fever, malaise, myalgia:* These flu like symptoms often precede dry cough and dyspnoea in Legionella pneumonia.
- *Bilateral basal consolidation:* Chest X-ray showing bilateral basal consolidation is feature of Legionella pneumonia.

CONFUSA

There should be no confusion in this question. This is very commonly asked in PLAB.

Investigation of Choice
Chest X-ray and legionella serology.

Treatment of Choice
High dose erythromycin.

Your notes:

119. A woman 10 days following hysterectomy complaints of severe left sided chest pain and breathlessness. Chest X-ray and ECG failed to relieve any abnormality.

Diagnosis: Pulmonary embolism.

Clinchers

- *10 days following hysterectomy:* Any cause of immobility or hypercoagulability, e.g. recent surgery (in this case hysterectomy), recent stroke or MI, disseminated malignancy, thrombophilia/antiphospholipid syndrome, prolonged bed-rest and pregnancy.
- *Severe left chest pain/breathlessness:* Symptoms of pulmonary embolism are—acute breathless, pleuritic chest pain, haemoptysis, dizziness and syncope.
- *Chest X-ray and ECG show no abnormality:* Chest X-ray and ECG is generally normal in pulmonary embolism.

Investigation of Choice

- *Screening:* V/Q scan or spiral CT.
- *Definitive:* CT pulmonary angiography. This shows clots down to 5th order pulmonary arteries.

Immediate Management
Screen for DVT.

Treatment of Choice
Anticoagulation.

Your notes:

126. This test of lung function is characteristically not involved in asthmatic patients.

Diagnosis: Asthma.

Clinchers

- Amongst all the options given in this question only vital capacity is not a criteria to assess an asthmatic patient. Vital capacity refers to the largest amount of air that can be expired after a maximal inspiratory effort. It is an index of pulmonary function. The fraction of vital capacity expired during the first second of a forced expiration (FEV_1, timed vital capacity) is reduced in diseaes like asthma, in which airway resistance is increased because of bronchial constriction, but the vital capacity remains unaffected.
- *Important tests in asthmatic patients:* Pulmonary expiratory flow rate (PEFR) monitoring (It correlates well with the forced expiratory volume in 1 sec, i.e. FEV_1 and used as an estimate of airway calibre).

CONFUSA

PEFR should be monitored regularly in asthmatics to monitor response to therapy and disease control. Spirometry: Obstructive defects (¯FEV_1/FVC, -residual volume), *Aspergillus* serology, and hyperinflation on chest X-ray. In acute attack arterial blood gases analysis and blood culture may be helpful besides other regular tests.

Investigation of Choice

Spirometry for obstructive defects (FEV1, FVC_1 and - residual volume), PEFR.

Immediate Management

In acute attack—Sit patient up and give O_2 (100% via non-rebreathing bag) followed by salbutamol nebulization and hydrocortisone 200 mg IV/prednisolone 30 mg go for chest X-ray to exlclude pneumothorax.

Your notes:

127. This substance is released by mast cells and causes flushing.

Diagnosis: Asthma

Clinchers

- Histamine, the richest source being the mast cells, released by degranulation of mast cells in response to variety of stimuli.

  Along with serotonin, histamine is available from preformed stores and is among the first mediators to be released during inflammation.

  In humans, histamine causes dilatation of the arterioles and increases vascular permeability of the venules (it, however, constricts large arteries) causing venular gaps and hence flushing.

CONFUSA

A direct question with no scope for any confusion.

Immediate Management

Of asthma discussed in Question 126.

Your notes:

128. This substance is characteristically found in the sputum of most asthma patients.

Diagnosis: Raised eosinophil count.

Clinchers

- Sputum examination of asthmatic patients reveals
  - Eosinophilia
  - Curschmann's spirals (costs of small airways)
  - Charcot-Layden crystals
  - Large number of neutrophils (suggesting bronchial infection)
- Complete blood count may also show eosinophilia.
- IgE may show mild elevations in blood. Marked elevation of IgE suggests evidence of allergic bronchopulmonary *Aspergillosis.*

CONFUSA

There is no question of confusion in this question. IgA is predominant class of immunoglobulin in secretions (tear, saliva, nasal secretions, GIT fluid and human milk) not to be confused with this question.

Immediate Management

Of asthma is discussed in question 126.

Your notes:

129. This test is done as a diagnostic test for asthma.

Diagnosis: Asthma

Clinchers

- The diagnosis of asthma is established by demonstrating reversible airway obstruction. Though there are various tests to diagnose asthma, traditionally 15% or greater improvement of FEV_1 following two puffs of keto adrenergic agonist is considered to be diagnostic of asthma.
- *Other tests for asthma:* Pulmonary expiratory flow rate (PEFR) monitoring (If correlates well with the forced expiratory volume in 1 sec, i.e. FEV_1 and used as an estimate of airway calibre).

CONFUSA

No confusion in this question.

Immediate Management

Of asthma is discussed in question 126.

Your notes:

130. Blocking of these can cause worsening of asthma.

Diagnosis: Asthma

Clinchers

- The walls of bronchi and bronchioles are innervated by the autonomic nervous system. There are abundant muscarinic receptors and cholinergic discharge causes bronchoconstriction. There are β_1 and β_2 adrenergic receptor in bronchial epithelium and smooth muscles. Some are located on cholinergic endings and ganglia where they inhibit acetylcholine release. In humans, β_2 receptors predominate. Therefore if β_2 receptors are blocked, there will be increased stimulation of cholinergic system which will lead to bronchoconstriction, worsening asthma.
- Here we can discuss role of β_2 agonists in asthma. β_2 agonists relax bronchial smooth muscle acting within minutes. Salbutamol is best given by inhalation, but can be given per oral or IV.

CONFUSA

No confusion in this question.

Immediate Management

Given in question 126.

Your notes:

PAPER 4

16. First line drug used in treating mild asthma.

Diagnosis: Asthma

Clinchers

Guidelines laid by the British Thoracic Society should be followed here.

In mild asthma, first line of drugs used is short acting inhaled β_2-agonists (as and when required for symptom relief). But this should be used only once daily. If used more than once daily add standard dose inhaled steroid, beclometasone or budesonide. Cromoglycate or nedocromil can be tried but if they do not control symptoms change to inhaled steroids.

β_2 adrenoreceptor agonists relax bronchial smooth muscle, acting within minutes. Salbutamol is best given by inhalation, but can be given PO or IV (do not use regular short acting β-agonists as maintenance).

CONFUSA

Since British Thoracic Society has laid down strict guidelines, there should be no confusion in this question. For guidelines refer page 172 (OHCM), 5th edn.

Immediate management (in acute severe asthma)

- Sit patient up and give high dose O_2
- Salbutamol 5 mg/terbutaline 10 mg nebulized with O_2
- Hydrocortisone 200 mg IV or prednisolone 30 mg PO (if very ill)
- Exclude pneumothorax (CXR).

Your notes:

20. A nine-year-old boy has a mild cough and wheeze after playing football in the cold weather.

Diagnosis: Exercise-induced asthma

Clinchers

- *A 9-year-old boy:* Exercise-induced asthma is most commonly present in childhood.
- *Mild cough and wheeze:* These are the diagnostic symptoms of asthma.
- *After playing football in cold weather:* Cold weather and exercise are both precipitants of asthma. Exercise is one of the most common precipitants of acute episodes of asthma. Exercise probably provokes bronchospasm to some extent in every asthmatic patients, and in some it is the only trigger that produces symptoms. There is a significant interaction between the ventilation produced by exercise, the temperature, and the water content of the inspired air and the magnitude of the postexertional obstruction.

CONFUSA

Cromoglycate is used prophylaxis is mild and exercised asthma (always inhaled), especially in children. Note that it may precipitate asthma. Exercise induction differs from other naturally occurring provocations of asthma, such as antigens or viral infections, in that it does not evoke any long-term sequelae nor does it change airway reactivity.

Investigation of Choice
PEFR

Immediate Management
Nebulisation

Treatment of Choice
Prophylactic inhaled sodium cromoglycate.

Your notes:

47. Chronic smoker 1 day after splenectomy presents with chest pain and dyspnea.

Diagnosis: Pulmonary collapse.

Clinchers

- *Chronic smoker:* Smokers are at particular risk, with increased secretions and ineffective cilia.
- *Splenectomy:* Some degree of pulmonary collapse occurs after almost every abdominal or transthoracic procedure.
  Mechanism: Mucus is retained in the bronchial tree
  ↓
  Blocks smaller bronchi
  ↓
  Alveolar air is then absorbed
  ↓
  Collapse of the supplied lung segments (usually the basal lobes)
  ↓
  Collapsed lung continued to be perfused and acts as a shunt
  ↓
  This reduced oxygenation
  ↓
  Secondary infection of collapsed segment
  ↓
  Abscess formation
- *1 day after:* Pulmonary collapse occurs within the first postoperative 48 hours. Also this excludes other conditions which occurs:
  - Pulmonary embolism—10th postoperative day
  - Infection—5th postoperative day
- *Chest pain and dyspnoea:* The patient is dyspnoeic with a rapid pulse and elevated temperature. There may be cyanosis. The patient attempt to cough, but this is painful.

CONFUSA

To relieve chest pain or abdominal pain (of operative scar), intercostal nerve blocks and epidural anaesthesia are preferred over opiate analgesia as the latter causes respiratory depression and worsens the already reduced O_2 saturation.

Fruity cough is typical pulmonary collapse and results from the sound of the bronchial secretions rattling within the chest (A good clinicians should be able to make the diagnosis while skill several yards away from the patient)

Investigation of Choice
CXR (mediastinal shift + opacity of involved segment—usually basal or mid zone)
+
Pulse oximetry (reduced saturation)

Immediate Management
Referral to a physiotherapist

Treatment of Choice
Symptomatic + breathing exercises.

Your notes:

49. Man with COPD presents with central cyanosis postoperatively.

Diagnosis: Pulmonary collapse.

Clinchers

- *COPD:* Pre-existing chronic pulmonary disease like emphysema or COPD is a risk factor for complicated pulmonary collapse after surgery.
- *Central cyanosis:* Cyanosis may or may not be present depending upon the severity of pulmonary collapse. In pre-existing diseases it tends to be severe enough to produce cyanosis.

Risk factors for pulmonary collapse

- Preoperative
  - Pre-existing acute or chronic pulmonary infection
  - Smokers
  - Chronic inflammatory diseases
  - Chest wall diseases, e.g. ankylosing spondylitis
- Operative
  - Anaesthetic drugs
  - Atropine
- Postoperative
  - Pain

Investigation of Choice
Pulse oximetry (as cyanosis is the main feature; if dyspnoea is the main feature; CXR will be done first).

Immediate Management
Referral to a physiotherapist.

Treatment of Choice
See Q 47.

Your notes:

111. A 40-year-old man underwent removal of tooth under anaesthesia, presents after one month with coughing up of blood.

Diagnosis: Inhaled foreign body

Clinchers

- *Removal of tooth under anaesthesia:* Tooth removal may have a complication of aspiration of a piece of tooth, especially when it is done under anaesthesia.
- *Coughing up of blood after one month:* The foreign body may lodge in the right main bronchus or upper basal lobe (most common sites because approach to them is wider, straighter and almost in line with the trachea). Inside the lung it can trigger a granulomatous reaction or infection which can then lead to haemoptysis and other symptoms.

CONFUSA

If the hemoptysis in this case is due to infection by foreign body, it would have presented much earlier (i.e. within a week) and the predominant symptom would have been of a swinging pyrexia. The given presentation is thus more indicative of a granulomatous reaction which will present usually after one month and with haemoptysis mainly.

Investigation of Choice

Chest X-ray.

Immediate Management

Contact dental surgeon who has operated upon him for a detailed history.

Treatment of Choice

Removal (endoscopic).

Your notes:

112. Female with cough, copious blood tinged sputum for more than a month. She is from south-east Asia.

Diagnosis: Pulmonary tuberculosis.

Clinchers

- *Cough:* Pulmonary TB may be silent but it causes cough more commonly.
- *Copious blood tinged sputum:* Copious sputum is a typical feature of tuberculosis. It may be blood tinged or associated with frank haemoptysis. Other associated presenting features can be:
  - Pneumonia
  - Pleurisy
  - Pleural effusion
- *South-east Asia*: Tuberculosis is most prevent in Indian subcontinent and is mostly seen in UK among immigrants from there (Pakistan, India, Bangladesh).

CONFUSA

Primary TB is usually asymptomatic, but there may be fever, lassitude, sweats, anorexia, cough, sputum, erythema nodosum or phlyctenular conjunctivitis. The most common nonpulmonary infection is GI, most commonly affecting the ileocaecal junction and associated lymph nodes.

Investigation of Choice

- *Screening:* CXR (consolidation, cavitation, fibrosis, calcification)
- *Definitive:* Sputum culture.

Immediate Management

Trace family contacts for prophylaxis

Treatment of Choice

Directly observed therapy (DOT) with rifampicin, isoniazid, pyrazinamide ± ethambutol x 2 months, and then only with rifampicin and isoniazid for next for months.

Your notes:

113. Female presents with acute pleuritic chest pain, haemoptysis after undergoing hysterectomy.

Diagnosis: Pulmonary embolism.

Clinchers

- *Acute pleuritic chest pain:* It is the usual presenting feature of pulmonary embolism. Other common associated presenting features can be:
  - Acute breathlessness
  - Haemoptysis
  - Dizziness
  - Syncope
- *Haemoptysis:* Haemoptysis occurs in 30%, often three or more days after the initial event.
- *After undergoing hysterectomy:* Any cause of immobility, i.e. postoperative immobility can increase the risk of pulmonary embolism. This risk is much more in middle-aged females on oral contraceptive pills (it induces hypercoagulability).

CONFUSA

Peluritic chest pain is common with small or medium sized pulmonary embolism. A massive pulmonary embolism give rise to severe central pain because of cardiac ischaemia due to lack of coronary blood flow.

Investigation of Choice

- *Screening*
  - If patient stable = V/Q scan
  - If unable to undergo the above test = spiral CT
- *Definitive:* Pulmonary angiogram.

Immediate Management

Anticoagulation with LMW heparin

Treatment of Choice

Oral warfarin 10 mg PO x 3 months.

Your notes:

114. A middle-aged woman develops a purulent cough with some haemoptysis. A chest X-ray reveals right upper lobe shadows.

Diagnosis: Pulmonary tuberculosis (PTB)

Clinchers

- *Middle-aged women:* Usually symptomatic primary tuberculosis develops due to reactivation of a primary complex years after the exposure.
- *Purulent cough with some haemoptysis:* Sputum in PTB may be mucoid, purulent or blood-stained.
- *CXR reveals right upper lobe shadows:* The CXR typically shows patchy or nodular shadows in the upper zones, loss of volume, and fibrosis with or without cavitation.

CONFUSA

Reactivation of tuberculosis is usually due to:

- DM
- Malnutrition
- Immunosuppression
- Drugs
  - Cytotoxins
  - Steroids
- Lymphoma
- AIDS

Investigation of Choice

- *Screening:* CXR
- *Definitive:* Sputum culture and microscopy.

Immediate Management

Find out cause of reactivation (often none found).

Treatment of Choice

Directly observed therapy (DOT) x 6 months

Your notes:

118. A woman 10 days following hysterectomy complaints of severe left sided chest pain and breathlessness. Chest X-ray and ECG failed to relieve any abnormality.

Diagnosis: Pulmonary embolism.

Clinchers

- *10 days following hysterectomy:* Any cause of immobility or hypercoagulability, e.g. recent surgery (in this case hysterectomy), recent stroke or MI, disseminated malignancy, thrombophilia/antiphospholipid syndrome, prolonged bed-rest and pregnancy.
- *Severe left chest pain/breathlessness:* Symptoms of pulmonary embolism are—acute breathless, pleuritic chest pain, haemoptysis, dizziness and syncope.
- *Chest X-ray and ECG show no abnormality:* Chest X-ray and ECG is generally normal in pulmonary embolism.

Investigation of Choice

- *Screening:* V/Q scan or spiral CT.
- *Definitive:* CT pulmonary angiography. This shows clots down to 5th order pulmonary arteries.

Immediate Management
Screen for DVT.

Treatment of Choice
Anticoagulation.

Your notes:

PAPER 5

34. A 29-year-old motorist, in the Accident and Emergency Department resuscitation room, appears to be stable after an accident. While standing up, he becomes progressively dyspnoeic. There is reduced air entry on the left side of his chest.

Diagnosis: Tension pneumothorax

Clinchers

- *A 29-year-old motorist:* The incidence of RTA is maximum in young motorcyclists. The accident must have caused chest trauma and hence a rib fracture which could've been easily missed in presence of other serious and more evident injuries.
- *Progressively dyspnoeic:* Progressive dyspnoea suggests a tension pneumothorax. It is a medical emergency and can lead to a fatal outcome if not treated urgently.
- *While standing up:* The process of mobilisation might have pushed the sharp end of a fractured rib against the pleura and thereby puncturing it to produce this condition.
- *Reduced air entry on left side of chest:* This confirms our diagnostic suspicion, or at least provide as enough clinical ground to proceed a head with management of tension pneumothorax.

CONFUSA

Traumatic pneumothoraxes can result from both penetrating and nonpenetrating chest trauma. Tension pneumothorax usually occurs during mechanical ventilation or resuscitative efforts. Tension pneumothorax must be treated as a medical emergency. If the tension in the pleural space is not relieved, the patient is likely to die from inadequate cardiac output or marked hypoxaemia. A large bore needle should be inserted into the pleural space through the second anterior intercostal space. If large amounts of gas escape from the needle after insertion, the diagnosis is confirmed. The needle should be left in place until a thoracostomy tube can be inserted.

Investigation of Choice
CXR (but after needle thoracocentesis).

Immediate Management
Immediate needle thoracocentesis.

Treatment of Choice
Chest drain (must in all cases of traumatic pneumothorax).

186. A tall young woman developed sharp pain on one side of his chest two days ago. Since then he has been short of breath on exertion.

Diagnosis: Pneumothorax after spontaneous primary rupture

Clinchers

- *Tall*: It increases the risk of having apical bullae became of increased negative intrathoracic pressure.
- *Young*: Spontaneous pneumothorax is predominantly seen in "tens and twenties".
- *Man*: Incidence of spontaneous pneumothorax is more in males.
- *Sharp pain*: It is the characteristic pleuritic pain of pneumothorax.
- *Unilateral*: It is characteristic of pneumothorax as there are two pleural cavities.
- *Shortens of breath on exertion*: It confirms the diagnosis of pneumothorax.
- *Two days ago*: Spontaneous primary rupture of bullae is usually mild.

CONFUSA

Insertion of large gauge open bore cannula (16-17 G) is only done for tension pneumothoraces. All other pneumothoraces are treated with water seal.

Investigation of Choice

CXR

Immediate Management

Serial radiographic observation.

Treatment of Choice

Aspiration or underwater seal drainage if necessary.

Your notes:

188. A 23-year-old woman on the oral contraceptive pill suddenly gets tightness in her chest and becomes very breathlessness.

Diagnosis: Pulmonary venous thromboembolism (PE).

Clinchers

- *A 23-year-old woman:* She belongs to the typical OCP user age group.
- *OCP*: They increase the risk of pulmonary embolism by producing a hypercoagulable state.
- *Sudden tightness and breathlessness*: Chest pain and shortness of breath are the two most usual symptoms in PE. The pain is most often pleuritic in nature; sharp and worse with deep inspiration and couphing. There may be haemoptysis.

CONFUSA

Sometimes collapse is the presenting symptom. A sudden urge to defaecate may herald the onset of symptoms. Signs are very variable and often absent. There may be tachycardia and tachypnoea. Areas of crepitus or a pleural rub are sometimes heard, as is a pulmonary flow murmur. Thrombosis of the deep veins is rarely clinically apparent.

Investigation of Choice

V/Q scan

Immediate Management

High flow O_2 + 10 mg IV morphine + anticoagulation

Treatment of Choice

Heparin (loading dose of 5000-10000 units of standard heparin IV followed by a continuous infusion of 1000-2000 units per hour).

Your notes:

191. Tuberculosis.

Diagnosis: Sputum culture.

Clinchers

- Tuberculosis is caused by bacteria belonging to *Myobacterium tuberculosis* complex. Usually affects lungs, though in one-third cases other organs may be involved.
- Tuberculous spinal disease in Egyptian mummies proves, that it is one of the oldest diseases known to affect humanity.
- The key to diagnosis of tuberculosis is high index of suspicion. Go for CXR, followed by AFB microscopy and mycobacterial culture.

CONFUSA

Though in suspected tuberculosis, the first investigation to be done is CXR (shows upper lobe infiltrates with cavitations), sputum culture is the most definitive investigation, where the organism can be isolated and cultured.

Investigation of Choice

Sputum culture.
— Sputum microscopy
— CXR

Immediate Management

If sputum positive, isolate the patient, and start Antitubercular therapy (ATT) immediately.

Treatment of Choice

Five major drugs are considered the first line agents for treatment of tuberculosis.

- Isoniazid (5 mg/kg), max 300 mg daily
- Rifampicin (10 mg/kg), max 600 mg daily
- Pyrazinamide (15-30 mg/kg) max 2 g daily
- Ethambutol (15-25 mg/kg)
- Streptomycin (15 mg/kg) in max 1 gm daily.

Your notes:

192. Carcinoma of the right main bronchus.

Diagnosis: Fiberoptic bronchoscopy

Clinchers

- Fiberoptic bronchoscopy in the procedure of choice for visualizing an endobronchial tumour and collecting cytologic and histologic specimens. Inspection of the tracheobronchial mucosa can demonstrate and endobronchial granulomas often seen in sarcoidosis, and endobronchial biopsy of such lesions or transbronchial biopsy of the lung interstition can confirm the diagnosis.
- Inspection of the airway mucosa by bronchoscopy can also demonstrate the characteristic appearance of endobronchial Kaposi's sarcoma in patient with AIDS.
- Symptoms of bronchial carcinoma are cough (80%), haemoptysis (70%), dyspnoea (60%), chest pain (40%), anorexia, weight loss.

CONFUSA

Bronchoscopy gives histological diagnosis and assess operatility. CT stages the tumour, CXR for bony secondaries can be seen besides peripheral circular opacity, hilar enlargement, consolidation and pleural effusion.

Investigation of Choice

Fiberoptic bronchoscopy.

Immediate Management

Look for complications (local metastatic, endocrine) and treat.

Treatment of Choice

Nonsmall cell tumour: Excision for peripheral tumours, with no metastatic spread.

Small cell tumour: These are almost always disseminated at presentation. May respond to chemotherapy.

Your notes:

193. Pulmonary embolism.

Diagnosis: Already stated as the question.

Clinchers

Since the question, has not given any clinical profile, let us see the most common 'clinchers', that GMC uses in their exams for this condition.

- *Precipitants:* Air travel, recent operation, pregnancy, OCP, hormone replacement therapy, disseminated malignancy, DVT.
- *Symptoms:* Acute breathlessness, pleuritic chest pain, haemoptysis.
- *Signs:* Tachypnoea, tachycardia, hypotension, raised JVP, pleural rub.
- *CXR:* Usually normal (in GMC questions).
- *ECG:* Usually normal (in GMC questions), $S_I Q_{III} T_{III}$ pattern, sinus tachycardia, right bundle branch block.

CONFUSA

Pulmonary embolism produces central cyanosis due to decreased oxygen saturation. Which is produced by only three other common conditions, i.e.
- Pulmonary oedema
- Severe respiratory disease
- Congenital cyanotic heart disease.

Investigation of Choice

Investigation of pulmonary embolism is a point of major confusion in PLAB examination. Consider following points while choosing the investigation for PE:
- *Screening*
  - V/Q scan—only if the patient is stable and not severely breathless
  - Spiral CT with contrast—if facilities are available patient's general state do not allow a V/Q scan to be done
- *Definitive:* Pulmonary angiogram—but not usually done because of risk of complications and it being an invasive test.

Note: Always look in the "instructions" to the theme about the type of investigation being asked for, i.e. is it "definitive" or "screening". It is important as the answer is usually different for both and you will end up losing marks for something you know.

Immediate Management

Anticoagulation with LMW heparin (Dalteparin 200 U/kg/24 hr SC; max dose 18,000 IU/24h)
- Stop when INR > 2

Treatment of Choice

Oral warfarin 10 mg for minimum 3 months

194. Bronchiectasis.

Diagnosis: Already stated as the question.

Clinchers

Bronchiectasis is a frequent question in PLAB exam. The most frequent 'clinchers' used by GMC to describe this condition are:

- *Secondary to:* Cystic fibrosis, kartageneger's syndrome, pertussis in the childhood, allergic bronchopulmonary aspergillosis.
  "Non-GMC" conditions—Young's syndrome (primary ciliary dyskinesia), measles, bronchiolitis, pneumonia, TB, HIV, bronchial obstruction (tumour, foreign body), hypogammaglobulinaemia, rheumatoid arthritis, ulcerative colitis, idiopathic.
- *Symptoms:* Persistent cough, copious purulent sputum, intermittent haemoptysis.
- *Signs:* Finger clubbing, coarse inspiratory, crackles, wheeze.
- *Complications:* Pneumonia, pleural effusion, pneumothorax, haemoptysis, cerebral abscess, amyloidosis.

CONFUSA

Spirometry is bronchiectasis shows an obstructive pattern. Reversability should be assessed to differentiate from asthma.

Investigation of Choice
- *Screening:* CXR—Tramline and ring shadows.
- *Definitive:* High resolution CT chest—to assess extent and distribution.

Immediate Management

Antibiotics if infection (usually pseudomonas) is present.

Treatment of Choice

Postural drainage + bronchodilators (if asthma, COPD, cystic fibrosis, ABPA present) + steroids (if ABPA present).

Indications for surgery are:
- Localized bronchiectasis
- To control severe haemoptysis.

Your notes:

195. Bronchial carcinoid.

Diagnosis: Already stated as the question.

Clinchers

Questions about bronchial carcinoids are a rarity in PLAB exam. Still let us review some salient features of them.

- Usually follow a benign course
- May secrete other hormones, effects of whom constitute the common presenting complaints of this condition. They can secrete
  - ACTH
  - Arginine vasopressin
- Carcinoid syndrome is only produced when any carcinoid has liver metastases. It is characterised by:
  - Cutaneous flush
  - Bronchoconstrition
  - Diarrhoea.

CONFUSA

Bronchial carcinoids and small cell carcinoma both develops from the same cells (kulchitsky cell in bronchial epithelium). But carcinoid can be differentiated by presence of carcinoid syndrome (only in presence of liver metastases) and cardiac valvular lesions—both of these are absent in small cell carcinoma of lung. Paraneoplastic syndromes are not a criteria for differentiation as both can cause them (especially ACTH).

Investigation of Choice

- *Screening:* 24 hour urine 5HIAA increase.
- *Definitive:* CXR/CT—usually done only if liver metastases are absent as only then a curative resection is possible.

Immediate Management

High dose octreotide for crises + careful fluid balance.

Treatment of Choice

- Crises—Octreotide
- Flushing—Ketanserin
- Diarrhoea—Loperamide/cyproheptadine
- Hepatic metastases—embolisation
- Bronchial obstruction—surgical debulking

Your notes:

PAPER 6

71. A man who has been worked as boiler worker for 20 years presents with dyspnoea and pleurisy.

Diagnosis: Asbestosis

Clinchers

- *Boiler worker for 20 years:* Exposure to asbestos occurred particularly in naval ship building yards and in power stations, especially boiler workers. There is a considerable time lag between exposures and development of the disease, particularly mesothelioma (20-40 years).
- *Dyspnoea:* It is due to progressive airflow limitation due to fibrosis in this condition.
- *Pleurisy:* It denotes a pleural lesion which is most probably a mesothelioma in this case.

CONFUSA

Asbestosis is defined as fibrosis of the lungs caused by asbestos dust, which may or may not be associated with fibrosis of the parietal or visceral layers of the pleura. It is a progressive disease characterised by breathlessness and accompanied by finger clubbing and bilateral basal end expiratory crackles. Fibrosis, not detectable on chest X-ray, may be revealed.

Investigation of Choice

CXR/CT scan (screening)
Pleural biopsy (definitive)

Immediate Management

Legal advise, as he may be entitled for compensation in UK.

Treatment of Choice

No treatment is known to alter the progress of the disease, though corticosteroids are often prescribed.

Your notes:

72. Female with cough, copious blood tinged sputum for more than a month. She is from south-east Asia.

Diagnosis: Pulmonary tuberculosis.

Clinchers

- *Cough:* Pulmonary TB may be silent but it causes cough more commonly.
- *Copious blood tinged sputum:* Copious sputum is a typical feature of tuberculosis. It may be blood tinged or associated with frank haemoptysis. Other associated presenting features can be:
  - Pneumonia
  - Pleurisy
  - Pleural effusion
- *South-east Asia*: Tuberculosis is most prevent in Indian subcontinent and is mostly seen in UK among immigrants from there (Pakistan, India, Bangladesh).

CONFUSA

Primary TB is usually asymptomatic, but there may be fever, lassitude, sweats, anorexia, cough, sputum, erythema nodosum or phlyctenular conjunctivitis. The most common nonpulmonary infection is GI, most commonly affecting the ileocaecal junction and associated lymph nodes.

Investigation of Choice

- *Screening:* CXR (consolidation, cavitation, fibrosis, calcification)
- *Definitive:* Sputum culture.

Immediate Management

Trace family contacts for prophylaxis

Treatment of Choice

Directly observed therapy (DOT) with rifampicin, isoniazid, pyrazinamide ± ethambutol x 2 months, and then only with rifampicin and isoniazid for next for months.

Your notes:

73. A middle-aged woman develops a purulent cough with some haemoptysis. A chest X-ray reveals right upper lobe shadows.

Diagnosis: Pulmonary tuberculosis (PTB)

Clinchers

- *Middle-aged women:* Usually symptomatic primary tuberculosis develops due to reactivation of a primary complex years after the exposure.
- *Purulent cough with some haemoptysis:* Sputum in PTB may be mucoid, purulent or blood-stained.
- *CXR reveals right upper lobe shadows:* The CXR typically shows patchy or nodular shadows in the upper zones, loss of volume, and fibrosis with or without cavitation.

CONFUSA

Reactivation of tuberculosis is usually due to:

- DM
- Malnutrition
- Immunosuppression
- Drugs
  - Cytotoxins
  - Steroids
- Lymphoma
- AIDS

Investigation of Choice

- *Screening:* CXR
- *Definitive:* Sputum culture and microscopy.

Immediate Management

Find out cause of reactivation (often none found).

Treatment of Choice

Directly observed therapy (DOT) x 6 months

Your notes:

74. Female presents with acute pleuritic chest pain, haemoptysis after undergoing hysterectomy.

Diagnosis: Pulmonary embolism.

Clinchers

➢ *Acute pleuritic chest pain:* It is the usual presenting feature of pulmonary embolism. Other common associated presenting features can be:
- Acute breathlessness
- Haemoptysis
- Dizziness
- Syncope

➢ *Haemoptysis:* Haemoptysis occurs in 30%, often three or more days after the initial event.

➢ *After undergoing hysterectomy:* Any cause of immobility, i.e. postoperative immobility can increase the risk of pulmonary embolism. This risk is much more in middle-aged females on oral contraceptive pills (it induces hypercoagulability).

CONFUSA

Pleuritic chest pain is common with small or medium sized pulmonary embolism. A massive pulmonary embolism give rise to severe central pain because of cardiac ischaemia due to lack of coronary blood flow.

Investigation of Choice
- *Screening*
  - If patient stable = V/Q scan
  - If unable to undergo the above test = spiral CT
- *Definitive:* Pulmonary angiogram.

Immediate Management

Anticoagulation with LMW heparin

Treatment of Choice

Oral warfarin 10 mg PO x 3 months.

Your notes:

76. Patient with acute shortness of breath, wheeze. Chest X-ray—normal, low oxygen, $PaCO_2$. PEFR-120 ml/minute.

Diagnosis: Asthma.

Clinchers

➢ *Acute shortness of breath, wheeze:* These are the characteristic of asthma may be associated with cough (often nocturnal) symptoms and sputum.

➢ *CXR normal:* In asthma CXR may be normal or hyperinflation may be observed. This helps to rule out other chronic lung pathologies.

➢ *Low oxygen, low $PaCO_2$:* Arterial blood gases (ABG) analysis in asthma usually shows a normal or slightly reduced PaO_2 and low $PaCO_2$ (hyperventilation). If $PaCO_2$ is raised, transfer the patient to ITU for ventilation.

➢ *PEFR—120 ml/min:* PEFR < 50% of predicted is seen in severe attack of asthma. PEFR < 33% along with silent chest, cyanosis, bradycardia is life-threatening.

Predicted PEFR: Predicted values of PEFR vary with age, sex and height, and typically 450-600 ml/min in men and 350-500 ml/min in women. Values under 100-200 ml/min indicate severe ventilatory dysfunction.

CONFUSA

Differentiate asthma from the following:
- COPD (often coexists with asthma)
- Pulmonary oedema (cardiac asthma)
- Large airway obstruction (e.g. foreign body, tumour)
- SVC obstruction (wheeze/dyspnoea not episodic)
- Pneumothorax
- Pulmonary embolism/bronchiectasis
- Obliterative bronchiolitis (in elderly).

Investigation of Choice
- PEFR
- ABG
- Spirometry: obstructive defects (ˉFEV_1, FVCM - residual volume).

Immediate Management
- Sit patient up and give high dose O_2
- Nebulize with salbutamol 5 mg or terbutaline 10 mg.

Treatment of Choice

Once patient starts improving reduce nebulized salbutamol and switch to inhaled β_2-agonists.
- Initiate inhaled steroids and stop oral steroids if possible
- Continue to monitor PEFR.

77. Bilateral hilar opacities, ACE is high.

Diagnosis: Sarcoidosis

Clinchers

- *Bilateral hilar opacities:* Respiratory symptoms are the most common presentation of sarcoidosis, with bilateral hilar opacities (bilateral hilar lymphadenopathy) being characteristic feature. This can be detected on routine chest X-ray.

  Sarcoidosis is a multisystem granulomatous disorder, that presents with bilateral hilar lymphadenopathy, pulmonary infiltration and skin or eye lesions. Diagnosis is confirmed histologically.
- *ACE is high:* In sarcoidosis, serum level of angiotensin converting enzyme is high. Though raised levels of ACE are also seen with patients.

CONFUSA

Differential diagnosis of this bilateral hilar lymphadenopathy includes:
- Lymphoma—though it is rare for this to affect only hilar lymph nodes.
- *Pulmonary tuberculosis:* Though it is rare for the hilar lymph nodes to be symmetrically enlarged
- *Carcinoma of bronchus with malignant spread to the contralateral hilar lymph nodes:* Though rare for this to give rise to typical symmetrical picture.

Investigation of Choice

Serum ACE + CXR.

Immediate Management

None.

Treatment of Choice

Patients with bilateral hilar opacities alone do not require treatment since the majority recover spontaneously.

Your notes:

79. An alcoholic admitted semi-comatose. ABG shows low oxygen saturation.

Diagnosis: Aspiration pneumonia.

Clinchers

Aspiration of liquid (foreign material), into the tracheobronchial tree results from various disorders that impair normal deglutition, especially disturbances of consciousness and esophageal dysfunction.

- *Alcoholic admitted semicomatose:* Consumption of alcohol, cigarette smoking, and use of theophylline are known to relax lower esophageal sphincter. This allows reflux of gastric contents into the esophagus and predisposes to pulmonary aspiration especially at night. But in this question the presentation appears to be acute, and therefore in an alcoholic with disturated consciousness, aspiration of alcohol can be the likely cause, which led to abrupt onset of respiratory distress, thus low oxygen,

CONFUSA

Since the question is incomplete, lefts discuss the differential diagnosis:
- *Alcoholic intoxication:* In severe cases alcohol overdose is marked by respiratory depression, stupor, seizures, shock syndrome, coma and death.
- *Subdural haemorrhage:* Subdural haemorrhage is a common cause of semicomatose presentation in alcoholics, due to fall.
- *Hypoglycaemia:* Alcohol related hypoglycaemia is due to hepatic glycogen depletion combined with alcohol-mediated inhibition of gluconeogenesis.

Investigation of Choice

- Arterial blood gases (ABG) analysis.
- Blood sugar.
- CT scan to rule out subdural haemorrhage.

Immediate Management

- Maintain airway with high flow oxygen.

Treatment of Choice

O_2 to maintain PaO_2 > 8 kPa. With aspiration there is risk of aspirating oropharyngeal anaerobes.

Streptococcus pneumonia: Cefuroxime 1.5 g/h IV + Metronidazole 500 mg/8 h IV.

Your Notes

80. Patient with recent MI, develops acute breathlessness and haemoptysis. CXR shows dilated pulmonary artery and wedge shaped area of infarction. Decreased PaO_2 and decreased $PaCO_2$.

Diagnosis: Pulmonary embolism (PE).

Clinchers

- *Recent MI:* Though most commonly pulmonary embolism arises from venous thrombosis in pelvis or legs, recent stroke or MI may also lead to PE (right ventricular thrombus).
- *Acute breathlessness/haemoptysis:* These are along with pleuritis chest pain, dizziness and family history of thromboembolism are important symptoms of pulmonary embolism.
- *CXR:* In pulmonary embolism. CXR may be normal or may show
  - Oligemia of affected segment
  - Dilated pulmonary artery
  - Linear atelectasis
  - Small pleural effusion
  - Wedge-shaped opacities or cavitations (rare) (wedge-shaped area of infarction).

Decreased PaO_2 and $PaCO_2$

Arterial blood gases (ABG) analysis shows hyperventilation + gas exchange $^-$, thereby $^-$ PaO_2 and $^-PaCO_2$.

Investigation of Choice

- U and E, ECG
- CT pulmonary angiography (determines emboli in pulmonary arteries
- V/Q scan (ventilation/perfusion scan) may show mismatched defects.

Immediate Management

- Oxygen 100%
- Morphine 10 mg IV (if in pain).

Treatment of Choice

- Heparin for ≥ 5 days, and until INR > 2.
- If obvious remedial cause, 6 weeks treatment with Warfarin. Otherwise continue for 3-6 months. Patients with recent MI, are at risk of developing DVT and PE and therefore they should be prophylactically heparinized (50000/12 h SC) until fully mobile.

Your Notes

81. A tall young woman developed sharp pain on one side of his chest two days ago. Since then she has been short of breath on exertion.

Diagnosis: Pneumothorax after spontaneous primary rupture

Clinchers

- *Tall*: It increases the risk of having apical bullae became of increased negative intrathoracic pressure.
- *Young*: Spontaneous pneumothorax is predominantly seen in "tens and twenties".
- *Man*: Incidence of spontaneous pneumothorax is more in males.
- *Sharp pain*: It is the characteristic pleuritic pain of pneumothorax.
- *Unilateral*: It is characteristic of pneumothorax as there are two pleural cavities.
- *Shortens of breath on exertion*: It confirms the diagnosis of pneumothorax.
- *Two days ago*: Spontaneous primary rupture of bullae is usually mild.

CONFUSA

Insertion of large gauge open bore cannula (16-17 G) is only done for tension pneumothoraces. All other pneumothoraces are treated with water seal.

Investigation of Choice

CXR

Immediate Management

Serial radiographic observation.

Treatment of Choice

Aspiration or underwater seal drainage if necessary.

Your notes:

183. A woman 10 days following hysterectomy complaints of severe left sided chest pain and breathlessness. Chest X-ray and ECG failed to relieve any abnormality.

Diagnosis: Pulmonary embolism.

Clinchers

- *Ten days following hysterectomy:* Any cause of immobility or hypercoagulability, e.g. recent surgery (in this case hysterectomy), recent stroke or MI, disseminated malignancy, thrombophilia/antiphospholipid syndrome, prolonged bed-rest and pregnancy.
- *Severe left chest pain/breathlessness:* Symptoms of pulmonary embolism are—acute breathless, pleuritic chest pain, haemoptysis, dizziness and syncope.
- *Chest X-ray and ECG show no abnormality:* Chest X-ray and ECG is generally normal in pulmonary embolism.

Investigation of Choice

- *Screening:* V/Q scan or spiral CT.
- *Definitive:* CT pulmonary angiography. This shows clots down to 5th order pulmonary arteries.

Immediate Management

Screen for DVT.

Treatment of Choice

Anticoagulation.

Your notes:

PAPER 7

17. Patient with acute shortness of breath, wheeze. Chest X-ray—normal, low oxygen, $PaCO_2$. PEFR-120 ml/minute

Diagnosis: Asthma.

Clinchers

- *Acute shortness of breath, wheeze:* These are the characteristic of asthma may be associated with cough (often nocturnal) symptoms and sputum.
- *CXR normal:* In asthma CXR may be normal or hyperinflation may be observed. This helps to rule out other chronic lung pathologies.
- *Low oxygen, low $PaCO_2$:* Arterial blood gases (ABG) analysis in asthma usually shows a normal or slightly reduced PaO_2 and low $PaCO_2$ (hyperventilation). If $PaCO_2$ is raised, transfer the patient to ITU for ventilation.
- *PEFR—120 ml/min:* PEFR < 50% of predicted is seen in severe attack of asthma. PEFR < 33% along with silent chest, cyanosis, bradycardia is life-threatening. *Predicted PEFR:* Predicted values of PEFR vary with age, sex and height, and typically 450-600 ml/min in men and 350-500 ml/min in women. Values under 100-200 ml/min indicate severe ventilatory dysfunction.

CONFUSA

Differentiate asthma from the following:

- COPD (often coexists with asthma)
- Pulmonary oedema (cardiac asthma)
- Large airway obstruction (e.g. foreign body, tumour)
- SVC obstruction (wheeze/dyspnoea not episodic)
- Pneumothorax
- Pulmonary embolism/bronchiectasis
- Obliterative bronchiolitis (in elderly).

Investigation of Choice

- PEFR
- ABG
- Spirometry: Obstructive defects (¯FEV$_1$, FVCM - residual volume).

Immediate Management

- Sit patient up and give high dose O_2
- Nebulize with salbutamol 5 mg or terbutaline 10 mg.

Treatment of Choice

Once patient starts improving reduce nebulized salbutamol and switch to inhaled β_2-agonists.

- Initiate inhaled steroids and stop oral steroids if possible
- Continue to monitor PEFR.

19. An alcoholic admitted semi-comatose. ABG shows low oxygen saturation.

Diagnosis: Aspiration pneumonia.

Clinchers

Aspiration of liquid (foreign material), into the tracheobronchial tree results from various disorders that impair normal deglutition, especially disturbances of consciousness and esophageal dysfunction.

- *Alcoholic admitted semicomatose:* Consumption of alcohol, cigarette smoking, and use of theophylline are known to relax lower esophageal sphincter. This allows reflux of gastric contents into the esophagus and predisposes to pulmonary aspiration especially at night. But in this question the presentation appears to be acute, and therefore in an alcoholic with disturated consciousness, aspiration of alcohol can be the likely cause, which led to abrupt onset of respiratory distress, thus low oxygen,

CONFUSA

Since the question is incomplete, lefts discuss the differential diagnosis:

- *Alcohol intoxication:* In severe cases alcohol overdose is marked by respiratory depression, stupor, seizures, shock syndrome, coma and death.
- *Subdural haemorrhage:* Subdural haemorrhage is a common cause of semicomatose presentation in alcoholics, due to fall.
- *Hypoglycaemia:* Alcohol related hypoglycaemia is due to hepatic glycogen depletion combined with alcohol-mediated inhibition of gluconeogenesis.

Investigation of Choice

- Arterial blood gases (ABG) analysis.
- Blood sugar.
- CT scan to rule out subdural haemorrhage.

Immediate Management

- Maintain airway with high flow oxygen.

Treatment of Choice

O_2 to maintain $PaO_2 > 8$ kPa. With aspiration there is risk of aspirating oropharyngeal anaerobes.

Streptococcus pneumoniae: Cefuroxime 1.5 gh IV + Metronidazole 500 mg/8 h IV.

Your Notes:

20. Patient with recent MI, develops acute breathlessness and hemoptysis. CXR shows dilated pulmonary artery and wedge shaped area of infarction. Decreased PaO_2 and decreased $PaCO_2$.

Diagnosis: Pulmonary embolism (PE).

Clinchers

- *Recent MI:* Though most commonly pulmonary embolism arises from venous thrombosis in pelvis or legs, recent stroke or MI may also lead to PE (right ventricular thrombus).
- *Acute breathlessness/haemoptysis:* These are along with pleuritis chest pain, dizziness and family history of thromboembolism are important symptoms of pulmonary embolism.
- *CXR:* In pulmonary embolism. CXR may be normal or may show
  - Oligemia of affected segment
  - Dilated pulmonary artery
  - Linear atelectasis
  - Small pleural effusion
  - Wedge-shaped opacities or cavitations (rare) (wedge-shaped area of infarction).

Decreased PaO_2 and $PaCO_2$

Arterial blood gases (ABG) analysis shows hyperventilation + gas exchange ↓, thereby ↓ PaO_2 and ↓$PaCO_2$.

Investigation of Choice

- U and E, ECG
- CT pulmonary angiography (determines emboli in pulmonary arteries
- V/Q scan (ventilation/perfusion scan) may show mismatched defects.

Immediate Management

- Oxygen 100%
- Morphine 10 mg IV (if in pain).

Treatment of Choice

- Heparin for ≥ 5 days, and until INR > 2.
- If obvious remedial cause, 6 weeks treatment with Warfarin. Otherwise continue for 3-6 months. Patients with recent MI, are at risk of developing DVT and PE and therefore they should be prophylactically heparinized (50000/12 h SC) until fully mobile.

Your Notes:

21. Patient involved in road traffic accident (RTA), neck immobilised. Has massive head and facial injuries, together with noisy breathing despite administration of 100% oxygen.

Diagnosis: Partial upper airway obstruction.

Clinchers

- *RTA:* It usually causes polytrauma requiring ICU maintenance.
- *Neck immobilised:* It means that cervical spine has been protected.
- *Massive head and facial injuries:* These require continuous observation and monitoring till a definitive diagnosis of any specific injury is made. Facial injuries often produce upper respiratory obstruction due to discontinuing in respiratory tract.
- *Noisy breathing despite 100% oxygen:* High flow 100% oxygen is the second step in primary survey after protecting the neck. Noises from the upper airway indicate airway obstruction. There may be snoring, rattles, stridor or other sounds.

CONFUSA

Any partial upper airway obstruction require urgent intubation as there is high-risk of development of a complete obstruction.

Investigation of Choice

Skull and face X-rays.

Immediate Management

Intubate and PPV under expert care.

Treatment of Choice

As per the diagnosis.

Your Notes:

23. Known asthmatic patient involved in road traffic accident (RTA). Has a right-sided chest pain. On auscultation, right side is hyper-resonant. Trachea is deviated to the left.

Diagnosis: Tension pneumothorax (right side).

Clinchers

- *Asthmatic patient:* In patients over 40 years of age, COPD most commonly predisposes to pneumothorax. Rarer causes include bronchial asthma, carcinoma, a lung abscess breaking down and leading to bronchopulmonary fistula and severe pulmonary fibrosis with cyst formation.
- *RTA:* A simple pneumothorax in a patient of trauma may develop into a tension pneumothorax—particularly when the patient receives IPPV.
- *Right sided chest pain:* This is pleuritic pain which is variably in intensity.
- *Hyper-resonance on same side:* This rules out cardiac tamponade and confirms pneumothorax.
- *Trachea is deviated to left:* Signs of tension pneumothorax are:
  - Hypotension
  - Distended neck veins
  - Trachea deviated away from the side of pneumothorax
  - Severe respiratory distress.

CONFUSA

A CXR should not be performed if a tension pneumothorax is suspected as it will delay immediate necessary treatment. The clinical picture of tension pneumothorax may be mistaken for that of a cardiac tamponade. However, tension pneumothorax is more common and may be differentiated by the hyperresonance over the affected side.

Investigation of Choice

CXR but only after needle thoracocentesis.

Immediate Management

Needle thoracocentesis urgently.

Treatment of Choice

Chest drain (always required in a traumatic pneumothorax irrespective of its size).

Your Notes:

41. Patient stabbed in right chest. Ultrasound showed no free fluid perabdominally, patient is breathless, pale.

Diagnosis: Haemothorax.

Clinchers

- *Stabbed in right chest:* A stab wound may cause profound bleeding from the internal thoracic artery or other intrathoracic structures.
- *USG showed no free fluid per-abdominally:* This rules out intraperitoneal bleed after injury to any abdominal viscera.
- *Breathless:* Dyspnoea and reduced breath sounds are characteristic.
- *Pale:* It signifies blood loss and hence haemothorax.

CONFUSA

Haemothorax is usually a result of intercostal or internal thoracic vessel damage. The bleeding is often brisk and continuous from the high pressure of the intercostal arteries. In contrast, bleeding from the low-pressure pulmonary vessels usually stops with the collapse of the lung.

Investigation of Choice

CXR (blunting of costophrenic angles).

Immediate Management

High concentration oxygen by mask.

Treatment of Choice

Chest drain (always required in a stab wound).

Your notes:

45. A known asthmatic on treatment with inhaled Beta-2-agonist and steroid. Now presents with hypotension, breathlessness and distended neck veins.

Diagnosis: Tension pneumothorax.

Clinchers

- *Asthmatic:* Asthma and other chronic lung diseases predispose to spontaneous pneumothorax. However, the most common disease implicated is COPD.
- *On treatment with inhaled beta-2 agonist and steroid:* This is the standard treatment to moderate to severe asthma. The presence of steroids in treatment regimen suggests a long-standing history and hence a comparatively higher risk of pneumothorax.
- *Hypotension, breathlessness and distended neck veins:* The six cardinal signs of a tension pneumothorax are:
  1. Air hunger + respiratory distress
  2. Pulse - + BP ¯
  3. Tracheal deviation
  4. Breath sounds ¯ on one side
  5. Cyanosis
  6. Neck vein distension.

CONFUSA

Insertion of a needle does not always decompress a tension pneumothorax as the underlying pleura and lung are "sucked" into the needle and occlude it. If this happens, a second attempt should be made failure to achieve decompression at this point indicates the need to proceed immediately to rapid insertion of a chest drain.

Note: Never use nitrous oxide mixtures (e.g. Entonox) for pain relief in pneumothorax as it may result in expansion of a gas filled space.

Investigation of Choice

CXR (after needle thoracocentesis).

Immediate Management

Needle thoracocentesis (urgent).

Treatment of Choice

Chest drain.

Your notes:

131. 25-year-old patient now has to use inhaled β2 agonists 2-3 times a day.

Best management: Inhaled steroids

Clinchers

For the management of chronic asthma, certain steps/ guidelines have been formulated by the British Thoracic Society.

According to these guidelines, occasional short acting inhaled β_2 agonists is the first step for symptom relief. If used more than once daily, or night time symptoms present, add standard dose *inhaled steroids:* beclometasone or budesonide 100-400 µg/12 h.

For British Thoracic Society Guidelines refer the high yield section of this book.

CONFUSA

Cromoglycate or nedocromil can also be tried after inhaled β_2 agonists, but they are no substitute to inhaled steroids, if symptoms are aggravate.

Investigation in chronic asthma

- PEFR monitoring
- CXR: hyperinflation
- Spirometry: obstructive defects (¯FEV_1/FVC, -residual volume).

Investigations in acute asthma

PEFR, sputum culture, blood culture, FBC, U and E, CRP.

Your notes:

132. 35-year-old uses β2 agonist + low dose steroid but symptoms still uncontrolled.

Best management: Inhaled long acting β_2 agonist

Clinchers

According to British Thoracic Society Guidelines, if symptoms do not get relieved by inhaled short acting β_2 agonist + low dose steroids, then increase the dose of inhaled steroids. Alternatively we can try *long-acting* β_2 *agonist* (Salmeterol 50 mg/12 h). For these guidelines refer page 172 (OHCM), 5th edn.

β_2 adrenoreceptor agonists relax bronchial smooth muscle, acting within minutes.

Salmeterol is a long-acting inhaled β_2 agonist, that can help nocturnal symptoms and reduce morning dips.

CONFUSA

If the symptoms still persist, give combination of drugs or add regular oral prednisolone (1 daily dose) and refer to asthma clinic.

Immediate Management

Inhaled long-acting β_2 agonist.

Your notes:

133. 37-year-old female presents with breathlessness, high RR.

Best management: Nebulized β_2 agonist

Clinchers

Features of acute attack of asthma are:
- *Breathlessness* (unable to complete sentences)
- *Respiratory rate > 25/min*
- Pulse rate > 110 beats/min
- Peak expiratory flow less than 50% of predicted or best.

Aerosolized (nabulized) β_2 agonists are the primary therapy of acute episodes of asthma. In emergency, give every 20 minute subsides for 3 doses, then every 2 hours until attack.

Nebulize with: Salbutamol 5 mg or terbutaline 10 mg made upto 5 ml with normal saline and nebulized in air.

Investigation of Choice

PEFR, spirometry, CXR (rule out pneumothorax), sputum culture and full blood count.

Immediate Management
- Sit patient up and give high dose O_2
- Nebulized β_2 agonist
- Hydrocortisone 200 mg IV or prednisolone 30 mg PO (both if very ill).

Your notes:

134. A patient who was on 1000 microgram of beclomethasone has now developed oral thrush.

Best management: Reduce steroid

Clinchers
- *1000 mg of beclomethasone:* Standard dose of beclomethasone is 100-400 µg/12 hr. According to British Thoracic Society Guidelines, if the symptoms are not relieved by short-acting inhaled β_2 agonists and standard dose inhaled steroids, then high-dose inhaled steroids are given.
- *Developed oral thrush:* High-dose steroids can weaken host defence, hence susceptibility to infection increases.

If high dose steroids create problems like in this question, reduce the dose of steroid and if symptoms persist, add either long-acting β_2 agonists or modified release oral theophylline.

Always rinse mouth after inhaled steroids to prevent oral candidiasis.

CONFUSA

Oral steroids are used acutely (high dose, short courses, e.g. prednisolone 30-40 mg/24 h PO for 7d) and longer term in lower doses (e.g. 5-10 mg/24 h), if control is not optimal on inhalers.

Immediate Management

Reduce steroids

Your notes:

135. An asthmatic patient of presents to A and E department with sudden onset, dyspnoea. On examination there is reduce, expansion, and diminished breathsounds on one side of chest. Trachea is deviated towards otherside.

Diagnosis: Tension pneumothorax

Clinchers

- *Asthmatic patient with sudden onset dyspnoea:* Patients with chronic lung disease are more prone to tension pneumothorax.
- *Reduce expansion, diminished breath sounds, and deviation of trachea* are all signs of tension pneumothorax. It is a medical emergency, and has to be dealt with immediately, else the patient may die.

CXR should not be performed if a tension pneumothorax is suspected, as it will delay immediate necessary treatment.

CONFUSA

Ensure that the suspected pneumothorax is not a large emphysematous bulla.

Investigation of Choice

Arterial blood gas analysis

Immediate Management

Aspiration of pneumothorax without waiting for CXR.

Treatment of Choice

Surgical advice

- If bilateral pneumothoraces
- If lung fails to expose after intercoastal drain insertion
- If 2 or more previous pneumothoraces on the same side
- If history of pneumothorax on other side.

Your notes:

23 Surgery

PAPER 1

Serial No. 10

Subject: Surgery

Topic: Oncology

Question: A young baby is brought with a paravaginal mass. Biopsy of the mass was done to come to a diagnosis of rhabdomyosarcoma.

Diagnosis: Rhabdomyosarcoma

Clinchers

- *Young baby*: Rhabdomyosarcoma occurs most frequently in the first two years of life.
- *Paravaginal mass:* This tumour can occur virtually anywhere throughout the body.
  The four major sites in which rhabdomyosarcoma is found are:
  -head and neck; around the eyes—35-40%
  -genitourinary tract—20%
  -extremities—15-20%
  -trunk (chest and lungs)—10-15%
- *Biopsy reveals rhabdomyosarcoma:* Rhabdomyosarcoma tumours arise from a cell called a "rhabdomyoblast", which is a primitive muscle cell. Instead of differentiating into striated muscle cells, the rhabdomyoblasts grow out of control. Since this type of muscle is located throughout the body, the tumours can appear at numerous locations.

Depending on the "histology" of the cells (how they look under a microscope), the tumours are classified as one of the following:

- Embryonal rhabdomyosarcoma: Most common type, usually found in children under 15 and in the head and neck region and genitourinary tract.
- Botryoid type: A variant of the embryonal type; the tumour arises as a grape-like lesion in mucosal-lined hollow organs such as the vagina and urinary bladder.
- Alveolar type: A more aggressive tumour which usually involves the muscles of the extremities or trunk.
- Pleomorphic type: Usually seen in adults and arises in muscles of the extremities.

CONFUSA

Rhabdomyosarcoma is one of the small, round, blue cell tumours of childhood. Occasionally, these types of tumours can be difficult to differentiate. Rhabdomyosarcoma cells tend to have variable differentiation along the myogenesis pathway and may appear as strap cells or myotubes, sometimes containing muscle cross-striations. Rhabdomyosarcoma cells may demonstrate positive immunohistochemistry results for muscle-specific markers, such as myoglobin, actin, and desmin. Cells from the Rhabdomyosarcoma subtypes have the following distinctive features:

- Botryoid: The cambium layer is characteristic.
- Alveolar: Cells line up along membranes that may be imperceptibly thin or may be obvious collagen bands, resembling the lung alveoli. A tumour should be classified into this type if it appears to be alveolar at any point in time.
- Undifferentiated: Usually, no evidence of myogenesis differentiation is present.

Investigation of Choice

Biopsy of the mass.
For Head & Neck and orbital tumours, MRI is required to know the exact extent of the mass.

Immediate Management

Local mass effect can be managed by radiotherapy or chemotherapy which causes rapid shrinkage of the mass.

Treatment of Choice

Treatment is by surgical excision after chemotherapeutic reduction of size.

A rhabdomyosarcoma that arises in childhood may be treated by a combination of surgery—either excision or biopsy, high dose radiotherapy and chemotherapy (commonly used agents are vincristine, cyclophosphamide, dactinomycin, adriamycin, ifosfamide).

Your notes:

Serial No. 49

Subject: Surgery

Topic: Urology

Question: A 60-year-old lady complaints of continuous dribbling of urine. She underwent hysterectomy few months back.

Diagnosis: Urinary fistula

Clinchers

- *60 year old lady:* Urinary incontinence is twice as prevalent in older women as in older men. Age itself is not a cause of incontinence; however, age-related changes may predispose or contribute to it.
- *Continuous dribbling of urine:* Signifies that she is having absolutely no control on her continence; suggesting True Incontinence. Occurs mostly due to formed fistulas which continuously drain urine.
- *Hysterectomy few months back:* Most acquired fistuals are due to obstetric causes (prolonged obstructed labour), pelvic surgical procedures or pelivic carcinoma/tuberculosis. A positive history of pelvic surgery which preceded the symptoms of incontinence in this lady is making the possibility of a vesicovaginal fistual (more common) or ureterovaginal fistula strong.

CONFUSA

- If a patient complains of passing urine during periods of 'stresses' (viz, coughing, lifting weight and the like)—think of Stress Incontinence.
- If a patient complains of 'incontinence' after a sudden overwhelming 'urge' or desire to pass urine—think of Urge Incontinence.
- If incontinence is associated with dysuria—rule out infectious causes—urinary tract infections, cystitis.

Investigation of Choice

Cystogram to confirm the presence and delineate the fistula.

Double dye test to differentiate between vesicovaginal and ureterovaginal fistula.

Rule out concurrent UTI.

Immediate Management

Personal Hygiene

Treat any concurrent UTI with appropriate antibiotics.

Treatment of Choice

Surgical repair

Serial No. 50

Subject: Surgery

Topic: Urology

Question: A lady after child birth complains of passing urine on coughing and stressing.

Diagnosis: Stress incontinence

Clinchers

- *Lady:* Stress incontinence more common in females.
- *After child birth*: Perhaps the most common cause of stress incontinence is pelvic floor injury/weakness following child birth. Stress incontinence occurs when the proximal urethra drops below the pelvic floor because of pelvic relaxation defects.
- *Complains of passing urine on coughing and stressing:* Typical picture of presentation of stress incontinence. Intra-abdominal pressure is no longer transmitted equally to the bladder and proximal urethra and the patient ends up passing urine during periods of raised intraabdominal pressure.

CONFUSA

- Pregnancy, labour and delivery may all cause mechanical and denervation injury to the normal supports of the bladder neck and proximal urethra and lead to stress incontinence.
- Stress incontinence is also after the menopause and occurs due to decreased intraurethral pressure due to lack of estrogen.
- Imperfect sphincter control also complicates epispadias which show a widened bladder neck, shortened urethra and separation of the symphysis pubis.

Investigation of Choice

Urodynamic studies

Immediate Management

incontinence pads—useful if urinary leakage is small

Treatment of Choice

- Pelvic floor exercises are the first line treatment for those with postpartum symptoms.
- Oestrogens improve stress incontinence in post menopausal women.
- Intravaginal devices: These provide support the bladder neck and urethral and may be an acceptable alternative in women unfit for surgery.
- Surgery—indicated if failure of conservative treatment. All methods aim to correct the relaxation defect and to restore the proximal urethra above the level of the pelvic floor.

Serial No. 51

Subject: Surgery

Topic: Urology

Question: A young girl with history of visual loss and bilateral lower limb weakness, complains of not able to pass urine at all.

Diagnosis: Multiple Sclerosis (MS)

Clinchers

- *Young girl:* MS is more common in females than males and onset is usually between 16-50 years with a peak at 20-40 years.
- *History of visual loss:* Though the natural progress of the disease is characterised by multiple neurological deficits, optic neuritis is one most consistent finding in most patients. It presents as retrobulbar pain and patchy loss of vision.
- *Bilateral lower limb weakness:* This is signifying spinal cord involvment by the disease process.
- *Not able to pass urine at all:* She is presenting with acute retention of urine. Both incontinence and retention are commonly seen in bladder dysfunction associated with multiple sclerosis.

CONFUSA

Bladder dysfunction associated with multiple sclerosis can take various forms:

- Disinhibition of detrusor muscle—produces a combination of urgency and incontinence.
- Complete urinary retention.
- Retention associated with urinary tract infection—the resulting cystitis exacerbates the urgency and incontinence, and so a vicious cycle occurs.
- Also note that, spinal cord lesions may necessitate prolonged catheterization and cause urethral stricture in the long run.

Investigation of Choice

Confirm multiple sclerosis by CSF examination (typical oligoclonal bands).

MRI will shows areas of patchy demyelination.

Immediate Management

Catheterize

Treatment of Choice

- Disease modifying agents (beta interferon, glatiramer acetate and azathioprine).
- Urinary frequency and incontinence treated by anti-cholinergics (oxybutynin) and tricyclic antidepressants (amitriptyline)
- Urinary retention: offer intermittent self-catheterisation

Your notes:

Serial No. 52

Subject: Surgery

Topic: Urology

Question: A 47-year-old lady with frequency and unavoidable desire to urinate at a few seconds' notice but no dysuria.

Diagnosis: Detrusor Instability

Clinchers

- *A 47-year-old lady:* Any sort of incontinence is more common in females and age-related changes may predispose or contribute to it.
- *Frequency:* The unstable detrusor is not able to withstand the normal filling pressure and starts to contract even when partially filled.
- *Unavoidable desire to urinate at a few seconds' notice:* occurs due to and uninhibited contraction of the detrusor muscle during bladder filling.
- *No dysuria:* This rules out any infectious causes of the presenting complaints.

CONFUSA

- Detrusor instability presents with features of urge incontinence.
- It usually occurs in elderly, may complicate multiple sclerosis or a stroke.
- Detrusor instability refers to overactive bladder symptoms without neurologic impairment. External sphincter functions normally, in synergy.
- Neurogenic bladder is a malfunctioning bladder due to any type of neurologic disorder.
- Autonomous bladder is a type of neurogenic bladder characterised by large residual volume of urine and no desire to micturate; is caused by LMN cord lesions above S2, 3, 4

Investigation of Choice
Urodynamic studies show involuntary contraction of bladder during filling.

Immediate Management
Bladder training

Treatment of Choice
Anticholinergics: oxybutynin, propiverine, tolterodine, trospium chloride, Antispasmodic: flavoxate
Sacral nerve stimulation in patients who do not respond to other treatments.

Serial No. 95

Subject: Surgery

Topic: Prostate

Question: A 72-year-old man with poor stream, hesitancy and dribbling.

Diagnosis: Bladder outflow obstruction.

Clinchers

- *A 72-year-old man:* The most common cause of bladder outflow obstruction is benign prostatic hyperplasia. However, in all cases carcinoma prostate should be ruled out.
- *Poor stream:* This suggest that flow of urine is weaker, and it takes longer to empty the bladder.
- *Hesitancy:* The patient may have to wait at the toilet for a while before urine starts to flow.
- *Dribbling:* Some urine may trickle out soon after finishing at the toilet.

CONFUSA

Levels of Prostate Specific Antigen (PSA) change with age. The following cut off levels indicates further investigation:

AGE (YEARS)	PSA CUT OFF (ng/ml)
50-59	>=3.0
60-69	>=4.0
70 and over	>5.0

Investigation of Choice
Prostate specific antigen—if PSA is high, perform a transrectal ultrasound with an ultrasound-guided biopsy.
Other investigations like: FBC, urea and electrolytes, MSU to exclude UTI.

Immediate Management
UTI requires immediate antibiotics.
Hydronephrosis or bladder stone require immediate management.

Treatment of Choice
Depending on the cause identified.

Your notes:

Serial No. 96

Subject: Surgery

Topic: Urology

Question: A 30 year old man comes with acute retention of urine following blow to perineum. On examination, perineum is swollen and bruised.

Diagnosis: Urethral Injury

Clinchers

- *A 30-year-old man:* Most urethral injuries bear a close relationship to trauma, and follows the same incidence pattern as trauma, being highest in males of 15-25 years of age. However, a significant amount of urethral injury do occur due to various iatrogenic causes and can appear in any age for that matter.
- *Acute retention of urine:* An njury to urethra usually presents as acute retention as the urine is not able to drain because of the discontinuation in the path.
- *Blow to the perineum:* Injury to the perineum appears to be one of the most common mode of injury to the anterior urethra. Urtethral injuries associated with pelvic fractures are usually posterior, while those due to instrumentation and prostatic surgeries are most commonly at the level of the sphincter.
- *Perineum is swollen and bruised:* This indicates the rupture of the Buck's Fascia alongwith the anterior urethra, allowing the haematoma to extend beyond the shaft, with Colle's Fascia acting as the lower limiting membrane. This results in a characteristic butterfly pattern of bruising in the perineum.

CONFUSA

- Anterior urethral injuries are suspected when there is blood at the meatus, inability to pass water or rapid development of a perineal urinoma/hematoma, forming down the sleeve of Buck's Fascia.
- Diagnosing posterior urethral injuries require high index of suspicion, more so in a patient with associated pelvic fracture involving the displacement of pubic rami. This, in association with blood a urethral meatus, inability to pass urine or distended bladder and a high riding prostate on rectal examination is suggestive of posterior urtehral injury.

Investigation of Choice:
Diagnosed clinically. Pass a suprapubic catheter to confirm.

USG (per rectal) can be used in rare cases.

Immediate Management
Avoid any per urethral catheter.
Ask for expert urological help.

Treatment of Choice
Surgical repair

Your notes:

Serial No. 102

Subject: Surgery

Topic: Venous Thrmobosis

Question: A young child with abscess near upper lip.

Diagnosis: Cavernous sinus thrombosis

Clinchers

- *Young child:* All ages and sexes can be equally affected by cavernous sinus thrombosis. However, infectious causes are more common among the young and those in immunocompromised states and diabetics.
- *Abscess near upper lip:* The area on the face in distribution of the maxillary and ophthalmic nerves is known as the "dangerous area of the face", and is most important as the extracranial connections of cavernous sinus drain the face in these areas of trigeminal nerve and communicate with the veins around the ear via the pterygoid plexus.
- The affected patients usually have sinusitis or a midface infection (most commonly a furuncle) and in most cases, theres is a history of manipulating the furuncle in some fashion either, squeezing or surgical incision. Cavernous sinus thrombosis may also follow trauma and fracture skull.
- Patient classically presents with headache, fever, and malaise followed by development of ocular findings viz, orbital pain and fullness accompanied by periorbital edema and visual disturbances.

CONFUSA

- A carotid cavernous fistula is a very close differential diagnosis for cavernous sinus thrombosis. It usually follows trauma to the base of the skull or from the rupture of a saccular aneurysm.
- The clinical features for both the condition essentially remain the same, the only distinguishing feature being the rapidity of symptoms which is seen in carotid cavernous fistula.

Investigation of Choice

It's a clinical diagnosis.

However, CT is the modality of choice to confirm the diagnosis and to differentiate it from alternatives such as orbital cellulitis, which may have a similar clinical presentation.

MRI angiography is the gold standard.

Immediate Management

High dose dexamethasone to reduce cerebral edema.

Anticonvulsants may be required to control seizures.

Rule out the exact cause for thrombosis.

Perform surgical drainage of sinuses if these are the source of infection.

Mastoidectomy may be indicated in case the precipitating cause is acute mastoiditis.

Treatment of Choice

The mainstay of therapy is early and aggressive antibiotic administration. Although *S. aureus* is the usual cause, broad-spectrum coverage for gram-positive, gram-negative, and anaerobic organisms should be instituted pending the outcome of cultures.

For, primary thrombosis, treatment of choice is anticoagulants.

Your notes:

Serial No. 104

Subject: Surgery

Topic: Trauma

Question: A laceration near the angle of mandible in front of masseter with profuse bleeding.

Diagnosis: Facial Artery Injury

Clinchers

- *laceration:* Lacerations are the most common type of facial injury especially encountered in the athletic setting. When blunt trauma occurs over a bony prominence of the facial skeleton, a linear or stellate laceration may result, known as burst-type laceration. Most common sites for 'burst-lacerations' being mandible and zygomatic prominences.
- *near angle of mandible in front of masseter:* This typically describes the location and path of facial artery. The facial artery passes over the lower border of mandible at the anterior border of the masseter (known as 'Groove for facial artery').
- *profuse bleeding:* Because of the abundant blood supply to the facial soft tissues, bleeding from facial soft tissue injuries are usually brisk, copious and profuse.

CONFUSA

- While repairing the injured vessel, ligation should only be performed under direct visualization and after careful identification of the bleeding vessel. Blind clamping of bleeding areas should be avoided, because critical structures like facial nerve and parotid duct are susceptible to injury.
- Associated fractures of mandible, maxilla or the orbit should always be ruled out.

Investigation of Choice

Carefully identify the bleeding vessel.
Rule out associated fractures
Rule out cervical spine injury

Immediate Management

Apply direct pressure over the involved area with a sterile gauze pad. Once hemostasis is achieved, the wound is cleaned with sterile saline delivered under pressure via an 18-gauge needle attached to a 20-mL syringe. This adequately removes bacteria and other debris from the wound.

Treatment of Choice

Small and superficial lacerations may be closed using adhesive bandages or by applying a skin adhesive such as butyl cyanoacrylate.

Larger lacerations require to be closed in layers within 24 hrs of injury. Facial skin sutures are usually removed within 5 days, followed by the application of adhesive bandages and a liquid adhesive for another 7 days.

Your notes:

Serial No. 106

Subject: Surgery

Topic: Head and Neck Injury

Question: A 42-year-old man with fracture petrous temporal bone and confusion.

Diagnosis: Superficial Temporal artery Injury.

Clinchers

- *42 year old man:* There is no age prediliction for the rupture or injury of superficial temporal artery, however, the fracture of petrous temporal bone requires considerable force and is usually seen in road traffic accidents or as a part of sports injuries like during boxing; hence, these type of injuries is more common in male sex.
- *Fracture petrous temporal:* Most temporal bone fractures are longitudinal (80%); only 20% being transverse. This is usually associated with significant ear injury and CSF otorrhea, hemotympanum and Battle's sign (hematoma over mastoid) are common findings. The superficial temporal artery ascends in front of the auricle and supplies the scalp over the temporal region. This is the most commonly injured vessel in the temporal region.
- *Confusion:* Fracture of temporal bone requires considerable force, and hence is usually associated with concussion injuries of the brain or vasogenic cerebral oedema which can be the cause of the confusion.

CONFUSA

- Middle Meningeal artery is a dural vessel and hence, any fracture in the temporal region which is associated with a dural nick or stripping can be associated with injury to middle meningeal artery and thus, extradural haemorrhage.
- Any trauma to the temporal region should carefully rule out any extradural haemorrhage with the characteristic history of 'lucid Interval' and unequal pupils (dilated on the side of the injury).

Investigation of Choice

CT scan

Immediate Management

Rule out associated head injury.

Rapid detoriation of consciousness signifying extradural haemorrhage require immediate burring of skull.

Treatment of Choice

Follow head injury protocol.

CSF otorrhoea and rhinorrhoea usually resolve spontaneously.

Facial nerve exploration and microneural repair may be necessary and ossiculoplasty may be required to restore hearing.

Your notes:

Serial No. 107

Subject: Surgery

Topic: Haematemesis

Question: A patient with haematemesis following 40% burns. His vitals are stable; aesophago-duodenoscopy shows multiple superficial ulcers in stomach.

Diagnosis: Curling's Ulcer

Clinchers

- *Hematemesis following 40% burns:* Curling's Ulcer is a stress ulcer associated with severe burns. The mechanism of ulcer formation is loss of plasma volume leading to sloughing of the gastric mucosa.
- *Vitals stable:* Most patients admitted to hospital following an acute upper gastrointestinal bleed will stop bleeding without the need for early drug. However, regular monitoring of the vitals are required and IV fluids and blood transfusion should form the important line of management.
- *Esophagoduodenoscopy shows multiple superficial ulcers in stomach:* This confirms the cause bleeding is Curling's Ulcer and not any other pathology.

CONFUSA

- In people with severe burns, Curling's Ulcer can be prevented by early initiation of oral feeds. However, in cases of severe burns omeprazole should be intiated as preventive therapy.
- A similar stress ulcer is seen in conjunction with raised intracranial pressure and is known by the name Cushing's Ulcer.

Investigation of Choice

Esophagogastroduodenoscopy

Immediate Management

IV fluids and blood transfusion depending upon the vitals.

Control of bleed by endoscopic adrenaline (if actively bleeding).

Urgent Endoscopy.

Treatment of Choice

IV Omeprazole 20 mg daily for 3 days rapidly reverse the gastric mucosal changes and reduces the risk of rebleed.

Your notes:

Serial No. 108

Subject: Surgery

Topic: Haematemesis

Question: A 47-year-old female comes with haematemesis. Her vitals are now stable. She was on treatment for rheumatoid arthritis.

Diagnosis: NSAIDs induced gastric erosions

Clinchers

- *A 47-year-old female:* Rheumatoid arthritis is three times more common in women than men and usually presents at the age of 40-60 years.
- *Haematemesis:* NSAIDs being the most common first line of drug used in the pain relief associated with rheumatoid arthritis, over use or over aggressive long term treatment usually results in upper gastrointestinal haemorrhages.
- *Vitals stable:* This signify that the primary resucitation has been performed, with controlled bleeding and stable vitals.
- *On treatment for rheumatoid arthritis:* This confirms NSAIDs as the most likely cause for haematemesis in this case.

CONFUSA

- Urgent specialist referral for endoscopy is indicated for patients of any age with dyspepsia when presenting with any of the following:
  - chronic gastrointestinal bleeding
  - progressive unintentional weight loss
  - progressive difficulty swallowing
  - persistent vomiting
  - iron deficiency anaemia
  - epigastric mass or suspicious barium meal

Investigation of Choice

Urgent upper GI endoscopy

Immediate Management

Fluid resuscitation

Control bleeding

Treatment of Choice

Stop NSAIDs.

If cannot be stopped, offer long-term gastric protection, usually with misprostol.

Your notes:

Serial No. 115

Subject: Surgery

Topic: Oesophagus

Question:
Temp 37 ºC
JVP decreased
PR 120 bpm regular
BP 90/60
CXR shows left sided effusion
Surgical emphysema present on neck palpation

Diagnosis: Rupture Oesophagus

Clinchers

- *Temp 37 ºC:* Most oesophageal rupture are iatrogenic (Esophagogastroduodenoscopy being the most common procedure associated). Spontaneous rupture usually follow forceful vomiting which increase the intramural pressure (Boerhaave's syndrome). Patient becomes febrile later in the process as infection ensues.
- *JVP decreased, PR 120 bpm regular, BP 90/60:* The parameters signify the shocked state of the patient. Esophageal rupture is a surgical emergency and patient goes into shock in couple of minutes.
- *CXR shows left sided effusion:* This is characteristic of esophageal rupture. The hydrothorax is seen in 90% of cases on CXR and is usually on the left side.
- *Surgical emphysema present on neck palpation:* subcutaneous emphysema in the neck again making the possibility of esophageal rupture strong. It characteristically gives a 'cracking feel' on palpation.

CONFUSA

- The classic presentation of spontaneous esophageal rupture is in a middle-aged man with a history of dietary overindulgence and overconsumption of alcohol, with chest pain and subcutaneous emphysema after recent vomiting or etching (Mackler triad).
- Intramural rupture of the oesophagus is a rare form of spontaneous rupture where the tear passes deep to the mucosa but does not reach to the surface of the oesophagus. A large intramural hematoma at endoscopy is diagnostic. Treatment is conservative.

Investigation of Choice

Definitive diagnosis made with Gastrograffin Swallow to show the site of the perforation.

Don't go for Barium Swallow as it can cause severe chemical mediastinitis in case, perforation is present.

Immediate Management

Surgical Emergency—Arrange blood, fluid resusciation, inform surgeons.

Treatment of Choice

Surgery within 6 hours of diagnosis. After this time, the metabolic effects and damage to the oesophagus make survival less likely.

Your notes:

Serial No. 120

Subject: Surgery

Topic: Neck swellings

Question: An infant with brilliantly transilluminable swelling at the base of his neck.

Diagnosis: Cystic Hygroma

Clinchers

- *An infant:* This is a congenital lesion comprised of lymph-filled spaces which arise from an embryonic remnant of the jugular lymph sac. Cystic hygroma are invariably present at birth, smaller masses may be missed and present later in childhood as an expanding lump.
- *Brilliantly transilluminable swelling:* It is not a true cyst but rather a lymphatic hamartoma which forms multilocular cyst-like spaces. Which contain clear fluid and this make them transilluminate brilliantly.
- *At the base of his neck:* Most occur in the base of the neck, both in the anterior and the posterior triangle, and may extend up to the jaw, over the anterior chest wall, and down into the axilla. Rarely, it occurs alone in the axilla, pelvis, or groin.

CONFUSA

- Cystic hygromas are common associations with Turner's and Noonan's syndrome.
- Branchial cyst is a close differential, usually presenting in young adults as a smooth swelling in front of the anterior border of the sternomastoid at the junction of its upper and middle thirds. The position is characteristic. It is usually fluctuant and may transilluminate.

Investigation of Choice

Clinical diagnosis.

Immediate Management

Rule out associated syndromes.
Rule out active infection.

Treatment of Choice

Surgical excision
(can be difficult because of infiltration of vital neck structures)

Your notes:

Serial No. 126

Subject: Surgery

Topic: Crush Injuries

Question: A person develops anuria and pulmonary edema after severe crushing injuries. His blood urea level at 60 mmol/L and serum potassium 7.5 mmol/L.

Diagnosis: Rhabdomyolysis (Crush Syndrome or Bywater's syndrome)

Clinchers

- *Severe crushing injuries:* Rhabdomyolysis is breakdown of muscle fibres and leakage of toxic contents from injured myocytes into the systemic circulation. It most commonly follows severe crush injuries, but may also be an important side effect of statins. It may also occur in infants with inherited enzyme deficiencies of carbohydrate or lipid metabolism.
- *Develops anuria:* Liberated myocyte contents are severely toxic (especially cytochrome c) which kidney tubules or cause renal artery spasm, precipitating acute renal failure.
- *Blood urea level at 60 mmol/L:* such severely raised urea signify severe renal injury demanding emergency treatment.
- *Serum potassium 7.5 mmol/L:* This level of hyperkalemia is a medical emergency capable of producing life threatening arrhythmias. It occurs due to release of intracellular potassium into the systemic circulation.

CONFUSA

- In case of proceeding for amputation of the involved limb in the crush injury, remember that any amputation must be carried out above the site of compression and before the crushing force is removed.
- In case, the compression force has already be removed then the limb must be cooled and the patient first treated for renal failure and shock.
- A limb which has had a tourniquet on for more than 6 hours also needs to be amputated.

Investigation of Choice

Serum creatinine kinase is the most useful investigation.
Monitor serum potassium levels closely.
Blood urea and electrolytes to monitor renal functions.

Immediate Management

Immediate renal dialysis

Indications for haemodialysis:
- Hyperkalemia >7.0 mmol/L
- Severe acid-base disturbances
- Refractory pulmonary oedema
- Progressive renal failure.

Get venous access.
Start saline infusion of 1000-1500 ml/h.
When a urine flow has been established, a forced mannitol-alkaline diuresis up to 8 L/day should be maintained (urine pH greater than 6.5).
Once the patient reaches hospital, 5% dextrose should be alternated with normal saline to reduce the potential sodium load.

Treatment of Choice

Fasciotomy in case of compartment syndrome. It may be necessary to amputate the crushed limbs.

Your notes:

Serial No.142

Subject: Surgery

Topic: Renal

Question: A 47-year-old female with bilateral pelvic masses and terminal haematuria.

Diagnosis: Bladder Calculi

Clinchers

- *47-year-old female:* Bladder stones are common in developing countries and rare in UK. It usually affects males more than females with peak at 20 years. A later peak at around 50 years is observed in females and is attributed to infective stones.
- *Bilateral pelvic masses:* The site of impaction if being at the neck of bladder, it can cause back pressure and reflux leading first to bilateral hydronephrosis and later when infection ensues, bilateral pyelonephritis.
- *Terminal haematuria:* This is the most important sign of bladder stone. The haematuria is usually at the end of the micturiation, when the stone tries to follow the urethral tract with the flow of the urine and injuring the mucosa on its way.

CONFUSA

The presence of upper urinary tract calculi is not necessarily a predisposition to the formation of bladder stones. Stones in the bladder are often formed in situ, rather than originating from the upper tracts. Stones that do reach the bladder from the upper tracts are likely to pass easily down the urethra.

Investigation of Choice

X-ray KUB - Screening
Abdominal Ultrasound—to rule out complications like pyelonephritis/ hydronephrosis.

Immediate Management

Urinary analysis to know the nature of stones—oxalate, uric acid or pigment stones.
Analgesics to control associated pain.
Adequate fluid to maintain hydration.

Treatment of Choice

- The only potentially effective medical treatment for bladder calculi is urinary alkalinization for the dissolution of uric acid stones. Stone dissolution may be possible if the urinary pH is greater than or equal to 6.5. Potassium citrate at 60 mEq/d is commonly used.

- Endoscopy is the surgical intervention of choice. Small stones may simply be washed out of the bladder via a cystoscope. Larger stones must first be fragmented. Traditionally, this is done by litholapaxy or ESWL (requires full bladder).

Your notes:

Serial No. 143

Subject: Surgery

Topic: Acute Abdomen

Question: A man underwent sigmoidoscopy after which he develops severe pain abdomen and guarding.

Diagnosis: Acute Peritonitis (following hollow viscus perforation).

Clinchers

- *Underwent sigmoidoscopy:* Diagnostic procedures such as colonoscopy, sigmoidoscopy and the like hold a high probability to perforate the hollow viscus and cause acute peritonitis. Other causes of perforation include perforated peptic ulcer, perforated diverticulum, stab wounds, inflammatory bowel disease.
- *Develops severe pain abdomen:* The pain associated with peritonitis is severe and is made worse by slightest movements; patient tends to lie as still as possible to avoid worsening of pain. (compare with that of biliary or renal colic, where patients can never lie still and rolls over in an attempt to find the most comfortable position).
- *Guarding:* This is due to contraction of abdominal muscles because of irritation by the underlying inflamed periotoneum, more so when palpation is attempted. Abdomen is classical described as 'Wood-like' because of this guarding.

CONFUSA

- Peritonitis is often localised in early stages because omentum and the surrounding structures try to limit the infection. However, later this doesn't suffice to contain the inflammation and a condition that initially presented with localised peritonitis may eventually develop into generalised peritonitis.

Investigation of Choice

Plain X-ray abdomen (Erect) or erect Chest X-ray will show gas under diaphragm.

Immediate Management

- Correct fluid balance—rapid IV infusion of Hartmann's solution, 2.5-3.0 litres over 3 hours in a 70 kg adult, with monitoring of central venous pressure (especially in elderly).
- Insert a urinary catheter to monitor urinary output
- Take blood for culture, then give parenteral antibacterial treatment, e.g. metronidazole for anaerobes and cephalexin for aerobes.

- Analgesic
- Oxygen via a face mask as diaphragmatic movements are likely to be reduced
- Nasogastric tube to keep the stomach empty.

Treatment of Choice

Laparotomy with peritoneal lavage and closing the perforation.

Your notes:

Serial No. 144

Subject: Surgery

Topic: Acute Abdomen

Question: A man with features of peritonitis; Erect CXR shows gas under diaphragm.

Diagnosis: Acute Peritonitis

Clinchers

- *Features of peritonitis:* Peritonitis usually presents with features of abdominal pain, made worse by movement of the abdomen. This is associated with localized/generalised tenderness, guarding, rebound tenderness, rectal tenderness along with features of systemic toxicity like malaise, low-grade fever, tachycardia, leucocytosis on FBC.
- *Erect CXR shows gas under diaphragm:* This confirms that the features present in the patient is due to peritonitis and is due to perforation of some hollow viscus.

CONFUSA

- Peritonitis is often localised in early stages because omentum and the surrounding structures try to limit the infection. However, later this doesn't suffice to contain the inflammation and a condition that initially presented with localised peritonitis may eventually develop into generalised peritonitis.

Investigation of Choice

Plain X-ray abdomen (Eerct) or erect Chest X-ray will show gas under diaphragm.

Immediate Management

- Correct fluid balance—rapid IV infusion of Hartmann's solution, 2.5-3.0 litres over 3 hours in a 70kg adult, with monitoring of central venous pressure (especially in elderly).
- Insert a urinary catheter to monitor urinary output.
- Take blood for culture, then give parenteral antibacterial treatment, e.g. metronidazole for anaerobes and cephalexin for aerobes.
- Analgesic
- Oxygen via a face mask as diaphragmatic movements are likely to be reduced.
- Nasogastric tube to keep the stomach empty.

Treatment of Choice

Laparotomy with peritoneal lavage and closing the perforation.

Serial No. 145

Subject: Surgery

Topic: Acute Abdomen

Question: A child with abdominal pain and current jelly stools. A sausage shaped mass is palpable per abdomen.

Diagnosis: Acute intussusception

Clinchers

- *A child:* Intussusception occurs most commonly in children 5-18 months, affecting male children almost 3 times more than the females.
- *Abdominal pain:* Symptoms usually start abruptly in a previously healthy child with paroxysms of abdominal colic, with screaming and pallor. During each episode the infant becomes pale and draws up the legs. Spasms occur at intervals of about ten to 15 minutes, lasting two to three minutes, increasing in frequency.
- *Current jelly stools:* This is a late feature; passage of blood mixed with mucous give the appearance of 'red current jelly'.
- *Sausage shaped mass is palpable per abdomen:* This is seen in most cases with the mass usually seen in the right upper quadrant.

CONFUSA

- In most cases, the intussusception is Ileo cecal (75% cases)—Here the apex of intussusception is the ileocecal valve. Other types include ileo-ileal, ileo-colic and colo-colic.
- In most cases Peyer's patch hypertrophy is noted at surgery, leading to the suggestion that there may be an infective aetiology for this condition. Adenovirus, rotavirus and HHV 6 are most commonly blamed. has been suggested. The enlarged Peyer's patches create an axis on which the process of invagination can occur.

Investigation of Choice

Barium enema—'stack' of coins sign.

Immediate Management

Fluid Resuscitation—"drip and suck" Regimen, Insert NG tube and administer iv fluids.

Treatment of Choice

Reduction by barium enema under radiological control Barium enema is contraindicated if there are features of perforation or generalised peritonitis.

Surgical reduction is indicated in cases of:
- Peritonitis
- Child <3 months or >2 years
- Severe dehydration
- Failure of reduction by barium enema.

Your notes:

Serial No. 149

Subject: Surgery

Topic: Intestinal Obstruction

Question: A lady underwent debulking surgery for ovarian carcinoma few years back, now presents with signs of intestinal obstruction.

Diagnosis: Intestinal Obstruction

Clinchers

- *Underwent debulking surgery for ovarian carcinoma few years back:* The history of surgery makes this patient high risk for intestinal obstruction, as adhesions (especially, post-operative) are the most common cause for the development of intestinal obstruction. The underlying cause for operation being carcinoma, again makes the risk more strong, as such cases are prone for extensive adhesions because of the recurring carcinomatous growth.
- *Now presents with signs of intestinal obstruction:* The clinical features of intestinal obstruction includes mainly abdominal pain, usually diffuse and colicky. Proximal obstruction appears with more epigastric pain and distal is more periumbilical. Constant pain signify strangulation or perforation and peritonitis. This is associated with vomiting in proximal obstruction, constipation in distal obstruction.

CONFUSA

- Most cases of intestinal obstruction are initially managed on 'Drip and Suck' regimen. However, surgery is indicated if features of obstruction do not resolve, if there is general deterioration of the patient's condition with onset of abdominal tenderness and a tachycardia.
- Immediate surgery is indicated in cases of severe increasing pain, localised peritonism, complete colonic obstruction with competent ileocaecal valve and caecum dilated to greater than 8 cm, "closed loop" seen radiologically, obstruction occurring as a result of hernial incarceration.

Investigation of Choice

Abdominal radiographs:
Supine—shows the site of obstruction
Erect—shows fluid levels

Immediate Management

Nil by mouth
Rehydrate the patient—start IV fluids
Aspirate gastrointestinal contents—Put Nasogastric Tube (the 'Drip and Suck' regimen).
Analgesics for pain relief
Antibiotic prophylaxis should be considered.

Treatment of Choice

Surgery

Your notes:

Serial No. 162

Subject: Surgery

Topic: Trauma

Question: A man comes to A and E after high speed automobile injury. CXR shows widened mediastinum.

Diagnosis: Aortic rupture

Clinchers

- *High speed automobile injury:* Aortic rupture is a medical emergency caused by decelerating forces or blunt chest injuries as common with high speed automobile injuries, fall from height or diresct assault on chest wall.
- *CXR shows widened mediastinum:* Classic Chest X-ray findings seen in aortic rupture are widened mediastinum, obliteration of aortic knob, deviation of trachea to right, loss of space between pulmonary artery and aorta, depression of left mainstem bronchus, deviation of esophagus to the right, widened paratracheal stripe, widened paraspinal interfaces, pleural or apical cap present, left hemothorax.

CONFUSA

Pericardial tamponade can be easily confused with aortic rupture in this setting. However, do not forget that an acute pericardial tamponade doesn't produces widened mediastinum. The typical 'flask shaped' heart associated with pericardial tamponade is the description of long standing cases of gradually accumulating fluid in the pericardium. Morever, in the absence of acute of features of pericardial tamponade, viz., hypotension, jugular venous distension with distant heart sounds (Beck's Traid), aortic rupture seems a more favourable diagnosis.

Investigation of Choice

Aortogram is the Gold standard.

However, a transesophageal ECHO may provide immediate diagnosis in an acute setting.

Immediate Management

Arrange blood

Inform surgeons

Treatment of Choice

Surgical repair

Your notes:

Serial No. 163

Subject: Surgery

Topic: Trauma

Question: A lady after road traffic accident comes with hypotension and rigid abdomen. She has broken left ribs 10-12.

Diagnosis: Splenic rupture

Clinchers

- *Road traffic accident:* Spleen appears to be the most common organ injured in cases of blunt injury abdomen. It can become evident immediately after the assault or may present days-weeks later.
- *Hypotension and rigid abdomen:* Spleen being a highly vascular organ, its rupture leads to enormous blood loss in the free cavity of abdomen. This leads to hemodynamic instability with features of hypotension, shock, tacvhycardia and pallor. The presence of blood in the peritoneal cavity elicits a chemical peritonitis, causing rigidity and guarding.
- *Broken left ribs 10-12:* This is the most common associated injury seen with spleen rupture, as otherwise it is well protected under these lower ribs on the left side.

CONFUSA

Although rib fracture, commonly seen with splenic injuries, it is not always necessary for the offending force to fracture the ribs as splenic rupture are quite commonly seen due to rapid deceleration or even a trivial trauma can cause splenic rupture in diseased spleen. Spleen in cases of infectious mononucleosis, malaria and hematological malignancies are typically prone for this.

Investigation of Choice

CT scan - in stable patients

Diagnostic peritoneal lavage (DPL) - in hemodynamically unstable patients (largely replaced by bedside USG now).

Immediate Management

Resuscitate- IV fluids, blood transfusion

Treatment of Choice

Splenectomy - if bleeding continues

Your notes:

Serial No. 164

Subject: Surgery

Topic: Trauma

Question: A lady after road traffic accident presents with increased pulse decreased BP.

Diagnosis: Acute blood loss (Hypovolemic Shock)

Clinchers

- *Road traffic accident:* Road traffic accidents are associated with variety of injuries most of which relate to acute blood loss and patient requiring immediate resuscitation with IV fluids to support circulation and maintain perfusion. Most injuries either cause bleeding into the abdominal cavity (spleen rupture, being most common here) or fracture of long bones, especially of lower limbs and that of pelvis are associated with profuse bleeding.
- *Increased pulse decreased BP:* This is the initial compensated stage of hypovolemic shock where the baroreceptor reflexes aim to increase the myocardial contractility, tachycardia and vasoconstriction. All is done to maintain cardiac output and blood pressure;

CONFUSA

Physiologically three stages of hypovolaemic shock are recognised:

- *Compensated*—baroreceptor reflexes result in increase in myocardial contractility, tachycardia and vasoconstriction. They maintain cardiac output and blood pressure; release of vasopressin, aldosterone and renin;
- *Progressive/uncompensated*—myocardial depression, failure of vasomotor reflexes and failure of the microcirculation with increase in capillary permeability, sludging and thrombosis resulting in cellular dysfunction and lactic acidosis;
- *Irreversible*—unrecoverable failure of vital organs.

Investigation of Choice

Thorough clinical examination to find out the source of bleeding.

Immediate Management

IV fluids till blood can be arranged
Blood transfusion

Treatment of Choice

According to the cause of bleeding identified

Clinial Staging of Blood Loss

Class I: 10-15% blood loss; physiological compensation and no clinical changes appear.

Class II: 15-30% blood loss; postural hypotension, generalized vasoconstriction and reduction in urine output to 20-30 ml/hr.

Class III: 30-40% blood loss; hypotension, tachycardia over 120, tachypnoea, urine output under 20 ml/hr and the patient is confused.

Class IV: 40% blood loss, marked hypotension, tachycardia and tachypnoea. No urine output and the patient is comatose.

Your notes:

PAPER 2

Serial No. 1

Subject: Surgery

Topic: Breast

Question: Female with breast carcinoma 3 yrs back, was treated with mastectomy & lymph node clearance on the left side. She now presents with a swollen right arm and decreased hand movements.

Diagnosis: Lymphedema

Clinchers

- *Breast carcinoma 3 yrs back:* The long duration of cancer and the present lymphedema, suggest recurrence of the cancer. (see Confusa).
- *Treated with mastectomy & lymph node clearance:* Destructive surgeries especially those involving the lymph nodes, interfere with the lymphatic drainage of the arm and lead to accumulation of the lymph. The edema is more severe when the node clearance is combined with radiotherapy, as it further causes fibrosis of the remaining lymphatic channels.
- *Swollen right arm and decreased hand movements:* This occurs due to accumulation of lymph; in late stages, secondary changes on the skin of the arm can also occur leading to induration.

CONFUSA

The time course of the oedema is predictive of the cause:
- within 1-2 weeks—axillary vein thrombosis
- within 1-2 months and progressing rapidly—constriction of the axillary vein by scar tissue or lymphatic obstruction
- months or years later—recurrent carcinoma in the lymph nodes.

Investigation of Choice
Lymphangiography

Immediate Management
Rule out local recurrence of the carcinoma

Treatment of Choice

General measures
-Arm elevation,
-Compression bandaging,
-Exercise and massage
-Maintain good skin hygiene
-Antibiotics, if infection is present

Serial No. 21

Subject: Surgery

Topic: Trauma

Question: A boy was riding his bicycle when he was hit by a car. After examination in the A & E, he was found to have left upper quadrant tenderness.

Diagnosis: Spleen Rupture

Clinchers

- *A boy was.... hit by a car:* Spleen appears to be the most common organ injured in cases of blunt injury abdomen. It can become evident immediately after the assault or may present days-weeks later.
- *Left upper quadrant tenderness:* The typical setting of blunt trauma to the abdomen followed by left upper quadrant tenderness signify splenic injury. It is especially common in such type of injuries which are associated with rapid deceleration.

CONFUSA

Although rib fracture, commonly seen with splenic injuries, it is not always necessary for the offending force to fracture the ribs as splenic rupture are quite commonly seen due to rapid deceleration or even a trivial trauma can cause splenic rupture in diseased spleen. Spleen in cases of infectious mononucleosis, malaria and haematological malignancies are typically prone for this.

Investigation of Choice
CT scan—in stable patients
Diagnostic peritoneal lavage (DPL)—in hemodynamically unstable patients (largely replaced by bedside USG now).

Immediate Management
Resuscitate—IV fluids, blood transfusion

Treatment of Choice
Splenectomy—if bleeding continues

Your notes:

Serial No. 22

Subject: Surgery

Topic: Trauma

Question: A man fell off a ladder, has diffuse pain on right side of the trunk. IVU shows no excretion on right side.

Diagnosis: Renal pedicle avulsion

Clinchers

- *Man fell off a ladder:* While direct blow to the abdomen may result in renal contusion and hematoma formation, these type of decelerating injuries (as, falling off from a ladder with a sudden deceleration on reaching the ground, on one's trunk) is associated with avulsion injuries of the renal pedicle.
- *Diffuse pain on right side of the trunk:* This signify local peritonitis, perhaps due to the accumulation of blood in the retroperitoneal space from the avulsed pedicle.
- *IVU shows no excretion on right side:* This IVU picture is typical for an absent kidney on the right side. The man most probably has had avulsed his renal pedicle due to which the contrast fails to reach the affected kidney.

CONFUSA

The process of injury may also result in renal contusion, however, a renal contusion would show a dense and delayed nephrogram with minor distortion of the entire collecting system with puddling of contrast in adjacent parenchyma.

Investigation of Choice

CT is the most informative radiologic study and the method of choice in cases of severe renal trauma.

Immediate Management

Rule out any other associated injury to abdominal organs.

Correct shock, if any.

Treatment of Choice

Injury to the renal pedicle requires immediate surgical intervention.

Your notes:

Serial No. 23

Subject: Surgery

Topic: Trauma

Question: A man was stabbed with a 10 cm knife in the left upper quadrant, stable for 20 min after which BP falls to 90/60 mmHg. On USG, no free fluid seen in abdomen.

Diagnosis: Splenic Injury

Clinchers

- *Stabbed with a 10 cm knife in the left upper quadrant:* The site is typical for injury to spleen and a 10 cm knife can go just deep enough to harm this organ, apparently safe behind the ribs.
- *Stable for 20 min after which BP falls to 90/60 mmHg:* A rapid fall in BP following injury in left upper quadrant makes spleen the most likely injured organ. The fall in BP can be delayed in spleen injuries due to initial haematoma formation.
- *No free fluid seen in abdomen:* A negative finding on USG may be due to the bleeding contained in the splenic capsule or even localisation of the bleeding by initial haematoma formation.

CONFUSA

The picture can easily be confused with cardiac tamponade as the left upper quadrant injury and no free fluid in the abdomen would also suggest a thoracic injury rather than abdominal injury. However note that, a cardiac tamponade would have given us more hints like raised JVP or distant heart sounds along with haemodynamic compromise. Considering these close possibilities in diagnosis, the question is open for further discussion at **www.rxpgonline.com**

Investigation of Choice

CT scan—in stable patients

Diagnostic peritoneal lavage (DPL)—in haemodynamically unstable patients (largely replaced by bedside USG now).

Immediate Management

Resuscitate—IV fluids, blood transfusion

Treatment of Choice

Splenectomy—if bleeding continues

Your notes:

Serial No. 24

Subject: Surgery

Topic: Trauma

Question: A 25-year-old woman car driver is involved in a front impact accident. She develops central, epigastric and shoulder tip pain three hours later and is noted to have linear transverse bruising from the lap belt above the umbilicus.

Diagnosis: Mesenteric vascular injury (Seat Belt Injury)

Clinchers

- *25-year-old woman car driver:* Road traffic accidents are comparatively more common in males; The patients on the driver seat are more prone for all sorts of injury because of front wheel and the backward pressure due to worn seat belts during rapid deceleration.
- *Front impact accident:* This produces rapid deceleration and thus the associated injuries.
- *Central, epigastric and shoulder tip pain three hours later:* The gradual (not immediate) deteoriation is suggesting mesenteric vascular injury which causes ischaemia of the bowel and subsequent injury and symptoms.
- *Linear transverse bruising from the lap belt above the umbilicus:* The seat belt syndrome consists of skeletal, soft-tissue, and visceral injuries associated with use of two- and three-point restraints in patients involved in motor vehicle accidents.
- Skin abrasions of the neck, chest, and abdomen—the classic seat belt sign—indicate internal injury in 30% of cases.
- Neck abrasions are associated with injuries to the carotid artery, larynx, and cervical spine; chest abrasions, with fractures of the sternum, ribs, and clavicles and injuries to the heart and thoracic aorta; and abdominal abrasions, with mesenteric tears, bowel perforation and haematoma, chance fractures, and injuries to the abdominal aorta. The seat belt sign should prompt a diligent search for related injuries.

CONFUSA

The process of the injury and presentation can also be confused with pancreatic contusion. However, in the absence of hints at raised serum amylase levels or pain radiating to back or the like, its safest to go with mesenteric vascular tears.

Investigation of Choice

USG and CT abdomen to search for related injuries.

Immediate Management

Treat Shock

Treatment of Choice

Surgical Repair

Your notes:

Serial No. 25

Subject: Surgery

Topic: Trauma

Question: A 32-yr-old man has a kick in the loin region, developed haematuria. There is no blood seen at the urethral meatus, no perineal injury seen.

Diagnosis: Renal Contusion

Clinchers

- *32 yr old man:* Renal trauma in children is more common than in adults, possibly because children tend to have less developed musculoskeletal protection and proportionally larger kidneys than adults.
- *Kick in the loin region:* A direct blow to the flank or back is the most common mechanism of injury, and 80% of all renal injuries occur as a result of blunt trauma.
- *Developed haematuria:* Haematuria is the most common sign following renal injury. It may also be accompanied by flank pain and ecchymosis.
- *No blood seen at the uretheral meatus:* This rules out any urethral injury which can be accounted for the present haematuria.
- *No perineal injury seen:* This rules out any injury to bladder or the adjacent strictures.

CONFUSA

Haematuria in athletes following vigorous activity is not uncommon (don't forget rhabdomyolysis and transient haematuria which is also commonly associated with athletes). The first time an athlete is evaluated for this condition, whether it be gross or microscopic in nature, a serial urinalysis at 24 and 48 hours is important. If the urine clears, no further evaluation is necessary. Those with progressive symptoms such as flank pain, haematuria lasting more than 48 hours, gross haematuria, prolonged oliguria, or urinary casts need further evaluation with urine culture, imaging studies, and serum renal studies.

Investigation of Choice

CT is the most informative radiologic study and the method of choice in cases of severe renal trauma.

Immediate Management

Rule out any other associated injury to abdominal organs.

Treatment of Choice

Most urologists generally advocate conservative management of renal injury for haemodynamically stable patients who do not have concomitant organ involvement.

Conservative management consists of monitoring the patient's vital signs in a controlled hospital environment.

If coexisting intraperitoneal trauma is present, surgical intervention may be recommended.

Injury to the renal pedicle requires immediate surgical intervention.

Your notes:

Serial No. 42

Subject: Medicine

Topic: Constipation

Question: A 32-year-old female presents with acute onset constipation with abdominal pain and vomiting. She is noted to have a small swelling in her groin.

Diagnosis: Intestinal Obstruction

Clinchers

- *32 year old female:* Intestinal obstruction can present at any age and can affect men and women equally. In children the most common cause include congenital anomalies and congenital hernias; while in the adults the common causes are post-operative adhesions or acquired hernias.
- *Acute onset constipation:* The acute presentation of intestinal obstruction usually presents with abdominal pain and an inability to pass faeces or flatus with gradually worsening abdominal distension.
- *Abdominal pain and vomiting:* The abdominal pain is usually colicky and felt in mid abdomen. Vomiting becomes a more prominent feature with a proximal obstruction.
- *Small swelling in her groin:* This is apparently inguinal hernia or femoral hernia through the neck of which the bowel has been obstructed.

CONFUSA

In small bowel obstruction, vomiting occurs earlier, distension is less, pain is higher in the abdomen. The abdominal X-ray (AXR) plays a key role in diagnosis. In small bowel obstruction, AXR shows central gas shadows and no gas in the large bowel. Small bowel is identified by valvulae conniventes that completely cross the lumen (large bowel haustoral folds do not cross all the lumen's width). In large bowel obstruction, pain is more constant; AXR shows gas proximal to the block(e.g. in caecum) but not in the rectum. If the ileocaecal valve is competent, pain may be felt over a distended caecum.

Investigation of Choice

Supine and upright abdominal X-rays (see confusa above).

Barium studies can help distinguish ileus from obstruction and locate specific area of obstruction (should not be done in suspected perforation).

Immediate Management

'Drip and suck' regime—Correct dehydration by Intravenous fluid administration and aspirate intestinal contents with a nasogastric tube to relieve distention.

Treatment of Choice

Surgery in cases of worsening symptoms or signs of strangulation. Hernial defect should be corrected appropriately after relieving obstruction.

Your notes:

Serial No. 45

Subject: Medicine

Topic: Gastro

Question: A 25-year-old teacher complains that she has had central abdominal discomfort of six-month duration, intermittent abdominal distension and alteration in bowel habit. On examination, there is a palpable swelling in the right iliac fossa. A Barium enema carried out showed no abnormality.

Diagnosis: Mesenteric Adenitis

Clinchers

- *A 25-year-old teacher:* Patients with mesenteric adenitis is usually under 30 years of age. It occurs due to non-specific inflammation of the mesenteric lymph nodes which provokes a mild peritoneal reaction and stimulates painful peristalsis in the terminal ileum.
- *Central abdominal discomfort.... alteration in bowel habit:* Patients usually present with abdominal pain, usually in the right iliac fossa. There is little guarding or rebound, and moderate tenderness. The patient may be pyrexial and there may be diarrhoea, with or without vomiting, or a recent upper respiratory tract infection.
- *Palpable swelling in the right iliac fossa:* This further confirms the diagnosis of mesenteric adenitis.
- *A Barium enema carried out showed no abnormality:* The pathology is extra-luminal; hence barium enema is very unlikely to be helpful. Also, a normal barium enema rules out possibility of carcinomas which can have similar presentations.

CONFUSA

The important differential for mesenteric adenitis is acute appendicitis, but the clinical picture of this condition can usually be discriminated from the absence of rectal tenderness, and a temperature higher than 38.5 degrees C. However, if there is uncertainty, a laparotomy may be performed. Adenitis is confirmed by a normal appendix and large inflamed, fleshy lymph nodes in the mesentery.

Investigation of Choice
Abdominal CT scan

Immediate Management
None; carefully rule out appendicitis

Treatment of Choice
None required; its a self limiting process

Serial No. 111

Subject: Surgery

Topic: Trauma

Question: A 40-year-old man sitting in a passenger seat met an accident where the car is hit from the left side. He now complains of pain in the left side abdomen. There is also bruising of that side.

Diagnosis: Rupture Spleen

Clinchers

- *A 40-year-old man:* Road traffic accidents (RTA) are more common in males and peak incidence is seen in age group 20-50 years of age.
- *Sitting in a passenger seat:* This hints towards the mode of the injury. A person in the driving seat most commonly sustains injuries due to the crushing force against the steering wheel, seat belt and the rapid deceleration forces, a passenger seat occupier mainly sustains injury due to the compressive forces of the seat belt.
- *Car is hit from the left side:* This again emphasises towards the most likely site of injury. A hit from the left side, throws the passenger towards right and with the seat belt, it's the left side of the abdomen which experiences maximum compression from the seat belt.
- *Pain, bruising on left side of abdomen:* The most likely intra-abdominal organ to be injured by blunt forces is the spleen and the mode of injury and the symptoms are all in favour of the same.

CONFUSA

Hypovolemia, hypotension and shock are the most important leading signs of intrabdominal bleed, especially when the picture is combined with an immediate history of trauma. Per abdominal swelling or features of peritonitis, though observed in typical cases, their absence does not rule out presence of intrabdominal bleed.

Investigation of Choice
CT scan—in stable patients
Diagnostic peritoneal lavage (DPL)—in haemodynamically unstable patients (largely replaced by bedside USG now).

Immediate Management
Resuscitate—IV fluids, blood transfusion

Treatment of Choice
Splenectomy—if bleeding continues

Serial No. 112

Subject: Surgery

Topic: Trauma

Question: A patient involved in an RTA comes to A&E complaining of pain in upper abdomen and breathlessness. On X-ray the nasogastric tube is seen coiled up in the chest region.

Diagnosis: Diaphragm Rupture

Clinchers

- *Involved in RTA:* Road traffic accident (RTA) can lead to a variety of injuries, which can present either immediately or late.
- *Pain in the upper abdomen and breathlessness:* While breathlessness hints that something wrong with the lungs or any part of the respiratory system, the upper abdominal pain hints towards either an intrathoracic or intra-abdominal pathology.
- *Nasogastric tube is seen coiled up in the chest region:* This is suggesting that intestines are occupying the chest region, a picture which occurs following diaphragmatic rupture. The coils of the intestines in the chest cause mediastinal shift and compression of lungs (same side) resulting in respiratory compromise and breathlessness.

CONFUSA

A similar picture can be observed in newborns where the condition occurs due to patent pleuro-peritoneal membrane resulting in Congenital diaphragmatic hernia. This is usually seen on the left side with the heart shifted to right and left lung is severely hypoplastic. The child presents with breathlessness, cyanosis and an 'empty abdomen'. Face mask is absolutely contraindicated in these cases as this will inflate the intestines even more and increase respiratory compromise. Ventilation only after intubation should be performed.

Investigation of Choice

CXR with NG tube in situ.

Immediate Management

Intubate and ventilate in cases of severe respiratory compromise.
Symptomatic support while awaiting surgery.
Rule out other concomitant injuries to other intrabdominal organs.

Treatment of Choice: Surgical Repair

Serial No. 113

Subject: Surgery

Topic: Trauma

Question: A woman had met with an RTA in the car she was driving. She went and hit to the windscreen and now developed epigastric pain.

Diagnosis: Pancreatic Injury

Clinchers

- *Met with an RTA:* Road traffic accident (RTA) can lead to a variety of injuries, which can present either immediately or late.
- *Car she was driving:* Driving seat injuries occur mainly due to the seat belt, steering wheel or the whiplash injury.
- *She went and hit the windscreen:* This sudden effect of the decelerating forces compresses the intra-abdominal organs against the seat belt, and thence the resulting injury.
- *Now developed epigastric pain:* Epigastric pain with radiation to the back, associated with vomiting or haemorrhagic bruises on the abdomen, suggest in favour of pancreatic injury.

CONFUSA

Although, the hints given in the question is not specific for pancreatic injury, the only other injury in this setting would be mesenteric pedicle avulsion. However mesenteric pedicle avulsion is not a common injury and would usually present with diffuse abdominal pain, shock and bleeding PR (in extreme cases).

Investigation of Choice

Raised pancreatic enzymes (Serum amylase levels)

Immediate Management

Fluid resuscitation
High flow oxygen

Treatment of Choice

Conservative

Your notes:

Serial No. 114

Subject: Surgery

Topic: Trauma

Question: A man had met with a RTA and he developed shock and bruising of the flanks.

Diagnosis: Pancreatic Injury

Clinchers

- *Man, met with RTA:* Road traffic accidents (RTA) are four times more common in males than females, perhaps due to indulgence in more outdoor activities by the males.
- *Developed shock:* Injury to pancreas causes release of enzymes rich in proteases, elastases and collagenases, which cause widespread tissue damage leading to profound shock.
- *Bruising of flanks:* This is one of the characteristic signs due to haemorrhagic necrosis caused by the pancreatic enzymes.

CONFUSA

I think this question is very straight forward and there arises very little possibility of confusing this picture with any other injuries. However, always remember to read the question carefully and look for signs for injury to other intrabdominal organs. For e.g., this same question when presented like, '*A man met with a RTA, now in profound shock state*' will most likely point towards a splenic injury, rather than pancreatic. Similarly, while a hit from left side would cause a splenic rupture and shock, similar picture, but from the *right side* would be most likely due to a liver injury.

Investigation of Choice
Bed side USG

Immediate Management
Fluid Resuscitation
High flow oxygen (ARDS is an imminent complication of pancreatic injury).

Treatment of Choice
Conservative

Your notes:

Serial No. 127

Subject: Medicine

Topic: GIT

Question: A 32-year-old female presents with acute onset constipation with abdominal pain and vomiting. She is noted to have a small swelling in her groin.

Diagnosis: Intestinal Obstruction

Clinchers

- *A 32-year-old female:* Intestinal obstruction can present at any age and can affect men and women equally; In children the most common cause include congenital anomalies and congenital hernias; while in he adults the common causes are post-operative adhesions or acquired hernias.
- *Acute onset constipation:* The acute presentation of intestinal obstruction usually presents with abdominal pain and an inability to pass faeces or flatus with gradually worsening abdominal distension.
- *Abdominal pain and vomiting:* The abdominal pain is usually colicky and felt in mid abdomen. Vomiting becomes a more prominent feature with a proximal obstruction.
- *Small swelling in her groin:* This is apparently inguinal hernia or femoral hernia through the neck of which the bowel has been obstructed.

CONFUSA

In small bowel obstruction, vomiting occurs earlier, distension is less, pain is higher in the abdomen. The abdominal X-ray (AXR) plays a key role in diagnosis. In small bowel obstruction, AXR shows central gas shadows and no gas in the large bowel. Small bowel is identified by valvulae conniventes that completely cross the lumen (large bowel haustral folds do not cross all the lumen's width). In large bowel obstruction, pain is more constant; AXR shows gas proximal to the block (e.g. in caecum) but not in the rectum. If the ileocaecal valve is competent, pain may be felt over a distended caecum.

Investigation of Choice
Supine and upright abdominal X-rays (see confusa above).

Barium studies can help distinguish ileus from obstruction and locate specific area of obstruction (should not be done in suspected perforation).

Immediate Management

'Drip and suck' regime—Correct dehydration by Intravenous fluid administration and aspirate intestinal contents with a nasogastric tube to relieve distention.

Treatment of Choice

Surgery in cases of worsening symptoms or signs of strangulation. Hernial defect should be corrected appropriately after relieving obstruction.

Your notes:

Serial No. 128

Subject: Medicine

Topic: GIT

Question: A 40 year old patient comes with two year history of epigastric pain after food and tarry stools.

Diagnosis: Peptic Ulcer

Clinchers

- *A 40-year-old:* Peptic ulcers is a common condition with a lifetime incidence of up to 10%, occurring four times more commonly in men than women and most common in middle age with peak at 30-50 years.
- *Two year history of epigastric pain after food*: This is the most usual symptom seen in peptic ulcers. The patient usually complains of localized epigastric pain, described as burning or gnawing, for which the patient can characteristically point to the location of maximum intensity. The pain is associated with meals. Gastric ulcers give rise to pain 15-20 minutes after meals, whereas duodenal ulceration causes pain 1-3 hours after a meal.
- *Tarry stools:* This is signifying complication of long standing peptic ulcer—gastrointestinal bleeding. It occurs in 25% to 33% of cases and accounts for 25% of ulcer deaths. Haemorrhage arises from the small blood vessels at the base of the ulcer.

CONFUSA

Peptic ulcer is a broad term including both duodenal and gastric ulcers. While duodenal ulcer is most commonly related to infection by *Helicobacter pylori*, gastric ulcer owe their existence to the factors which are related with increased serum gastrin levels and inadvertent use of NSAIDs.

Investigation of Choice

Upper GI Endoscopy with biopsy.

Immediate Management

Urgent admission to hospital is required in cases of actively bleeding peptic ulcer.

Treatment of Choice

According to the cause identified:

HP eradication for duodenal ulcer

Stopping the offending drug (NSAIDs)

Proton pump inhibitors or Surgical resection for Zollinger-Ellison syndrome

Serial No. 129

Subject: Medicine

Topic: GIT

Question: A 55-year-old woman presents with a six-month history of severe central abdominal pain, which comes on 30-minutes after meals. She has lost 10-kg in weight, and on examination of her abdomen there is a bruit in the epigastrium. She also suffers from intermittent claudication.

Diagnosis: Intestinal Claudication (Abdominal Angina)

Clinchers

- *55-year-old woman:* Atherosclerosis is the leading cause of morbidity in the Western world, accounting for more than half of all deaths. It affects nearly all adults, with a variable pattern and severity. Increases with age; more common in males than in females, particularly in younger age groups—aged 35 to 44 the prevalence in males is six times that of females, compared to just two times in 65 to 74-year-old.
- *Six-month history... After meals:* The patient typically is presenting with features suggesting of mesenteric ischaemia. Patients may present with a history of postprandial pain, typically starting 20-30 minutes after their last meal, that may last up to 60-90 minutes.
- *Lost 10 kg in weight:* Because of this typical relation of symptoms with food, they develop food fear and experience subsequent weight loss. Patients may be severely malnourished upon presentation.
- *Bruit in the epigastrium:* This is again suggesting the narrowed mesenteric artery due to probable athero-sclerosis.
- *Intermittent claudication:* Atherosclerosis of aorta and internal iliac arteries can cause intermittent claudi-cation. Presence in this patient suggests widespread atherosclerosis.

CONFUSA

Patient can also present with acute mesenteric ischaemia due to embolic or thrombotic occlusion of the mesentric artery. Look carefully for hints such as a prosthetic heart valve or atrial fibrillation which can be the source of the offending embolus. Such patients will present acutely with sudden onset of symptoms. Palpation of the abdomen would reveal no peritoneal signs and pain is usually out of proportion to examination. Auscultation of the abdomen may reveal a bruit.

Investigation of Choice
Mesenteric angiogram

Immediate Management
Correct dehydration

Treatment of Choice
Surgery

Your notes:

Serial No. 130

Subject: Medicine

Topic: GIT

Question: A 25-year-old teacher complains that she has had central abdominal discomfort of six-month duration, intermittent abdominal distension and alteration in bowel habit. On examination, there is a palpable swelling in the right iliac fossa. A Barium enaema carried out showed no abnormality.

Diagnosis: Mesenteric Adenitis

Clinchers

- *25-year-old teacher:* Patients with mesenteric adenitis is usually under 30 years of age. It occurs due to non-specific inflammation of the mesenteric lymph nodes which provokes a mild peritoneal reaction and stimulates painful peristalsis in the terminal ileum.
- *Central abdominal discomfort.... alteration in bowel habit:* Patients usually present with abdominal pain, usually in the right iliac fossa. There is little guarding or rebound, and moderate tenderness. The patient may be pyrexial and there may be diarrhoea, with or without vomiting, or a recent upper respiratory tract infection.
- *Palpable swelling in the right iliac fossa:* This further confirms the diagnosis of mesentric adenitis.
- *A Barium enaema carried out showed no abnormality:* The pathology is extraluminal; hence barium enaema is very unlikely to be helpful. Also, a normal barium enaema rules out possibility of carcinomas which can have similar presentations.

CONFUSA

The important differential for mesenteric adenitis is acute appendicitis, but the clinical picture of this condition can usually be discriminated from the absence of rectal tenderness, and a temperature higher than 38.5 degrees C. However, if there is uncertainty, a laparotomy may be performed. Adenitis is confirmed by a normal appendix and large inflamed, fleshy lymph nodes in the mesentery.

Investigation of Choice
Abdominal CT scan

Immediate Management
None; carefully rule out appendicitis

Treatment of Choice
None required; its a self limiting process

Serial No. 149

Subject: Surgery

Topic: Neck swellings

Question: An infant with brilliantly transilluminable swelling at the base of his neck.

Diagnosis: Cystic Hygroma

Clinchers

- *An infant:* This is a congenital lesion comprised of lymph-filled spaces which arise from an embryonic remnant of the jugular lymph sac. cystic hygroma are invariably present at birth, smaller masses may be missed and present later in childhood as an expanding lump.
- *Brilliantly transilluminable swelling:* It is not a true cyst but rather a lymphatic hamartoma which forms multilocular cyst-like spaces. which contain clear fluid and this make them transilluminate brilliantly.
- *At the base of his neck:* Most occur in the base of the neck, both in the anterior and the posterior triangle, and may extend up to the jaw, over the anterior chest wall, and down into the axilla. Rarely, it occurs alone in the axilla, pelvis, or groin.

CONFUSA

- Cystic hygromas are common associations with Turner's and Noonan's Syndrome.
- Branchial cyst is a close differential, usually presenting in young adults as a smooth swelling in front of the anterior border of the sternomastoid at the junction of its upper and middle thirds. The position is characteristic. It is usually fluctuant and may transilluminate.

Investigation of Choice
Clinical diagnosis.

Immediate Management
Rule out associated syndromes.
Rule out active infection.

Treatment of Choice
Surgical excision
(can be difficult because of infiltration of vital neck strictures)

Your notes:

PAPER 3

11. A 28-year-old woman after cholescystectomy following a perforated gallbladder has a raised right diaphragm with a temperature of 38°C and a pulse of 120 beats per minute.

Diagnosis: Subphrenic abscess (right sided).

Clinchers

- *Woman:* The incidence of cholelithiasis (which sometimes lead to perforated gallbladder) in much more in females. Although its maximum incidence is seen in forties (fair, fat, fertile female in forties).
- *Perforated gallbladder:* Usually the underlying cause of subphrenic abscess is a peritonitis involving the upper abdomen, i.e. leakage following biliary or gastric surgery or perforation.
- *After cholecystectomy:* Subphrenic infection usually follows general peritonitis after 10-21 days, although if antibiotics have been given as abscess may be disguised and may only become manifest weeks or even months after the original episode.
- *Raised right diaphragm:* It occurs if the abscess is of a significant size.
- *Temperature of 38°C:* Along with a mild persisting/swinging pyrexia, other features can be anaemia, malaise, nausea and loss of weight. Tachycardia usually occurs in response to pyrexia (as is in this case).

CONFUSA

There may be no localising symptoms of a subphrenic abscess if it is small enough (hence the aphorism—pus somewhere, pus nowhere, pus under the diaphragm).

Investigation of Choice

- *Screening:* Ultrasound/Chest X-ray.
- *Definitive:* CT scan (it also locates any other peritoneal collections of pus).

Immediate Management

Broad spectrum antibiotics.

Treatment of Choice

- Percutaneous drainage (USG/CT guided)
- Surgical drainage is done if:
  - Percutaneous drainage fails
  - Abscess is loculated

Your notes:

14. A middle-aged man with acute pancreatitis develops hypotension. On CT he is found to have peripancreatic fluid and a lack of enhancement of the pancreatic tail.

Diagnosis: Hypotensive shock secondary to acute pancreatitis.

Clinchers

- *Middle-aged man:* Most common cause of acute pancreatitis in a middle-aged is alcohol. In females it is gallstones. (Note: But alcohol more commonly is responsible for chronic pancreatitis).
- *With acute pancreatitis:* The usual symptoms are epigastric pain which radiates to back between the scapula. The pain vary from mild discomfort to excruciating in severe disease. It is usually accompanied by nausea and vomiting. Sitting forward may help.
- *Develops hypotension:* It is because of third space accumulation of fluid in the peripancreatic region early in the disease. It can produce hypotensive shock which may be compounded by episodes of vomiting. So fluid resuscitation is of utmost importance.
- *Peripancreatic fluid and a lack of enhancement of the pancreatic tail:* Contrast enhances dynamic CT scanning is the most valuable technique in diagnosis of acute pancreatitis. It can detect swelling of the pancreas and the presence of pancreatic necrosis, peripancreatic fluid collections or diffuse inflammatoy changes in the retroperitoneum (which explains the lack of enhancement of the pancreatic tail).

CONFUSA

If there is doubt about the diagnosis, explorative laparotomy must be performed in all but mild cases to excluded a potentially fatal but treatable non-pancreatic lesion.

Investigation of Choice

- *Screening:* Serum amylase (five times increase).
- *Definitive:* USG/CT/ERCP.

Immediate Management

- Fluids (plasma expander + normal saline)
- Analgesia (pethidine + prochlorperazine)
- Monitoring of vitals

Treatment of Choice

- Conservative if mild
- ERCP + gallstone removal if progressive jaundice
- A recent study using the platelet activating factor antagonist (lexipafant) showed a reduction in complications and overall mortality if given within 48 hours.

15. Following a perforated bowel, a middle-aged man develops severe shock and septicaemia as well as a central dark discoloration on his abdomen, which is growing larger.

Diagnosis: Generalised peritonitis.

Clinchers

- *Severe shock and stepticaemia:* Any delay in treatment of peritonitis secondary to a perforation produces profound toxaemia and septicemia. Since this stage takes some time to develop, it means that perforation is 10-15 hours old.
- *Central dark discoloration on his abdomen, which is growing larger:* This is a feature of generalised peritonitis which is by chemical irritation due to leakage of intestinal contents and superadded infection by *E. coli* and bacteroides. Basically it rules out localised peritonitis in this patient and hence rules out any need for conservative management only.

CONFUSA

Conservative treatment is indicated, at least initially, where the infection has been localised (appendix mass), or where the primary focus is irremovable (pancreatitis). Surgery is indicated if the source of infection can be removed or closed, e.g. the repair of a perforated ulcer or removal of a gangrenous, perforated appendix.

Investigation of Choice

- Chest X-ray (erect)
- Findings: Free gas under diaphragm

Immediate Management

Morphine + fluids + antibiotics.

Treatment of Choice

Generalised peritonitis is always treated surgically after adequate resuscitation with the re-establishment of a good urinary output.

Your notes:

67. Following a motorcyle accident a young man has a pulse rate of 110 and a blood pressure that falls to 90/50. On examination of the CXR he is noted to have fractures of the lower ribs on the left.

Diagnosis: Splenic rupture

Clinchers

- *Motorcyle accident:* The main injuries in a motorcycle accident are sustained on head, thorax and legs.
- *Young man:* Young men are more involved in motorcycle accidents.
- *Pulse rate of 110:* A pulse >100 and systolic BP < 100 signifies hypovolaemic shock.
- *Blood pressure falls to 90/50:* This signifies a massive blood loss.
- *Fractures of the lower ribs on the left:* Fracture of ribs does not lead to a significant fall in BP as the blood loss is very minimal. It could fall to 90/50 only if there is rupture of spleen which lies beneath lower left ribs.

CONFUSA

Haemothorax can present with same profile but that would be visible on CXR.

Investigation of Choice

- Peritoneal lavage if patient is shocked
- Otherwise USG

Immediate Management

Fluid resuscitation + cross-match.

Treatment of Choice

Urgent laparotomy (with splenic preservation wherever possible).

Your notes:

142. An elderly gentleman with left iliac fossa pain and tenderness and rectal bleeding.

Diagnosis: Diverticulitis.

Clinchers

- *Elderly gentleman:* Diverticulitis is unusual before 40 years. Sex distribution is roughly equal.
- *Left iliac fossa pain:* Acute diverticulitis is well nick-named left-sided appendicitis. Here abdominal pain shifts to left iliac fossa (LIF) accompanied by fever, vomiting, local tenderness and guarding.
- *Rectal bleeding:* In chronic cases passage of mucosa or bright red blood per rectum or malaena or occult bleeding is present. There may be diarrhoea alternating with constipation.

Bleeding from a diverticulum is the most likely cause of a sudden perfuse, bright red bleed in an elderly, often hypertensive patient.

Diverticulitis may lead to

- Perforation
- Chronic infection
- Haemorrhage.

CONFUSA

The symptoms and presentation in this question may very much be confused from neoplasm of the colon. It is imposible to be certain of this differentiation clinically or even on special investigations, unless positive biopsy is obtained by flexible sigmoidoscopy or colonoscopy.

Investigation of Choice

Sigmoidoscopy (fibre optic-flexible)—can be performed to visualize colonic diverticula and to take a biopsy. This is an investigation of choice. Barium enaema should not be performed in the acute phase to prevent iatrogenic perforation of friable and inflamed bowel, rather in acute cases CT scan may be useful to exclude other causes of lower abdominal pain.

Treatment of Choice

This case should be managed conservatively. Perform flexible sigmoidoscopy and place the patient on fluid diet and antibiotics. In chronic cases bowels are regulated by means of lubricant laxative (e.g., Milpar) and prescribe high roughage diet (fruit, vegetables, whole meal bread and barley).

Your notes:

143. A middle-aged woman with recurrent right upper abdominal pain radiating to the right shoulder. She is tender in this region.

Diagnosis: Cholelithiasis.

Clinchers

- *Middle-aged woman:* Always remember the five F's of cholelithiasis: fair, fat, fertile, female of fourty (40). But this is just an approximation to the truth. The incidence of cholelethiasis is higher in overweight, middle-aged women.
- *Recurrent right upper abdominal pain:* Recurrent bouts of pain occur due to mild cholecystitis, which may or may not be accompanied by fever. In acute cases upper abdomen is extremely tender and often a palpable mass develops in the region of the gall-bladder.

Though stones may be absent from the duct system, a tinge of jaundice may be produced due to pressing of common bile duct by sudden gallbladder.

Fatty meals cause discomfort, as they stimulate release of cholecystokinin which causes the gallbladder to contract onto stones.

CONFUSA

Differentiate it from pancreatitis, chronic dyspepsia, including peptic ulceration and hiatus hernia. So for serum amylase to exclude pancreatitis, and chest X-ray to rule out pneumonia.

Investigation of Choice

Ultrasonography—show presence of stones in inflamed gallbladder with oedema around the gallbladder wall.

Immediate Management

Conservative management.

Treatment of Choice

Conservative treatment followed by cholecystectomy.

Your notes:

144. Middle-aged chronic alcoholic presents with severe pain in upper abdomen, radiating to the back.

Diagnosis: Pancreatitis

Clinchers

- *Middle-aged chronic alcoholic:* Pancreatitis is more commonly seen in obese and middle-aged or elderly, women being affected more than male.
  Alcoholism is the main cause of chronic pancreatitis. Acute cases are associated with either gallstones or alcohol.
- *Severe pain (upper abdomen) radiating to back:* In pancreatitis the pain severe, constant, usually epigastric and often radiates to back. Pain is sometime relieved on bending forward. Abdomen is tender with positive guarding.
  To diagnose pancreatitis go for serum amylase. Amylase is liberated into circulation by damaged pancreas. Amylase may be raised in variety of other conditions like—renal failure, salivary gland diseases (like parotitis) severe diabetic ketoacidosis, morphine administration (causing sphincter of Oddi spasm), perforated' peptic ulcer, acute cholecystitis, intestinal obstruction and many more.

Investigation of Choice

Serum amylase.

Immediate Management

Conservative consists of analgaesia with pethidine (avoid morphine, which may produce sphincter spasm) and fluid replacement.

Treatment of Choice

In acute cases, conservative management is done. Surgery is indicated if diagnosis is not certain, but should be avoided. In chronic pancreatitis—analgesia and diet control is advised. Surgery if very frequent attacks or severe pain—partial pancreatectomy or pancreaticojejunostomy.

Your notes:

145. A fit 17-year-old man present with a 12 hour history of central abdominal pain localising to his right iliac fossa. He is pyrexical with tenderness, guarding and rebound tenderness in the right iliac fossa.

Diagnosis: Acute appendicitis

Clinchers

- *A 17-year-old man:* Acute appendicitis may occur at any age but is most common between the ages of 15 and 30 years and is uncommon under the age of 2 years.
- *12 hour history of central abdominal pain localising to his right iliac fossa:* The pain in appendicitis is initially periumbilical or epigastric, later radiating to right iliac fossa.
- *Pyrexical with tenderness, guarding and rebound tenderness in RIF:* Right iliac fossa is usually most tender and guarded part of the abdoman in appendicitis. Rebound tenderness points towards peritonitis. Pyrexia and tachycardia are usual.

CONFUSA

Differentiate it from other causes of acute abdomen. Refer page 196, lecture notes on general surgery, 9th edn.

Investigation of Choice

Diagnostic laparoscopy. This is the best answer amongst all the options given. Though it is important to note that the diagnosis of acute appendicitis is made on the basis of history and examination. No special investigation is indicated unless alternative diagnosis is being considered.

Immediate Management

The treatment of acute appendicitis is appendicectomy, except in following conditions.

- Patient is morifund with advanced peritonitis
- Attack has already resolved, in such a case appendicectomy can be adviced as an elective procedure.

Your notes:

162. An elderly male develops pain in his thigh and leg when walking for approximately 20 metres. This pain resolves with rest. He is a long time smoker. In examination his dorsalis pedis pulse on the affected side is absent.

Diagnosis: Buerger's disease (thromboangiitis obliterans).

Clinchers

- *Elderly:* The disorder develos most frequently in men under 40. The prevalence is higher in Asians and individual of eastern european descent.
- *Pain in his thigh and leg when walking for approximately 20 meters:* This is claudication and 20 meters is the claudication distance. Buerger's disease presents as a triad of claudication of the affected extremity, Raynaud's phenomenon, and migratory superficial vein thrombophlebitis. Claudication is usually confined to the lower calves and feet or the forearms and hands, because this disorder primarily affects distal vessels.
- *Pain resolves with rest:* A hallmark of claudication.
- *Long-time smokers:* While the cause of Buerger's disease is unknown there is a definite relationship to cigarette smoking and an increased incidence of HLA-B5 and A9 antigens in patients with this disorder.
- *Dorsalis pedis pulse absent:* The physical examination shows normal branchial and popliteal pulses but reduced or absent radial, ulnar, and/or tibial and dorsalis pedis pulses.

CONFUSA

Buerger's disease can be clinically indistinguishable from atheromatous peripheral vascular disease.

Investigation of Choice

- *Screening:* Arteriography
- *Definitive:* Biopsy

Immediate Management

Local debridement if gangrene is present.

Treatment of Choice

Advise stop smoking and exercise. The prognosis is worst in patients who continue to smoke.

Your notes:

163. A 70-year-old with known atrial fibrillation on treatment dvelops a sudden cold leg. Pulses are absent in the level at and below the knee.

Diagnosis: Femoral artery emboli.

Clinchers

- *Known atrial fibrillation:* Emboli commonly arise from the heart secondary to atrial fibrillation and infarcts.
- *Develops a sudden cold leg:* Sings or symptoms of acute leg ischaemia due to emboli are described by six Ps—the part is pale, pulseness, painful, paralysed, paraesthetic and perishing with cold. All these symptoms can be explained by occlusion of the arterial supply.
- *Pulses are absent in the levell at and below the knee:* it indicates that the site of occlusion by emboli is above popliteal artery, i.e. in superficial femoral artery.

CONFUSA

The other common source of leg emboli an aneurysm (aorta, femoral or popliteal). So perform an extensive clinical examination to rule it out.

Investigation of Choice

Urgent arteriography (only if diagnosis in doubt).

Immediate Management

Urgent surgical referral.

Treatment of Choice

Femoral embolectomy (Fogarty catheter)
or
Local thrombolysis (t-PA)

Your notes:

164. A 67-year-old male with a history of peripheral vascular disease develops sever ulceration and cellulitis in his left foot and extending up his left leg above the left ankle. The popliteal pulse is absent on that side. He has a history of ulceration on the contralateral side which resolved following a bypass graft operation on that side.

Diagnosis: Peripheral vascular disease (PVD) with gangrene.

Clinchers

- *A 67-year-old male:* It chiefly occurs over the age of 50 years, chiefly in men.
- *Severe ulceration and cellulitis in his left foot and extending up his left leg above the left ankle:* Ulceration and gangrene of the affected limb is present in severe disease. It usually start at the toes.
- *Popliteal pulse absent:* There are diminished or absent pulses to diseased areas. The limb is cold with dry skin and lack of hair due to chronic ischaemia.
- *History of ucelration on contralateral side which resolved following a bypass graft operation:* Aortoiliac bypass grafts give good results in PVD. Aslo PVD is usually bilateral.

CONFUSA

Atherosclerotic PVD can be easily confused clinically with Buerger's diseases, but in Buerger's disease, the popliteal pulse is almost always present. Also patients with atherosclerotic PVD usually have symptomatic ischaemic heart disease.

Investigation of Choice

Arteriography.

Immediate Management

Urgent surgical referral.

Treatment of Choice

Amputation is necessary for severely ischaemic limbs, usually those with gangrene (as in this case).

Note: Bypass operations are not done till 3 months after an acute attack (to let a collateral circulation develop).

Your notes:

165. A 55-year-old man complains of intermittent pain in his toe on walking. He says that in addition it looks 'white'.

Diagnosis: Peripheral vascular disease (PVD).

Clinchers

- *A 55-year-old:* Patients with arterial disease tend to be elderly and have generalised atherosclerosis.
- *Intermittent pain on walking:* This is intermittent claudication, the hallmark of PVD. It is typically relieved by rest (except in severe disease, where it may be present at rest).
- *Toe looks 'white':* It is due to arterial narrowing and decreased perfusion of the toe.

CONFUSA

Arterial diseases produces white toes or feet, while venous disease will produce blue extremities (cyanosis). Arterial diseases, when minimal can be demonstrated by mild exercise. Exercise produces vasodilatation below the obstructing lesion and the arterial, inflow, reduced by the lesion, cannot keep pace with the increasing vascular shape, arterial pressure falls and the pulse disappears producing the white limb or toe.

Some important points in PVD differential diagnosis:

- PVD symptoms in young females—suspect Raynaud's disease
- PVD symptoms in young males—suspect Buerger's disease
- PVD symptoms in migraine patient—suspect ergotamine overdose
- PVD symptoms in TIA patient—suspect atherosclerosis

Investigation of Choice

- *Screening:* Ankle branchial pressure index (ABPI)
  - Resting value is 1.0
  - < 0.9 signify some degree of arterial obstruction
  - < 0.5 signify severe ischaemia
  - < 0.3 signify imminent necrosis
- *Definitive:* Arteriography.

Immediate Management

Detailed work up to rule out diabetes and coronary artery disease.

Treatment of Choice

If claudication is a significant handicap to the patient, the possibility of reconstructive surgery or angiographic intervention should be considered.

167. An 18-year-old man who has sustained stab wounds to his abdomen and trunk. His respiratory rate is 23 breaths/min, his breath sounds appear normal but his pulse is 142/min and his BP is only 80/40 mm Hg.

Diagnosis: Hypovolaemic shock.

Clinchers

- *Stab wounds in abdomen and trunk:* Haemothorax and haemoperitoneum are the two conditions producing hypovolaemic shock by internal bleeding. This person is at risk of both.
- *Respiratory rate is 23 breaths/min:* Tachypnoea is an early feature of hypovolaemic shock.
- *Breath sounds normal:* This rules out haemothorax which can lead to absence of breath sounds on affected side.
- *Pulse rate is 142/min:* Tachycardia is also a characteristic feature of circulatory failure due to shock.
- *BP is only 80/40 mm Hg:* This signifies that the blood loss is significant and requires urgent resuscitation.

CONFUSA

It is very important to remember that in a young and fit person (like this man of 18 years age), BP can remain stable even upto loss of 30% of circulating blood volume (though the pulse pressure will fall).

Investigation of Choice
Ultrasound (abdomen)
Note: Peritoneal lavage is often indicated in older textbooks but rarely indicated.

Immediate Management
Colloid infusion followed by infusion of crossmatched blood (or "O-ve" blood in emergency).

Treatment of Choice
Urgent explorative laparotomy.

Your notes:

176. A 23-year-old woman develops an acute pain in her right chest radiating to her right shoulder associated with a fever. She is vomiting and has mild yellowing of her skin.

Diagnosis: Acute cholecystitis

Clinchers

- *A 23-year-old woman:* Female sex is a definitive risk factor for gallstones. Acute cholecystitis follows stone impaction in the neck of gallbladder.
- *Acute pain:* The pain may begin suddenly but is then constant and very severe.
- *Pain in right chest radiating to her right shoulder:* There is constant right upper quadrant pain referred to back and shoulder.
- *Fever:* Pyrexia and malaise are commonly part of the presentation.
- *Vomiting:* Nausea and vomiting are almost always present.
- *Mid yellowing of skin:* Obstructive jaundice may be present as the common causes of acute cholecystitis in a female are biliary calculi.

CONFUSA

Acute pancreatitis usually do not occur as commonly in young females. Pyrexia is uncommon in it. It is more characterised by tachycardia and cyanosis due to hypovolaemic shock (third space sequestration of fluids).

Investigation of Choice
Early USG

Immediate Management
Analgaesia and admission.

Treatment of Choice
Cefuroxime 1.5 g/8 h IV.

In suitable cases, do cholecystectomy within 48 hours (laparoscopic if no question of GB perforation). Otherwise operate after 3 months.

Your notes:

180. Minutes after upper GI endoscopy a 57-year-old man develops chest pain. When you examine him, he has a crackling feeling under the skin around his upper chest and neck.

Diagnosis: Ruptured oesophagus

Clinchers

- *Minutes after upper GI endoscopy:* Oesophageal injury is a well recognised complication of upper GI endoscopy. The most common site of perforation is the level of cricopharyngeus.
- *A 57-year-old man:* Elderly people have a lax musculature of oesophagus which is more prone to perforation by instrumentation or rupture by repeated vomiting against a closed glottis (Boerhaave's syndrome).
- *Chest pain:* After instrumentation, perforation is suspected if the patient complains of pain in the neck, chest or upper abdomen. Pyrexia and dysphagia are also present. Consider oesophageal performation if there is:
  - Inexplicable shock after trunk injury
  - Left pneumothorax without rib fracture
  - Gastric contents in a chest drain
- *Crackling feeling under the skin around his upper chest and neck:* This is subcutaneous emphysema and its location (i.e. supraclavicular) is pathognomic of oesophageal rupture. It is due to the gas escaping into the mediastinum.

CONFUSA

Since the site of pain in this patient is chest, this is most probably a thoracic rupture (usually instrumentation produce perforation in the neck). It is important to differentiate a thoracic rupture from a rupture in neck as the latter can be conservatively managed.

Investigation of Choice

- *Screening:* Chest X-ray (mediastinal gas)
- *Definitive:* Gastrograffin swallow (a water soluble contrast fluid) will confirm the perforation and define its position.

Immediate Management

Crossmatch 10 units blood and inform surgeons.

Treatment of Choice

Thoractomy and suturing of oesophagus (or resection if a carcinoma is instrumentally perforated).

Your notes:

PAPER 4

36. Man rescued from burning building. Burns on face and anterior chest, soot in pharynx and singed nasal hair, asking about his family members.

Diagnosis: Inhalation injury.

Clinchers

- *Rescued from burning building:* Inhalation of hot smoke and fumes is common in patients exposed to house fires.
- *Burns on face and anterior chest:* Burns around the lips, mouth, throat or nose suggest high likely hood of inhalation injury.
- *Soot in pharynx:* Soot in pharynx and production of carboniferous (black) sputum is virtually diagnostic inhalation injury.
- *Signed nasal hair:* It should always arouse the suspicious of inhalation injury. One should always check a burns patient for singeing of nasal vibrissa to rule out inhalation injury.
- *Asking about his family members:* This rules out impaired consciousness or confusion which is a common complication after inhalation injury. It is caused by a combination of hypoxia, carbon monoxide poisoning and hydrogen cyanide poisoning.

CONFUSA

Fumes may contain gases which impair surfactant activity and irritate the respiratory mucosa. Early bronchospasm may occur but there may be no obvious evidence of damage until pulmonary oedema develops some hours later. Airway obstruction may also rapidly result from delayed sloughing of tracheal or bronchial mucosa.

Beware of conventional blood gas analyser readings in patients who may have high carboxy- or methaemoglobin levels. The oxygen electrode measure oxygen dissolve in plasma only and oxygen saturation in then calculated assuming all haemoglobin to be normal. PaO_2 and oxygen saturation may thus appear to be satisfactory despite very low total blood oxygen content.

Investigation of Choice

Fibreoptic bronchoscopy + ABG + COHb

Immediate Management

- High concentration O_2
- Ask for senior anaesthetic advice about intubation

Treatment of Choice

Early intubation (late intubation is difficult because of oedema).

Note: Endotracheal tubes should be left long and uncut to allow for swelling.

37. Baby with less than 3 per cent burns on chest and shoulders [scald due to tea falling on him] is irritable, crying, not allowing examination.

Diagnosis: Superficial small burns.

Clinchers

- *Less than 3 per cent burns:* This patient does not require a referral for admission to burns unit. The criteria for admission are:
  - Children and elderly—>10% burns
  - Adults—>15% burns
  - Other—facial, hand, perineal burns.
- *Scald due to tea falling on him:* A scald from hot fluid with produce a cascade effect, with streaks of burnt skin following the path of the falling fluid, possibly with increasing depth of injury where its flow has been held up by constricting clothes such as waistbands or socks.
- *Irritable, crying*: That means the burn is painful. This is significant as full thickness burns are painless because of destruction of nerve endings.
- *Not allowing examination:* To perform examination, analgesia need to be given.

CONFUSA

Simple erythema is extremely painful. Even patients expected to go home after treatment may need parenteral analgesia. A scald with a glove or stocking distribution is unusual and suggests abuse (non-accidental injury) in children.

Investigation of Choice
Determination of depth of burn.

Immediate Management
IV opioid (analgesia must be given as soon as possible, especially to children. The beneficial effects of morphine is small children greatly outweigh any haemodynamic side effects).

Treatment of Choice
Dressing with medication and discharge with follow up instructions.

Your notes:

38. Man was electrocuted. Full thickness burn on fingers complainting of pain.

Diagnosis: Electric burns.

Clinchers

- *Electrocuted:* Electric burns are of two types:
  1. *High voltage injury:* Produce ECG changes (RBBB and/or ST changes ± SVT) and are usually fatal. The causes include lightning.
  2. *Low voltage injury:* These are usually sustained from the domestic electricity supply and usually localised without cardiac complications. The case described in question is most probably of this type.
- *Full thickness burns on fingers with pain:* Local burns even in low voltage injury are almost always full-thickness and much deeper than it appears. Pain may be present in adjoining ischaemic area which usually also necrose within few days.

CONFUSA

The fingers quickly stiffen up and conventional bandages become very dirty, with an increased risk of infection. These complications are avoided if plastic gloves are used initially instead of standard dressings. Silver sulphadiazine cream is applied and a loosely fitting examination glove is fitted in place with tape around the wrist. The gloves tend to burst, so patients must be given a supply to apply themselves.

Investigation of Choice
ECG.

Immediate Management
Escharotomy.

Treatment of Choice
Early excision and grafting.

Your notes:

39. Man with 40 per cent burns over trunk and limbs.

Diagnosis: Burns requiring admission to burns unit.

Clinchers

- *40% burns:* The criteria for admissions are:
  - Adults—>*15%* burns
  - Child (<10 yr)—>10% burns
  - Elderly (>70 yr)—>10% burns

  The admission is required as these patients require IV fluid resuscitation to correct haemodynamic changes.
- *Over trunk and limbs:* This rules out inhalation injury (but sill check ABG and nasal vibrissae singeing).

CONFUSA

Fluid replacement must be calculated from the time of burns and not from the time of admission. This is so because exudative fluid loss start immediately after burns. Fluid given in the first time band has to be given at a faster rate if there is a delay between time of burns and time of arrival at hospital.

Investigation of Choice
U and E.

Immediate Management
IV fluids + referral for admission to burns unit.

Treatment of Choice
Monitoring + care in specialist burns care unit
± skin grafting later on.

Your notes:

40. Man, slept while sunbathing comes with redness, and pain all over his body. Otherwise well.

Diagnosis: Sunburns.

Clinchers

- *Sunbathing:* It can cause sunburns if prolonged, but these are usually not serious.
- *Redness:* It is superficial erythema and is never taken into accounting when calculating the area of burn.
- *Pain:* Simple erythema is extremely painful. Even patients expected to go home after treatment may need parenteral analgesia.
- *Otherwise well:* This rules out any other injury or fluid compromise. Since simple erythema do not require active treatment, he can be safely discharged home.

CONFUSA

Unprotected exposure to UV radiation can cause extremely painful, blistering, oedematous skin. In general the treatment is as for any other burn.

Investigation of Choice
None required.

Immediate Management
Oral analgesia if required.

Treatment of Choice
Reassure and discharge
+
Regular application of hydrocortisone 1% cream.

Your notes:

46. Woman after open cholecystectomy presents with fever, redness and tenderness of wound.

Diagnosis: Wound infection.

Clinchers

- *Open cholecystectomy:* Wound infections are especially common when the alimentary, biliary or urinary tract is opened during surgery, allowing bacterial contamination to occur.
- *Fever with redness and tenderness of wound:* The onset of would infection is usually a few days after operations; this may be delayed still further, even upto weeks, if antimicrobial chemotherapy has been employed. The patient complaints of
  - pain and swelling in the wound
  - general effects of infection, e.g.
    - malaise
    - anorexia
    - vomiting
  - runs a swinging, pyrexia.

The wound is red, swollen, hot and tender.

CONFUSA

The principal causes of wound infection are the penicillin resistant *Staphylococcus aureus*, together with *Streptococcus faecalis, Pseudomonas,* coliform bacilli and other bowel bacteria including bacteroides. With continued use of antibiotics, mothicillin resistant *Staphylococcus aureus* (MRSA) and the vancomycin resistant enterococcus (VRE) becoming more common.

Investigation of Choice

Wound swab.

Immediate Management

Removal of sutures of probing of the wound to release the contained pus.

Treatment of Choice

Established infection is treated by drainage. Antibiotics are given, if there is, in addition, a spreading cellulitis.

Your notes:

50. Man after appendicectomy presents with spiking fever with rigors, tenesmus, diarrhoea.

Diagnosis: Pelvic abscess.

Clinchers

- *Appendicectomy:* Pelvic abscess formation is an occasional complication of appendicitis and can occur irrespective of the position of the appendix within the peritoneal cavity.
- *Spiking fever with rigors:* The most common presentation is a spiking pyrexia several days following appendicitis (the patient may have been discharged from hospital).
- *Tenesmus and diarrhoea:* Pelvic pressure or discomfort associated with loose stool or tenesmus is common.

CONFUSA

A pelvic abscess may follow any general peritonitis, but it is particularly common after acute appendicitis (75%), or after gynaecological infections. In the male the abscess lies between the bladder and the rectum, in the female between the uterus and posterior fornix of the vagina anteriorly, and the rectum posteriorly (pouch of Douglas). Left untreated the abscess may burst into the rectum or vagina or may discharge onto the abdominal wall, particularly if there has been previous abdominal laparotomy incision at the time of the original episode of peritonitis (as in this case).

Investigation of Choice

- *Screening:* Per rectal examination (foggy mass in pelvis, anterior to rectum, at the level of peritoneal reflection).
- *Definitive:* Pelvic USG/CT scan.

Immediate Management

Antipyretics + short course chemotherapy.

Treatment of Choice

Transrectal drainage under GA.

Note: Very often even this is not required, as firm pressure by the finger in the rectum may be followed by rupture of the abscess through the rectal wall.

Your notes:

71. A boy was riding his bicycle when he was hit by a car. After examination in A and E, he was found to have left upper quadrant tenderness. He is pale.

Diagnosis: Probable splenic rupture.

Clinchers

- *Riding bicycle when he was hit by a car:* Road traffic accidents (RTA) are the most common cause of traumatic splenic rupture. Usually the patient has sustained a blunt trauma to the abdomen.
- *Left upper quadrant pain:* This is the anatomical site of spleen. Always rule out splenic rupture by USG in RTA with LUQ pain.
- *Tenderness:* Most probably due to associated rib fractures.
- *Pale:* If a patient is abnormally pale following an injury always suspect splenic rupture if no other bleeding sites or cause of blood loss is evident.

CONFUSA

There is an increasing trend to preserve the spleen after rupture, if its salvageable, in children. It is so because of the risk of sudden, overwhelming sepsis which can occur at any time of lift after splenectomy.

Investigation of Choice
USG (early).

Immediate Management
Resuscitation + crossmatch blood.

Treatment of Choice
Urgent laparotomy.

Your notes:

72. A man fell off a ladder,has diffuse pain on right side of the trunk. IVU shows no excretion on right side.

Diagnosis: Avulsion of renal pedicle.

Clinchers

- *Fell of a ladder*: Injuries to the loins are common after all and assault.
- *Diffuse pain on right side of trunk:* Local pain and tenderness are invariably present in renal injury. Haematuria is characteristically absent in complete avulsion of renal pedicle.
- *IVU shows no excretion on right side:* This is characteristic of pedicle avulsion (see confusa below). It may also suggest absence of kidney on right side due to previous nephrectomy. In that case a history will exclude this diagnosis. Absence of one kidney may be due to congenital aplasia which can be confirmed by USG. Also in this case the other kidney will be hypertrophied. An absent or grossly atrophic kidney is found in about 1: 1400 individuals.

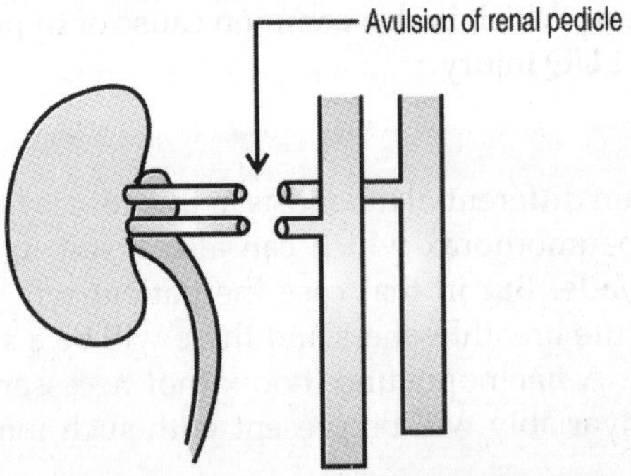

CONFUSA

Superficial soft tissue bruising may testify to the severity of the blow but is often absent. The main differential diagnosis is from renal contusion but an IVU will differentiate that. In contusion injuries there is at least some uptake of the contrast and there may be extravasation of contrast media outside the renal outline. Haematuria is the main symptom in renal contusion which will be completely absent in avulsion of renal pedicle. In avulsion injuries, the detachment may be partial or complete. There may be complete detachment of a pole of kidney.

Investigation of Choice
USG to confirm the existence of kidney.

Immediate Management
Fluid resuscitation and crossmatch.

Treatment of Choice
Urgent nephrectomy is the only course of treatment.

73. Man was stabbed with a 10 cm knife in the left upper quadrant, stable for 20 min after which BP falls to 90/60 mmHg. On USG, no free fluid seen in abdomen.

Diagnosis: Cardiac tamponade.

Clinchers

- *Stabled with 10 cm knife:* A long blade is invariably required to produce cardiac lacerations. A shorter knife may only result in open haemopneumothorax.
- *LUQ:* That is the anatomical site of the heart.
- *Stable for 20 min:* A small laceration to the heart will be asymptomatic till the leak fills up the pericardial cavity.
- *BP falls to 90/60 mmHg:* Cardiac tamponade is characterised by a rise in venous pressure and fall in arterial pressure. Overall BP falls due to blood loss and restricted heart function.
- *No free fluid in abdomen:* This rules out splenic rupture, which is also common cause of hypotension after LUQ injury.

CONFUSA

The main differential diagnosis in this case is from tension pneumothorax which can also result in cardiac tamponade. But in that case the patient will present with acute breathlessness and there will be a suckling wound. A haemopneumothorax (not necessarily tension) invariably will be present with such injuries.

Investigation of Choice

CXR (enlarged cardiac shadow)

Immediate Management

Crossmatch blood + careful fluid resuscitation.

Treatment of Choice

Pericardiotomy (urgent)

↓

evacuation of blood

↓

Suturing of cardiac laceration

Your notes:

74. Known asthmatic patient involved in road traffic accident (RTA). Has a right-sided chest pain. On auscultation, right side is hyper-resonant. Trachea is deviated to the left.

Diagnosis: Tension pneumothorax (right side).

Clinchers

- *Asthmatic patient:* In patients over 40 years of age, COPD most commonly predisposes to pneumothorax. Rarer causes include bronchial asthma, carcinoma, a lung abscess breaking down and leading to bronchopulmonary fistula and severe pulmonary fibrosis with cyst formation.
- *RTA:* A simple pneumothorax in a patient of trauma may develop into a tension pneumothorax—particularly when the patient receives IPPV.
- *Right sided chest pain:* This is pleuritic pain which is variably in intensity.
- *Hyper resonance on same side:* This rules out cardiac tamponade and confirms pneumothorax.
- *Trachea is deviated to left:* Signs of tension pneumothorax are:
  - Hypotension
  - Distended neck veins
  - Trachea deviated away from the side of pneumothorax
  - Severe respiratory distress.

CONFUSA

A CXR should not be performed if a tension pneumothorax is suspected as it will delay immediate necessary treatment. The clinical picture of tension pneumothorax may be mistaken for that of a cardiac tamponade. However, tension pneumothorax is more common and may be differentiated by the hyper-resonance over the affected side.

Investigation of Choice

CXR but only after needle thoracocentesis.

Immediate Management

Needle thoracocentesis urgently.

Treatment of Choice

Chest drain (always required in a traumatic pneumothorax irrespective of its size).

Your notes:

75. A 19-year-old girl has fallen off her horse. Neck is immobilised + 100% oxygen. Has left upper abdominal pain, is pale and tachycardiac.

Diagnosis: Splenic rupture (hypotensive shock).

Clinchers

- *19-year-old has fallen off her house:* Falls in a young person usually produce polytrauma and blunt injuries.
- *Neck is immobilized + 100% O_2:* This means that the airway and breathing in primary survey is taken care of. Now there is a need to assess the circulation (ABC approach).
- *Left upper abdominal pain:* This could be due to rib fracture or blunt impact over this area. Such a finding should make one strongly suspicious of splenic rupture.
- *Pale and tachycardiac:* This suggest that patient is in hypotensive shock (most probably due to massive blood loss into peritoneum after splenic rupture).

CONFUSA

In hypotensive shock after massive blood loss, give colloid (Haemacoel) fast IV until BP -, pulse ¯, urine flows (> 30 mL/h) and crossmatched blood arrives.

Investigation of Choice

USG/peritoneal lavage.

Immediate Management

Crossmatch blood and inform surgeons after starting IV fluids.

Treatment of Choice

Immediate laparotomy.

Your notes:

171. Female with bilateral varicose veins, lipodermatosclerosis. She is using compression stockings. Despite that increase in itching and eczema. BMI is 27.

Diagnosis: Bilaterally symptomatic varicose veins.

Clinchers

- *Females:* Females are most frequently affected than man. Inheritance is also a major factor. Women in whom neither parent has varicose veins have a 10 percent risk of developing varices, but when both parents are affected there is an 80 percent chance.
- *Bilateral varicose veins:* Bilaterality of the condition rules out any local cause or obstruction producing them in one limb.
- *Using compression stockings:* Graded compression stockings are indicated for minor varicosities and is the first line of management. They may also be indicated in:
  - Elderly
  - Pregnant
  - Unfit people for surgery.

  The stocking is elasticated and specially fitted to ensure that it delivers gradual compression along its length such that at the ankle the elastic compression of the leg is much higher than that at the thigh.
- *Increased itching and eczema:* A proportion of patients develops skin complications. These range from mild eczema to severe ulceration. Since the condition is occurring in this female, despite using graded compression stockings, it implies failure of first line of management and that the disease is progressive. Surgery is definitely indicated now as the patient is symptomatic and this eczema may lead to severe venous ulceration.
- BMI is 27: She is mildly overweight. Varicose veins usually benefit by losing weight in the initial stages (more difficult to improve now in this patient). Although, still help the patient in losing weight as it may be beneficial in preventing recurrence after treatment. Also a normal weight reduces risk of other disease.

CONFUSA

Sclerotherapy will not be used in this patient because it is mainly indicated for:

- Cosmetic reasons (acid not symptomatic)
- Small and moderate sized varices below the knee
- It may complicate the already existing eczema.

Investigation of Choice

Venography or Duplex scanning

Immediate Management

Loose weight

Treatment of Choice

- For cosmetic reasons—sclerotherapy
- For symptomatic condition—surgery (as is this case)

Note: Varicose vein surgery is one of the most commonly performed elective surgical procedures in UK.

Your notes:

172. 75-year-old ,underwent 2 operations for varicose veins, presents with painful legs, has history of heart failure. On examination bilateral gross varicose veins, lipodermatosclerosis, no ulcers.

Diagnosis: Complicated varicose veins.

Clinchers

- *75-year-old:* Incidence of varicose vein increases with age, as accumulation of environmental factors also contribute to its pathogenesis.
- *Underwent 2 operations for varicose veins:* This means the condition is recurrent and another operation will be useless.
- *History of heart failure:* A relative contraindication for surgery now.
- *Lipodermatosclerosis:* It is a late and serious complication in which palpable indication develops in the skin and subcutaneous tissues. This particularly affects the gaitre area of the leg, just above the malleoli, and may be precursor for leg ulceration. Contraction of the skin and subcutaneous tissues is seen and the ankle becomes narrower (*champagne bottle leg).*
- *No ulcers:* This rules out a relative contraindication for sclerotherapy. Hence it can be safely given.

CONFUSA

The basis of sclerotherapy is that a solution which destroys the endothelial lining of the veins is injected. In the UK the most widely employed drug is sodium tetradecyl (STD), which chemically is a soap. To be effective the sclerosant has to be given into an empty vein that is compressed immediately after the injection has been given to avoid the development of thrombosis with vein. Sclerotherapy is treatment of choice for recurrent varicose veins because:

- The vein sclerose to form a fibrous cord incapable of recanalisation and recurrence
- Remove the risk and damage produce by repeated operations
- Easily manageable as an OPD treatment.

Investigation of Choice

Venography/Duplex scanning

Immediate Management

Gradual compression stockings (not if ulcers are present)

Treatment of Choice

Graded compression stockings.

Indications for graded compression stockings:

- Minor varicosities (no skin manifestation and below the knee) no clinical features of DVT.
- Elderly
- Pregnant
- Unfit

Your notes:

173. Female with BMI 33, comes with complaints of varicose veins and eczema.

Diagnosis: Varicose veins due to obesity.

Clinchers

- *Female:* Varicose veins are twice as common in females as in males.
- *BMI 33:* She is grossly overweight. She should loose weight and aim for a BMI of 20-25. Obesity is a definitive risk factor. Other risk factors are:
  - Family history
  - Prolonged standing
  - Female sex
- *Bilateral:* Thus rules out any local pathology in one leg leading to this condition.
- *Eczema:* This is the first stage of development of complication. She may not require invasive treatment later on if she act now to lose weight.

CONFUSA

Pregnancy per se is not a risk factor. It only accentuates an existing condition and may bring to notice the insignificant varicosities. It is partly as a result of enlarged uterus or the iliac veins and partly due to relaxation of smooth muscle under the influence of hormones such as progesterone.

Investigation of Choice

Doppler USG/venography

Immediate Management

Counselling to loose weight

Treatment of Choice

Aim for BMI of 20-25 by loosing weight.

Your notes:

174. Man with varicose veins has to fly for 20 hours. His father has a history of pulmonary embolism after flying.

Diagnosis: High-risk case for pulmonary embolism.

Clinchers

- *Varicose veins:* Thrombosis is a common complication for varicose veins and is referred to as superficial thrombophlebitis. Usually this remain in the superficial veins and only cause considerable discomfort. Sometimes thrombosis extends into the deep venous system to cause deep vein thrombosis (DVT) although this in infrequent. DVT is the most common risk factor for pulmonary embolism (PE).
- *Fly for 20 hours:* Prolonged sitting as in a long flight increases the risk for DVT considerably in a predisposed.
- *Father has a history of PE after flying:* This increases the risk of family history is also positive.

CONFUSA

Since in this case three definite risk factors for PE are present, this person need to take precautions. He should be prescribed graded compression stocking for the period of immobility and should be given a proper advice on how to keep himself mobile during flight.

Investigation of Choice

Patients with a family history of thromboembolism should be investigated for thrombophilia.

Immediate Management

Counselling

Treatment of Choice

Graded compression stockings.

Note: Prophylactic anticoagulation is only indicated if the patient himself had any past history of PE or DVT.

Your notes:

175. A patient presents with a shallow ulcer, with no in rolled edges, situated over the medical malleolus. It has been reducing in size with compression bandaging. There is some evidence of lipodermatosclerosis and varicose veins in the distribution of the greater saphenous veins.

Diagnosis: Venous ulcer

Clinchers

- *Shallow ulcer:* Venous ulcers are always shallow and superficial.
- *No in rolled edges:* Rules out basal cell carcinoma which has rolled out edges.
- *Situation over the medical malleolus:* Venous ulcers are typically found in gaitre area of the leg, especially around the medial malleolus.
- *Reducing in size with compression bandaging:* It is due to improving deep venous competence due to compression bandaging. Note that compression bandaging is absolutely contraindication in arterial ulcers as it will worsen the condition. So preferably avoid them in all ulcers.
- *Lipodermatosclerosis:* It is a late complication of varicose veins and signify that the disease is longstanding.
- *Varicose veins in the distribution of greater saphenous vein:* This explains the anatomical location of ulcer over the medial malleolus.

CONFUSA

- *Venous ulcers*—painless, shallow, over medial malleolus (i.e. gaitre area of leg)
- *Arterial ulcers*—painless, deep and punched out, over dorsum of foot and toes.

Investigation of Choice

Venography or duplex scan

Immediate Management

Calculate BMI

Treatment of Choice

Sclerotherapy

(surgery is reversed for more symptomatic conditions).

Your notes:

177. An 80-year-old man has never been out of UK, one month history of epigastric pain, dark urine, pale stools, jaundice.

Diagnosis: Common bile duct obstruction (CBD obstruction).

Clinchers

- *An 80-year-old man:* The age point more towards malignancy than a stone as the cause of obstruction of CBD.
- *Never been out of UK:* Rules out infective causes like cholangitis or hepatitis.
- *One month history:* It signify that the symptomatology is chronic and rules out infective causes and acute cholecystitis.
- *Epigastric pain:* Gallbladder pathologies produce continuous picture of any obstructive jaundice. Dark urine is due to bilirubinuria and pale stools due to decreased bile pigments.

CONFUSA

A young person is more likely to have hepatitis, so questions should be asked about drug and alcohol se, and sexual behaviour. An elderly person with gross weight loss is more likely to have a carcinoma. All patients may complain of malaise. Abdominal pain occurs in patients with biliary obstruction by gallstones and sometimes with an enlarged liver there is pain resulting from distension of the capsule.

Investigation of Choice

ERCP

Immediate Management

Heme test of stools (if positive, suspect malignancy)

Treatment of Choice

Depends on diagnosis

- Stones—cholecystectomy
- Malignancy—surgery/palliation.

Your notes:

178. Female with fever, rigors, right upper quadrant pain, jaundice, USG is normal.

Diagnosis: Acute cholecystitis.

Clinchers

- *Female:* Female sex is a risk factor for cholesterol stones in gallbladder, which is the usual cause for acute cholecystitis. The disease can occur at any age.
- *Fever, rigors:* The patient is usually ill with a fever and shallow respirations.
- *Right upper quadrant (RUQ) pain:* The main symptoms are severe pain in the epigastrium and right hypochondrium. The pain is continuous, increasing in intensity over 24 hours. It can radiate to back and shoulder. It may be accompanied by nausea and vomiting. Right hypochondrium tenderness is present, being worse on inspiration (Murphy's sign). There is guarding and rebound tenderness.
- *Jaundice:* Mild jaundice occurs in 20% of cases owing to accompanying common duct stones or to surrounding oedema occluding the CBD.
- *USG is normal:* Although can accurately diagnose stones as small as 2 mm, it may be false negative in 2-4 percent of cases.

CONFUSA

A less severe case of acute pancreatitis simulates acute cholecystitis. The fever in acute cholecystitis is more marked than pancreatitis and is in range of 38-39° C with marked toxaemia and leucocytosis. Rigors are almost nerve seen in acute pancreatitis.

Investigation of Choice

Oral cholecystography (OCG)

OCG is a useful procedure for diagnosis of gallstones but has been diagnosis replaced by USG. However, OCG is still useful for

- Selection of patients for nonsurgical therapy of gallstone disease such as
  - Lithotripsy
  - Bile duct dissolution therapy
- When USG is inconclusive.

Immediate Management

Nil by mouth + analgesia

Treatment of Choice

Cefuroxime 1.5 g/8 h IV

In suitable candidates do cholecystectomy (laparoscopic if no question of GB perforation).

186. Condition that can cause necrosis, formation of fluid-filled spaces that can get infected.

Diagnosis: Acute pancreatitis.

Clinchers

- *Necrosis formation of fluid filled space that can get infected:* Acute pancreatitis is an unpredictable disease which if not treated early can become severe and fatal. Due to self-perpetuating pancreatic inflammation (and of other retroperitoneal tissues). Litres of extracellular fluid are trapped in the gut, peritoneum and retroperitoneum. There may be a rapid progress from a phase of mild oedema to one of necrotising pancreatitis. In fulminating cases the pancreas is replaced by black fluid. Death may be from shock, renal failure, sepsis, or respiratory failure, with contributory factors being protease-induced activation of complement, kinin, and the fibrinolytic and coagulation cascades.

CONFUSA

Acute pancreatitis may present as a hypovolaemic shock which may confuse a fresh SHO as there is no evident source of bleed or blood loss. Also the serum amylase levels should be more than 1000 IU/mL as many other disease processes may produce mild rise in it.

Investigation of Choice

Serum amylase (> 1000 IU/ml)

Immediate Management

Plasma expanders (Haemaccel) and 0.9% saline until vital signs are satisfactory and urine flow at > 30 mL/h.

Treatment of Choice

Laparotomy ± debridement on suspect abscess formation or pancreas necrosis.

Your notes:

188. Condition associated with epigastric pain radiating to the back, pale loose stools, associated with alcohol consumption.

Diagnosis: Chronic pancreatitis.

Clinchers

- *Epigastric pain radiating to the back:* In chronic pancreatitis the epigastric pain 'bores' through to the back. It is relieved by:
  - Sitting forward
  - Hot water bottles on epigastrium/back: look for *erythema abignes* dusky greyness here.
- *Pale loose stools:* These signify steatorrhoea a common finding in this condition. It is due to pancreatic insufficiency and also results in malabsorption (hence bloating) and weight loss.
- *Alcohol consumption:* Chronic alcohol intake is the most common cause of chronic pancreatitis. Although rarely it can be produced by:
  - Cystic fibrosis
  - Haemochromatosis
  - Pancreatic duct obstruction
    - Stones
    - Pancreatic cancer
  - Hyperparathyroidism
  - Familial.

CONFUSA

Serum amylase estimations performed during attacks of pain may be elevated, but in long-standing disease are often normal, there being insufficient pancreatic tissue remaining to cause a large rise. The differential diagnosis of chronic pancreatitis from a pancreatic carcinoma is usually possible only at laparotomy.

Investigation of Choice

USG (dilated biliary tree; stones)

Note: If USG is normal consider CT or ERCP

Immediate Management

Blood glucose (as chronic pancreatitis can produce diabetes)

Treatment of Choice

Stop alcohol

+

Analgesia

+

Low fat diet with pancreatic enzyme (pancreatin) by mouth

Pancreatico-jejunostomy/total pancreatectomy for refractive cases.

192. **Old lady with smooth neck swelling, bradycardia, spare coarse hair, macrocytic anemia.**

Diagnosis: Hashimoto's thyroiditis.

Clinchers

- *Old lady:* It usually occurs in women aged 60-70 years.
- *Smooth neck swelling:* The gland is usually uniformly enlarged and firm, although it may occasionally be a symmetrical and irregular.
- *Bradycardia:* It is due to hypothyroidism which may be a feature of Hashimoto's thyroiditis (although the patient is mostly euthyroid).
- *Sparse coarse hair:* The patients of hypothyroidism have a slow, deep voice and are usually overweight and apathetic, with a dry, coarse skin and thin hair, especially in the lateral third of the eyebrows.
- *Macrocytic anemia:* Hypothyroid patients often have normochromic macrocytic anemia.

CONFUSA

It is important to diagnose the condition correctly by demonstrating the presence of thyroid antibodies and if necessary, by biopsy, because thyroidectomy will precipitate severe hypothyroidism in these cases. Occasionally lymphoma occurs in such glands. Note that in

- Graves' disease—TSH autoantibody -
- Hashimoto's thyroiditis—thyroglobulin autoantibody increased

Investigation of Choice

Autoantibody titres (thyroglobulin)

Immediate Management

Exclude lymphoma in thyroid and other autoimmune diseases.

Treatment of Choice

T_4 replacement therapy upto 0.3 mg/day will shrink the gland and the symptoms of myxoedema should disappear.

Your notes:

PAPER 5

33. **A 30-year-old man is involved in a fight. He has a bruise on the cheek. He complains of an acute abdominal pain and is vomiting. He had a herniorraphy two weeks ago. He is conscious and fundoscopy has not been done.**

Diagnosis: Wound dehiscence

Clinchers

- *30-year-old is involved in a fight:* This necessiates the exclusion of occult head or abdominal injuries to rule out serious trauma.
- *Bruise on cheek:* Most probably this signifies no fatal head injury.
- *Acute abdominal pain:* It could be due to blunt abdominal trauma or wound dehiscence.
- *Herniorraphy two weeks ago:* This suggests that the wound of the operation, though sealed by now, is weak and prove to dehiscence.
- *Conscious:* Rules out head injury for the moment but continuous observation is required.

CONFUSA

Fundoscopy has not been done in this patient. It is usually done to rule out raised ICT which is represented by papilloedema. But since our suspicioun of head injury or haematoma formation is minimal and abdominal injury is high, this investigation can be postponed or even excluded in the order of priorities.

Investigation of Choice

USG.

Immediate Management

Take the patient to OT.

Treatment of Choice

Surgical repair.

Your notes:

41. Chest X-ray shows raised right diaphragm with small pleural effusion above.

Diagnosis: Subphrenic abscess.

Clinchers

➢ *Chest X-ray shows....:* In subphrenic abscess the chest X-ray may show the following:
- Elevation of the diaphragm on the affected side.
- Pleural effusion and/or collapse of the lung base.
- Gas and fluid level below the diaphragm.

CONFUSA

A localised collection of pus may occur in the subphrenic region following general peritonitis. Usually the underlying cause is a peritonitis involving the upper abdomen—leakage following biliary or gastric surgery or a perforated peptic ulcer. Rarely, infection occurs from haematogenous spread or from direct spread from a primary chest lesion, e.g. emphysema.

Investigation of Choice
- *Screening:* CXR (already done in this case)
- *Definitive:* CT scan.

Immediate Management

Find the cause (evident in this case).

Treatment of Choice

Broad spectrum antibiotics
↓
If fails
↓
Ultrasound/CT guided percutaneous drainage

Your notes:

42. Ultrasound scan shows intra-abdominal free fluid with paralytic ileus.

Diagnosis: Biliary peritonitis.

Clinchers

➢ *Intra-abdominal free fluid:* In advanced peritonitis the abdomen becomes distended and tympanitic, signs of free fluid are present, the patient becomes increasingly, toxic with a rapid, feeble pulse, vomiting is faeculent and the skin is moist, cold and cyanosed (the Hippocratic Facies).

➢ *Paralytic ileus:* Because of it the abdomen is silent in peritonitis or the transmitted sounds of the heart-beat and respiration may be detected.

CONFUSA

Bile peritonitis is only a rare accompaniment of acute cholecystitis, because unlike the appendix, which when inflamed rapidly undergoes gangrene, the inflamed gallbladder is usually thickened and walled off by adhesions. In addition, again unlike the appendix, which only receives an end-artery supply from the ileo-colic artery, the gallbladder has an additional blood supply from the liver bed, therefore, frank gangrene of the inflamed gallbladder is unusual.

Investigation of Choice

Erect CXR.

Immediate Management

IV morphine.

Treatment of Choice

Laparotomy (required to deal with the underlying cause, but the mortality is approximately 50%).

Your notes:

46. A 50-year-old woman underwent an anterior resection for carcinoma of the rectum one week ago. Has low grade fever and with complaint of pain in the calf + tenderness in the calf.

Diagnosis: Deep vein thrombosis.

Clinchers

- *50-year-old:* Incidence of this complication is particularly more in:
  - Elderly
  - Obese
  - Those with malignant disease
  - Who have varicose veins
  - History of previous DVT
  - Those undergoing
    - Abdominal surgery
    - Pelvic surgery
    - Hip surgery (most common)
  - Women on
    - OCP
    - HRT
  - Presence of predisposing factors
    - Reduced levels of endogenous anticoagulants
      - protein C
      - protein S
      - antithrombin III
    - Possession of the Leiden mutation of coagulation factor V.
- *Anterior resection for carcinoma of rectum:* Pelvic surgeries have the highest incidence of DVT postoperatively.
- *One week ago:* DVT typically occurs in the second postoperative week (see confusa also).
- *Low grade fever:* DVT is often associated with a mild pyrexia. The skin temperature of the affected calf is invariably raised (due to dilatation of the superficial veins of the leg and inflammatory reaction).
- *Complaint of pain in calf:* It is the major presenting feature and is usually associated with swelling and redness.
- *Tenderness in calf:* This confirm that pain is due to DVT only.

CONFUSA

DVT usually occurs during the second postoperative week. Earlier thrombosis particularly occurs when the patient has already been in hospital for some time preoperatively. Radioiodine studies have confirmed that the thrombotic process usually commence at, or soon after, the operation. The classical *Homan's sign* (- resistance to forced foot dorsiflexion, which may be painful) is positive in less than 20% cases and cannot be relied upon. On the contrary, it may dislodge thrombus giving rise to thromboembolism.

Investigation of Choice

Doppler USG/venogram.

Immediate Management

Enoxapain 1 mg/kg bd or 1.5 mg/kg/od.

Treatment of Choice

Heparin for 3 months.

Your notes:

47. A young woman underwent emergency appendicectomy 6 days ago for perforated appendix. She appeared to be making a good recovery but has developed intermittent pyrexia (up to 39°C). On examination—no obvious cause found, but she is tender anteriorly on rectal examination.

Diagnosis: Anterior pelvic abscess.

Clinchers

- *Appendicectomy:* A pelvic abscess may follow any general peritonitis, but it is particularly common after acute appendicitis (75%), or after gynaecological infections.
- *Perforated appendix:* This increases the chances of development of the abscess manifold as there is direct exposure of the septic load.
- *Good recovery:* Rules out any systemic involvement.
- *Intermittent pyrexia (upto 39°C):* This is the characteristic swinging pyrexia and points towards an abscess somewhere in body.
- *Tender anteriorly on rectal examination:* This suggests that the abscess in situated anteriorly between the uterus and posterior fornix of vagina.

CONFUSA

In the male the abscess lies between the bladder and the rectum, in the female between the uterus and posterior fornix of the vaginal anteriorly, and the rectum posteriorly (pouch of Douglas). An early pelvic cellulitis may respond rapidly to a short cause of chemotherapy, but there is the risk that the prolonged antibiotic treatment of an unresolved infection may produce a chronic inflammatory mass. It is safer therefore, where there is an established pelvic abscess, to withhold chemotherapy and await pointing into the vagina (as in this case) or rectum through which surgical drainage can be carried out.

Investigation of Choice

USG/CT scan.

Immediate Management

Chemotherapy (see confusa also).

Treatment of Choice

Drainage of abscess.

Your notes:

49. An elderly woman underwent emergency laparotomy for peritonitis. Fourth postoperative day she is noted to have serosanguinous discharge from the wound, but there is no erythema or tenderness around the wound.

Diagnosis: Impending burst abdomen.

Clinchers

- *Elderly women:* Incidence of wound dehiscence is more in elderly patients because of poor wound healing and weak abdominal muscles.
- *Peritonitis:* It implies a high septic load in the peritoneal cavity. It can have a significance in aetiology of burst abdomen indirectly by inducing wound infection (not likely in this case).
- *Fourth postoperative day:* The abdomen usually dehiscence on about the 10th day. But the warning signs may be visible much before.
- *Serosanguineous discharge from the wound:* This is the blood-tinged serous effusion (which is always present during the first week or two within the abdominal cavity after operation). It usually seeps through the breathing-down wound and serves as a warning of impending burst abdomen.
- *No erythema or tenderness around the wound:* This rules out wound infection and leaves us with only the above diagnosis.

CONFUSA

Sometimes, the deep layer of the abdominal incision gives way but the skin sutures hold; such cases result in a massive incisional hernia.

Investigation of Choice

Clinical diagnosis, no investigation required.

Immediate Management

Place a sterile dressing over the wound + call seniors.

Treatment of Choice

Reassessment of wound in OT.

Your notes:

96. A 35-year-old woman comes to the clinic for screening of her breasts.

Diagnosis: Normal

Clinchers

- *35-year-old:* The UK national health service offers 3 yearly single view of mammography to those between 55 and 64-years-old. (Other age groups above 30 years may be screened if they want, but are not sent for).
- *Screening:* Mammography uses negligible radiation and cancer pick-up rate is 5 per 1000 'healthy' woman screened. It is a good screening examination. The patient should also be taught monthly self-examination and advised to report if she finds and discrete lump.

CONFUSA

Mammogram is a soft tissue X-ray of the breast, which may reveal small carcinomas that typically show as an area of speckled calcification. It may also be helfpul in reassuring the patient that a lesion is benign. Mammograms may reveal malignancies that are impalpable, but may mislead in some malignant lesions and inter a benign nature and vice-versa. Biopsy is the safest policy in any doubtful case.

Investigation of Choice

Mammography.

Immediate Management

Teach local self examination.

Treatment of Choice

Depends on the investigation result.

Your notes:

97. A 45-year-old woman presents with a mass in the right upper quadrant of her right breast. A round smooth mass is found in the axilla.

Diagnosis: Breast mass (suspected malignancy)

Clinchers

- *45-year-old:* There is an increased incidence of breast cancer with age. Any age may be affected, but it is rare below the age of 30 years.
- *Mass in the right upper quadrant of her right breast:* This is the most common site of a breast malignancy.
- *Woman:* Females are 100 times more likely to have a breast carcinoma than men.
- *Round smooth mass in axilla:* The main lymphatic drainage of breast is through axillary nodes, so this could be a metastatic node. Lymph node metastases usually present as smooth, firm, painless, swelling.

CONFUSA

There is a high degree of clinical error (around 25%) in estimating whether a tumour is stage I or II—axillary lymph nodes may be involved, although they cannot be felt. Conversely axillary nodes that are palpable may prove free from tumour. However, it does not make much of a difference in management as both stages I and II lesions are usually submitted to curative surgery (III and IV—palliative surgery).

Investigation of Choice

FNAC.

Immediate Management

Examine contralateral axilla.

Treatment of Choice

Curative surgery if FNAC shows malignant cells.

Your notes:

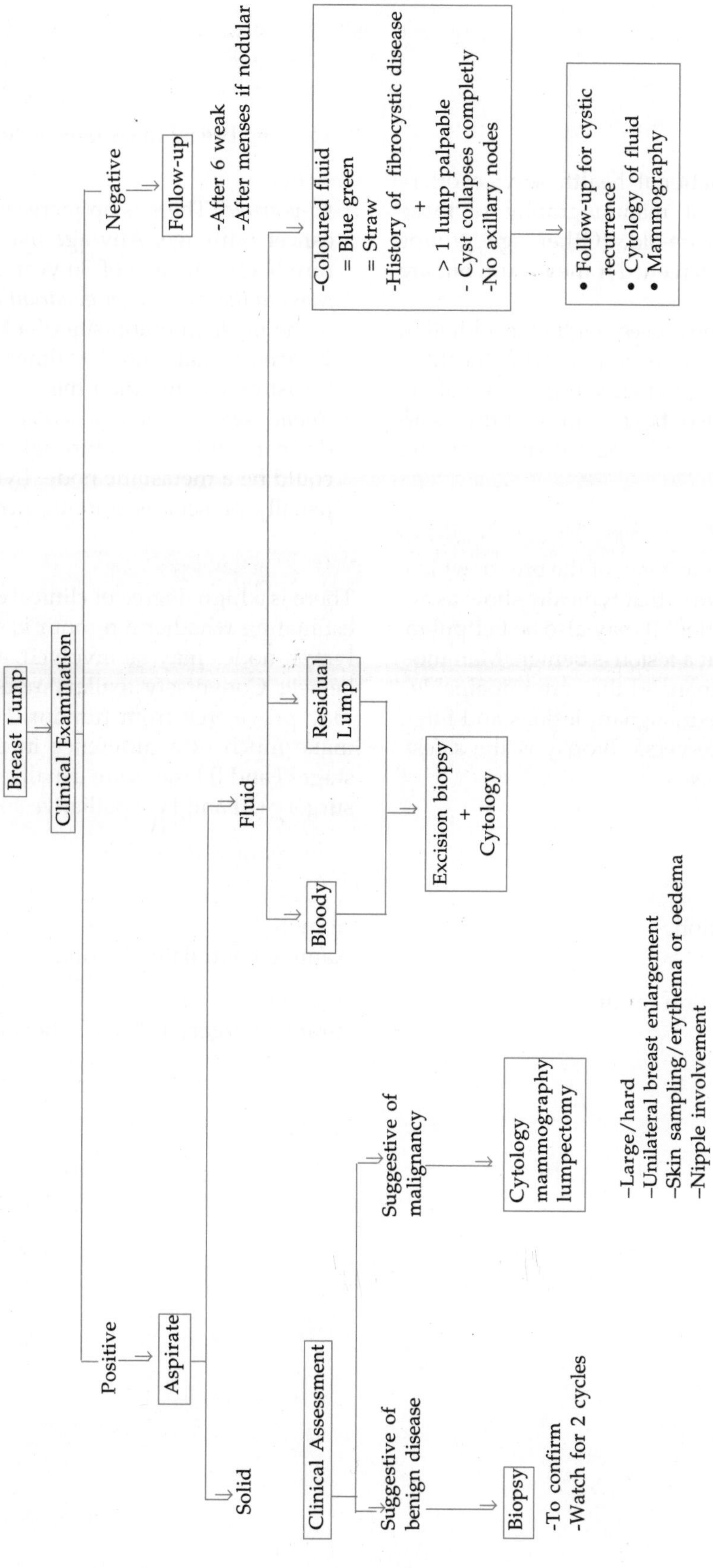
Breast Lump
Clinical Examination
Negative
Follow-up
-After 6 weak
-After menses if nodular
Positive
Aspirate
Fluid
-Coloured fluid
= Blue green
= Straw
-History of fibrocystic disease
+
> 1 lump palpable
- Cyst collapses completly
-No axillary nodes
• Follow-up for cystic recurrence
• Cytology of fluid
• Mammography
Residual Lump
Bloody
Excision biopsy
+
Cytology
Solid
Clinical Assessment
Suggestive of benign disease
Biopsy
-To confirm
-Watch for 2 cycles
Suggestive of malignancy
Cytology
mammography
lumpectomy
-Large/hard
-Unilateral breast enlargement
-Skin sampling/erythema or oedema
-Nipple involvement

98. A 36-year-old woman comes with a hard mass in her breast. The skin is tethered. Ultrasound and mammography were inconclusive. The patient wants to be satisfied that this is not malignant.

Diagnosis: Breast mass (probable malignancy)

Clinchers

- *36-year-old:* There is an increased incidence of breast cancer with age. Any age may be affected, but it is rare below the age of 30 years.
- *Hard mass:* Usually malignant tumours are hard in feeling on palpation.
- *Skin is tethered:* Involvement of skin and subcutaneous tissues leads to skin dimpling, retraction of the nipple and eventually ulceration.
- *USG and mammography where inconclusive:* These are preliminary noninvasive screening tests. If these are inconclusive and the condition is suggestive of malignancy, cytological diagnosis (through FNAC) is the only option left.
- *Patient wants to be satisfied:* This also necessiates FNAC as the patient is demanding the proof.

CONFUSA

Skin fixation is a strong supporting evidence of carcinoma, although it may be seen rarely over an area of fibroadenosis and may accompany fat necrosis or follow chronic abscess.

Investigation of Choice

FNAC.

Immediate Management

Respect the patient's wishes and proceed for FNAC

Treatment of Choice

Surgery according to cytological diagnosis and staging.

Your notes:

99. A 36-year-old woman presents with itching of her left nipple. On examination, no ulceration is seen, but a scaly lesion around the nipple is observed.

Diagnosis: Eczema/fungal infection

Clinchers

- *36-year-old:* It can occur in any age group after puberty as it is a primarily allergic disorder.
- *Itching of her left nipple:* It is invariably associated with any eczematous disease.
- *No ulceration:* It is usually absent. Its presence in eczema may signify the excerations due to scratching.
- *Scaly lesion around the nipple:* This confirms our diagnostic suspicion somewhat. But a fungal infection can also present in the same way.

CONFUSA

Eczema of nipple is rare and is usually bilateral. It is usually associated with eczema elsewhere on body whereas in case of fungal infection, the lesion might be solitary. Paget's disease always needs to be ruled out before dignosing eczema (Paget's disease also have an additional feature of discharge from surface). Psoriasis can also be a diagnosis but it is never so localized.

Investigation of Choice

KOH examination of smear.

Immediate Management

Reassurance

Treatment of Choice

As per the diagnosis.

Your notes:

100. A 23-year-old woman says she feels lumps in her breasts during the time of her periods. She also feels anxious and irritable.

Diagnosis: Fibrocystic breast disease (FCBD)

Clinchers

- *23-year-old:* FCBD are more common in the young females.
- *Feels lumps in her breasts:* This is a complaints that require a complete evaluation to rule out any disease (see confusa).
- *During the time of her periods:* This is characteristic of FCBD and is due to cyclical developmental changes in young women.
- *Anxious and irritate:* This could be secondary to FCBD or primarily due to the accompanying pre-menstrual syndrome (PMS).

CONFUSA

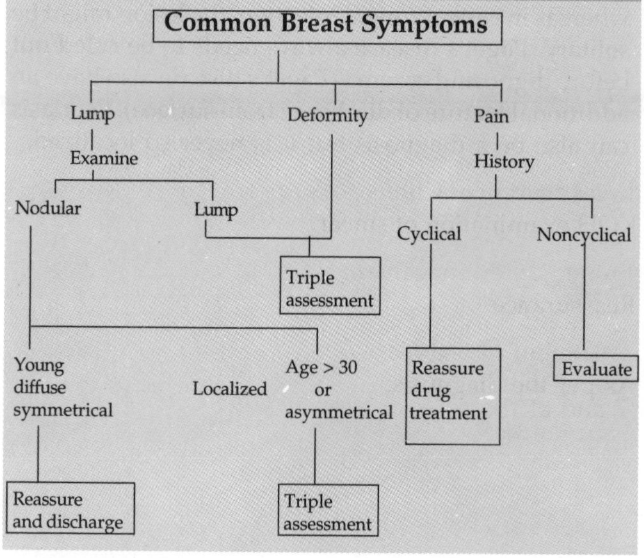

Investigation of Choice

Clinical examination

Immediate Management

Mammography (Mammography is a best screening procedure, and especially important over 35 years).

Treatment of Choice

None required. Dischage her after proper evaluation

129. Condition associated with epigastric pain radiating to the back, pale loose stools, associated with alcohol consumption.

Diagnosis: Chronic pancreatitis.

Clinchers

- *Epigastric pain radiating to the back:* In chronic pancreatitis the epigastric pain 'bores' through to the back. It is relieved by:
  - Sitting forward
  - Hot water bottles on epigastrium/back: look for *erythema ab ignes* dusky greyness here.
- *Pale loose stools:* These signify steatorrhoea a common finding in this condition. It is due to pancreatic insufficiency and also results in malabsorption (hence bloating) and weight loss.
- *Alcohol consumption:* Chronic alcohol intake is the most common cause of chronic pancreatitis. Although rarely it can be produced by:
  - Cystic fibrosis
  - Haemochromatosis
  - Pancreatic duct obstruction
    - Stones
    - Pancreatic cancer
  - Hyperparathyroidism
  - Familial.

CONFUSA

Serum amylase estimations performed during attacks of pain may be elevated, but in long-standing disease are often normal, there being insufficient pancreatic tissue remaining to cause a large rise. The differential diagnosis of chronic pancreatitis from a pancreatic carcinoma is usually possible only at laparotomy.

Investigation of Choice

USG (dilated biliary tree; stones)

Note: If USG is normal consider CT or ERCP.

Immediate Management

Blood glucose (as chronic pancreatitis can produce diabetes).

Treatment of Choice

Stop alcohol

+

Analgesia

+

Low fat diet with pancreatic enzyme (pancreatin) by mouth

Pancreatico-jejunostomy/total pancreatectomy for refractive cases.

130. Female with fever, rigors, right upper quadrant pain, jaundice, USG is normal.

Diagnosis: Acute cholecystitis.

Clinchers

➢ *Female:* Female sex is a risk factor for cholesterol stones in gallbladder, which is the usual cause for acute cholecystitis. The disease can occur at any age.

➢ *Fever, rigors:* The patient is usually ill with a fever and shallow respirations.

➢ *Right upper quadrant (RUQ) pain:* The main symptoms are severe pain in the epigastrium and right hypochondrium. The pain is continuous, increasing in intensity over 24 hours. It can radiate to back and shoulder. It may be accompanied by nausea and vomiting. Right hypochondrium tenderness is present, being worse on inspiration (Murphy's sign). There is guarding and rebound tenderness.

➢ *Jaundice:* Mild jaundice occurs in 20% of cases owing to accompanying common duct stones or to surrounding oedema occluding the CBD.

➢ *USG is normal:* Although can accurately diagnose stones as small as 2 mm, it may be false negative in 2-4 per cent of cases.

CONFUSA

A less severe case of acute pancreatitis simulates acute cholecystitis. The fever in acute cholecystitis is more marked than pancreatitis and is in range of 38-39° C with marked toxaemia and leucocytosis. Rigors are almost nerve seen in acute pancreatitis.

Investigation of Choice

Oral cholecystography (OCG)

OCG is a useful procedure for diagnosis of gallstones but has been diagnosis replaced by USG. However, OCG is still useful for

- Selection of patients for nonsurgical therapy of gallstone disease such as:
  - Lithotripsy
  - Bile duct dissolution therapy
- When USG is inconclusive.

Immediate Management

Nil by mouth + analgesia

Treatment of Choice

Cefuroxime 1.5 g/8 h IV

In suitable candidates do cholecystectomy (laparoscopic if no question of GB perforation).

165. A 25-year-old woman with a family history of deep vein thrombosis was prescribed a combined oral contraceptive pill six months ago and has not missed any tablets.

Diagnosis: Inherited clotting abnormality.

Clinchers

➢ The oral contraceptive pill is contraindicated in those with a tendency of deep vein thrombosis, as suggested in this case by a family history of DVT.

CONFUSA

Contraindications to the pill

— any disorder predisposing to venous or arterial problems
  - abnormal lipids
  - prothrombotic disorders
    —APC resistance

— Many cardiovascular problems

Except:
  - Mild non-pill related hypertension
  - Varicose veins

— Liver disease

— Migraine
  - Status migranosus
  - Requiring ergotamine

— Gross obesity

— Immobility

— Undiagnosed uterine bleeding.

Investigation of Choice

PT and aPTT

Immediate Management

Discontinue OCP.

Treatment of Choice

Prescribe alternative methods of contraception, i.e. condoms by male partner.

Your notes:

187. After a heavy bout of drinking a 56-year-old man vomits several times and develops chest pain. When you examine him, he has a crackling feeling under the skin around his neck.

Diagnosis: Pneumomediastinum after oesophageal rupture.

Clinchers

- *Heavy bout of drinking*: It is a risk factor for Boerhaare's syndrome (oesophageal rupture)
- *56-years-old*: Older age cames weakness of oesophageal musculature and hence increases the chances of rupture.
- *Vomits several times*: Recurrent vomiting, especially against a closed glottis (common after a heavy bout of drinking) can produce oesophageal rupture.
- *Chest pain*: Always suspect oesophageal perforation of chest pain follows vomiting.
- *Cracklin feeling*: This is subcutaneous emphysema which is characteristically present in suprasternal region after oesophageal rupture. It confirms our diagnosis.

CONFUSA

On more examination Hamman's sign can be found in this patient, i.e.

- Crunching/clicking noise synchronous with heart beat.
- Best heard in left lateral decubitus.

Drinking is also associated with Mallory Weiss syndrome (MWS). It can be differentiated from Boerhaave's syndrome as:

- MWS has gastric tear in 90% cases (Below squamocolumnar junction) and oesophageal tear in 10% cases
- MWS present with haemetemesis which is not mentioned here.
- Complete tear (perforation) is very rare in MWS
- MWS—forceful vomiting in a chronic alcoholic BS—Recurrent vomiting after bout of alcohol drinking

NOTE:

- Weakest portion of oesophagus is its lower third
- If it is only pneumomediastinum without oesophageal rupture, high flow oxygen (100%) can help in early resorption of air. No surgery is required then.

Investigation of Choice CXR

Immediate Management Crossmatch blood and inform surgeons.

Treatment of Choice Surgical repair (Though oesophageal rupture can also be managed in Boerhaave's syndrome because of high septic load).

PAPER 6

82. After a heavy bout of drinking a 56-year-old man vomits several times and develops chest pain. When you examine him, he has a crackling feeling under the skin around his neck.

Diagnosis: Pneumomediastinum after oesophageal rupture.

Clinchers

- *Heavy bout of drinking*: It is a risk factor for Boerhaave's syndrome (oesophageal rupture).
- *56-years-old*: Older age cames weakness of oesophageal musculature and hence increases the chances of rupture.
- *Vomits several times*: Recurrent vomiting, especially against a closed glottis (common after a heavy bout of drinking) can produce oesophageal rupture.
- *Chest pain*: Always suspect oesophageal perforation of chest pain follows vomiting.
- *Cracklin feeling*: This is subcutaneous emphysema which is characteristically present in suprasternal region after oesophageal rupture. It confirms our diagnosis.

CONFUSA

On more examination Hamman's sign can be found in this patient, i.e.

- Crunching/clicking noise synchronous with heart-beat.
- Best heard in left lateral decubitus.

Drinking is also associated with Mallory Weiss syndrome (MWS). It can be differentiated from Boerhaave's syndrome as:

- MWS has gastric tear in 90% cases (Below squamocolumnar junction) and oesophageal tear in 10% cases
- MWS present with haemetemesis which is not mentioned here.
- Complete tear (perforation) is very rare in MWS
- MWS—forceful vomiting in a chronic alcoholic BS—Recurrent vomiting after bout of alcohol drinking

NOTE:

- Weakest portion of oesophagus is its lower third
- If it is only pneumomediastinum without oesophageal rupture, high flow oxygen (100%) can help in early resorption of air. No surgery is required then.

Investigation of Choice CXR

Immediate Management Crossmatch blood and inform surgeons.

Treatment of Choice Surgical repair (Though oesophageal rupture can also be managed in Boerhaave's syndrome because of high septic load).

83. A 23-year-old woman on the oral contraceptive pill suddenly gets tightness in her chest and becomes very breathlessness.

Diagnosis: Pulmonary venous thromboembolism (PE).

Clinchers

- *23-year-old woman:* She belongs to the typical OCP user age group.
- *OCP*: They increase the risk of pulmonary embolism by producing a hypercoagulable state.
- *Sudden tightness and breathlessness*: Chest pain and shortness of breath are the two most usual symptoms in PE. The pain is most often pleuritic in nature; sharp and worse with deep inspiration and coughing. There may be haemoptysis.

CONFUSA

Sometimes collapse is the presenting symptom. A sudden urge to defaecate may herald the onset of symptoms. Signs are very variable and often absent. There may be tachycardia and tachypnoea. Areas of crepitus or a pleural rub are sometimes heard, as is a pulmonary flow murmur. Thrombosis of the deep veins is rarely clinically apparent.

Investigation of Choice

V/Q scan

Immediate Management

High flow O_2 + 10 mg IV morphine + anticoagulation.

Treatment of Choice

Heparin (loading dose of 5000-10000 units of standard heparin IV followed by a continuous infusion of 1000-2000 units per hour).

Your notes:

97. A 40-year-old male has a lump in the supero-posterior area of the anterior triangle.

Diagnosis: Parotid tumour.

Clinchers

- *40 years old:* Ninety per cent parotid tumours present before the age of 50 although any age may be affected.
- *Male:* Sex distribution is equal.
- *Lump in superoposterior area of anterior triangle:* In a > 40-year-old patient, a lump in this area is most likely to be a parotid tumour (498, OHCM, 5th edn). Although the swelling can be anywhere within the parotid gland, but usually in the lower pole and in the region of the angle of the jaw. The lump is well defined, usually firm or hard but sometimes cystic in consistency.

CONFUSA

The facial nerve is never involved in parotid tumours, except by frankly malignant tumours. Its integrity, however, should always be confirmed. Although slow growing, there tumours cannot be considered benign because of the lack of encapsulation, the occasional wide infiltration of the surrounding tissues and the tendency to recur.

Investigation of Choice

Biopsy

Immediate Management

Check the integrity of facial nerve.

Treatment of Choice

Superficial parotidectomy.

98. A 16-year-old female has a midline lump in the neck which moves on protrusion of the tongue and is below the hyoid bone.

Diagnosis: Thyroglossal cyst

Clinchers

- *16-year-old:* Thyroglossal cyst almost always presents before 20 years of age.
- *Female:* The sex ratio is nondiscriminatory.
- *Midline lump:* It is a fluctuant swelling in the midline of the neck.
- *Moves on protrusion of tongue:* It is diagnosed by its characteristic physical signs:
  - It moves upwards when the patient protrudes the tongue because of its attachment to the tract of the thyroid descent
  - It moves on swallowing because of its attachment to the larynx by the pretracheal fistula.
- *Below the hyoid bone:* This is its most common location.

CONFUSA

Thyroglossal cyst may be present in any part of the thyroglossal tract. The common situations, in order of frequency are:

1. Beneath the hyoid
2. In the region of thyroid cartilage
3. Above the hyoid bone

Such a cyst occupies the midline, except in the region of the thyroid cartilage, where the thyroglossal tract is pushed to one side, usually to the left.

Investigation of Choice

Entirely clinical diagnosis. USG may help.

Immediate Management

Rule out an infected cyst which indicates a delay in surgery.

Treatment of Choice

Excision (because infection is inevitable).

99. A 19-year-old male has a cystic mass under the anterior border of sternomastoid at the junction of upper 1/3 and middle 1/3 of the muscle. Aspiration revealed fluid containing cholesterol crystals.

Diagnosis: Branchial cyst (BC).

Clinchers

- *19-year-old:* BC usually presents in early adult life.
- *Male:* The sex ratio is nondiscriminatary.
- *Cystic mass:* BC forms a soft swelling like a "half-filled hot water bottle."
- *Under the anterior border of sternomastoid at the junction of upper 1/3 and middle 1/3 of the muscle:* This is the typical location of the branchial cyst and it bulges forward from beneath the anterior border of sternomastoid.
- *Fluid containing cholesterol crystals:* This confirms the diagnosis of BC as it always contains pus like material, which is in fact cholesterol crystals. These are demonstrated under the microscope.

CONFUSA

BC often presents following an upper respiratory tract infection. Occasionally the cyst may be infected. It signifies the persistence of remnants of the second branchial arch. A rare first branchial arch cyst may present just below the external auditory meatus at the angle of the jaw, with extension closely related to VII nerve.

Investigation of Choice

Aspiration and microscopy (already done in this case).

Immediate Management

Rule out cyst infection but is an indication for delay in surgery.

Treatment of Choice

Surgical excision.

100. An infant present with a transilluminant swelling in the lower third of neck.

Diagnosis: Cystic hygroma (CH).

Clinchers

- *Infant:* CH usually manifests itself in the neonate or in early infancy and occasionally may be present at birth and be so large as to obstruct labour.
- *Transilluminant swelling:* The characteristic that distinguishes CH from all other neck swellings is that it is brilliantly transilluminant.
- *Lower third of neck:* Swelling in CH usually occurs in the lower third of the neck and as it enlarges it passes upwards towards the ear. Often the posterior triangle of the neck is mainly involved.

CONFUSA

As a result intercommunication of its many compartments, the swelling of CH is soft and partially compressible. It visibly increases in size when the child coughs or cries. The cheek, axilla, groin and mediastinum are other, although less frequent, sites for a cystic hygroma.

Investigation of Choice
Transillumination test.

Immediate Management
Rule out infection of the cyst.

Treatment of Choice
Excision of all the cyst at an early stage.

Your notes:

101. Patient after escaping from fire in a building has singed nostrils.

Diagnosis: Inhalation injury.

Clinchers

- *After escaping from fire in a building:* Incapacity, which occurs quickly in domestic and industrial fires, is caused by a combination of:
  - Hypoxia
  - Carbon monoxide poisoning (caused by incomplete combustion)
  - Hydrogen cyanide poisoning

  Soft furnishing are a particular hazard, producing many topic substances, including highly irritant and lethal hydrogen chloride.
- *Signed nostrils:* Burns around the lips, mouth, throat or nose, including singeing of nasal hairs invariably points towards associated inhalation injury.

CONFUSA

Beware of conventional blood gas analyser readings in patients who may have high carboxy or methemoglobin levels. The oxygen electrode measures oxygen dissolved in plasma only and oxygen saturation is then calculated assuming all haemoglobin to be normal. PaO_2 and oxygen saturation may thus appear to be satisfactory despite very low total blood oxygen content.

Investigation of Choice
Carboxy haemoglobin (CoHb).

Immediate Management
High concentration O_2 + early intubation.

Treatment of Choice
Admit and observation for 24 hours (even if burns appear minimal).

102. Patient has a large tense blister.

Diagnosis: Dermal burns.

Clinchers

➢ *Large tense blister:* Small blisters can be left alone. Large ones can be slit open at the dependent edge to allow drainage. Alternatively they can be aspirated with a needle.

CONFUSA

Complete derooting of any blister is unnecessary and leaves a painful base. So avoid it. Blisters are absent in epidermal burns. Superficial dermal burns with blistering are usually dressed to absorb exudate, prevent desiccation, provide pain relief, encourage epithelialisation and prevent infection.

Investigation of Choice
None required.

Immediate Management
Drainage of blister/aspirate blister.

Treatment of Choice
Regular dressing.

103. An adult patient has partial thickness burns on the anterior chest and upper thighs

Diagnosis: Significant burns requiring admission

Clinchers

➢ *Partial thickness burns:* They can be managed by cleaning the wound and covering with a non adherent dressing such as paraffin gauze or with silver sulfadiazine (flamazine cream).

➢ *On anterior chest and upper thighs:* According to Lund and Browder chart anterior chest is 7½ and upper thigh = 4). So the total area is 7½ + 4) + 4 = 17%. A burn of more than 15% in adults (>10% in children) require IV fluids and hence an admission to the hospital and treatment in a burns unit.

CONFUSA

Infection can easily convert a partial thickness burn to a full thickness burn, so ensure proper prevention from infection. For IV fluid resuscitation, the priming fluid can be isotolic saline. Thereafter a colloid is used. The choice of colloid includes synthetic sugars, gelatin and starch, albumin, plasma protein fraction and reconstitute plasma. Whole blood will be required if there is a significant element of full thickness skin loss.

Investigation of Choice
Urine output.

Immediate Management
Admit and refer to burns unit after starting IV fluids and maintaining airway.

Treatment of Choice
- Regular dressing
- Grafting and contracture release after healing.

104. An adult patient has full thickness circumferential burns (from the elbow to the fingers, covering them completely.

Diagnosis: Circumferential full thickness burns over limb.

Clinchers

- *Circumferential full thickness burns:* These can contract and impair blood flow to the hand and forearm. Such contractions must be excised acutely to save the limb (escharotomy).
- *From elbow to fingers:* Face, hands and the joint flexures and priority areas for immediate skin grafting as scanning or contractures at these sites will obviously produce considerable deformity and disability.

CONFUSA

Eschar is a completely burnt and coagulated skin. Apart from limbs they can cause mechanical obstruction is present around the chest (by restricting chest movements they impair respiration). Moreover, they become a culture medium for bacteria such as *Streptococcus pyogenes* and *Pseudomonas aeruginosa.*

Investigation of Choice
Urine output.

Immediate Management
Escharotomy.

Treatment of Choice
Immediate excision and split skin grafting.

PAPER 7

12. A 1-year-old child presents with vomiting, crying and lifting her legs. Nappy is stained red. On examination sausage-shaped mass is palpated per abdominally.

Diagnosis: Intussusception.

Clinchers

- *1-year-old:* Patients may be of any age but usually of 5-12 months.
- *Presents with vomiting, crying and lifting her legs:* Patients usually present with episodic intermittent inconsolable crying with drawing the legs up (colic) ± vomiting.
- *Nappy is stained red:* The child must have passed blood per rectally as it is a feature of this condition. The bleed is like red-currant jam or merely flecks.
- *Sausage-shaped abdominal mass:* It is a characteristic finding in this condition.

CONFUSA

Children older than 4 years present differently with intussusception:

- Rectal bleeding is less common
- More likely to have a long history (> 3 weeks)
- More likely to have some contributing pathology, e.g. HSP, Peutz-Jeghers syndrome, cystic fibrosis, scariasis, nephrotic syndrome.

Investigation of Choice
USG.

Immediate Management
PR examination (always indicated when rectal bleeding is present intussusception).

Treatment of Choice
Reduction by air enema
If it fails, reduction at laparoscopy or laparotomy is needed.

Your Notes:

24. A 19-year-old girl has fallen off her horse. Neck is immobilised + 100% oxygen. Has left upper abdominal pain, is pale and tachycardiac.

Diagnosis: Splenic rupture (hypotensive shock).

Clinchers

- *19-year-old has fallen off her house:* Falls in a young person usually produce polytrauma and blunt injuries.
- *Neck is immobilized + 100% O_2:* This means that the airway and breathing in primary survey is taken care of. Now there is a need to assess the circulation (ABC approach).
- *Left upper abdominal pain:* This could be due to rib fracture or blunt impact over this area. Such a finding should make one strongly suspicious of splenic rupture.
- *Pale and tachycardiac:* This suggest that patient is in hypotensive shock (most probably due to massive blood loss into peritoneum after splenic rupture).

CONFUSA

In hypotensive shock after massive blood loss, give colloid (Hemaccel) fast IV until BP -, pulse ¯, urine flows (> 30 ml/h) and crossmatched blood arrives.

Investigation of Choice

USG/peritoneal lavage.

Immediate Management

Crossmatch blood and inform surgeons after starting IV fluids.

Treatment of Choice

Immediate laparotomy.

Your Notes:

30. After an abdominal operation, a patient presents with subfebrile state and abdominal distention. There is associated abdominal tenderness, constipation. On auscultation no bowel sounds are heard.

Diagnosis: Paralytic ileus.

Clinchers

- *Abdominal operation:* Paralytic ileus is most commonly seen in the postoperative stage of peritonitis or of major abdominal surgery.
- *Subfebrile state:* It is quite common after major surgeries.
- *Abdominal distension, associated abdominal tenderness, constipation:* There is abdominal distension, absolute constipation and effortless vomiting. Pain is not present, apart from the discomfort of the laparotomy wound and the abdominal distension.

CONFUSA

The distension that occurs on the first and second postoperative day is probably produced by swallowed air. The air passes through the small intestine (where peristalsis usually returns quickly) to the colon, which is atonic and produces a functional hold up.

Investigation of Choice

X-ray (usually not required).

Immediate Management

Pethidine (as it has little effect on bowel motility).

Treatment of Choice

Nasogastric suction (to remove swallowed air and prevent gaseous distension).

Your notes:

52. Patient on antacids for extensive epigastric pain presents with acute abdominal pain, rigidity and is pale.

Diagnosis: Perforated peptic ulcer.

Clinchers

- *Patient on antacids for extensive epigastric pain:* Points forwards peptic ulcer disease. Epigastric pain is a characteristic feature of peptic ulcer disease. Both gastric and duodenal ulcers are helped by antacids.
- *Acute abdominal pain, rigidity, pale:* Since it is a case of peptic ulcer, these signs point towards perforation of peptic ulcer. Duodenal ulcer perforate more commonly than gastric ulcers, usually into the peritoneal cavity. Look for acute abdomenal conditions (e.g. cholecystitis, pancreatitis, etc).

CONFUSA

Check serum amylase to rule out pancreatitis. Avoid laparotomy if pancreatitis is diagnosed. Look for other acute gastrointestinal condition (e.g. cholecystitis). Non GI conditions (e.g. myocardial infarction).

Investigation of Choice

- X-ray abdomen/USG
- Serum amylase
- ECG.

Immediate Management

Investigate. If perofation diagnosed—laparotomy.

Treatment of Choice

Immediate laparotomy.

Your notes:

53. Female patient with 24 hours history of severe abdominal pain and vomiting. She is restless and afebrile. She has a history of chronic alcoholism.

Diagnosis: Acute pancreatitis.

Clinchers

- *Female:* Women are more affected than men. The patient is often obese and middle aged or elderly.
- *24 hours history of severe abdominal pain:* The pain is severe, constant usually epigastric and often radiates into the back.
- *Vomiting:* Vomiting is early, profuse and prominent sign. The patient often sits forward, and repeated setching is common.
- *Restless:* It is due to the severe pain which is relieved in certain positions, e.g. sitting forward.
- *Afebrile:* The temperature may either be subnormal or riased upto 39.5° C (103°F).
- *Chronic alcoholism:* The majority of non-gallstone pancreatitis is alcohol related. This is particularly common in France and North America. Alcohol is also the most common cause of recurrent pancreatitis. The mechanism is unlcear, and it may follow either chronic alcohol abuse or finge drinking.

CONFUSA

Causes of acute pancreatitis: mnemonic *"GET SMASHED"*.

G —Gallstones
E —Ethanol
T —Trauma
S —Steroids
M —Mumps
A —Autoimmune (PAN)
S —Scorpion venom
H —Hyperlipidemia
Hypercalcaemia
Hypothermia
E —ERCP
Emboli
D —Drugs = azathioprine
= asparaginase
= mercaptopurine
= pentamidine
= didanosine

Investigation of Choice

Serum amylase > 1000 μ/ml.

Immediate Management Nil by mouth.

Treatment of Choice Symptomatic

55. A 50-year-old chronic alcoholic presents with a sudden onset difuse abdominal pain. It is radiating to the back. He has generalised abdominal tenderness with vomiting and rigidity.

Diagnosis: Acute pancreatitis.

Clinchers

Note: See Q 53 of this theme also

- *50-year-old:* The patient is often obese and middle-aged or elderly.
- *Sudden onset:* The pain may be gradual or sudden onset but is severe and constant.
- *Diffuse abdominal pain:* The pain may be epigastric or central or diffuse.
- *Radiates to back:* It radiates to back characteristically.
- *Generalised abdominal tenderness with vomiting and rigidity:* On examination the abdomen reveals generalised tenderness and guarding.

CONFUSA

The symptoms of acute pancreatitis may be mild in severe disease. There may be periumbilical discoloration (Cullen's sign) or flank bruising (Grey turner's sign) later on. About 30% of cases have a tinge of jaundice due to oedema of the pancreatic head obstructing the common bile duct.

Investigation of Choice

Serum amylase > 1000 μ/ml.

Immediate Management

Nil by mouth.

Treatment of Choice

Symptomatic.

Your notes:

71. Patient after escaping from fire in a building has singed nostrils.

Diagnosis: Inhalation injury.

Clinchers

- *After escaping from fire in a building:* Incapacity, which occurs quickly in domestic and industrial fires, is caused by a combination of:
  - Hypoxia
  - Carbon monoxide poisoning (caused by incomplete combustion)
  - Hydrogen cyanide poisoning

  Soft furnishing are a particular hazard, producing many topic substances, including highly irritant and lethal hydrogen chloride.
- *Signed nostrils:* Burns around the lips, mouth, throat or nose, including singeing of nasal hairs invariably points towards associated inhalation injury.

CONFUSA

Beware of conventional blood gas analyser readings in patients who may have high carboxy or methemoglobin levels. The oxygen electrode measures oxygen dissolved in plasma only and oxygen saturation is then calculated assuming all haemoglobin to be normal. PaO_2 and oxygen saturation may thus appear to be satisfactory despite very low total blood oxygen content.

Investigation of Choice

Carboxy haemoglobin (CoHb).

Immediate Management

High concentration O_2 + early intubation.

Treatment of Choice

Admit and observation for 24 hours (even if burns appear minimal).

Your notes:

73. An adult patient has partial thickness burns on the anterior chest and upper thighs.

Diagnosis: Significant burns requiring admission

Clinchers

- *Partial thickness burns:* They can be managed by clearning the wound and covering with a non adherent dressing such as paraffin gauze or with sliver sulfadiazine (flamazine cream).
- *On anterior chest and upper thighs:* According to Lund and Browder chart anterior chest is 7½ and upper thigh = 4). So the total area is 7½ + 4) + 4 = 17%. A burn of more than 15% in adults (>10% in children) require IV fluids and hence an admission to the hospital and treatment in a burns unit.

CONFUSA

Infection can easily convert a partial thickness burn to a full thickness burn, so ensure proper prevention from infection. For IV fluid resuscitation, the priming fluid can be isotolic saline. Thereafter a colloid is used. The choice of colloid includes synthetic sugars, gelatin and starch, albumin, plasma protein fraction and reconstitute plasma. Whole blood will be required if there is a significant element of full thickness skin loss.

Investigation of Choice

Urine output.

Immediate Management

Admit and refer to burns unit after starting IV fluids and maintaining airway.

Treatment of Choice

- Regular dressing
- Grafting and contracture release after healing.

Your notes:

74. An adult patient has full thickness circumferential burns (from the elbow to the fingers, covering them completely.

Diagnosis: Circumferential full thickness burns over limb.

Clinchers

- *Circumferential full thickness burns:* These can contract and impair blood flow to the hand and forearm. Such contractions must be excised acutely to save the limb (escharotomy).
- *From elbow to fingers:* Face, hands and the joint flexures and priority areas for immediate skin grafting as scanning or contractures at these sites will obviously produce considerable deformity and disability.

CONFUSA

Eschar is a completely burnt and coagulated skin. Apart from limbs they can cause mechanical obstruction is present around the chest (by restricting chest movements they impair respiration). Moreover, they become a culture medium for bacteria such as *Streptococcus pyogenes* and *Pseudomonas aeruginosa.*

Investigation of Choice

Urine output.

Immediate Management

Escharotomy.

Treatment of Choice

Immediate excision and split skin grafting.

Your notes:

24 Toxicology

PAPER 1

Serial No. 25

Subject: Medicine

Topic: Toxicology

Question: A child living with his grandmother presents with nausea, vomiting and features of heart block.

Diagnosis: Digoxin Toxicity

Clinchers

- *Child:* poisoning and overdosages of drugs is fairly common in growing children who get attracted to unattended medicaments and ingest them out of curiosity.
- *Living with grandmother:* This especially stresses the fact that the activities of child can easily be ignored. Also, living with elderly means access to various medications.
- *Nausea, vomiting and features of heart block:* These features of gastrointestinal symptoms associated with heart block is typical of digoxin toxicity. Associated features can also be yellow vision and various arrhythmias.

CONFUSA

- Tricyclic Antidepressants can also produce arrhythmias, however they are usually also associated with cholinergic symptoms like dilated pupils, dry mouth and urinary retention.
- In case of features of digoxin toxicity in an adult, always rule out hypokalemia.

Investigation of Choice
Blood electrolytes

Immediate Management
See Flow chart 24.1: Management of digoxin toxicity

Treatment of Choice
Digoxin neutralizing antibodies

Your notes:

Flow chart 24.1: Management of digoxin toxicity

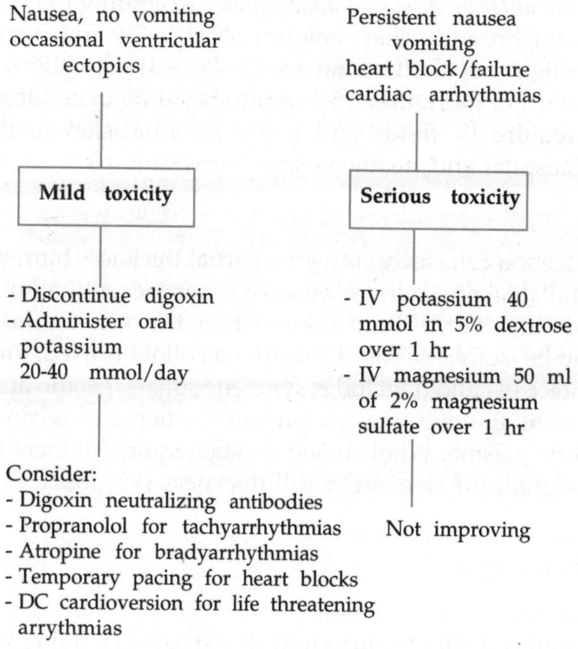

Serial No. 26

Subject: Medicine

Topic: Toxicology

Question: A farmer presents with excessive sweating, abdominal pain and small pupils and bradycardia.

Diagnosis: Organophosphorus poisoning

Clinchers

- *Farmer:* Organophosphorus poisoning is more common among the farmers because of the commonly used pesticides which contain organophosphates as common constituents.
- *Excessive sweating:* This is due to excessive stimulation of glands due to accumulation of acetylcholine. Also there is excessive sweating. Both by stimulating muscarinic receptors.
- *Abdominal pain:* Excessive stimulation of gastro-intestinal muscarinic receptors causes Increased salivation, nausea and vomiting, abdominal pain, diarrhoea, and foecal incontinence.
- *Small pupils:* Due to miosis induced by acetylcholine.
- *Bradycardia:* Due to stimulation of postganglionic receptors on heart, bradycardia and hypotension are important features.

CONFUSA

- As there are no clinical features specific to organophosphorus poisoning, diagnosis requires a high index of suspicion. The combination of a history of exposure (especially occupational exposure, as farmer, here) and the typical clinical features, are typical clues for diagnosis.
- However, remember that history of exposure may be denied by patients who have attempted suicide, or unavailable in unconscious patients.
- Helpful signs of poisoning include the pungent garlic- like odour of organophosphorus in breath and vomitus, miosis, bradycardia and muscle fasciculations. Excessive salivation, excessive respiratory tract secretions and lacrimation are other helpful signs.
- It should be remembered that some patients may present with the nicotinic effects of tachycardia, hypertension and mydiasis (rather than the anticipated bradycardia and hypotension).

Investigation of Choice

Diagnosis is mainly clinical.

Lab diagnosis is done by measurement of cholinesterase activity.

Immediate Management

- Secure airway; may require intubation in severe respiratory distress.
- Remove soiled clothes
- Wash skin
- Avoid contaminating yourselves (wear gloves before you start on anything).

Treatment of Choice

- Atropine IV 2 mg every 10 minutes till full atropinization is achieved.
- Pralidoxime 30 mg/kg slowly IV
- Even if fits not occurring diazepam 5-10 mg IV seems to control the CNS effects of poisoning (viz anxiety, restlessness, confusion).

Your notes:

Serial No. 27

Subject: Medicine

Topic: Toxicology

Question: A man comes to accident and emergency with complains of sore mouth. He is also having pulmonary edema, raised creatinine and oliguria.

Diagnosis: Paraquat Poisoning

Clinchers

- *Sore mouth:* Ingestion of paraquat causes painful oral blisters and soreness of skin.
- *Pulmonary edema:* The main pathology is alveolitis, induced by paraquat which is reversible in small doses. In larger doses, this can progress to pulmonary fibrosis and later long-term respiratory impairment.
- *Raised creatinine and oliguria:* These signify renal toxicity of the offending agent, usually characterised by proteinuria, raised urea and creatinine and oliguria.

CONFUSA

- The risk is largely dependent on route of exposure as well as dose. Ingestion being producing maximum damage.
- The target organs are: lungs, kidneys, liver and myocardium.
- "Redox Cycling" is the primary reaction responsible for the toxicity of paraquat. Paraquat is thought to cause cell death by lipid peroxidation or NADPH depletion, as in the lung where there is selective accumulation.
- The final outcome depends on the lung lesion which is dose related.

Investigation of Choice

The diagnosis of paraquat in vomit or urine may be performed with sodium dithionate as follows:

- Add alkali — sodium hydroxide or sodium bicarbonate — to 10 ml urine or gastric aspirate— until pH above 9
- Add sodium dithionate and shake gently
- Blue or green colour is positive for paraquat

Immediate Management

- Remove contaminated clothing. Wash thoroughly with soap and water.
- Immediate copious irrigation of eyes (in case, exposure suspected), followed by prophylactic topical antibiotics. Topical steroids to aid resolution of granulation tissue.
- Perform gastric lavage
- Instill into stomach Fuller's Earth 30% suspension down the lavage tube with 5% magnesium sulphate as a purgative; alternatively, activated charcoal can be used.
- Repeat Fuller's earth and magnesium sulphate four hourly until faecal samples are negative to testing with alkaline Na dithionate

Treatment of Choice

- Haemoperfusion and haemodialysis may help to lower paraquat levels but neither appears to affect prognosis.
- The prevention of pulmonary complications using cyclophosphamide and dexamethasone has been advocated, but the effectiveness of this regime has not as yet been proven.

Your notes:

Serial No. 28

Subject: Medicine

Topic: Toxicology

Question: A 13-year-old girl with hyperventilation and acidosis.

Diagnosis: Salicyalte Poisoning

Clinchers

- *13-year-old girl:* Patient age is one important factor in salicylate poisoning. Over the age of 12 years, there is a characteristic sequence of respiratory alkalosis caused by an initial direct stimulation of the respiratory centre followed by metabolic acidosis. In children, metabolic acidosis develops more rapidly, but below the age of 4 years, preceding respiratory alkalosis is rare.
- *Hyperventilation:* Salicylates causes both direct and indirest stimulation of respiratory centres leading to both increase in rate as well as depth of breaths. This ultimately leads to respiratory alkalosis.
- *Acidosis:* Salicylates also interfere with the Krebs cycle, limit production of ATP, and increase lactate production, leading to ketosis and a wide anion-gap metabolic acidosis.

CONFUSA

Salicylate poisoning can produce varied confusing pictures:

- Phase 1 of the toxicity is characterized by hyperventilation leading to respiratory alkalosis and compensatory alkaluria. Both potassium and sodium bicarbonate are excreted in the urine. This phase may last as long as 12 hours.
- In phase 2, paradoxic aciduria in the presence of continued respiratory alkalosis occurs when sufficient potassium has been lost from the kidneys. This phase may begin within hours and may last 12-24 hours.
- Phase 3 includes dehydration, hypokalemia, and progressive metabolic acidosis. This phase may begin 4-6 hours after ingestion in a young infant or 24 hours or more after ingestion in an adolescent.
- Tinnitus is another important characteristic of salicylate toxicity.
- Hyperthermia is an indication of severe toxicity.

Investigation of Choice

- Plasma salicylate level - take sample at 6 hours or earlier if indicated; repeat at 4 hourly intervals to ensure that level is not rising due to slow absorption.
- Blood gases - initially, respiratory alkalosis, followed by metabolic acidosis (different in children)
- Chest X-ray - pulmonary oedema, ARDS
- Full blood count
- Prothrombin time - may be increased
- Urea and electrolytes - possible hypokalaemia
- Blood glucose - possible hypoglycaemia

Immediate Management

- Gastric lavage with suitable airway protection (within 24 hrs of intake).
- Activated charcoal
- Ensure adequate fluids/electrolytes with special attention to hypokalemia, hypoglycemia and hypoprothrombinemia.
- Monitor urine output with urinary catheter

Treatment of Choice

- Mild poisoning — ensure adequate fluid and electrolyte replacement
- Moderate poisoning - Forced alkaline diuresis. This is at levels of salycilate of 500 mg per litre and over.
- Severe poisoning (levels more than of 750 mg/L) - consider for haemodialysis or haemoperfusion.

Your notes:

Serial No. 29

Subject: Medicine

Topic: Toxicology

Question: A 15-year-old girl presents with right upper quadrant pain and raised liver enzymes.

Diagnosis: Paracetamol Poisoning

Clinchers

- *15-year-old girl:* Paracetamol is the most commonly abused drug because of its easy availability; Drug abuse and suicidal tendency being more common among adolescents.
- *Right upper quadrant pain:* Right upper quadrant pain and tender hepatomegaly are signify hepatic toxicity due to paracetamol.
- *Raised liver enzymes:* Aspartate aminotransferase (AST) and alanine aminotransferase (ALT) begin to rise within 24 hours postingestion and peak at about 72 hours. Toxicity is defined as serum AST or ALT levels greater than 1000 IU/L.

CONFUSA

- Toxicity is increased in patients with induction of the P450 system, through drugs such as rifampicin, phenobarbital, isoniazid, phenytoin, carbamazepine and alcohol, or patients with low glutathione reserves as a product of genetic variation, HIV+ve, malnutrition, and alcohol-related or other liver disease.
- Pediatric patients under the age of five years seem to fare better after paracetamol poisoning, perhaps due to a greater capacity to conjugate with sulfate, enhanced detoxification of NAPQI or greater glutathione stores. However, the treatment principles remain the same as adults.

Investigation of Choice

- Emergency blood paracetamol level should be taken, at least 4 hours after ingestion.(The level reaches a peak at 4 hours and measurements before this are of little benefit.)
- Check for prothrombin time:
  - a prothrombin time > 45 sec indicates severe liver damage
  - a prothrombin time > 25 sec after 46 hr is prognostically ominous.
- Salicylate level is usually measured together with paracetamol (most intentional ingestions are mixed medications)
- Urea and electrolytes, creatinine
- Liver function tests
- Glucose (hourly)
- INR (12 hourly)

Immediate Management

- Perform gastric lavage if >12 g ingested within 1 hr.
- Give activated charcoal if <8 hr since ingestion

Treatment of Choice

- N acetylcysteine (NAC) remains the antidote of choice.
  Check 4 hr plasma levels; if level above the normal treatment line on graph administer NAC IV infusion (150 mg/kg in 200 ml of 5% dextrose over 15 min).
- In case of late presentations (>8 hrs) and suspected high dose, don't wait for plasma levels, start NAC immediately. NAC can be stopped if INR and ALT are normal.
- An alternative to NAC is methionine.

Your notes:

Serial No. 30

Subject: Medicine

Topic: Toxicology

Question: A 25-year-old male presents in coma metabolic acidosis, dilated pupil, elevated serum amylase and hypoglycemia.

Diagnosis: Ethanol toxicity

Clinchers

- *25-year-old male:* Ethanol remains the most commonly abused substance among children, adolescents or adults.
- *Coma:* Alcohol is major CNS depressant and coma can be due to this direct depressant action. However, in all such cases of a possibility of head injury should always be kept in mind.
- *Metabolic acidosis:* Acidosis is due to hepatic metabolism of alcohol and release of large amounts of acetaldehyde and acetic acid. However, presence of a large anion gap or severe acidosis should suggest the ingestion of another substance, such as methanol or ethylene glycol.
- *Dilated pupil:* Rule out head injury, so commonly associated with and ignored in alcohol intoxication.
- *Elevated serum amylase:* The finding of hyperamylasemia in acutely intoxicated patients is common. This is most frequently due to a rise in the salivary (nonpancreatic) isoamylase.
- *Hypoglycemia:* Hypoglycemia is a common association of alcohol intoxication and occurs secondary to ethanol's inhibition of gluconeogenesis and more pronounced in those with poor glycogen reserves.

CONFUSA

Methanol intake can also present similar features of acidosis, coma and hyperamylasemia. However, early visual disturbances are the classic findings that are associated with methanol intoxication and include decreased vision or blurred vision. Patients may complain of a 'snowstorm' in front of the eyes or photophobia. The pupils may be fixed and dilated with the funduscopic exam revealing retinal oedema with hyperemia of the optic disc.

Investigation of Choice

Toxicology screen
Blood ethanol levels
Blood glucose levels
Serum electrolytes
CT scan to rule out head injury
Blood gases if the patient is in coma

Immediate Management

Maintain airway
Access intravenous line, correct dehydration
correct hypoglycemia

Treatment of Choice

Supportive
Intravenous naloxone has reversed coma in a proportion of cases.

Your notes:

Serial No. 36

Subject: Medicine

Topic: Epilepsy

Question: An epileptic patient on treatment develops nausea vomiting with oliguria and raised levels of urea and creatinine.

Diagnosis: Carbamazepine side effect

Clinchers

- *Epileptic on treatment:* Carbamazepine is an anticonvulsant and analgesic drug that is used in the treatment of pain associated with trigeminal neuralgia and in epilepsy, especially in partial seizures, particularly of the temporal lobe type, and in major tonic-clonic epilepsy.
- *Nausea and vomiting:* Carbamazepine is associated with acute renal failure. Nausea, vomiting and anorexia being non-specific signs of uremia, occurs due to nitrogenous substances irritating chemoreceptor trigger zone (CTZ).
- *Oliguria:* Acute renal failure should be immediately suspected on any patient on carbamazepine, developing oliguria or anuria.
- *Raised levels of urea and creatinine:* Confirms the diagnosis of acute renal failure.

CONFUSA

- Diagnosis of acute renal failure due to carbamazepine should always be supported by laboratory evidence as the anuria can also be due to anticholinergic side effect of carbamazepine.
- In a patient on antiepileptics developing renal dysfunction, hepatic impairment, agranulocytosis or water intoxication/hyponatremia, think of the possibility of carbamazepine toxicity.

Investigation of Choice

BUN and other renal function tests.
Serum levels of carbamazepine.

Immediate Management

Supportive

Treatment of Choice

Withdraw drug under coverage of another antiepileptic and diazepam.

Your notes:

Serial No. 37

Subject: Medicine

Topic: Epilepsy

Question: A boy on treatment for generalized tonic-clonic epilepsy, develops features of hepatic failure in few weeks of starting treatment.

Diagnosis: Valproate-induced liver failure

Clinchers

- *Boy on treatment for generalized tonic-clonic epilepsy:* Valproate is the first drug of choice, according to NICE guidelines, in patients who have tonic-clonic seizures as part of idiopathic generalised epilepsy.
- *Features of hepatic failure:* Liver dysfunction (including fatal hepatic failure) has occurred in association with valproate, especially in children under 3 years of age.
- *Within few weeks of starting treatment:* Valproate induced liver dysfunction is usually seen in the first 6 months of therapy.

CONFUSA

- Raised liver enzymes are not uncommon during valproate treatment and are usually transient. Patients should be reassessed clinically and liver function (including prothrombin time) monitored until return to normal.
- An abnormally prolonged prothrombin time (particularly in association with other relevant abnormalities) requires discontinuation of treatment.
- Any concomitant use of salicylates should be stopped.

Investigation of Choice

Liver Function Tests - Prothrombin Time

Immediate Management

Regularly monitor liver functions till it returns to normal.

In case of deterioration or abnormally prolongation of prothrombin time, discontinue valproate under coverage of 2nd line anti-convulsants.

Treatment of Choice

Discontinue valproate under coverage of 2nd line anticonvulsants.

Your notes:

PAPER 4

31. A 10-year-old girl, unconscious, brought to A and E. She is found to be dehydrated on examination and respiratory rate is 40/min.

Diagnosis: Salicylate poisoning

Clinchers

- *A 10-year-old girl:* Children can accidentally consume household drugs, often in large amounts. Salicylates are a common drug to be taken in this way as they are easily available in almost every household.
- *Unconscious:* In severe poisoning, convulsions and coma may occur.
- *Dehydrated:* It is a marked and potentially fatal symptom of salicylates poisoning. It also differentiates it from paracetamol poisoning.
- *Respiratory rate is 40/min:* Hyperventilation is due to direct stimulation of the central respiratory centres and produce respiratory alkalosis initially in salicylate poisoning. It also differentiates the clinical condition from that of paracetamol poisoning.

CONFUSA

In salicylate poisoning, initial stimulation of the respiratory centre causes a respiratory alkalosis. As more of the drug is absorbed a metabolic acidosis supervenes. In between the two phases there may be a transitory period with a relatively normal blood gas picture.

Investigation of Choice

Blood glucose immediately (plasma salicylates concentration measured usually 4 hours after ingestion).

Immediate Management

Toxicology screen + Correct dehydration

Treatment of Choice

Gastric lavage—if present with 1 hr
+ Activated charcoal
+ Intensive monitoring
+ Dialysis if plasma level > 700 mg/L
or forced alkaline diuresis if > 300 mg/L (500 mg/L for adults).

Your notes:

PAPER 5

73. A man was found in his car with a hose directed from the exhaust. What would you give?

Diagnosis: Carbon monoxide poisoning
I would give: 100% O_2

Clinchers

In CO poisoning despite hypoxaemia skin is pink (or pale), not blue as carboxyhemoglobin (COHb) displaces O_2 from Hb binding sites. These are tachycardia, tachypnoea. If COHb >50%, fits, coma and cardiac arrest.

Investigation of Choice

Confirm diagnosis with heparinized blood sample (CO Hb > 10%) quickly (as levels become normal quickly)

Immediate Management

Remove the source
Give 100% O_2
Treatment of choice
In severe cases, anticipate cerebral oedema. Give mannitol IV

- Monitor ECG
- Hyperbaric O_2
- Discuss with poisons service.

Your notes:

75. This interferes with metabolism at the mitochondrial level.

Diagnosis: Cyanide poisoning

Clinchers

Cyanide blocks electron transport, resulting in decreased oxidative metabolism and oxidative utilization, decreased ATP production and lactic acidosis.

Lethal dose

- Sodium cyanide 200-300 mg
- Hydrocyanic acid 500 mg

Early effects: Headache, vertigo, excitement, anxiety, burning of mouth and throat, dyspnoea, tachycardia, hypertension.

Later effects: Coma, seizures, opisthotonus, trismus, paralysis, respiratory, arrhythmia, hypotension and death.

Immediate Management

100% O_2 and GI decontamination.

Treatment of Choice

Amyl nitrite inhaled for 30 sec each min.

Sodium nitrite 3% solution IV, 2.5-50 ml/min then 50 ml of 25% sodium thiosulphate is given IV over 1-2 min, producing sodium thiocyanide, excreted in urine.

If symptom persists, repeat half the dose of sodium nitrite and sodium thiosulphate.

Your notes:

PAPER 6

16. Condition in which patient was found with nasal involvement and nasal hairs sighing. He presents with myalgia, malaise and headache.

Diagnosis: Carbon monoxide poisoning.

Clinchers

➢ *Nasal involvement and nasal hairs sighing:* This may signify smoke inhalation.

Carbon monoxide poisoning may occur due to:

- Deliberate self-harm (45%)
- Faulty domestic heating (33%)
- Smoke inhalation in fires (20%)

Symptoms of CO poisoning include myalgia, malaise and headache. There may be confusion, coma, dysphagia, hypotension, LVF, metabolic acidosis, hypokalemia.

CONFUSA

This under-recognized condition causes about 1800 deaths every year in the UK. Acidosis in CO poisoning will resolve with oxygenation. It should never be treated with bicarbonate.

Investigation of Choice

- Blood gases: metabolic acidosis
- ECG (ischaemia)
- Plasma electrolytes and
- Carboxy haemoglobin levels

Immediate Management

High concentration oxygen therapy for 120 minutes, given via an endotracheal tube or tight fitting mask.

Treatment of Choice

- High concentration oxygen.
- Consider the need for hyperbaric oxygen therapy
- Unresponsive patients should be intubated and ventilated.
- Acidosis will resolve with oxygenation and should not be treated with bicarbonates.

Your notes:

17. Condition in which vitamin K is given to improve patient.

Diagnosis: Warfarin Overdosage

Clinchers

Warfarin has a narrow therapeutic range, that varies with the condition being treated. Warfarin inhibits the reductase enzyme responsible for regenerating the active form of vitamin K, thus producing a state analogous to vitamin K deficiency.

If major bleed, treat with IV vitamin K, or FFP.

CONFUSA

If normally on warfarin and not bleeding, but INR dangerously high, give either vitamin K or FFP.

Investigation of Choice

Measure INR (a ratio of warfarin compared with a standard prothrombin time).

Vitamin K levels.

Immediate Management

If bleeding, treat with vitamin K or FFP. DEFIX® if life threatening (it has factors II, IX, X).

Cholestyramine 4 g/6 h PO aids elimination. Warfarin can normally be restarted within 2-3 days but take expert help.

Your notes:

18. A 7-year-old boy accidentally swallowed some unknown white tablets and now complaining of right hypochondrial pain after 12 hours.

Diagnosis: Paracetamol poisoning.

Clinchers

- *Swallowed white tablets, now complaining of right hypochondrial pain:* In this question, tablet was taken accidentally, even otherwise paracetamol is the most common drug involved in self-poisoning. Only early feature of poisoning are nausea and vomiting.
- *Right hypochondrial pain:* Following paracetamol intake, usually signifies the development of hepato-cellular necrosis, or there may be renal tubular necrosis.
- Paracetamol 150 mg/kg (12 g or 24 standard tablets for adults) constitutes a significant ingestion of the drug.

CONFUSA

Patient presenting 12 hours or longer after ingestion tend to be more severely poisoned and at a greater risk of serious liver damage.

Investigation of Choice

- Plasma paracetamol concentration
- Simultaneously measure plasma salicylates
- LFT

Immediate Management

Depends upon the presentation, and time of ingestion. Here let us discuss the management of patient who presents 8-15 hours after ingestion.

- Measure plasma paracetamol concentration
- Consider gastric decontamination with charcoal if the timing is in doubt or if other drugs may be involved.
- Give IV N-acetylcysteine (NAC) while waiting for paracetamol concentration results. The efficacy of the antidote declines from 8 hours after ingestion.
- Assess the possibility of liver damage.
- Arrange medical admission of psychiatric referral.

Your notes:

19. The side effect is urinary retention, heart block and ringing of ear.

Diagnosis: Quinine overdose

Clinchers

Toxicity of quinine is high and dose related 8-10 g taken in a single dose may be fatal. Large single dose or higher therapeutic doses taken for few days produce a clinical syndrome called cinchonism (ringing of ear, nausea, headache, mental confusion, vertigo, visual defects, etc).

Higher doses may cause respiratory depression, hypotension, cardiac arrhythmias.

Quinine occasionally causes haemolysis specially in pregnant women, resulting in haemoglobinuria (black water fever), and kidney damage.

CONFUSA

During pregnancy quinine should be used only for life-threatening infection, with special care to prevent hypoglycaemia.

Investigation of Choice

U and E, ECG, plasma quinine levels.

Immediate Management

Foley's catheterization

Treatment of Choice

Stop quinine and manage the complications.

Your notes:

20. A patient who has overdosed on an unknown medication presents with palpitations. What is the most likely cause?

Diagnosis: Tricyclic antidepressants overdose.

Clinchers

Acute poisoning due to overdose of tricyclic antidepressant is not infrequent and it may endanger life. It is usually self-attempted by the depressed patients.

Manifestations include ECG changes, ventricular arrhythmia, tachycardia.

Excitement, delirium and other anticholinergic symptom as seen in atropine poisoning along with respiratory depression with low BP may be present.

CONFUSA

Atropine poisoning should be kept in mind, as it also presents with anticholinergic symptoms.

Investigation of Choice

Blood tests

ECG

Immediate Management

Physostigmine (0.5-2 mg IV), reversed central and peripheral anticholinergic effects.

Treatment of Choice

Treatment is primary supportive

- Correct acidosis by bicarbonate infusion
- Physostigmine
- Propranolol/lidocaine (for arrhythmias)
- Diazepam IV (for convulsions and delirium).

Your notes:

22. A homeless patient presents to A and E with drowsiness. On examination, abrasions and puncture marks were found on his arm. He has pin-point pupil.

Diagnosis: Opioid poisoning

Antidote: **Naloxone**

Clinchers

- *Homeless patient:* Risk factor for drug addiction.
- *Drowsiness:* Stupor, coma, fall in BP, shallow and occasional breathing are all signs of acute opioid poisoning.
- *Abrasions and puncture marks:* Further support the diagnosis of drug injection.
- *Pin-point pupil:* This confirms the diagnosis of opioid poisoning.

CONFUSA

Drowsiness, coma can be caused by benzodiazepines, alcohol, opiates, tricyclic or barbiturates.

Constricted pupils are seen opiates or insecticides (organophosphates). On the other hand dilated pupils are seen in amphetamines, cocaine, quinine or tricyclic.

Investigation of Choice

Take blood. Always check for paracetamol and salicylate levels. Diagnosis is mainly from history.

Immediate Management

Naloxone e.g. 0.8-2 mg IV repeat every 2 minutes, until breathing adequate.

Treatment of Choice

Advocate supportive measures

Start the antidote

Referral to psychiatrist.

Your notes:

PAPER 7

121. Interferes with glutathione (reversible by methionine and acetyl cysteine).

Diagnosis: Paracetamol poisoning

Clinchers

- *Interferes with glutathione:* Paracetamol is partly converted into a toxic metabolite, N-acetyl-p-benzoquinonimine, which is normally inactivated with glutathione. After a large overdose, glutathione is depleted and the toxic metabolite binds covalently with sulphydryl groups on liver cell membranes, initiating a sequence of changes which leads to hepatocyte necrosis. Marked liver necrosis can occur with as little as 7.5 g (15 tablets), and death with 15 g.
- *Reversible by methionine and acetyl cysteine:* N-acetyl cysteine provides sulphydryl groups that increase the availability of hepatic glutathione. Oral methionine is an alternative and is significantly cheaper than N-acetyl cysteine but absorption and efficacy are unreliable if patient is vomiting (which is usual in such cases).

CONFUSA

Patients with lower reserve of glutathione are more susceptible to liver damage and should be treated in paracetamol poisoning if there plasma concentration is above the high risk treatment line. Such patients are:

- Malnourished people
- Have taken alcohol with overdose
- Alcohol dependent
- Taking enzyme-inducing drugs
- HIV positive or with AIDS.

Investigation of Choice

Plasma paracetamol concentration.

Immediate Management

Toxicology screen for associated poisons

Treatment of Choice

N-acetylcysteine IV.

Your notes:

122. Interferes with haemoglobin.

Diagnosis: Carbon monoxide poisoning

Clinchers

➤ *Interferes with haemoglobin:* Carbon monoxide (CO) combines readily with haemoglobin to form carboxy haemoglobin, thus preventing the formation of oxyhaemoglobin. CO has a special affinity for fetal Hb and so babies and pregnant women present a special risk. This severity of poisoning is related to:
- The concentration of CO inhaled
- The length of exposure
- The level of activity during the exposure.

CONFUSA

The classic pink colour of the skin due to carboxy-haemoglobin is rarely seen before death. (It is paradoxical to be pink despite hypoxemia). The symptoms of CO poisoning may persist or reoccur and are not well related to COHb level. This is probably because the intracellular half-life of CO is bound to the respiratory enzymes is upto 48 hours, as opposed to 280 minutes in the blood, as COHb. Patients with coexisting medical problems, i.e.
- Heart disease
- Respiratory disease
- Anaemia.

and children are usually the worst affected. Usual treatment is with high concentration O_2 but hyperbaric O_2 should be given if:
- Symptoms of poisoning + COHb > 40%
- Last trimester of pregnancy + FCTG changes + COHb > 20%
- Loss of unconsciousness
- Severe cardiovascular complications
- Unresolved neurological signs after 2 hours of treatment with high-concentration O_2.

Investigation of Choice

Early blood gas analysis (as levels may soon return to normal).

Immediate Management

If the poisoning is severe, anticipate cerebral oedema and give mannitol IVI.

Treatment of Choice

High concentration O_2 for 120 minutes given via endotracheal tube or tight-fitting mask.

+

Consider hyperbric O_2 therapy (i.e. if COHb > 40%).

125. This interferes with metabolism at the mitochondrial level.

Diagnosis: Cyanide poisoning

Clinchers

Cyanide blocks electron transport, resulting in decreased oxidative metabolism and oxidative utilization, decreased ATP production and lactic acidosis.

Lethal dose
- Sodium cyanide 200-300 mg
- Hydrocyanic acid 500 mg

Early effects: Headache, vertigo, excitement, anxiety, burning of mouth and throat, dyspnoea, tachycardia, hypertension.

Later effects: Coma, seizures, opisthotonos, trismus, paralysis, respiratory, arrhythmia, hypotension and death.

Immediate Management

100% O_2 and GI decontamination.

Treatment of Choice

Amyl nitrite inhaled for 30 sec each min.

Sodium nitrite 3% solution IV, 2.5-50 ml/min then 50 ml of 25% sodium thiosulphate is given IV over 1-2 min, producing sodium thiocyanide, excreted in urine.

If symptom persist, repeat half the dose of sodium nitrite and sodium thiosulphate.

Your notes:

25 Urology

PAPER 2

Serial No.81, 95

Subject: Urogenital

Topic: Incontinence Urine

Question: A 47-year-old lady presents with urinary incontinence and recurrent urinary tract infections. She continues to soil her clothes with urine even after being catheterized.

Diagnosis: Urinary Fistula

Clinchers

- *47-year-old lady:* Urinary incontinence is twice as prevalent in older women as in older men. Age itself is not a cause of incontinence; however, age-related changes may predispose or contribute to it.
- *Urinary incontinence and recurrent urinary tract infections:* recurrent urinary tract infection is a common finding associated with urinary incontinence because of inability to maintain proper personal hygiene, increased instrumental interventions and catheterization. Rare cases of incontinence associated with urinary fistulas are also associated with typically severe and recurrent urinary tract infection which is usually resistant to urinary antiseptics.
- *Continues to soil her clothes with urine even after being catheterized:* This signifies that she is leaking urine from some tract other than the normal urinary tract. Pointing towards urinary fistula.

CONFUSA

- If a patient complains of passing urine during periods of 'stresses' (viz, coughing, lifting weight and the like) - think of Stress Incontinence.
- If a patient complains of 'incontinence' after a sudden overwhelming 'urge' or desire to pass urine—think of Urge Incontinence.
- If incontinence is associated with dysuria—rule out infectious causes—urinary tract infections, cystitis.

Investigation of Choice

Cystogram to confirm the presence and delineate the fistula.

Double dye test to differentiate between vesicovaginal and ureterovaginal fistula.

Rule out concurrent UTI.

Immediate Management

Personal Hygiene

Treat any concurrent UTI with appropriate antibiotics.

Treatment of Choice

Surgical repair

Your notes:

Serial No. 82

Subject: Urogenital

Topic: Incontinence Urine

Question: A 28-year-old multipara complains of passing urine on coughing and stressing.

Diagnosis: Stress Incontinence

Clinchers

- *28-year-old:* stress incontinence more common in females and at this young age, is most commonly due to obstetric injuries.
- *Multipara:* Perhaps the most common cause of stress incontinence is pelvic floor injury/weakness following child birth. Stress incontinence occurs when the proximal urethra drops below the pelvic floor because of pelvic relaxation defects.
- *Complains of passing urine on coughing and stressing:* Typical picture of presentation of stress incontinence. Intra-abdominal pressure is no longer transmitted equally to the bladder and proximal urethra and the patient ends up passing urine during periods of raised intra-abdominal pressure.

CONFUSA

Pregnancy, labour and delivery may all cause mechanical and denervation injury to the normal supports of the bladder neck and proximal urethra and lead to stress incontinence.

Stress incontinence is also common after the menopause and occurs due to decreased intraurethral pressure due to lack of estrogen.

Investigation of Choice

Urodynamic studies

Immediate Management

Incontinence pads - useful if urinary leakage is small

Treatment of Choice

Pelvic floor exercises are the first line treatment for those with postpartum symptoms.

Oestrogens improve stress incontinence in post menopausal women.

Intravaginal devices: These provide support the bladder neck and urethral and may be an acceptable alternative in women unfit for surgery.

Surgery-indicated if failure of conservative treatment. All methods aim to correct the relaxation defect and to restore the proximal urethra above the level of the pelvic floor.

Serial No. 84, 94

Subject: Urogenital

Topic: Incontinence Urine

Question: A 47-year-old lady with frequency and unavoidable desire to urinate at a few seconds' notice but no dysuria.

Diagnosis: Detrusor Instability

Clinchers

- *47-year-old lady:* Any sort of incontinence is more common in females and age-related changes may predispose or contribute to it.
- *Frequency:* The unstable detrusor is not able to withstand the normal filling pressure and starts to contract even when partially filled.
- *Unavoidable desire to urinate at a few seconds' notice:* Occurs due to and uninhibited contraction of the detrusor muscle during bladder filling.
- *No dysuria:* This rules out any infectious causes of the presenting complaints.

CONFUSA

Detrusor instability presents with features of urge incontinence. It usually occurs in elderly, may complicate multiple sclerosis or a stroke. Detrusor instability refers to overactive bladder symptoms without neurologic impairment. External sphincter functions normally, in synergy. Neurogenic bladder is a malfunctioning bladder due to any type of neurologic disorder. Autonomous bladder is a type of neurogenic bladder characterised by large residual volume of urine and no desire to micturate; is caused by LMN cord lesions above S2,3,4.

Investigation of Choice

Urodynamic studies show involuntary contraction of bladder during filling.

Immediate Management

Bladder training

Treatment of Choice

Anticholinergics: oxybutynin, propiverine, tolterodine, trospium chloride.

Antispasmodic: flavoxate

Sacral nerve stimulation in patients who do not respond to other treatments.

Your notes:

Serial No. 85, 91

Subject: Urogenital

Topic: Incontinence Urine

Question: A 60-year-old lady complains of continuous dribbling of urine. She underwent hysterectomy few months back.

Diagnosis: Urinary Fistula

Clinchers

- *60-year-old lady:* Urinary incontinence is twice as prevalent in older women as in older men. Age itself is not a cause of incontinence; however, age-related changes may predispose or contribute to it.
- *Continuous dribbling of urine:* Signifies that she is having absolutely no control on her continence; suggesting True Incontinence. Occurs mostly due to formed fistulas which continuously drain urine.
- *Hysterectomy few months back:* Most acquired fistulas are due to obstetric causes (prolonged obstructed labour), pelvic surgical procedures or pelvic carcinoma/tuberculaosis. A positive history of pelvic surgery which preceded the symptoms of incontinence in this lady is making the possibility of a vesicovaginal fistula (more common) or ureterovaginal fistula strong.

CONFUSA

- If a patient complains of passing urine during periods of 'stresses' (viz, coughing, lifting weight and the like) - think of Stress Incontinence.
- If a patient complains of 'incontinence' after a sudden overwhelming 'urge' or desire to pass urine - think of Urge Incontinence.
- If incontinence is associated with dysuria- rule out infectious causes - urinary tract infections, cystitis.

Investigation of Choice

Cystogram to confirm the presence and delineate the fistula.
Double dye test to differentiate between vesicovaginal and ureterovaginal fistula.
Rule out concurrent UTI.

Immediate Management

Personal Hygiene
Treat any concurrent UTI with appropriate antibiotics.

Treatment of Choice

Surgical repair

Serial No. 92

Subject: Urogenital

Topic: Incontinence Urine

Question: A lady after child birth complains of passing urine on coughing and stressing.

Diagnosis: Stress Incontinence

Clinchers

- *Lady:* stress incontinence more common in females.
- *After child birth:* Perhaps the most common cause of stress incontinence is pelvic floor injury/weakness following child birth. Stress incontinence occurs when the proximal urethra drops below the pelvic floor because of pelvic relaxation defects.
- *Complains of passing urine on coughing and stressing:* Typical picture of presentation of stress incontinence. Intra-abdominal pressure is no longer transmitted equally to the bladder and proximal urethra and the patient ends up passing urine during periods of raised intra-abdominal pressure.

CONFUSA

- Pregnancy, labour and delivery may all cause mechanical and denervation injury to the normal supports of the bladder neck and proximal urethra and lead to stress incontinence.
- Stress incontinence is also common after the menopause and occurs due to decreased intraurethral pressure due to lack of oestrogen.
- Imperfect sphincter control also complicates epispadias which show a widened bladder neck, shortened urethra and separation of the symphysis pubis.

Investigation of Choice

Urodynamic studies

Immediate Management

Incontinence pads - useful if urinary leakage is small

Treatment of Choice

Pelvic floor exercises are the first line treatment for those with postpartum symptoms.
Oestrogens improve stress incontinence in post-menopausal women.
Intravaginal devices: These provide support the bladder neck and urethral and may be an acceptable alternative in women unfit for surgery.
Surgery - indicated if failure of conservative treatment. All methods aim to correct the relaxation defect and to restore the proximal urethra above the level of the pelvic floor.

Serial No. 96

Subject: Urogenital

Topic: Retention Urine

Question: A patient of multiple sclerosis has had urinary catheterization for 4 years with intermittent obstruction.

Diagnosis: Urethral Stricture

Clinchers

- *Multiple sclerosis:* Multiple sclerosis is associated with variety of neurological bladder dysfunction which can present in the form of urgency, frequency, incontinence or retention. While the overactive bladder symptoms (viz urgency, frequency) are treated with anticholinergics, retention is usually managed by teaching self-catheterization to the patient.
- *Urinary catheterization for 4 years:* The single most important cause of urethral stricture in UK is catheterization or an otherwise instrumentation of the urinary tract. The risk for formation of stricture directly related to the duration of catheter left in situ.
- *Intermittent obstruction:* Catheterization or instrumentation traumatizes the urethral wall and causes a zone of ischaemia, which later heals with scar formation. The process recurs again and again with prolonged catheterization, narrowing the urethral lumen with each episode, until the patient finally presents with acute urethral obstruction.

CONFUSA

Multiple sclerosis can itself present with the features of acute urinary retention, when the spinal cord is affected and the bladder looses all its tone. However, the history of prolonged catheterization in this patient with intermittent obstruction, fits well in the picture of gradually developing stricture.

Investigation of Choice

Urine flow studies for screening

Immediate Management

Opiate analgesics to relive pain.
Suprapubic catheter

Treatment of Choice

Urethral dilatation and urethrotomy are most commonly used procedures.
Urethroplasty is indicated for recurrent strictures.

Serial No. 99

Subject: Urogenital

Topic: Prostate

Question: A 65-year-old man presents with history of frequency, urgency and decreased urinary flow.

Diagnosis: Benign Prostatic Hyperplasia (BPH)

Clinchers

- *65-year-old:* The most common cause of bladder outflow obstruction is benign prostatic hyperplasia. However, the possibility of carcinoma prostate should be kept in mind and ruled out. It is unusual before 50 years of age and is most common between 60 and 70.
- *Frequency, urgency:* These suggest irritation of bladder, either due to the impinging enlarged prostate or due to co-existent urinary tract infection.
- *Decreased urinary flow:* This suggests that flow of urine is weaker, and it takes longer to empty the bladder, pointing to obstruction at the bladder outlet and below.

CONFUSA

Carcinoma prostate also presents in the elderly with similar features of bladder outlet obstruction. However, hints such as grossly raised PSA or back pain are usually given in the question, if the diagnosis of carcinoma prostate is expected. Note that PSA can be raised in cases of BPH, prostatitis or after sexual intercourse. Only levels more than 10 ng/ml require biopsy.

Investigation of Choice

Prostate specific antigen-if PSA is high, perform a transrectal ultrasound with an ultrasound-guided biopsy.

Other investigations like: FBC, urea and electrolytes, MSU to exclude UTI.

Immediate Management

Urinary retention- Catheterize
Urinary Infection - Antibiotics

Treatment of Choice

Mild -moderate symptoms - watchful waiting
Severe symptoms:
1st durg of choice - alpha-adrenoceptor blockers
Finasteride - indicated in very large prostates
Transurethral resection of prostate (TURP) is the surgery of choice wherever feasible.

Serial No. 106

Subject: Medicine

Topic: Infections

Question: A 30-year-old man complains of severe burning on passing urine like 'passing a broken glass'. He also has a penile discharge. Gram stain of the urethral swab is negative.

Diagnosis: Non-Gonococcal Urethritis (NGU)

Clinchers

- *30-year-old man:* Urethritis is predominantly a disease of adult men.
- *Severe burning on passing urine, like 'passing a broken glass', penile discharge:* Most patients with NGU are asymptomatic and if present, symptoms are predominantly dysuria, thin mucoid urethral discharge and pruritus at the meatus.
- *Gram stain of the urethral swab is negative:* This is the statement in the question which actually suggests that our patient is not suffering from gonococcal infection. Gram stain of urethral discharge in case of a gonococcal infection would typically show multiple gram negative diplococci

CONFUSA

Non-gonococcal urethritis is a syndrome with multiple microbial etiology and is diagnosed when *N. gonorrhoeae* cannot be isolated. The most common organisms are *Chlamydia trachomatis* and *Ureaplasma urealyticum*. Other causes also incude Trichomonas vaginalis and herpes infection. Gram stain of the urethral discharge will typically reveal no organisms and multiple polymorphonuclear leukocytes.

Investigation of Choice
Gram stain of the urethral discharge

Immediate Management
Refer to GUM clinic

Treatment of Choice
Empirical Treatment of NGU includes ofloxacin 200 mg twice a day.
Sexual partner(s) should be treated with the same regime.

Your notes:

Serial No. 115

Subject: Urology

Topic: Trauma

Question: A 25-year-old man had fallen from scaffolding astride. He now complains of pain and swelling in the scrotum.

Diagnosis: Urethral Injury

Clinchers

- *A 25-year-old man:* Most urethral injuries bear a close relationship to trauma, and follows the same incidence pattern as trauma, being highest in males of 15-25 years of age. However, a significant amount of urethral injury do occur due to various iatrogenic causes and can appear in any age for that matter.
- *had fallen from scaffolding astride:* This appears to be the most common mode of injury to the anterior urethra. Urtethral injuries associated with pelvic fractures are usually posterior, while those due to instrumentation and prostatic surgeries are most commonly at the level of the sphincter.
- *Complains of pain and swelling in the scrotum:* This indicates the rupture of the Buck's Fascia alongwith the anterior urethra, allowing the haematoma to extend beyond the shaft, with Colles' fascia acting as the lower limiting membrane. This results in a characterisitic butterfly pattern of bruising in the perineum.

CONFUSA

- Anterior urethral injuries are suspected when there is blood at the meatus, inability to pass water or rapid development of a perineal urinoma/haematoma, forming down the sleeve of Buck's Fascia.
- Diagnosing posterior urethral injuries require high index of suspicion, more so in a patient with associated pelvic fracture involving the displacement of pubic rami. This,in association with blood a urethral meatus, inability to pass urine or distended bladder and a high riding prostate on rectal examination is suggestive of posterior urethral injury.

Investigation of Choice:
Diagnosed clinically. Pass a suprapubic catheter to confirm.
USG (per rectal) can be used in rare cases.

Immediate Management
Avoid any per urethral catheter.
Ask for expert urological help.

Treatment of Choice: Surgical repair

PAPER 3

35. A 23-year-old man who sustained a pelvic fracture is unable to pass urine. On examination he has abdominal tenderness and fullness and blood on the urethral meatus.

Diagnosis: Injury to membranous urethra.

Clinchers

- *Pelvic fracture:* Membranous urethra is most commonly injured in pelvic fractures, especially those involving dislocation of a portion of the pelvis. It is usually form at its junction with the prostatic urethra.
- *Abdominal tenderness and fullness:* It signifies distended bladder which can be painful and tender. It is due to discontinuity of the outflow system due to injury.
- *Blood on the urethral meatus:* The presence of bleeding from the meatus, or a fracture of the pelvis, combined with urinary retention, should alert to the possibility of extravasation of urine which could lead to secondary infection.

CONFUSA

Injury to bulbous urethra is usually not associated with pelvic fractures and is commonly seen after direct blows to perineum. It is characterised by severe perineal pain, bruising and fresh blood dripping from external meatus. In any suspected urethral injury, a Foley's catheter should never be passed before obtaining an urethrogram.

Investigation of Choice

Urethrogram with water soluble contrast (to identify any extravasation, loss of continuity and to localise site of injury).

Immediate Management

Per rectal examination to palpate prostate. An absent or high prostate implies a complete rupture of the membranous urethra and warrants urgent exploration.

Treatment of Choice

Suprapubic catheterisation
+
Repair

PAPER 2

105. A 70-year-old woman, confusion, constipation, frequency of urine.

Diagnosis: Urinary tract infection (UTI)

Clinchers

- *70-year-old:* UTIs are more common in the elderly, in whom impaired bladder emptying due to prostatic disease in males and neuropathic bladder—especially common in females—is frequently found.
- *Woman:* Impaired bladder emptying due to neuropathic bladder is common in elderly females and produce urinary stasis which can then lead to UTI especially proteus infections.
- *Confusion:* May be due to dementia of elderly or due to severe debilitating illness. Or it may be due to secondary bacteremia from UTI.
- *Constipation:* Quite common in elderly due to impaired mobility or poor nutrition. Note that constipation produces urinary incontinence in elderly.
- *Frequency of urine:* Incontinence, nocturia, smelly urine or vague changes in well-being are often the only symptoms of UTI in an elderly patient.

CONFUSA

This is a question from GMC PLAB booklet. Repetition of this question in the actual exam shows that GMC has a very limited question bank.

Investigation of Choice

MSU

Immediate Management

Consider a PR examination to rule out faecal impaction.

Treatment of Choice

Systemic treatment of UTI in elderly is required if bacteremia is present. Otherwise focus on local hygiene.

Your notes:

166. An 85-year-old with 14 children, severe heart failure, complains of dysuria, feeling of pressure in lower abdomen.

Diagnosis: Genital prolapse

Clinchers

- *85-year-old:* Prolapse is more evident in older age (i.e. late after menopause) when there is general weakening and shrinking of the supports of the pelvic organs.
- *With 14 children:* Each labour increases the risk of prolapse. It is due to overstretching of the uterine supports during labour.
- *Severe heart failure:* This patient is unfit for operation on medical grounds. So pessary treatment is indicated here.
- *Dysuria:* Urinary symptoms in genital prolapse are:
  - *Frequency of* micturition is common and is often only at day time. Nocturnal frequency may be present if there is added cystitis
  - *Urgency* of micturition due to weakness of the bladder sphincter mechanism and urge incontinence may occur in some cases
  - *Difficulty in emptying:* The bladder completely
  - *Retention of urine* following urethral overstretch
  - *Stress incontinence.*
- *Feeling of pressure in lower abdomen:* A dragging sensation or bearing down in the back or lower abdomen is a common complaint in prolapse. Other associated complaints can be:
  - A feeling of fullness of vagina
  - A lump coming down

CONFUSA

Symptoms similar to those of prolapse may be caused by:

- Varicose veins of the vulva
- Haemorrhoids
- Rectal prolapse
- Cystitis
- Vaginitis with congestion of vulva
- Pressure form a large abdominal tumour

There are a few cases where a ring pessary fails to control prolapse and operation cannot be performed. In these cases use: *Cup and stem pessary.*

Investigation of Choice

- Colposcopy
- Urine microscopy and culture if UTI is also suspected

Immediate Management

Reassurance that the condition is treatable

Treatment of Choice

Plastic ring pessary.

167. Female with well-controlled diabetes mellitus type 2 with recurrent urinary tract infection (UTI).

Diagnosis: Chlamydial UTI

Clinchers

- *Well-controlled diabetes:* Infections in persons with diabetes may not occur more frequently than in non-diabetics but they tend to be more severe, possibly because of impaired leucocyte function, a frequent accompaniment of poor control. But since this case has a well-controlled diabetes, this is also ruled out. Most probably this is a case of recurrent UTI with no identifiable source.
- *Recurrent UTI:* Females have a higher incidence of UTI because of a short urethra which is prone to entry of bacteria during intercourse poor perineal hygiene and the occasional inefficient voiding ability (due to diabetic neuropathy).

CONFUSA

In women with recurrent acute urinary symptoms, pyuria and urine that is sterile (even when obtained by suprapubic aspiration), sexually transmitted urethritis—producing agents such as *Chlamydia trachomatis, Neisseria gonorrhoeae,* and herpes simplex virus are etiologically important.

Investigation of Choice

- *Screening:* MSU—nitrate stick test
- *Definitive:* MSU—culture (pure growth of more than 10^5 organisms per ml urine).

Immediate Management

Rule out diabetic neuropathy (i.e. bladder involvement) and pyelonephritis).

Treatment of Choice

Recurrent UTI for which an identifiable source has not been found may be managed by long-term low dose antimicrobial therapy, such as trimethoprim. Ciprofloxacin or norfloxacin can be alternatives.

Your notes:

181. Man after trip to Asia presents with red, swollen scrotum.

Diagnosis: Epididymo-orchitis

Clinchers

- *Trip to Asia:* He might have caught gonococcal infection from sex workers in Thailand. Or it could be TB also but that needs a primary infection somewhere else.
  Chlamydia can also cause epididymo-orchitis in < 35 years old.
- *Red, swollen scrotum:* The patient will have a very painful swelling of the epididymis, often with a secondary hydrocele and constitutional effects (pyrexia, headaches and leucocytosis). There may be a history of dysuri suggesting a UTI, or urethral discharge suggesting a sexually transmitted organism.

CONFUSA

Examination of urine may reveal the presence of organisms and pus cells, but the urine need not be abnormal. Rectal examination of the prostate may reveal coexistent prostatitis. Always look for urethral discharge in a patient of epididymo-orchitis. A 'first-catch' is more likely to show abnormalities than MSU.

Investigation of Choice

Urethral swab for culture

Immediate Management

Rule out torsion of testis which usually present like epididymo-orchitis

- If the patient is in his teens, torsion is more likely; if he is in his twenties and sexually active, epidymitis is more likely.
- In torsion the testes like high in scrotum and pain is a bit relieved by lifting testes (worsens in epididymo-orchitis).

Treatment of Choice

Erythromycin for chlamydia
For others—ciprofloxacin.

Your notes:

182. Man with painful red scrotum and vomiting.

Diagnosis: Torsion of testis.

Clinchers

- *Painful red scrotum:* The differential diagnoses are:
  - Mumps orchitis
  - Epididymo-orchitis
  - Torsion of testes
  - Torsion of testicular appendage
- *Vomiting:* Of all the above conditions, only torsion produces a pain severe enough to produce vomiting. There may be associated abdominal pain also which is because the nerve supply of the testis is mainly from T_{10} sympathetic pathway.

CONFUSA

Torsion of the testis can also present as a pain in lower abdomen (can mimic appendicitis if on right side) torsion of appendicular appendage can present in similar way but on examination the testis does not lie high in scrotum and a dark blue pea like swelling may be visible through the scrotal skin. Torsion may also mimic a strangulated inguinal hernia.

Investigation of Choice

The diagnosis is entirely clinical. The only investigation is to see whether the testis is still viable or not and that is possible only on surgical exploration (usually viability maintained till 6 hours).

Immediate Management

Inform surgeons.

Treatment of Choice

Urgent surgical exploration.

Your notes:

183. Man with painless testicular swelling since 2 months.

Diagnosis: Suspected testicular tumour.

Clinchers

➢ *Painless testicular swelling:* Tumours of the testes usually present as a painless, swollen testicle or lump on a testicle which is hard and may be associated with an overlying secondary hydrocele, which sometimes contains blood stained fluid.

➢ *Since two months:* Tumours usually become noticeably in a considerable time and one to two months after appearance are taken by the patient to realise that it is abnormal. Age of the man is not specified in this question otherwise a clinical differentiation between suspected seminoma (30-40 years) and teratoma (20-30 years) might have been possible.

CONFUSA

Tumours of testes may present with a misleading history of recent trauma, and rarely it may present having undergone torsion. Occasionally gynaecomastia may be a presenting feature, due to production of paraneoplastic hormones.

Investigation of Choice

Scrotal USG may reveal a solid tumour in a hydrocele but a negative finding cannot exclude malignancy. Also

- Seminomas—β hCG
- Teratomas—AFP

Immediate Management

Staging is essential. Conduct all necessary investigations. (CXR, CT and excision biopsy).

Treatment of Choice

Orchidectomy.

Your notes:

184. Man with a swelling of scrotum since 3 years.

Diagnosis: Sebaceous cyst (most probably)

Clinchers

➢ *Swelling of scrotum:* Since the question is not about testicular swelling but only a scrotal swelling, we are left with a handful of diagnosis, i.e.

- *Filarial elephantiasis of the scrotum:* It is due to obstruction of pelvic lymphatics by *Wuchereria bancrofti*. But it is rarely seen in UK and is associated with penile swelling also. So it can be safely excluded as a diagnosis.
- *Sebaceous cysts:* These are common in scrotal area. Although they are often multiple, a solitary scrotal sebaceous cyst is not an infrequent finding.

CONFUSA

A sebaceous cyst can remain as it is (i.e. with no increase in size) for many years. In scrotal area, they are often small (unlike-skull) and thus do not produce any problem to the patient (except cosmetic). They are painful only when they are infected.

Investigation of Choice

The diagnosis of a sebaceous cyst is entirely clinical.

Immediate Management

None

Treatment of Choice

Complete excision along with cyst wall if:

- Patient ask for it
- Cosmetic reasons
- Infected
- Producing discomfort.

Your notes:

185. Man with no history of unsafe sex presents with dysuria and urinary frequency.

Diagnosis: Urinary tract infection (UTI)

Clinchers

- *History of unsafe sex:* It is the main risk factor for acquisition of UTI in sexually active population. Exposure to commercial sex workers increases the risk much more.
- *Dysuria:* It is a feature of cystitis. Other features of cystitis are:
  - Frequency
  - Urgency
  - Strangury
  - Haematuria
  - Suprapubic pain
- *Urinary frequency:* Also a feature of cystitis in UTI.

CONFUSA

The most common organism causing UTI is *E. coli.* (>70% in community but ≤ 41% in hospital). Among sexually transmitted diseases (like this one) *Chlamydia* is the main culprit (in < 35 years).

Investigation of Choice

MSU—send it for lab culture if urine dipsticks show leucocytes, nitrite, proteinuria or haematuria.

Immediate Management

Take a detailed history.

If this is not the first UTI of his life, try to differentiate between:

- Recurrent UTI: Further infection with new organisms
- Relapse of UTI: Further infection with same organisms

Treatment of Choice

Trimethoprim 200 mg/12 h PO × 3 days is the DOC for cystitis.

Alternative: Cephalexin.

Your notes:

PAPER 3

92. A young mother with chronic bronchitis says that every time she coughs, she pees, and she would like you to do something about it. She is on a course of antibiotics at the moment.

Diagnosis: Genuine stress incontinence (GSI)

Clinchers

- *Chronic bronchitis:* This gives a repetitive stress factor to the patient, i.e. cough.
- *Everytime she coughs, she pees:* On clinical examination. GSI may be demonstrated when the patient coughs. It occurs when the bladder pressure exceeds the maximum uretheral pressure in the absence of any detrusor contraction.
- *On a course of antibiotics:* This suggests that her bronchitis is severe. Also it suggests that she is undergoing treatment for the basic cause and now we need to treat the incontinence.

CONFUSA

The aetiology of GSI after child birth is due to damage to the nerve supply of the pelvic floor and uretheral sphincter (caused by child birth). It leads to progressive changes in these structures resulting in altered function. In addition, mechanical trauma to the pelvic floor musculature and endopelvic fascia and ligaments occurs as a consequence of vaginal delivery. Prolonged second stage, large bodies and instrumental deliveries cause the most damage.

Investigation of Choice

Urodynamic studies

Immediate Management

Clinical examination by an expert

Treatment of Choice

Pelvic floor exercises/physiotherapy

±

Surgery

Your notes:

93. A middle aged woman complains of having to urinate frequently. She says that unless she rushes to the toilet she wets herself and she finds wetting herself most embarrassing.

Diagnosis: Urge incontinence (UI)

Clinchers

- *Middle aged woman:* The most common cause of urge incontinence in such females is bladder unstability following child births.
- *Having to urinate frequently:* This is "frequency", a common finding in UI. It is due to detrusor instability.
- *Unless she rushes to toilet she wet herself:* This is "urgency" which is characteristic of urge incontinence. It is due to contraction of bladder while the patient is attempting to inhibit micturition.
- *Embarrassing:* Since the condition is symptomatic and embarrassing, it requires urgent treatment.

CONFUSA

Urge incontinence can be present alone or association with GSI in which case it is called mixed incontinence. The cause of the unsuppressible or unhibited bladder contractions is usually idiopathic, but bacterial cystitis, bladder tumour, bladder outlet obstruction and neurogenic bladder must be excluded.

Investigation of Choice

Urodynamic studies

Immediate Management

Exclude UTI and glycosuria

Treatment of Choice

Bladder training (gradually increasing the time interval between voiding).

Your notes:

94. A 36-year-old sales executive says she wets herself without warning all the time. Before the birth of her third child she had no complaints but now she says she has no control whatsoever.

Diagnosis: True incontinence

Clinchers

- *36-year-old:* True incontinence presenting in this age is due to acquired causes, i.e. obstetric injuries.
- *Wets herself without warning all the time:* In true incontinence of urine, due to a vesicovaginal or ureterovaginal fistula, the urine is discharged involuntarily and continuously so that the patient is constantly wet.
- *No complaints before birth of her third child:* This suggests obstetric trauma to be the cause, i.e. prolonged labour, forceps application etc.

CONFUSA

The bladder is always empty without residual urine in the case of a vesicovaginal fistula and only contains half the expected normal in the case of a ureterovaginal fistula.

Investigation of Choice

Micturition cysto-uretherography

Immediate Management

Detailed obstetric history

Treatment of Choice

Surgery.

Your notes:

95. A 27-year-old travel guide wants something done about the pain she feels on micturition, especially when it is cold. Repeated urine cultures have all been negative. Sometimes, she says, going to the toilet is very painful for her.

Diagnosis: Urethral syndrome (US)

Clinchers

- *27-year-old:* US is mostly seen in the sexually active females and is often associated with intercourse.
- *Pain she feels on micturition, especially when it is cold:* This is dysuria, a common manifestation of cystitis.
- *Repeated urine cultures have all been negative:* Characteristically MSU are all negative in cystitis causing US. It may be due to subinfective numbers of organisms being massaged into the urethra during the intercourse.
- *Going to the toilet is very painful:* This suggests a symptomatic cystitis and hence an indication for active treatment.

CONFUSA

Mildly symptomatic US can be managed by using proper lubrication during the intercourse. Micturating before and after intercourse, different coital positions (her on top) can help.

Investigation of Choice

None

Immediate Management

Exclude glycosuria

Treatment of Choice

Trimethoprim.

Your notes:

108. A 32-year-old woman presents with dysuria, swinging fever and loin pain.

Diagnosis: *Escherichia coli* (urinary tract infection)

Clinchers

- *32-year-old:* UTI are common in sexually active females.
- *Dysuria:* The most typical symptoms of UTI are:
  - Frequency of micturition by day and night
  - Painful voiding (dysuria)
  - Suprapubic pain and tenderness
  - Haematuria
  - Smelly urine
- *Swinging fever and loin pain:* Swinging fever typically represents a foci of pus in the body. Loin pain and tenderness, with fever and systemic upset, suggest extension of the infection to the pelvis and kidney, known as pyelitis and pyelonephritis.

CONFUSA

Organisms causing UTI in domicilliary practice:

• *E. coli* and other coliforms	68%+
• *Proteus mirabilis*	12%
• *Klebsiella aerogenes*	4%
• *Enterococcus faecalis*	6%
• *Staphylococcus saprophyticus* or epidermidis	10%

Investigation of Choice

- *Screening:* MSU
- *Definitive:* IVU (as pyelonephritis is suspected)

Immediate Management

Rule out complicated disease

Treatment of Choice

Trimethoprim.

Your notes:

136. Uncomplicated urinary tract infection (UTI)

Diagnosis: Stated as the question itself.

Clinchers

In acute uncomplicated cases, more than 80% of infections are due to *E. coli* and although resistance patterns vary geographically, most strains are sensitive to many antibiotics. Single doses of trimethoprim-sulfamethoxazole (four single strength tablets), trimethoprim alone (400 mg), sulfa alone (2.0 g), and most fluoroquinolones (norfloxacin, ciprofloxacin, ofloxacin) have been used successfully to treat acute uncomplicated episodes.

CONFUSA

The advantages of single dose therapy include less expense, ensured compliance, fever side effects and perhaps less intense pressure following the selection of resistant organisms in the intestinal, vaginal or perianal flora.

Investigation of Choice

MSU culture

Immediate Management

Exclude STD

Treatment of Choice

Trimethoprim.

Your notes:

PAPER 6

42. Man with painful red scrotum and vomiting.

Diagnosis: Torsion of testis.

Clinchers

- *Painful red scrotum:* The differential diagnoses are:
  - Mumps orchitis
  - Epididymo-orchitis
  - Torsion of testes
  - Torsion of testicular appendage
- *Vomiting:* Of all the above conditions, only torsion produces a pain severe enough to produce vomiting. There may be associated abdominal pain also which is because the nerve supply of the testis is mainly from T_{10} sympathetic pathway.

CONFUSA

Torsion of the testis can also present as a pain in lower abdomen (can mimic appendicitis if on right side) torsion of appendicular appendage can present in similar way but on examination the testis does not lie high in scrotum and a dark blue pea like swelling may be visible through the scrotal skin. Torsion may also mimic a strangulated inguinal hernia.

Investigation of Choice

The diagnosis is entirely clinical. The only investigation is to see whether the testis is still viable or not and that is possible only on surgical exploration (usually viability maintained till 6 hours).

Immediate Management

Inform surgeons.

Treatment of Choice

Urgent surgical exploration.

Your notes:

43. Man with painless testicular swelling since 2 months.

Diagnosis: Suspected testicular tumour.

Clinchers

- *Painless testicular swelling:* Tumours of the testes usually present as a painless, swollen testicle or lump on a testicle which is hard and may be associated with an overlying secondary hydrocele, which sometimes contains blood stained fluid.
- *Since two months:* Tumours usually become noticeably in a considerable time and one to two months after appearance are taken by the patient to realise that it is abnormal. Age of the man is not specified in this question otherwise a clinical differentiation between suspected seminoma (30-40 years) and teratoma (20-30 years) might have been possible.

CONFUSA

Tumours of testes may present with a misleading history of recent trauma, and rarely it may present having undergone torsion. Occasionally gynaecomastia may be a presenting feature, due to production of paraneoplastic hormones.

Investigation of Choice

Scrotal USG may reveal a solid tumour in a hydrocele but a negative finding cannot exclude malignancy. Also

- Seminomas—β hCG
- Teratomas—AFP

Immediate Management

Staging is essential. Conduct all necessary investigations. (CXR, CT and excision biopsy).

Treatment of Choice

Orchidectomy.

Your notes:

44. Man with a swelling of scrotum since 3 years.

Diagnosis: Sebaceous cyst (most probably)

Clinchers

- *Swelling of scrotum:* Since the question is not about testicular swelling but only a scrotal swelling, we are left with a handful of diagnosis, i.e.
  - *Filarial elephantiasis of the scrotum:* It is due to obstruction of pelvic lymphatics by *Wuchereria bancrofti*. But it is rarely seen in UK and is associated with penile swelling also. So it can be safely excluded as a diagnosis.
  - *Sebaceous cysts:* These are common in scrotal area. Although they are often multiple, a solitary scrotal sebaceous cyst is not an infrequent finding.

CONFUSA

A sebaceous cyst can remain as it is (i.e. with no increase in size) for many years. In scrotal area, they are often small (unlike-skull) and thus do not produce any problem to the patient (except cosmetic). They are painful only when they are infected.

Investigation of Choice

The diagnosis of a sebaceous cyst is entirely clinical.

Immediate Management

None

Treatment of Choice

Complete excision along with cyst wall if:

- Patient ask for it
- Cosmetic reasons
- Infected
- Producing discomfort.

Your notes:

45. Man with no history of unsafe sex presents with dysuria and urinary frequency.

Diagnosis: Urinary tract infection (UTI)

Clinchers

- *History of unsafe sex:* It is the main risk factor for acquisition of UTI in sexually active population. Exposure to commercial sex workers increases the risk much more.
- *Dysuria:* It is a feature of cystitis. Other features of cystitis are:
  - Frequency
  - Urgency
  - Strangury
  - Haematuria
  - Suprapubic pain
- *Urinary frequency:* Also a feature of cystitis in UTI.

CONFUSA

The most common organism causing UTI is *E. coli.* (>70% in community but ≤ 41% in hospital). Among sexually transmitted diseases (like this one) *Chlamydia* is the main culprit (in < 35 years).

Investigation of Choice

MSU—send it for lab culture if urine dipsticks show leucocytes, nitrite, proteinuria or haematuria.

Immediate Management

Take a detailed history.

If this is not the first UTI of his life, try to differentiate between:

- Recurrent UTI: further infection with new organisms
- Relapse of UTI: further infection with same organisms

Treatment of Choice

Trimethoprim 200 mg/12 h PO × 3 days is the DOC for cystitis.

Alternative: cephalexin.

Your notes:

48. A 30-year-old female, insulin-dependent diabetic, presents with failure to pass urine.

Diagnosis: Autonomic neuropathy

Clinchers

- *IDDM patient:* Such patients are more prone to autonomic neuropathy.
- *Failure to pass urine:* Retention of urine is suggestive of autonomic involvement of the bladder. That occurs with a long-standing history of diabetes. Since the patient is now 30-year-old and IDDM usually have a juvenile onset, one must be having a long history to substantiate our diagnosis.

CONFUSA

Diabetic neuropathy may affect every part of the nervous system, with the possibel exception of brain. While rarely a direct cause of death, neuropathy is a major cause of morbidity. Most common picture is that of a peripheral polyneuropathy.

Investigation of Choice

Pelvic USG.

Immediate Management

Urinary catheterisation.

Treatment of Choice

Chronic catheter drainage.

Your notes:

162. Female with well-controlled diabetes mellitus type 2 with recurrent urinary tract infection (UTI).

Diagnosis: Chlamydial UTI

Clinchers

- *Well-controlled diabetes:* Infections in persons with diabetes may not occur more frequently than in non-diabetics but they tend to be more severe, possibly because of impaired leucocyte function, a frequent accompaniment of poor control. But since this case has a well-controlled diabetes, this is also ruled out. Most probably this is a case of recurrent UTI with no identifiable source.
- *Recurrent UTI:* Females have a higher incidence of UTI because of a short urethra which is prone to entry of bacteria during intercourse poor perineal hygiene and the occasional inefficient voiding ability (due to diabetic neuropathy).

CONFUSA

In women with recurrent acute urinary symptoms, pyuria and urine that is sterile (even when obtained by suprapubic aspiration), sexually transmitted urethritis—producing agents such as *Chlamydia trachomatis*, *Neisseria gonorrhoeae*, and herpes simplex virus are etiologically important.

Investigation of Choice

- *Screening:* MSU—nitrate stick test
- *Definitive:* MSU—culture (pure growth of more than 10^5 organisms per ml urine).

Immediate Management

Rule out diabetic neuropathy (i.e. bladder involvement) and pyelonephritis).

Treatment of Choice

Recurrent UTI for which an identifiable source has not been found may be managed by long-term low dose antimicrobial therapy, such as trimethoprim. Ciprofloxacin or norfloxacin can be alternatives.

Your notes:

PAPER 7

6. A 3-year-old boy has a first confirmed urinary tract infection. Abdominal ultrasound is normal.

Diagnosis: UTI

Clinchers

- *3-year-old:* New renal scars appear in 43% of those less than 1-year-old, 84% of those aged 1-5, and 80% of those less than 5-year-old.
- *Boy:* Annual incidence of UTI in UK is:
  Boys: 0.17-0.23%
  Girls: 0.31-1%
  Sex ratios are reversed in neonates.
- *First confirmed UTI:* This suggests that it is an uncomplicated case of UTI. Also it rules out need for MCU (see confusa).
- *Abdominal USG is normal:* USG is worthwhile even in first UTI. It has 99% specificity and 43% sensitivity. It may miss reflux and scarring.

CONFUSA

Almost all the significant lesions missed by USG either occur in infants < 2 years, or occurs with fever and vomiting, so if these are present and USG is normal, proceed not to IVU, which is radiation rich and unreliable but to:

- ^{99}Technetium renography—static for scarring.
- Isotope cystography—dynamic for obstructive uropathy.
- Isotope cystography—Micturating cystourethrogram (MCU) is still the best way of excluding reflux but it is not done if:
  - Pyelonephritis is unlikely
  - There is no family history of reflux
  - There are no recurrent UTIs

Since this case is just a first episode of UTI, MCU is not indicated.

Investigation of Choice

MSU (midstream urine).

Immediate Management

Start antibiotics.

Treatment of Choice

Trimethoprim 50 mg/5 mL and follow up MSU after 3 week to find response to treatment.

Your Notes

7. A female presents with frequent dysuria. This is the third episode. At this time *E. coli* confirmed.

Diagnosis: UTI

Clinchers

- *Female:* The vast majority of acute symptomatic UTI involve young women. Such infections are unusual in men under the age of 50.
- *Frequent dysuria:* Approximately 30% of women with acute dysuria have midstream urine cultures that show either no growth or insignificant bacterial growth.
- *Third episode:* Gross haematuria, suprapubic pain, an abrupt onset of illness, a duration of illness of less than 3 days and a history of previous UTI favour the diagnosis of *E. coli* infection.
- *E. coli confirmed: E. coli* is the most common pathogen in UTI accounting for > 70% cases in community (but ≤ 41% cases in hospitals) frequent relapses suggest P-strain of *E. coli* that infect individuals with P positive erythrocytes.

CONFUSA

Not all strains of *E. coli* are equally able to infect the intact urinary tract. Only the uropathogenic *E. coli* (with P-pilus and haemolysin secretion) produce persistent infections.

Investigation of Choice

IVU (always indicated for relapsing/recurrent UTI).

Immediate Management

Blood group P antigen testing (not always required-optional).

Treatment of Choice

Trimethoprim.

Your Notes:

8. A 70-year-old with prostatic symptoms. Urine culture is negative.

Diagnosis: Bladder outflow obstruction.

Clinchers

- *70-year-old:* This person can have prostatic enlargement either by prostatic carcinoma or benign hyperplasia.
  Note: 70% of the men have benign hyperplasia by the age of 70 years.
- *Prostatic symptoms:* These can hesitancy, terminal dribbling frequency, urgency, nocturia and acute retention.
- *Urine culture negative:* This rules out UTI which can either produce similar symptoms or can be secondary to bladder outflow obstruction.

CONFUSA

USG will demonstrate bladder enlargement, hydronephrosis and hydroureter following voiding it can be used to estimate the amount of residual urine in the bladder. Normally these is none; however, in the presence of bladder outflow obstruction the bladder cannot be completely emptied. USG has replaced the IVU in the routine investigation of patients with outflow obstruction.

Investigation of Choice

USG

Immediate Management

Exclude carcinoma prostate.

Treatment of Choice

- TURP/finasteride + prazosin—if BHP
- Prostatectomy/chemotherapy—if carcinoma.

Your Notes:

9. A 25-year-old male has a first confirmed urinary tract infection. IVU is normal.

Diagnosis: Uncomplicated UTI

Clinchers

- *25-year-old male:* Although UTI is unusual in adults males below 50 years of age they may occur in certain conditions, e.g.
  - renal stones
  - instrumentation.
- *First confirmed UTI:* This signifies that there is low-risk of resistant infection and trimethoprim will work.
- *IVU is normal:* This rules out any renal tract malformation or abnormality and thus makes the diagnosis of uncomplicated UTI.

CONFUSA

A UTI in a young adult male with normal GU tract should prompt one to initiate investigations for any underlying immunosuppression or diabetes mellitus.

Investigation of Choice
None required.

Immediate Management
Blood sugar (to rule out diabetes).

Treatment of Choice
Trimethoprim
and follow up MSU after 3 weeks.

Your Notes:

31. A patient of multiple sclerosis has had urinary catheterisation for 4 years with intermittent obstruction.

Diagnosis: Multiple sclerosis (MS) with spinal cord lesions.

Clinchers
Sphincter disturbances such as urinary urgency or hesitancy which disappear after few days or weeks, to come again (relapsing/remitting disorder), weakness, numbness, tingling, or unsteadiness in a limb, unilateral optic neuritis are the symptoms of multiple sclerosis. First presentations are usually monosymptomatic MS consists of plaques of demyelination throughout the CNS.

CONFUSA

In MRI, initially individual plaques (e.g. in optic nerve, brainstem or cord) may cause diagnostic difficulty. They must be distinguished from compressive, inflammatory or vascular lesions.

Investigation of Choice
In MS investigations only support and do not make the diagnosis. MRI is sensitive but not specific for plaque defection. It is the first line of investigation.

Treatment of Choice
There is no curative treatment, but dietary polyunsaturated fats may help.

Your notes:

34. 65-year-old man with history of frequency, urgency and decreased urinary flow.

Diagnosis: Benign prostatic hypertrophy (BPH).

Clinchers

- *65-year-old man:* BPH occurs in men over 50 years of age. By 60 years 50% of men home histological evidence of BPH.
- *Frequency, urgency, decreased urinary flow:* These are the symptoms of benign prostatic hypertrophy (BPH) due to bladder outflow obstruction (BOO). Relationships between BPH, BOO (urodynamically proven) and symptoms of prostatism
- *Rectal examination:* In benign enlargement, posterior surface of prostate is smooth, convex and elastic (sometimes firm because of fibrous element of prostate)
  - Rectal mucosa can be made to more over the prostate
  - Sometimes fluctuating swelling over the prostate (this is residual urine).

CONFUSA

All these symptoms of disturbed voiding in ageing men should not be always attributed to BPH causing BOO. These symptoms may owe to impairment of smooth muscles function and neurovesical coordination. Rule out prostatic carcinoma, refer to Q-32 (July 2001).

Investigation of choice

- PSA (rule out carcinoma)
- Flow rate measurement: Typical history and flow rate < 10 ml/second (for voided volume of > 200 ml) alarms treatment
- *Cystourethroscopy:* Before prostatectomy
- Serum creatinine/electrolytes

Treatment of choice

- Transurethral resection of the prostate (TURP)
- Transurethral incision of the prostate (TUIP)
- Retropubic prostatectomy
- Drugs (in mild cases)
  - *a blockers (terazosin or indoramin):* Decrease smooth muscle tone (prostate and bladder)
  - *a reductase inhibitor (finasteride):* It is conversion of testosterone to dihydrotestosterone.

54. Patient with presenting complaint of severe flank pain. He is now restless. He says that the pain is radiating to the groin he is passing reddish urine.

Diagnosis: Ureteric colic

Clinchers

- *Severe flank pain:* Impaction of the stone at the pelvi-ureteric junction, or migration down the ureter itself, produces the deadful agony of ureteric colic.
- *Restless:* The pain is of great severity and is accompanied by typical restlessness of the patient, who is quite unable to lie still in bed.
- *Radiating to groin:* The pain typically radiates from groin to loin.
- *Reddish urine:* Haematuria, which may be microscopic or macroscopic, is frequently present so that detection of blood in the urine is an extremely helpful means of confirming the clinical diagnosis.

CONFUSA

Unlike the usual textbook description the pain is not usually intermittent, but is continuous, although quite often with sharp exacerbations on a background of continued pain. There is often accompanying vomiting and sweating. Pain is the presenting feature of the great majority of kidney stones, but if the calculus is embedded within the solid substance of the kidney it may be entirely symptom-free. Within the minor or major calyx system the stone produces a dull loin pain.

Investigation of Choice

- *Screening:* Abdominal KUB film.
- *Definitive:* IVU.

Immediate Management

See urgent urological help.

Analgesia: Diclofenac suppository 100 mg (single dose).

Treatment of choice

Lithotripsy or open surgery.

Your notes:

26 Single Best Answers (SBAs)—Explanatory Notes

PAPER 1

Serial No. 170

Subject: ENT

Topic: Foreign Body

Question: A mentally retarded child puts a green pea in his ear while having his dinner. The carer confirms this. Otoscopy shows a green coloured object in the ear canal.

Most appropriate single best approach to remove this:

a. By a magnet
b. Syringing
c. Under GA
d. By hook
e. By instilling olive oil

Correct Answer: (D) by hook

Explanation:

Children or mentally disturbed adults are the most common group presenting to ENT OP with foreign body in the ear. Forceps should be avoided in spherical foreign bodies (as here in this case), because of poor gripping. Hook is the most appropriate method for the removal of spherical foreign bodies. Magnet can be used for metallic small chip-like foreign bodies, while syringing is usually unsuccessful and best avoided. Uncooperative patients or previous unsuccessful attempts at removal (leading to edematous passage) may necessitate the use of general anesthesia. Live insects are usually removed by 1st drowning in olive oil and then syringing.

Serial No. 171

Subject: Surgery

Topic: Anatomy

Question: During laparoscopy the first trocar is inserted midway between umbilicus and anterior superior iliac spine.

The structures most likely to be pierced by the inserted trocar are:

a. Rectus abdominis muscle
b. Linea alba
c. External oblique aponeurosis and internal oblique muscle
d. External oblique and internal oblique muscles
e. Conjoint tendon

Answer: (C) External oblique aponeurosis and internal oblique muscle

Explanation:

The external oblique muscle is the outermost muscle the anterior abdominal wall, originating from the lower eight ribs, and then curves down on itself forming a tough aponeurosis which gets inserted into the outer anterior crest of the ileum. The internal oblique lies below external oblique, originating from the inguinal ligament finally getting inserted into the linea alba. Now, at the point of insertion of this trocar, i.e. midway between anterior superior iliac spine and umbilicus, it is almost the point of origin of internal oblique and the point of insertion of external oblique. Hence, external oblique aponeurosis and internal oblique muscle are the most appropriate structure to get pierced. Linea alba lies in the midline, and rectus abdominis lies laterally on both sides of the linea alba, both unlikely to be pierced by the trocar in question.

Serial No. 172

Subject: Medicine

Topic: Gastro

Question: A 47-year-old man comes with 2 episodes of grossly bloody stools. He is a chronic alcoholic taking 10 units of alcohol per day. On examination he has raised alkaline phosphatase and bilirubin.

Single most likely diagnosis could be:

a. Alcoholic hepatitis
b. Chronic hepatitis
c. Viral hepatitis
d. Primary sclerosing cholangitis
e. Autoimmune hepatitis

Answer: (B) Chronic hepatitis

Explanation:
The patient is typically presenting with features of chronic liver disease secondary to alcohol consumption. While alcoholic hepatitis is an acute affection of liver following a bout of heavy alcohol consumption, repeated episodes of alcoholic hepatitis produces irreversible damage leading to alcoholic cirrhosis or chronic hepatitis. The 2 episodes of grossly bloody stools are suggesting portal hypertension and rectal varices (similar to esophageal varices, which can be the cause of life-threatening hematemesis). Grossly, the five sites of portosystemic anastomosis are in the regions of: lower end of oesophagus, upper end of anal canal, bare area of the liver, periumbilical region and retroperitoneal areas.

Serial No. 173

Subject: Pediatrics

Topic: Respiratory System

Question:
A boy is brought to A and E with complaints of barking cough associated with inspiratory and expiratory stridor; A diagnosis of laryngotrachebronchitis is reached.

What is the single most likely prognosis of the disease if left untreated ?

a. Bronchiectasis
b. Complete resolution
c. Lung abscess
d. Pneumonia
e. Bronchial asthma

Answer: (B) Complete resolution

Explanation:
Laryngotracheobronchitis or croup is a viral infection of the upper respiratory tract commonly affecting infants and toddlers. Parainfluenza viruses are the most common causative agent. A barking cough, stridor, and fever are characteristic. The disease is self-limited and the child only requires proper monitoring to prevent the development of respiratory obstruction from laryngeal edema. Treatment is aimed at keeping the patient well hydrated and preventing respiratory failure. To avoid confusion, bronchiectasis is a long-term complication of whooping cough (pertusis), not laryngotracheobronchitis.

Serial No. 174

Subject: Pediatrics

Topic: Renal

Question:

A boy develops generalized oedema with proteinuria +++1. He is started on steroids and improves.

What is the single best long-term prognosis of the disease?

a. Complete resolution
b. Recurrence with gradual resistant to steroids
c. Recurrence with full response to steroids
d. Chronic renal failure
e. Acute renal failure

Answer: (C) Recurrence with full response to steroids

Explanation:

The child most probably is suffering from minimal change disease, the most common cause of nephrotic syndrome in children, which usually presents with heavy proteinuria, generalized oedema and hypercholesterolemia. Minimal change disease is steroid responsive and usually does not lead to chronic renal failure. However, frequent relapses are common. Most relapses respond favourably to steroids curing more than 90% children. Frequent relapsers can become steroid dependent (*not* resistant). For steroid resistant cases the diagnosis should be reconsidered.

Serial No. 175

Subject: Medicine

Topic: Diabetes

Question:

A diabetic with blood pressure 140/90 and proteinuria 0.2 gm/litre.

The single most likely agent to offer him benefit is:

a. ACE inhibitors
b. Angiotensin inhibitors
c. Betablockers
d. Fibrates
e. Statins

Answer: (A) ACE inhibitors

Explanation:

The patient is clearly showing microalbuminuria which is described pathological albuminuria in the 30-200 mg/litre range which is not detectable by qualitive chemical dip sticks. Microalbuminuria is the earliest indicator of renal disease (nephropathy) attributable to diabetes. NICE recommends that if the screening is positive for microalbuminuria in a type 1 diabetic, then an ACE inhibitor should be used even if the patient is normotensive. For low risk cases, target BP is <= 140/80 mmHg and for high risk cases, target BP is 135/75 mmHg. According to NICE, 'LOW RISK' cases are those without proteinuria or microalbuminuria, and 'High Risk' cases are those with (microalbuminuria - albumin/creatinine ratio > = 2.5 mg/mmol (men) or 3.5 mg/mmol (women), or albumin concentration > = 20 mg/L and/or albumin/creatinine ratio greater than or equal to 30 mg/mmol or albumin concentration > = 200 mg/L). ACE inhibitors are single most strongly supported drugs prescribed as first line for renal as well as cardiovascular protection in the diabetics.
URL: **http: //www.nice.org.uk**

Serial No. 176

Subject: Gynaecology

Topic: Gynaecological malignancies

Question: A 30-year-old lady was treated successfully for CIN 2 two years back. She was a heavy smoker and discontinued smoking few months back. She was on oral contraceptives all these years, but now her partner uses condoms. She is anxious as her aunt died of ovarian carcinoma at the age of 48. The most important factor which puts her at the risk of ovarian cancer is:

a. Age
b. Family history
c. CIN 2
d. Smoking
e. Oral contraceptives

Answer: (B) Family history

Explanation:
Ovarian cancer is the 5th most common malignancy in females in the UK and causes the maximum number of deaths due to gynecological malignancies. Out of all the risk factors, family history is most strongly linked to the development of ovarian carcinomas. It follows an autosomal dominat inheritance and is linked to the BRCA 1 and 2 locus on chrmosome 17. One close relative affected - mother, sister - is associated with a three-fold increased risk of ovarian cancer, corresponding to a 2.5% risk of death from ovarian cancer by the age of 70 years; for two or more affected close relatives, the lifetime risk may be 30-40%. Other risk factors associated with ovarian cancer are nulliparity, first child after the age of 35 years, late age of menopause and white race. Oral contraceptives are protective by suppressing ovulation

Serial No. 177

Subject: Medicine

Topic: Electrolyte abnormality

Question:
A 59-year-old man underwent surgery for rectal carcinoma, has not yet opened his bowels. He complains of abdominal distension and NG tube is aspirating large amount of fluids.

Single most likely cause for his condition is:

a. Calcium 2.2 mmol/l
b. Potassium 2.4 mmol/litre
c. Sodium 128 mmol/litre
d. Chloride 94 mmol/litre
e. Bicarbonate 22.5 mmol/litre

Correct Answer: (B) Potassium 2.4 mmol/litre

Explanation:
The patient in question is apparently suffering from paralytic ileus, as is evident by abdominal distension, failure to pass flatus/faeces and the NG tubes aspirating large volumes of fluids. Any intra-abdominal surgery is likely to cause paralytic ileus because of transient ischaemia produced to the nerves supplying the gut wall. Moreover, opiates used in the postoperative period are also implicated in the causing ileus. Hypokalaemia is the single most common electrolyte abnormality known to cause paralytic ileus. Recall that the normal potassium level ranges between 3.5-5.0 mmol/L. Rest of the electrolyte values mentioned in the question are within normal limits.

Serial No. 178

Subject: Medicine

Topic: Headache

Question:

A 62-year-old lady comes with unilateral weakness of arm and headache. On examination the affected arm has brisk reflexes and increased tone. Rest all examination appears normal.

The single best investigation required to be done here:

a. Skull X-ray
b. CT scan head
c. Lumbar puncture
d. X-ray limb
e. Electromyography

Answer: (B) CT scan head

Explanation:

The presence of unilateral limb weakness along with brisk reflexes and increased tone are suggesting an upper motor neuron lesion. The accompanying headache is pointing in the direction of raised intracranial tension. All this providing a cumulative evidence of some intracranial mass, which is compressing the cortex representative area of the affected limb. CT scan head is the most likely to yield the mass occupying the cerebral hemispheres. The most likely cause in an aged female is metastasis from an extracranial malignancy.

Serial No. 179

Subject: Medicine

Topic: Electrolyte Imbalance

Question:

A 47-year-old female with carcinoma breast complains of intense thirst, polyuria and confusion.

The single best way to manage is by administrating:

a. Dexamethasone
b. Palmidronate
c. Fluid restriction
d. Insulin therapy
e. Calcium gluconate

Answer: (B) Palmidronate

Explanation:

Malignancy with osteolytic metastatic deposits (like, carcinoma breast, here) is the most common cause of hypercalcaemia in an elderly. In the young, primary hyperparathyroidism is the most important cause. The symptoms of hypercalcaemia are lethargy, bone pain, abdominal pain, peptic ulceration, constipation, dementia, depression, polyuria and polydypsia. In hypercalcaemia of malignancy, bisphosphonates are the treatment of choice, e.g. pamidronate, clodronate, etridonate. Pamidronate is the most potent and the commonly used one. This should be accompanied with adequate fluids (Normal saline). Oral steroids can be used as an adjunct in severe hypercalcaemia.

Serial No. 180

Subject: Ortho

Topic: Spine injuries

Question:

A man fell from scaffold to injure his spine. Investigation revealed damage to S1.

Which single symptom will correspond to this level of injury:

a. Bladder dysfunction
b. Bowel dysfunction
c. Limb weakness
d. Numbness of sacral area
e. Loss of ankle jerk

Answer: (E) Loss of ankle jerk

Explanation:

For an injury to cause lower limb weakness, the level of injury should be above L1. S1 is mainly concerned with the sensory innervation of the ankle (Fig. 26.1).

Impingement of the S1 nerve can lead to weakness with the large gastronemius muscle in the back of the calf, causing difficulty with foot push off. The S1 nerve root also supplies innervation for the ankle jerk, and a loss of this reflex indicates S1 impingement, although it does not create loss of function.

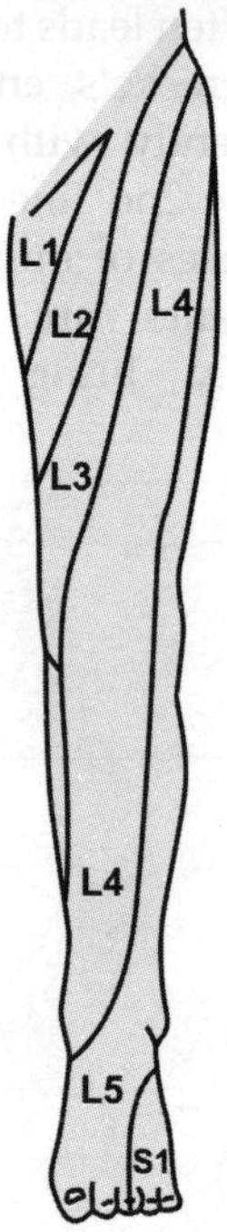

Fig. 26.1: Lower limb: Level of injury

Serial No. 181

Subject: Medicine

Topic: Dysphagia

Question:

A male complains of sudden onset dysphagia after eating bread which gets relieved by vomiting. He had 2 similiar episodes in last 3 years while having steaks. His BMI is 32.

The single most likely investigation which would lead to the diagnosis of his condition is:

a. Barium swallow
b. Chest X-ray
c. Motility studies
d. Esophgaoscopy
e. 24 hour esophageal pH monitoring

Answer: (A) Barium swallow

Explanation:

His BMI being on the higher side, he could have developed a benign stricture as a long-term complication of his being overweight (due to gastric relux), which could have caused this presenting symptom of intermittent dysphagia, which got relieved by vomiting. Esophageal spasm is another possibility but it should have presented more acutely, with chest pain on eating either very cold/hot food, which most likely induces spasm. In either case, a barium swallow is the most appropriate next diagnostic step, which would reveal a stricture or a 'corckscrew esophagus' (in case of esophageal spasm) or even achalasia cardia. Further tests for confirmation of diagnosis will be based on the findings observed on the barium swallow.

Serial No. 182

Subject: Medicine

Topic: Substance Abuse

Question:

A vagrant man, disheveled, sweating and fizzy. He is brought to A&E with seizures and dilated pupil.

Which is the single most likely substance he could be abusing:

a. Alcohol
b. Heroine
c. Cocaine
d. Cannabis
e. Solvent abuse

Answer: (C) Cocaine

Explanation:

Cocaine causes significant release of catecholmaines and the abuser usually presents with features similar to that seen in pheochromocytoma, viz excitement, flightiness, emotional instability, restlessness, irritability, apprehension, inability to sit still, teeth grinding, cold sweats, tremors, twitching of small muscles (especially of face, fingers, feet), muscle jerks, hallucinations (cocaine bugs, snow lights, voices and sounds, smells), and cocaine psychosis. Cocaine also lowers down the threshold for seizures and the patient often presents with extreme restlessness, seizures and dilated pupils. Note that alcohol *withdrawal* can also produce similar symptoms as that of cocaine abuse. The question has stressed specifically on *abuse* than withdrawal.

Serial No. 183

Subject: Medicine

Topic: Alcohol

Question:

A chronic alcoholic is brought to A/E in agitated state, picking at imaginary things. He is started on chlordiazepoxide.

The other single most important agent to be added to his treatment regimen should be:

a. Chlormethiazole
b. Thiamine
c. IV Glucose
d. Phenobarbitone
e. Phenothiazines

Answer: (B) Thiamine

Explanation:

The patient is showing features of alcohol withdrawal, typically delirium tremens which is a state of acute confusion characterized by restlessness, sweating, disorientation and often visual/aural hallucinations. Chlordiazepoxide is the preferred benzodiazepine for treating alcohol detoxification, because of its long half-life, and also because there is less likelihood of 'diversion' into the illicit drug scene. Diazepam is often a avoided because it often leads to abuse. Detoxification may precipitate Wernicke's encephalopathy, which must be treated urgently with parenteral thiamine. Chlormethiazole is the 2nd line of drug in inpatients and is not used in cases of outpatient detoxification. Routine anticonvulsants are not indicated and antipsychotics usually bring down the seizure threshold.

Serial No.184

Subject: Surgery

Topic: Head Injury

Question:

A female experienced sudden intense headache, while painting her bathroom wall. She fainted and hit her head. She was brought to A&E, where she regained her consciousness and is well otherwise, except for a small laceration on her skull.

The single most important investigation to be done at this stage is:

a. CT scan
b. Skull X-ray
c. Doppler
d. EEG
e. ECG

Answer: (A) CT scan

Explanation:

Although the patient appears to be fine now, leaving apart the small laceration on the skull, mentioned, we need to investigate the lady for the sudden headache, which had caused this fall and subsequent injuries. With the nature of the headache being sudden and intense in a previously healthy individual it is likely to be a subarachnoid bleed. A CT scan head is indicated to rule out the same.

Serial No. 185

Subject: Surgery

Topic: Trauma

Question:

A 27-year-old man is brought to A and E, with severe breathlessness following RTa. His breathlessness not relieved even after putting chest drain.

The single most likely cause could be:

a. Tension pneumothorax
b. Bronchial rupture
c. Aortic rupture
d. Simple Pneumothorax
e. Hemothorax

Answer: (B) Bronchial rupture

Explanation:

Tension pneumothorax or simple pneumothorax could have immediately responded to chest drain placement, which could have immediately helped in re-expansion of the collapsed lung. However, if the pneumothorax is communicating with the exterior (which happens in the cases of bronchial rupture), the atmospheric pressure in the pleural cavity equalizes with that of the atmosphere, and the amount of the air which is sucked out by the chest drain, is again sucked in by the bronchial communication, and the lungs remaining in the collapsed state. This is a rare injury and is usually associated with subcutaneous emphysema. CXR classically shows, 'Drop Lung Sign". Bronchoscopy and localization of the tear is the most useful investigation. Treatment is directed at suturing of the torn bronchial mucosa.

Serial No. 186

Subject: Pediatrics

Topic: Infection

Question:

A 20-day-old neonate is brought to A and E with temperature of 38.5ºC. He is otherwise appearing normal.

The single best next step should be:

a. Reassurance
b. Discharge with broad spectrum antibiotics
c. Admit for full infection screen
d. Admit for full infection screen and start broad spectrum antibiotics
e. Admit and observe

Answer: (C) Admit for full infection screen

Explanation:

The physical exam in a neonate is unreliable and the risk associated with an undetected severe infection is significant. A complete sepsis evaluation, antibiotic treatment, and hospital admission is recommended for febrile neonates. A full sepsis screen should be performed, including:

- Full blood count
- Urea and electrolytes, with glucose estimation
- Blood culture
- Chest radiology
- Lumbar puncture
- Bag urine or suprapubic aspirate of urine

No antibiotic therapy should be initiated in a stable patient until all cultures are obtained.

Serial No. 187

Subject: Medicine

Topic: Cardiology

Question:

A man with chronic atrial fibrillation develops features of pulmonary oedema.

Single best next step would be:

a. DC cardioversion
b. Anticoagulation and digoxin
c. Digoxin
d. Frusemide
e. Dopamine

Answer: (A) DC cardioversion

Explanation:

In a patient with chronic atrial fibrillation, DC cardioversion is indicated if the patient develops haemodynamic compromise. This patient being developing pulmonary oedema is signifying his compromised state and hence, DC cardioversion is most appropriate. Anticoaglution is definitely needed for a chronic AF patient, but here the immediate need is to restore the normal rhythm as fast as possible. Anticoagulation would provide only prophylaxis from embolic events and digoxin would take sometime(days to week) to act (because it takes at least a week for this dosage to build up to an effective therapeutic amount in the body, and that is why, digoxin is usually administered in haemodynamically stable patients).

Serial No. 188

Subject: Medicine

Topic: GIT

Question:

A patient with a long history of GORD, underwent esophago-duodenoscopy and a diagnosis of Barret's oesophagus was reached.

The single most appropriate term to define this condition would be:

a. Squamous metaplasia
b. Columnar metaplasia
c. Dysplasia
d. Neoplasia
e. Hyperplasia

Answer: (B) Columnar Metaplasia

Explanation:

Barret's oesophagus is a long-term complication of gastro-oesophageal reflux disease where, the normal squamous lining of the lower end of oesophagus is replaced by columnar epithelium (hence, columnar metaplasia). It is also known as intestinal or gastric metaplasia. It is a pre-malignant condition, leading to adenocarcinoma of the oesophagus, if left untreated.

Serial No. 189

Subject: Surgery

Topic: Varicose veins

Question:

A 30-year-old heavy smoker with previous history of treatment for DVT and varicose veins develops swelling and ulcer just above her medial malleolus surrounded by lipodermarosclerosis and induration on her right foot. She is currently on OCPs.

The single most likely cause for her foot condition is:

a. Varicose veins
b. DVT
c. Peripheral vascular disease
d. OCPs
e. Smoking

Correct Answer: (A) Varicose veins

Explanation:

She is classically presenting with a venous ulcer. Venous ulcers are usually found within the "gaiter" region of the lower leg i.e., below the bulge of the gastrocnemius and above the lower border of the malleoli of the ankle. The pigmentation, induration and lipodermatosclerosis, again confirming a venous ulcer due to venous stasis. The positive history of previous varicose veins and she being a chronic smoker as well as on OCPs, makes the picture complete. Moreover, varicose veins is more commonly seen in females because of muscle relaxing effects of progesterone, which decrease the tones in the venous channels causing venous stasis.

Serial No. 190

Subject: Medicine

Topic: GIT

Question:

A young girl complains of abdominal pain whenever in school. She is otherwise normal in public holidays and when her school is closed. Her epigastric pain is associated with nausea and no vomiting. She was also, needed to be sent home from school because of this abdominal pain on a number of occasions.

The single most likely diagnosis could be:

a. Abdominal Migraine
b. Coeliac disease
c. Appendicitis
d. Mesenteric adenitis.
e. Intussusception

Correct Answer: (A) Abdominal migraine

Explanation:

Abdominal migraine is a rare variant of classical migraine, which is characterized by recurrent excruciating abdominal pain which gets precipitated by triggers known or unknown to the patient. Common food triggers include chocolate, alcohol and red wine, certain cheeses, pickled meats containing nitrites or amines, and certain beans. Many non-food triggers also exist like emotional states, menstruation, hunger, intense sexual activity, smoking, computer screens and sleep deprivation can all trigger migraines. Abdominal migraine is typically more common in the adolescents where the triggering factor most commonly recognized is intense study or educational pressures.

Serial No. 191

Subject: Ortho

Topic: Fractures

Question:

A patient after a fall on his outstretched hands complains of pain in his wrist. X-ray of the wrist appears normal. No fracture is seen.

The single most appropriate next step should be:

a. Discharge with reassurance
b. Scaphoid cast for 6 weeks
c. Take X-ray at a later date
d. Plaster and review after 2 weeks
e. Open reduction

Answer: (D) Plaster and review after 2 weeks

Explanation:

Scaphoid fractures should be suspected in any cases pain wrist presenting after sustaining fall on outstretched hands. For cases where a fracture is suspected from clinical signs but not confirmed on X-ray, require complete immobilisation in a scaphoid cast. For a confirmed fracture, the cast is retained for 6 weeks. For a suspected fracture, the cast should be removed after 10 days and the injury re-evaluated with a repeat oblique X-ray.

Serial No. 192

Subject: Psychiatry

Topic: Anti-psychotics

Question:

A 25 years old man was recently admitted with severe depression complicated by psychosis now came in emergency because of worsening mental status and fever. He is unable to give history because he is profoundly confused and claimed to be on Mars. He was taking haloperidol and amitryptline. On examination: temperature 105° C, muscle rigidity and dry skin. (A) cooling blanket is ordered.

Which single most important agent should be ordered at this time?

a. Bromocriptine
b. Atropine
c. Lavretrenol
d. Chlorpheniramine
e. Methyl-prednisolone

Answer: (A) Bromocriptine

Explanation:

The patient is apparently suffering from neuroleptic malignant syndrome which was precipitated by haloperidol, he was started on for his psychosis. Discontinuation of the causative agent is the single most important step in treating neuroleptic malignant syndrome. Fluid replacement, fever reduction, and support of cardiac, respiratory, and renal function is required. Dopaminergic drugs such as bromocriptine or amantadine are used to counteract the presumed dopamine blockade that produces the symptoms of NMS. Dantrolene (skeletal muscle relaxant) can be used to decrease rigidity and, possibly, fever.

Serial No. 193

Subject: ENT

Topic: Tonsils

Question:

A man comes to OPD with earache. On examination his left tonsil is ulcerated with rolled out edges.

Single most likely diagnosis could be:

a. Carcinoma tonsil
b. Quinsy
c. Lymphoma
d. Abscess
e. Follicular tonsilitis

Answer: (A) Carcinoma tonsil

Explanation:

Squamous cell cancer is the most common neoplasm of the tonsil. Cigarette smoking and heavy drinking are common risk factors. Patient commonly presents with oropharyngeal pain, otalgia, dysphagia, weight loss and cervical lymphadenopathy. Surgery followed by radiation is the standard treatment for squamous cell carcinoma of the tonsil.

Serial No. 194

Subject: Psychiatry

Topic: Personality disorders

Question:

A patient comes again and again to his general physician saying that he is suffering from AIDs. His all results for HIV are negative, checked thrice.

The single most likely condition which describes his symptoms best is:

a. OCD
b. Hypochondriasis
c. Munchhausen's syndrome
d. Body dysmorphic disorder
e. Briquet syndrome

Answer: (B) Hypochondriasis

Explanation:

In hypochondriasis the patient is preoccupied with fancied bodily illness. The condition is defined in ICD 9 as a neurotic disorder in which the conspicuous features are excessive concern with one's health in general, in the integrity and functioning of some part of one's body or, less frequently, one's mind. Preoccupation occurs despite reassurance and showing all proofs against patients belief for the particular illness.

Munchausen syndrome is the habitual seeking of hospital or other medical treatment for apparent self inflicted, 'acute' illness giving a plausible and dramatic history. In body dysmorphic disorder patient has false belief that a part of his body is grossly dysmorphed. Briquet syndrome is hypochondriasis or somatization disorder with >13 unexplained symptoms in various organs.

Serial No. 195

Subject: Surgery

Topic: Postoperative complications

Question:

A 42-year-old man develops fever 48 hours after undergoing surgery. He has mild abdominal distension.

The single most likely cause for his fever could be:

a. Pleural effusion
b. UTI
c. Thrombophlebitis
d. Sepsis
e. DVT

Answer: (B) UTI

Explanation:

Mild pyrexia is common in postoperative period especially within 24 hr because of tissue damage and necrosis. However, a persistent high fever should initiate an infection screen. Most common causes which can present in with 48 hr with fever are pulmonary atelectasis and urinary tract infection (especially in catheterized patients). Pleural effusion is a very late complication and is usually associated with decreased chest movement than abdominal distension. Thrmobophlebitis and sepsis typically occur after 3-5 days. DVT would present with fever and calf pain. Fever with mild abdominal distension on 2nd postoperative day, goes more in favor of UTI as lower abdominal pain and distension are not uncommon association with UTI.

Serial No. 196

Subject: Surgery

Topic: Testes

Question:

A tall young guy is brought with acute onset scrotal pain associated with vomiting.

The single most likely diagnosis can be:

a. Testicular torsion
b. Torsion of appendicular appendage
c. Epididymo-orchitis
d. UTI
e. Scrotal abscess

Answer: (A) Testicular torsion

Explanation:

This is the classical presentation of torsion testes, which is apparently more common in tall visceroptic males, as the long stalk of testes give them more mobility and increase the chances of torsion. Presentation is typically with an acutely swollen and painful testis, lower abdominal pain and sometimes, vomiting. Acute epididymo-orchitis is typically associated with fever and local infection (urethritis). For torsion of testicular appendages, pain develops gradually over days and is not associated with systemic symptoms like nausea/ vomiting. Testes are not tender to palpation. The presence of a paratesticular nodule at the superior aspect of the testicle, with its characteristic blue-dot appearance, is pathognomonic for the torsion of testicular appendages.

Serial No. 197

Subject: Psychiatry

Topic: Mood disorders

Question:

A woman on postnatal period on being visited by midwife on the 4th day, is extremely worried about her kid. Her husband says she is showing mood changes and is extremely tearful sometimes. She is caring normally for the child.

The single most likely diagnosis is:

a. Postpartum psychosis
b. Postnatal blues
c. Postpartum depression
d. Mania
e. OCD

Answer: (B) Postnatal blues

Explanation:

Postnatal blues is characterized by rapidly fluctuating mood, tearfulness, irritability, and anxiety. Symptoms typically peak on the fourth or fifth day after delivery and last for several days, but they are generally time-limited and spontaneously remit within the first 2 postpartum weeks. Symptoms do not interfere with a mother's ability to function and to care for her child.

Serial No. 198

Subject: Psychiatry

Topic: Mood disorders

Question:

A 27-year-old female 7-10 days postpartum, is feeling depressed, worried and tearful. Recurring thoughts of harming baby disturbs her. She expresses her anxiety if she can take care of her baby properly.

The single most likely diagnosis is:

a. Postpartum psychosis
b. Postnatal blues
c. Postpartum depression
d. Mania
e. OCD

Answer: (C) Postpartum depression

Explanation:

Typically, postpartum depression develops insidiously over the first 3 postpartum months. Signs and symptoms are clinically indistinguishable from major depression that occurs in women at other times. Symptoms may include depressed mood, tearfulness, anhedonia, insomnia, fatigue, appetite disturbance, suicidal thoughts, and recurrent thoughts of death. Anxiety is prominent, including worries or obsessions about the infant's health and well-being. The mother may have ambivalent or negative feelings toward the infant. She may also have intrusive and unpleasant fears or thoughts about harming the infant. Postpartum depression often interferes with the mother's ability to care for herself or her child.

Postpartum psychosis is the most severe form of postpartum psychiatric illness, having a dramatic onset, emerging as early as the first 48-72 hours after delivery. The condition resembles a rapidly evolving manic or mixed episode with symptoms such as restlessness and insomnia, irritability, rapidly shifting depressed or elated mood, and disorganized behaviour. The mother may have delusional beliefs that relate to the infant (e.g., baby is defective or dying, infant is Satan or God), or she may have auditory hallucinations that instruct her to harm herself or her infant.

Serial No. 199

Subject: Medicine

Topic: Syncope

Question:

A 37-year-old lady experiences dizziness while looking back as she was reversing her car.

The single most likely cause for her presenting symptoms could be:

a. Vertebrobasilar insufficiency
b. Carotid artery insufficiency
c. Thoracic outlet syndrome
d. Migraine
e. Stroke

Answer: (A) Vertebrobasilar insufficiency

Explanation:

Carotid artery insufficiency would most likely produce symptoms corresponding to anterior circulation compromise viz, confusion, homonymous hemianopia, dysphasia. This lady is presenting with symptoms which is more characteristic of a posterior circulation compromise. More so, the mode by which the symptoms are precipitated is quite typical for vertebrobasilar insufficiency. Thoracic outlet syndrome would present with neurovascular compressive symptoms on the ulnar border of the arm on the affected side. Migraine or stroke, are not posture related, unlikely to be precipitated on turning head.

Serial No. 200

Subject: Paediatrics

Topic: Infectious diseases

Question:
Child after taking his MMR vaccination 2 weeks back comes with fever, headache, photophobia and a rapidly spreading purpuric rash.

The single most likely diagnosis is:

a. Anaphylaxis
b. Meningococcemia
c. Vaccine side effect
d. Aseptic meningitis
e. Measles

Answer: (B). Meningococcemia

Explanation:
Anaphylaxis or vaccine side effect is unlikely to present this way, more so when 2 weeks have already passed. The triad of fever, headache and photophobia is pointing towards meningitis, and the associated rapidly spreading purpuric rash is suggesting Neisseria meningitis as the causative organism. It is the most common cause of pyogenic meningitis in UK. Aseptic meningitis will not be associated with purpura.

PAPER 2

Serial No 171

Subject: Medicine

Topic: Drug Side effect

Question: A 42-year-old male expatriate is admitted semi-conscious being feverish with sweats. He is noted to have a temperature of 39.0°C and some neck stiffness. Thick blood film is positive for *Falciparum malaria* and he is started on medication.

The single most likely cause for his present condition is:

a. Septicemia
b. Aspirin overdosage
c. Quinine Therapy
d. Alcoholic binge
e. Postprandial hypoglycaemia

Correct Answer: (C) Quinine therapy

Explanation
Although all the listed options above can precipitate hypoglycaemia, the most important hint in the question is suggested by the fact that he is recently being diagnosed with Falciparum malaria and have been started on medications. For falciparum malaria, the treatment is usually aggressive and sudden surge of high levels of quinine in circulation is more likely to produce the side effects, hypoglycaemia being one of the most common ones. However, for future questions on this topic, don't forget that *Falciparum malaraia* can itself produce coma and coma-like states.

Serial No. 172

Subject: Pharmacology

Topic: Teratogenicity

Question: A 28-year-old lady in 20 weeks of gestation suffered a severe upper respiratory tract infection which she could manage to treat herself by taking high doses of azithromycin.

The single most likely theoretical risk to her baby could be:

a. VI Nerve damage
b. VII Nerve damage
c. VIII Nerve damage
d. II Nerve damage
e. I Nerve damage

Correct Answer: (C) VIII Nerve damage

Explanation

Aminoglycosides are known for long for their nephrotoxicity and ototoxicity, and thus their use is particularly contraindicated during pregnancy, for the fear of cause renal damage and VIII Nerve damage of the developing fetus. Most of the antiepileptics, Lithium and ACE- inhibitors are the common drugs which require reconsideration during pregnancy because of their imminent teratogenic effects.

Serial No. 173

Subject: Medicine

Topic: Hematology

Question: A 35-year-old man has an appendicectomy. 48 hours late he becomes febrile, hypotensive and unwell. Hb 12.8 g/dl , WBC 19.4 x 109/l , platelets 48 x 109/l Blood film shows a neutrophilia.

The single most likely cause of the thrombocytopenia could be:

a. Immune thrombocytopenia
b. Disseminated intravascular coagulation
c. Post-transfusion purpura
d. Heparin induce thrombocytopenia
e. Aplastic anaemia

Correct Answer: (B) Disseminated intravascular coagulation

Explanation

Infection, disseminated malignancy and obstetric complications are few common of the several causes that can precipitate DIC. This particular patient apparently developed septicaemia postoperatively which is evident by his raised temperature, hypotension and neutrophilia. The coagulation casacade once getting activated leads to the consumption of the clotting factors and also the platelets. This picture suggests DIC and demands immediate infusion of fresh frozen plasma while expert advice is sought.

Serial No. 174

Subject: Obstetrics and Gynaecology

Topic: Disorders of mensturation

Question: A 31-year-old woman complains of abdominal pain which seems to increase during her periods. Over the last year, she has noticed difficulty in breathing and chest pain associated with occasional haemoptysis, following her periods. She has been unable to conceive. On examination she is found to have an enlarged and tender uterus. Her BMI is 20.

The single most likely diagnosis is:

a. Possible malignancy
b. Polycystic ovarian disease
c. Adenomyosis
d. Endometriosis
e. Pulmonary tuberculosis

Correct Answer: (D). Endometriosis

Explanation

The characteristic abdominal pain which increases with her periods along with history of infertility goes in favour of the diagnosis of endometriosis. Her cyclical haemoptysis can be explained on the basis of being lungs also affected by the disease process. Adenomyosis is the most close differential diagnosis here, but cyclical haempotysis and infertility cant be explained on the basis of adenomysis. Widespread organ involvment is seen most characteristically with endometriosis. A typical description of adenomyosis would have been a multiparous female in late 30s-40s, presenting with gradually worsening dysmenorrhoea.

Serial No. 175

Subject: Medicine

Topic: Edocrinology

Question: A 45-year-old man complains of headaches, excessive thirst and frequent urination. On examination he is noted to have bad acne, coarse skin and has a goitre. He has moved his wedding band to the 5th finger.

The single most likely diagnosis is:

a. Hypothyroidism
b. Cushing's syndrome
c. Hysterical neurosis
d. Autonomic side effects
e. Acromegaly

Correct Answer: (E) Acromegaly

Explanation

The patient is clearly showing signs of excess soft tissue growth as evidenced by bad acne, coarse skin and moving his wedding band to the little finger. The presence of headache and features of diabetes insipidus hints towards some pituitary tumour, which in the presence of the above said features points towards a growth hormone secreting tumour. Goitre is due to secondary hypothyroidism seen in acromegaly.

Serial No. 176

Subject: Medicine

Topic: Infections

Question: A 35-year-old lady delivered a baby at term. She had Hepatitis B infection during pregnancy and is worried for the baby.

For the baby, it is required to give:

a. Hepatitis B Immunoglobulin alone
b. Hepatitis B Immunoglobulin and vaccine
c. Hepatitis B vaccine only
d. Interferon
e. None

Correct Answer: (B) Hepatitis B Immunoglobulin and vaccine

Explanation

Infection during preganancy exposes the fetus to high levels of viremia and it warrantes immediate protection. While it is of less important in a mother who already have had hepatitis B in the past and has efficient immunoglobulin levels to pass on to her baby, a mother who suffers an attack during pregnancy cant afford the same. Thus, it requires that the baby should be provided with both active and passive immunization at birth, for maximum protection.

Serial No. 177

Subject: Medicine

Topic: Chest

Question: A young thin man suddenly become breathless.On examination, air entry is reduced in left side and no movement in right side.Trachea is deviated to left.

The single most important initial management should be:

a. Chest drain to right lung
b. Chest drain to left lung
c. Wide bore needle to right pleural cavity
d. Wide bore needle to left pleural cavity
e. Take a chest X-ray immediately

Correct Answer: (D) Wide bore needle to right pleural cavity

Explanation

The diminished air entry on the left side is apparently due to the mediastinal shift which is caused by the tension pneumothorax on the right, which is suggested by absent movement on the right side. The condition requires immediate insertion of a wide bore needle on the side of the pneumothorax which is later replaced by an under water drainage of the residual air.

Serial No 178

Subject: Medicine

Topic: Infections

Question: An 18-year-old student has come back from Ghana. He was taking anti-malarials for 2 weeks after he returned home. He has a temp of 39.5 C and is vomiting. He is now sensitive to light and has a stiff neck.

The single most useful investigation would be:

a. CT scan
b. MRI
c. Lumbar puncture
d. Thick and thin smear
e. Blood culture

Correct Answer: (D) Thick and thin smear

Explanation

It is most important in this case is to rule out a possibility of Falciparum malaraia, taking in view his recent travel to an endemic region and that he did not take the anti malarial prophylaxis for the required duration. A thick and thin smear at this stage would be the most appropriate investigation at this stage. Although his presenting feature is that of meningitis, a lumbar puncture would not reveal much info, as most likely we are dealing with a case of cerebral malaria.

Serial No. 179

Subject: Medicine

Topic: Haematology

Question: A woman has had severe rheumatoid arthritis for 12 years. She has been on long-term methotrexate and naproxen for years. Her blood investigations reveal Hb 9.8, MCV 72, Reticulocytes 6% . The most likely diagnosis is:

a. Macrocytic anaemia
b. Folic acid deficiency
c. Chronic gastrointestinal blood loss
d. Anaemia of chronic disease
e. Haemolytic anaemia

Correct Answer: (C) Chronic gastrointestinal Blood Loss

Explanation

Although it is very alluring to go for a diagnosis of Anaemia of chronic disease in this case, however, do not forget that we do not get reticulocytosis in anemia of chronic disease. Morever, a MCV of 72 is pointing towards a Microcytic anaemia rather than a Normocytic anaemia (as it would have been expected in anaemia of chronic disease). For Normocytic anaemia, MCV range between 80 and 100 fl. while, for microcytic anaemia it is usually <80 fl. This lady is probably suffering from iron deficiency anaemia secondary to chronic GI blood loss owing to her long-term NSAIDs use.

Serial No. 180

Subject: Paediatrics

Topic: Neonatal jaundice

Question: A 4-week-old baby is noticed to have breast milk jaundice. Otherwise the baby is well and developing.

The single most appropriate mode of action would be to:

a. Continue breast milk
b. Increased fluid intake
c. Phototherapy
d. Exchange transfusion
e. Stop breast milk

Correct Answer: (A) Continue breast milk

Explanation

The main aim of treaing a neonatal jaundice is to avoide neuronal damage due to high levels of bilirubin. As because this baby is thriving well and is otherwise healthy, little or no intervention is required, apart from keeping a vigilant eye on the bilirubin levels. Breast milk jaundice can sometimes occur due to immature enzymes in the baby. This gradually resolves by itself and seldom requires discontinuation of the breast milk.

Serial No. 181

Subject: Medicine

Topic: GIT

Question: A 24-year-old woman has had 24 hours of vomiting and diarrhoea 'which she thinks followed eating reheated take away food. There was fresh blood in the last three vomitus. Vital signs are stable.

The single most likely diagnosis is:

a. Gastric erosions
b. Acute gastroenteritis
c. Oesophageal varices
d. Mallory Weiss tear
e. Bleeding diathesis

Correct Answer: (D) Mallory Weiss tear

Explanation

Remember that, whenever there is a history of repeated vomiting and then hematemesis, the most likely diagnosis is Mallory Weiss tear. This lady was vomiting since 24 hr and now blood in vomitus - its mallory Weiss, straight! A similar picture is also presented when the patient is usually an alcoholic or a teenager with a diagnosis of bulimia. Just be aware of the general sequence of the events.

Serial No.182

Subject: Surgery

Topic: Head injury

Question:

A female experienced sudden intense headache, while painting her bathroom wall. She fainted and hit her head. She was brought to A and E, where she regained her consciousness and is well otherwise, except for a small laceration on her skull.

The single most important investigation to be done at this stage is:

a. CT scan
b. Skull X-ray
c. Doppler
d. EEG
e. ECG

Answer: (A) CT scan

Explanation:

Although the patient appears to be fine now, leaving apart the small laceration on the skull, mentioned, we need to investigate the lady for the sudden headache, which had caused this fall and subsequent injuries. With the nature of the headache being sudden and intense in a previously healthy individual it is likely to be a subarachnoid bleed. A CT scan head is indicated to rule out the same.

Serial No. 183

Subject: Medicine

Topic: Electrolyte imbalance

Question:

A 47-year-old female with carcinoma breast complains of intense thirst, polyuria and confusion.

The single best way to manage is by administrating:

a. Dexamethasone
b. Palmidronate
c. Fluid restriction
d. Insulin therapy
e. Calcium gluconate

Answer: (B) Palmidronate

Explanation:

Malignancy with osteolytic metastatic deposits (like, carcinoma breast, here) is the most common cause of hypercalcaemia in an elderly. In the young, primary hyperparathyroidism is the most important cause. The symptoms of hypercalcaemia are lethargy, bone pain, abdominal pain, peptic ulceration, constipation, dementia, depression, polyuria and polydypsia. In hypercalcaemia of malignancy, bisphosphonates are the treatment of choice, e.g. pamidronate, clodronate, etridonate. Pamidronate is the most potent and the commonly used one. This should be accompanied with adequate fluids (Normal saline). Oral steroids can be used as an adjunct in severe hypercalcaemia.

Serial No. 184

Subject: Medicine

Topic: Substance Abuse

Question:

A vagrant man, disheveled, sweating and fizzy. He is brought to A and E with seizures and dilated pupil.

Which is the single most likely substance he could be abusing:

a. Alcohol
b. Heroine
c. Cocaine
d. Cannabis
e. Solvent abuse

Answer: (C) Cocaine

Explanation:

Cocaine causes significant release of catecholmaines and the abuser usually presents with features similar to that seen in pheochromocytoma, viz excitement, flightiness, emotional instability, restlessness, irritability, apprehension, inability to sit still, teeth grinding, cold sweats, tremors, twitching of small muscles (especially of face, fingers, feet), muscle jerks, hallucinations (cocaine bugs, snow lights, voices and sounds, smells), and cocaine psychosis. Cocaine also lowers down the threshold for seizures and the patient often presents with extreme restlessness, seizures and dilated pupils. Note that alcohol *withdrawal* can also produce similar symptoms as that of cocaine abuse. The question has stressed specifically on *abuse* than withdrawal.

Serial No. 185

Subject: Medicine

Topic: Cardiology

Question:

A man with chronic atrial fibrillation develops features of pulmonary oedema.

Single best next step would be:

a. DC cardioversion
b. Anticoagulation and digoxin
c. Digoxin
d. Frusemide
e. Dopamine

Answer: (A) DC cardioversion

Explanation:

In a patient with chronic atrial fibrillation, DC cardioversion is indicated if the patient develops hemodynamic compromise. This patient being developing pulmonary oedema is signifying his compromised state and hence, DC cardioversion is most appropriate. Anticoagulation is definitely needed for a chronic AF patient, but here the immediate need is to restore the normal rhythm as fast as possible. Anticoagulation would provide only prophylaxis from embolic events and digoxin would take sometime (days to week) to act (because it takes at least a week for this dosage to build up to an effective therapeutic amount in the body, and that is why, digoxin is usually administered in hemodynamically stable patients).

Serial No. 186

Subject: Surgery

Topic: Trauma

Question: A butcher cut himself in the groin area. He used a towel, which is full of blood. On examination the BP was 80/60 and pulse rate 130.

The estimated amount of blood loss is:

a. 250 ml
b. 500 ml
c. 750 ml
d. 1000 ml
e. 1500 ml

Correct Answer: (E) 1500 ml

Explanation

This person is showing tachycardia with a fall in both systolic and diastolic blood pressure, seen in a Class III hypovolemic shock, where the blood loss is usually between 1500 and 2000 ml.

Classification of hypovolemic shock

Class I	*Class II*	*Class III*	*Class IV*
Loss upto 750 ml	Loss of 750-1500 ml	Loss of 1500-2000 ml	Loss >2 litres
Minimal tachycardia No changes in BP, pulse respiratory rate	PR > 100 bpm Decreased pulse pressure Increased diastolic BP	Marked Tachypnoea and tachycardia Decreased systolic BP	Life threatening Class III features with markedly decreased urine output and obtunded consciousness

Serial No. 187

Subject: Medicine

Topic: Cardiology

Question: A 45-year-old man has developed left ventricular failure 2 weeks after an attack of myocardial infarction, which was successfully controlled by diuretics. The ECHO shows poor left ventricular function.

The single most proven drug class beneficial for this patient would be:

a. Beta blockers
b. Calcium channel blockers
c. ACE inhibitors
d. Aspirin
e. Clopidogrel

Correct Answer: (C) ACE Inhibitor

Explanation:

It is a standard practice to start an ACE inhibitor drug on all patients who demonstrate a compromised left ventricular function post MI. Studies have shown that acute large anterior myocardial infarctions have favourable mortality experience if Captopril 6.25 mg four times a day is begun even at the time of thrombolysis.

Serial No. 188

Subject: Obstetrics and Gynaecology

Topic: Ca Cervix

Question: A lady presents for follow-up six months after cervical smear was done showing mild atypia (CIN II) on the previous smear. On examination, ulcerated cervix found.

The single most appropriate step at this stage would be to go for:

a. Another cervical smear
b. Colposcopy
c. Urgent colposcopy
d. Urgent Biopsy
e. Urgent colposcopy and biopsy

Correct Answer: (E) Urgent colposcopy and biopsy

Explanation:

Previous history of CIN II with ulceration on the cervix now places this lady at a higher risk for invasive carcinoma cervix. Another cervical smear wont be of any help, as it would show only more atypia. What is required is careful inspection of the involved area and if small, the biopsy will help both, diagnostically and therapeutically.

Serial No. 189

Subject: Surgery

Topic: Acute abdomen

Question: A 60-year-old patient presents with fever and pain in the left iliac fossa. He appears flushed and takes care to remain still. On examination, there is a tender mass palpable in the left iliac fossa.

The single best procedure that would be of help to diagnose the condition would be:

a. Abdominal ultrasound
b. Sigmoidoscopy
c. Colonoscopy
d. CT scan abdomen and pelvis
e. Barium enema

Correct Answer: (D) CT scan abdomen and pelvis

Explanation:

This patient is apparently suffering from acute diverticulitis. The pain usually starts suddenly and is exacerbated even by slightest movement. However, diverticular disease is a diagnosis of exclusion. Other conditions especially Inflammatory Bowel Disease and carcinoma colon should be carefully ruled out. Barium meal, barium enema and sigmoidoscopy are the usual first line investigations. However, all these invasive investigations should be deferred until the acute stage gets settled, for the risk of perforation remains very high. A bedside ultrasound, although would be useful in excluding peritonitis or perforation, however, a CT scan would be just perfect at this stage to confirm the diagnosis as well as rule out other possible diagnosis.

Serial No. 190

Subject: Pharmacology

Topic: Antibiotics

Question: Trimethoprim was advised for a child weighing 10 kg, in a dose 4 mg/kg twice daily. The available pharmacological preparation contains 50 mg/5 ml.

The single most appropriate prescription for the drug would be:

a. 0.4 ml twice daily
b. 4 ml twice daily
c. 0.8 ml twice daily
d. 1 ml twice daily
e. 2 ml twice daily

Correct Answer: (B) 4 ml Twice daily

Explanation:
A child weighing 10 kg, when prescribed a drug at 4 mg/kg, would need:

- (10 X 4) mg of the drug twice daily
- 40 mg twice daily.

  Now, 50 mg drug is present in 5 ml of solution,
- 40 mg drug should be present in (5/50) X 40 ml
- 4 ml

So, as he needs 40 mg twice daily, 4 ml twice daily would be just appropriate.

Serial No. 191

Subject: Ophthalmology

Topic: Conjunctiva

Question: A 25-year-old farmer complains of redness and grittiness in his eyes. On examination, no foreign body is found.

The single most useful agent for him would be:

a. Local antibacterial
b. Local antihistaminic
c. Local antifungal
d. Local anesthetic
e. Local antibiotic

Correct Answer: (B) Local antihistaminic

Explanation:
This is an obvious case of conjunctivitis as is evidenced by redness and grittiness in the eyes in the absence of any foreign bodies. The only other clue in the question is the patient being a 'farmer'. Allergic conjunctivitis is usually suspected in patients with occupational exposure to pollen or hay. Look also for hints such as seasonal recurrence of symptoms, presence of any other allergic diseases viz, asthma, hay fever, eczema. Treatment is usually by topical antihistamine drops. Drops such as sodium cromoglycate can be used to prevent the allergic response and they need to be used for many weeks in order to give any result. Corticosteroid drops are occasionally used, but should only be used under the supervision of an ophthalmologist. The main treatment should be identifying what is triggering off the allergic response and removing this source of allergen.

Serial No. 192

Subject: Obstetrics and Gynaecology

Topic: Cervix

Question: A 38-year-old lady, mother of 4 children and now in 30th week of pregnancy, presents with blood tinged watery discharge from vagina 3 weeks duration. On examination, there appears a 'raw' ring around the Os.

The single most likely diagnosis is:

a. Cervical carcinoma
b. Genital herpes
c. Cervical ectropion
d. Vaginitis
e. Marginal sinus bleed

Correct Answer: (A) Cervical Ectropion

Explanation:

Cervical erosion or ectropion is a common condition, especially in high estrogenic stages. The squamous epithelium of the cervix is replaced by the columnar epithelium of the endocervix and appears as a red ring or 'raw' area around the Os. A pregnant cervix is very soft and is prone to bleed very easily. Usually the condition resolves by itself, however, a pap smear is necessary to rule out a possibility of infections or cervical carcinoma.

Serial No. 193

Subject: Obstetrics and Gynaecology

Topic: Cervix

Question: A 16-year-girl with multiple sexual partners presents with painless post coital bleeding.

The single most important investigation required at this stage is:

a. Pap smear
b. Biopsy
c. Colposcopy and biopsy
d. Speculum examination
e. Gram staining

Correct Answer: (D) Speculum examination

Explanation:

Although the clinical presentation looks more like a carcinoma cervix, it's a very rare possibility at 16 years of age. We ought to rule out other possibilities like cervical erosion (possibility of regular OCPs cannot be ruled out) and infections. The best thing to do at this stage will be to have look at the cervix and then take a smear or do a gram staining, if required.

Serial No. 194

Subject: Medicine

Topic: CNS/CVS

Question: A lady over 40 years of age presents with repeated episodes of amaurosis fugax, with complete recovery after the attacks. What is the single most appropriate investigation that would diagnose the condition:

a. CT scan
b. Carotid Doppler
c. Echocardiography
d. MRI
e. Transcranial Doppler

Correct Answer: (B) Carotid Doppler

Explanation:

Amaurosis fugax (AF) is a painless, monocular loss of vision, which may be total or sectorial. This is a traditional blackout of the patient's vision. Vision loss typically lasts only seconds, but may last for hours and will resolve completely. There are no other neurological symptoms or findings in association with AF. AF result from either an embolic, thrombotic, vasospastic, or hematological phenomenon. Such patients usually require referral to a neurologist since other neurological areas are involved in the attack. They are required to be sent for carotid artery studies, such as Doppler imaging or magnetic resonance angiography to check if there is significant stenosis of the carotid artery, and then to consider for a possible endarterectomy. However, these patients are typically medicated with blood thinners such as aspirin and they do quite well. Typically, this patient requires carotid endarterectomy. Amaurosis fugax in elderly patients may be the initial sign of giant cell arteritis. The single most important *haematological* cause for AF is Sickle cell anaemia.

Serial No. 195

Subject: Medicine

Topic: Chest

Question: A 60-year-old man presents with progressive dyspnoea and massive left-sided pleural effusion.

The single best diagnostic procedure that would diagnose the condition is:

a. CXR
b. Pleural biopsy
c. Aspiration
d. Ultrasound
e. Bronchoscopy

Correct Answer: (C) Aspiration

Explanation:

This is a controversial question. While some students are in favour of pleural biopsy, others are in favour of aspiration. The case is most likely a case of lung or pleural malignancy. Progressive dyspnoea and massive pleural effusion can be present in either of the two. Considering his massive pleural effusion, which anyway would be required to be aspirated, in my opinion, aspiration would be the best possible investigation as it will help us both diagnostically and therapeutically. Moreover, a blind pleural biopsy is more likely to miss the pathology if not guided by a CT, especially if the malignancy is arising from lungs rather than pleura.

Serial No. 196

Subject: Psychiatry

Topic: Personality Disorders

Question: A 20-year-old student after being transferred to a new school has insomnia and loses weight. He does not mix with people and does not attend programmes as he thinks there will be a lot of germs over there. He lags behind in school work as he does all his work very perfectly.

The single most likely diagnosis is:

a. Adjustment disorder
b. Obsessive compulsive disorder
c. Post-traumatic stress disorder
d. Depression
e. Autism

Correct Answer: (B) Obsessive Compulsive Disorder

Explanation

Obsessive compulsive disorder (OCD), is the diagnosis here based on the hints of this patient's 'perfect' behaviour and avoiding mixing with people and going to places because of the fear of getting contaminated. Although this question is not giving us direct hint that this patient washes his hands very frequently, careful eliciting of the history would always reveal that. Insomnia and loosing weight is signifying depression, which is again a usual association with OCD. It cannot be adjustment disorder, as the 'fear of germs' doesn't really fit in there. It cannot be Post-traumatic stress disorder as it needs to be followed by some major life event. Autism is associated with stereotyped behaviour not 'perfection' or fear of germs.

Serial No. 197

Subject: Surgery

Topic: Acute Abdomen

Question: A 76-year-old known hypertensive comes to the casualty ward with a painful abdominal mass. On examination, he has a pulsatile abdominal mass and is having a BP of 70/40 and a pulse rate of 120 bpm.

The single most appropriate management option for this patient would be:

a. CT scan abdomen
b. Transfuse till systolic BP 90 mmHg
c. Transfuse till systolic BP 120 mmHg
d. Per abdomen examination
e. Diagnostic peritoneal lavage

Correct Answer: (B) Transfuse till systolic BP 90 mmHg

Explanation

This is a case of abdominal aortic aneurysm (AAA) and hypotension with tachycardia is signifying that the aneurysm has ruptured. The idea is to maintain perfusion by transfusing blood till systolic BP 90 is attained. A higher systolic BP would confer excess fluid load, excess work by the heart and increases the risk of dissection. Any manipulation of the abdomen, in the form of per abdominal examination or DPL would only prove drastic to this already compromised patient.

Serial No 198

Subject: Medicine

Topic: Anaphylaxis

Question: A 14-year-old boy suddenly develops difficulty in breathing with red oedematous lips after eating peanuts.

The single most likely diagnosis is:

a. Aspiration
b. Asthma
c. Meckel's syndrome
d. Anaphylaxis
e. Shock

Correct Answer: (D) Anaphylaxis

Explanation:

The symptoms clearly signify anaphylactic reaction and the precipitating factor here is peanuts. Although not so widely known, peanut allergy is prevalent in appreciable number of population. The patients with recognized peanut allergy should be treated like any other allergies. These patients should be clearly informed to avoid food, which might contain peanuts. Opening peanut packets or even handling peanuts can sometimes precipitate an anaphylaxis especially when in a closed space like an aircraft. All necessary precautions should be taken to tackle anaphylaxis at anytime.

Serial No. 199

Subject: Pharmacology

Topic: Drug Side effect

Question: A 25-year-old patient on lithium now comes to you with tremors of hand.

The single most helpful investigation would be:

a. Thyroid function test
b. Lithium levels
c. ECHO
d. Doppler
e. USG

Correct Answer: (B) Lithium levels

Explanation:

Although its very alluring to go with thyroid function tests as answer to this question, however, two important facts should be kept in mind. First, that the thyroid manifestation of lithium therapy usually presents as hypothyroidism. Hyperthyroidism, especially thyrotoxicosis is an uncommon manifestation of lithium therapy. Second important fact is that, lithium has a very narrow therapeutic range and lithium toxicity usually presents as tremor and labile blood pressure. Hence, the most important step in this patient will be to rule out lithium toxicity.

Serial No. 200

Subject: Paediatrics

Topic: Metabolic Diseases

Question: A six months old child, can smile, but has head lag.

The single most likely diagnosis is:

a. Fragile X syndrome
b. Tay-Sachs disease
c. Ducchene's muscular atrophy
d. Foetus alcohol syndrome
e. Hypothyroidism

Correct Answer: (B) Tay-Sachs Disease

Explanation

The presenting features are typical of Tay-Sachs disease. Here, early development is normal but at around the age of 4-6 months, the child does not sit up, loses head control and takes no interest in the environment.

For Fragile X syndrome, hints like large ears, testis with mental retardation in the child and similar history in the male members of the family would have been given. Ducchene's muscular dystrophy mainly presents with gradual muscular weakness and typical 'Gower's Sign.' Fetal alcohol syndrome will have facial abnormalities, with impaired development of midline structures (viz, cleft lip, cleft palate). Congenital hypothyroidism would have presented with coarse skin, shriek voice and overall developmental delay.

Section 4

Single Best Answers—Question Bank

1. A homeless alcoholic with a chronic productive cough, presents with haemoptysis. The chest X-ray shows a cavitating lesion.

   What is the single most likely causative organism?
   A. *Chlamydia psittaci*
   B. *Mycobacterium tuberculosis*
   C. *Staphylococcus aureus*
   D. *Haemophilus influenzae*
   E. *Streptococcus pneumoniae*

2. A 50-year-old man became suddenly breathless whilst eating. He has marked stridor and is choking and drooling.

   What is the single most next appropriate step in management?
   A. IV aminophylline
   B. Pleural aspiration
   C. Heimlich maneuver
   D. Chest drain
   E. IV frusemide

3. A 60-year-old man presents with acute breathlessness and a cough productive of frothy, pink sputum. He cannot lie flat. On examination he has crackles in both midzones and a few scattered wheezes.

   What is the single most next appropriate step in management?
   A. Chest drain
   B. IV frusemide
   C. Rapid infusion of saline
   D. Forced alkaline diuresis
   E. Intramuscular adrenaline

4. A 20-year-old woman is too breathless to speak. Her pulse is 120/min respiratory rate 30/min and PEFR is 100 L/min. Examination reveals a very quiet chest and CXR is normal.

   What is the single most next appropriate step in management?
   A. Nebulisd salbutamol
   B. IV aminophylline
   C. Pleural aspiration
   D. Heimlich maneuver
   E. Chest drain

5. A chronic smoker with COPD develops a fever. He reports bringing up green phlegm on coughing.

   What is the single most likely causative organism?
   A. *Staphylococcus aureus*
   B. *Haemophilus influenzae*
   C. *Streptococcus pneumoniae*
   D. *Chlamydia trachomatis*
   E. *Mycoplasma pneumoniae*

6. A young male homosexual with Kaposi's sarcoma complains of increasing breathlessness and a dry cough.

   What is the single most likely causative organism?
   A. *Chlamydia trachomatis*
   B. *Mycoplasma pneumoniae*
   C. *Pneumocystis carinii*
   D. *Legionella pneumoniae*
   E. *Klebsiella pneumoniae*

7. A 25-year-old man has a 3 day history of shivering, general malaise and productive cough. The X-ray shows right lower lobe consolidation.

   What is the single most likely causative organism?
   A. *Mycobacterium tuberculosis*
   B. *Mycoplasma pneumoniae*
   C. *Pneumocystis carinii*
   D. *Staphylococcus aureus*
   E. *Streptococcus pneumoniae*

8. A 26-year-old man presents with severe shortness of breath and dry cough which he has had for 24hrs. He is very distressed. He has been on IV drug abuser. The X-ray shows perihilar fine mottling.

   What is the single most likely causative organism?
   A. Mixed growth of organisms
   B. *Mycobacterium tuberculosis*
   C. *Mycoplasma pneumoniae*
   D. *Pneumocystis carinii*
   E. *Staphylococcus aureus*

9. A 35-year-old previously healthy man returned from holiday five days ago. He smokes 10 cigarettes per day. He presents with mild confusion, a dry cough and mild pyrexia. His chest is normal. The X-ray shows widespread upperzone shadowing.

   What is the single most likely causative organism?
   A. *Legionella pneumophila*
   B. Mixed growth of organisms
   C. *Mycobacterium tuberculosis*
   D. *Mycoplasma pneumoniae*
   E. *Pneumocystis carinii*

10. A 20-year-old previously healthy woman presents with general malaise, severe cough and breahlessness, which has not improved with a 7 day course of amoxicillin. There is nothing significant to find on examination. The X-ray shows patchy shadowing throughout the lung fields. The blood film shows clumping of red cells with suggestion of cold agglutinins.

What is the single most likely causative organism?

A. Mixed growth of organisms
B. *Mycobacterium tuberculosis*
C. *Mycoplasma pneumoniae*
D. *Pneumocystis carinii*
E. *Staphylococcus aureus*

11. A 35-year-old woman presents with 4-month history of cough, productive and recent haemoptysis. She has lost 5 kg in weight. The CXR shows right upper lobe consolidation.

What is the single most likely diagnosis?

A. *Streptococcus pneumoniae*
B. Influenza
C. Tuberculosis
D. *Klebsiella pneumoniae*
E. Viral

12. A previously well 18-year-old has had influenza for the last 2 weeks. She is deteriorating and has a swinging fever. She is coughing up copious purulent sputum. CXR shows cavitating lesions.

What is the single most likely diagnosis?

A. Influenza
B. Tuberculosis
C. *Klebsiella pneumoniae*
D. Viral
E. Lung cancer

13. A 65-year-old man currently undergoing chemotherapy of chronic leukemia has felt unwell with fever and unproductive cough for 2 weeks despite treatment with broad-spectrum IV antibiotics. The CXR shows an enlarging right sided mid zone consolidation.

What is the single most likely diagnosis?

A. Fungal
B. *Streptococcus pneumoniae*
C. Influenza
D. Tuberculosis
E. *Klebsiella pneumoniae*

14. A 27-year-old male prostitute has felt generally unwell for 2 months with some weight loss. Over the last 3 weeks he has noticed a dry cough with increasing breathlessness. Two courses of antibiotics from the GP have produced no improvement. The CXR shows bilateral interstitial infiltrates.

What is the single most likely diagnosis?

A. *Streptococcus pneumoniae*
B. *Haemophilus influenzae*
C. Tuberculosis
D. *Klebsiella pneumoniae*
E. *Pneumocystis carinii*

15. On return to university, a 20-year-old student presented with the onset of fever, malaise and a dry cough. The student health service gave him amoxicillin. After a week he felt no better and his CXR showed patchy bilateral consolidation.

What is the single most likely diagnosis?

A. *Klebsiella pneumoniae*
B. Viral
C. Lung cancer
D. *Legionella pneumoniae*
E. *Mycoplasma pneumoniae*

16. A 64-year-old man with COPD presents with pneumonia. Clinically he improves with antibiotics. In the out patient clinic 4 weeks later, the consolidation on his CXR has not resolved.

What is the single most likely diagnosis?

A. *Haemophilus influenzae*
B. Tuberculosis
C. *Klebsiella pneumoniae*
D. Viral
E. Lung cancer

17. A 27-year-old male patient has just returned from holiday abroad presents with flu like illness, headache, high fever prior to this, he had complained of abdominal pain, vomiting, diarrhoea associated with blood per rectum.

What is the single most likely diagnosis?

A. *Klebsiella pneumoniae*
B. Viral
C. Lung cancer
D. *Legionella pneumoniae*
E. *Mycoplasma pneumoniae*

18. A 30-year-old obese man complains of retrosternal chest pain worse at night and after meals.
What is the single most appropriate investigation?
A. Pulmonary angiography
B. Gastroscopy
C. Cardiac catheterization
D. Oesophagoscopy
E. Indirect laryngoscopy

19. A 32-year-old woman who works in a pet shop complains of fever, a dry cough and increasing breathlessness.
What is the single most likely causative organism?
A. *Chlamydia psittaci*
B. *Mycoplasma tuberculosis*
C. *Staphylococcus aureus*
D. *Haemophilus influenzae*
E. *Streptococcus pneumoniae*

20. A 30-year-old woman has just returned from a holiday in Cyprus. She complains of a dry cough, fever, malaise. A CXR shows patchy consolidation.
What is the single most likely causative organism?
A. *Mycoplasma pneumoniae*
B. *Pneumocystis carinii*
C. *Legionella pneumoniae*
D. *Klebsiella pneumoniae*
E. *Mycobacterium tuberculosis*

21. A 34-year-old man presents with history of chest pain radiating to the jaw, brought on by exercise and relieved by rest.
What is the single most appropriate investigation?
A. CT scan
B. ECG
C. USG
D. ECHO
E. Pulmonary angiography

22. A 67-year-old woman presents with a 2 hr history of chest pain radiating to the left shoulder. He is sweating and feels sick.
What is the single most appropriate investigation?
A. CXR
B. CT scan
C. EEG
D. ECG
E. ECHO

23. A tall young man presents with history of sudden chest pain radiating to the back and interscapular area.
What is the single most appropriate investigation?
A. CT scan
B. USG
C. ECG
D. ECHO
E. Pulmonary angiography

24. A 52-year-old woman on HRT presents with swollen left calf, chest pain and shortness of breath.
What is the single most likely disease process?
A. Pulmonary embolism
B. Pneumonia
C. Bronchial asthma
D. Pleural effusion
E. Cryptogenic fibrosing alveolitis

25. A 78-year-old man has been short of breath for a few weeks. His chest radiography shows a right basal shadow rising towards axilla.
What is the single most likely disease process?
A. Pulmonary embolism
B. Pneumonia
C. Bronchial asthma
D. Pleural effusion
E. Cryptogenic fibrosing alveolitis

26. A 45-year-old woman presents with progressive breathlessness and cyanosis. Clinical examination reveals clubbing and bilateral inspiratory crackles.
What is the single most likely disease process?
A. Pulmonary embolism
B. Pneumonia
C. Bronchial asthma
D. Pleural effusion
E. Cryptogenic fibrosing alveolitis

27. A 27-year-old farmer presented with fever, malaise, cough and breathlessness which he has had for a few days. His symptoms were worse in the evening. Clinical examination demonstrated coarse end inspiratory crackles.
What is the single most likely disease process?
A. Anaemia
B. Pulmonary oedema
C. Bronchogenic carcinoma
D. Extrinsic allergic alveolitis
E. Pneumothorax

28. A 34-year-old tall slim porter presents with sudden onset chest pain and breathlessness. He has had similar episodes in the past.

What is the single most likely disease process?

A. Anaemia
B. Pulmonary oedema
C. Bronchogenic carcinoma
D. Extrinsic allergic alveolitis
E. Pneumothorax

29. A 76-year-old man presents with acute breathlessness, cough, frothy blood stained sputum and palpitations. He is apyrexial. ECG shows sinus tachycardia.

What is the single most likely disease process?

A. Anaemia
B. Pulmonary oedema
C. Bronchogenic carcinoma
D. Extrinsic allergic alveolitis
E. Pneumothorax

30. A 37-year-old man presents with dyspnoea, cough, weight loss and night sweats. His CXR shows diffuse bilateral infiltrates.

What is the single most likely causative organism?

A. *Pneumocystis carinii*
B. *Chlamydia psittaci*
C. *E. Coli*
D. *Pseudomonas aeruginosa*
E. *Mycobacterium tuberculosis*

31. A 48-year-old man presents with fever, rigors, headache and diarrhoea. He recently had been on a holiday abroad. CXR shows consolidation.

What is the single most likely causative organism?

A. *Staphylococcus aureus*
B. *Cryptococcus*
C. *Streptococcus pneumoniae*
D. *Legionella pneumophilia*
E. *Mycobacterium avium-intracellulare*

32. A 45-year-old farmer presents with flu like illness, anorexia and dry cough. His CXR shows patchy consolidation.

What is the single most likely causative organism?

A. *Legionella pneumophilia*
B. *Mycobacterium avium-intracellulare*
C. *Mycoplasma pneumoniae*
D. *Pneumocystis carinii*
E. *Chlamydia psittaci*

33. A 41-year-old drug abuser presents with fever, cough and breathlessness. This was preceded by viral influenza. Chest radiograph shows multiple abscesses.

What is the single most likely causative organism?

A. *Pneumocystis carinii*
B. *Chlamydia psittaci*
C. *Escherichia coli*
D. *Pseudomonas aeruginosa*
E. *Mycobacterium tuberculosis*

34. A 14-year-old student with cystic fibrosis rapidly deteriorated and developed acute respiratory failure while in hospital.

What is the single most likely causative organism?

A. *Cryptococcus*
B. *Streptococcus pneumoniae*
C. *Legionella pneumophilia*
D. *Mycobacterium avium-intracellulare*
E. *Mycoplasma pneumoniae*

35. A 55-year-old smoker with a long history of recurrent chest infection presents with haemoptysis and greenish sputum. On examination he has clubbing and coarse crepitations over the bases of both lungs.

What is the single most likely disease process?

A. Pulmonary infarction
B. Pneumonia
C. Tuberculosis
D. Bronchiectasis
E. Mitral stenosis

36. A 69-year-old woman who had a total hip replacement a week ago presents with severe chest pain, shortness of breath and haemoptysis.

What is the single most likely disease process?

A. Pulmonary infarction
B. Pneumonia
C. Tuberculosis
D. Bronchiectasis
E. Mitral stenosis

37. A 52-year-old diabetic presents with fever, pleuritic pain and rusty coloured sputum.
What is the single most likely disease process?
A. Pneumonia
B. Tuberculosis
C. Bronchiectasis
D. Mitral stenosis
E. SLE

38. A 45-year-old bank manager presents with cough, pleuritic chest pain and haemoptysis. This was preceded by rhinitis, recurrent epistaxis and haematuria, CXR shows multiple nodular masses.
What is the single most likely disease process?
A. Foreign body inhalation
B. Wegener's granulomatosis
C. Haemorrhagic telangiectasia
D. Polyarteritis nodosa
E. Bronchogenic carcinoma

39. A 70-year-old smoker presents with cough, haemoptysis and weight loss. On examination, there is clubbing and gynaecomastia.
What is the single most likely disease process?
A. Foreign body inhalation
B. Wegener's granulomatosis
C. Haemorrhagic telangiectasia
D. Polyarteritis nodosa
E. Bronchogenic carcinoma

40. A 72-year-old Asian immigrant presents with cough, haemoptysis, night fever and sweating.
What is the single most likely disease process?
A. Tuberculosis
B. Bronchiectasis
C. Mitral stenosis
D. SLE
E. Foreign body inhalation

41. A 50-year-old man presents with progressive burning pains in the sole of his left foot, bilateral cramps in both calves, and left foot drop. He is known asthmatic and suffers from recurrent sinusitis. FBC shows eosinophilia.
What is the single most likely disease process?
A. Acute myocardial infarction
B. Churg-Strauss syndrome
C. Pulmonary embolism
D. Pneumothorax
E. Allergic bronchopulmonary

42. A 33-year-old man presented with breathlessness at rest, cough and haemoptysis all of which he has had for a few days. On examination he is cyanosed and there are bilateral inspiratory and expiratory wheezes. His PEFR is normal. Blood investigations show evidence of renal failure.
What is the single most likely disease process?
A. Extrinsic allergic alveolitis
B. *Pneumocystis carinii*
C. Cystic fibrosis
D. Cryptogenic fibrosing alveolitis
E. Goodpasture's syndrome

43. A 73-year-old man presents with pneumonia which he has had for 2 weeks and which was resistant to antibiotics. He has had asthmatic bronchitis for more than 50 years. CXR shows consolidation of the right upper zone and the left perihilar consolidation. Blood tests show neutrophilia.
What is the single most likely disease process?
A. Acute myocardial infarction
B. Churg-Strauss syndrome
C. Pulmonary embolism
D. Pneumothorax
E. Allergic bronchopulmonary

44. A 29-year-old farmer presented with worsening cough breathlessness and flu like symptoms which he had each winter for 3 years. CXR showed fine miliary shadows. Pulmonary function tests showed evidence of restrictive lung disease.
What is the single most likely disease process?
A. Extrinsic allergic alveolitis
B. *Pneumocystis carinii*
C. Cystic fibrosis
D. Cryptogenic fibrosing alveolitis
E. Goodpasture's syndrome

45. A 30-year-old woman presents with fever, pharyngitis and cough. The CXR shows widespread bilateral patchy consolidation. Erythema multiforme is present.
What is the single most likely disease process?
A. *Mycoplasma pneumoniae*
B. Bilateral bronchopneumonia
C. Adult respiratory distress syndrome
D. Sarcoidosis
E. Pulmonary contusion

46. A 40-year-old alcoholic presents with repeated small haemoptysis and cough of mucoid sputum. His CXR shows right upper lobe consolidation and a large central cavity. Heaf test is positive.
What is the single most likely disease process?
A. Bilateral bronchopneumonia
B. Adult respiratory distress syndrome
C. Sarcoidosis
D. Pulmonary contusion
E. Tuberculosis

47. A 60-year-old man presents with dyspnoea and cough. The CXR shows extensive pulmonary fibrosis, bilateral pleural thickening and pleural calcifications.
What is the single most likely disease process?
A. Pneumoconiosis
B. Carcinoma bronchus
C. Cystic fibrosis
D. Pancoast's tumor
E. Mycoplasma pneumoniae

48. A 14-year-old boy presents with repeated lower respiratory infections. On examination he is noted to have finger clubbing and suffers from weight loss and steatorrhoea. The CXR shows bronchial wall thickening, ring shadows of bronchiectasis and wide spread ill-defining shadowing.
What is the single most likely disease process?
A. Cystic fibrosis
B. Pancoast's tumour
C. Mycoplasma pneumoniae
D. Bilateral bronchopneumonia
E. Adult respiratory distress syndrome

49. A 40-year-old man presents with cough and haemoptysis. The CXR shows a right hilar mass and a patch of consolidation in the right upper lobe laterally.
What is the single most likely disease process?
A. Carcinoma bronchus
B. Cystic fibrosis
C. Pancoast's tumour
D. Mycoplasma pneumoniae
E. Bilateral bronchopneumonia

50. A 20-year-old woman presents with a week's history of fever, rigors and productive rusty cough. CXR shows right lower lobe consolidation.
What is the single most appropriate treatment?
A. Tetracycline
B. Flucloxacillin
C. Benzyl penicillin
D. Cefotaxime
E. Prednisolone

51. A 12-year-old boy with cystic fibrosis presents with persistent productive cough. The CXR shows spherical shadow containing a central lucency. An air fluid level is also seen.
What is the single most appropriate treatment?
A. Erythromycin
B. Tetracycline
C. Flucloxacillin
D. Benzyl penicillin
E. Cefotaxime

52. A 50-year-old man presents with shortness of breath and dry cough. CXR shows widespread pulmonary shadowing. He takes azathioprine for resistant rheumatoid arthritis.
What is the single most appropriate treatment?
A. Pyridoxine and ethambutol
B. Isoniazid alone
C. Cotrimoxazole
D. Salbutamol inhaler
E. Ciprofloxacin

53. A 20-year-old woman presents with malaise, cough and progressive shortness of breath. The CXR shows symmetrical lobulated bilateral hilar gland enlargement.
What is the single most appropriate treatment?
A. Tetracycline
B. Flucloxacillin
C. Benzyl penicillin
D. Cefotaxime
E. Prednisolone

54. A 50-year-old diabetic presents with a productive cough and malaise. CXR shows right upper lobe consolidation and hilar lymphadenopathy.
What is the single most appropriate treatment?
A. Rifampicin + Isoniazid
B. Pyridoxine and ethambutol
C. Isoniazid alone
D. Cotrimoxazole
E. Salbutamol inhaler

55. A 35-year-old pet shop owner presents with high fever, excruciating headache and a dry hacking cough. The CXR shows patchy consolidation.

What is the single most likely causative organism?

A. *Chlamydia psittaci*
B. Actinomycosis
C. *Pneumocystis carinii*
D. *Streptococcus pneumoniae*
E. *Mycoplasma pneumoniae*

56. A 40-year-old man who works in an abattoir presents with sudden onset of fever, myalgia, headache, dry cough and chest pain. CXR shows patchy consolidation of the right lower lobe giving a ground glass appearance.

What is the single most likely causative organism?

A. Tuberculosis
B. *Pseudomonas aeruginosa*
C. *Coxiella burnetti*
D. *Legionella pneumophilia*
E. Aspergillosis

57. A 44-year-old travelling insurance salesman presents with high fever, myalgia, abdominal pain, and haemoptysis. CXR shows diffuse patchy lobar shadows. The cough progresses from a modest nonproductive cough to producing mucopurulent sputum. The fever persists for 2 weeks.

What is the single most likely causative organism?

A. Tuberculosis
B. *Pseudomonas aeruginosa*
C. *Coxiella burnetii*
D. *Legionella pneumophilia*
E. Aspergillosis

58. A 10-year-old man with HIV presents with a productive cough and haemoptysis. CXR shows a round ball in the right upper lobe surmounted by a dome of air.

What is the single most likely causative organism?

A. Tuberculosis
B. *Pseudomonas aeruginosa*
C. *Coxiella burnetii*
D. *Legionella pneumophilia*
E. Aspergillosis

59. A 20-year-old male IV drug abuser presents with breathlessness and cough. CXR reveals patchy areas of consolidation with abscess formation.

What is the single most likely causative organism?

A. *Streptococcus pneumoniae*
B. *Mycoplasma pneumoniae*
C. *Haemophilus influenzae*
D. *Staphylococcus aureus*
E. *Legionella pneumophilia*

60. A 12-year-old boy with cystic fibrosis presents with a chest infection. The boy also suffers from mild renal failure.

What is the single most appropriate treatment?

A. Tobramycin and Carbenicillin
B. Plasmaphoresis
C. Ciprofloxacin
D. Tetracycline
E. Cotrimoxazole

61. A 30-year-old presents with haemoptysis, dyspnoea and haematuria. CXR reveals bilateral alveolar infiltrates. Urine analysis reveals presence of protein and red cell casts.

What is the single most appropriate next investigation?

A. 12 lead ECG
B. Tissue biopsy
C. ANA
D. Sputum cytology
E. Antiglomerular basement antibodies

62. A 60-year-old man presents with a chronic cough and mild haemoptysis. On examination he has digital clubbing with pain and swelling around his wrists. CXR reveals a single nodule.

What is the single most appropriate next investigation?

A. Pulmonary angiogram
B. 12 lead ECG
C. Tissue biopsy
D. ANA
E. Sputum cytology

63. A 30-year-old IV drug abuser presents with dyspnoea and haemoptysis. His CXR is unremarkable and ECG shows sinus tachycardia with a mean P axis shift to the right. ABG show a low $PaCO_2$ and an elevated pH.

What is the single most appropriate next investigation?
A. Heaf test
B. Bronchography
C. Urinalysis
D. Chest X-ray
E. Pulmonary angiogram

64. A 40-year-old mental patient with dry cough and confusion. Blood tests reveal lymphopenia and hyponatremia. CXR shows right lobar shadowing.

What is the single most appropriate treatment?
A. Erythromycin
B. Cyclophosphamide
C. Tobramycin and Carbenicillin
D. Plasmaphoresis
E. Ciprofloxacin

65. A 10-year-old boy presents with wheezing attacks and episodic shortness of breath. His PEFR is 400 L/min.

What is the single most appropriate treatment?
A. Beta 2 agonist
B. Rifampicin + Isoniazid
C. IV aminophylline
D. Prednisolone
E. Erythromycin

66. A 40-year-old male presents with rhinorrhoea, cough, haemoptysis and pleuritic chest pain. CXR shows multiple nodules.

What is the single most appropriate treatment?
A. Erythromycin
B. Cyclophosphamide
C. Tobramycin and Carbenicillin
D. Plasmaphoresis
E. Ciprofloxacin

67. A 60-year-old farmer presents with fever, cough and shortness of breath. He had been forking hay that morning. CXR shows fatty nodular shadows in the upper zone.

What is the single most appropriate treatment?
A. Prednisolone
B. Erythromycin
C. Cyclophosphamide
D. Tobramycin and Carbenicillin
E. Plasmaphoresis

68. A 40-year-old man presents with recurrent epitaxis, haemoptysis and haematuria. On examination he has nasal septai perforation and nodules on CXR.

What is the single most appropriate next investigation?
A. Pulmonary angiogram
B. 12 lead ECG
C. Tissue biopsy
D. ANA
E. Sputum cytology

69. A 50-year-old man presents with occasional haemoptysis and chronic productive cough. He has a history of recurrent pneumonia. CXR reveals peri-bronchial fibrosis.

What is the single most appropriate next investigation?
A. FBC
B. CT chest
C. Clotting studies
D. Heaf test
E. Bronchography

70. 30-year-old woman: ABG - pH 7.51, pCO_2 3.7 kPa, pO_2 14.3 kPa, HCO_3- 28 mmol/l.

What is the single most likely diagnosis?
A. Pulmonary embolism
B. Panic attack
C. Sarcoidosis
D. Cystic fibrosis
E. Extrinsic tracheal compression

71. A 40-year-old Afro Caribbean woman: PFT - FEV1 2.51, FVC 2.91, FEV1/FVC 86%, Serum ACE levels - high.

What is the single most likely diagnosis?
A. Pneumonectomy
B. Pulmonary fibrosis
C. Pulmonary embolism
D. Panic attack
E. Sarcoidosis

72. A 60-year-old male non-smoker: PFTs - FEV 1.14 L, FVC 3.51, FEV1/FVC = 40%. After bronchodilator trial - FEV1/FVC = 50%. After 2 weeks of prednisolone 30 mg daily REV1/FVC = 65%.

What is the single most likely diagnosis?
A. Asthma
B. Pulmonary haemorrhage
C. Emphysema
D. Extrinsic allergic alveolitis
E. Chronic bronchitis

73. A 29-year-old teacher is 7 months pregnant. She presents with sudden collapse and breathlessness. On examination, she is afebrile, severely cyanosed and hyperventilating. Her pulse is 140/min and BP 70/30 mmHg.

What is the single most appropriate next investigation?

A. CT brain
B. Blood count and film
C. Spiral CT with contrast
D. ECHO
E. Arterial blood gases

74. A 74-year-old woman presents to casualty with acute breathlessness. She has had 3 similar admissions in last few months. She has a past history of rheumatic fever. On examination, she has an irregular pulse of 110/min. She has a non-displaced tapping apex beat with no evidence of left ventricular dysfunction. No murmurs are audible. There are crepitations heard in both lower lung fields.

What is the single most likely cause of pulmonary oedema?

A. Adult respiratory distress syndrome
B. Mitral stenosis
C. Anaemia
D. Aortic stenosis
E. Acute renal failure

75. A 67-year-old man has had an elective total knee replacement. He has no significant medical history. 36 hrs after operation he complains of increasing breathlessness. He is cyanosed and has crackles up to midzones of both lung fields. His ECG is normal and CXR shows pulmonary oedema with normal cardiac dimensions. His urine output since the operation has been poor and he has been persistently hypotensive with a BP of around 90/60 mmHg.

What is the single most likely cause of pulmonary oedema?

A. Myocardial infarction
B. Constrictive pericarditis
C. Myocarditis
D. Iatrogenic
E. Cardiomyopathy

76. A 50-year-old farmer PFTs: FEV1 2.81, FVC 3.51, FEV1/FVC 80%. Reduced TLCO and KC Bronchoalveolar lavage - lymphocytes and mast cells. Precipitins to Microspora faeni - positive.

What is the single most likely diagnosis?

A. Emphysema
B. Extrinsic allergic alveolitis
C. Chronic bronchitis
D. Pneumonectomy
E. Pulmonary fibrosis

77. A 35-year-old woman ABG: pH 7.4, pCO_2 4.4, pO_2 9.4, TLCO 90% of predicted, KCO 160% of predicted. All results were normal 24 hours ago.

What is the single most likely diagnosis?

A. Pulmonary haemorrhage
B. Emphysema
C. Extrinsic allergic alveolitis
D. Chronic bronchitis
E. Pneumonectomy

78. A 26-year-old nurse is brought to casualty as an emergency. She is hyperventilating but drowsy, She has been complaining of nausea and tinnitus and had an episode of haematemesis.

What is the single most appropriate next investigation?

A. Salicylate levels
B. Serum lactose
C. CT brain
D. Blood count and film
E. Spiral CT with contrast

79. A 21-year-old motorcycle courier was involved in an head on collision with a van. He had an obvious deformity of his left thigh and knee. X-ray confirmed communited fracture of the shaft of the femur that was reduced and placed in traction. Five days later he suddenly deteriorates becomes drowsy, confused and febrile. He is hyperventilating and cyanosed. There are crackles at both lung bases and petechiae over his chest and neck.

What is the single most appropriate next investigation?

A. Blood count and film
B. Spiral CT with contrast
C. ECHO
D. Arterial blood gases
E. V/Q scan

80. A 15-year-old school girl was out with her friends at a party last night. When she returned home this morning she was drowsy unwell and vomiting. She has lost 5 kg over last 2 months. On arrival at hospital, she is drowsy, confused and hyperventilating but not cyanosed. Her breath smells of pear drops.

What is the single most appropriate next investigation?

A. Blood glucose
B. Salicylate levels
C. Serum lactose
D. CT brain
E. Blood count and film

81. A 24-year-old car mechanic is brought to casualty by his girlfriend. She describes a 2 day history of rigors, sweats and intermittent confusion. On examination he is agitated, sweaty and pyrexial with 38.6°C temp. He is hyperventilating and cyanosed despite receiving O_2 by face mask. There is dullness to percussion and bronchial breathing at the left lung base.

What is the single most appropriate next investigation?

A. None required
B. Urea and electrolytes
C. Chest X-ray
D. Blood glucose
E. Salicylate levels

82. A 14-year-old boy presents to casualty complaining of severe chest pain and difficulty in breathing. He hyperventilating and pale but not cyanosed. He has had 4 similar admissions in last year and his older brother also attends the hospital frequently.

What is the single most appropriate next investigation?

A. Blood glucose
B. Salicylate levels
C. Serum lactose
D. CT brain
E. Blood count and film

83. A 21-year-old man has become increasingly breathless over a period of 4 days. He has also had severe central chest pain and a fever. He was previously fit and well. On examination, he looks unwell, cyanosed and dyspnoeic. Pulse is 120/min, regular BP 90/40 mmHg. JVP elevated and he has a gallop rhythm with no murmurs. There are crackles in both lung bases. CXR shows pulmonary oedema and a normal heart rate. ECG shows extensive ST elevation in the anterior and inferior leads without Q waves.

What is the single most likely cause of pulmonary oedema?

A. Myocarditis
B. Iatrogenic
C. Cardiomyopathy
D. Hypoalbuminemia
E. Mitral regurgitation

84. A 38-year-old woman was admitted to hospital two days ago with abdominal pain and vomiting. She was tender in the epigastrium and was found to have a very high serum amylase level. She has been treated with large volumes of IV fluids and has maintained a good urine output. Nonetheless she has been persistently hypoxic and is deteriorating rapidly. She now has crackles throughout both lung fields and a pO_2 of 5.1 kPa despite receiving 60% O_2 by mask. CXR shows massive bilateral pulmonary oedema. Her serum albumin is 30 mmol/l.

What is the single most likely cause of pulmonary oedema?

A. Adult respiratory distress syndrome
B. Mitral stenosis
C. Anaemia
D. Aortic stenosis
E. Acute renal failure

85. A 30-year-old lady complains increasing breathlessness, tiredness, malaise, poor appetite and weight loss.

What is the single most likely cause of breathlessness?

A. Asthma
B. Tuberculosis
C. Angioneurotic oedema
D. Thyroiditis
E. Branchial cyst

86. A 56-year-old man wheezes and coughs. He has tried to give up smoking, but he finds it very difficult. He is thin and healthy looking with a rounded chest. His breathing is noisy. His cough is unproductive.

What is the single most appropriate next step in management?

A. Ipratropium
B. Amoxycillin
C. Aminophylline
D. Prednisolone
E. Salbutamol

87. A 37-year-old man who has had recurrent chest infections since a serious bout of influenza 3 years ago presents with chronic productive cough. His sputum is tenacious and blood stained, On auscultation you find crackling.

What is the single most appropriate next step in management?

A. Postural drainage B. Aspiration
C. Chest wall drain D. Bronchoscopy
E. Pleurectomy

88. A woman who has been treated for hypothyroidism cannot breathe. At night she must sit propped up and she has a constant dull chest pain. On examination of her chest you find stony dullness and bronchial breathing.

What is the single most appropriate next step in management?

A. Postural drainage B. Aspiration
C. Chest wall drain D. Bronchoscopy
E. Pleurectomy

89. A healthy young woman comes to you complaining of a swelling in front of the neck and diarrhoea. She also has palpitations and is short of breath.

What is the single most likely cause of breathlessness?

A. Asbestosis
B. CML
C. Erysipelas
D. Primary thyrotoxicosis
E. Hay fever

90. A 50-year-old train conductor complains of chronic productive cough. He is also a heavy smoker.

What is the single most likely diagnosis?

A. Erysipelas
B. Primary thyrotoxicosis
C. Hay fever
D. Depression
E. Bronchogenic carcinoma

91. A 14-year-old girl is brought into A and E with very difficult and noisy breathing.

What is the single most likely cause of breathlessness?

A. Bronchogenic carcinoma
B. Sinusitis
C. Asthma
D. Tuberculosis
E. Angioneurotic oedema

92. A young woman complains of sore eyes, a dull chest pain, malaise and a low grade fever. She thinks she has had a recurrent low grade fever for 4 months. A CXR shows bilateral hilar enlargement.

What is the single most likely diagnosis?

A. Sarcoidosis B. Asthma
C. Histiocytosis D. Emphysema
E. *Aspergillus fumigatus*

93. A middle aged pharmaceutical engineer presents with increasing breathlessness and cough. He doesn't smoke. On CXR you find diffuse bilateral mottling and multiple small cystic lesions. Six months ago he had a pneumothorax.

What is the single most likely diagnosis?

A. Sarcoidosis B. Asthma
C. Histiocytosis D. Emphysema
E. *Aspergillus fumigatus*

94. For the last 3 years a young man has complained of recurrent bouts of pneumonia with wheeziness, cough, fever and malaise. His sputum is tenacious. Peripheral blood shows a very high ESR and Ige.

What is the single most likely diagnosis?

A. Aspergillus fumigatus
B. Lung fibrosis
C. Idiopathic thrombocytopenia
D. Pleurisy
E. Polyarteritis nodosa

95. A 30-year-old computer engineer with a long history of asthma and rhinitis presents with wheezing cough and fever. A CXR shows patchy consolidation. Physical examination shows multiple tender subcutaneous nodules and purpura.

What is the single most likely diagnosis?

A. Pleurisy B. Polyarteritis nodosa
C. Lung collapse D. Hyperparathyroidism
E. Tuberculosis

96. A 43-year-old man presents with chest pain and cough. He complains of fullness and pressure in the chest and a sharp pain affecting 2 or 3 ribs on the right side. A CXR shows a right sided hilar enlargement.

What is the single most likely diagnosis?

A. Lung collapse
B. Hyperparathyroidism
C. Tuberculosis
D. Silent MI
E. Bronchogenic carcinoma

97. A middle aged woman brings her husband into your surgery. She complains of his heavy snoring. Also in the middle of the night he stops breathing, gags and wakes up. Also his performance at work has been declining and he is being threatened of retirement.

What is the single most appropriate next step in management?

A. Surgical excision
B. CPAP
C. Ipratropium
D. Amoxycillin
E. Aminophylline

98. A young man with chronic hepatitis develops chest complaints. He has become breathless and coughs. He has lost weight and his joints bother him. On physical examination you note mild cyanosis.

What is the single most appropriate next step in management?

A. Ipratropium
B. Amoxycillin
C. Aminophylline
D. Prednisolone
E. Salbutamol

99. A middle aged woman complains of dyspnoea. Over the past year she had to give up her gardening. An ECG shows right ventricular hypertrophy and strain.

What is the single next most appropriate step in management?

A. Lobectomy
B. Antidepressants
C. A healthy diet
D. Anticoagulants
E. Contraception

100. An elderly woman cannot carry on her household chores but has to sit down every few minutes. A CXR shows diffuse reticular nodular shadows especially in her lower lobes.

What is the single next most appropriate step in management?

A. Oxygen therapy
B. Thymectomy
C. Chemotherapy
D. Change occupation
E. Radiotherapy

101. A middle aged housewife presents with exertional dyspnoea. She also has a dry cough, general malaise and is mildly cyanosed. On auscultation of chest you find crepitations. She has a history of arthritis.

What is the single most likely diagnosis?

A. Respiratory failure
B. Bronchitis
C. Bronchial asthma
D. Emphysema
E. Rheumatoid lung

102. A 35-year-old accountant presents with a chronic cough, dyspnoea and wheezing. He produces copious sputum. His arterial carbon dioxide is low and his arterial oxygen is normal.

What is the single most likely diagnosis?

A. Rheumatic heart disease
B. Respiratory failure
C. Bronchitis
D. Bronchial asthma
E. Emphysema

103. A middle aged smoker presents with chronic cough and phlegm. His sputum is tenacious but not yellow or blood stained. His chest is hyperinflated. His arterial carbon dioxide is high and is arterial oxygen is low.

What is the single most likely diagnosis?

A. Bronchitis
B. Bronchial asthma
C. Emphysema
D. Rheumatoid lung
E. Fibrosing alveolitis

104. A 53-year-old smoker with chronic cough and copious yellow sputum presents in a state of agitation. He is confused. His pulse is bounding. He has a terrible headache and you find papilloedema on fundoscopy.

What is the single most likely diagnosis?

A. Tuberculosis
B. Pulmonary embolism
C. Rheumatic heart disease
D. Respiratory failure
E. Bronchitis

105. A young woman complains of wheeze, dyspnoea and cough. She cannot sleep at night because of a chronic cough. She and her mother love animals and together they have 14 cats. Her PEFR is normal but her CXR suggests hyperinflation.
What is the single most likely diagnosis?
A. Respiratory failure
B. Bronchitis
C. Bronchial asthma
D. Emphysema
E. Rheumatoid lung

106. A 36-year-old woman presents "with increasing breathlessness over a period of 10 months. She now finds herself unable to climb stairs. Also she has just had her 3rd child in 3 years and complains of feeling depressed.
What is the single next most appropriate step in management?
A. Blood transfusion B. Lobectomy
C. Antidepressants D. A healthy diet
E. Anticoagulants

107. A 43-year-old shipyard worker complains of gasping for breath. On physical examination you discover mild cyanosis and restricted chest movements.
What is the single next most appropriate step in management?
A. Oxygen therapy B. Thymectomy
C. Chemotherapy D. Change occupation
E. Radiotherapy

108. A 62-year-old man says he can't get enough air. Over the past few months he has become increasingly breathless. Also, he has noticed he has had difficulty in finishing his dinner. His jaw tires.
What is the single next most appropriate step in management?
A. Edrophonium chloride
B. Iron supplements
C. Oxygen therapy
D. Thymectomy
E. Chemotherapy

109. A 65-year-old warehouse man is admitted with severe wheeze and breathlessness. He has had to sleep propped up. And during the past few days his legs have become swollen.
What is the single next most appropriate step in management?
A. Furosemide
B. Oxygen therapy
C. GTN
D. Morphine
E. Nasal IPPV

110. A 50-year-old taxi driver and heavy smoker complains that his feet swell up at the end of the day. He has also noticed increasing shortness of breath.
What is the single next most appropriate step in management?
A. Sputum culture
B. Pericardial aspiration
C. Streptokinase
D. Furosemide
E. Oxygen therapy

111. A middle-aged woman complains of a chronic cough and purulent sputum. Recently she has become very wheezy and dyspnoeic. An ECG gives a low voltage trace and a CXR shows a large heart shadow.
What is the single next most appropriate step in management?
A. Antibiotics
B. Sputum culture
C. Pericardial aspiration
D. Streptokinase
E. Furosemide

112. An elderly woman complains of acute chest pain, breathlessness and haemoptysis. A month ago she had pain and swelling in the legs but did not go to the doctor with these complaints.
What is the single next most appropriate step in management?
A. Antibiotics
B. Sputum culture
C. Pericardial aspiration
D. Streptokinase
E. Furosemide

113. His friends bring in a 48-year-old businessman. He is very distressed, breathless, cold and clammy. He has severe chest pain and he has vomited 3 times.
What is the single next most appropriate step in management?
A. Morphine
B. Nasal IPPV
C. Venesection
D. Advise stop smoking
E. Beta agonists

114. A 4-year-old child has severe cough and fever. She appears acutely ill and cyanosed.
What is the single most likely diagnosis?
A. Bronchogenic carcinoma
B. Parainfluenzae
C. Respiratory syncytial virus
D. Rhinovirus
E. Pleurisy

115. A 6-year-old child complains of a very sore throat. He has a mild fever and red fauces.
What is the single most likely diagnosis?
A. Bronchogenic carcinoma
B. Parainfluenzae
C. Respiratory syncytial virus
D. Rhinovirus
E. Pleurisy

116. A 33-year-old bus driver complains of a persistent cough and blood stained sputum. He does not smoke. He has a fever and supraclavicular glands. A CXR shows a dense irregular hilar expansion.
What is the single most likely diagnosis?
A. Tuberculosis
B. MI
C. Asthma
D. Meningitis
E. Bronchiectasis

117. A 32-year-old lecturer has had a fever for a week with no cough. Her fever came on suddenly and she says half her department is similarily ill. She has fine rales and a positive chest X-ray.
What is the single most likely diagnosis?
A. Parainfluenzae
B. Respiratory syncytial virus
C. Rhinovirus
D. Pleurisy
E. Pneumococci

118. A 40 year man complains of swollen legs and breathlessness. Examination reveals hepatosplenomegaly. And a chest X-ray shows a normal but dense heart shadow and clear lung fields.
What is the single next most appropriate step in management?
A. Pericardial resection
B. Radiotherapy
C. Furosemide
D. Anti-emetics
E. Aspirin

119. A middle aged decorator complains of severe chest pain radiating to the neck. The pain came on after dinner and as he was retiring for the night.
What is the single next most appropriate step in management?
A. Diamorphine
B. Diazepam
C. Combination antibiotics
D. Anxiolytics
E. Lobectomy

120. An elderly housewife was operated on for gall-stones and at operation a gangrenous gallbladder was removed. A couple of days later she complained of nausea and feeling unwell.
What is the single next most appropriate step in management?
A. Diamorphine
B. Diazepam
C. Combination antibiotics
D. Anxiolytics
E. Lobectomy

121. A 62-year-old lifelong smoker has a dry cough, weight loss and haemoptysis. CXR and CT show right middle lobe collapse. He is sent to chest clinic for investigation.
What is the single next most appropriate investigation?
A. Bronchoalveolar lavage
B. ECHO
C. Serum precipitins
D. Fibreoptic bronchoscopy
E. Flow volume loop

122. A 54-year-old farmer with intermittent dry cough, fever and dyspnoea, progressive weight loss and fine crepitations on auscultation.
What is the single next most appropriate investigation?
A. Serum precipitins
B. Fibreoptic bronchoscopy
C. High resolution CT
D. Mantoux test
E. Seek immediate expertise help

123. A 24-year-old male develops sudden onset dyspnoea, chest pain on inspiration and haemoptysis whilst straining at stool. He had a cholecystectomy 10 days previously. He rapidly becomes cyanosed and loosed consciousness. On examination his blood pressure is 75/50, heart rate 156 and thready with a loud pulmonary heart sound. His jugular venous pressure is raised by 6 cm.

What is the single next most appropriate investigation?

A. Seek immediate expertise help
B. Arterial blood gases
C. EGG, blood gases and V/Q scan
D. Serum calcium, ACE levels
E. Static lung volumes

124. A 22-year-old barman presents with a dry cough of sudden onset. He complains of a chest pain and rusty sputum. He also has a very high fever, rapid breathing, cyanosis and crepitations.

What is the single most likely diagnosis?

A. Pleurisy
B. Pneumococci
C. Pleural effusion
D. Q fever
E. Chronic bronchitis

125. A young officer manager complains of palpitations for 2 months. He says that when he mounts the stairs he can feel his heart beating. His health history is unremarkable.

What is the single next most appropriate step in management?

A. Combination antibiotics
B. Anxiolytics
C. Lobectomy
D. Pericardial tap
E. Incision and drainage

126. A 37-year-old Nigerian woman develops clubbing, erythema nodosum, iritis, dyspnoea and lymphadenopathy on her CXR.

What is the single next most appropriate investigation?

A. Seek immediate expertise help
B. Arterial blood gases
C. EGG, blood gases and V/Q scan
D. Serum calcium, ACE levels
E. Static lung volumes

127. A 47-year-old Caucasian childminder in Glasgow presents with dry cough, night sweats and haemoptysis.

What is the single next most appropriate investigation?

A. Flow volume loop
B. Mantoux test
C. Seek immediate expertise help
D. Arterial blood gases
E. EGG, blood gases and V/Q scan

128. What is the single most characteristic lung function test picture in emphysema?

A. FEV1/FVC 62%, no reversibility to bronchodilators, gas trapping, hyperinflation and reduced transfer factor
B. Normal PFTs
C. FEV1/FVC 89%
D. FEV1/FVC 85%, globally reduced lung vols. Reduced inspiratory and expiratory mouth pressures
E. Reduced transfer factor alone

129. What is the single most characteristic lung function test picture in pneumonectomy?

A. FEV1/FVC 85%, globally reduced lung vols. Reduced inspiratory and expiratory mouth pressures
B. Reduced transfer factor alone
C. Inspiratory and expiratory fixed obstruction on volume loop
D. Spirometry, lung volumes and incorrected transfer factor 50% predicted. Corrected factor normal.
E. Increased transfer factor FEV1/FVC 58%, 25% reversibility to bronchodilators, normal transfer factor

130. What is the single most characteristic lung function test picture in Neuromuscular disease?

A. FEV1/FVC 85%, globally reduced lung vols. Reduced inspiratory and expiratory mouth pressures
B. Reduced transfer factor alone
C. Inspiratory and expiratory fixed obstruction on volume loop
D. Spirometry, lung volumes and incorrected transfer factor 50% predicted / Corrected factor normal.
E. Increased transfer factor FEV1/FVC 58%, 25% reversibility to bronchodilators, normal transfer factor

131. What is the single most characteristic lung function test picture in Interstitial lung disease?
A. FEV1/FVC ratio 90%, TLC reduced by 30%, Considerably reduced transfer factor
B. FEV1/FVC 62%, no reversibility to bronchodilators, gas trapping, hyperinflation and reduced transfer factor
C. Normal PFTs
D. FEV1/FVC 89%
E. FEV1/FVC 85%, globally reduced lung vols. Reduced inspiratory and expiratory mouth pressures

132. A 30-year-old woman presents with a 3 day history of pyrexia, rigors and sweats. This was preceded by a 1 week history of cough and increasing dyspnoea. She had a swinging fever and dullness to percussion at the left lung base.
What is the single most likely cause of pleural effusion in this case?
A. Emphysema
B. Rheumatoid arthritis
C. Tuberculosis
D. SLE
E. Bronchial carcinoma

133. A 12-year-old female presents with increasing breathlessness and abdominal swelling. She has a right sided pleural effusion. On examination she has generalised lymphadenopathy.
What is the single most likely cause of pleural effusion in this case?
A. Rheumatoid arthritis
B. Tuberculosis
C. SLE
D. Bronchial carcinoma
E. Yellow nail syndrome

134. A 31-year-old IV drug abuser presents with a 3 week history of cough, fever and general malaise with occasional haemoptysis. He has a right sided pleural effusion.
What is the single most likely cause of pleural effusion in this case?
A. Pneumonia
B. Pleural metastases
C. Emphysema
D. Rheumatoid arthritis
E. Tuberculosis

135. A 55-year-old retired builder has a 3 month history of cough and left sided chest pain. He has a pleural effusion on the left. On CXR there is evidence of pleural calcification.
What is the single most likely cause of pleural effusion in this case?
A. Cardiac failure
B. Mesothelioma
C. Hypoalbuminemia
D. Meig's syndrome
E. Pneumonia

136. A 25-year-old woman has just returned from a holiday in Kenya. She suddenly became breathless and is cyanosed. Her pulse is 120/min, BP 110/70 mmHg, PEFR 400 L/min. CXR is normal.
What is the single most next appropriate step in management?
A. IV Insulin
B. IV adrenaline
C. Rebreathing into paper bag
D. Heparin
E. Methylene blue

137. A 50-year-old with pulmonary fibrosis develops sudden left sided pleuritic chest pain and dyspnoea. He has reduced air entry in the left side of the chest and percussion is hyper resonant. O_2 saturation is 80%.
What is the single most next appropriate step in management?
A. Chest drain
B. IV furosemide
C. Rapid infusion of saline
D. Forced alkaline diuresis
E. Intramuscular adrenaline

138. A 58-year-old woman presents with intermittent breathlessness and cough. On examination, she has a right sided pleural effusion and discoloured nails.
What is the single most likely cause of pleural effusion in this case?
A. Rheumatoid arthritis
B. Tuberculosis
C. SLE
D. Bronchial carcinoma
E. Yellow nail syndrome

139. A 72-year-old woman presents with a 2 month history of increasing breathlessness and swollen legs. On examination, she has a raised JVP and a left sided pleural effusion.

What is the single most likely cause of pleural effusion in this case?

A. Cardiac failure
B. Mesothelioma
C. Hypoalbuminemia
D. Meig's syndrome
E. Pneumonia

140. A 70-year-old woman presents with confusion and productive cough. CXR shows right lower lobe consolidation.

What is the single most likely causative organism?

A. Actinomycosis
B. *Pneumocystis carinii*
C. *Streptococcus pneumoniae*
D. *Mycoplasma pneumoniae*
E. *Staphylococcus aureus*

141. A pet shop owner presents with high swinging fever, cough and malaise. He has scanty rose spots over his abdomen. CXR reveals diffuse pneumonia.

What is the single most likely causative organism?

A. *Chlamydia psittaci*
B. *Streptococcus pneumoniae*
C. *Mycoplasma pneumoniae*
D. *Haemophilus influenzae*
E. *Staphylococcus aureus*

142. A 70-year-old alcoholic man presents with sudden onset of purulent productive cough. CXR shows consolidations left upper lobe.

What is the single most likely causative organism?

A. *Pneumocystis carinii*
B. *Aspergillus fumigatus*
C. CMV
D. *Actinomyces israelii*
E. *Klebsiella pneumoniae*

143. A 10-year-old boy with cystic fibrosis presents with pneumonia.

What is the single most likely causative organism?

A. *Pseudomonas aeruginosa*
B. *Pneumocystis carinii*
C. *Aspergillus fumigatus*
D. CMV
E. *Actinomyces israelii*

144. A 30-year-old man with AIDS presents with fever, dry cough and dyspnoea, CXR shows diffuse bilateral alveolar and interstitial shadowing beginning in the perihilar regions and spreading outward.

What is the single most likely causative organism?

A. *Pseudomonas aeruginosa*
B. *Pneumocystis carinii*
C. *Aspergillus fumigatus*
D. CMV
E. *Actinomyces israelii*

145. What is the single best criterion for the diagnosis of asthma?

A. 10% reversibility
B. 5% reversibility
C. 15% reversibility
D. FVC
E. Positive pollen skin test

146. A 9-year-old boy has a mild cough and wheeze after playing football in the cold weather.

What is the single most appropriate treatment option?

A. Oral theophylline
B. Inhaled steroids
C. Regular inhaled bronchodilation
D. Intermittent inhaled bronchodilation
E. Regular oral bronchodilation

147. A 6-year-old girl with asthma uses her bronchodilator twice a day to relieve her mild wheeze. Her parents refuse to give her any treatment containing steroids.

What is the single most appropriate treatment option?

A. Desensitization
B. Oral steroids
C. Inhaled long acting bronchodilator
D. Nebulized bronchodilator
E. Inhaled sodium cromoglycate

148. A 9-year-old girl with chronic asthma presents to A and E with rapidly worsening wheeze not relieved with inhaled bronchodilator. Steroids have been given orally.

What is the single most appropriate treatment option?

A. Nebulized bronchodilator
B. Inhaled sodium cromoglycate
C. Oral theophylline
D. Inhaled steroids
E. Regular inhaled bronchodilation

149. A 4-year-old boy with eczema and recurrent wheeze whenever he gets a viral infection has now developed night cough. There has been no improvement in spite of using inhaled bronchodilator twice each night.

What is the single most appropriate treatment option?

A. Inhaled sodium cromoglycate
B. Oral theophylline
C. Inhaled steroids
D. Regular inhaled bronchodilation
E. Intermittent inhaled bronchodilation

150. A 14-year-old boy with well controlled asthma, using inhaled steroids and a bronchodilator comes to A and E with breathlessness and swollen lips after eating a peanut butter sandwich.

What is the single most appropriate treatment option?

A. As required bronchodilator
B. IV aminophylline
C. Adrenaline intramuscularly
D. Milk free diet
E. Desensitization

151. A 10-year-old boy is getting very poor grades at school and according to headmaster seems to think like a 2-year-old. The mother also says that he has a very short temper. On examination unusually large testes are found. The boy's elder brother and uncle had similar complaints.

What is the single most likely diagnosis?

A. Fetal alcohol syndrome
B. Normal finding
C. Familial predisposition
D. Fragile X syndrome
E. Tay-Sachs' disease

152. A 5-year-old girl was born after a normal delivery has been developing normally. After an acute illness a regression of milestones has been noticed.

What is the single most likely diagnosis?

A. Birth asphyxia
B. Meningoencephalitis
C. Duchenne's muscular dystrophy
D. Klinefelter's syndrome
E. Celiac disease

153. A 2-year-old girl was born weighing 4 kg after a labour that lasted 15 hrs in a mother of 2 children. She is able to stand but is yet to walk. The mother says her other child had a similar history.

What is the single most likely diagnosis?

A. Birth asphyxia
B. Meningoencephalitis
C. Duchenne's muscular dystrophy
D. Klinefelter's syndrome
E. Celiac disease

154. A 25-year-old bartender gives birth to a 2.9 kg baby boy. The baby is found to have a head circumference of 35 cm. She has had her job for last 6 years.

What is the single most likely diagnosis?

A. Celiac disease
B. Phenylketonuria
C. Fetal alcohol syndrome
D. Normal finding
E. Familial predisposition

155. A 5-year-old boy presents with a painful knee joint. His mother notices that he has started to limp. On examination all the movements of the hip joint are limited. X-ray of the femoral head shows patchy density.

What is the single most likely diagnosis?

A. Transient synovitis (Irritable hip)
B. Ankylosing spondylitis
C. Slipped upper femoral epiphyses
D. Perthes' disease
E. Congenital hip dislocation

156. A 3-year-old girl is brought to hospital by an anxious mother, who says the child is taking too long to walk normally. On examination her perineum appears wide and the lumbar lordosis appears to be increased. She complains of occasional hip pain and is seen to have a waddling gait.

What is the single most likely diagnosis?

A. Slipped upper femoral epiphyses
B. Perthes' disease
C. Congenital hip dislocation
D. Septic arthritis
E. Juvenile rheumatoid arthritis

157. A 5-year-old boy presents with painful right hip and is seen to be limping. There is no history of trauma. The SHO in-charge admits the boy and 24 hrs later, the boy has no complaints and is discharged. X-ray of the right hip appears normal and no other joints are involved.

What is the single most likely diagnosis?

A. Transient synovitis (Irritable hip)
B. Ankylosing spondylitis
C. Slipped upper femoral epiphyses
D. Perthes' disease
E. Congenital hip dislocation

158. A 3-year-old girl with a running nose, fever and loss of appetite, presents to hospital. This was followed by stridor and cough described by mother as 'barking'.

What is the single most likely diagnosis?

A. Laryngotracheobronchitis
B. Mediastinal tumor
C. Foreign body
D. Recurrent laryngeal nerve paralysis
E. Laryngomalacia

159. A 4-year-old boy presents to the A and E with severe difficulty in breathing and stridor. He was febrile and had a pulse of 200/min. Throat cultures done upon arrival revealed a growth of influenza type b.

What is the single most likely diagnosis?

A. Foreign body
B. Recurrent laryngeal nerve paralysis
C. Laryngomalacia
D. Acute epiglottitis
E. Laryngeal stenosis

160. A 2-day-old breastfed male infant is vomiting after each feed. Abdominal X-ray demonstrated a "double bubble".

What is the single most likely diagnosis?

A. Duodenal atresia
B. Pancreatitis
C. Gastro-esophageal reflux
D. Psychogenic vomiting
E. Gastroenteritis

161. A 6-week-old breast fed boy has had projectile vomiting after every feed for past 2 weeks. He is now lethargic, dehydrated and tachypnoeic.

What is the single most likely diagnosis?

A. Pyloric stenosis
B. Meconium ileus
C. UTI
D. Meningitis
E. Whooping cough

162. A 4-month old boy who is thriving has persistent vomiting, which is occasionally blood stained and is associated with crying.

What is the single most likely diagnosis?

A. Duodenal atresia
B. Pancreatitis
C. Gastro-esophageal reflux
D. Psychogenic vomiting
E. Gastroenteritis

163. An 8-year-old girl shows signs of moderated dehydration. She has vomited all fluids for 24 hrs and the vomit is not bile stained. Her abdomen is now soft and non-tender. She has had 2 similar episodes in the past year.

What is the single most likely diagnosis?

A. Mesenteric adenitis
B. Cyclical vomiting
C. Overfeeding
D. Duodenal atresia
E. Pancreatitis

164. A 12-week-old thriving baby is vomiting after every feed. He is developmentally normal and is fed by the bottle at 260 ml/hg day.

What is the single most likely diagnosis?

A. Mesenteric adenitis
B. Cyclical vomiting
C. Overfeeding
D. Duodenal atresia
E. Pancreatitis

165. A 15-year-old boy has very poor grades at school despite being very attentive and hard working. His mother reckons its because he is teased at school because his breasts look like a girl's. On further examination he is found to have a small testes. He is mildly asthmatic.

What is the single most likely diagnosis?

A. Klinefelter's syndrome
B. Sickle cell trait
C. Patau syndrome
D. Beta thalassemia
E. Down's syndrome

166. A 5-year-old South African boy is brought to the A and E deeply jaundiced. He is found to have mildly swollen, tender feet and hands. His mucosae are pale.

What is the single most likely diagnosis?

A. Di George syndrome
B. Fragile X syndrome
C. Acute myeloid leukemia
D. Sickle cell disease
E. Edward's syndrome

167. A 6-year-old Asian boy gets regular blood transfusions for his hematological abnormality. His mucosae are pale and skull is grossly bossed. Haematological investigations were done and are as follows:

MCHC 25 g/dl
Hb 8 g/dl
MCV 74 fl

What is the single most likely diagnosis?

A. Patau syndrome B. Beta thalassaemia
C. Down's syndrome D. William's syndrome
E. Turner's syndrome

168. A 10-year-old boy is brought to the A and E with a swollen right arm. His temperature is 38.5°C and is unable to move his arm due to severe pain. Blood cultures confirm salmonella osteomyelitis. This is his second presentation this month and earlier presented with an acute onset hepatosplenomegaly associated with severe pallor. The SHO does a sodium metabisulphite test on the patient's blood, which turns out to be positive.

What is the single most likely diagnosis?

A. Di George syndrome
B. Fragile X syndrome
C. Acute myeloid leukemia
D. Sickle cell disease
E. Edward's syndrome

169. A 39-year-old male is getting progressively forgetful and is later found to have Alzheimer's disease. He has small ears and an IQ score of 67.

What is the single most likely diagnosis?

A. Klinefelter's syndrome
B. Sickle cell trait
C. Patau syndrome
D. Beta thalassaemia
E. Down's syndrome

170. A 4-year-old girl looks wasted and appears short for her age. The mother reports the daughter has been vomiting on several occasions in the past with associated diarrhea. The SHO thinks she has an enteropathy and on serology, anti-endomysial antibodies were found.

What is the single most likely diagnosis?

A. Chronic non-specific diarrhoea
B. Irritable bowel syndrome
C. Celiac disease
D. Endometriosis
E. Ulcerative colitis

171. A mother brings her 5-year-old son who has been passing bloody stool associated with severe abdominal pain. On examination he is found to have mildly swollen tender wrists and red nodular tender lesions were found on his forearms.

What is the single most likely diagnosis?

A. Endometriosis
B. Ulcerative colitis
C. Acute on chronic appendicitis
D. Giardiasis
E. Enterobius vermicularis infection

172. An 8-year-old girl has got repeated episodes of diarrhoea. On each occasion the stool contains segments of undigested vegetables. The pediatrician recommends restricting fluids to meal times. The girl's condition improves and she is thriving.

What is the single most likely diagnosis?

A. Chronic non-specific diarrhea
B. Irritable bowel syndrome
C. Celiac disease
D. Endometriosis
E. Ulcerative colitis

173. A mother and her daughter have just returned from a tropical holiday and the mother is concerned that her daughter has an STD, since she complains of constant perianal and vulval irritation. There is no associated vaginal discharge.
What is the single most likely diagnosis?
A. Endometriosis
B. Ulcerative colitis
C. Acute on chronic appendicitis
D. Giardiasis
E. Enterobius vermicularis infection

174. A 15-year-old girl complains of episodic diarrhea, which typically starts in the morning with a constant urge to go to the toilet on waking and after breakfast. She says there is associated abdominal pain in the right iliac fossa relieved by defecation or flatus. She has had the symptoms for 3 months.
What is the single most likely diagnosis?
A. Hirschsprung's disease
B. Acrodermatitis enteropathica
C. Intussusception
D. Chronic non-specific diarrhoea
E. Irritable bowel syndrome

175. A 5-month-old baby presents with vomiting, following a 2 hr history of abdominal pain associated with drawing up of legs. The mother says her baby has passed reddish stool.
What is the single most likely diagnosis?
A. Acute cholecystitis
B. Cyclical vomiting
C. Duodenal atresia
D. Necrotizing enterocolitis
E. Intussusception

176. A 12-year-old girl presents with fever, flank pain. An abdominal mass is found on examination. Urine microscopy shows no haematuria.
What is the single most likely diagnosis?
A. Wilms' nephroblastoma
B. UTI
C. Mesenteric thrombosis
D. Acute pancreatitis
E. Gastro-esophageal reflux

177. An 8-year-old girl shows signs of moderate dehydration. She has vomited all fluids for 24 hrs and the vomit is not bile stained. Her abdomen is now soft and non-tender. She has had 2 similar episodes in the past year.
What is the single most likely diagnosis?
A. Meconium ileus
B. Acute cholecystitis
C. Cyclical vomiting
D. Duodenal atresia
E. Necrotizing enterocolitis

178. A 6-week old breastfed girl has projectile vomiting after every feed for the past 2 weeks. She is now lethargic, dehydrated and tachypnoeic.
What is the single most likely diagnosis?
A. Hirschsprung's disease
B. Meningitis
C. Pyloric stenosis
D. Meconium ileus
E. Acute cholecystitis

179. A 1-day-old breastfed infant is vomiting after each feed. Abdominal X-ray shows a double-bubble sign.
What is the single most likely diagnosis?
A. Cyclical vomiting
B. Duodenal atresia
C. Necrotizing enterocolitis
D. Intussusception
E. Psychogenic vomiting

180. A 6-year-old febrile child is drowsy and vomiting. She is being treated for otitis media by her GP.
What is the single most likely diagnosis?
A. Meningitis
B. Pyloric stenosis
C. Meconium ileus
D. Acute cholecystitis
E. Cyclical vomiting

181. Eight days after a premature birth, a mother notices her baby crying excessively and has passed blood and mucus per rectum. The infant is still in the special care baby unit.
What is the single most likely diagnosis?
A. Acute cholecystitis
B. Cyclical vomiting
C. Duodenal atresia
D. Necrotizing enterocolitis
E. Intussusception

182. A 15-year-old boy who is thriving has a mild abdominal pain and is passing "rice water" stools. She had been at a mates' birthday party the night before.

What is the single most likely diagnosis?

A. UTI
B. Mesenteric thrombosis
C. Acute pancreatitis
D. Gastroesophageal reflux
E. Gastroenteritis

183. A 15-month boy is admitted to A and E shocked. There is no history of diarrhoea, but he has been passing large amounts of melanotic stools. On examination he is anaemic.

What is the single most likely diagnosis?

A. Meckel's diverticulum
B. Ulcerative colitis
C. Eosinophilic colitis
D. Crohn's disease
E. Intussusception

184. A 4-year-old girl presents with bloody diarrhoea and crampy abdominal pain. Blood tests show anaemia and thrombocytopenia.

What is the single most likely diagnosis?

A. Haemorrhoids
B. Haemolytic-uraemic syndrome
C. Hirschsprung's disease
D. Lymphonodular hyperplasia
E. Anal fissure

185. A 5-week-old infant presents with scanty streaks of fresh blood mixed with normal coloured stools.

What is the single most likely diagnosis?

A. Meckel's diverticulum
B. Ulcerative colitis
C. Eosinophilic colitis
D. Crohn's disease
E. Intussusception

186. A 7-year-old boy presents with streaks of fresh blood on the side of normal coloured stools and drops of fresh blood in the toilet. There is no history of abdominal pain or rectal pain.

What is the single most likely diagnosis?

A. Haemolytic-uraemic syndrome
B. Hirschsprung's disease
C. Lymphonodular hyperplasia
D. Anal fissure
E. Juvenile polyps

187. A 3-year-old boy is admitted to A and E after passing several grossly bloody stools. There is no history of abdominal pain, fever or vomiting. On examination he is markedly pale.

What is the single most likely diagnosis?

A. Meckel's diverticulum
B. Ulcerative colitis
C. Eosinophilic colitis
D. Crohn's disease
E. Intussusception

188. A 12-year-old girl presented with a 4-week history of rectal bleeding and frequent loose motions. She reported lower abdominal cramping during defaecation but denied fever, rash, weight loss, arthritis or vomiting. Investigations showed anaemia but normal ESR, albumin and liver enzymes.

What is the single most likely diagnosis?

A. Ulcerative colitis
B. Eosinophilic colitis
C. Crohn's disease
D. Intussusception
E. Haemorrhoids

189. A 20-year-old first time mother with severe weight loss, anorexia and believes that her husband is interested in killing her and their baby son and feels completely worthless.

What is the single most appropriate treatment option?

A. Electroconvulsive therapy
B. Imipramine
C. Flupenthixol
D. NO action
E. Psychodynamic psychotherapy

190. A 40-year-old man has been treated for depression for 6 months. He is now beginning to lose weight and getting 'suicidal thoughts more frequently than before.

What is the single most appropriate treatment option?

A. Electroconvulsive therapy
B. Imipramine
C. Flupenthixol
D. NO action
E. Psychodynamic psychotherapy

191. A 29-year-old woman presents with inability to sleep and aggressiveness and increased libido. Her husband says prior to this, she was markedly with drawn and blamed herself for their daughter's death due to cancer, threatening to join her.

What is the single most appropriate treatment option?

A. Behavioural therapy
B. Abreaction
C. Marital therapy
D. Counselling
E. Lithium

192. A 12-year-old boy refuses to go to school because of constant failure to get grade. He is threatening to starve himself to death.

What is the single most appropriate treatment option?

A. Psychodynamic psychotherapy
B. Psychosurgery
C. Cognitive therapy
D. Hypnotherapy
E. Behavioural therapy

193. A 16-year-old girl with a BMI of 16 complains of 3-month history of amenorrhoea. She is not on the pill and the pregnancy test is negative. She wants to be a model.

What is the single most appropriate treatment option?

A. Hypnotherapy
B. Behavioural therapy
C. Abreaction
D. Marital therapy
E. Counselling

194. A 20-year-old man keeps cleaning his hands every time he shakes his partner's hands. He was a high achiever in high school.

What is the single most likely diagnosis?

A. Borderline personality disorder
B. Obsessive compulsive disorder
C. Schizotypal personality disorder
D. Avoidant personality disorder
E. Schizoid personality disorder

195. A 56-year-old farmer believes that his neighbour is killing his farm animals despite the local veterinary's advice that the death is due to an outbreak of anthrax. He spends hours watching his neighbour through pair of binocular lens, hoping to catch him in the act.

What is the single most likely diagnosis?

A. Histrionic personality disorder
B. Paranoid personality disorder
C. Borderline personality disorder
D. Obsessive compulsive disorder
E. Schizotypal personality disorder

196. A 16-year-old girl is described as 'queer' by her mates. She is unfriendly and has no close friends despite numerous attempts by boys in her college. She lacks empathy and is largely introspective.

What is the single most likely diagnosis?

A. Schizotypal personality disorder
B. Avoidant personality disorder
C. Schizoid personality disorder
D. Antisocial personality disorder
E. Panic attack disorder

197. A 16-year-old girl in high school always comes late to class wearing strong perfume in a vain attempt to attract attention. She laughs loudly at jokes, many of her mates don't find particularly hilarious.

What is the single most likely diagnosis?

A. Histrionic personality disorder
B. Paranoid personality disorder
C. Borderline personality disorder
D. Obsessive compulsive disorder
E. Schizotypal personality disorder

198. A 32-year-old man always gives in to his wife over any decision even when he knows that this isn't right. He insists on having his wife prepare his every meal, wash him and put him to sleep. He cries whenever his wife is away.

What is the single most likely diagnosis?

A. Avoidant personality disorder
B. Schizoid personality disorder
C. Antisocial personality disorder
D. Panic attack disorder
E. Dependant personality disorder

199. A 23-year-old student presents with insomnia, headaches, sweating, palpitations, chest pain and poor appetite.
What is the single most likely diagnosis?
A. Chronic alcoholism
B. Hysteria
C. Phobia
D. Paranoid state
E. Anxiety neurosis

200. A 35-year-old single woman presents with weight loss, poor appetite, decreased ability to concentrate and guilt feelings.
What is the single most likely diagnosis?
A. Depression
B. Mania
C. Post-traumatic stress disorder
D. Obsessional neurosis
E. Schizophrenia

201. A 19-year-old female student presents with sudden blindness. Neurological examination reveals no abnormality.
What is the single most likely diagnosis?
A. Obsessional neurosis
B. Schizophrenia
C. Depersonalization
D. Chronic alcoholism
E. Hysteria

202. A 20-year-old man presents with disinhibition, hyperactivity, increased appetite and grandiose delusions.
What is the single most likely diagnosis?
A. Depression
B. Mania
C. Post-traumatic stress disorder
D. Obsessional neurosis
E. Schizophrenia

203. A 30-year-old man presents with auditory hallucinations, social withdrawal and delusions of persecution.
What is the single most likely diagnosis?
A. Schizophrenia
B. Depersonalization
C. Chronic alcoholism
D. Hysteria
E. Paranoia

204. A 21-year-old man presents with compulsions and rituals, which he resists.
What is the single most likely diagnosis?
A. Post-traumatic stress disorder
B. Obsessional neurosis
C. Schizophrenia
D. Depersonalization
E. Chronic alcoholism

205. A 70-year-old retired engineer experiences changes in personality and impaired social skills. His family, who describe him as forgetful and not as sharp, corroborates this. There are no objective features of depression.
What is the single most likely diagnosis?
A. Dementia
B. Grief reaction
C. Panic attacks
D. Schizophrenia
E. Postnatal psychosis

206. A 20-year-old man is noted to be withdrawn, isolated and 'peculiar'. He experiences persecutory delusions and auditory hallucinations.
What is the single most likely diagnosis?
A. Dementia
B. Grief reaction
C. Panic attacks
D. Schizophrenia
E. Postnatal psychosis

207. A 60-year-old widow is noted by her family to be restless, disorganized, crying and frequently expresses her wish to join her deceased partner.
What is the single most likely diagnosis?
A. Suicidal risk
B. Opioid abuse
C. Alcohol abuse
D. Depression
E. Anxiety

208. A 40-year-old Irishman complains of frequent episodes of chest pains, sweating, palpitations, a sense of impending doom and trembling that lasts for minutes at a time.
What is the single most likely diagnosis?
A. Anxiety
B. Delirium
C. Dementia
D. Grief reaction
E. Panic attacks

209. A 25-year-old man presents with miosis, slurred speech, disorientation, and respiratory depression.
What is the single most likely diagnosis?
A. Opioid abuse B. Alcohol abuse
C. Depression D. Anxiety
E. Delirium

210. A 70-year-old man presents with progressive forgetfulness and mood changes. He has a shuffling gait. The head CT scan shows cortical atrophy and enlarged ventricles.
What is the single most appropriate treatment option?
A. Propranolol
B. Donepezil
C. Disulfiram
D. Levodopa + carbidopa
E. Methadone

A 60-year-old man presents with a disturbance of voluntary motor function. His face is expressionless. On examination he has cogwheel rigidity and bradykinesia.
What is the single most appropriate treatment option?
A. Disulfiram
B. Levodopa + carbidopa
C. Methadone
D. Diazepam
E. Prozac

212. A 10-year-old boy presents with brief repetitive motor tics and is brought in by his parents for shouting obscenities at school.
What is the single most appropriate treatment option?
A. Levodopa + carbidopa
B. Methadone
C. Diazepam
D. Prozac
E. Haloperidol

213. A 40-year-old man presents with ataxia. His wife states that it runs in her husband's family. He is difficult to live with, very irritable, clumsy and suffers from jerky movements of the legs.
What is the single most appropriate treatment option?
A. Long-term psychotherapy
B. Tetrabenzine
C. Lithium
D. Propranolol
E. Donepezil

214. A 20-year-old man presents with sweating, muscle twitching and abdominal cramps. On examination he had dilated pupils.
What is the single most appropriate treatment option?
A. Propranolol
B. Donepezil
C. Disulfiram
D. Levodopa + carbidopa
E. Methadone

215. A 23-year-old female complains of irritability and constant depression. She has thought about suicide. She has trouble sleeping and has lost her appetite.
What is the single most likely diagnosis?
A. Major depression
B. Porphyria
C. Drug-induced depression
D. Manic-depressive disorder
E. Bereavement reaction

216. A 20-year-old female complains of episodes of irritability and depression. She also complains of monthly bloating and tension.
What is the single most likely diagnosis?
A. Premenstrual syndrome
B. Cushing's syndrome
C. Puerperal affective disorder
D. Hyperparathyroidism
E. Major depression

217. A 30-year-old female complains of depression, lethargy, constipation, and weight gain. She also suffers from menorrhagia.
What is the single most likely diagnosis?
A. Manic-depressive disorder
B. Bereavement reaction
C. Drug abuse
D. Hypothyroidism
E. Vitamin and mineral disorders

218. A 40-year-old woman presents with depression and weight gain. She complains of back pain and excessive thirst. Her menstrual period lasts for 3 days and sometimes she skips a cycle. On examination she is obese with acne and peripheral edema.
What is the single most likely diagnosis?
A. Cushing's syndrome
B. Puerperal affective disorder
C. Hyperparathyroidism
D. Major depression
E. Porphyria

219. A 30-year-old female on OC pills presents with colicky abdominal pain, vomiting, and depression. She is noted to be hypertensive. On standing, the urine turns deep red.
What is the single most likely diagnosis?
A. Porphyria
B. Drug induced depression
C. Manic-depressive disorder
D. Bereavement reaction
E. Drug abuse

220. A 25-year-old man has no close friends. He avoids social situations. He is unable to express tender emotions. He has no overt signs of hallucination or delusional behaviour.
What is the single most likely diagnosis?
A. Schizoid
B. Multiple personality
C. Borderline
D. Histrionic
E. Narcissistic

221. A 17-year-old boy is brought to his GP by his parents for abusive behaviour. He is delinquent from school and has been arrested for assault and theft.
What is the single most likely diagnosis?
A. Antisocial
B. Avoidant
C. Schizotypal
D. Passive-aggressive
E. Paranoid

222. A 23-year-old man believes that he is perfect. He is unable to empathize and manipulates people and situations. He sees everyone else as flawed. His relationships are shallow.
What is the single most likely diagnosis?
A. Borderline
B. Histrionic
C. Narcissistic
D. Antisocial
E. Avoidant

223. A 33-year-old female presents to the GP with chronic feelings of boredom and depression. She shops excessively and is sexually promiscuous. She has cut herself in the past to relieve her anxiety.
What is the single most likely diagnosis?
A. Schizoid
B. Multiple personality
C. Borderline
D. Histrionic
E. Narcissistic

224. A 25-year-old anxious female presents to her GP. She suffers from low self-esteem and doesn't take risks in life. She seems extremely sensitive to criticism.
What is the single most likely diagnosis?
A. Avoidant
B. Schizotypal
C. Passive-aggressive
D. Paranoid
E. Obsessive-compulsive

225. A 40-year-old man insists that his wife is unfaithful and sleeping with an entire neighbourhood. He is hypersensitive, argumentative and litigious, his wife has left him due to his behaviour. He functions well at work.
What is the single most likely diagnosis?
A. Delusional disorder
B. Major depression
C. Paranoid schizophrenia
D. Body dysmorphic disorder
E. Postpartum depression

226. A 25-year-old woman presents with personality changes. She is noted by her friends initially to be anxious, irritable and an insomniac and weeks later she becomes profoundly depressed with low self-esteem and contemplates suicide. In consultation she has pressured speech with boundless energy.
What is the single most likely diagnosis?
A. Schizoaffective disorder
B. Bipolar disorder
C. Delusional disorder
D. Major depression
E. Paranoid schizophrenia

227. A 20-year-old woman has a mental breakdown. She has recently broken up with her boyfriend. She has dramatic mood swings, memory loss and incoherent speech. This lasts for a month.
What is the single most likely diagnosis?
A. Post-traumatic stress disorder
B. Brief reactive psychosis
C. Schizoaffective disorder
D. Bipolar disorder
E. Delusional disorder

228. A 20-year-old woman presents to her GP complaining of feeling depressed ever since she can remember. Her parents died in a car crash 10 years ago. She sees herself as a failure but functions well at work. She has trouble falling asleep.
What is the single most likely diagnosis?
A. Paranoid schizophrenia
B. Body dysmorphic disorder
C. Postpartum depression
D. Panic disorder
E. Dysthymia

229. A 50-year-old woman complains of sudden episodes of feeling impending doom. During these episodes she feels choked and sweats profusely.
What is the single most likely diagnosis?
A. Paranoid schizophrenia
B. Body dysmorphic disorder
C. Postpartum depression
D. Panic disorder
E. Dysthymia

230. A 2-year-old boy presents with anemia and abdominal pain. His mother states that she has seen him peeling paint chips off the wall and wonders if he has been eating this ?
What is the single most likely diagnosis?
A. Pica
B. Algophobia
C. Formication
D. Delirium
E. Alcohol withdrawal

231. A 23-year-old woman becomes afraid to leave her home. She functions normally except will not step outside the house.
What is the single most likely diagnosis?
A. Schizophrenia
B. Opioid withdrawal
C. Xenophobia
D. Drug toxicity
E. Agoraphobia

232. An 18-year-old man presents with nausea, vomiting and diaphoresis. His pupils are dilated and his blood pressure is elevated. He has a history of drug addiction.
What is the single most likely diagnosis?
A. Alcohol intoxication
B. Cocaine intoxication
C. Schizophrenia
D. Opioid withdrawal
E. Xenophobia

233. A 30-year-old woman is found in an amnesic state. Her husband reports that she had been missing for a few days after she has been served with divorce papers.
What is the single most likely diagnosis?
A. Alcohol withdrawal
B. Fugue
C. Alcohol intoxication
D. Cocaine intoxication
E. Schizophrenia

234. A 30-year-old man with bipolar disorder is taking lithium. He was recently started on thiazide diuretics for mild hypertension. He is now confused with ataxia, blurred vision and a coarse tremor.
What is the single most likely diagnosis?
A. Cocaine intoxication
B. Schizophrenia
C. Opioid withdrawal
D. Xenophobia
E. Drug toxicity

235. A 28-year-old female presents with lower abdominal pain. On examination she has multiple surgical scars over her abdomen. Her abdominal and pelvic examinations are normal. She insists, she needs a laparoscopy.
What is the single most likely diagnosis?
A. Munchausen's syndrome
B. Dissociative disorder
C. Alcohol withdrawal delirium
D. Malingering disorder
E. Extra-pyramidal side effect

236. A 50-year-old schizophrenic is started on haloperidol. A month later he is noted to be drooling saliva and walking with a shuffling gait. He also suffers from involuntary chewing movements.
What is the single most likely diagnosis?
A. Malingering disorder
B. Extra-pyramidal side effect
C. Parkinson's disease
D. Hypothyroidism
E. Cushing's syndrome

237. A 40-year-old female complains of dry mouth, blurry vision, and constipation. On examination she had dilated pupils. She was started on amitriptyline for major depression.
What is the single most likely diagnosis?
A. Cushing's syndrome
B. Hysterical neurosis
C. Autonomic side effect
D. Acromegaly
E. Anticholinergic side effect

238. A 45-year-old man complains of headaches, excessive thirst, and frequent urination. On examination he is noted to have bad acne, coarse skin and has a goitre. He has moved his wedding band to the 5th finger.
What is the single most likely diagnosis?
A. Hypothyroidism
B. Cushing's syndrome
C. Hysterical neurosis
D. Autonomic side effect
E. Acromegaly

239. A 30-year-old man presents to casualty with a dislocated shoulder. On examination, the shoulder is found not to be dislocated. The patient insists it is dislocated.
What is the single most likely diagnosis?
A. Munchausen's syndrome
B. Dissociative disorder
C. Alcohol withdrawal delirium
D. Malingering disorder
E. Extra-pyramidal side effect

240. A 28-year-old woman lost her job 3 months ago. She attends her GP complaining of difficulty in sleeping. She feels tired, has a poor appetite and has lost some weight. She feels worthless. She says before she was fired from her job her boss used to record her phone calls and also heard him talking ill about her to her colleagues. She thought of committing suicide and says that her husband would not miss her if she were dead.
What is the single most appropriate treatment option?
A. Temazepam
B. Fluoxetine
C. Zopiclone
D. Buspirone
E. Risperidone

241. A 41-year-old man has been brought to casualty after being found in the street acting in a bizarre fashion. He was exposing his genitals to passers-by. In casualty he was angry and abusive. He refuses to have any tests in the hospital.
What is the single most appropriate treatment option?
A. Risperidone
B. Lithium carbonate
C. Thioridazine
D. Haloperidol
E. Drug treatment not appropriate

242. A 21-year-old single woman gave birth to her first child 2 days ago. Since the birth she has been unable to sleep and is reluctant to hold her baby or feed her. She is very tearful and cries for no reason. She denies thoughts of harming the baby.
What is the single most appropriate treatment option?
A. Risperidone
B. Lithium carbonate
C. Thioridazine
D. Haloperidol
E. Drug treatment not appropriate

243. A 64-year-old woman has a 3 year history of increasing confusion, loss of mobility and tremor. She has recently developed frequent visual hallucinations and tends to cry out for no reason, particularly at night. There is no evidence of an acute medical cause for her confusion. On examination she is alert but disorientated and quite agitated. She has a coarse resting tremor, increased tone in her limbs and normal reflexes.

What is the single most appropriate treatment option?

A. Temazepam
B. Fluoxetine
C. Zopiclone
D. Buspirone
E. Risperidone

244. A mother is worried about her 25-year-old son. He seems to jump from I topic to another, make up words, laugh at inappropriate things and talk to someone imaginary. He has blacked out his windows and complains that someone else is controlling his thoughts.

What is the single most likely diagnosis?

A. Anorexia nervosa
B. Schizophrenia
C. Mania
D. Depression with psychomotor
E. Hypomania retardation

245. A 40-year-old man presents to his GP with headaches, insomnia and weight gain. He is slow and sluggish when he speaks. He describes a loss of interest in everything, a feeling of worthlessness and often cries alone.

What is the single most likely diagnosis?

A. Anorexia nervosa
B. Schizophrenia
C. Mania
D. Depression with psychomotor
E. Hypomania retardation

246. A 23-year-old woman presents with an episode of generalized paraesthesia, "flapping" limbs, loss of urinary incontinence and abnormal posturing of the hands. These episodes are preceded by chest tightness and difficulty swallowing. Recently she has been feeling that parts of her are made of cotton wool.

What is the single most likely diagnosis?

A. Obsessive compulsive disorder
B. Cyclothymic disorder
C. Phobia
D. Hyperventilation syndrome
E. Acute confusional state

247. A wife cannot cope up with her husband's moods. She says he is very labile. He goes from being full of energy and happy one day to being so pessimistic about everything the next day.

What is the single most likely diagnosis?

A. Obsessive compulsive disorder
B. Cyclothymic disorder
C. Phobia
D. Hyperventilation syndrome
E. Acute confusional state

248. A 35-year-old lady has a persistent abnormality of mood continually alternating between euphoria and depression.

What is the single most likely diagnosis?

A. Obsessional personality
B. Immoral personality
C. Sociopathic personality
D. Asthenic personality
E. Affective disorder

249. A 36-year-old gentleman who is a perfectionist to a rigid degree.

What is the single most likely diagnosis?

A. Schizoid personality
B. Suicidal personality
C. Obsessional personality
D. Immoral personality
E. Sociopathic personality

250. A 45-year-old serial killer who shows no remorse for crimes he has committed.

What is the single most likely diagnosis?

A. Schizod personality
B. Suicidal personality
C. Obsessional personality
D. Immoral personality
E. Sociopathic personality

251. A 24-year-old lady whom has had a number of failed relationships and has a tendency to dramatize limb pains.

What is the single most likely diagnosis?

A. Hysterical personality
B. Manic personality
C. Schizoid personality
D. Suicidal personality
E. Obsessional personality

252. A shy 27-year-old man who is shy of advances and tends to be aloof.
What is the single most likely diagnosis?
A. Manic personality
B. Schizoid personality
C. Suicidal personality
D. Obsessional personality
E. Immoral personality

253. A 56-year-old woman says that she sees her deceased husband in and around the house.
What is the single most appropriate treatment option?
A. Behavioural therapy
B. Anti-psychotic therapy
C. Bereavement counseling
D. Anti-depressive medication
E. Chlorpromazine treatment

254. A 19-year-old female university student undertakes hand washing up to 30 times in one day; this is getting in the way of her work.
What is the single most appropriate treatment option?
A. Benzodiazepine medication
B. Cognitive therapy
C. Hypnotherapy
D. Group therapy
E. Behavioural therapy

255. A 50-year-old vagrant thought to be alcoholic is admitted to the ward where is being unruly and thinks the nurses are going to kill him.
What is the single most appropriate treatment option?
A. Lithium
B. Emergency care order
C. Electroconvulsive therapy
D. Benzodiazepine medication
E. Cognitive therapy

256. A 24-year-old man says that aliens are talking to him and controlling his thoughts.
What is the single most appropriate treatment option?
A. Behavioural therapy
B. Anti-psychotic therapy
C. Bereavement counseling
D. Anti-depressive medication
E. Chlorpromazine treatment

257. A 40-year-old woman is scared of flying.
What is the single most appropriate treatment option?
A. Benzodiazepine medication
B. Cognitive therapy
C. Hypnotherapy
D. Group therapy
E. Behavioural therapy

258. A mother brings her child to you with chronic diarrhoea. You have strong grounds to suspect a fractious illness because the nursing staff have found a number of packets of laxatives in her bag.
What is the single most appropriate management option?
A. Inform the police
B. Reassure
C. Inform social services
D. Imipramine
E. Refer to a dietician

259. A 25-year-old lady arrives at the local accident and emergency department after ingesting an unknown amount of an unknown drug.
What is the single most appropriate management option?
A. Refer to a dietician
B. Counselling
C. Refer to a psychiatrist
D. Contact the GP
E. Refer to general medical team

260. You get a call to visit a patient's house. The patient had been missing for last 4 days. The patient's neighbour tells you that 4 days back the patient's GP had come to visit him.
What is the single most appropriate management option?
A. Refer to a dietician
B. Counselling
C. Refer to a psychiatrist
D. Contact the GP
E. Refer to general medical team

261. A 30-year-old man presents with dizziness and irritability. In the A and E the patient behaves aggressively and abuses the nursing staff. On examination you find him to be febrile. Mild neck rigidity is present.

What is the single most appropriate management option?

A. Refer to a dietician
B. Counselling
C. Refer to a psychiatrist
D. Contact the GP
E. Refer to general medical team

262. A young lady who use to be an IV drug abuser has now completely stop taking drugs. She comes to you saying that her boyfriend is now forcing her to take drugs again.

What is the single most appropriate management option?

A. Inform the police
B. Reassure
C. Inform social services
D. Imipramine
E. Refer to a dietician

263. A 32-year-old lady is afraid to go out in the market. Whenever she goes out of the house she comes home running and gasping for breath. She immediately locks her doors and windows after reaching home. She is otherwise normal in the house.

What is the single most appropriate management option?

A. Inform social services
B. Imipramine
C. Refer to a dietician
D. Counselling
E. Refer to a psychiatrist

264. A 25-year-old woman finds it difficult to leave her home. She becomes very agitated in supermarkets and describes palpitations and difficulty breathing when in crowds.

What is the single most likely diagnosis?

A. Bipolar affective disorder
B. Panic attacks
C. Anxiety neurosis
D. Post-traumatic stress disorder
E. Agoraphobia

265. A 40-year-old man complains of low mood and fatigue. He has a poor appetite and has loss of libido. He wakes at 2 am and is unable to return to sleep. He feels guilty about the death of his mother 2 years ago.

What is the single most likely diagnosis?

A. Depression
B. Social phobia
C. Bipolar affective disorder
D. Panic attacks
E. Anxiety neurosis

266. A 30-year-old man is seen in dermatology outpatients with very sore hands. He has dry, cracked skin on all his fingers. He says he has to wash his hands at least 30 times a day and is unable to sleep of he has not done so.

What is the single most likely diagnosis?

A. Anxiety neurosis
B. Post-traumatic stress disorder
C. Agoraphobia
D. Specific phobia
E. Obsessive compulsive disorder

267. A 20-year-old woman attends A and E complaining of sudden breathlessness and anxiety. She describes palpitations and paraesthesia of her hands, feet and lips. ECG shows sinus tachycardia and O_2 saturation is normal.

What is the single most likely diagnosis?

A. Depression
B. Social phobia
C. Bipolar affective disorder
D. Panic attacks
E. Anxiety neurosis

268. A 35-year-old train driver is on sick leave after an incident in which a child ran onto the tracks. He is unable to go near railways and takes excessively long route to avoid them. He is troubled by flashbacks of the accident, which frequently disturbs his sleep.

What is the single most likely diagnosis?

A. Anxiety neurosis
B. Post-traumatic stress disorder
C. Agoraphobia
D. Specific phobia
E. Obsessive compulsive disorder

269. A 35-year-old man is agitated and euphoric. He claims to be helping the Prime Minister with economic policy, although this is not true when checked.

What is the single most likely diagnosis?

A. Paraphrenia
B. Mania
C. Drug-induced
D. Toxic confusional state
E. Personality disorder

270. A 20-year-old man complains that all his movements are being watched. Sometimes he feels as though his actions are being controlled by his radio. At other times he is aware of voices describing what he is doing.

What is the single most likely diagnosis?

A. Schizophrenia
B. Korsakoff's psychosis
C. Psychotic depression
D. Paraphrenia
E. Mania

271. A 50-year-old man complains of being pursued by the police for a crime he denies committing. He has poor concentration and impaired short-term memory. He admits to drinking large amounts of alcohol.

What is the single most likely diagnosis?

A. Korsakoff's psychosis
B. Psychotic depression
C. Paraphrenia
D. Mania
E. Drug-induced

272. A 65-year-old woman says that she dies 3 months ago and is very distressed that nobody has buried her. When she is outdoors she hears people say that she is evil and needs to be punished.

What is the single most likely diagnosis?

A. Korsakoff's psychosis
B. Psychotic depression
C. Paraphrenia
D. Mania
E. Drug-induced

273. A 40-year-old teetotal woman is recovering from a hysterectomy 2 days ago. At night she becomes agitated and complains of seeing animals and children walking around the wards.

What is the single most likely diagnosis?

A. Paraphrenia
B. Mania
C. Drug-induced
D. Toxic confusional state
E. Personality disorder

274. A 30-year-old male slides slowly into a severe depression over a number of months for no particular reason. His hobbies and interests are dropped, his social contact diminishes and his mood lower. He visits a psychiatrist for the first time because he is becoming increasingly distressed with disturbed sleep patterns and no appetite. He feels his future is hopeless.

What is the single most appropriate treatment option?

A. Tricyclic depressants
B. MAOI
C. Reserpine
D. Carbamazepine
E. Sodium valproate

275. A 40-year-old has repeated episodes of depressed mood in response to feeling rejected and a craving for sweets and chocolates. These reactive mood changes are accompanied by hypersomnia, lethargy and increased appetite particularly with a preference for carbohydrates.

What is the single most appropriate treatment option?

A. Tricyclic depressants
B. MAOI
C. Reserpine
D. Carbamazepine
E. Sodium valproate

276. A 55-year-old woman has mania associated with cyclic and frequent depressive features.

What is the single most appropriate treatment option?

A. Tricyclic depressants
B. MAOI
C. Reserpine
D. Carbamazepine
E. Sodium valproate

277. An 18-year-old previously healthy girl waiting for her college exam result. The result is arriving that day by post and she is suffering from acute anxiety due to the importance of the results for her future career. Her mother consults her GP.

What is the single most appropriate treatment option?

A. SSRI
B. Lorazepam
C. St Johns Wort
D. Electroconvulsive therapy
E. Lithium

278. A 30-year-old female patient with suspected manic depression suffers from severe mood swings.

What is the single most appropriate treatment option?

A. Electroconvulsive therapy
B. Lithium
C. Tricyclic depressants
D. MAOI
E. Reserpine

279. A 64-year-old man with bronchoscopically confirmed squamous cell carcinoma of the right upper lobe has a normal FEV1 of 2.5 L and normal serum biochemistry.

What is the single most appropriate investigation to assess operability?

A. Bone scan
B. Chest CT scan
C. Differential perfusion lung scan
D. Measurement of total lung capacity
E. Sputum cytology

280. A 55-year-old female is admitted with a chest infection. Investigations reveal consolidation in the right base on the chest X-ray and urinary legionella antigen is found to be positive.

What is the single most appropriate treatment?

A. Cefotaxime
B. Clarithromycin
C. Co-amoxiclav
D. Minocycline
E. Vancomycin

281. A 17-year-old boy attends the Accident and Emergency Department having been taken ill whilst playing football. He gives a history of sudden onset of left-sided chest pain followed by severe and persistent breathlessness.

What is the single investigation most likely to provide a definitive diagnosis?

A. Blood gases
B. Chest X-ray
C. Echocardiogram
D. Electrocardiogram (ECG)
E. Pulmonary function tests

282. An 85-year-old man who weighs 80 kg is admitted as an emergency with fever and delirium. He gives a history of dysuria and frequency. His blood pressure (BP) is 70/50 mmHg and temperature 38.6°C. His serum creatinine is 620 μmol/l and his serum urea is 46 mmol/l. The microbiologist recommends the prescription of gentamicin.

What is the single most appropriate dose of gentamicin?

A. 40 mg single dose
B. 40 mg once daily
C. 80 mg 8 hourly
D. 80 mg 12 hourly
E. 160 mg single dose

283. A 55-year-old man presents having recently noticed a lump in his right groin. He smokes heavily, has a persistent cough and has previously had an appendicectomy.

What is the single most likely diagnosis?

A. Epigastric hernia
B. Femoral hernia
C. Incisional hernia
D. Inguinal hernia
E. Spigelian hernia

284. A 58-year-old postmenopausal woman presents with one week history of vaginal bleeding. Digital vaginal examination is normal.

What is the single most appropriate diagnostic test?

A. Cervical smear
B. Endometrial aspiration
C. Plasma oestrogen
D. Serum FSH/LH levels
E. Transvaginal ultrasound scan

285. A two-year-old boy is brought to the Accident and Emergency Department by his mother. He has been unable to bear weight since a fall from a chair last night. He is tender over the mid-tibia but there is no obvious limb deformity.

What is the single most likely radiographic appearance of the fracture?

A. Angulated fracture
B. Compound fracture
C. Epiphyseal fracture
D. No fracture likely
E. Spiral fracture

286. An 83-year-old woman admitted with a chest infection becomes confused with poor concentration. She is restless and frightened. She is verbally abusive and has perceptual abnormalities. There is no significant previous psychiatric history.

What is the single most likely diagnosis?

A. Acute confusional state
B. Drug-induced psychosis
C. Lewy body dementia
D. Multi-infarct dementia
E. Psychotic depression

287. A 32-year-old woman was painting her bathroom when she experienced a sudden, severe headache, vomited and collapsed hitting her head. She has been brought to the Accident and Emergency Department. She now has a Glasgow Coma Scale (GCS) score of 15, temperature of 37.7°C, blood pressure of 145/85 mmHg and pulse rate of 70 beats/minute. Her physical examination is normal apart from an abrasion over her right temple.

What is the single most appropriate initial management?

A. Admit for head injury observation
B. Carboxyhaemoglobin level
C. Computed tomography (CT) brain scan
D. Lumbar puncture
E. Skull X-ray

288. A patient with dilated cardiomyopathy and permanent atrial fibrillation (AF) has a resting heart rate of 110 bpm. Twenty four hour taped recordings show even higher uncontrolled rates, particularly associated with exercise. He is already taking 187.5 mg of digoxin and has a normal creatinine.

What is the single most beneficial treatment?

A. Addition of beta blocker
B. Addition of verapamil
C. AV node ablation and permanent pacemaker insertion
D. DC cardioversion
E. Increase digoxin to 250 mg

289. A 60-year-old lady presents with increasing swelling of ankles, abdominal distension and dyspnoea. She has a past medical history of pulmonary tuberculosis as a child and a left mastectomy and subsequent radiotherapy 5 years previously. On examination she is apyrexial, with a sinus tachycardia of 100 bpm and blood pressure of 110/60 (paradox 8 mmHg). She has significant peripheral oedema and ascites. Her JVP is elevated at 8 cm above the sternal angle and demonstrates a rapidly descent.

What is the single most likely diagnosis?

A. Cardiac tamponade
B. Constrictive pericarditis
C. Intra-abdominal neoplasm
D. Severe tricuspid incompetence
E. Superior vena cava obstruction

290. What is the single most likely physiological variables to have the greatest influence toward increasing cardiac output during the latter stages of strenous exertion in a healthy adult?

A. Coronary vasodilatation
B. Decrease in systemic vascular resistance
C. Increased alveolar ventilation
D. Increased stroke volume
E. Increased ventricular rate

291. A 15-year-old girl presents with a short history of fever, malaise and a flitting polyarthritis. Clinical examination reveals a soft apical systolic murmur and pericardial rub. Investigations demonstrate elevated inflammatory markers (CRP and ESR).

What is the single most likely diagnosis?

A. Acute rheumatic fever
B. Atrial myxoma
C. Kawasaki disease
D. Subacute bacterial endocarditis
E. Systemic lupus erythematosus

292. A 45-year-old man is referred to you because of breathlessness. You diagnose a pleural effusion, which you aspirate and find to have an eosinophilia.

What is the single least likely diagnosis?

A. Asbestos pleural effusion
B. Drug reaction
C. Fungal infection
D. Haemopneumothorax
E. Malignant pleural effusion

293. A 24-year-old male has noted for the last two months that his face is swollen in the morning. He has lost 10 kg in weight over six months. He has no other complaints. On examination his external jugular veins are dilated. His chest X-ray shows a mediastinal mass.

What is the single most likely diagnosis of his superior venacaval obstruction?

A. Adenocarcinoma of the lung
B. Hodgkin's disease
C. Sarcoidosis
D. Seminoma
E. Tuberculosis

294. A 6-year-old boy with a birth head circumference of 29 cm and short palpebral fissure is found to be mentally retarded. The boy's mother is on acamprosate.

What is the single most likely diagnosis?

A. Duchenne's muscular dystrophy
B. Klinefelter's syndrome
C. Celiac disease
D. Phenylketonuria
E. Fetal alcohol syndrome

295. A 70-year-old man presents with history of weight loss, pain on eating and abdominal distension. Plain abdominal X-ray films show the 'coffee bean' sign. Most likely diagnosis is:

A. Carcinoma of the caecum
B. Colonic polyp
C. Diverticulitis
D. Sigmoid volvulus
E. Ulcerative colitis

296. A young female presents with a 4-day history of frequency, and dysuria:

A. Cystoscopy
B. Frequency/volume chart
C. Midstream urinary sample
D. Pad test
E. Ultrasound scan of the bladder

297. A 60-year-old man with presents to you with brief collapse at home. Earlier he complained of epigastric discomfort. He is now alerts with some mild back pain and tachycardia:

A. Acute salpingitis
B. Adhesive small bowel obstruction
C. Leaking aortic aneurysm
D. Mesenteric ischaemia
E. Perforated peptic ulcer

298. A young female presents with right iliac fossa pain for 4 days, associated with nausea A dipstick urine test is normal and she also complains of an offensive vaginal discharge:

A. Appendicitis
B. Acute salpingitis
C. Ureteric colic
D. Cervical erosion
E. UTI

299. An old chronic cigarette smoker complains of worsening right sided earache, a sore tongue and difficulty talking. Most likely diagnosis is:

A. Bell's palsy
B. Myringitis bullosa
C. Ramsay Hunt syndrome
D. Squamous cell carcinoma of the ear canal
E. Squamous cell carcinoma of the tongue

300. A 21-year-old female with a 7 weeks history of amenorrhoea with lower abdominal pain she fainted twice. Most likely diagnosis is:

A. Threatened abortion
B. Abruptio placenta
C. Ectopic pregnancy
D. Insertio velamentosa
E. Molar pregnancy

301. A 30-year-old woman in advanced labour and normal vital signs with the foetal heart rate dropping steadily:

A. Insertio velamentosa
B. Placenta praevia
C. Molar pregnancy
D. Abruptio placenta
E. Threatened abortion

302. An HIV-positive man on retroviral treatment presents with painless lymphadenopathy fevers, drenching night sweats and weight loss:

A. Acute myeloid leukaemia
B. Acute promyelocytic leukaemia
C. Chronic myeloid leukaemia
D. Hodgkin's lymphoma
E. Non-Hodgkin's lymphoma

303. An old man undergoes Hartmann's procedure On the 8th postoperative day he develops a high spiking fever. Most likely cause is:
A. Basal lung collapse
B. CVP line infection
C. Subphrenic abscess
D. Urinary tract infection
E. Wound infection

304. A 14-year-old girl presents with a long history of up to five painful oral ulcers occurring at intervals of 1-2 months. She is otherwise well, most likely diagnosis is:
A. Erythema multiforme
B. Oral mucositis
C. Recurrent oral ulceration
D. Shingles
E. Squamous cell carcinoma

305. A 62-year-old obese, diabetic and hypertensive woman presents with two episodes of postmenopausal bleeding. Investigation of first choice will be:
A. CT abdomen and pelvis
B. Cytology
C. Hysteroscopy and D and C
D. Diagnostic laparoscopy
E. Examination under anaesthesia and representative biopsies

306. A thin 17-year-old girl with thickened calluses on the dorsum of her hand and has bilateral parotid swelling. Most likely cause is:
A. Bulimia nervosa
B. Crohn's disease
C. Mumps
D. Sarcoidosis
E. Sjögren's syndrome

307. A 28-year-old obese female presents in early labour. On vaginal examination there is an 'empty' pelvis. Most appropriate step of management is:
A. CTG monitoring
B. Fetal blood sampling
C. Oxygen supply
D. Ultrasound scan
E. Pregnancy test

308. CTG is showing variable decelerations in a multiparous woman in advanced labour. The next appropriate step will be:
A. Foetal blood sampling
B. Emergency caesarean section
C. Instrumental vaginal delivery
D. Oxygen supply
E. Ultrasound scan

309. A 8-month-old girl passing large offensive stools since 3 months of age. She feeds well but her weight has gradually fallen across the centiles She has had persistent 'chest infections needing frequent antibiotics:
A. Cystic fibrosis
B. Gluten enteropathy
C. Hirschsprung disease
D. Milk protein intolerance
E. Ulcerative colitis or chronic inflammatory bowel disease

310. An asymptomatic 18-year-old girl with normal secondary characteristics and normal endocrine results has a negative progesterone challenge test:
A. Absent uterus
B. Constitutional
C. Prolactinoma
D. Sheehan's syndrome
E. XO-karyotype

311. A 62-year old female presents with lethargy, thinning hair and loss of the outer third of her eyebrows:
A. Androgenetic alopecia
B. Hypothyroidism
C. Iron deficiency
D. Malnutrition,
E. Telogen effluvium

312. A 33-year-old multiparous woman is admitted with a blood pressure of 160/96 mmHg and 1+ protein excretion. First investigation you would do will be:
A. 24 hours urine protein excretion
B. Doppler ultrasound of the umbilical artery
C. Glucose tolerance test
D. Kleihauer test
E. Ultrasound whole abdomen

313. **The triple test of a 23-year-old female showed that her baby was in increased risk of developing Down's syndrome. Your next step to confirm will be:**
A. Amniocentesis
B. Doppler ultrasound of the umbilical artery
C. Kleihauer test
D. Ultrasound whole abdomen
E. Bile acids

314. **A 52-year-old obese woman complains of a burning retrosternal discomfort on lying down and on eating:**
A. Achalasia
B. Carcinoma of the oesophagus
C. Chronic benign stricture
D. Myasthenia gravis
E. Plummer-Vinson syndrome

315. **A 38-year-old female who is pale complains that food is sticking in the back of her throat. She is found to have spoon-shaped nails, a smooth tongue and angular cheilitis:**
A. Achalasia
B. Carcinoma of the oesophagus
C. Myasthenia gravis
D. Plummer-Vinson syndrome
E. Reflux oesophagitis

316. **A young man presents with groups of small intensely itchy vesicles affecting the skin on his knees, buttocks, elbows and scalp:**
A. Dermatitis herpetiformis
B. Eczema
C. Lichen planus
D. Liver disease
E. Scabies

317. **A 20-year-old boy presents to clinic with painless cervical lymphadenopathy which he noticed while taking bath. He has been feeling lethargic for some time with night sweats and itchy skin:**
A. Lymphoma
B. Liver disease
C. Tuberculosis
D. Dermatitis herpetiformis
E. Polycythaemia

318. **A 48-year-old female has developed increase in abdominal girth alongside with constipation and weight loss:**
A. Irritable bowel syndrome
B. Ovarian cancer
C. Pelvic endometriosis
D. Ruptured ovarian cyst
E. Torsion of an ovarian cyst

319. **A patient complains of difficulty opening the eyes on waking with a purulent discharge and discomfort from both eyes. He has inflamed conjunctivae. There is no loss of visual acuity:**
A. Acute angle closure glaucoma
B. Bacterial conjunctivitis
C. Chlamydial conjunctivitis
D. Scleritis
E. Viral conjunctivitis

320. **A 32-year-old dentist complains of a painful, red eye and photophobia with watery discharge. Dendritic corneal ulceration are seen with fluorescein drops:**
A. Ulcerative keratitis
B. Acute angle closure glaucoma
C. Viral conjunctivitis
D. Bacterial conjunctivitis
E. Anterior uveitis

321. **Following the removal of his plaster for a fracture of the distal radius and ulna after 2 weeks a 15-year-old boy notes a deformity of his right wrist. Which one of the following is the most likely cause:**
A. Compartment syndrome
B. Growth plate disturbance/damage
C. Malunion
D. Muscle haematoma
E. Tendon rupture

322. **Erb's point is formed by the confluence of BDC 26:**
A. C7, C
B. C5, C6
C. C8, C6
D. C2, C3
E. C4, C5

323. **Warfarin-induced skin necrosis is due to:**
A. Protein C deficiency
B. Protein S deficiency
C. Antithrombin III defect
D. Increased factor VII
E. Increased platelet count

324. True about supraglottic carcinoma:
A. Cigarette smoking is the most important predisposing factor
B. Rarely presents with neck nodes
C. Hot potato voice is a feature
D. Treatment is surgery with adjuvant chemotherapy
E. More common in females

325. All of the following are true about Ludwig's angina *except:*
A. It is an infection of the floor of the mouth
B. It may involve the sublingual and submandibular spaces
C. It is caused by *H. Influenzae*
D. Treatment is with antibiotics
E. Caused by anaerobic organisms

326. Cephalic index is useful for determination of:
A. Age
B. Sex
C. Race
D. Religion
E. Caste

327. Prolongation of rigor mortis is seen in:
A. Lead
B. Arsenic
C. Mercury
D. Copper

328. Which of the following conditions is associated with decreased levels of serum alpha-fetoprotein in the mother:
A. Pre-eclampsia
B. IUGR
C. Trisomy 21
D. Multiple pregnancy
E. Large baby

329. A 26-year-old woman with a dead foetus in transverse lie and with hand prolapse is now in second stage of labour. The management would include:
A. Craniotomy
B. Decapitation
C. Cleidotomy
D. Caesarian section
E. Amniotomy

330. In brow presentation, the engaging diameter is:
A. Submentovertical
B. Mentovertical
C. Submentobregmatic
D. Suboccipitofrontal
E. Suboccipitobregmatic

331. Signs of heart disease in pregnancy:
A. Diastolic murmur
B. Systolic murmur
C. Tachycardia
D. Dyspnoea on exertion
E. Nervousness or syncope on exertion

332. All of the following cells are seen in Hodgkin's *except*:
A. Hodgkin cells
B. L and H cells
C. Langerhans' cells
D. Lacunar cells
E. Reed-Sternberg cells

333. When hypoglycemic coma is suspected, then glucose is to be infused based on:
A. Clinical assessment only
B. After consulting endocrinologist
C. After blood glucose estimation
D. After seeing for urine glucose
E. After ruling out electrolyte imbalance

334. Causes of palpable purpura include:
A. HUS
B. DIC
C. Henoch-Schönlein purpura
D. TTP

335. The Schilling test:
A. Requires marrow to be aspirated from the sternum
B. Involves labelling with radioactive chromium
C. Can determine the rate at which red cells are destroyed D may confirm a diagnosis of pernicious anaemia
D. Sometimes indicates the need for splenectomy

336. In a patient with lower ulnar nerve palsy which of the following would be seen:
A. Loss of extension at carpometacarpal
B. Sensory loss over dorsal surface of medial 4 fingers
C. Loss of abduction at thumb
D. Weakness of hand movements
E. Thenar wasting

337. All of the following are autosomal recessive *except:*
A. Phenylketonuria
B. Alpha 1 antitrypsin deficiency
C. Hereditary spherocytosis
D. Gaucher's disease
E. Hereditary hemochromatosis

338. Causative agent for pseudomembranous colitis include:
A. Staphylococci
B. *Clostridium difficile*
C. Streptococcus
D. Pseudomonas
E. *Candida albicans*

339. Adventitial bursitis due to tuberculosis is found in which of the following sites commonly:
A. Prepatellar
B. Greater trochanter of femur
C. Subacromial
D. Metatarsal
E. Subolecranon

340. True about etiopathogenesis of Alzheimer's disease include:
A. APP gene defect
B. Prion disease
C. Autoantibody formation
D. Herpes infection

341. Call exner bodies are seen in:
A. Leydig's cell tumor
B. Granulosa cell tumor
C. Embryonal cell carcinoma
D. Endodermal sinus tumor
E. Brenner's tumor

342. True regarding physiological jaundice includes:
A. It occurs due to increased RBC destruction
B. Indication to stop breastfeeding
C. Lasts up to 3 weeks
D. Appears before 24 hours
E. Due to biliary obstruction

343. What is the age of the child when he can follow horizontally 180° has got almost full head control and cannot sit without support:
A. 2 months
B. 3 months
C. 6 months
D. 9 months
E. 10 months

344. Infant with Down's syndrome have all *except:*
A. VSD
B. Duodenal atresia
C. Leukemia
D. Normal intelligence
E. Delayed skeletal maturation

345. Antagonists to opium poisonings include:
A. Neostigmine
B. Nalorphine
C. Buprenorphine
D. Pyridostigmine
E. Meptazinol

346. In a normal person at resting condition GFR in mL/min is:
A. 125
B. 90
C. 60
D. 150
E. 2000

347. Flight of ideas is seen in which of the following diseases:
A. Depression
B. Schizophrenia
C. Mania
D. Obsessive disorders
E. Hysteria

348. A homosexual person feels that he is imposed by female body and persistent discomfort with his sex. The diagnosis is:
A. Gender identity disorder
B. Transvestitism
C. Voyeurism
D. Paraphilia

349. In a patient with intestinal obstruction which of the following investigations would be required:
A. X-ray abdomen
B. Barium meal
C. Upper GI endoscopy
D. Ultrasonography
E. CT abdomen

350. Henoch-Schönlein purpura may be distinguished from post-streptococcal nephritis by the following finding:
A. Swollen joints
B. High temperature
C. Red cell casts in the urine
D. Arthralgia
E. Melaena

ANSWERS

1 B	2 C	3 B	4 A	5 B	6 C	7 E
8 D	9 A	10 C	11 C	12 A	13 A	14 E
15 E	16 E	17 D	18 D	19 A	20 A	21 B
22 D	23 A	24 A	25 D	26 E	27 D	28 E
29 B	30 B	31 A	32 A	33 D	34 A	35 D
36 D	37 A	38 B	39 E	40 A	41 B	42 E
43 E	44 A	45 A	46 E	47 A	48 A	49 A
50 C	51 C	52 B	53 E	54 A	55 A	56 C
57 D	58 E	59 D	60 C	61 E	62 C	63 E
64 A	65 A	66 B	67 A	68 C	69 E	70 B
71 E	72 A	73 C	74 B	75 D	76 B	77 A
78 A	79 D	80 A	81 C	82 E	83 A	84 A
85 B	86 E	87 A	88 B	89 D	90 E	91 B
92 A	93 C	94 A	95 B	96 E	97 A	98 D
99 D	100 C	101 E	102 E	103 A	104 D	105 C
106 A	107 A	108 D	109 C	110 D	111 C	112 D
113 A	114 C	115 D	116 A	117 A	118 A	119 A
120 C	121 D	122 A	123 A	124 B	125 B	126 D
127 B	128 A	129 D	130 A	131 A	132 A	133 E
134 E	135 B	136 E	137 A	138 E	139 A	140 C
141 A	142 E	143 A	144 B	145 C	146 D	147 E
148 A	149 A	150 C	151 D	152 B	153 A	154 D
155 D	156 C	157 A	158 A	159 D	160 A	161 A
162 C	163 B	164 C	165 A	166 D	167 B	168 D
169 E	170 C	171 B	172 A	173 E	174 E	175 E
176 A	177 C	178 C	179 B	180 A	181 D	182 E
183 A	184 B	185 C	186 E	187 A	188 A	189 B
190 A	191 E	192 C	193 B	194 B	195 B	196 C
197 A	198 E	199 E	200 A	201 E	202 B	203 A
204 B	205 A	206 D	207 A	208 E	209 A	210 B
211 B	212 E	213 B	214 E	215 A	216 A	217 D
218 A	219 A	220 A	221 A	222 C	223 C	224 A
225 A	226 B	227 B	228 E	229 D	230 A	231 E
232 B	233 B	234 E	235 A	236 B	237 E	238 E

239 D	240 B	241 D	242 E	243 E	244 B	245 D
246 D	247 B	248 E	249 C	250 E	251 B	252 B
253 C	254 E	255 D	256 B	257 E	258 C	259 E
260 D	261 E	262 A	263 B	264 E	265 A	266 E
267 E	268 B	269 B	270 A	271 A	272 B	273 C
274 A	275 B	276 E	277 B	278 B	279 B	280 B
281 B	282 E	283 D	284 E	285 E	286 A	287 C
288 E	289 B	290 E	291 A	292 E	293 B	294 E
295 D	296 C	297 C	298 A	299 E	300 C	301 A
302 E	303 C	304 C	305 C	306 A	307 D	308 A
309 A	310 A	311 B	312 A	313 A	314 E	315 A
316 A	317 A	318 B	319 B	320 A	321 C	322 B
323 A	324 A	325 A	326 C	327 B	328 C	329 B
330 B	331 A	332 C	333 A	334 C	335 D	336 D
337 C	338 B	339 B	340 A	341 B	342 B	343 C
344 D	345 B	346 A	347 C	348 A	349 A	350 E

Section 5

Data Base of High Yield Study Material

HIGH YIELD TOPIC ONE

CHILD IMMUNISATION CLINICS IN UK

AIMS

1. For all children aged 8 weeks to 4 years 3 months in the practice population to be fully immunised against:
   - Diphtheria
   - Tetanus
   - Whooping cough
   - Hib meningitis
   - Polio
   - Measles
   - Mumps
   - Rubella
2. For the provision of a smooth running, safe clinic, which is easily accessible to families, and in which waiting times are held to a standard. (Suggested standard: no longer than 20 minutes beyond appointment time).

TARGET GROUP

- All children aged between 8 weeks and 5 years.
- Those children over 5 years who for some reason have not been immunised yet.
- Parents of children in receipt of the polio vaccine who have not had a course of vaccine themselves at all.

In order to achieve this target, newly registered infants and children will have to have their immunisation status established at registration with practice.

IDENTIFICATION OF PATIENTS

Patients to be identified by:

1. Birth register held by health visitors and the clerical assistant.
2. Practice computer search monthly.
3. Appointments will be made using an appointment book designed solely for use at the immunisation clinics
4. For new births, the appointment for first immunisation will be given to parents at the health visitor's primary visit or at the 6 week check.
5. Appointments for the second and third immunisations will be given following attendance at the clinic for the previous injection.
6. For the MMR, due at 13-15 months of age, the health visitor's clerical assistant will send patients an appointment by post, 7-14 days
7. For the pre-school booster dose of diphtheria, tetanus, polio and MMR, the health visitor's clerical assistant will send patients an appointment by post 7-14 days before hand.
8. Health visitors will give opportunistic advice about immunisation at antenatal visits and onwards. This advice is reinforced by good quality, easily understood information either in the book birth to five years or child health record.
9. Specific advice on the care of a child following immunisation will be given to parents, both verbally and in written form, following each immunisation.
10. Patients who fail to attend will be sent one further appointment by post by the clerical assistant. If this is not successful, the health visitor concerned will contact the family and negotiate a new appointment.

PROTOCOL

Consent

Consent must always be obtained before immunisation. It is the responsibility of the health visitor to ensure that this is informed consent and that all parents' questions have been answered and concerns about immunisation have been sensitively considered. Written consent provides a permanent record, but consent, either written or verbal is required at the time of each immunisation after the child's fitness and suitability have been established.

Consent before the occasion on which the child is brought for immunization is only an agreement for the child to be included in the programme.

Bringing a child for immunisation after an invitation to attend for this purpose will be viewed as acceptance that the child may be immunised. When a child is brought for this purpose, and fitness and suitability have been established , consent to immunisation will be implied in the absence of any expressed reservation to the immunisation proceeding at that stage.

Childhood Vaccinations

All Vaccinations

1. Child's name and date of birth.
2. Is the child well?-if you are uncertain or think the child is unfit for vaccination ask the doctor to see.
3. Have the child's notes available plus claim forms.
4. Check immunisation to be given
   - In notes. (Write in notes which batch no.)
   - In immunisation record
   - With parents.

Before the administration of any injection, the contra indications and side effects must be discussed with the parents.

Second and third vaccinations and pre-school booster

1. Child's name and date of birth.
2. Is child well? Any diarrhoes? (polio)
3. Was there any reaction to previous vaccination?
4. Has the child have been well since previous vaccination?
5. Any of polio vaccine contraindications?

IMMUNISATION SCHEDULE IN UK

Primary Course	8 weeks 2 months	First Diphtheria Pertussis, Tetanus Polio, Hib and Men C	Hib, Diphtheria, Pertussis, Tetanus is given currently as a single injection, whilst Polio is given as drop of liquid on the tongue
	12 Weeks 3 months	Second Diphtheria, Pertussis, Tetanus, Polio, Hib and Men C	Triple
	16 Weeks 4 months	Third Diphtheria, Pertussis, Tetanus, Polio, Hib and Men C	
Measles, Mumps and Rubella (MMR)	13-15 months Not 9 months as in India	MMR vaccine	Given as a single injection
Pre School Booster	Age 4	Diphtheria, Tetanus, Polio and MMR + Acellular Pertussis Vaccine Since Oct 2001	Injections of Diphtheria Tetanus and MMR are given as two separate injections at the same clinic appointment. Polio is given as drops at liquid on the tongue. Children are sent appointments shortly after their fourth birthday.
	15-18 yrs	DT + Polio booster	
	>65 yrs	Flu vaccine (annually)	*Parents should get OPV at time of their children's vaccine

Polio

Contraindications (Live)

1. Febrile illness.
2. Vomiting, and diarrhoea.
3. Suppression of immune system, e.g. drugs, steroids, radiation, tumours, leukaemia, lymphoma and Hodgkin's disease.
4. Siblings of immunosuppressed children, (but can have inactivated polio vaccine).
5. When live vaccine has been given if second live vaccine is needed, there must be an interval of 3 weeks.

Pertussis

Contraindications

1. Neonatal cerebral damage-evolving neurological problems until condition is stable.
2. Febrile illness.

Special Consideration—discuss with doctor

1. Severe local or general reaction to previous pertussis vaccination
2. Epilepsy in parents or siblings.
3. Personal or family history of febrile convulsion.

Measles; Mumps and Rubella

Contra-indications (Live)

1. Acute febrile illness
2. True egg allergy (anaphylaxis).
3. Immunosuppression-drugs, steroids, irradiation, malignancy.
4. Allergy to neomycin or kanamycin (would have had serious) had any illness to have these.
5. Within three weeks of previous live vaccination or 3 months of immunoglobulin.

Advice

"About 5-10 days after MMR vaccination some children are slightly unwell with fever and occasionally a rash. This is not serious. It is like a very mild form of measles and your child is not infections. It is important to give paracetamol paediatric suspension- one teaspoon four times a day to prevent a high temperature and keep your child cool."

N.B You can give DPT and Polio or Polio or DT and Polio at the same time as MMR, i.e. if child comes late for 3rd DPT and Polio but is at least one year old. When recording- white batch No. of vaccine and injection site.

Convulsions

The parents of children with a tendency to have convulsions should be counselled on the management of any fever developing after immunisation. Febrile convulsions may occur 5-10 days after measles immunisation (or MMR) whereas

they may take place in the first 72 hours after pertussis immunisation. Suggestions may include paracetamol, sponge with repid water, give extra-fluids, dress in thin clothing and place in a cool room. In high risk children, an antipyretic drug may be suggested routinely for the first 72 hours after immunisation. Where the tendency is severe, the parents may be instructed on rectal diazepam administration.

Therefore ask about:

1. Was the birth normal?
2. Did the baby need any special attention ?
3. Has the baby been well since birth?
4. Is there FH of epilepsy? In who?
5. Has the baby had any fits?

Discuss any queries with doctor or if parents are not happy about baby having pertussis vaccination, encourage parent to report any reaction to first vaccination and give Paracetamol Paediatric Suspension—leaflet and prescription.

Anaphylactic Shock

No Absolute contraindication to use adrenaline in life threatening conditions.

HIGH YIELD TOPIC TWO

WHAT IS NEW IN BNF NO. 43?

Note: BNF is *British National Formulary* and every PLAB giving student is required to keep himself aware of the latest developments and recent changes from here.

Vaccines

The Chief Medical Officer's letter (PL/CMO/2002/1 of 4 January 2002) gives details about extending meningococcal C vaccination to adults aged between 20 and 24 years because meningoccal infection occurs more frequently in these young adults than in order adults.

Pneumoccocal vaccinations is recommended for those at particular risk (because of immunodeficiency, diabetes, or heart, lung or liver disease). Unfortunately, the 2-3 valent pneumococcal vaccine is not suitable for children under 2 years. In order to protect younger children at particular risk, the CMO advises a 7-valent conjugated pneumococcal vaccine in those aged between 2 months and 2 years. Section 14.4 of the BNF reflects the CMO's advice.

BNF 43 also includes changes to the schedule for immunisation against pertussis (announced in CMO's letter PL/CMO/2001/5 of 15 October 2001). The new arrangement advises a booster dose of diphtheria, tetanus and acellular pertussis vaccine before starting school or nursery school. Using the acellular pertussis component (rather than the whole-cell pertussis components) as a booster minimises reactions)

Myasthenia gravis

Corticosteroids have an important role in the management of all the but milder forms of myasthenia gravis. Prednisolone is generally used but it should be introduced carefully to minimise the risk of an initial worsening of symptoms. Interestingly, summaries of product characteristics of some corticosteroids warm that they can reduce the effects of anticholinesterases in myasthenia gravis. Whereas this statement might be identified as an 'interaction' in some sources, the BNF, having taken expert advice, carefully omits it form High Yield Topic 1.

Notes on the use of drugs, including anticholinesterases, corticosteroids and immunosuppressants, have been revised in BNF 43 to better reflect their place in the management of myasthenia gravis (see section 10.2.1).

Aspirin and children

Healthcare professionals are aware of the association between Reye's syndrome and the use of aspirin in children. The incidence of this devastating condition –uncommon as it was-declined sharply when the use of aspirin in children under 12 years was restricted. The BNF has warned about the link between aspirin and Reye's syndrome since 1986.

Recent reports have linked Reye's syndrome with the use of aspirin in children older than 12 years (*BMJ* 2001; 322: 1591-2 and *N Engl J Med* 1999; 341: 845-7).In all, fewer than 20 cases have been reported in the UK in the last 15 years, but the reports suggest a tiny possibility of aspirin-associated Reys's syndrome in older children. BNF 43 (section 4.7.1) therefore advises that aspirin should preferably also be avoided in teenagers during a feverish illness.

Anthrax

The Public Health Laboratory Service has issued guidelines for action in case of deliberate release of the anthrax organism. Also, the marketing authorisation of ciprofloxacin now includes the treatment of inhalational anthrax in adults and children. BNF 43 contains advice on the management of anthrax as well as licensed and unlicensed doses of antibacterials used for the infection (see section 5.1.12).

Multiple sclerosis

BNF 43 summarises guidance from the National Institute for Clinical Excellence on interferon beta and glatiramer for multiple sclerosis. (Technology Appraisal Guidence No-32 issued in January 2002). NICE does not recommendal use of these drugs. In order to collect more data on the role of disease-modifying drugs for multiple sclerosis, the UK health departments have agreed to share the risk of research with manufacturers of interferon beta and glatiramer (Health Service Circular HSC 2002/004). More information is included in BNF 43 (section 8.2.4).www.bnf.org

HIGH YIELD TOPIC THREE

TUMOUR MARKERS (Reference 652-OHCM)

Marker	*Generally Elevated in*	*May also cause elevation*
α FP (Alpha Foeto Protein-adult)	Hepatoma, germ-cell tumour HCC, cirrhosis	Pregnancy, Neonates (call for data) Open neural tube defect
CA 125 (F)	Ca Ovary, Breast, Hepatoma, HCC	Pregnancy,Cirrhosis, Peritonitis
CA 15-3	Ca Breast	Benign Breast Disease
CA-19-9 (GIT)	Ca Pancreas, Colorectal Ca	Cholestasis
CEA (GIT)	Ca Colon and GI tract (Breast)	Cirrhosis, Pancreatitis, Smoking
hCG (urine)	Pregnancy, Germ-cell Tumour	
NSE (Neurone-Specific Enolase)	Small-Cell Ca Lung	
PLAP (Placental Alk. Phos'tase)	Seminoma, Ca ovary,	Smoking, Pregnancy
PSA (Prostate-Specific Antigen)	Ca Prostate	BPH, Digital Rectal Examination
SCC (Squamous Cell Ca)	Ca Cervix, Lung, Buccal Cavity	

HIGH YIELD TOPIC FOUR

EVIDENCE BASED CLINICAL PRACTICE IN PSYCHIATRY GUIDELINES (BRIEF VERSION)

PSYCHOLOGICAL THERAPIES AND COUNSELLING

Introduction

The recommendations in this guideline are relevant to the following presenting problems: depression, including suicidal behaviour, anxiety, panic disorder, social anxiety and phobias, post-traumatic disorders, eating disorders, obsessive compulsive disorders, personality disorders, including repetitive self harm, and some somatic complaints (e.g. chronic pain, chronic fatigue).

The following condition for which psychological therapies may be helpful are excluded from this guideline: Disorders in childhood and adolescence, psychoses including schizophrenia, mania and bipolar disorder, alcohol and other drug addictions, sexual dysfunction and paraphilias, organic.

Brain syndromes, and learning disabilities. The guideline does not consider pharmacological treatments, but in general, there is no reason.

Why medication and psychotherapy should not be used together.

This document may be photocopied freely.

The recommendations are weighted as follows:

A. Based on a consistent finding in a majority of studies in high quality systematic reviews or evidence from high quality studies.
B. Based on at least one high quality trial, a weak or inconsistent finding in high quality reviews or a consistent finding in reviews that do not meet all the criteria of "high quality."
C. Based on evidence from individual studies that do not meet all the criteria of 'high quality.'
D. Based on evdence from structured expert consensus.

General Principles

Effectiveness of all types of therapy depends on the patient and the therapist forming a good working relationship. (B) The patient's age, sex, social class or ethnic group should not determines access to therapy. (C) In considering psychological therapies, more severe or complex mental health problems should receive secondary, specialist assessment. (D) Therapies of fewer than eight sessions are unlikely to be optimally effective for most moderate to severe mental health problems. Often 16 sessions are required for symptomatic relief, and more for lasting change. (C) Counselling is not recommended as the main intervention for sever and complex mental health problems or personality disorders. (D) A co-existing personality disorder may take treatment of most disorders more difficult and possibly less effective; indications of personality disorder include forensic history, severe relationship difficulties, and recurrent complex problems. (D) Patient preference should inform treatment choice, particularly where the research evidence does not indicate a clear choice of therapy. (D) Interest in self-exploration and capacity to tolerate frustration in relationships may be particularly important for success in psychoanalytic and psychodynamic therapies.(C) The skill and experience of the therapist should also be taken into account. More complex problems, and those where patients are poorly motivated, require the more skilful therapist. (D) ***Psychological Therapies and Counselling***

SESSIONAL REQUIRED

8 sessions	for any effect
16 sessions	for symptomatic relief
more	for lasting effect

PRINCIPAL RECOMMENDATIONS

Psychological therapy should be routinely considered as an option when assessing mental health problems. (B) Patients who are adjusting to life events, illness, disabilities or counselling losses may benefits from brief therapies such as counselling. (B) post-traumatic stress symptoms may be helped by psychological therapy, with most evidence for cognitive behavioural methods. Routine debriefing following traumatic events is not recommended. (A) Depression may be treated effectively with cognitive therapy or interpersonal therapy. A number of other brief structured therapies for depression may be of benefit, such as psychodynamic therapy. (A) Anxiety disorders with marked symptomatic anxiety (panic disorder, agoraphobia, social phobia, obsessive compulsive disorders, generalised anxiety disorders) are likely to benefit from cognitive behavior therapy (A) Psychological intervention should be considered for somatic complaints with a psychological component with most evidence for CBT in the treatment of chronic pain and chronic fatigue. (C) Eating disorders can be treated with psychological therapy. Best evidence in bulimia nervosa is for CBT, IPT and family therapy for teenagers. Treatment usually includes psychoeducational methods. There is little strong evidence on the best therapy type for anorexia. (B) Structured psychological therapies delivered by skilled paractitioners can contribute to the longer-term treatment of personality disorders. (C)

- PTSD—Cognitive behavioural therapy (Psychological therapy)
- Depression—Cognitive therapy/Interpersonal/ Psychodynamic therapy brief standard therapy)
- Anxiety disorders (Includes OCD) - Cognitive behaviour therapy.
- Somatic complaints - Psychological interven therapy with psychological components (max in-chronic pain).
- Chronic fatigue rating disorder—Psychological therapy

EVIDENCE

Psychological therapy shows benefits over no treatment for a wide range of mental health difficulties. There is evidence of counselling effectiveness is mixed anxiety/depression, most effective when used with specified client groups, e.g. postnatal mothers, bereaved groups. CBT has been found helpful. Some evidence of efficacy has been shown for other forms of psychological therapy. Single session debriefing appears to be unhelpful in preventing later disorders. CBT and IPT effectively reduce symptoms of depression. Benefits has also been found for other forms of psychological therapy, including focal psychodynamic therapy, Psychodynamic interpersonal therapy and counselling. CBT effectively reduces symptoms of panic and anxiety. Behaviour therapy and cognitive therapy both appear effective in treatment of obsessional problems. Psychological therapies have benefit in a range of somatic complaints including gastrointestinal and gynaecological problems. CBT has been found more effective than control in improving functioning in chronic fatigue and chronic pain. Etiology of CBT and IPT in bulimia has been established. Individual therapies have shown some benefit in anorexia, with little to distinguish treatment types. Early onset of anorexia may indicate family therapy, and later onset, broadly based individual therapy. A number of therapy approaches have shown some success with personality disorders, including dialectical behaviour therapy, psychoanalytic day hospital programme and therapeutic communities.

TYPES OF PSYCHOLOGICAL THERAPY

- **Cognitive behaviour therapy (CBT)** This refers to the pragmatic combination of concepts and techniques from cognitive and behaviour therapies, common in clinical practice. Cognitive techniques (such as challenging negative automatic thoughts) and behavioural techniques (such as graded exposure and activity scheduling) are used to relieve symptoms by changing maladaptive thoughts, beliefs and behaviour.
- **Psychoanalytic therapies** A number of different therapies draw on psychoanalytic theories. Focal psychodynamic therapy identifies a central conflict arising from early experience that is being re-enacted in adult life producing mental health problems. It aims to resolve this through the vehicle of the relationship with the therapist giving new opportunities for emotional assimilation and insight. Psychoanalytic psychotherapy is a longer-term process (usually a year or more) of allowing unconscious conflicts opportunity to be re-enacted and interpreted in the relationship with the therapist.
- **Systemic and family therapy** (whether treating individuals, couples or families) focuses on the relational context addresses patterns of interaction and meaning aims to facilitate personal and interpersonal resources within a system as a whole. Therapeutic work may include consultation to wider networks such as other professionals working with the individual or the family.
- **Other** This list is not comprehensive. Many others types of therapy are practised in the NHS including cognitive-analytic, existential, humanistic, feminist, personal construct, art therapy, drama therapy, transactional analysis, group analysis and interpersonal therapy (IPT).
- **Counselling** A form of psychological therapy that gives individuals an opportunity to explore, discover, and clarify ways of living more resoucefully, with a greater sense of well being. Counsellors practise within the main therapeutic approaches listed above.

KEY IMPLEMENTATIONS POINTS

Recommendations are given to inform first treatment choice. Patients may choose not to accept this, and further treatment options may be considered if the first line treatment is unacceptable or inappropriate. Guidelines may be adapted to take account of the availability and organisation of local services, but not at the expense of changing the main recommendations. User involvement in local implementation and adult of the guideline is recommended.

Key Audit Criteria

Has access to the recommended range of psychological therapies been identified for the primary care group? Has psychological therapy been considered as one option for all patients with these presenting problems? Has patients preference and motivation been assessed? Do more severe and complex problems receive specialist assessment? Are adequate lengths of psychological therapies offered? Are patients'ethnic and cultural background considered? The full guideline is available at:

www.doh.gov.UK/mental health/treatment guideline

Psychological therapies are provided by mental health professionals from a range of disciplines, including clinical and counselling psychologists, psychiatrists, psychotherapists, art and drama therapists, and counsellors.

HIGH YIELD TOPIC FIVE

DETECTION OF DELIBERATE RELEASES—CARDINAL SIGNS FOR CASE DETECTION

Note: Although such questions have never been asked in PLAB exam, but with increasing threat of terrorism, these may be asked in future.

In a previously healthy person any of the following four clinical pictures requires urgent attention:

1. Inhalational (Pulmonary) Anthrax and Plague

- Rapid onset severe sepsis with respiratory failure, not due to a predisposing illness.
- Sudden, severe, unexplained febrile illness or febrile death

Note: The cardinal sign for anthrax is mediastinal widening on chest X-ray.

2. Cutaneous Anthrax

- Commonly affects hands, forearms and head
- Cardinal feature is painless swelling of skin
- Originally a small bump which then ulcerates and becomes weepy
- Pronounced swelling (oedema of skin) frequently surrounds the lesion
- Ulcer develops a black centre in 2-6 days.

For microbiologists the unexpected finding of non-motile positive bacilli in normally sterile or fluids or from wound sites require urgent consideration of the possibility of B. *anthracis.*

3. Botulism

- Acute onset of bilateral cranial nerve involvement
- Descending weakness or paralysis which may extend to complete flaccid paralysis, but the patient remains alert.
- Fever is unusual, as is loss of sensation.

4. Smallpox

In the events of a deliberate release in the UK population (mostly nonimmune), it is extremely unlikely that single, mild cases of feverish, pox-like illnesses will occur, it is much more likely that clusters of moderate to severe disease would be seen, i.e. clusters of cases of:

- An abrupt onset moderate fever (up to 39°C), with extreme prostration.
- A characteristic vesicular rash most dense on the extremities and face begins on the third to fourth day of illness. Skin lesions over one area of body are generally of the same stage of development. New and enlarging vesicles coalesce to form soft, flaccid bullae covered by skin, which easily rubs off.
- Less commonly, an erythematous or purpuric rash may appear earlier in the illness and is associated with a poorer prognosis.

If a patient is seen with any of these four pictures, expert clinical opinion should be sought urgently. In addition in England, Wales and Northern Ireland the local Consultant in Communicable Disease Control (or their counterpart in Scotland) and the CDSC Duty Doctor (020-8200-6868) should also be contracted urgently and given details.

HIGH YIELD TOPIC SIX

ASTHMA GUIDELINES—CHRONIC MANAGEMENT

- *BTS Guidelines Thorax 1997;52 Suppl 11-21*

Adults and School Children		Symptoms
• Step 1 PEFR=100%	Occasional use of relief bronchodilators Inhaled short acting β agonists if > once daily—stage 2	Occasional symptoms less frequent than day
• Step 2 (≤ 80%)	Regular inhaled anti-inflammatory agents Inhaled β-agonist + Budesonide/beclomethasone 100-400 μg b.d. Or Cromoglycate, but start steroid if control not achieved	Daily symptoms
• Step 3 (50-80%)	High dose inhaled steroids or low dose steroids + long acting β-agonist e.g. Budesonide/beclomethasone 800-2000 μg daily Or Salmeterol 50*ug bd+ budesonide/beclomethasone 100-400*ug	Severe symptoms
• Step 4 (50-80%)	High dose inhaled steroids and regular bronchodilators Budesonide/beclomethasone 800-2000 μg daily plus • Inhaled long acting β-agonist • SR theophylines • Inhaled ipratropium bromide • Long acting β-agonist tablets • High dose inhaled bronchodilators • Cromoglycate	Severe symptoms uncontrolled with high dose inhaled corticosteroid
• Step 5 (< 50%)	Addition of regular steroids tablets Education Inhaler technique Avoidance of provoking factors PEFR monitoring at home	Severe symptoms deteriorating
• Step 6 (PEFR<30%)	Sever symptoms deteriorating inspite or oral Prednisolone	Hospital Admission
Children under 5 years old		
• Step 1	Occasional use of relief bronchodilators Short acting inhaled β-agonists prn Mild cases oral β-agonists prn	
• Step	Regular inhaled preventer therapy Inhaled short acting β-agonist+ Cromoglycate as powder via MDI Becotide/beclomethasone<400 μg [IFP<200 μg] Consider 5/7 oral prednisolone/high dose inhaled steroid to achieve control	

Contd....

Contd...

• Step 3	Increased dose inhaled steroids Inhaled β-agonists + Becotide/beclomethasone < 800 mg [FP < 500 μg] Consider regular long acting β-agonists b.d.
• Step 4	High dose inhaled steroids and bronchodilators Inhaled steroids up to 200 μg Slow release xanthines or nebulised β-agonists

Leukotriene Antagonists

Oral treatment of atopic conditions

LT antagonists	montelukast and zafirlukast
5 lipoxygenase inhibitor	Zieluton

HIGH YIELD TOPIC SEVEN

FITNESS TO DRIVE

The patient must inform the DVLA, the doctor must advise the patient

• Vision		
Acuity	6/9 6/10 corrected 3/60 without correction	
Monocular vision	No need to notify it field is full	
Field defect	Banned if <120°	
Diplopia	Banned unless mild	
Night blindness	Banned if fails to meet the field and acuity regulations at all times	
Colour blindness	No need to notify	
• Neurology	All epileptics should inform the DVLA	
Epilepsy	Single fit	Banned for 1 year
	Awake	Fit-free for 2 years
	Asleep	Fit-free for 3 years
	HGV	10 years fir-free, no treatment
LOC	Cease driving 1 year, restored until 70 years	
CVA	Cease driving 3/12 if full clinical recovery	
TIAs	Cease driving until 3/12 free from attacks	
• Diabetes	All diabetics should inform the DVLA	
IDDM/Type I	hypo awareness and visual acuity standards	
	1, 2 or 3 years licence	
NIDDM/Type II	Tablets	Limit by end-organ complications
	Diet	No need to notify
Frequent Hypo's Cease driving		
• Cadiology		
Angina	If at the wheel cease driving	
QMI	Cease driving for 4/52	
Angioplasty	Cease driving for 4/52	
PPM/Catheter	Cease driving for 4/52	
CABG	Cease driving for 4/52	
Transport	Cease driving for 8/52	
Arrhythmias	Cease driving if no capacitate restart 4/52 after control established	
ICD	Cease driving	
	Re-issue if no discharge in 6/12	
	No incapacitating arrythmia in 5 years	
• Drugs	Banned if any chemical, drug alcohol dependency	

HIGH YIELD TOPIC EIGHT

DRUGS IN PREGNANCY

	I TM	*II TM*	*III TM*	*Complications*
ACE inhibitors	C/I	C/I	C/I	
Warfarin	C/I	safe	C/I	
Heparin	Safe	Safe	Safe	
Trimethoprim Sulfonamides			C/I	Kernictercus
Tetracycline	C/I	C/I/(safe?)	C/I	I-TM-bone and teeth III TM-Decompensation of liver
Gilibenclamide	Safe	Safe	C/I (late)	
Metformin	C/I	C/I	C/I	
Trimethoprim-sulflame thoxazole			C/I	
Chloramphemicol	C/I	C/I	C/I	Grey baby syndrome
Streptomycin	Restricted	restricted	restricted	To only complicated case of pregnancy
Erythromycin	Safe	Safe	Safe	
Penicillin	Safe	Safe	Safe	
Nitrofurantoin	Specific C/I	Specific C/I	Specific C/I	in G6PD defcy

* C/I = Contraindication
TM = Trimester

HIGH YIELD TOPIC NINE

BRITISH NOMENCLATURE FOR DRUGS

A number of drugs are known by different names in the UK to other countries, particularly the USA. Spellings often differ from accepted international spellings. Many of the British approved names are to be changed in line with the recommended international non-proprietary names. There are a number of exceptions where the British name or spelling is so well established that either name may be used interchangeably. A few British names have been retained for drugs used in emergency settings, where confusion might be dangerous. In this book, I have mostly used the International name, except for emergency drugs. The lists below are not exhaustive but cover most drugs in common use. A full list may be found in the British National Formulary (BNF).

Drugs where the British Name has been retained

British approved name	*Recommended international non-proprietary name*
adrenaline	epinephrine
bendrofluazide	bendroflumethiazide
chlorpheniramine	chlorphenamine
frusemide	furosemide
lignocaine	lidocaine
methylene blue	methylthioninium chloride
noradrenaline	norepinephrine

Drugs where the British spelling remains in common usage

British approved name	*Recommended international non-proprietary name*
amoxycillin	amoxycillin
beclomethasone	beclometasone
cephalexin	cefalexin
chlormethiazole	chlomethiazole
cholecalciferol	colecalciferol
cholestyramine	colestyramine
corticotrophin	corticotropin
indomethacin	indometacin
phenobarbitone	phenobarbital
sodium cromoglycate	sodium cromoglicate
sulphasalazine	sulfasalazine

HIGH YIELD TOPIC TEN

GMC GUIDELINES ABOUT MEDICAL ETHICS

SERIOUS COMMUNICABLE DISEASES

Use of term 'serious communicable disease'

In this guidance the term serious communicable disease applies to any disease which may be transmitted from human to human and which may result in death or serious illness. It particularly concerns, but is not limited to, infections such as human immunodeficiency virus (HIV), tuberculosis and hepatitis B and C.

Providing a good standard of practice and care

1. All patients are entitled to good standards of practice and care from their doctors, regardless of the nature of their disease or condition.
2. You must not deny or delay investigation or treatment because you believe that the patient's actions or lifestyle may have contributed to their condition. Where patients pose a serious risk to your health or safety you may take reasonable, personal measures to protect yourself before investigating a patient's condition or providing treatment. In the context of serious communicable diseases these will usually be infection control measures. You must follow the guidance in paragraph 4 on consent to testing.
3. You must keep yourself informed about serious communicable diseases, and particularly their means of transmission and control. You should always take appropriate measures to protect yourself and others from infection. You must make sure that any staff for whom you are responsible are also appropriately informed and co-operate with measures designed to prevent transmission of infection to other patients.

Consent to testing for a serious communicable disease

4. You must obtain consent from patients before testing for a serious communicable disease, except in the rare circumstances described in paragraphs 6, 7, 9, 11 and 17 below. The information you provide when seeking consent should be appropriate to the circumstances and to the nature of the condition or conditions being tested for. Some conditions, such as HIV, have serious social and financial, as well as medical, implications. In such cases you must make sure that the patient is given appropriate information about the implications of the test, and appropriate time to consider and discuss them.

Children

5. When testing patients under 16 for a serious communicable disease, you must follow the guidance in paragraph 4 if you judge that they have sufficient maturity to understand the implications of testing.
6. Where a child cannot give or withhold consent, you should seek consent from a person with parental responsibility for the child. If you believe that that person's judgement is distorted, for example, because he or she may be the cause of the child's infection, you must decide whether the medical interests of the child override the wishes of those with parental responsibility. Whenever possible you should discuss the issues with an experienced colleague before making a decision. If you test a child without obtaining consent, you must be prepared to justify that decision.

Unconscious patients

7. You may test unconscious patients for serious communicable diseases, without their prior consent, where testing would be in their immediate clinical interests—for example, to help in making a diagnosis. You should not test unconscious patients for other purposes.

Injuries to health care workers

8. If you or another health care worker has suffered a needlestick injury or other occupational exposure to blood or body fluids and you consider it necessary to test the patient for a serious communicable disease, the patient's consent should be obtained before the test is undertaken. If the patient is unconscious when the injury occurs consent should be sought once the patient has regained full consciousness. If appropriate, the injured person can take prophylactic treatment until consent has been obtained and the test result is known.
9. If the patient refuses testing, is unable to give or withhold consent because of mental illness or disability, or does not regain full consciousness within 48 hours, you should reconsider the severity of risk to yourself, or another injured health care worker, or to others. You should not arrange testing against the patient's wishes or without consent other than in exceptional circumstances, for example where you have good reason to think that the patient may have a condition such as HIV for which prophylactic treatment is available. In such cases you may test an existing blood sample, taken for other purposes, but you should consult an experienced colleague first. It is possible that a decision to test an existing blood without consent could be challenged in the courts, or be the subject of a complaint to your employer or the GMC. You must, therefore, be prepared to justify your decision.
10. If you decide to test without consent, you must inform the patient of your decision at the earliest opportunity. In such cases confidentiality is paramount: only the

patient and those who have been exposed to infection may be told about the test and its result. In these exceptional circumstances neither the fact that test has been undertaken, nor its result, should be entered in the patient's personal medical record without the patient's consent.

11. If the patient dies you may test for a serious communicable disease if you have good reason to think that the patient may have been infected, and a health care worker has been exposed to the patient's blood or other body fluid. You should usually seek the agreement of a relative before testing. If the test shows the patient was a carrier of the virus, you should follow the guidance in paragraphs 21 - 23 of these guidelines on giving information to patients' close contacts.

Testing in laboratories

12. It is the responsibility of the doctor treating the patient to obtain consent to testing for diagnostic purposes. If you work in a laboratory you may test blood or other specimens for serious communicable diseases only for the purposes for which the samples have been obtained, or for closely related purposes which are in the direct interests of the patient. See paragraph 14 for guidance on testing undertaken for research purposes.

Unlinked anonymised screening

13. In unlinked anonymised surveillance programmes for serious communicable diseases, you should make sure that patients are provided with information which covers:
    - Their right to refuse inclusion of the sample in the programme.
    - The fact that their blood sample cannot be identified and there is no way of tracing it back to them.
    - The benefits of seeking a test if they think they have been exposed to infection.

Research

14. You may undertake research only where the protocol has been approved by the appropriate, properly constituted research ethics committee. It remains your responsibility to ensure that research does not infringe patients' rights.

Deceased patients

15. When a patient who is brain stem dead is being considered as an organ donor, you should explain to relatives that assessing the suitability of organs for transplantation will involve testing for certain infections, including HIV.

Post-mortem testing

16. Where a post-mortem has been authorised or ordered you may test the deceased patient for communicable diseases where relevant to the investigation into the causes of death.

17. You should not routinely test for serious communicable diseases before performing post-mortems; but you should take precautions to protect yourself and other health care workers. If you have reason to believe the deceased person had a serious communicable disease, you should assume the body to be infectious.

Confidentiality

Informing Other Health Care Professionals

18. If you diagnose a patient as having a serious communicable disease, you should explain to the patient:
    a. The nature of the disease and its medical, social and occupational implications, as appropriate.
    b. Ways of protecting others from infection.
    c. The importance to effective care of giving the professionals who will be providing care information which they need to know about the patient's disease or condition. In particular you must make sure that patient understands that general practitioners cannot provide adequate clinical management and care without knowledge of their patients' conditions.

19. If patients still refuse to allow other health care workers to be informed, you must respect the patients' wishes except where you judge that failure to disclose the information would put a health care worker or other patient at serious risk of death or serious harm. Such situations may arise, for example, when dealing with violent patients with severe mentally illness or disability. If you are in doubt about whether disclosure is appropriate, you should seek advice from an experienced colleague. You should inform patients before disclosing information. Such occasions are likely to arise rarely and you must be prepared to justify a decision to disclose information against a patient's wishes.

Disclosures to others

20. You must disclose information about serious communicable diseases in accordance with the law. For example, the appropriate authority must be informed where a notifiable disease is diagnosed. Where a communicable disease contributed to the cause of death, this must be recorded on the death certificate. You should also pass information about serious communicable diseases to the relevant authorities for the purpose of communicable disease control and surveillance.

21. As the GMC booklet confidentiality makes clear, a patient's death does not of itself release a doctor from the obligation to maintain confidentiality. But in some circumstances disclosures can be justified because they protect other people from serious harm or because they are required by law.

Giving information to close contacts

22. You may disclose information about a patient, whether living or dead, in order to protect a person from risk of death or serious harm. For example, you may disclose

information to a known sexual contact of a patient with HIV where you have reason to think that the patient has not informed that person, and cannot be persuaded to do so. In such circumstances you should tell the patient before you make the disclosure, and you must be prepared to justify a decision to disclose information.

23. You must not disclose information to others, for example relatives, who have not been, and are not, at risk of infection.

Doctors' responsibilities to protect patients from infection

24. You must protect patients from unnecessary exposure to infection by following safe working practices and implementing appropriate infection control measures. This includes following the Control of Substances Hazardous to Health Regulations 1994 and other health and safety at work legislation. These regulations may require you to inform your employer, or the person responsible for health and safety in your organisation, if there are any deficiencies in protection measures in your work place. Failure to do so may amount to a criminal offence.
25. You must follow the UK Health Departments' advice on immunisation against hepatitis B. If you are in direct contact with patients you should protect yourself and your patients by being immunised against other common serious communicable diseases, where vaccines are available.
26. You must always take action to protect patients when you have good reason to suspect that your own health, or that of a colleague, is a risk to them.
27. You must consider how any infection you have may put patients at risk. You must take particular care if you work with patients for whom exposure to infection may be serious, for example, pregnant women or immuno-suppressed patients.
28. You must comply promptly with appropriate requests to be tested for serious communicable diseases when there is an investigation into an outbreak of disease amongst patients.

Responsibilities of doctors who have been exposed to a serious communicable disease

29. If you have any reason to believe that you have been exposed to a serious communicable disease you must seek and follow professional advice without delay on whether you should undergo testing and, if so, which tests are appropriate. Further guidance on your responsibilities if your health may put patients at risk is included in our booklet Good Medical Practice.
30. If you acquire a serious communicable disease you must promptly seek and follow advice from a suitably qualified colleague—such as a consultant in occupational health, infectious diseases or public health on:
    - Whether, and in what ways, you should modify your professional practice.
    - Whether you should inform your current employer, your previous employers or any prospective employer, about your condition.
31. You must not rely on your own assessment of the risks you pose to patients.
32. If you have a serious communicable disease and continue in professional practice you must have appropriate medical supervision.
33. If you apply for a new post, you must complete health questionnaires honestly and fully.

Treating colleagues with serious communicable diseases

34. If you are treating a doctor or other health care worker with a serious communicable disease you must provide the confidentiality and support to which every patient is entitled.
35. If you know, or have good reason to believe, that a medical colleague or health care worker who has or may have a serious communicable disease, is practising, or has practised, in a way which places patients at risk, you must inform an appropriate person in the health care worker's employing authority, for example, an occupational health physician, or where appropriate, the relevant regulatory body. Such cases are likely to arise very rarely. Wherever possible you should inform the health care worker concerned before passing information to an employer or regulatory body.

CONFIDENTIALITY: PROTECTING AND PROVIDING INFORMATION

The new guidance on confidentiality is the result of extensive discussion and debate with professional and patient groups. It places new responsibilities on doctors to keep patients informed about, and get agreement to, the disclosure of information. It sets out a framework for respecting patients' rights while ensuring that information needed to maintain and improve health care is passed to those who need it.

The additional duties to obtain consent and to anonymise data tie in with developments in the law, including the Data Protection Act 1998. The Data Protection Commissioner sees our guidance 'as a sound basis for establishing privacy-friendly relationships between patients and doctors assisting doctors in complying with their obligations under the Data Protection Act 1998.'

The guidance will have far-reaching effects on some areas of practice, for example, in research and public health and drug safety monitoring. The Medicines Control Agency's Yellow Card scheme, which has provided invaluable information on the safety of medicines in clinical use since 1964, asked doctors for identifiable data. The MCA said 'We recognise the need to adopt a privacy enhancing approach while maintaining the effectiveness of the scheme in the interests of public health. We are, therefore, introducing an updated Yellow Card which no longer requests patient personal identifiers so that doctors can continue to report suspected adverse drug reactions with confidence.'

Dr Declan Mulkeen, of MRC, also welcomed the GMC's principles on disclosing information for medical research, as 'striking the right balance in a difficult area.' MRC will issue more detailed guidelines for research in the Autumn.

Frequently Asked Questions

Deciding whether to disclose information is often difficult. Our guidance sets out the principles which you should follow. The notes which follow explain how those principles apply in circumstances which doctors often meet, or find hard to deal with.

My health authority wants to conduct a post-payment verification (PPV) for claims I have made. Can I give them free access to the records?

Some disclosures, for example to the police or employers, may cause significant harm or distress to patients, but others, such as disclosures for audit or planning, are unlikely to affect patients. In these cases consent based on the patients' understanding and acceptance of the disclosure will be sufficient.

It is good practice to tell patients how their records might be used to help the running of the NHS or the development of medical care. You should make sure patients know they have a right to object to such disclosures and provide clear instructions about how they can do so. You can do this by providing leaflets for those attending the surgery, clinic or hospital; discussing the issues at a suitable consultation or at clinics or when new patients join a practice or attend a hospital for the first time; or by writing to your patients.

Where a health authority asks for access to your records for PPV you should:

- Review whether you have already given patients information about the use of records for audit and administration and about their right to object.
- Identify any patients who have expressed objections.
- If you are not satisfied that patients have had this information, ask your HA whether the patients whose records will be checked have been identified, and if so whether the HA has asked their permission to look at the records. If not, ask the HA to do so, or contact the patients yourself and ask whether they object to their records being examined.

When the PPV audit takes place:

- Make sure that you disclose only the minimum information necessary for the audit.
- Check with the health authority that staff have had training in confidentiality and have a contractual or professional duty to respect patients' privacy.

A patient of mine suffers from a serious mental illness. He is often erratic and unstable. I know that he drives, although I have warned him that it is often unsafe for him to do so. He insists that his illness does not affect his judgment as a driver. Should I tell the DVLA?

If you think the patient may be a danger to himself or others when driving and you cannot persuade him to stop driving or to inform the DVLA himself, then you should disclose the information to a Medical Adviser at DVLA . You should let him know of your decision.

I work with sex offenders who are transferred from prison to hospital during their custodial sentence. A patient has recently been discharged, but I know he does not intend to register his new address with the police, as he is required to do by law. Should I tell the police he has been discharged?

The Sex Offenders Act 1997 requires the offender to register his name and address with the police. However, disclosures without consent are justified when a failure to disclose information may put the patient, or someone else, at risk of death or serious harm. If you believe that the patient poses a risk to others, and you have good reason to believe that he does not intend to notify the police of his address, then disclosure of the patient's discharge would be justified.

Sometimes administrative staff in my practice need access to patients' records. At present they can call up the whole record on screen. Is that all right?

It is best practice to ensure that administrative staff have immediate access to information only on a need to know basis. When using computerised records, make sure that administrative data, such as names and addresses, can be accessed separately from clinical information, so that sensitive data is not automatically displayed. This will also help to reduce the risk of accidental breaches of confidentiality in reception areas or other areas to which patients have access. In addition, all staff who have access to clinical information must have a full understanding of their duty of confidentiality, and understand their responsibilities. Make sure new staff receive proper training.

A patient of mine is a doctor; I am concerned that he has a drinking problem which could affect his judgment. It has taken me a long time to get him to admit to any problems, and if I disclose the information to his employer or the GMC now he will probably deny everything and find another doctor. What should I do?

This patient has the same right to good care and to confidentiality as other patients. But, there are times when the safety of others must take precedence. If you are concerned that his problems mean that he is an immediate danger to his own patients, you must tell his employing authority or the GMC straight away. If you think the problem is currently under control, you must encourage him to seek help locally from counselling services set up for doctors or for the public generally. You must monitor his condition and ensure that if the position deteriorates you take immediate action to protect the patients in his care.

A child in my practice has recently been taken to hospital suffering serious injuries from abuse. His father is now being prosecuted. I have been asked to provide information about the child and her family for a Part 8 Review. I am the GP to the child's father and he would not give consent to the release of information, what should I do?

Part 8 Reviews are intended to identify why a child has been seriously harmed, to learn lessons from mistakes and to improve systems and services for children and their families. The overall purpose can reasonably be regarded as serving to protect other children from a risk of serious harm. You should, therefore, co-operate with requests for information, even where the child's family does not consent or if it is not practicable to ask for their consent. Exceptionally, you may see a good reason not to disclose information; in such cases you should be prepared to explain your decision to the GMC.

GMC Confidentiality: Key Principles

Confidentiality is central to trust between doctors and patients. Without assurances about confidentiality, patients may be reluctant to give doctors the information they need in order to provide good care. If you are asked to provide information about patients you should:

- Seek patients' consent to disclosure of information wherever possible, whether or not you judge that patients can be identified from the disclosure.
- Anonymise data where unidentifiable data will serve the purpose.
- Keep disclosures to the minimum necessary.

Are you complying with the Data Protection Act 1998?

The Act requires everyone who processes personal information about living individuals to notify the commissioner. GP practices, individual GPS and other doctors who control records about patients or staff must notify the commissioner and comply with the data protection principles.

To start the notification process telephone the Commissioner's notification department on 01625 545740 or visit http://www.dpr.gov.uk

Glossary: This defines the terms used within this document. These definitions have no wider or legal significance.

Anonymised Data: Data from which the patient cannot be identified by the recipient of the information. The name, address, and full post code must be removed together with any other information which, in conjunction with other data held by or disclosed to the recipient, could identify the patient. NHS numbers or other unique numbers may be included only if recipients of the data do not have access to the 'key' to trace the identity of the patient using this number.

Consent: Agreement to an action based on knowledge of what the action involves and its likely consequences.

Express Consent: Consent which is expressed orally or in writing (except where patients cannot write or speak, when other forms of communication may be sufficient).

Health Care Team: The health care team comprises the people providing clinical services for each patient and the administrative staff who directly support those services.

Patients: Competent patients and parents of, or those with parental responsibility for, children who lack maturity to make decisions for themselves. (Adult patients who lack the capacity to consent have the right to have their confidentiality respected. Guidance on disclosure of information about such patients is included in paragraphs 38-39).

Personal Information: Information about people which doctors learn in a professional capacity and from which individuals can be identified.

Public Interest: The interests of the community as a whole, or a group within the community or individuals.

Section 1—Patients' right to confidentiality

1. Patients have a right to expect that information about them will be held in confidence by their doctors. Confidentiality is central to trust between doctors and patients. Without assurances about confidentiality, patients may be reluctant to give doctors the information they need in order to provide good care. If you are asked to provide information about patients you should:
   a. Seek patients' consent to disclosure of information wherever possible, whether or not you judge that patients can be identified from the disclosure.
   b. Anonymise data where unidentifiable data will serve the purpose.
   c. Keep disclosures to the minimum necessary.

   You must always be prepared to justify your decisions in accordance with this guidance.

Protecting Information

2. When you are responsible for personal information about patients you must make sure that it is effectively protected against improper disclosure at all times.
3. Many improper disclosures are unintentional. You should not discuss patients where you can be overheard or leave patients' records, either on paper or on screen, where they can be seen by other patients, unauthorised health care staff or the public. Whenever possible you should take steps to ensure that your consultations with patients are private.

Section 2—Sharing information with patients

4. Patients have a right to information about the health care services available to them, presented in a way that is easy to follow and use.
5. Patients also have a right to information about any condition or disease from which they are suffering. This should be presented in a manner easy to follow and use, and include information about diagnosis, prognosis, treatment options, outcomes of treatment, common and/or serious side-effects of treatment, likely time-scale of treatments and costs where relevant. You should always give patients basic information about treatment

you propose to provide, but you should respect the wishes of any patient who asks you not to give them detailed information. This places a considerable onus upon health professionals. Yet, without such information, patients cannot make proper choices, as partners in the health care process.

6. It is good practice to give patients information about how anonymised information about them may be used to protect public health, to undertake research and audit, to teach or train medical staff and students and to plan and organise health care services.

Section 3—Disclosure of information

Sharing information with others providing care

7. Where patients have consented to treatment, express consent is not usually needed before relevant personal information is shared to enable the treatment to be provided. For example, express consent would not be needed before general practitioners disclose relevant personal information so that a medical secretary can type a referral letter. Similarly, where a patient has agreed to be referred for an X-ray physicians may make relevant information available to radiologists when requesting an X-ray. Doctors cannot treat patients safely, nor provide the continuity of care, without having relevant information about the patient's condition and medical history.
8. You should make sure that patients are aware that personal information about them will be shared within the health care team, unless they object, and of the reasons for this. It is particularly important to check that patients understand what will be disclosed if it is necessary to share personal information with anyone employed by another organisation or agency providing health or social care. You must respect the wishes of any patient who objects to particular information being shared with others providing care, except where this would put others at risk of death or serious harm.
9. You must make sure that anyone to whom you disclose personal information understands that it is given to them in confidence, which they must respect. Anyone receiving personal information in order to provide care is bound by a legal duty of confidence, whether or not that they have contractual or professional obligations to protect confidentiality.
10. Circumstances may arise where a patient cannot be informed about the sharing of information, for example because of a medical emergency. In these cases you should pass relevant information promptly to those providing the patients' care.

Section 4—Disclosure of information other than for treatment of the individual patient

Principles

11. Information about patients is requested for a wide variety of purposes including education, research, monitoring and epidemiology, public health surveillance, clinical audit, administration and planning. You have a duty to protect patients' privacy and respect their autonomy. When asked to provide information you should follow the guidance in paragraph 1, that is:
    a. Seek patients' consent to disclosure of any information wherever possible, whether or not you judge that patients can be identified from the disclosure.
    b. Anonymise data where unidentifiable data will serve the purpose.
    c. Keep disclosures to the minimum necessary.
12. The paragraphs which follow deal with obtaining consent, and what to do where consent is unobtainable, or it is impracticable to seek consent.

Obtaining consent

13. Seeking patients' consent to disclosure is part of good communication between doctors and patients, and is an essential part of respect for patients' autonomy and privacy.

Consent where disclosures will have personal consequences for patients

14. You must obtain express consent where patients may be personally affected by the disclosure, for example when disclosing personal information to a patient's employer. When seeking express consent you must make sure that patients are given enough information on which to base their decision, the reasons for the disclosure and the likely consequences of the disclosure. You should also explain how much information will be disclosed and to whom it will be given. If the patient withholds consent, or consent cannot be obtained, disclosures may be made only where they can be justified in the public interest, usually where disclosure is essential to protect the patient, or someone else, from risk of death or serious harm.

Consent where the disclosure is unlikely to have personal consequences for patients

15. Disclosure of information about patients for purposes such as epidemiology, public health safety, or the administration of health services, or for use in education or training, clinical or medical audit, or research is unlikely to have personal consequences for the patient. In these circumstances you should still obtain patients' express consent to the use of identifiable data or arrange for members of the health care team to anonymise records (see also paragraphs 16 and 18).
16. However, where information is needed for the purposes of the kind set out in paragraph 15, and you are satisfied that it is not practicable either to obtain express consent to disclosure, nor for a member of the health care team to anonymise records, data may be disclosed without

express consent. Usually such disclosures will be made to allow a person outside the health care team to anonymise the records. Only where it is essential for the purpose may identifiable records be disclosed. Such disclosures must be kept to the minimum necessary for the purpose. In all such cases you must be satisfied that patients have been told, or have had access to written material informing them:

a. That their records may be disclosed to persons outside the team which provided their care.
b. Of the purpose and extent of the disclosure, for example, to produce anonymised data for use in education, administration, research or audit.
c. That the person given access to records will be subject to a duty of confidentiality.
d. That they have a right to object to such a process, and that their objection will be respected, except where the disclosure is essential to protect the patient, or someone else, from risk of death or serious harm.

17. Where you have control of personal information about patients, you must not allow anyone access to them for the purposes of the kind set out in paragraph 15, unless the person has been properly trained and authorised by the health authority, NHS trust or comparable body and is subject to a duty of confidentiality in their employment or because of their registration with a statutory regulatory body.

Disclosures in the public interest

18. In cases where you have considered all the available means of obtaining consent, but you are satisfied that it is not practicable to do so, or that patients are not competent to give consent, or exceptionally, in cases where patients withhold consent, personal information may be disclosed in the public interest where the benefits to an individual or to society of the disclosure outweigh the public and the patient's interest in keeping the information confidential.
19. In all such cases you must weigh the possible harm (both to the patient, and the overall trust between doctors and patients) against the benefits which are likely to arise from the release of information.
20. Ultimately, the 'public interest' can be determined only by the courts; but the GMC may also require you to justify your actions if we receive a complaint about the disclosure of personal information without a patient's consent.

SECTION 5—Putting the principles into practice

21. The remainder of this booklet deals with circumstances in which doctors are most frequently asked to disclose information, and provides advice on how the principles in paragraphs 14 Ò 20 should be applied.

Disclosures which benefit patients indirectly

Monitoring public health and the safety of medicines and devices including disclosures to cancer and other registries

22. Professional organisations and government regulatory bodies which monitor the public health or the safety of medicines or devices, as well as cancer and other registries, rely on information from patients' records for their effectiveness in safeguarding the public health. For example, the effectiveness of the yellow card scheme run by the Committee on Safety of Medicines depends on information provided by clinicians. You must co-operate by providing relevant information wherever possible. The notification of some communicable diseases is required by law (see also paragraph 43), and in other cases you should provide information in anonymised form, wherever that would be sufficient.
23. Where personal information is needed, you should seek express consent before disclosing information, whenever that is practicable. For example, where patients are receiving treatment there will usually be an opportunity for a health care professional to discuss disclosure of information with them.
24. Personal information may sometimes be sought about patients with whom health care professionals are not in regular contact. Doctors should, therefore, make sure that patients are given information about the possible value of their data in protecting the public health in the longer-term, at the initial consultation or at another suitable occasion when they attend a surgery or clinic. Patients should be given the information set out in paragraph 16: it should be clear that they may object to disclosures at any point. You must record any objections so that patients' wishes can be respected. In such cases, you may pass on anonymised information if asked to do so.
25. Where patients have not expressed an objection, you should assess the likely benefit of the disclosure to the public and commitment to confidentiality of the organisation requesting the information. If there is little or no evident public benefit, you should not disclose information without the express consent of the patient.
26. Where it is not practicable to seek patients' consent for disclosure of personal information for these purposes, or where patients are not competent to give consent, you must consider whether disclosures would be justified in the public interest, by weighing the benefits to the public health of the disclosure against the possible detriment to the patient.
27. The automatic transfer of personal information to a registry, whether by electronic or other means, before informing the patient that information will be passed on, is unacceptable save in the most exceptional circumstances. These would be where a court has already decided that there is such an overwhelming public interest in the disclosure of information to a registry that patients' rights to confidentiality are overridden; or where you are willing and able to justify the disclosure, potentially before a court or to the GMC, on the same grounds.

Clinical audit and education

28. Anonymised data will usually be sufficient for clinical audit and for education. When anonymising records you should follow the guidance on obtaining consent in paragraphs 15-17 above. You should not disclose non-anonymised data for clinical audit or education without the patient's consent.

Administration and financial audit

29. You should record financial or other administrative data separately from clinical information, and provide it in anonymised form, wherever that is possible.
30. Decisions about the disclosure of clinical records for administrative or financial audit purposes, for example where health authority staff seek access to patients' records as part of the arrangements for verifying NHS payments, are unlikely to bring your registration into question, provided that, before allowing access to patients' records, you follow the guidance in paragraphs 15-17. Only the relevant part of the record should be made available for scrutiny.

Medical research

31. Where research projects depend on using identifiable information or samples, and it is not practicable to contact patients to seek their consent, this fact should be drawn to the attention of a research ethics committee so that it can consider whether the likely benefits of the research outweigh the loss of confidentiality. Disclosures may otherwise be improper, even if the recipients of the information are registered medical practitioners. The decision of a research ethics committee would be taken into account by a court if a claim for breach of confidentiality were made, but the court's judgement would be based on its own assessment of whether the public interest was served. More detailed guidance is issued by the medical royal colleges and other bodies.

Publication of case-histories and photographs

32. You must obtain express consent from patients before publishing personal information about them as individuals in media to which the public has access, for example in journals or text books, whether or not you believe the patient can be identified. Express consent must therefore be sought to the publication of, for example, case-histories about, or photographs of, patients. Where you wish to publish information about a patient who has died, you should take into account the guidance in paragraphs 40-41 before deciding whether or not to do so.

Disclosures where doctors have dual responsibilities

33. Situations arise where doctors have contractual obligations to third parties, such as companies or organisations, as well as obligations to patients. Such situations occur, for example, when doctors:
    a. Provide occupational health services or medical care for employees of a company or organisation.
    b. Are employed by an organisation such as an insurance company.
    c. Work for an agency assessing claims for benefits.
    d. Provide medical care for patients and are subsequently asked to provide medical reports or information for third parties about them.
    e. Work as police surgeons.
    f. Work in the armed forces.
    g. Work in the prison service.
34. If you are asked to write a report about and/or examine a patient, or to disclose information from existing records for a third party to whom you have contractual obligations, you must:
    a. Be satisfied that the patient has been told at the earliest opportunity about for the purpose of the examination and/or disclosure, the extent of the information to be disclosed and the fact that relevant information cannot be concealed or withheld. You might wish to show the form to the patient before you complete it to ensure the patient understands the scope of the information requested.
    b. Obtain, or have seen, written consent to the disclosure from the patient or a person properly authorised to act on the patient's behalf. You may, however, accept written assurances from an officer of a government department that the patient's written consent has been given.
    c. Disclose only information relevant to the request for disclosure: accordingly, you should not usually disclose the whole record. The full record may be relevant to some benefits paid by government departments.
    d. Include only factual information you can substantiate, presented in an unbiased manner.
    e. The Access to Medical Reports Act 1988 entitles patients to see reports written about them before they are disclosed, in some circumstances. In all circumstances you should check whether patients wish to see their report, unless patients have clearly and specifically stated that they do not wish to do so.
35. Disclosures without consent to employers, insurance companies, or any other third party, can be justified only in exceptional circumstances, for example, when they are necessary to protect others from risk of death or serious harm.

Disclosures to protect the patient or others

36. Disclosure of personal information without consent may be justified where failure to do so may expose the patient or others to risk or death or serious harm. Where third parties are exposed to a risk so serious that it outweighs the patient's privacy interest, you should seek consent to disclosure where practicable. If it is not practicable,

you should disclose information promptly to an appropriate person or authority. You should generally inform the patient before disclosing the information.

37. Such circumstances may arise, for example:
    a. Where a colleague, who is also a patient, is placing patients at risk as a result of illness or other medical condition. If you are in doubt about whether disclosure is justified you should consult an experienced colleague, or seek advice from a professional organisation. The safety of patients must come first at all times. (Our booklet Serious Communicable Diseases gives further guidance on this issue.)
    b. Where a patient continues to drive, against medical advice, when unfit to do so. In such circumstances you should disclose relevant information to the medical adviser of the Driver and Vehicle Licensing Agency without delay. Fuller guidance is given in High Yield Topic 2.
    c. Where a disclosure may assist in the prevention or detection of a serious crime. Serious crimes, in this context, will put someone at risk of death or serious harm, and will usually be crimes against the person, such as abuse of children.

Children and other patients who may lack competence to give consent

38. Problems may arise if you consider that a patient is incapable of giving consent to treatment or disclosure because of immaturity, illness or mental incapacity. If such patients ask you not to disclose information to a third party, you should try to persuade them to allow an appropriate person to be involved in the consultation. If they refuse and you are convinced that it is essential, in their medical interests, you may disclose relevant information to an appropriate person or authority. In such cases you must tell the patient before disclosing any information, and, where appropriate, seek and carefully consider the views of an advocate or carer. You should document in the patient's record the steps you have taken to obtain consent and the reasons for deciding to disclose information.
39. If you believe a patient to be a victim of neglect or physical, sexual or emotional abuse and that the patient cannot give or withhold consent to disclosure, you should give information promptly to an appropriate responsible person or statutory agency, where you believe that the disclosure is in the patient's best interests. You should usually inform the patient that you intend to disclose the information before doing so. Such circumstances may arise in relation to children, where concerns about possible abuse need to be shared with other agencies such as social services. Where appropriate you should inform those with parental responsibility about the disclosure. If, for any reason, you believe that disclosure of information is not in the best interests of an abused or neglected patient, you must still be prepared to justify your decision.

Disclosure after a patient's death

40. You still have an obligation to keep personal information confidential after a patient dies. The extent to which confidential information may be disclosed after a patient's death will depend on the circumstances. These include the nature of the information, whether that information is already public knowledge or can be anonymised, and the intended use to which the information will be put. You should also consider whether the disclosure of information may cause distress to, or be of benefit to, the patient's partner or family.
41. There are a number of circumstances in which you may be asked to disclose, or wish to use, information about patients who have died. For example:
    a. To assist a Coroner, Procurator Fiscal or other similar officer in connection with an inquest or fatal accident inquiry. In these circumstances you should provide relevant information (see also paragraph 19 of Good Medical Practice).
    b. As part of National Confidential Enquiries or other clinical audit or for education or research. The publication of properly anonymised case studies would be unlikely to be improper in these contexts.
    c. On death certificates. The law requires you to complete death certificates honestly and fully.
    d. To obtain information relating to public health surveillance. Anonymised information should be used unless identifiable data is essential to the study.
42. Particular difficulties may arise when there is a conflict of interest between parties affected by the patient's death. For example, if an insurance company seeks information in order to decide whether to make a payment under a life assurance policy, you should release information in accordance with the requirements of the Access to Health Records Act 1990 or with the authorisation of those lawfully entitled to deal with the person's estate who have been fully informed of the consequences of disclosure. It may also be appropriate to inform those close to the patient.

Section 6—Disclosure in connection with judicial or other statutory proceedings

43. You must disclose information to satisfy a specific statutory requirement, such as notification of a known or suspected communicable disease.
44. You must also disclose information if ordered to do so by a judge or presiding officer of a court. You should object to the judge or the presiding officer if attempts are made to compel you to disclose what appear to you to be irrelevant matters, for example matters relating to relatives or partners of the patient, who are not parties to the proceedings.
45. You should not disclose personal information to a third

party such as a solicitor, police officer or officer of a court without the patient's express consent, except in the circumstances described at paragraphs 36-37, 39 and 41.

46. You may disclose personal information in response to an official request from a statutory regulatory body for any of the health care professions, where that body determines that this is necessary in the interests of justice and for the safety of other patients. Wherever practicable you should discuss this with the patient. There may be exceptional cases where, even though the patient objects, disclosure is justified.

If you decide to disclose confidential information you must be prepared to explain and justify your decision.

SEEKING PATIENTS' CONSENT: THE ETHICAL CONSIDERATIONS

Introduction

1. Successful relationships between doctors and patients depend on trust. To establish that trust you must respect patients' autonomy - their right to decide whether or not to undergo any medical intervention even where a refusal may result in harm to themselves or in their own death1. Patients must be given sufficient information, in a way that they can understand, to enable them to exercise their right to make informed decisions about their care.
2. This right is protected in law, and you are expected to be aware of the legal principles set by relevant case law in this area 2. Existing case law gives a guide to what can be considered minimum requirements of good practice in seeking informed consent from patients.
3. Effective communication is the key to enabling patients to make informed decisions. You must take appropriate steps to find out what patients want to know and ought to know about their condition and its treatment. Open, helpful dialogue of this kind with patients leads to clarity of objectives and understanding, and strengthens the quality of the doctor/patient relationship. It provides an agreed framework within which the doctor can respond effectively to the individual needs of the patient. Additionally, patients who have been able to make properly informed decisions are more likely to co-operate fully with the agreed management of their conditions.

Consent to investigation and treatment

Providing sufficient information

4. Patients have a right to information about their condition and the treatment options available to them. The amount of information you give each patient will vary, according to factors such as the nature of the condition, the complexity of the treatment, the risks associated with the treatment or procedure, and the patient's own wishes. For example, patients may need more information to make an informed decision about a procedure which carries a high risk of failure or adverse side effects; or about an investigation for a condition which, if present, could have serious implications for the patient's employment, social or personal life 3.
5. The information which patients want or ought to know, before deciding whether to consent to treatment or an investigation, may include:
   - Details of the diagnosis, and prognosis, and the likely prognosis if the condition is left untreated;
   - Uncertainties about the diagnosis including options for further investigation prior to treatment;
   - Options for treatment or management of the condition, including the option not to treat;
   - The purpose of a proposed investigation or treatment; details of the procedures or therapies involved, including subsidiary treatment such as methods of pain relief; how the patient should prepare for the procedure;and details of what the patient might experience during or after the procedure including common and serious side effects;
   - For each option, explanations of the likely benefits and the probabilities of success; and discussion of any serious or frequently occurring risks, and of any lifestyle changes which may be caused by, or necessitated by, the treatment;
   - Advice about whether a proposed treatment is experimental;
   - How and when the patient's condition and any side effects will be monitored or re-assessed;
   - The name of the doctor who will have overall responsibility for the treatment and, where appropriate, names of the senior members of his or her team;
   - Whether doctors in training will be involved, and the extent to which students may be involved in an investigation or treatment;
   - A reminder that patients can change their minds about a decision at any time;
   - A reminder that patients have a right to seek a second opinion;
   - Where applicable, details of costs or charges which the patient may have to meet.
6. When providing information you must do your best to find out about patients' individual needs and priorities. For example, patients' beliefs, culture, occupation or other factors may have a bearing on the information they need in order to reach a decision. You should not make assumptions about patients' views, but discuss these matters with them, and ask them whether they have any concerns about the treatment or the risks it may involve. You should provide patients with appropriate information, which should include an explanation of any risks to which they may attach particular significance. Ask patients whether they have understood the information and whether they would like more before making a decision.

7. You must not exceed the scope of the authority given by a patient, except in an emergency 4. Therefore, if you are the doctor providing treatment or undertaking an investigation, you must give the patient a clear explanation of the scope of consent being sought. This will apply particularly where:
   - Treatment will be provided in stages with the possibility of later adjustments;
   - Different doctors (or other health care workers) provide particular elements of an investigation or treatment (for example anaesthesia in surgery);
   - A number of different investigations or treatments are involved;
   - Uncertainty about the diagnosis, or about the appropriate range of options for treatment, may be resolved only in the light of findings once investigation or treatment is underway, and when the patient may be unable to participate in decision making.

   In such cases, you should explain how decisions would be made about whether or when to move from one stage or one form of treatment to another. There should be a clear agreement about whether the patient consents to all or only parts of the proposed plan of investigation or treatment, and whether further consent will have to be sought at a later stage.
8. You should raise with patients the possibility of additional problems coming to light during a procedure when the patient is unconscious or otherwise unable to make a decision. You should seek consent to treat any problems which you think may arise and ascertain whether there are any procedures to which the patient would object, or prefer to give further thought to before you proceed. You must abide by patients' decisions on these issues. If in exceptional circumstances you decide, while the patient is unconscious, to treat a condition which falls outside the scope of the patient's consent, your decision may be challenged in the courts, or be the subject of a complaint to your employing authority or the GMC. You should, therefore, seek the views of an experienced colleague, wherever possible, before providing the treatment. And you must be prepared to explain and justify your decision. You must tell the patient what you have done and why, as soon as the patient is sufficiently recovered to understand.

Responding to questions

9. You must respond honestly to any questions the patient raises and, as far as possible, answer as fully as the patient wishes. In some cases, a patient may ask about other treatments that are unproven or ineffective. Some patients may want to know whether any of the risks or benefits of treatment are affected by the choice of institution or doctor providing the care. You must answer such questions as fully, accurately and objectively as possible.

Withholding information

10. You should not withhold information necessary for decision making unless you judge that disclosure of some relevant information would cause the patient serious harm. In this context serious harm does not mean the patient would become upset, or decide to refuse treatment.
11. No-one may make decisions on behalf of a competent adult. If patients ask you to withhold information and make decisions on their behalf, or nominate a relative or third party to make decisions for them, you should explain the importance of them knowing the options open to them, and what the treatment they may receive will involve. If they insist they do not want to know in detail about their condition and its treatment, you should still provide basic information about the treatment. If a relative asks you to withhold information, you must seek the views of the patient. Again, you should not withhold relevant information unless you judge that this would cause the patient serious harm.
12. In any case where you withhold relevant information from the patient you must record this, and the reason for doing so, in the patient's medical records and you must be prepared to explain and justify your decision.

Presenting information to patients

13. Obtaining informed consent cannot be an isolated event. It involves a continuing dialogue between you and your patients which keeps them abreast of changes in their condition and the treatment or investigation you propose. Whenever possible, you should discuss treatment options at a time when the patient is best able to understand and retain the information. To be sure that your patient understands, you should give clear explanations and give the patient time to ask questions. In particular, you should:
    - use up-to-date written material, visual and other aids to explain complex aspects of the investigation, diagnosis or treatment where appropriate and/or practicable;
    - Make arrangements, wherever possible, to meet particular language and communication needs, for example through translations, independent interpreters, signers, or the patient's representative;
    - Where appropriate, discuss with patients the possibility of bringing a relative or friend, or making a tape recording of the consultation;
    - Explain the probabilities of success, or the risk of failure of, or harm associated with options for treatment, using accurate data;
    - Ensure that information which patients may find distressing is given to them in a considerate way. Provide patients with information about counselling services and patient support groups, where appropriate;

- Allow patients sufficient time to reflect, before and after making a decision, especially where the information is complex or the severity of the risks is great. Where patients have difficulty understanding information, or there is a lot of information to absorb, it may be appropriate to provide it in manageable amounts, with appropriate written or other back-up material, over a period of time, or to repeat it;
- Involve nursing or other members of the health care team in discussions with the patient, where appropriate. They may have valuable knowledge of the patient's background or particular concerns, for example in identifying what risks the patient should be told about;
- Ensure that, where treatment is not to start until some time after consent has been obtained, the patient is given a clear route for reviewing their decision with the person providing the treatment.

Who obtains consent

14. If you are the doctor providing treatment or undertaking an investigation, it is your responsibility to discuss it with the patient and obtain consent, as you will have a comprehensive understanding of the procedure or treatment, how it is carried out, and the risks attached to it. Where this is not practicable, you may delegate these tasks provided you ensure that the person to whom you delegate:
    - Is suitably trained and qualified;
    - Has sufficient knowledge of the proposed investigation or treatment, and understandsthe risks involved;
    - Acts in accordance with the guidance in this booklet.

    You will remain responsible for ensuring that, before you start any treatment, the patient has been given sufficient time and information to make an informed decision, and has given consent to the procedure or investigation.

Ensuring voluntary decision making

15. It is for the patient, not the doctor, to determine what is in the patient's own best interests. Nonetheless, you may wish to recommend a treatment or a course of action to patients, but you must not put pressure on patients to accept your advice. In discussions with patients, you should:
    - Give a balanced view of the options;
    - Explain the need for informed consent.

    You must declare any potential conflicts of interest, for example where you or your organisation benefit financially from use of a particular drug or treatment, or treatment at a particular institution.
16. Pressure may be put on patients by employers, insurance companies or others to undergo particular tests or accept treatment. You should do your best to ensure that patients have considered the options and reached their own decision. You should take appropriate action if you believe patients are being offered inappropriate or unlawful financial or other rewards.
17. Patients who are detained by the police or immigration services, or are in prison, and those detained under the provisions of any mental health legislation may be particularly vulnerable. Where such patients have a right to decline treatment you should do your best to ensure that they know this, and are able to exercise this right.

Emergencies

18. In an emergency, where consent cannot be obtained, you may provide medical treatment to anyone who needs it, provided the treatment is limited to what is immediately necessary to save life or avoid significant deterioration in the patient's health. However, you must still respect the terms of any valid advance refusal which you know about, or is drawn to your attention. You should tell the patient what has been done, and why, as soon as the patient is sufficiently recovered to understand.

Establishing capacity to make decisions

19. You must work on the presumption that every adult has the capacity to decide whether to consent to, or refuse, proposed medical intervention, unless it is shown that they cannot understand information presented in a clear way5. If a patient's choice appears irrational, or does not accord with your view of what is in the patient's best interests, that is not evidence in itself that the patient lacks competence. In such circumstances it may be appropriate to review with the patient whether all reasonable steps have been taken to identify and meet their information needs (see paragraphs 5-17). Where you need to assess a patient's capacity to make a decision, you should consult the guidance issued by professional bodies 6.

Fluctuating capacity

20. Where patients have difficulty retaining information, or are only intermittently competent to make a decision, you should provide any assistance they might need to reach an informed decision. You should record any decision made while the patients were competent, including the key elements of the consultation. You should review any decision made whilst they were competent, at appropriate intervals before treatment starts, to establish that their views are consistently held and can be relied on.

Mentally incapacitated patients

21. No-one can give or withhold consent to treatment on behalf of a mentally incapacitated patient 7. You must first assess the patient's capacity to make an informed decision about the treatment. If patients lack capacity to decide, provided they comply, you may carry out an

investigation or treatment, which may include treatment for any mental disorder 8, that you judge to be in their best interests. However, if they do not comply, you may compulsorily treat them for any mental disorder only within the safeguards laid down by the Mental Health Act 1983 9, and any physical disorder arising from that mental disorder, in line with the guidance in the Code of Practice of the Mental Health Commission10. You should seek the courts' approval for any non-therapeutic or controversial treatments which are not directed at their mental disorder.

Advance statements

22. If you are treating a patient who has lost capacity to consent to or refuse treatment, for example through onset or progress of a mental disorder or other disability, you should try to find out whether the patient has previously indicated preferences in an advance statement ('advance directives' or 'living wills'). You must respect any refusal of treatment given when the patient was competent, provided the decision in the advance statement is clearly applicable to the present circumstances, and there is no reason to believe that the patient has changed his/her mind. Where an advance statement of this kind is not available, the patient's known wishes should be taken into account - see paragraph 25 on the 'best interests' principle.

Children

23. You must assess a child's capacity to decide whether to consent to or refuse proposed investigation or treatment before you provide it. In general, a competent child will be able to understand the nature, purpose and possible consequences of the proposed investigation or treatment, as well as the consequences of non-treatment. Your assessment must take account of the relevant laws or legal precedents in this area11. You should bear in mind that:
    - At age 16 a young person can be treated as an adult and can be presumed to have capacity to decide;
    - Under age 16 children may have capacity to decide, depending on their ability to understand what is involved12;
    - Where a competent child refuses treatment, a person with parental responsibility or the court may authorise investigation or treatment which is in the child's best interests. The position is different in Scotland, where those with parental responsibility cannot authorise procedures a competent child has refused. Legal advice may be helpful on how to deal with such cases.
24. Where a child under 16 years old is not competent to give or withhold their informed consent, a person with parental responsibility may authorise investigations or treatment which are in the child's best interests13. This person may also refuse any intervention, where they consider that refusal to be in the child's best interests, but you are not bound by such a refusal and may seek a ruling from the court. In an emergency where you consider that it is in the child's best interests to proceed, you may treat the child, provided it is limited to that treatment which is reasonably required in that emergency.

'Best interests' principle

25. In deciding what options may be reasonably considered as being in the best interests of a patient who lacks capacity to decide, you should take into account:
    - Options for treatment or investigation which are clinically indicated;
    - Any evidence of the patient's previously expressed preferences, including an advance statement;
    - Your own and the health care team's knowledge of the patient's background, such as cultural, religious, or employment considerations;
    - Views about the patient's preferences given by a third party who may have other knowledge of the patient, for example the patient's partner, family, carer, tutor-dative (Scotland), or a person with parental responsibility;
    - Which option least restricts the patient's future choices, where more than one option (including non-treatment) seems reasonable in the patient's best interest.

Applying to the court

26. Where a patient's capacity to consent is in doubt, or where differences of opinion about his or her best interests cannot be resolved satisfactorily, you should consult more experienced colleagues and, where appropriate, seek legal advice on whether it is necessary to apply to the court for a ruling. You should seek the court's approval where a patient lacks capacity to consent to a medical intervention which is non-therapeutic or controversial, for example contraceptive sterilisation, organ donation, withdrawal of life support from a patient in a persistent vegetative state. Where you decide to apply to a court you should, as soon as possible, inform the patient and his or her representative of your decision and of his or her right to be represented at the hearing.

Forms of consent

27. To determine whether patients have given informed consent to any proposed investigation or treatment, you must consider how well they have understood the details and implications of what is proposed, and not simply the form in which their consent has been expressed or recorded.

Express consent

28. Patients can indicate their informed consent either orally or in writing. In some cases, the nature of the risks to which the patient might be exposed make it important

that a written record is available of the patient's consent and other wishes in relation to the proposed investigation and treatment. This helps to ensure later understanding between you, the patient, and anyone else involved in carrying out the procedure or providing care. Except in an emergency, where the patient has capacity to give consent you should obtain written consent in cases where:

- The treatment or procedure is complex, or involves significant risks and/or side effects;
- Providing clinical care is not the primary purpose of the investigation or examination;
- There may be significant consequences for the patient's employment, social or personal life;
- The treatment is part of a research programme.

29. You must use the patient's case notes and/or a consent form to detail the key elements of the discussion with the patient, including the nature of information provided, specific requests by the patient, details of the scope of the consent given.

Statutory requirements

30. Some statutes require written consent to be obtained for particular treatments (for example some fertility treatments). You must follow the law in these areas.

Implied consent

31. You should be careful about relying on a patient's apparent compliance with a procedure as a form of consent. For example, the fact that a patient lies down on an examination couch does not in itself indicate that the patient has understood what you propose to do and why.

Reviewing consent

32. A signed consent form is not sufficient evidence that a patient has given, or still gives, informed consent to the proposed treatment in all its aspects. You, or a member of the team, must review the patient's decision close to the time of treatment, and especially where:
    - significant time has elapsed between obtaining consent and the start of treatment;
    - there have been material changes in the patient's condition, or in any aspects of the proposed treatment plan, which might invalidate the patient's existing consent;
    - new, potentially relevant information has become available, for example about the risks of the treatment, or about other treatment options.

Consent to screening

33. Screening (which may involve testing) healthy or asymptomatic people to detect genetic predispositions or early signs of debilitating or life threatening conditions can be an important tool in providing effective care. But the uncertainties involved in screening may be great, for example the risk of false positive or false negative results. Some findings may potentially have serious medical, social or financial consequences not only for the individuals, but for their relatives. In some cases the fact of having been screened may itself have serious implications.
34. You must ensure that anyone considering whether to consent to screening can make a properly informed decision. As far as possible, you should ensure that screening would not be contrary to the individual's interest. You must pay particular attention to ensuring that the information the person wants or ought to have is identified and provided. You should be careful to explain clearly:
    - The purpose of the screening;
    - The likelihood of positive/negative findings and possibility of false positive/negative results;
    - The uncertainties and risks attached to the screening process;
    - Any significant medical, social or financial implications of screening for the particular condition or predisposition;
    - Follow up plans, including availability of counselling and support services.

    If you are considering the possibility of screening children, or adults who are not able to decide for themselves, you should refer to the guidance at paragraphs 19-25. In appropriate cases, you should take account of the guidance issued by bodies such as the Advisory Committee on Genetic Testing 14.

Consent to research

35. Research involving clinical trials of drugs or treatments, and research into the causes of, or possible treatment for, a particular condition, is important in increasing doctors' ability to provide effective care for present and future patients. The benefits of the research may, however, be uncertain and may not be experienced by the person participating in the research. In addition, the risk involved for research participants may be difficult to identify or to assess in advance. If you carry out or participate in research involving patients or volunteers, it is particularly important that you ensure:
    - as far as you are able, that the research is not contrary to the individual's interests;
    - that participants understand that it is research and that the results are not predictable.
36. You must take particular care to be sure that anyone you ask to consider taking part in research is given the fullest possible information, presented in terms and a form that they can understand. This must include any information about possible benefits and risks; evidence that a research ethics committee has given approval; and advice that they can withdraw at any time. You should ensure that participants have the opportunity to read and consider the research information leaflet. You must allow them sufficient time to reflect on the implications of

participating in the study. You must not put pressure on anyone to take part in research. You must obtain the person's consent in writing. Before starting any research you must always obtain approval from a properly constituted research ethics committee.

37. You should seek further advice where your research will involve adults who are not able to make decisions for themselves, or children. You should be aware that in these cases the legal position is complex or unclear, and there is currently no general consensus on how to balance the possible risks and benefits to such vulnerable individuals against the public interest in conducting research. (A number of public consultation exercises are under way.) You should consult the guidance issued by bodies such as the Medical Research Council and the medical royal colleges16 to keep up to date. You should also seek advice from the relevant research ethics committee where appropriate.

HIGH YIELD TOPIC ELEVEN

SIX DEVELOPMENT (DENVER SCREENING) AND MOTOR MILESTONES

Mean age	*Eye/Hand coordination*	*Locomotor skills*	*Speech/Communication skills*	*Social/Personal skills*
6 weeks	Follow a moving face with eyes	Holds head but some head lag	Cooing noise begins	Smiles when spoken to
3 months	Hand regard brings hand to midline Follows horizontally and vertically	Minimal or no head-lag Lift head upon prone	Stills to mother's voice. Coos reciprocally with mother	Friendly response to attention Initiates smile
6 months	Transfers cube from one hand to others Reaches nut and grasps a rattle or toy	Up on extended forearms in prone. Sits without lateral support	Squeals and starts to bubble (blow bubbles)	Discriminates family from stangers. Laughs out loud
9 months	Picks up cube with fine pincer grasp Looks for a fallen body	Stands holding on to furniture. Pulls self to stand	Babbles Ma-Ma/Da-Da/ Ba-Ba. understands 'No' and shakes head for 'No'	Waves good-bye. Finger feeds self
1 years	Bangs bricks together when shown. Picks up pellet with pincer grasp	Cross round the furniture. Pulls self to stand	Mama, Dada and Baba with meaning 2-3 other words reported	Finds toy under cup. Claps hands. Begins to point
15 months	Holds two 1″ cubes in one hand Stop casting toys	Walks with one hand held. Walk unsupported	3-4 clear words heard Beginning to point to what he wants	Manages cup or transfer cup Helps with dressing
1½ years	Scribbles freely on paper. Builds 3 × 1″ cube tower when shown	Climbs up stairs, (hand held). Kneels with support	Points to three parts of the body. Single word vocabulary 6-20 words	Spoon feeds self Manages cup on own. Know parts of body like eye and nose
2 years	Vertical line/circular scrible Builds 6 7 × 1″cube tower	Up and down stairs, hand held, two feet per step. Runs and kick a ball	Simple 3-4 word combi- nations. Names 6-8 familiar pictures/toys	Aware when wet/dirty May use potty Worries if mother leave room
3 years	Builds a brige of 3 cubes Copies line	Walk on tip toes. Walks up stairs, one foot per step	Talks in 6-syllable sentences. Able to give name, age and sex	Washes hands/undresses self imagenative play/ cooperates with friends
4 years	Draws a recognisable man. Copies a square	Hops on one foot. Walks down stairs, one foot per step.	Clear, grammatical conversation. Knows primary colours and big/small	Dresses self (not laces/ fastenings) Play with friends separate from parents
	WARNING SIGNS: 1. Presistent fisting of hands. 2. Handedness before 15 months 3. Casting all toys after 18 months	*WARNING SIGNS:* 1. Scissoring at any age 2. Mark hypotonia 3. Persistent moro reflex reflex after 4 months 4. Unexpected limp	*WARNING SIGNS:* 1. No babble at 8 months 2. Persistent drooling after 18 months 3. No comprehension of situation of single command by 18 months 4. No words by 18 months 5. Marked echolalia after 2½ years 6. Speech unintelligiable by 3 years	*WARNING SIGNS:* 1. Persistent high pitched screaming 2. Marked eye contact avoidance 3. Persistent hand regard 5 months 4. Repetitive movement (stereotypes) 5. Persistent mouthing after 18 months 6. Persistent tantrums after 3 years

NOTE: Not all children develop at same rate.

HIGH YIELD TOPIC TWELVE

NEW CPR GUIDELINES IN UK

The adult basic and advanced algorithms and paediatric resuscitation algorithms have been updated to reflect changes in the guidelines.

Rescuers begin CPR if the victim is unconscious or unresponsive and not breathing normally (ignoring occasional gasps). A single compression-ventilation (CV) ratio of **30:2** is used by the single rescuer of an adult or child (excluding neonate) out of hospital, and for all adult CPR. This single ratio is designed to simplify teaching, promote skill retention, increase the number of compressions given, and decrease interruption to compressions. Once a defibrillator is attached, if a shockable rhythm is confirmed, a single shock is delivered. Irrespective of the resultant rhythm, chest compressions and ventilations (two minutes with a CV ratio of 30:2) are resumed immediately after the shock to minimise the 'no-flow' time.

Recent evidence indicates that unnecessary interruptions to chest compressions occur frequently both in and out of hospital. Resuscitation instructors must emphasise the importance of minimising interruptions to chest compression.

ADULT BASIC LIFE SUPPORT

Introduction

This section contains the guidelines for out-of-hospital, single rescuer, adult basic life support (BLS). Like the other guidelines in this publication, it is based on the document 2005 International Consensus on Cardiopulmonary Resuscitation and Emergency Cardiovascular Care Science with Treatment Recommendations *(CoSTR), which was published in November 2005. Basic life support implies that* no equipment is employed other than a protective device.

Guideline Changes

There are two main underlying themes in the BLS section of CoSTR: the need to increase the number of chest compressions given to a victim of cardiac arrest, and the importance of simplifying guidelines to a id acquisition and retention of BLS skills, particularly for lay persons. It is well documented that interruptions in chest compression are common and are associated with a reduced chance of survival for the victim.2 The 'perfect' solution is to deliver continuous compressions whilst giving ventilations independently. This is possible when the victim has an advanced airway in place, and is discussed in the adult advanced life support (ALS) section. Chestcompression-only CPR is another way to increase the number of compressions given and will, by definition, eliminate pauses. It is effective for a limited period only (about 5 min) 3 and is not recommended as standard management of out-ofhospital cardiac arrest.

The following changes in the BLS guidelines have been made to reflect the greater importance placed on chest compression, and to attempt to reduce the number and duration of pauses:

1. Make a diagnosis of cardiac arrest if a victim is unresponsive and not breathing normally.
2. Teach rescuers to place their hands in the centre of the chest, rather than to spend more time using the 'rib margin' method.
3. Give each rescue breath over 1 sec rather than 2 sec.
4. Use a ratio of compressions to ventilations of 30:2 for all adult victims of sudden cardiac arrest. Use this same ratio for children when attended by a lay rescuer.
5. For an adult victim, omit the initial 2 rescue breaths and give 30 compressions immediately after cardiac arrest is established.

Adult Basic Life Support

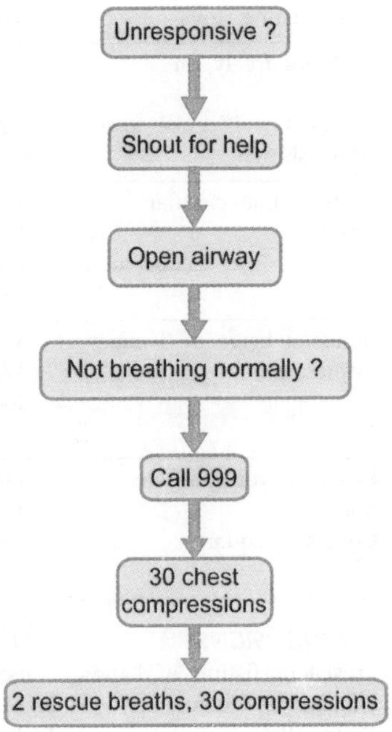

Index

A

I

Published by

Jitendar P Vij
Jaypee Brothers Medical Publishers (P) Ltd
EMCA House, 23/23B Ansari Road, Daryaganj
New Delhi 110 002, India
Phones: +91-11-23272143, +91-11-23272703, +91-11-23282021, +91-11-23245672
Fax: +91-11-23276490, +91-11-23245683 e-mail: jaypee@jaypeebrothers.com
Visit our website: www.jaypeebrothers.com

Branches

- 2/B Akruti Society, Jodhpur Gam Road, Satellite
  Ahmedabad 380 015, Phone: +91-079-30988717, +91-079-26926233
- 202 Batavia Chambers, 8 Kumara Krupa Road, Kumara Park East
  Bangalore 560 001, Phones: +91-80-22285971, +91-80-22382956, +91-80-30614073
  Tele Fax: +91-80-22281761 e-mail: jaypeemedpubbgl@eth.net
- 282 IIIrd Floor, Khaleel Shirazi Estate, Fountain Plaza, Pantheon Road
  Chennai 600 008, Phones: +91-44-28193265, +91-44-28194897
  Fax: +91-44-28193231 e-mail: jpchen@eth.net
- 4-2-1067/1-3, Ist Floor, Balaji Building, Ramkote, Cross Road
  Hyderabad 500 095, Phones: +91-40-66610020, +91-40-24758498
  Fax: +91-40-24758499 e-mail: jpmedpub@rediffmail.com
- "KURUVI BUILDING", 1st Floor, Plot/Door No. 41/3098-B &B1, St. Vincent Road
  Kochi 682 018, Ph: +91-0484-4036109 e-mail: jaypeekochi@rediffmail.com
- 1A Indian Mirror Street, Wellington Square
  Kolkata 700 013, Phones: +91-33-22456075, +91-33-22451926
  Fax: +91-33-22456075 e-mail: jpbcal@dataone.in
- 106 Amit Industrial Estate, 61 Dr SS Rao Road, Near MGM Hospital, Parel
  Mumbai 400 012, Phones: +91-22-24124863, +91-22-24104532, +91-22-30926896
  Fax: +91-22-24160828 e-mail: jpmedpub@bom7.vsnl.net.in
- "KAMALPUSHPA", 38 Reshimbag, Opp. Mohota Science College, Umred Road
  Nagpur 440 009, Phones: +91-712-3945220, +91-712-2704275
  e-mail: jaypeenagpur@dataone.in

RPG PLAB

First Edition: 2003
Second Edition: 2005
Third Edition: 2007

ISBN 81-8061-817-X

Typeset at JPBMP typesetting unit
Printed at Rajkamal Electric Press, G.T.Karnal Road, Industrial Area, Delhi-33

RxPG SERIES
(www.RxPG.com)

Based on Latest PLAB Pattern

RxPG PLAB

PART I Exam

International Edition

THIRD EDITION

Himanshu Tyagi
Senior House Officer
St Mary's General Psychiatry Training Scheme
London

Ankush Vidyarthi
Senior House Officer
Royal Free Hospital, Training Scheme in Psychiatry
London

Rashmi Yadav
Senior House Officer
Cardiothoracic Surgery, Leeds General Infirmary
Leeds

JAYPEE BROTHERS
MEDICAL PUBLISHERS (P) LTD
NEW DELHI

Disclaimer

Medicine is an ever changing science. As new research and clinical experience broaden our knowledge, changes in existing treatment and drug therapies are required. The authors and the publisher of this book have checked with sources believed to be reliable in their efforts to provide information that is complete and generally in accordance with the standards accepted at the time of publication. However, in view of the possibility of human error or changes in medical sciences, neither the authors not the publisher nor any other party who has been involved in the publication of this work warrants that the information contained herein is in every respect accurate or complete, and they disclaim all responsibility for any errors or omissions or for the results obtained from use of the information contained in this book. Readers are encouraged to confirm the information contained herein with other sources. Moreover, the authors and the publisher do not claim any responsibility for the accuracy or even existence of any question in this book in the exam quoted. All the questions have been reproduced solely on the basis of the memory of the appearing students and there can be wide variations from the actual questions or their options.

℞PG PLAB

Part I Exam